Common Chest Diseases

Dr RS Bhatia
MMBS, DTM & HAB, MNAS, FCCP, FACCP, FICA (USA)
Physician–Pulmonologist–Diabetologist
Diplomate App. Medicine
Member National Advisory Board, JAPI
Model Town, Ludhiana - 141002

PEEPEE
PUBLISHERS AND DISTRIBUTORS (P) LTD.

Common Chest Diseases

Published by
Pawaninder P. Vij and Anupam Vij

Peepee Publishers and Distributors (P) Ltd.
Head Office: 160, Shakti Vihar, Pitam Pura
Delhi-110034 (India)

Correspondence Address: 7/31, First Floor, Ansari Road
Daryaganj, New Delhi-110002 (India)
Ph: 41512412, 23246245, 9811156083
e-mail: peepee160@yahoo.co.in
e-mail: peepee160@gmail.com
www.peepeepub.com

First Edition: **2016, Reprint 2023**

ISBN : 978-81-8445-202-0

Dedicated to

My Respected Parents

FOREWORD

Chest diseases cause a significant morbidity and mortality all over the world. In India, while Tuberculosis is the major respiratory illness, other problems including asthma, pneumonias, environmental and occupational lung diseases and lung cancer are also as frequent as anywhere else in the world. Unfortunately, the prevalence of most lung diseases is increasing. This can be attributed to increasing air pollution, overcrowding, industrialization and the spread of tuberculosis and HIV infections. We are likely to face some of these problems in an epidemic fashion in the near future. But there is relative lack of awareness about the diagnosis and treatment of common lung ailments.

There are several textbooks on respiratory diseases meant for students of medicine and pulmonologists. Dr Bhatia has written this text for the benefit of physicians practising chest medicine. It covers most of the topics in lung diseases. He has also tried to include the references on Indian experience in some of his chapters. This shall give the book an Indian flavour. I do hope that the readers will find the material useful.

S.K. Jindal
Prof. and Head
Department of Pulmonary Medicine
PGIMER, Chandigarh

PREFACE

Patients with chest ailments form an important part of outdoor patients in most of the Indian hospitals. At the same time, specialization is a hallmark of modern times; respiratory medicine is no exception. With the recognition of chest medicine as a speciality, apart from better diagnosis and treatment of tuberculosis, which had earlier been overshadowing other chest diseases, more and more non-tuberculous pulmonary disorders have been recognized in the recent decades, through application of advanced diagnostic procedures. The advancement has helped chest physicians to better understand the pathophysiology of diseases, thereby creating possibilities to provide better chest care to the community.

The book provides current information regarding tropical pulmonary disorders in a simple language. Bronchial asthma has since been recognised as an inflammatory problem, the role of inhaled corticosteroids has been stressed as the first line of treatment. Similarly, setting up of convenient and economic high-tech pulmonary functional laboratories to provide proper evaluation and management of other airflow limitation disorders has been suggested. Management of bronchial carcinoma reaffirms the physician's stress to create tobacco-free global atmosphere as the only answer to this dreadful fatal disease. Current topics on lung transplantation, drug induced pulmonary disorders and lungs in connective tissue disorders have also been, though precisely touched, yet with full justice and completeness.

The book is an attempt to provide precise and to the point information, that is essential for medical students and practitioners regarding common respiratory diseases and disorders. It may look exacerbated to anticipate that the material provided in a concise manner may serve as a valuable teaching tool as well, since hardly any comparable compendium of information on chest medicine with Indian reference is available. The book may serve as a medium to allow certain outstanding academicians to exchange and crossfertilize ideas, thus encouraging the new investigators in respiratory medicine to initiate further research in this field. Most of the chapters are based on my short experiences in pulmonology that I gained through medical literature and through my clinical practice, while being in close association and direct communication with professors like Dr PS Shankar, Dr SK Jindal and Sir J Crofton respectively. I am grateful to Dr PS Shankar and salute him for his critical evaluation and wise comments. In fact, nothing could pass through his wise eye without scrutiny; that shows the masterly class that he has achieved through his academic career. I express my indebtedness to Professor PS Kalsi for kindly arranging the publication of the book.

I express my deep sense of gratefulness to my family members, who have always encouraged and supported me to prepare the manuscript. I would be glad if this book is accepted as a modest contribution towards an easy understanding of respiratory medicine.

RS Bhatia
Model Town
Ludhiana (PB)

Special Thanks To

Dr Rajbir Singh
KDDC, Mathura

Dr Surya Kant
HOD, Department of Respiratory Medicine
King's George Medical University, Lucknow

Dr BL Bharadwaj
Prof., Department of Medicine
GMC & H, Patiala

Dr SS Shergill
Principal, GMC & H, Amritsar

Dr Subhash Batta
CMO, Ludhiana

Dr Jaikishan
Director, Research and Medical Education, Punjab

Dr AK Janmeja
HOD, Department of Respiratory Medicine
GMC & H, Chandigarh

Dr P Bhattacharya
Director, Institute of Pulmocare and Research, Kolkata

Dr R Seth
Director, Seth Hospital, Ludhiana

Dr Sanjeev Mehta
Pulmonologist, Leelawati Hospital, Mumbai

Dr Soumya Swaminathan
Head, AIDS Division, TRC, Chennai

Dr NK Jain
(Ex) Head, Department of Chest Diseases, SMS Medical College, Jaipur

Dr LS Chawla
Foudner VC, Baba Farid Medical University, Punjab

Dr BM Hegde
Former VC, Manipal Medical Unviersity, Manipal

Dr GC Ahir
Principal, GMC & H
Faridkot

Dr NC Kajal
HOD, Department of Chest Diseases
GMC & H, Amritsar

Dr Virendra Singh
HOD, Department of Pulmonary Medicine
SMS Hospital, Jaipur

Dr SK Luhadia
Former, HOD, Department of Resp Medicine
Medical College, Udaipur

Prof. CN Deivanayagam
(Former) Medical Supdt. Hospital for Thoracic Medicine Chennai

Prof. PS Shankar
Emeritus Prof. of Medicine, Director, MR Medical College
Gulbarga

Prof. VK Vijayan
(Former) Director, VP Chest Institute, Delhi University, Delhi

Prof. SK Jindal
HOD, Department of Pulmonary Medicine, PGIMER, Chandigarh

Dr YP Munjal
Director, Diabetes Institute, Delhi
Past President, API, Mumbai
Editor-API Book of Medicine

Dr SS Sibia
Director, Sibia Medical Centre, Ludhiana

Dr SS Arora
Director, Batra Hospital Delhi

Dr Raj Bahadur
Principal, CMC & H, Chandigarh

CONTENTS

CONTENTS

Common Respiratory Symptoms, Clinical Examination and Applied Investigations in Respiratory Medicine

1

History[1]

History is very important in the diagnosis of pulmonary diseases. Personal history, occupational history, history of smoking and extramarital contact, history of previous residence or visit to a particular place and history of a drug intake for a short or long period, are quite helpful in reaching a conclusive diagnosis of a chest ailment. Common symptoms due to pulmonary diseases and disorders are discussed below:

SYMPTOMS

Cough[2-7]

Next to pain, cough is the most common symptom encountered in clinical practice. Cough as such is not a separate disease entity, but is a symptom of variety of conditions in the respiratory or extra-respiratory passages. It is also an indicator of environmental pollution. The causes of cough may vary between wax in the ear or a psycho-neurosis to a life-threatening malignancy. In fact, cough is a nature's way of protecting the lungs (a protective reflex) against aspiration or inhalation of a foreign material. It aids in the removal of bronchial secretions which are either infected or produced in excess. Mild cough is useful as well as harmless and does not require any remedies, severe coughing may be harmful and has to be suppressed and dealt with. However, under circumstances of a suppressed cough reflex, coughing has to be encouraged or induced by regular physiotherapy of chest in order to cleanse the lungs and remove the excessive secretions.

The Cough Reflex

Cough reflex has an afferent limb, the medullary centre and an efferent limb. The highest density of cough receptors is found in the larynx, trachea, bronchi, and further down in the acini. The afferent fibres travelling in the vagus transmit sensory impulses to the cough centre in the medulla. Other afferent pathways are in the trigeminal nerve, from receptors in the nose and paranasal sinuses; the glossopharyngeal nerve from receptors in the pharynx; the vagus from receptors in the pleura, stomach and ear passages, and the phrenic nerve from receptors in the pericardium and diaphragm. The efferent functional pathways in cough include the vagus nerves, which transmit impulses to the larynx, trachea and bronchi, and the phrenic and spinal nerves, which transmit impules to the diaphragm and respiratory muscles.

The Act of Coughing

Direct stimulation of the cough receptors occurs by physical agents like inhaled particulate matter, cigarette smoke, irritant gases, vapour and fumes from the environment at home or at work, inflammation due to viral, bacterial, allergic or non-specific origin, granulomatous changes, foreign body, and neoplasia. Indirect stimulation of these receptors can also occur due to inspiratory traction on the bronchial walls in pulmonary fibrosis, oedema, atelectasis and distortion of the tracheo-bronchial tree due to increased intrathoracic pressure swings.

The reflex response consists of contraction of respiratory muscles against a closed glottis causing rise in intrathoracic pressure (may be upto 100 mm Hg) followed by opening of the glottis and forced expiration with very high flow rates in the upper airways. This sweeps out all materials in the lumen of the respiratory passages.

Effectiveness of Coughing

The effectiveness of coughing as a protective reflex depends directly upon the physiological soundness of the neurogenic reflex as well as of the mucociliary action. The receptors get adapted to the stimuli. For instance, cough in response to smoking and inhalation of other pollutants is more forceful in the beginning but waves off with time to a weaker reflex. Contrarily, the constant presence of secretions in the airways reduces the stimulation of receptors. The second important component of cough reflex is the medullary centre which is depressed during sleep, respiratory failure, general anesthesia, coma, administration of sedative drugs, head injury and stroke. The third component is the efferent nerves and muscles. Its functions may be impaired in neuromuscular disorders like Guillain-Barré syndrome poliomyelitis, myasthenia gravis etc. The fourth important component is the state of the airways. The presence of airflow limitation reduces the generation of high expiratory flow rates ratio. Such patients may have prolonged wheezy bouts of cough and all the efforts fail to effectively expel secretions from the airways.

Causes of Persistent Cough

The common causes of cough differ at different ages. In neonates, cardiac disease and tracheo-oesophageal fistula should be excluded. During later childhood, chronic maxillary sinusitis, enlarged inflammed tonsils, adenoids, asthma and inhaled foreign body are common causes. Nocturnal coughing in children is almost pathognomonic of asthma. Viral infections may cause cough lasting for several months. Psychogenic cough, sometimes related to maternal anxiety, may occur in children. In adults, persistent cough is most commonly due to cigarette smoking. Carcinoma of lung should be suspected in cases of smokers whenever there is a change in the pattern of coughing. In non-smoker adults, asthma is the most common cause, though viral infections may also cause persistent cough lasting for months. Some causes of cough are given in Tables 1.1, 1.2 and 1.3. Ref: [Murray and Nadel, in Respiratory Medicine, 1988, W.B. Saunders].

Table 1.1: Some causes of cough

Exogenous irritants	**Restrictive lung disease**
Tobacco smoke	Pulmonary fibrosis
Smog	Congestive heart failure
High levels of atmospheric SO_2	Pneumoconiosis
Noxious gases at the work place	Collagen vascular disease
Mechanical irritants	Granulomatous disease
Retained bronchopulomonary secretions	**Infections**
Foreign body within the airways	Acute laryngitis
Voice strain	Acute bronchitis
Postnasal drip	Pneumonia
Aspiration of gastric contents	Pericarditis
Abnormally long uvula	Tuberculosis
Enlarged tonsils	**Pulmonary vascular disease**
Allergic	Pulmonary emboli
Inflammatory	Pulmonary hypertension
Asthma	**Neoplastic**
Airway hyperresponsiveness	Laryngeal tumour
Milk product intolerance	Endobronchial tumour
Loffler's pneumonia	Extrinsic compression of airways by tumour
Obstructive airway disease	Psychogenic
Chronic bronchitis	**Drugs**
Emphysema	ACE inhibitors therapy
Cystic fibrosis	
Bronchiectasis	

Rare Causes of Cough

1. Those associated with impaction of serumen in the external auditory canal or irritation of the ear drum by hair which have been reported to cause cough.
2. Cough may occur because of globus hystericus or anxiety reaction, in Gilles de la Tourettes disease—a neurogenic disorder associated with abnormality of neural transmission of the face and shoulders, as well as in echolalia and corpolalia. In these conditions, it has been suggested that afferent pathways from higher centres are in appropriately stimulated. Sometimes, idiopathic self-sustaining cough occurs in persons with superimposed anxiety or depression.

Complications of Severe Coughing

Cough syncope is well-known in patients with whoop or severe paroxysmal cough, more so in the elderly people and with a severe bout of cough. Syncope occurs because of sustained rise in the intrathoracic pressure (Valsalva Manoeuvre) which impedes venous return to heart and lowers the cardiac output. This effect is potentiated by the cough induced reflex vasodilatation in the skeletal muscles resulting in *bleed in the legs.* The consequent cerebral hypoperfusion on account of cardiovascular effects is worsened by the simultaneous increase in the CSF pressure. The cough syncope has a short span. Other potential complications occurring as a result of coughing are pulmonary interstitial oedema and pneumomediastinum, rupture of subconjunctival nasal and anal veins, bradycardia and heart block, rupture of rectus abdominis muscle, abdominal wall haematoma, prolapse of intervertebral disc and rib fractures in the axillary line. Chronic cough leads to inguinal herniae (Table 1.4).

Management of Cough

The management of cough considering the most diverse nature of its aetiology, should be done on firm footing, keeping in view the sound clinical evaluation. As cough is a manifestation of a disease, every effort should be made towards identifying the cause. Since most coughs are transient and related to upper respiratory infections, the latter may be treated first before investigating further. Clinical history, occupational site exposures, chest radiograph, WBC count, bacteriology of sputum, nasal and throat secretion smear examination, Mantoux reaction, spirometry and residual volume measurements and in rare cases diffusion test would in most cases give the clue to

Table 1.2: Cough

Acute *(Cough for less than 3 weeks)*	*Subacute* *(Cough lasting for 3-8 weeks)*	*Chronic* *(Cough for 8 weeks or more)*
• Pneumonia • Left ventricular failure asthma • Aspiration of foreign matter • Common cold, allergic rhinitis, sinusitis • Exacerbation of COPD • Bordetella pertussis infection	• Post infectious cough • B. pertussis infection • Subacute bacterial sinusitis • Asthma	**I (95% of cases)** • Asthma • GERD • Smokers • Chronic bronchitis • Eosinophilic bronchitis • ACE-inhibitors • Postnasal drip in a variety of rhinosinus conditions **II (5% of cases)** • Bronchogenic carcinoma • Carcinomatosis • Tuberculosis • Sarcoidosis • Left ventricular failure • Aspiration from pharyngeal dysfunction

Table 1.3: Common causes of cough in paediatric patients

Acute cough	*Chronic cough*
1. Upper respiratory infections like common cold, sinusitis, rhinitis, tonsilitis, adenitis, pharyngitis, laryngitis and bronchitis 2. Nasobronchial allergy 3. Asthma 4. Whooping cough 5. Foreign body in respiratory passage	1. Chronic rhinitis, sinusitis, adenitis etc. 2. Chronic asthmaticus bronchitis 3. Bronchiectasis 4. Lung abscess 5. Loffler's syndrome 6. Tuberculosis 7. Tracheal pressure due to lymph nodes, abscess or tumour 8. Tracheoesophageal fistula 9. Enterofenous cyst or duplication of eosophagus

Table 1.4: Cardiopulmonary complications of cough

- Pneumothorax, pneumomediastinum
- Loss of consciousness (modified valsalva manoeuvre)
- Rupture of anal, nasal or subconjunctival veins
- Bradycardia

aetiology. In difficult cases however, cardiovascular assessment, Casoni's test, bronchoscopy, CAT scan of thorax etc, may be needed. Treatment of cough means treating the cause although sometimes it may be necessary to suppress the cough when a paroxysmal non-productive, sleep disturbing, apprehending cough becomes a personal and social nuisance. Also, in case of bronchial carcinoma, cough adds to the misery of a terminally ill patient. In some cases with persistent cough, suppression of cough may break the vicious circle of the cough receptor stimulation. The use of small regulated doses of chlorpheniramine and codeine linctus, supplemented by steam inhalation and for more severe cough, a course of methadone linctus may be justified. People have been using honey alone or in combination with ginger juice/black pepper as a cough remedy. In terminal disease cases, small but frequent doses of heroin are often advisable.

Chronic Cough in Children

Chronic cough in a child of preschool age is more difficult and frustrating. It is often viewed as difficult problem for its diagnostic dilemmas and treatment failures. Many of diagnostic tests, such as pulmonary functions, cannot be performed. Nevertheless, if one can obtain a careful and detailed history, perform relevant diagnostic tests, and occasionally provide trials of medications, usually the symptoms can be adequately controlled.[4] Exposure to airborne irritants such as cigarette smoke or to potential allergens such as house dust mites, furry animals, or fungal spores can aggravate any respiratory inflammatory process. A careful environmental history combined with immediate hypersensitivity skin testing help to identify potentially important allergens. Ongoing postnasal drainage is a common cause of cough, with or without sinusitis. The worsening of symptoms in the supine position supports this association. Sinus X-ray films will be abnormal as well. It is increasingly becoming apparent, however, that plain films of the paranasal sinuses may not correlate with findings on coronal computed tomographic scan.[5] If the diagnosis of sinusitis remains a question, this *gold standard* study should be performed. If the cough is worsened by exercise or exposure to cold air, the diagnosis of asthma may be inferred. Although children of this age cannot reliably perform pulmonary function tests, provocation test a simple method of performing methacholine challenges in this age group can allow the diagnosis of asthma to be made.[6] This test can be performed in OPD. The diagnosis of gastroesophageal reflux can be considered, as an uncommon cause of cough in this age group. However, a more sensitive diagnostic test would be direct monitoring of esophageal pH for a 12 to 24 hours period. Pulmonary infections may be responsible, but very unlikely given the chronic nature of the symptoms. Other diagnostic possibilities, such as a foreign body, cystic fibrosis, or a congenital anomaly can well be excluded as differential diagnosis. ACE inhibitors have also been implicated.[7]

From a therapeutic standpoint, first focus on the upper airways should be kept. Nasal steroids have been attempted, salbutamol or beclomethasone has no effect on cough frequency, irrespective of airway hyperresponsiveness. Nasal irrigations with saline may be extremely helpful in flushing the nasal passages of obstructing and irritating mucus. Topical nasal decongestants for 3 to 5 days may also be helpful. If the computed tomograph scan suggests sinusitis, aggressive antibiotics should be used. Given the protracted nature of his symptoms, an antibiotic that provides coverage for β-lactamase-producing organisms as well as anaerobes (e.g., amoxicillin-clavulanate, 40 mg/kg per day for 3 to 4 weeks) should be used. Although bronchodilators, cromolyn, and anti-cholinergics have not been successful, more aggressive treatment for asthma may be needed. Oral corticosteroids (e.g., prednisone, 1 mg/kg per day) for 1 week in conjunction with inhaled corticosteroids (e.g., beclomethasone, three sprays three times a day) for 3 to 4 weeks should be attempted. Metered-dose preparations can usually be adequately administered in this age group if spacing devices (e.g., aero spacer with mask) are used. Trials of antacids or H_2 antagonists may be considered. In order to break the cycle of airways irritation, antitussive agents, including narcotics, may be of help for a short period of time.[5,6]

Dyspnoea[8,9]

Breathlessness is an important symptom of cardiorespiratory ailment. Dyspnoea of cardiac origin usually has evidence of heart enlargement and failure; cardiac murmur or gallop rhythm. Nocturnal attacks of dyspnoea pose difficulty in differentiating pulmonary oedema of cardiac origin or bronchial asthma. Relationship of dyspnoea with rest or exertion and associated chest pain or cough and the type of cough and expectoration commonly help physician to differentiate the type of dyspnoea. MRC scale is shown in Table 1.5.

Table 1.5: Medical Research Council (MRC) scale of dyspnoea

Grade I	Breathlessness on strenuous exertion
II	Dyspnoea on hurrying up on the level
III	Patient has to stop walking on level after a mile or 1/2 hour
IV	Has to stop after few minutes of walking or after 100 yards
V	Patient is too breathless to leave the house

The actual mechanism of dyspnoea is not properly understood, but the severity of dyspnoea is directly related to the gravity of cardiopulmonary dysfunction. The mechanism involves abnormal activation of respiratory centres through stimulation via different somatic nerves from respiratory muscles as well as from skeletal muscles and joints, intrathoracic receptors via vagi, chemoreceptors in brain, carotid bodies and elsewhere in the circulatory system, cortical centres and different fibres in the phrenic nerves.

Acute airways, obstruction by aspiration, allergic oedema, acute intermittent obstruction as asthma and chronic bronchitis and bronchiectasis can cause dyspnoea.

Parenchymal pulmonary disorders, like different types of pneumoconiosis and vascular occulusive diseases such as pulmonary embolism have dyspnoea as a presenting symptom.

Involvement of chest wall or respiratory muscles may have gradually progressive dyspnoea in correspondence to developing respiratory failure. At the same time, dyspnoea of psychogenic origin must be kept in mind as a differential. Different causes are shown in Tables 1.6 and 1.7.

Table 1.6: Orthopnoea

Mitral stenosis
LVF

Table 1.7: Dyspnoea (Shortness of breath)

Respiratory tract	Pharyngeal abscess, laryngeal tumour or oedema
Pulmonary	Asthma, atelectesis, anthrax, bronchiolitis, bronchiectasis, croup, COPD, emphysema with bronchitis, Goodpasture's syndrome, pleural effusion, pneumonia, pneumothorax, pressure on larynx from abscess

Chest Pain

It is an important cardinal manifestation of pulmonary diseases, especially when there is an inflammation of lung parenchyma, pleura, tubercular infection, pulmonary thromboembolism, malignancy etc. Pain is generally of pleuritic origin, often related to respiratory movement. Mediastinal involvement generally gives a local discomfort while parenchymal involvement doesn't produce pain. The radiation of the pain may also provide a clue. Superficial pain may occur from extrathoracic reasons, as neuritis in herpes zoster. Other causes of thoracic pain include myositis, costochondral involvements, angina pectoris, pericarditis, aortic dissection and aneurysm, oesophageal affections etc. Superficial pains can be readily distinguished by palpation as they get aggravated. Differentiation between pleuropulmonary and myocardial chest pain sometimes poses a great difficulty. Common causes especially the cardio-pulmonary have been shown in Table 1.8.

Table 1.8: Cardiopulmonary causes of chest pain

Cardiac	Anaemia, Angina pectoris, Aortic aneurysm, Cardiac neurosis, Congenital heart disease, Myocardial infarction, Myocarditis, Mitral valve prolapse, Pericarditis, Pericardial effusion
Pulmonary	Bronchiectasis, Hyperventilation (Tetany), Pulmonary thromboembolism, Pulmonary infections, Pleurisy, Pneumonitis, Pneumothorax, Pneumomediastinum, Tracheitis
Others	Thoracic malignancy, Mediastinal and thymic tumours, Melioidosis, Sarcoidosis
Chest wall (Musculoskeletal)	Trauma, Superficial chest infections, Tietze's syndrome, Bornholm's syndrome, Vertebral arthritis and Vertebral malignancy

Haemoptysis[10-13]

Haemoptysis is usually frightening and brings the patient immediately to his family physician, but may not always be serious. Any blood in the sputum from minor streaks to massive haemorrhage (600-800 ml) per 24 hours called haemoptysis is a commonly encountered feature which can be differentiated from haemetemesis as it is bright red and frothy compared to the latter which is dark red in colour. Incidence varies from 2-40% and 5-15% of cases with massive haemoptysis generally remain undiagnosed. Haemoptysis is generally scanty in pneumonitis and viral respiratory infections and is a rare observation in metastatic malignant lung disease. Various causes are listed in Table 1.9.

Apart from acute infections like bronchiectasis, tuberculosis, pulmonary thromboembolism, lung cancer, mitral stenosis are other known causes. Frothy pinkish diluted secretions show acute pulmonary odema while haemoptysis with pusy material goes in favour of pneumonia, abscess or bronchiectasis. Diffuse alveolar hemorrhage in rheumatoid arthritis may present with hemoptysis, having radiographic appearance of pulmonary edema. Frank haemoptysis is seen in pulmonary thromboembolism. Highly vascular tumour such as mediastinal schwannoma may rupture into adjacent bronchus producing massive haemoptosis. Haemoptysis is a cardinal respiratory symptom, occurring in 50% of patients with multiple pulmonary tuberculous cavities. Even it may occur in 1/5th of cases who have been adequately treated for pulmonary tuberculosis. Hence, haemoptysis is not to be taken as a sign of reactivation of healed residual pulmonary tuberculous lesion.

Table 1.9: Causes of haemoptysis

Inflammatory	Bronchitis Bronchiectasis Pneumonitis Lung abscess Pulmonary tuberculosis
Neoplastic	Bronchial adenoma , Lung cancer
Miscellaneous	
a. Pulmonary	Pulmonary thromoboembolism Chest trauma Primary pulmonary hypertension Congenital A.V. Malformations, Wegener's granuloma, Pulmonary amyloidosis, Good-pasture's syndrome, Pulmonary hemosiderosis
b. Cardiac	Mitral stenosis Left ventricular failure
c. Systemic	Haemorrhagic diathesis Anticoagulant therapy

Usually bleeding stops by itself without specific therapy. Massive haemorrhage may require surgical intervention. Bronchoscopy is useful only prior to surgery to locate the site of bleeding, otherwise it is better to avoid for several days as it may precipitate bleeding. Surgically unfit candidates can be managed by use of laser therapy.

Fever

It is a common symptom and requires to be differentiated from various causes. Physical examination[1,14] of chest is quite useful in reading most of the commonly known diseases, if history is correlated with proper stepwise examination of thorax, starting with inspection, palpation, percussion and auscultation. On general physical examination of the chest, cervical lymphadenopathy, may be found. General comatosed stage with smell of phosphine may point towards aluminium phosphide poisoning. Leukoplakic lips and inter finger strains in smokers, cutaneous lesions in sarcoidosis and infected oral hygiene in lung abscess may contribute towards clinching the ultimate diagnosis of pulmonary disorder. Thin, emaciated, coughing patient, running low grade persistent fever is likely to be suffering from pulmonary tuberculosis in countries like India.

Cyanosis[1,15,16]

Bluish colour of skin and mucosal membranes due to an increased amount of reduced haemoglobin is called cyanosis, which may not be accurately quantitatively detected clinically as proved by oximetric studies, but generally it is clinically detected as the arterial saturation falls below 85% (the red cyanosis is a different entity, seen in polycythemia vera and is caused by carboxyhaemoglobin) and the absolute quantity of reduced haemoglobin exceeds 5 gms/dl.

Cyanosis becomes evident in the presence of non-functional haemoglobin such as methaemoglobin and sulphemoglobin.

The central type affects both skin and mucosa while peripheral cyanosis spares tongue and buccal mucosa and is seen in cases of shock, congestive failure, peripheral vascular disease, cold exposure etc. In case of cardiogenic shock with pulmonary oedema, type differentiation of cyanosis becomes quite difficult.

Central cyanosis may be seen in pneumonitis, pulmonary odema, chronic brochitis with emphysema, congenital heart disease like Fallot's tetralogy, methaemoglobinemia etc. as shown in Table 1.10.

While diagnosing cyanosis, history of exposure to drugs, gas or chemicals is important. Gentle warming or massage of the cyanotic extremity will abolish peripheral cyanosis due to improved circulation and not the central cyanosis. Clubbing is not a feature of acutely developing central cyanosis and peripheral cyanosis.

Clubbing

Clubbing and osteoarthropathy may be seen in suppurative disorders or bronchogenic carcinoma, and congenital heart disease with pulmonary AV fistulae. Various causes of clubbing are shown in Table 1.11.

Clubbing occurs in association with a variety of pulmonary diseases.[17] The prevalence of clubbing in pulmonary tuberculosis is reported by different authors varies from 1% to 90%.[17,18] Clubbing has been present in tuberculosis and is usually associated with destructive disease and high mortality, with wide variation depending on the methods used and groups of patients studied.[19]

Table 1.11: Common causes of clubbing

Cardio-pulmonary
Bronchogenic carcinoma, Lung abscess, empyema, bronchiectasis, Pulmonary tuberculosis, ILD, Benign Mesothelioma, SABE, Primary pulmonary hypertension, congenital cyanotic heart disease, pulmonary AV fistula.

Gastrointestinal
Primary biliary cirrhosis, ulcerative colitis, Crohn's disease.

Differential clubbing
PDA with reverse shunt (clubbing of toes and in left hand only)

Unilateral clubbing
Arterial/aorticaneurysms, Pan coast's syndrome, venous varices, Trauma of peripheral nerves.

Finger clubbing may be associated with more severe pulmonary damage as indicated by presence of grade II disease and giant cavities in significantly larger number of patients, though number of patients having haemoptysis may not be significantly higher. This does not confirm the finding of Mcfarlane *et al.*[20] Haemoptysis with clubbing cannot be correlated because haemoptysis can be present in fresh, minimal and even healed cases.[19]

Patients with chronic tuberculosis tend to have clubbing more often than those without.[21] Patients with clubbing are found to be more anaemic as compared to patients without clubbing. Whether this anaemia could be due to the disease process itself or is a contributory factor to the occurrence of the disease is difficult to explain.

Since patients with chronic tuberculosis, giant cavities and bronchiectasis tend to have clubbing more commonly than the patients having minimal disease, clubbing can be used as an indicator to distinguish between patients having more severe pulmonary damage from those with less pulmonary damage. Differential diagnosis for clubbing must be kept in mind like ulcerative colitis, regional enteritis, biliary cirrhosis, etc.

Clinical examination of pulmonary system includes detailed examination of cardiovascular system as well. At the same time, physical examination can detect fluid in small amounts in the pleural cavities or mediastinum, bronchospasm and deviation of trachea more efficiently than by chest radiographic film.

Table 1.10: Causes of cyanosis

Central cyanosis		*Peripheral cyanosis*
Pulmonary causes	*Other causes*	
Pulmonary vein anomalies (shunts and fistulae) Pneumonia	Sulf haemoglobinemia	Diminished cardiac output
Respiratory failure, acute bronchical asthma Bronchiectasis	Methaemoglobinemia	Cold exposure
Emphysema Chronic lung disease like chronic bronchitis, COPD, ILD	Haemochromatosis	Vascular obstruction

CLINICAL EXAMINATION OF RESPIRATORY SYSTEM[22]

General Physical Examination may reveal an underweight, and emaciated patient as in emphysema, advanced pulmonary tuberculosis, lung cancer or a swollen, apparently heavy looking patient as in corpulmonale or the bloated upper half of the body as in obstruction of superior veva cava.

Clinical anemia may point towards the diagnosis of suppurative lung diseases, pulmonary tuberculosis and lung cancer.

Cervical lymphadenopathy may be noticed in tubercular involvement while generalised lymphadenopathy may help to search for diagnosis like sarcoidosis, lymphomas and fungal infections. An unusual single supraclavicular lymph node may fetch the attention towards lung cancer.

Raised jugular venous pressure is a feature of congestive heart failure secondary to corpulmonale, while a pulsus paradoxus of more than 10 mm Hg is seen in patients of acute bronchial asthma and acute exacerbations of COPD.

Severe anaemia, cyanosis, clubbing etc. have already been discussed. Following text space provide a detailed examination of respiratory system.

Anatomy

The respiratory system though a continuous tract has been divided into two parts, the upper and the lower respiratory passages, using the cricoid cartilage as the separating landmark. On surface anatomy, the right lung consists of three lobes and the left two. A greater portion of the front of the chest corresponds to the upper and middle lobes on the right and the upper lobe on the left. On the back, the lower lobes occupy the area below the spine of the scapula and the apex belongs to the upper lobe. In the axilla parts, all the lobes are closely situated. The apices of the lung rise, about two to three cms above the middle of the clavicle on each side. The shoulder girdle and its musculature cover the apical and the posterior segments of the right upper lobe and the apicoposterior segment of the left upper lobe. The major interlobar (oblique) fissure corresponds to a line drawn from the spine of the second thoracic vertebra downwards and medially to the sixth costal cartilage in front. It crosses the fifth rib at the midaxillary line. The lower lobe is situated below this line. The minor interlober (horizontal) fissure on the right side corresponds to a horizontal line drawn from the fourth costal cartilage to the posterior axillary line where it meets the first line at the fifth rib. The region bounded by these two lines on the right side corresponds to the middle lobe. The lower border of the lung begins at the level of the 6th costal cartilage. On the left side because of the situation of the cardia the lower margin of the lung takes a turn laterally in an arc-like manner to reach the 6th rib. The lower margin of the lung crosses the 8th rib in the mid axillary region the 10th rib in the scapular line and ends at the 10th thoracic spine.

The pleural sac extends beyond the lower limits of the lung and reaches the 8th, 10th and 12th ribs in the mid clavicular, mid axillary and scapular lines respectively. The cervical pleura follows closely the surface marking of the lung. The trachea divides into two main bronchi, the right and the left—at carina at the level of the disc between the 4th and the 5th thoracic vertebrae. It corresponds to the lower border of the manubrium sterni infront. The roots of the lungs are situated in the interscapular region at the level of the spines of the 4th, 5th and 6th thoracic vertebrae. The right bronchus gives two side branches called lobar bronchi to the upper and middle lobes and then discends as the lower lobe bronchus. The left bronchus gives a branch—the upper lobe bronchus and then descends as lower lobe bronchus. These lober bronchi divide into segmental bronchi and supply a wedge shaped lung tissue (bronchopulmonary segments). Each lobe and each segment have a homologue in the other lung. The segmental bronchi are ten on the right side and nine on the left. On the right side, the upper lobe bronchus divides into apical, anterior and posterior segmental bronchi, the middle into medial and lateral segmental bronchi and the lower into the apical and four basal segmental bronchi, medial, lateral, anterior and posterior. On the left side the upper lobe bronchus divides into two divisions. The upper divisions give apicoposterior and anterior segmental bronchi and the lower divisions supplies the lingula (represents the middle lobe on the left side) as the superior and the inferior segmental bronchi. The lower lobe bronchus gives an apical, anterior, posterior and lateral segmental bronchi.

The bony landmarks are the sternal angle (formed by the junction of the manubrium with the body of the sternum and it corresponds with the attachment of the second costal cartilage on either side of the sternum spine of the 7th cervical vertebra (vertebre prominens) clavicle, sternum ribs, spine of the scapula (inferior angle overlies the 7th intercostal space and the vertebral spines. The ribs are counted down from the 2nd costal cartilage. The sternal angle (the angle louis) is recognised as a transverse bony ridge. The 5th thoracic vertebra, the bifurcation of the trachea and the upper limits of the atria and arc of the aorta lie at the level of manubriosternal angle. The lung borders meet at that site. The nipple is not satisfactory as a landmark because of its in constant location. The chest is examined by inspection, palpation, percussion and auscultation to recognise signs caused by changes in the physical properties of lungs and pleura.

Inspection

The chest is stripped of clothing upto the waist and the patient is seated in a well lighted place. The shoulders are allowed to drop and the body has to be relaxed. In the case of the woman breasts are covered and the chest is examined part by part preserving her modesty. The chest is inspected from the front, sides and back. If the patient is too ill to sit, the back may be examined by rolling him in each side, in turn. During the inspection it has to be ascertained whether the patient can lie down comfortably. Respiratory distress, if present, has to be observed carefully. The patient having an attack of asthma, or, in cardiac failure, prefers to sit up to increase the efficiency of the respiratory excursions. The patient adopts wherein the shoulders are kept in an abducted position with elbows drawn away from the chest. One may hear noisy breathing. A wheezing sound may be evident during expiration in airway obstruction (asthma, chronic bronchitis). In conditions of oedema of the glottis, or laryngeal obstruction there is obstruction to the entry of air resulting in a harsh respiration (stridor). Normally the ribs exhibit a slope and are situated at about 45 degree angle in relation to the spine. The anterior ribs move upwards and outwards during inspiration. There is expansion of the chest laterally. Posteriorly the scapulae are firmly applied to the underlying chest wall. The expansion of the chest is markedly limited in conditions of airflow limitation (during attacks of bronchial asthma, chronic bronchitis and emphysema) and the accessory muscles of respiration (scalenii, sternomastoids and trapezii) will be active and the patient appears obviously breathless. The sternomastoid muscles become taut with inspiratory contraction. There is also abnormal recession of the suprasternal and supraclavicular fossae and lower interspaces during inspiration due to increased intrathoracic negative pressure. The patient may breathe with pursed lips in chronic obstructive pulmonary diseases. The lips are held tightly opposed at the height of inspiration and they are held narrowly apart during expiration to interpose an expiratory resistance. This is perhaps to lengthen the expiratory time and to increase lung volume. The nostrils may show inspiratory flaring in pneumonia and bronchial asthma. During inspection of chest, the shape of the chest and respiratory movements are to be noted carefully. The underlying respiratory diseases rarely cause any abnormality of the skin. The skin is examined for the presence of petechiae, exanthema, dilated superficial veins, supernumerary nipples, gynaecomastia, sinus scars, pityriasis versicolor infection, distribution of hair, swellings, sternomastoid tendon, pulsations, apical impluse and lymph nodes. There may be scars secondary to operations (thoracotomy), empyema drainage or branding.

Shape of the Chest

The shape of the chest is largely dependent on the build of the person. It may be short or broad in stocky individuals or long and narrow in asthenic individuals. Normally the chest is bilaterally symmetrical. The intercostal spaces are broader in front than behind. The transverse diameter is greater than the posteroanterior diameter in the ratio of 7:5 and the cross-section of the chest is elliptical. The subcostal is less than 90 degree and it widens during inspiration because of the lateral expansion of the chest. In children the chest appears cylindrical with the transverse and posteroanterior diameters being equal. With the advancing age in elders the posteroanterior diameter increases due to a slight dorsal non-vexity in the upper thoracic region. The shape of the chest may alter due to the disease of the past or the present. The abnormalities may be symmetrical or asymmetrical.

Symmetrical Abnormalities

Flat Chest

The posteroanterior is markedly decreased resulting in an increase in the transverse diameter. The chest appears like a shield. The scapula may stand out prominently like wings on either side (alar chest). Phthisical chest was said to be a feature in tuberculosis.

Rachitic Chest

The bones are soft during childhood and they can yield to pressure resulting in various abnormalities of chest. This is seen in those who have suffered from rickets, respiratory diseases like chronic severe asthma or cardiomegaly in childhood. The deformed chest may have any of the following abnormalities:

a. *Pigeon chest:* A forward bulged sternum projecting beyond the frontal place of thorax, particularly noticeable in its upper part, with sloping ribs losing their curvature, and chest appears triangular in cross-section (Pectus carinatum).
b. *Funnel chest (Pectus exacavatum):* It is associated with funnel like depression of the lower two thirds of the sternum behind the frontal plain of the thorax with prominent costochondral junctions.
c. *Harrison's groove:* It appears as a horizontal groove or constriction in the lower anterior thorax along the line of attachment of the diaphragm on one or both sides with coved in lower ribs.
d. *Rickety rosary:* It is seen as a beaded appearance due to enlargement of the successive costochondral junctions.

Barrel Shaped Chest

It is seen in cases of chronic air flow limitation as in emphysema and during acute severe attacks of asthma. Lungs are distended and the chest becomes over inflated with an increase in anteroposterior diameter of the chest. The ribs are horizontal with retraction of intercostal spaces on inspiration indicating obstruction to the free inflow of air in the respiratory tract. The spine is concave forwards, the sternum is prominently arched and the chest appears circular on cross-section. The subcostal angle is greater than 90 degrees and it shows little respiratory variation. Anteroposterior diameter of the chest may be increased without any obstructive airway disease as in thoracic kyphosis.

Asymmetrical Chest

The asymmetry of the chest may be due to the deformity of the vertebral column or diseases of the chest, causing retraction or prominence of one side. The vertebral column may show dorsal curvature (kyphosis). It may be widespread as in senile osteoporosis and ankylosing spondylitis of localized (gibbus) as in T.B. of the spine. The lateral spinal curvature is referred to as scoliosis. Both deformities may coexist as kyphoscoliosis. The abnormality may be developmental or secondary to neuro muscular diseases or respiratory diseases in childhood. The forward bend of the lumbar spine is referred to as lordosis.

Retraction

The chest may be flattened or even retracted on one side due to fibrosis of the lung or pleural thickening. The term frozen chest refers to a sunken hemithorax which is immobile due to thickened pleura. Interspaces may retract on inspiration, in airflow obstructive diseases.

Bulging

In massive pleural effusion and pneumothorax, the intercostal spaces are full and the chest becomes prominent. Even intercostal spaces may bulge out in emphysema. A swelling on the side of the chest may have cough impulse in emphysema necessitans while pulsatile swelling is seen in aortic aneurysm. A cold abscess or a tumour of subcutaneous tissue or chest wall may be seen on the chest surface.

Movements of the Chest (Respiration Rate)

In a normal person the respiration rate is 16-20 per minute, with a definite ratio to pulse as 1:4. An increase in rate and decrease is referred to as tachypnoea and bradypnoea respectively. Former occurs in pneumonia, pleurisy, hypoxia, heart failure, excitement, during fever and after exercise. Rate and depth increase simultaneously but rate may increase at the cost of depth in cases of pleurisy and fibrosis. Bradypnoea may be present in cases of narcotic poisoning, coma and tumour of brainstem.

Rhythm

Normal respiration is quiet, regular and rhythmic, where inspiration is active and expiration is passive, with a short pause in between the two. Inspiration is generally longer than the expiration. The latter is prolonged in cases of airways obstruction, while inspiration is prolonged in cases of laryngeal obstruction and mediastinal tumors. Wheeze is present in asthma and a periodic form of respiration called Cheyne-Stokes breathing is seen in cases of narcotic poisoning, raised intracranial tension, severe pneumonia, heart failure and renal failure. An irregular respiration—Biot *respiration* is observed in meningitis. Normally two types of respiration are considered, Costal (thoracic) and Diaphragmatic (abdominal). Costal respiration is commonly seen in females and diaphragmatic in males. But generally a combination is seen in normal healthy person. Costal respiration is more prominent in peritonitis, diaphragmatic paralysis, and ascitis, while diaphragmatic respiration is commonly seen in pulmonary fibrosis, pleurisy, ankylosing, spondylitis and paralysis of intercostal muscles.

Movements and Chest Expansion

There is synchronous and uniform movements of the chest in a normal healthy person, with an expansion of 5-8 cm. Unilateral decrease of the chest movements is an indicator of some underlying disease. The chest expansion is decreased in lung diseases (consolidation, collapse, tumor, fibrosis), pleural diseases (effusion, pneumothorax, pleural thickening) and in obstructive diseases like tumor or foreign body in the bronchus. The chest expansion is markedly decreased in airways obstructive disorders while a little expansion with considerable chest movements may be observed in emphysema. The movements at lung apices are restricted in tuberculosis while immobile chest is seen in ankylosing spondylitis. Both rate and depth of respiration—air hunger—are increased in diabetic ketoacidosis and renal failure (Kussmaul's breathing). Rise in depth is present in respiratory alkalosis and decrease in respiratory amplitude is seen in narcotics.

The diaphragmatic movements can be seen in the form of a wave of motion in thinly built persons (Litten's sign). In hyperinflation, an indrawing of anterior rib margins during inspiration by horizontal, rather than downward contraction of the diaphragm occurs (Hoover's sign). The diaphragmatic movements are almost reduced during pleural effusion, phrenic nerve paralysis and subdiaphragmatic abscess.

Mediastinal position is assessed by prominence of sternomastoid muscle due to tracheal displacement to that side (Trail's sign).

An obstruction to superior vena cava or azygos vein will lead to prominence of superficial veins on the chest wall.

Palpation

Palpation supplements as well as confirms the findings of inspection, e.g., any chest pain should be worked for eliciting an area of tenderness, which may be due to cough, injury, fracture or malignant deposits. Tenderness at the site of pleurisy, costochondral junctions (Teitze's syndrome) and intercostal muscles (Intercostal fibrositis) may be observed. A crackling sensation of air-bubble underneath the skin may be present in subcutaneous emphysema. Fluctuation may be present in cases of abscess as well as emphysema necessitans. Three features of palpation include:

1. *Chest expansion:* It is restricted on the affected side.
2. *Chest vibration:* It is felt in the form of fremitus and is appreciated as follows:
   (a) *Vocal fremitus:* It is a sign to detect vibrations produced by phonation, which are transmitted to the palpating hand through the airways, lungs, pleura and chest wall. This is called tactile fremitus and is more clear over the areas of trachea and bronchi. It is increased in cases of consolidation, infarction and neoplasm and decreased in obstructive airways disorders, collapse, emphysema, fibrosis, pleural effusion, thickened pleura, pneumothorax, hydropneumothorax and after tracheostomy (Table 1.12).
   (b) *Friction fremitus:* A specific superficial sensation felt in infra-axillary or infrascapular regions in cases of pleurisy. This occurs due to rubbing of inflammed pleura against each other.
   (c) *Rhonchial fremitus:* Expiratory rhonchi which disappear on coughing, are actually felt all over the chest, in cases of airways obstructive diseases.
3. *Tracheal position (Table 1.13):* A centrally located trachea is felt in the suprasternal notch in a normal person. Trachea along with cardiac impulse may be pushed to opposite side in conditions like pleural effusion, empyema, hydropneumothorax, and pneumothorax as well as following single lung transplantation, and pulled to the same side in diseases like lung collapse and fibrosis. Simultaneous shift of the cardiac impulse indicates shift of the lower mediastinum, while cardiac impulse may not shift along with trachea in case of tumor or mass of upper mediastinum. Cardiac impulse is affected in cardiac diseases and boney cage abnormalities like scoliosis and funnel chest. However, in dorsal scoliosis, the mediastinum may deviate to the concavity side. In pleural effusion, where airways obstruction is co-existing due to bronchogenic carcinoma, tracheal deviation occurs to the same side, while apical impulse moves towards opposite side. In shallow pneumothorax and in minimal pleural effusion there may not be any shift of trachea or cardiac impulse.

Table 1.12: Vocal fremitus
• Ulnar border of hand is used to detect variations in vibrations transmitted from larynx through the airways and lungs to the chest wall when a patient repeats a phrase (Thirtyeight)
• Absent: Feeble voice, foreign body or tumour in the bronchus, collapsed lung, pleural effusion, pneumothorax
• Increased: Pneumonia, tuberculosis, consolidation around major bronchus.

Table 1.13: Tracheal displacement
Definition: Deviation of trachea from the midline to the suprasternal towards the lesion:
Pulmonary collapse, fibrosis, tuberculosis
Away from lesion:
Pleural effusion, pneumothorax

Percussion

When chest is percussed, both the lungs as well as the chest wall are set into vibration, resulting into a sound, the quality of which and the resistance offered by the chest during percussion gives information. Normally, a resonant note is elicited over an inflated lung. Chest percussion, provides information regarding the cardiac and hepatic dullness (topography) (Table 1.14), in addition to pathological chest conditions. Apical resonance is dereased in tuberculosis. The lower border of lung resonance ascends in cases of pleural effusion, fibrosis and collapse and descends in emphysema and pneumothorax. Traube's space (Liver on right, spleen on left and left costal margin from below) is increased in lung collapse and fibrosis, and decreased in pleural effusion, pericardial effusion, hepatosplenomegaly.

The mobility of the hemidiaphragm is hindered in pleural effusion, adhesions and over inflation. A dull note is elicited in conditions like consolidation, tumor, pleural effusion or empyema. The note is flat dullness, compared to impaired note felt in collapse or fibrosis. The dullness note is definite in consolidation (Woody dullness), while it is absolute dull in pleural effusion (Stony dullness). In these cases, the dullness is highest in the axilla, sloping down to the front and back (Ellis S-shaped curve) but pleural fluid is detected only when it is

Table 1.14: Topography
Chest percussion infers
• Cardiac dullness
• Hepatic dullness

more than 300 ml in volume. Louder and more vibrant note—hyper resonant note—occurs in conditions like emphysema, pneumothorax (Table 1.15) and may be present in cases like pleural effusions and consolidation from an area above these pathologies as a drum like sound from the areas of compensatory emphysema (Skodiac resonance).

Table 1.15: Thoracic tympany

- Higher pitch of percussion note on striking a flat finger on the chest with another index finger is thoracic tympany. This occurs because large air masses reflect sound more rapidly
- Positive: In case of overinflation of lung (asthma, emphysema), Cavitation of lungs, Pneumothorax

Coin sound, with the help of percussing with two coins instead of fingers can be heard in cases of pneumothorax.

Unlike pleural effusion, upper border of dullness is horizontal in conditions like pyopneumothorax and hydropneumothorax. Shifting dullness can be demonstrated by recording the upper border of dullness in a sitting position and then eliciting a resonant note at the same area when the patient is in the lying position.

Myodema or myotatic irritability can be demonstrated in cachexia by giving a direct light tap on the sternum, resulting into a transitory local swelling.

Auscultation

Chest sounds are auscultated by using a biaural stethoscope, to observe the entry of the air, the breath sounds, additional sounds and vocal resonance. The sound transmission is affected by pleural effusion and pneumothorax. Air entry may be decreased in cases of lung consolidation, collapse, fibrosis, and airway obstructive disorders. Massive effusions, pneumothorax and bronchial occlusion may allow minimal air entry.

Breath sounds in health and disease are described in details separately. However, percussion and auscultatory findings in few common diseases have been shown in Tables 1.16 and 1.17.

Table 1.16: Chest percussion

If percussion note is dull	Probable diagnoses include Consolidation, Extensive carcinoma, Fibrosis, Pleural effusion, Pneumonia, Tuberculosis

Table 1.17: Pulmonary crepitations (Moist rales)

On auscultation: Moist sounds can be: Coarse: Bronchiectasis, Bronchitis: Fine: Elderly, Lung collapse, Pneumonia, Tuberculosis	Bubbling (Coarse), Crackling (Medium), Inspiratory tinkling (Fine)

INVESTIGATIONS

X-ray chest forms an important diagnostic tool for a chest ailment. Interpretation of chest roentgenograph in the light of history, clinical examination and previous chest X-ray, if any, is always rewarding.[1] Chest X-ray[23-25] can detect diseases ofthe bony thoracic cage as well as variety of pleuropulmonary disorders. Even pulmonary lesions may be detected silently or accidentally in a clinically normal patient. Further growth of chest radiological examination has given us better understanding of chest ailments with the help of tomographic and magnetic resonance studies.[26]

Chest screening can be performed in cases of coal workers or workers with silica dust exposure, asbestoses etc. Those occupational disorders which cause asthma rather than pneumoconiosis, should be screened. Common causes of nodular and reticular radiological shadowing are shown in Table 1.18. And findings on plain chest X-ray in HIV positive patient are shown in Table 1.19.

Conventional chest tomographic studies[27] for hilar region evaluation is still used. Computed tomography[28] is being currently used to assess mediastinal lymph node size in the staging of lung cancer as well as to distinguish vascular and non-vascular lesions, mediastinal tumors, cyst or calcification. Since calcification is not visible by magnetic resonance imaging, mediastinal CT is best used for revealing fibrosing mediastinitis. Contrast material studies are not popular. Pleural CT help in diagnosing tumors like mesothelioma and metastatic adenocarcinoma, bronchopleural fistulae, pleural fluid, asbestos pleural plaques and calcification. CT of lung and airways[29] is useful in alveolar and interstitial lung diseases and to some extent to have parenchymal study in cases of carcinomatosis, emphysema, interstitial fibrosis etc. Its application in studying bronchial thickening, dilatation or mucoid infection is of enormous value.

High resolution CT[30] is useful in both bronchial and parenchymal studies, especially the interstitial lung diseases in deciding probable diagnosis, activity of the disease, its prognosis and even best site to biopsy and possibly may become the choice method in ruling out bronchiectasis. It helps in diagnosing tracheal masses and in assessing constrictive bronchiolitis that often co-exists with bronchiectasis. Different varieties of emphysema can be distinguished with HRCT.

CT Densitometry[12] is quite contributory in deciding the presence or absense of calcification in solitary pulmonary nodule (SPN), evaluation of pulmonary thromboembolism and pathologies of mediastinum. 3DCT is virtual endoscopy in evaluating subglottic and tracheal stenosis.

Table 1.18: Common causes of nodular and reticular shadowing on chest X-ray

Diagnosis	*Radiographic pattern*	*Distribution of shadows*	*Other features which may be seen*
1. Miliary tuberculosis	Small nodules of uniform size	Uniform	Mediastinal/hilar lymph nodes, one or patches of consolidation
2. Sarcoidosis	(a) Fine nodular	Uniform	Hilar and paratracheal lymph nodes
	(b) Reticulonodular	Often predominant in mid and upper zones	Hilar and paratracheal lymph nodes
3. Coal miners' pneumoconiosis	Nodular	Predominant in upper zones	Progressive massive fibrosis in the complicated form of the disease emphysema
4. Asbestosis	Fine reticulonodular	Predominant in lower zones	Pleural thickening and or calcification
5. Fibrosing alveolitis	Reticulonodular	Often predominant in lower zones, but may show a variety of patterns	Diaphragm often high and indistinct
6. Lymphangitis carcinomatosa	Reticulonodular	No predominant pattern	Septal lines bronchial wall thickening Hilar adenopathy Other signs of carcinoma
7. Pulmonary oedema	Ill-defined nodules	Often central predominance with clear zone at periphery of lobes	Cardiac enlargement, left atrial enlargement, septal lines

Table 1.19: Chest X-ray in HIV positive patient

A (Involvement)	*B (Diagnostic yield)*
1. Airway involvement	1. PcP—5-25%
(a) Acute bronchitis	2. Myco. TB—in late HIV disease
(b) Bronchiectasis	3. Histoplasmosis—20-30%
2. Parenchymal involvement	4. Nonspecific interstitial pneumonitis—15%
(a) Focal	
1. SPN	
2. Consolidation	
3. Cavity	
(b) Diffuse	
1. Reticulonodular pattern	
3. Pleural involvement	
(a) Pleural effusion	
(b) Pneumothorax	

Magnetic Resonance Imaging[31-34]

Mediastinal tumors can be analysed by T_1 and T_2 properties, but differentiation between inflammatory mode and the tumor cannot be made. Cost of MR imaging is approximately twice that of a contrast CT and has limitation compared with CT but is more sensitive than CT in distinguishing non-vascular tissue in hilar region and central part of the lung. MR imaging has been experimentally used to detect pulmonary intravascular emboli or thrombi. MR imaging is not of much value in pleuropulmonary studies. It cannot be used in patients with pace-makers. It can be of potential value in pulmonary oedema, pulmonary embolism, radiation fibrosis, fibrosing mediastinitis and aortic diseases.

Spectroscopy[1]

Spectroscopy with MR is a research method, which may have its future in future pneumology. Indications for different kind of radiological investigational methods have been tabulated in Table 1.20. Table 1.21 shows different chest diseases with normal chest X-rays as well.

Pulmonary Scintiphotography

Nuclear medicine studies, by injecting or inhalation of radioisotopes as revealed by gamma camera are of clinical utility in pulmonary thromboembolism and local assessment in obstructive lung diseases.

Chest ultrasound[35] is useful in detecting pericardial fluid cysts, bronchogenic cysts, pleural effusions and empyema. It is convenient method but accuracy is less as compared to CT or MR lung scanning using Gallium-67 is useful in neoplastic and inflammatory lung condition. It is useful in diagnosing mediastinal involvement of bronchogenic carcinoma, PcP in AIDS and other infections like cytomegalovirus and cryptococcus infections in AIDS.

Interventional Radiology

CT or ultrasound guided percutaneous biopsy and drainage is better technique over fluoroscopically guided percutaneous

Table 1.20: Radiological investigational methods

Indications of Conventional Tomography	1. To show the shape of an intrathoracic mass and to detect any calcification or cavitation within it. 2. To localise a mass prior to biopsy. 3. To clarify the presence of rib distraction. 4. To analyse hilar shadows. 5. To clarify an indefinite pulmonary lesion.
Indications of Computed Tomography (CT)	1. To show the presence and extent of mediastinal masses and other mediastinal abnormalities. 2. To demonstrate the presence of disease when the plane chest radiograph is normal, e.g., in the detection of pulmonary metastases; finding a primary carcinoma in patients whose sputum cytology shows neoplastic cells; and demonstrating thymic tumours in patients with myasthenia gravis. 3. To detect diffuse calcification in a pulmonary nodule.
Indications of Brochography	1. The only indication is for the assessment of bronchiectasis.
Indications of Pulmonary Angiography	1. To demonstrate pulmonary emboli. 2. To demonstrate congenital vascular anomalies.
Uses of Radionuclide lung scanning	1. To diagnose or exclude pulmonary embolism.

Table 1.21: The chest diseases with a normal chest radiograph

The chest diseases with a normal chest radiograph	1. **Obstructive Airways Disease** Asthma and acute bronchiolitis may produce overinflation of the lungs but in many cases the chest film is normal. Emphysema when moderate, the chest radiograph may be normal or very nearly so. Uncomplicated acute or chronic bronchitis does not produce any radiological signs. A small proportion of patients with productive cough due to bronchiectasis show no plain film abnormality. 2. **Small Lesions** It is impossible to see solitary lung masses or consolidation of less than six mm in diametre and it is very rare to see them if they are less than 1 centimetre in size. Endobronchial lesions such as carcinoma, cannot be diagnosed on routine films unless they cause collapse/consolidation or considerable obstructive emphysema. 3. **Pulmonary Emboli Without Infarction** The chest radiograph is usually normal in such patients even with life threatening emboli. 4. **Infections** The consolidation may only develop after the onset of symptoms in viral infections. Patients with active tuberculosis including miliary tuberculosis may initially have a normal chest film. 5. **Diffuse Pulmonary Infiltration** Particularly pulmonary fibrosis of many different aetiologies may be responsible for breathlessness with substantial alteration in lung function test before any radiological abnormalities are evident. 6. **Pleural Abnormalities** Dry pleurisy will not produce any radiological findings and even 300 ml of pleural fluid may be impossible to recognise on PA and lateral chest films.
Application of the silhouette sign	1. It often makes it possible to localise a shadow by observing which borders are lost, e.g., loss of the heart border must mean that the shadow lies in the anterior half of the chest. Alternatively, loss of a part of the diaphragm outline indicates disease of the pleura or lower lobes. 2. It makes it possible an occasion to diagnose disorders such as pulmonary consolidation even when one is uncertain as to the presence of an opacity. It is surprising that a wedge or lens shaped opacity may be very difficult to see because the way the shadow fades out at its margins, but if such a lesion is in contact with the mediastinum or diaphragm, it causes loss of their normally sharped boundries.

needle lung biopsy. CT controlled needle biopsy of large nodes in mediastinum has made mediastinoscopic node biopsy obsolete. This is also quite useful in drainage of pleural effusions, empyema, lung abscess, pneumothorax etc. and in bronchial artery embolization in intractable haemoptysis with high success rate.

High-Resolution Computed Tomography of Lungs (HRCT)[36-40]

Chest X-rays may have number of abnormalities that may prove to be non-specific in atleast 10% of cases, and a similar number of radiographs may be normal in patients with histologically proved infiltrative parenchymal pulmonary disease. HRCT appears to be more sensitive than routine CT, as HRCT is a non-interventional procedure in diagnosing diffuse lung diseases, and helps in evaluating fibrotic, granulomatory and cystic lung diseases and tumours. It determines the optimal site of lung biopsy, and many a times obviate the need for biopsy in cases like idiopathic pulmonary fibrosis. Hypersensitivity pneumonitis, pneumoconiosis, lymphangitic carcinomatosis and sarcoidosis.

Surgical intervention has been put aside in cases of massive haemoptysis and arteriovenous malformations of lung with the use of transcatheter embolization technique.

Sputum Examination[1]

It is a rapid and simple diagnostic procedure, which can easily be done in a side laboratory, even in the tropical countries. Specimen should be physically examined. Colour would guide about infection (yellow-green) and blood (haemoptysis); smell would guide about anaerobic infection (if smelling foul).

Specific stained slides may demonstrate fungi, mycobact. tuberculosis and pneumocystis carinii.

Eosinophils signify reversible airway disease and macrophages with hemosiderin suggestive of Goodpasture's syndrome.

Casual handling and incompetent examination may not yield any diagnostic clues. Culture of sputum has been replaced by more positive methods like catheter-brush sample, BAL fluid, transtracheal aspirate, percutaneous needle aspirate of the lung and transbronchial lung biopsy, because they represent the required lung secretions sample and are devoid of oropharyngeal contamination.

Bronchoscopy

Flexible fiberoptic bronchoscopy (FOB) was introduced by Ikeda and Colleagues in 1968.[41] Since then, it has reduced the importance of general anaesthesia, rigid bronchoscopy and surgery because of its efficacy and simplicity. Flexible FOB has almost revolutioned the therapeutics in pulmonology, through its life saving therapeutic utility, thereby reducing the morbidity significantly. This simple and safe bedside procedure has been extensively used with diagnostic and therapeutic aim in pulmonary cases for the last one and a half decade,[42-48] since its start in India in 1978. FOB is useful in almost all types of pulmonary disorders but has been mostly used for diagnosing lung cancer. Success of modalities such as lung transplantation cannot be imagined without the availability of FOB. Diagnostic value of transthoracic fine needle biospy under sophisticated guidance is more[49] yet FOB is a safe, quick and relatively economic procedure for diagnosing peripheral lung tumours.[50] It is of diagnostic value in opportunist infections like PcP, mycobacteria, herpes, cytomegalovirus, histoplasma, candida, cryptococcus and legionella organisms in AIDS. Therapeutic applications of FOB are as follows:

1. It is used to remove foreign body from the airways. In India only recently plastic whistles from the major bronchi of two young boys have been removed.[51] If foreign body is visualised through FOB, it is removed by alligator-type biopsy forceps, either piecemeal or by withdrawing the FOB with the forceps snug against the tip. Suction may be required through FOB repeatedly in case of patient with tetanus. Basket type of foreign body forceps have been suggested to be of value. Preanaesthetic endotracheal intubation guided by FOB is convenient and comfortable in case anatomical distortions of cervico facial tissue and vertebrae exists. Chevelier Jackson's dictum was that any object which can be inhaled, can be removed by bronchoscope, but it demands skill, experience and should never be attempted by the untrained.
2. To maintain airways patency and blind-suction of pharynx and tracheo-bronchial tree. The suction, of course, has to be performed under visible guidance.
3. Tracheostomy may be avoided by repeated FOB. In situations where maintenance of airways patency becomes difficult, repeated FOB has a role, and can prevent tracheostomy in accidental cases of poisoning, drainage of secretions, post-operative cases, multi-organ failure disease etc.
4. Patients on mechanical respirator, FOB can be safe in expert hands and yields a low morbidity. FOB has significant role in intensive care units, especially in removing, thickened secretions.
5. Untreated lobar or lung collapse can be avoided, especially in destroyed lungs in bronchiectasis by early intervention by FOB. Even instantaneous re-expansion of the collapsed lung can be obtained with pressure controlled air insufflation in the wedged segment.[52] In cases atelectasis is recognised and if FOB is used, delayed resolution as well as bronchiectasis can be avoided. In these cases, lung destruction is not the cause of collapse, rather it is the result of fibrosis or gangrene caused by unresolved infection.[53] Reflation has to be done with pressure graded air insufflation, keeping in mind the complication due to barotrauma, through FOB, in the wedged segment to re-expand the atelectic parenchyma, 10 litres/m of O_2 is insufflated for 5-10 minutes via the suction channel while monitoring airway pressure by around 30 cms pressure by a manometer.
6. FOB forms the first line of therapy in lung abscess, supplementing postural drainage and antimicrobial agents.

With polythene drainage tube, there occurs either recurrent blockage due to secretions or dislodgement of the tube itself, causing irritability and discomfort to the patient. FOB is convenient and simple method, and aids in early resolution due to interval incision drainage. As the lung abscess is localised radiologically, the scoope is wedged in the appropriate segment. Allignator biopsy forceps introduced through suction channel penetrates the cavity wall and the forceps is introduced into the abscess. The wall is incised by repeated opening and closure of the forceps and the secretions are aspirated and abscess drained.

Complications include bronchospasm, acute drop in arterial PaO_2, hypotension, bleeding, cardiac arrhythmias, cardiopulmonary arrest and death. FOB in children may not be done under general anaesthesia.

7. Haemoptysis can be controlled by pressure, using baloon forgarty's catheter or using FOB by infusing thrombin, fibrinogen-thrombin or batroxobin.[54,55] In the presence of thrombin, batroxobin, which is an enzyme, converts fibrinogen monomer to polymer which in turn polymerises to fibrin clot.[56]
8. Local treatment with chemotherapeutics, bronchoplasty, laser treatment and photodynamic therapy are the areas where role of therapeutic pulmonary flexible FOB is already broadening. The brachy therapy (endobronchial irradiation) is useful in treating both intraluminal malignant tumours and malignant extrinsic pressure compressions. Laser bronchoscopy reduces symptoms, improves respiratory functions and quality of life. Operative mortality is less than 1%. Complications include haemorrhage, hypoxaemia, infection, pneumothorax, bronchopleural fistula, non-cardiogenic pulmonary edema, cardiac arrhythmia and systemic embolism. ND-YAG laser can be used to open a lumen by brachytherapy in case of complete obstruction.

The prophylactic antibiotic to cover the risk of bacteremia in patients at risk of endocarditis[57] on nasal intubation (FOB is generally introduced through nose) has been put aside and no antibiotic propyhlaxis is warranted in these patients when undergoing fiberoptic bronchoscopy.[58-60] Standardization of methods of disinfection of scope to prevent spread of communicable diseases are being laid down.

Flexible FOB has attained a prominent place in pulmonary care and the therapeutic achievement has been quite significant in such a short duration.[61] Its judicial use in the hands of flawless bronchoscopic expertise has not only popularised the pulmonary therapeutic FOB, but also added years of life to pulmonology. A lot has been achieved, yet a lot remains to be accomplished. Transbronchial needle aspiration for early diagnosis of lung cancer and acute fluorescence technology are being looked forward having great potential. Brachytherapy, endobronchial surgery and upcoming gene therapy using FOB as most important vehicle. FOB is likely to face challenges from technological advances such as virtual bronchoscopy, transthoracic ultrasonography and VATS procedures. Rising cost could also become its Achilles' heel. Limitations of virtual bronchoscopy include cost, lack of quantitative information, use of surface rendering instead of volume rendering and need for substantial off-line display computation. Advantages and disadvantages of rigid as well as flexible bronchoscope are shown in Tables 1.22 and 1.23.

Table 1.22: Rigid bronchoscope

Advantages	*Disadvantages*
(Mainly due to wide internal lumen) It is more effective in	
1. Controlling the bleeding	1. General anaesthesia is required
2. Removing foreign body	2. Visual range is limited
3. Removing thick tenacious sputum	3. Causes more discomfort to the patient
4. Obtaining large biopsy specimen	4. It cannot negotiate mechanical abnormalities like torticollis
5. Allows good visual quality and good photography	

Table 1.23: Fiberoptic bronchoscope

Advantages	*Disadvantages*
General anaesthesia not necessary Causes less discomfort to the patient Extensive visual range Can negotiate mechanical abnormalities Biopsy and bronchial brushing help in diagnosing more peripheral lung lesions	(Mainly due to narrow lumen) Biopsy specimen is small. Difficult to remove thick and tenacious secretions. Difficulty in controlling bleeding.

Bronchography[1]

This is done by instillation of radio opaque material into the tracheobronchial tree through a catheter or bronchoscope, followed by positioning of the patient and chest roentgenograms. This is useful in the diagnosis of bronchiectasis and congenital or acquired tracheobronchial distortions. Barium sulphate was used previously.[62-64] Dionosil is being currently in use. However, due to the cost factor, barium sulphate carboxymethyl cellulose and arachis oil (BACAAO) has been tried,[65] 50% of patients may have delayed excretion. Bronchospasm may occur in some patients. Chest CT is fast replacing this technique.

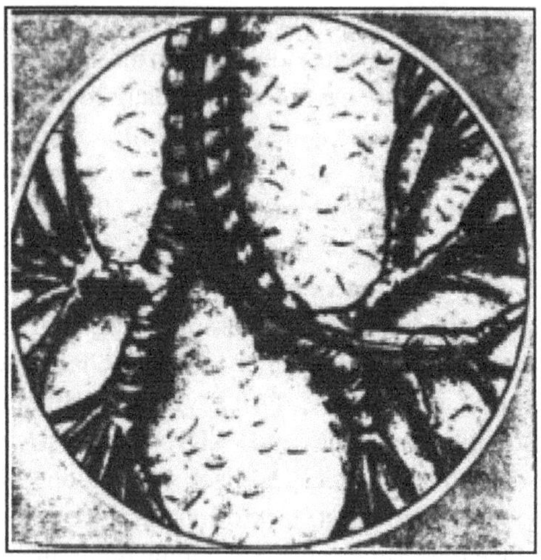

Fig.1.1: PRO-BAL diagnostic catheter

Bronchoalveolar Lavage (BAL)

Bronchoalveolar lavage (BAL) today is a useful and safe method of sampling cellular and biochemical components from the lung.[66,67]

BAL is a liquid biopsy of the contents of distal air spaces and has been of tremendous value in the diagnosis of pneumocystis pneumonia and other chest infections, alveolar proteinosis and interstitial pneumonitis. Technical excellence and expert sampling and processing of the fluid received, improves the diagnostic yield. BAL performance and BAL fluid processing has recently been standardised from technical aspect[68] which is being followed at various centres in India and abroad (Tables 1.24, 1.25).

BAL technique involves introduction of sterile saline into the lungs through fiberoptic bronchoscope to obtain secretions, cells and proteins from the lower respiratory tract (Table 1.26). The procedure of BAL has been described by Weinberger *et al.*[69] During fiberoptic bronchoscopy, 100 ml of saline is injected in aliquots of 20 ml each into a wedged segmental bronchus.[70] If a larger amount is injected for lavage, this may alter the cell counts.[51] After the lavage, the returning fluid is measured (which should be 2/3rd of the fluid in average)[7] filtered through the two layers of surgical gauze to remove mucus,[71] centrifuged at (1500 RPM) for 20 minutes. The cell pallets are pooled, re-suspended in 5 ml of normal saline. A small aliquot is further diluted one in 20 and total count is done with the help of haemocytometer.[73] A further aliquot is adjusted to 0.2×10^6 cells/ml using a special shandon filter cord and cyto-centrifuged at 500 RPM for 5 minutes. After air drying, slide is fixed with methanol for 5 minutes and differential count is done by microscopy glass cover technique.[74] Proximal the lavaged segment, lesser will be the cellular yield with or without increased number of epithelial cells.[75] Since first wash of BAL fluid is going to be from the distal bronchi and not the alveoli,[76] at least two sites are lavaged and recovered fluid is pooled for study. Behrens-Fischer test is done for statistical evaluation.[70] The usual tests of significance assume that two categories of samples have similar variances, if different Cochran's modification of Benrens-Fischer test can be applied.[70] Following BAL, crepitation at the bases may occur within 24 hours, for 3% patients may become pyrexic within few hours. In hypersensitive patients, wheezing may appear in 1-2 weeks.Transient decrease in VC, FEV_1 PEF and PaO_2 may occur. Bleeding or pneumothorax may occur when transbronchial biopsy is done.

Apart from cytologic profile, BAL fluid can be submitted for:

a. Examination of acid fast bacilli.
b. Examination for fungus by smear and culture.
c. Culture and sensitivity for pyogenic organisms.

This has been in use for many years in treating cystic fibrosis and severe asthma to remove mucus plugging in patients, not responding to other treatments.[67] It remains the only effective treatment for alveolar proteinosis.[66] BAL is a form of liquid biopsy, especially in non-expectorating patients, very useful in diagnosing occult stage of malignancy and smear negative pulmonary tuberculosis. BAL can be used to confirm asbestos exposure,[77] identification of reactivated tuberculosis and cytological diagnosis of tumours beyond the visual range of fiberoptic bronchoscope (FOB). Diagnosis of centrally situated lung tumour is improved with FOB[78] but diagnostic accuracy in peripheral lung lesions which is poor[79] with FOB, has improved with BAL.[80,81] A success rate of 65% diagnosis has been obtained[81] in an Indian study. BAL cellular analysis may help in identifying interstitial lung diseases.[83,84] Raised lymphocytes in BAL fluid are found in sarcoidosis and extrinsic alveolitis.[66] Lymphocytes increase in idiopathic alveolitis and sarcoidosis has been reported.[85,86] Higher neutrophills in rheumatoid lung disease, idiopathic interstitial lung disease,[75,87-89] pneumonitis, sarcoidosis and asbestosis,[90] have been reported. However,

BAL findings may be normal in asbestosis.[91] Extensive alveolitis type picture may be seen in methyl isocynate exposured subjects.[92] BAL does show increased total cell count in interstitial lung disease, but may not equal histology, although it provides a useful evidence of active alveolitis.[70] Raised neutrophils, macrophages and eosinophils are found in cryptogenic fibrosing alveolitis.[93] Similar changes are seen in collagen vascular disorders.[94,95] However, mast cells in extrinsic and lymphocytes in cryptogenic fibrosing alveolitis have also been reported.[96] The alteration in cell count may provide a clue to activity of the disease in sarcoidosis[97] and may guide the treatment in cryptogenic fibrosing alveolitis (Table 1.27).[98]

It can be used to understand pathogenesis of diseases like drug hypersensitivity, emphysema, occupational disease, adult respiratory distress syndrome and asthma.[66] BAL fluid shows increased eosinophils at base line,[99-102] Increased number of neutrophils in BAL fluid in patients with asthma before and after antigenic challenge confirms[103] inflammatory changes within the airways.[104]

More recently BAL technique has been used with good tolerability in establishing diagnosis of pneumocystis carinii,[105-107] cytomegalovirus,[105] Legionella pneumophilia[107] fungi[104] and mycobacterial infections.[107] Both cysts and trophozoites can readily be harvested from patients by BAL.[109] It was suggested in 1987 that sputum induction with nebulised saline may replace BAL in patients with HIV infection.[108] The choice method-BAL-till recently in the west,[110] has recently been pushed back by hypertonic saline nebulization for sputum induction to detect pneumocystis pneumonia (PCP). This is presently being considered far superior to unaided sputum[111,112] and its sensitivity increases upto 78% by addition of reducing agents such as dithiothreitol (DTT)[113] and use of monoclonal antibodies to pneumocystis carinii increases sensitivity to nearly 90%.[114] BAL has been extensively used to type and stage activity of alveolitis and assessing aetiology of various interstitial diseases.[115] Relatively non-invasive tool in rapid diagnosis of infections in immunocompromised patients, BAL cytology is more useful than microbial cultures. Whole lung lavage has been proposed in treating elveolar microlithiasis (Table 1.28).

Table 1.24: BAL: Primary information

1. First bronchoalveolar lavage was performed by Cantrell and colleagues in 1973, in normal volunteers.
2. BAL allows recovery of both cellular and non-cellular components from the epithelial surface of lower respiratory tract.
3. It differs from bronchial washings (which refer to aspiration of either secretions or small amounts of instilled saline from the large airways.
4. The analysis of cellular and molecular components help to elucidate the pathogenesis mechanisms.
5. It also help in assessing the activity of interstitial and other pulmonary diseases and disorders.

Table 1.25: BAL: Few facts

1. BAL is a safe procedure.
2. It is done under local anesthesia.
3. It is performed with a flexible fiberoptic bronchoscope.
4. Mild side effects include coughing during lavage, fever and chills few hours later and transient alveloar infiltration 24 hours after the procedure.
5. Supplemental oxygen, ear oximetry and ECG monitoring are advisable in selected cases with critical condition or severe underlying disease.

Table 1.26: Non-smoking adults: BAL fluid analysis: Cellular and soluble constituents

Cells	Mean ± SD
Total	10-15 × 10^6 cells/dl of BAL fluid
Macrophages %	84 ± 1
Lymphocytes %	11 ± 1
T cells	62 ± 2
Helper (CDA)	46 ± 3
Suppressor (CD4)	25 ± 2
B cell	05 ± 2
Neutrophils %	less than 1
Eosinophils %	less than 1
Basophils %	less than 1
Soluble factors	
IgG, IgA	
IgM	
C4, C3 factor B	
C5	

Ref: Daniel RP *et al.*, Annals of Internal Medicine 1985;102: 93-108.

Table 1.27: Diagnostic utility of BALF[118] in infectious and non-infectious diseases

Infectious diseases	Non-infectious diseases
Pneumocystis carinii (AIDS)	Alveolar proteinosis
Toxoplasma gondii	Histiocytosis X
Strongyloides	Pulmonary malignancies and pulmonary haemorrhage
Legionella	Cigarette smoking
Histoplasma	ARDS
Mycobact. tuberculosis	Bronchial asthma
Mycoplasma	Occupational disorders
Influenza	ILDs: Sarcoidosis, eosinophilic granuloma, scleroderma, hypersensitive pneumonitis, cryptogic fibrosing alveolitis
Respiratory syncytial virus	Cystic fibrosis

Table 1.28: Whole lung lavage (WLL):Therapeutic applications

1. It is useful in the treatment of alveolar proteinosis.
2. Mucus plugs can be removed in patients with status asthmaticus.
3. It can be used in removing irritating dust in acute form of silicosis, in order to prevent irreversible damage.
4. It has been proposed in the treatment of alveolar microlithiasis and exogenous lipoidosis.

BAL is a much preferred investigative tool over invasive procedures like transthoracic needle biopsy and exploratory thoracotomy,[82,116] which are poorly accepted by patients and have a significant morbidity, particularly in cases with advanced functional disability. It is a safe procedure but still a research tool, the exact evaluation of which as a diagnostic tool in clinical pulmonary medicine has to be made.[117]

ANGIOGRAPHY,[119] ECHOCARDIOGRAPHY AND BIOPSY

Pulmonary and Bronchial Angiography

Injection of radio opaque material into the pulmonary artery or its branches preferably cardiac catheterisation and then visualising by using magnification technique is called pulmonary angiography. It is used to detect pulmonary emboli as well as in vascular lesions of congenital or acquired nature. It has potential risk in pulmonary hypertension. Pulmonary angioscopy is in its infancy to visualise pulmonary arterial system and right sided chambers of the heart through a fiberoptic device via a peripheral view. Bronchial arteriography has its role in locating the site of bleeding, identifying bleeding and controlling the same by means of emboli (embolotherapy)[1] i.e., therapeutic embolization in massive haemoptysis. But bronchial arteriography has mainly been used as a research tool.

Contrast Echocardiography

Pulmonary arteriovenous fistulae cause extra cardiac right-to-left shunting of blood. This produces characteristic contrast echocardiographic features.[120] Contrast is visualized in left atrium and left ventricle after a delay of 2-4 cardiac cycles. Contrast echocardiography is a simple and reliable preliminary test.

The delayed appearance of contrast in left side of heart is diagnostic of pulmonary arteriovenous fistulae and incompatible with any other anomaly. It clearly distinguishes pulmonary arteriovenous fistulae from intracardiac shunts and also excludes persistent left superior vena cava draining to left atrium, a clinically similar condition.[121] Contrast echocardiography, however, has no extent to number of fistulae.[122] For this, angiography is required. Although contrast echocardiography is very sensitive for diagnosing right-to-left shunts,[123] whether smaller asymptomatic fistulae will be easily demostrated, is not clear. In asymptomatic patients, contrast echocardiography has been found to be negative in three of eleven patients.[124]

Mediastinoscopy and Mediastinotomy[1]

This procedure is very useful for inspection and biopsy of nodes in the mediastinum and has replaced scalene node biopsy, especially for the nodes of right side of mediastinum. Needle aspiration, mediastinoscopy and mediastinotomy (approach through a limited left anterior thoracotomy) are quite safe, low risk, high yield procedures, especially in staging of patients in suspected pulmonary carcinoma.

Medical Thoracoscopy

It is a diagnostic as well as therapeutic exploration of pleural cavity performed after an artificial pneumothorax. An old endoscopic technique introduced in 1910 by Swedish physician Von H.C. Jacobaens, present day thoracoscopy is most exciting diagnostic tool, allowing almost 7% of both visceral and parietal pleura's visualisation and helping in diagnosing disputed 25% of pleural effusion, with an almost 90-100% of diagnostic yield in tubercular and neoplastic pleural disorder. And results are well comparable with diagnostic accuracy of thoracoscopic lung biopsies and open lung biopsies. Its uses are listed in Table 1.29. Mortality rate is as low as 0.24%. Complications include bleeding, persistent air leak and infection in less than 2% of cases. Procedure is contraindicated in patients with obliterated pleural space. Relative contraindications are hypoxaemia, coagulation defects, and severe cardiac disease.

Table 1.29: Medical thoracoscopy
Diagnostic value
• Tuberculosis pleural effusion
• Malignant pleural effusion
• Spontaneous pneumothorax
• Diffuse pulmonary disorders
• Pulmonary infections
• Mineralogical study of asbestos fibre
Therapeutic value
• Empyema
• Spontaneous pneumothorax
• Malignant pleural effusion

Thoracoscopy/pleuroscopy is a minimally invasive procedure to have an access to pleural space, to diagnosis cause of effusion/thickening and to perform safe pleurodesis, and is different from video assisted thoracoscopic surgery. The sterile equipment allows visualization, exposure, manipulation and even biopsy can be taken if required, with a high-resolution video imaging system for better results.

The procedure in done in operating room with a dedicated team and patient is monitored in conscious sedation with a target of patient comfort and safety and yield. Procedure is contraindicated in case of lack of pleural space, uncorrected coagulopathy and haemodynamic instability. Complications are quite less; these can be bleeding pleural space infection, injury to intrathoracic organs, atelectasis and respiratory failure.

Scalene Node Biopsy[125]

It is a convenient method but diagnostic value is limited.

Superiority of scalene node biopsy, however, has been shown in an Indian study for histopathological diagnosis of lung cancer.[126]

Ultrasound

Ultrasound of chest has certain limitations but is of value in pleural effusion and mediastinal masses near the thoracic cage. It helps in differentiating the solids from liquid as well as localisation of loculated pleural collection. Advantages of ultrasound are convenient, cost-effective, non-imaginative and non-hazardous of any kind of dye, drug and radiations. Endobronchial ultrasound (EBUS) helps in deciding therapy for carcinoma in situ between photodynamic therapy and surgery. Also, it is useful in deciding in treatment plan by way of delineating the exact size, extent, spread, infiltration and relationship of a lesion with vascular structures. Common utility of EBUS include:

1. Diagnosing non-malignant thoracic lesions.
2. Assessing airway wall thickening in asthma.
3. Lung cancer staging.
4. Evaluating lung metastatic tumour.
5. Enhancing TBNA yield in sarcoidosis.

Being costly and lack of training has restricted is wide-spread use.

Tc-Diethylenetriamine Penta-acetate (DTPA) Scanning

Tc-DTPA aerosol clearance is an index of lung epithelial permeability increased permeability resulted from lung inflammation is seen in a variety of diffuse pulmonary lung diseases. A sensitive marker of inflammation, normal scan rules out lung parenchymal inflammation. However it cannot be used in tobacco smokers.

Lung Biopsy

It is described under 'practical procedures'. It is suggested that biopsy specimen should both be cultured and processed for pathologic examination.[1]

Transbronchial Lung Biopsy (TBLB)

Sampling is done via fiberoptic bronchoscope. Sampling error and too small or crushed specimen decrease the diagnostic yield. Multiple sampling achieves an overall good results. An outpatient procedure, pneumothorax (2-10%) and bleeding (9%).

Open Lung Biopsy (OLB)

OLB by limited thoracotomy provides larger specimen than transbronchial lung biopsy (TBLB), with respective diagnostic yield of 94% and 72%. Complication rate is 7% and mortality rate is less than 1%.

Video Assisted Thoracoscopic (VATS) Lung Biopsy or Thoracoscopic-Guided Lung Biopsy (TGLB)

It is done under general anesthesia, with a diagnostic yield of 86-95%. It is best avoided in conditions such as honey comb lung, pulmonary hypertension and vascular tumour are commonly encountered complications. Mortality is approximately 0.1%, which can further decrease of proper coagulation screaming prior to TBLB has been done. TBLB and BAL are crucial diagnostic methods presently available to evaluate pulmonary infiltrates in immunosuppressed patients[127] and in conjunction with conventional and molecular diagnostic methods, majority of the diagnoses are achieved. Strict adherence to the guidelines of disinfection of bronchoscopes to avoid norocomial transmission of infection is important.

PET

Fludeoxyglucose–PET imaging is evolving as powerful modality in diagnosing non-oncological disorders such as sarcoidosis, AIDS, environmental lung disorders, thus may play an important role in the management of inflammatory and other benign disorders.[127]

TB

Patient with persistent pyrexia in high burden countries like India, should not held for ATT for want of definite microbiological diagnosis.

REFERENCES

1. Cohen H.A., *et al.,* Effect of honey on nocturnal cough and sleep quality; A double blind randomized, placebo controlled study; Pediatrics 2012; 130: 1-7.
2. Singh N., Singh V., Combating cough–etiopathogenesis; JAPI 2013: 61(S): 6-7.
3. Smith J.A. *et al.,* Acoustic cough reflex association in chronic cough–potential triggers and mechanisms; Gastroenterology 2010; 139: 754-62.
4. Padma L., Current drugs for the treatment of dry cough; JAPI 2013; 61(S): 9-13.
5. Naik V., Role of bronchodilators in management of cough; JAPI 2013; 61 (S): 20-22.
6. Rai S.P. Chronic cough; JAPI 2013:61(S): 28-30.
7. Bhatia R.S., Enalapril precipitating an attack of asthmatics bronchitis, JAPI 1994; 42: 506.
8. Cherniack N.S. and Altose M.D., Mechanisms of dyspnoea, *Clin Chest. Med.* 1987; 8: 207.
9. Wasserman K. and Casaburi R., Dysopnea, physiological and pathophysiological mechanisms, *Ann. Rev. Med.* 1988, 39: 503.
10. Parmasivan R. *et al.* Haemoptysis and tuberculosis—analysis, Lung India 1994;12:192-94.
11. Adelman M. *et al.* Cryptogenic hemoptysis, clinical features, bronchoscopic findings and natural history in 67 patients; *An. Int. Med.* 1985; 102: 829.
12. Dua R, Rawat J; Diffuse alveolar hemorrhage in a patient of RA; Lung India 2014; 31:194-95.
13. Bandopadhyay S; *et al.,* Intrathoracic schwannoma presenting with massive haemoptysis; JAPI 2013:61:336.

14. Gopinathan VP; Uncommon presentations of a common disease—tuberculosis, IN; A Muruganathan; ed; Med update, API 2013;23;490-92.
15. Lupinetti F.M., *et al.*, Pathopysiology of chronic cyanosis in a Canine model: Functional and metabolic response to global ischemia, *J. Thorac. Cardiovas. Surg.* 1985; 90: 291.
16. Szidon J.P. and Fishman A.P., *Cyanosis and Clubbing in Pulmonary diseases* and *disorders,* 2nd Ed., Fishman (ED), Philadephia, Saunders 1988: 251.
17. Weirman W.H., Cleagett O.T. and Donald J.R., Articular Manifestations in Pulmonary Diseases, *J. Am. Med. Assoc.* 1954,155: 1459-63.
18. Neufeld O and Wallband W.L., Clubbed fingers, *Ohio Medical Journal* 1952, 48: 834-37.
19. Rao Sukhesh, Rau R.P. and Sahoo R.C., Clubbing in pulmonary tuberculosis: A clinico-radiological correlation, *Lung India* 1992, 10: 69-70.
20. Mc Farlane J.T., Ibrahim M. and Torr Agbidy S., Importance of Finger clubbing in Pulmonary Tuberculosis, *Tubercle* 1979, 60: 45-48.
21. Seaton A., Seaton D. and Gorden Leitch A., *Crofton and Douglas Respiratory Diseases.* Oxford University Press Delhi. 4th edition, 1989, Chapter 14, 407.
22. Shankar P.S., *Manual of clinical methods,* Oxford and TBH, New Delhi, 3rd Ed., 1992.
23. Freidman P.J., Practical radiology of the bita and mediastinum, *Post Grad. Radiol.* 1981,1:269.
24. Fraser R. *et al., Diagnosis of diseases of the chest,* 3rd Ed., Philadelphia, Saunders, 1988.
25. Shure D. (ed), *Diagnostic technics; Clinics in Chest Medicine,* Philadelphia, Saunders, 1987.
26. Sagel S.S. and Stanley R.J., *Computed body tomography with MRI correlation,* 2nd Ed., N. York, Raven, 1989.
27. Proto A.V., Mediastinal anatomy, Emphasis on conventional images with anatomic and computed tomographic correlations, *J. Thora. Imag.* 1987, 2:1.
28. Haaga J.R. and A.I. Fidi R.J. (Ed), *Computed Tomography of the whole body,* 2nd Ed., St. Louis Mosby, 1988.
29. Naidish P, *et al.* (Ed), *Computed Tomography of the Thorax,* N.York, Raven Press, 1984.
30. Wersetius L.J. *et al.*, Computer-assisted versus usual lung gallium-67 index in normals and patients with interstitial lung disorders, *Amer. Rev. Resp. Dis.* 1983, 128: 1084.
31. Carsoll F.E. Jr, *Lungs in Magnetic Resonance Imaging,* Partain C.L., *et al.* (Ed); Philadelphia, Saunders, 1988.
32. Higgins C.B. and Hricak H., *Magnetic resonance imaging of the body,* N. York, Raven Pub., 1987.
33. Webb W.R., Mediastinum and hila: IN: MRT: Partain C.L. *et al.*, (Ed); Philadelphia, Saunders, 1988.
34. Webb W.R., Magnetic resonance imaging of the hila and mediastinum, *Cardiovas Intervent. Radiol.* 1986,8: 306.
35. Van Sonnenberg E., *et al.*, CT and ultrasound-guided catheter drainage of empyemas after chest-tube failure, *Radiology* 1984,151:349.
36. Briglite A.H.A., *et al.*, Assessment of bronchiectasis; comparison of HRCT and spiral volumetric CT; J. Comp. Asst. Tomo 1996; 20: 15-19.
37. King I.Y., *et al.,* Bronchiectasis; comparison of preoperative thin section CT and pathologic findings in resected specimens; Radiol 1995; 195: 649-54.
38. Fenion H.M., *et al.*, High resolution chest CT in SLE; Amer J. Roentgen 1996; 166: 301-307.
39. Meyo J.R., HRCT: Technical aspects; Radiol. Clin. North Amer 1991; 29: 1043-49.
40. Optican R.J., *et al.*, HRCT in the diagnosis of miliary tuberculosis; Chest 1992; 102: 941-43.
41. Ikeda S., Yanui N. and I. Shikana S., Flexible broncho-fiberoscope, *Keio J. Med* 1968, 17: 1-16.
42. Shah A.C., Trivedi A.M.,Vishwanath N., *et al.* Intensive respiratory care service, organisation, orientation, system and failure; our experience of management of 288 cases; *JAPI* 1990, 30: 140-43.
43. Shah A.C., Flexible fibreoptic bronchoscopy in pulmonary medicine *JAPI* 1983, 32, 10: 659-61.
44. Shah A.C., Shroff C.F., Naber S.T., Pajankar S.P., Punjabi A.H., Deshmukh S.N.,Vaidya K.A., Trivedi A.M. and Merchant H.C., Flexible fibreoptic bronchoscopy as a diagnostic and therapeutic tool. *JAPI* 1987, 35, 2: 121-123.
45. Shah A.C., Fibreoptic bronchoscope as a therapeutic tool, present status and future in India, personal communication 1993.
46. Shah A.C., Role of flexible fibreoptic bronchoscopy in respiratory diseases. *Indian Chest Society, TNCRD* 1990.
47. Bhambure N.M., Abhyankar N.Y., Dalvi S.S., Salve A.A., Deshmukh S.N. and Shah A.C., Therapeutic Aspects of Flexible Fibre-optic bronchoscopy—our experience of 1586 cases. *Lung India* 1991, 9, 4: 136-140.
48. Abhyankar N.Y., Bhambure N.M., Kasekar S.C., Dalvoe S.S., Shah A.C. and Deshmukh S.N., Intensive Respiratory Care Service—Our Eight Years Experience; Ind. J. Chest. Dis. All Sci. 1992; 34(2): 65-72.
49. Pant M.C., *et al.*, Diagnosis of thoracic lesions; CT guided fine needle aspiration cytology; J Biol Chem Res 1992;11: 79-82.
50. Goel M.K., *et al.* FOB without fluoroscopic guidance in the diagnosis of peripheral lung tumours; Lung India 1996; 14(4): 161-64.
51. Kalra S., Bahera D., Jindal S.K. and Malik S.K., Removal of foreign bodies with FOBS, *The Ind. J. Chest. All. Scien* 1988, 30: 61-64.
52. Thomas Change-YaoTaso,Ying-Huang TSa, Ray-Shee Lan, Wen-Ben Shieh, Chong. Hue Lee, Treatment for collapsed lung in critically ill patients; Selective intrabronchial air insufflation using the FOB; *Chest* 1990, 97:435-38.
53. Deivanayagam C.N., *FOB-therapeutic applications* (personal communication) April 1993.
54. Abhyankar N.Y., Bhambure N.M., Gandhi Y.P., Patel Y.S., Shah A.C. and Deshmukh S.N. Management of haemoptysis by bronchoscopic infusion of batroxobin, *Lung India* 1990,4: 195-98.
55. James E.P., Raynolds Ed. Martindale, *The Extra Pharmacopea,* 29th Edition, The Pharmaceutical Press, London, 1989, p.1132.
56. Makona S., Use of reptilase with an endoscope against bronchial hemmorrhage; *Clin. Resp.* 1986,20: 228-35.
57. M.C. Shahe A.J., Hone R., Prevention of bacterial endocarditis: Does nasal intubation warrant prophylaxis? *BMJ* 1986, 292: 26-27.

58. Kane R.C., Cohen M.H., Fossiecki B.E. Jr. and Tvardzik A.V., Absence of bacteremia after FOB, *Amer. Rev. Resp. Dis.* 1975,111: 102-04.
59. Haynes J. and Greenstone M.A., FOB and use of antibiotics prophylaxis, *BMJ* 1987, 294: 1199.
60. Pereira W., Kovnat D.M., Zohn M.A., Iscovino J.R., Spivack M.L. and Snider C.L., Fever and pneumonia after flexible FOB, *Amer. Rev. Resp. Dis.* 1975, 112: 59-64.
61. Bhatia R.S. and Sibia S.S., FOB—Therapeutic applications, *Lung India* 1994,12: 138-39.
62. Nelson S.W., Christo-Foridis A.J. and Pratt P.C., Further experience with barium sulphate as a bronchographic contrast medium. *Am. J. Roentgenol Nuc. Med.* 1964, 92: 596-614.
63. Rath A.K., Motiani P.D., Gupta P.K., Agnihotri S.P. Barupal B.K. and Purohit G., Barium sulphate—A contrast medium in bronchography, *Lung India* 1988,6: 205-207.
64. Chaudhary B.S., Gupta N.K., Luhadia S.K., Jhamaria J.P., Gupta V.K. and Jain M.C., Comparison of barium sulphate and dionosil as contrast media for bronchography. *Ind. J. Chest. Dis. Allied Sci.* 1983,25: 96-100.
65. Sharma V.K., Jenaw A.K., Agnihotri S.P., *et al.* BACAAOM–A suggested replacement for dionosil in bronchography, *Lung India* 1992, 10: 107-109.
66. Reynolds H.Y., State of the art, BAL, *Amer. Rev. Resp. Dis.* 1987,135: 250-63.
67. Helmer R.A. and Hunnigahake G.W., BAL in the non-immunocompromised patient; *Chest* 1990, 96: 1184-90.
68. Klech H. and Pohl W., Technical recommendations and guidelines for BAL, Report of the European Society of Pneumonology, Task Group on BAL, *Eur. Resp. J.* 1989,2: 561-85.
69. Weingberger S.E., Kelman J.A., Elson N.A., Young R.C. Jr., Reynolds H.Y., Palmer J.P. and Crystal R.G., Bronchoalveolar lavage in interstitial lung disease. *Ann. Intern. Med.* 1978, 89: 459 -66.
70. Potdar P.V., Jain K., Prabha Karan L., *et al.*, Value of BAL in interstitial lung disease; JAPI 1989,37: 444-47.
71. Dohn M.N. and Baughman R.P., Effects of changing instilled volume for bronchoalveolar lavage in patients with interstitial lung diseases, *Am. Rev. Resp. Dis.* 1985, 132: 390-92.
72. Leigh T.R., Person P., Home C., *et al.*, Sputum induction for the diagnosis of Pneumocystis carinii pneumonia, *Lancet* 1989,11: 205-206.
73. Saltini C., Hance A.J., Ferrans V.J., Francoise Basset, Bitterman P.B. and Crystal R.G., Accurate quantification of cells recovered by bronchoalveolar lavage. *Am. Rev. of Res. Dis.* 1984,130: 650.
74. Laviolette M., Carreu M. and Coulombe R., Bronchoalveolar lavage cell differential on microscope glass cover technique. *Am. Rev. of Respir. Dis.* 1988,138:145.
75. Pingleton S.K., Harrison G.R., Stechschufe D.J., Wesselius L.J., Kerby G.R. and Ruth W.E., Effect of location, pH and temperature of instillate in bronchoalveolar lavage in normal subjects. *Am. Rev. Resp. Dis.* 1983, 128: 1035-37.
76. Crystal R.G., Reynolds H.Y. and Kalica A.R., Bronchoalveolar lavage, The Report of an International Conference, *Chest,* 1986, 90: 122.
77. Maubet A., Rodriguez-Roisin R., Bombi J.A. *et al.* Correlation of BAL and clinical and functional findings in asbestosis, *Amer. Rev. Resp. Dis.* 1986,133: 848-54.
78. Marsh B.R. and Wang *K., Bronchoscopy in Lung cancer, clinical diagnosis and treatment,* E.D., Strauss M.J., Grune and Stratton, New York 1983, 121-25.
79. Radke J.R., Conway W.A. and Eyler W.R., Diagnostic accuracy in peripheral lung lesions, factor predicting success with flexible FOB, *Chest.* 1975,76: 176-79.
80. Springmeryer S.C., Hackman R. and Carison J.J., Bronchoalveolar carcinoma diagnosed by BAL, *Chest.* 1983,83: 278-80.
81. Sestini P., Rottoll L. and Gotti G., BAL diagnosis of bronchoalveolar carcinoma; *Eur. J. Resp. Dis.* 1985, 66: 55-57.
82. Ajit Vigg, Role of BAL in diagnosis of peripheral lung cancer; *Lung India* 1991, 9: 61-62.
83. Reynolds H.Y., Interstitial lung diseases, classification, definition and correlation between clinical and histologic staging of interstitial lung diseases; Seminar in Resp. Dis. 1984; 6: 1-9.
84. Saltini C., Hance A.J., Ferrans V.J., *et al.* Accurate quantification of cells recovered by BAL; *Amer. Rev. Resp. Dis.* 1984,130: 650-58.
85. Haslam P.L., Turton C.W.G. and Lukoszo K.A., Broncho-alveolar lavage fluid cell counts in cryptogenic fibrosing alveolitis and their relation to therapy, *Thorax* 1980, 35: 328-39.
86. Garcia J.G., Wolven R.G., Garcia P.L. and Keogh B.A., Assessment of interlobar variation of bronchoalveolar lavage cellular differential in interstitial lung diseases, *Amer. Rev. Resp. Dis.* 1986,133: 444-49.
87. Hunninghake G.W., Gadek J.R., Kawamani O., Ferrans V.J. and Crystal R.G., Inflammatory and immune processes in the human lung in health and diseases, Evaluation by broncho-alveolar lavage, *Am. J. Pathol.* 1979, 97: 149-206.
88. Hunninghake G.W., Gadek J.R., Weinberger S., Kelman J., Fulmer J. and Crystal R.G., Comparison of the alveolities of sarcoidosis and idiopathic pulmonary fibrosis, *Chest.* 1979,75: 206-67.
89. Gupta R.K., Kulpati D.D.S, Hira H.S. and Chauhan M.R., Evaluation of bronchoalveolar lavage (BAL) in diffuse infiltrative lung diseases. *Indian J. Chest. Dis. All Sci.* 1985, 27: 207-10.
90. Zavala D.C. and Hunninghake G.W., *Lung lavage: In Recent advances in respiratory medicine;* Ed. Flenley D.C. and Petty TL; Churchill Livingstone, London 1983; 21-33.
91. Patel M.H., Bharathi H.S., Mahashur A.A.,Vaidya P.R. and Kamat S.R., A follow-up study of pulmonary asbestos is in Bombay, *Lung India* 1987, 5: 119-23.
92. Kamat S.R., Patel M.H., Kolhatkar V.P., Dave A.A. and Mahashur A.A., Sequential respiratory changes in those exposed to the gas leak at Bhopal. *Ind. J. Mal. Res.* 1987, 86: 20-38.
93. Haslam P., Furton C. and Heard B., BAL in pulmonary fibrosis, Comparison of cells obtained with lung biopsy and clinical features, *Thorax* 1980, 35: 9-18.
94. Garcia J.G.N., Parham N., Killam D., *et al.* BAL fluid evaluation in rheumatoid arthritis, *Amer. Rev. Resp. Dis.* 1986, 133: 450-54.

95. Wallaert B., Hatson P.Y., Grosbios J.M., *et al.* Subclinical pulmonary involvement in collagen vascular diseases assessed by BAL, Relationship between alveolitis and subsequent changes in lung functions, *Amer. Rev. Resp. Dis.* 1986,133: 574-80.
96. Bhatia R.S. and Sibia S.S., Intensive pulmonary care units; An urgent need; *Lung India* 1995,13:75-76.
97. Bauwer W., Gorny M.K., Baumann H.R., *et al.* I lymphocyte subsets and immunoglobulin concentrations in BAL of patients with sarcoidosis and high and low intensity alveolitis, *Amer. Rev. Resp. Dis.* 1985, 132: 1060-65.
98. Turner Warwick M. and Haslam P., The value of serial BALs in assessing the clinical progress of patients with cryptogenic fibrosing alveolitis, *Amer. Rev. Resp. Dis.* 1987,135: 26-34.
99. Godard P., Chaintreuil J., Damon M., Coupe M., Flandre O., Depaulet, *et al.* Functional assessment of alveolar macrophages, Comparison of cells from asthmatic and normal subject, *Allergy Clin. Immunol* 1982, 70: 38.
100. Metzer W.J., Moseley P., Nugent K., Richerson H.B. and Hunding Hake G.W., Local antigen challenge and broncho-alveolar lavage of allergic asthmatic lungs, *Chest.* 1985, 87(suppl): 155.
101. Kelly C.A.,Ward C., Bird G., Hendrick D.J. and Walter E.H., The effects of filtration on cell counts in bronchoalveolar lavage fluid (Abstract) *Thorax* 1986, 41: 727.
102. Raj B., Gupta K.B., Sharma R. and Sethi K.G., Cytologic profile in BAL of bronchial asthma patients, *Ind. J. Tuber.* 1991,38: 95-98.
103. D-Monchy J.G., Kauffman H., Venge P., *et al.* Bronchoalveolar eosinophilia during allergen induced late asthmatic reactions, *Am. Rev. Res. Dis.* 1985, 131: 373.
104. Kelly C.A., *et al.*, Number and activity of inflammatory cells in bronchoalveolar lavage fluid in asthma, *Thorax* 1988, 43: 684.
105. Milburn H.L., Prentic H.G. and Dubois R.M., Role of BAL in evaluation of interstitial pneumonitis in recipients of bone marrow transplants, *Thorax* 1987,42: 766-72.
106. Stover D.E., White D.A., Romani P.A., *et al.* Diagnosis of pulmonary disease in AIDS, *Amer. Rev. Resp. Dis.* 1984, 130: 659-72.
107. Hopkin J.M., Turney J.H., Young, J.A., *et al.* Rapid diagnosis of obscure pneumonia in immunosuppressed renal patients by cytology of alveolar lavage fluid, *Lancet* 1983: 299-301.
108. de Blic J., Mc Kelvie P., Le Bowrgeois M. *et al.* Value of BAL in the management of severe acute pneumonia and interstitial pneumonitis in immunocompromised child, *Thorax* 1987, 42: 759-65.
109. Stover D.E.,White D.A., Romeno P.A., Gellene R.A. and Roberson W.A., Spectrum of pulmonary diseases associated with AIDS, *Amer. J. Med.* 1985, 78: 429-37.
110. Sehegal S., Pneumocystis pneumonia, A time to shed complacence, JAPI 1993, 41: 5-7.
111. Pitchenik A.E., Ganje P., Torres A., Evens D.A., *et al.*, Sputum examination for diagnosis of PCP in AIDS; *Amer. Rev. Resp. Dis.* 1986,133: 226-29.
112. Leigh T.R., Person P., Home C., *et al.*, Sputum induction for the diagnosis of PCP, *Lancet* 1969, ii: 205-06.
113. Zaman M.K., Wooten O.J., Superhmanya B., Amkobiah W., *et al.* Rapid non-invasive diagnosis of pneumocystic carinii from induced liquified sputum. *Ann. Intern. Med.* 1988,109: 7-10.
114. Konacs J.A., Thiemez J.W., Mecher A.M., Stover D., *et al.*, PCP: A comparison between patients with AIDS and patients with other immunodeficiencies, *Ann Intern. Med.* 1984, 100: 663-71.
115. Mahashur A.A., Dave K.M., Kinare S.G., Kamat S.R., Shetye V.M. and Kolkattkar V.P., Diffuse fibrosing alveolitis—An Indian experience; *Lung India* 1983,5: 171-79.
116. Bhatia R.S., BAL, Therapeutic indications: Current status, *Lung India* 1994,12: 27-29.
117. Vijayan V.K., Current diagnostic status of BAL studies, *Ind. J. Clin. Pract.* 1993,3: 51-54.
118. American Thoracic Society, Clinical role of BAL in adults with pulmonary diseases, *Amer. Rev. Resp. Dis.* 1990,142: 481-86.
119. Nicod P., *et al.* (Ed) *Computed Tomography of the thorax;* N. York, Raven Press, 1984.
120. Talano J.V. and Gardian J.M., *Two-dimensional contrast Echocardiography in Text Book of Two-dimensional Echocardiography,* Grunn and Stratton 1983; p. 305-24.
121. Bajaj R., Kothari S.S., Behl V.K. *et al.* Role of contrast echography in diagnosis of pulmonary arteriovenous fistulas, *JAPI* 1988,36: 65-66.
122. Hemandez A., Stravess A.W., KcKnight R. and Hartmann A.F., Diagnosis of pulmonary arteriovenous fistula by contrast echocardiography. *J. Pediatr* 1978, 93: 258-60.
123. Valdes-Cruz L.M., Peironi D.R., Roland J. and Verghese P.J., Recognition of residual post operative shunts by contrast echo-cardiography techniques. *Circulation* 1977,55: 148-52.
124. Davis D.E., Seward J.B. and Bernatz. P.E., *Pulmonary arteriovenous fistulas.* Mayo clinic proceedings 1983, 58: 176-81.
125. Hassan M.I. *et al. An experience with scelene node biopsy in the diagnosis of intrathoracic lesions,* IN; Aziz A. and Ishaq M (ED): Tuberculosis and resp. diseases: IUAT & LD; Punjab T.B. Assn., Lahore, 1987.
126. Aryya N.C., Rastogi B.L., Lahiri T.K., *et al.* Significance of Bronchoscopic lymph nodal and Thoracotomy specimens and Pleural aspirate in diagnosis of Lung cancer, *Ind. J. Clin. Pract.* 1992, 2: 33-34.
127. Menon L.R., Divate S., Acharya V.N., *et al.*, Utility of BAL in diagnosis of immunosuppressed patients; JAPI 2002: 50: 1110-14.
128. Pradhan PK, Jain S; Empowerment of physicians to evaluate the molecular dynamics in the body with single photon emission CT and Position Emission Tomography; IN; A, Muruganathan; ED; Med Update API 2013;23:736-41.

PULMONARY SOUNDS IN COMMON PULMONARY DISEASES

Introduction

Listening lung sounds like wheeze or stridor at a distance from the patient was known to our ancestors since ages. Listening chest by directly applying the ear not only increased understanding but provided number of types of sounds related to different diseases. The science of auscultation, however, added another feather to our understanding. And this started with the invention of stethoscope by Laennec.[1] To settle the score regarding the use of different terms for the same lung sounds, a committee of the International Lung Sounds met in 1976 and after going through an acoustic analysis of tape recorded lung sounds by a variety of investigators, the

American Thoracic Society in 1977[2] adopted a new nomenclature of adventitious sounds. The word *Rales* in American Journals which was found to be virtually equivalent to *crepitations* in British Medical Journals[3] was recommended to be called *crackle.* An objective basis to use adjectives, time and course (fine or coarse) for crackle was provided by the work of Holford, by measuring time extended waveforms of individual crackles.[4]

Normal Breathing Lung Sounds

The normal breath sounds are transmitations of gas in the air pipe, the oscillations of which are offered resistance at acoustic frequencies which is carried across the lungs to the lung periphery due to generated turbulence during inspiration and fades away during expiration as the direction of the flow is reversed and expiration flow rate falls. The transfer of gas which has a wide range of evenly distributed frequencies from 200 to 2000 Hz, upto the mouth remains unaltered, followed by resistance by small bronchi and then beyond the segmental bronchi, breath sounds travel across the lung,[5] reaching the chest wall at a relatively narrow range of low frequencies with a steep fall in amplitude above 200 Hz.

Breath sounds were initially thought to be produced as a result of friction of air against airways' lining. Using a sheep lung preparation, it came to light that the sound was generated within the lung.[6] The breath sounds are generated at the larynx and conveyed to the chest wall through airways[7] was put aside by Kraman.[8] Although, the larynx produces a lot of noise but has no role in the production of vesicular lung sound, study of normal subjects by substraction phonopneumography concludes that trachea and main stem bronchi have no contribution in producing vesicular lung sounds.[9]

A sound spectrographical analysis revealed that inspiratory vesicular sound had maximum intensity at 200 Hz which decreased rapidly with increasing frequency and no sound energy could be detected at more than 500 HZ.[10] Another study demonstrated relationship between amplitude to inspiratory component of vesicular lung sound and regional ventilation within the lung.[11] Also there existed regional difference between the apex and the base of the lung.[12] Sounds are faint where ventilation is impaired.[13]

Bronchial Lung Sounds

These sounds are produced especially in conditions like consolidation, atelectasis or fibrosis.[4] The consolidated lung does not attenuate the transmitting sound unlike inflated lung, acting simply as a continuous acoustic conducting medium, because of lack of air in the lung tissue between the central airways and the chest wall. Clinically, the breath sounds are transmitted to the stethoscope practically without loss by attenuation or filtration, as if the stethoscope is placed over trachea. Graphic demonstration reveals higher frequency components in bronchial sounds than vesicular sounds. The site of origin of these sounds lies in the airways, 4 mm or more in diameter.[2] Bronchial breathing normally be heard over upper lobe because of proximity and contact with trachea from where the sound is directly transmitted to solid lung.[5] At the same time, bronchial breathing can be absent over the lower lobe in case it is both consolidated and atelectated or collapsed as a result of bronchial obstruction.[4]

Bronchovesicular Sounds

These intermediate lung sounds between bronchial and vesicular, may be present in normal healthy state, arising at the site of auscultation from different sources. In morbid stage, these are produced as a result of partial change in filteration characteristics.[4]

Voice Sounds

Oscillations of vocal cords, amplified by resonance of mouth, pharynx and paranasal sinuses, generate a low frequency fundamental note of sound of speech.

The interruption of flow, the turbulence in the mouth or the vibrations of the tongue help in articulation of consonants. Amplification of higher frequencies are moulded to give shape and resonance by the oropharynx. The fundamental note is 150 Hz in males and 230 Hz in females but the frequency of formants—a pair of partial tones which make a vowel—is same in both the sexes and is not dependent on fundamental note.[4] Different varieties[4] of voice sounds as transmitted can be detailed out as following:

1. *Bronchophony:* Low frequency upto 200 Hz is transmitted high above 200 Hz is attenuated. This happens in a normal lung where selective filteration removes most of the vowel formants and the speech heard over normal lung through stethoscope is a low pitched meaningless rumble. In case the lung between trachea and auscultatory area is airless, the higher frequency including the vowel formants are not filtered and transmitted as intelligible speech called bronchophony.
2. *Whispering Pectoriloquy (Table 1.30):* The low frequency component which can be transmitted, is lacking in whispering which is produced by turbulent air flow through pharynx, glottis and trachea and not by oscillations of vocal cords, and hence it is inaudible over a normal airy lung. These high frequency noise components along with formants of vowels get transmitted as intelligible speech through the airless lung as whispering pectoriloquy. The whispering pectoriloquy, bronchial breathing and bronchophony together form the triad of auscultatory signs of consolidation of lung.

Table 1.30: Whispering pectoriloquy
Identification of individual syllable on auscultating the chest, while patient whispers, e.g., thirty-eight. This occurs because solid lung tissue conducts sound better than an aerated one (Normal lung).
Positive: In cases of lung consolidation, cavitation, pneumonia, tuberculosis

3. *Aegophony:* Voice sounds become inaudible in pleural effusions and pneumothorax which are otherwise normally conducted through the chest wall. When a consolidation is separated by a thin layer of fluid from the chest wall, the attenuation becomes selective, permitting only high frequency formants of vowels and curtailing low frequency sound below 1000 Hz. Thus speech though remains intelligible, yet attains a nasal breathing quality of aegophony.

Continuous Adventitious Lung Sounds of the Lung

These sounds are usually of pathological origin. They may be superimposed over the breath sounds, louder and continuous. Continuous does not mean continuing throughout the inspiratory cycle, but signifies a duration of more than 250 ms along with several wheeze sounds which are produced due to interaction of airway wall with the gas moving within the airways.[5] Mechanism and sequences include, narrowing of airways leading to increase in the velocity of gas flow, causing fall in the lateral pressure due to venturi effect, causing narrowing or closure of the airways further. The venturi effect stops as the airway is closed, the airway lumen reopens and the cycle is reset into operation. This repeat sequence of self perpetuating pressure changes resulting in rapid oscillations of the airway wall to produce musical sound. A fall in lateral pressure during inspiration can produce stridor in stenosis of cervical part of trachea where outside pressure is atmospheric.[4] Absence of wheeze peaks over 1000 Hz over the lung has been demonstrated by digital respirosonography.[14] High-pitched wheeze may be heard over trachea, in case the lungs are hyperinflated, which may be useful auscultation in asthma patients.

Discontinuous Adventitious Lung Sounds (Crackles)

These include brief sounds of less than 20 ms duration. These are virtually explosive sounds of individual components. These are produced possibly as a result of more than one mechanism which involve:

a. Sudden opening of small airways with rapid equalisation of pressure causing implosive sound waves as seen in interstitial lung disease and conjestive cardiac failure.
b. The bubbling of air through secretions.

These sound waves radiate towards four directions rather than an expanding sphere.[15]

Tracings of time expanded crackles by waveform analysis describes[2] two types of crackles, i.e., fine and coarse, as shown in Table 1.31.

Table 1.31: Types of crackles	
a. Initial deflection width (IDW) – 0.9 ms	
b. Two cycle duration (2 CD) – 6.0 ms	
If a and b are more	Less
Coarse crackles	Fine crackles

LUNG SOUNDS—CLINICAL SIGNIFICANCE IN PATHOLOGICAL DISORDERS

Chronic Bronchitis

These crackles are low-pitched, evenly spaced, few, yet quite loud and clearly audible, especially during expiration and early inspiration due to widespread airflow obstruction. The cause of intermittent obstruction is uncertain and definitely not due to increased sputum within the large bronchi. The source of these sounds is in the central airways.[4]

Emphysema

The lung sounds in emphysema vary from breath to breath,[16] the sound at mouth is decreased in emphysema compared to be increased in bronchitis and asthma.[17] The variability in sounds in emphysema directly corresponds to transmission of sound through lung areas of relatively normal parenchyma, hyperinflation with airways obstruction (and less ventilation) and focal atelectasis and consolidation.[4]

Bronchial Asthma

High-pitched continuous lung sound is characteristic feature in bronchial asthma.[4] Wheeze may be auscultated over central airways during expiration in mild cases and distributed over the chest both in inspiration and expiration in severe forms of asthma. Absence of wheeze in asthma is an ominous sign and is indicative of so low the flow rate that the wheeze is not produced. Wheeze can be generated on forced expiration in a normal healthy person which can easily be distinguished from abnormal.[18] The wheeze may vanish or its frequency is decreased as the attack goes off spontaneously or after using bronchodilator therapy.[19]

Bronchiectasis

Crackles are classical in bronchiectasis, present in both phases of respiration, and can well be distinguished from those in chronic bronchitis and alveolitis[20] as shown in Table 1.32. They become less abundant after coughing. The inspiratory crackle

Table 1.32: Lung crackles[20]

Distinguishing features	*Obstructive chronic bronchitis*	*Bronchiectasis*	*Fibrosing alveolitis*
Time inspiratory crackle	Early phase	Early and mid phase	End phase
Number	Few	Moderate	Profuse ±
Effect of cough	No change	Temporarily decreased	No change
Effect of position	No change	No change	Abolished or modified
Intensity	Faint	Loud	Loud
Pitch	Coarse	Coarse	Fine
Expiratory crackle	May be present	Present	May be present
Transmission to mouth	Transmitted	Transmitted	Not transmitted

generates and fades away within the inspiration. However, there are expiratory crackles also.[4]

Interstitial Fibrosis

Fine crackles are characteristic in interstitial fibrosis. These are present in the end of inspiration in mild cases, best heard in an upright position at the lung bases, altered, or course, by change in position and may disappear as the patient bends forward. But in advanced stages, these crackles persist despite positional change and may be heard at above the bases at higher levels. As the disease advances, these may become *pan-inspiratory*, with an end inspiratory accentuation. These may be heard in the expiratory phase.[4,21] The suggested mechanism is as follows:

Initially patient's airways at the end of inspiration, close early in expiration and then reopen with the building of pressure of gas which is trapped within them, and which exceeds that of the adjacent airway during expiratory phases only to result in crackles.

Pulmonary fibrosis caused by asbestos exposure, result in end inspiratory crackles, which are present at the bases in midaxillary lines in the early stage, spreading to posterior bases[22] later on. It is believed to be an early sign of asbestosis.[23]

Pleuritis

Pleural rub is a classical feature of pleuritis.[24] Pleural layers are well lubricated smoothly over one another. The surface becomes rough due to deposition of fibrin, inflammatory or malignant cells infilteration and the frictional resistance thus occurs, interrupts the smooth sliding motion. Here comes the lung into action, acting like a bow of a string instrument. If the area involved is large, then large resonant oscillations are set in, resulting into a musical sound. Generally the jerky sliding pulmonary movements produce a series of non-musical sounds which are larger and low pitched than crackles called pleural rub. They arise from lung, heard during inspiration, often repeated in reverse sequence during expiration, giving a minor image effect.[4,25]

Pneumothorax

Loud crackles are heard in left side pneumothorax. These are generated due to sudden displacement of small air trapped in the mediastinal surface of the lung. These crackles are quite shallow and may disappear as the pneumothorax deepens or the lung re-expands.[25] Tables 1.33 to 1.36 show different types of breathing in different chest diseases.

Table 1.33: Bronchial breathing

Vesicular component of breath sound is suppressed when alveoli are not working, thus producing harsh, clear breath sound with equal inspiration and expiration, called bronchial breathing. Positive in:
Pulmonary consolidation
Pulmonary tumours
Pulmonary tuberculosis
Pneumonitis

Table 1.34: Cavernous breathing

When partially consolidated lung tissue is surrounded by lung cavity, hollow quality and low toned breath sound with equal inspiration and expiration is produced called cavernous breathing.
Positive in: Open pneumothorax
Lung cavities (Tuberculosis, Bronchiectasis, Lung abscess)

Table 1.35: Cheyne-Stokes respiration

Due to damaged cerebral respiratory centre, one full cycle equates to twice the circulation time, thereby producing a respiration that gradually decreases in frequency untill a temporary cessation occurs; Respiration then restarts and the frequency builds to maximum before the cycle repeats itself.
Positive in: CVA (Cerebro Vascular Accident)
Chronic diseases (Terminal stages)
Cardiac disease (Advanced), e.g., LVF (Left Ventricular Failure)
Cerebral tumours
Meningitis
Overdosage of barbiturates or narcotics
Raised intercranial pressure
Uremia

Table 1.36: Amphoric breathing
Breath sounds are similar to blowing over the top of a bottle producing high pitched, metallic toned bronchial breathing on auscultation.
Positive in:
Open pneumothorax
Tuberculous cavities

REFERENCES

1. Laennec R.T.H., *A treatise on the diseases of the chest (translated from the French).* New York: Hanar Publishing Co. 1962,319.
2. London R. and Murphy R.L.H. Lung sounds. State of art., *Am Rev. Respir. Dis.* 1984, 130: 663-673.
3. Bunin N.J. and Loudon R.G., Lung sounds terminology in case reports. *Chest* 1979, 76: 690-692.
4. Hira H.S., *Lung sounds*, J *Assn Phys India* 1993,41: 33-37.
5. Forgacs P., *Lung sounds.* Casell and Collar, Macmillan Publishers Ltd., 1978, London.
6. Bullar J.P., Experiments to determine the origin of respiratory sounds, *Proc. R. Soc., London* 1884,37: 411-422.
7. Bushnell G.E., The mode of production of the so-called vesicular murmur of respiration, *JAMA* 1921,77: 2104-2106.
8. Kraman S.S., Determination of the site of production of respiratory sounds by substraction phonopneumography. *Am. Rev. Respir. Dist.* 1980, 122: 303-309.
9. Kraman S.S., Does laryngeal noise contribute to the vesicular lung sound? *Am. Rev. Respir. Dist.* 1981,124: 292-294.
10. McKusick V.A., Jenkins J.T. and Webb G.H. The acoustic basis of the chest examination: Studies by means of sound spectrography, *Am. Rev. Tuberc.* 1966,72: 12-34.
11. Plysongsang Y, Macklem T and Ross W.R.D., Distribution of regional ventilation measured by breath sounds. *Am. Rev. Respir. Dist.* 1978,117: 657-664.
12. LeBlanc P, Macklem P and Ross W.R.D., Breath sounds and distribution of pulmonary ventilation. *Am. Rev. Respir. Dis.* 1970, 102: 10-16.
13. Ploysongsang Y, Martin R.R., Ross W.R.D., Loudon R.G. and Macklem P.T., Breath sounds and regional ventilation. *Am. Rev. Respir. Dis.* 1977, 116: 187-199.
14. Pasterkamp H., Carson Chris, Daien David and Oh Yunus, Digital respirosonography: New images of lung sounds. *Chest* 1989, 96: 1405-1412.
15. Fredberg J.J. and Holford S.K. Discrete lung sounds: Crackles (rales) as stress-relaxation quadruples. *J. Acoust. Soc. Am.* 1983, 73: 1036-1046.
16. Ploysongsang Y, Paze J.A.P. and Macklem P.T. Lung sounds in patients with emphysema. *Am. Rev. Respir. Dis.* 1981,124: 45-49.
17. Forgacs P., Noisy breathing, *Chest* 1973, 63: 385-415.
18. Forgacs P., The functional basis of pulmonary sounds. *Chest* 1978, 73: 399-405.
19. Martini J.J., Pierson D.J., Hudson L.D. and Lakshminarayanan S. The significance of wheezing in chronic airflow obstruction. *Am. Rev. Respir. Dis.* 1979, 120: 1069-1072.
20. Nath A.R. and Capel L.H. Lung crackles in bronchiectasis. *Thorax* 1980, 35: 694-699.
21. Walshaw M.J., Nisar M., Pearson M.G., Calverly P.M.A. and Earis J.R. Expiratory lung crackles in patients with fibrosing alveolitis, *Chest* 1990, 97: 407-409.
22. Smither W.G., Secular changes in asbestosis in an asbestos factory. *Ann. NY Acad. Sci.* 1965, 132: 166-181.
23. Shirai F., Kudoh S., Shibuya A., Sada K. and Mikami R., Crackles in asbestos workers; auscultation and lung sound analysis. *Br. J. Dis. Chest* 1981, 75: 386-396.
24. Forgacs P., Lung sounds, *Brit. J. Dis. Chest.* 1969, 63: 1-12.
25. Bhatia R.S., Pulmonary sounds in common pulmonary diseases: A short review, *Lung India* 1994, 12: 89-92.

PULMONARY FUNCTION TESTS IN HEALTH AND DISEASE

Recently, interest has been shown in the respiratory muscles[1] and the assessment of their power and strength has been stressed valuable in any comprehensive clinical evaluation of patients with neuromuscular disorders, dyspnoea and respiratory failure.[2,3]

Assessment of respiratory muscle function can be made by measuring maximal pressures generated at the mouth after full expiration, i.e., maximal expiratory pressure (MEP) and after full inspiration, i.e., maximal inspiratory pressure (MIP) using simple non-invasive methods, using mercury manometers and pressure gauges.[4,5] A meaningful interpretation of these values at a particular point of time can either be made by knowing the previous normal values of the person or comparing the values with those predicted for the particular individual based on physical parameters, as is done for spirometric indices, or as is being done for healthy children and young adults in the West.[5,6]

The predicting values for a community can be derived[7] by using MEP at TLC and MIP at RY as it is known that expiratory muscle contractility is highest at or near TLC whereas inspiratory muscle contractility is highest between functional residual capacity and RV.[8]

The values in males are comparable with previously published values in the West,[1,9] but may vary in females because of a lower muscle mass and lack of regular physical exercise in teenage girls as compared to the Western[9,10] women. The fall in respiratory muscle strength can be seen as the age advances in both sexes.[5,11]

PEFR recorded on the Wright's peak flow meter is quite useful both at the bed side and in field studies.[12-15] It has been recorded that in addition to age and sex,[16] higher values of PEFRS may be obtained in working class young adults from good socio-economic status, non-polluted urban localities, non-smokers and without any history of chronic chest ailments,[17] compared to other studies.[18-22] This has been further strengthened that rural and urban[23] growing children have similar PEFRs values while a steady decline in PEFR with age, especially in rural females has been documented possibly because of poor nutrition, recurrent chest infection[24] and lack of medical regard for respiratory illness.[25]

After discussing the various patterns of pulmonary function with regards to age, sex, rurality, environments etc., pulmonary function in few common diseases are discussed.

Pulmonary Function Test in COPD

Chronic obstructive pulmonary disease (COPD) is a major cause of morbidity and mortality in India.[26] Its prevalence varied from 1 per cent in urban non-smokers to 21 per cent in rural smokers.[27-29] The prevalence was even higher in smokers of hilly areas of Himachal (32%) and Chutta smokers of Orissa.[28,30-34]

There is limited information on the natural history of chronic bronchitis. Fletcher and colleagues,[35] identified two different forms (hypersecretory and obstructive) of chronic bronchitis. While mucus hypersecretion remained constant over many years, the obstructive disorder progressed further.[35] There is hardly any report on the natural history of COPD in the Indian population. Most Indian studies on prevalence of COPD do not differentiate the obstructive and hypersecretory disorders. Natural history of morbidity and mortality of COPD are now available for Western populations.[35-41]

Urban and rural men were smokers largely of cigarettes and bidis respectively. Similarly, the women differed with respect to the fuel used at home. Over 90 per cent of city women used liquefied petroleum gas (LPG) and/or kerosene, but most of the rural women used biomass fuels such as dried dung and wood.[42]

The overall COPD prevalence in smokers is 9.6 times higher than non-smokers. Also there is a high prevalence of respiratory symptoms in women using biomass fuels.[44] It is known that there is a age-related decline in PEFR and other lung functions in health.[45,46] This relationship with age is curvilinear showing an initial increase in the values and a gradual decline after the age of approximately 35 years.[46-48]

Presence of base-line airways obstruction is the other major determinant of the rate of fall of PEFR.[43] Age and base-line FEV_1were the best predictors of mortality.[37,38,41]

Pulmonary Function Tests in Ulcerative Colitis

The aetiology of chronic non-specific ulcerative colitis is still unknown. Autoimmune mechanism is considered to be the most possible cause.[49] Like the other well established autoimmune disorders such as systemic lupus erythematosus, rheumatoid arthritis, vasculitis, ulcerative colitis is also known to present with multisystem manifestations.[50-53] However, reports indicating direct or indirect involvement of lungs in ulcerative colitis are very few.

Apart from thrombotic changes in pulmonary arteries at autopsy[54] occurrence of pulmonary infiltrates due to vasculitis,[55] pulmonary functional abnormalities in ulcerative colitis have been observed. Obstructive defect of the lung functions may or may not be present.[48] Significant reduction in diffusing capacity in ulcerative colitis has been observed.[56] The severity of reduction is correlated with the extent and duration of the illness. The exact pathogenesis of reduction in diffusing capacity is difficult to offer. As such there is no consensus of views regarding the pathogenesis of other extra colonic manifestations of ulcerative colitis. The vasculitis may explain the pathogenesis and form the basis of further studies in this regard.[57]

Sulphasalazine is a drug widely used for the treatment of ulcerative colitis and pulmonary functional abnormalities have been described as side effects of this drug in ulcerative colitis.[58] Further studies to evaluate lung function to rule out changes in lung parenchyma and muscles are required.[49]

Pulmonary Functions in Tropical Pulmonary Eosinophilia

Lung function studies in tropical pulmonary eosinophilia (TPE) have received less attention as compared to its aetiological, pathological and radiological features. The conclusions of the few studies are conflicting.[59-62]

A significant reduction in all the ventilatory parameters is observed in both sexes.[59-62] Four types of ventilatory patterns like restrictive, mixed, obstructive and normal were noted. The predominantly restrictive pattern thus seems to be characteristic of the later stages of disease. Significant reduction in vital capacity found with increasing duration of symptoms indicates pulmonary fibrosis and disability as disease advances. Thus restriction may be present from the very onset of disease. Absence of obstruction in majority of patients with duration of symptoms of less than 3 months is reported.[61,62]

Significant decrease in MMFR value is observed even in those cases where FEV_1 and PEFR were normal, indicating small peripheral airway obstruction in TPE.[63] It is not clear why some patients develop predominantly obstructive ventilatory defect and others more restrictive defect. Perhaps the same aetiological agent is capable of eliciting both types of host response.[62]

Clinical response to drug usually starts in 2-4 days followed by haematological response.[64] Time taken for pulmonary functions to return to normal, if it does, is much longer.[60] Also haematological responses do not always reflect relief in clinical picture. After clinical, radiological and haematological response to DEC, some amount of residual lung function abnormality persists in TPE.[63]

Diabetic patients have reduced lung functions, possibly due to chronic complication of diabetes mellitus and is independent of smoking.[65]

REFERENCES

1. Wilson S.H., Cooke W.T., Edward R.H.T. and Spiro S.G., Predicted normal values for maximal respiratory pressures in Caucasian adults and children. *Thorax* 1984, 39: 535-38.
2. Black L.F. and Hyatt R.E., Maximal respiratory pressures in generalized neuromuscular disease. *Am. Rev. Respir. Dis.* 1971, 103: 641-50.
3. Byrd R.B. and Hyatt R.E., Maximal respiratory pressure in chronic obstructive lung disease. *Am. Rev. Respir. Dis.* 1968, 98: 848-56.

4. Brodey A.W., Wander HJ., O'Halloran R.S., Connolly J.J. and Schiverttey F.W., Correlations, normal standards and interdependence in tests of ventilatory strength and mechanics. *Am. Rev. Respir. Dis.* 1964, 89: 214-35.
5. Block L.F. and Hyatt R.E., Maximal respiratory pressures: Normal values and relationship to age and sex. *Am Rev. Respir. Dis.* 1969,99: 696-702.
6. Ringqvist T., The ventilatory capacity in healthy subject: Normal analysis of causal factors with special reference to the respiratory forces. *Scand J. Clin. Lab. Invest.* 1966, 18:(Suppl) 87-93.
7. Guleria R. and Jindal S.K., Normal maximal expiratory and inspiratory pressures in healthy teenagers, *JAPI* 1992,40: 108-109.
8. Rochester D.P., Tests for respiratory muscle function. *Clinics in Chest Medicine* 1988, 9: 249-61.
9. Leech J.A., Ghezzo H., Stevens D. and Becklaka M.R., Respiratory pressures and function in young adults. *Am. Rev. Respir. Dis.* 1983, 128: 17-23.
10. Jindal S.K. and Wahi P.L., *Pulmonary function laboratory in the tropics; needs, problems and solutions.* In: Sharma OP, Ed Lung Disease in the Tropics, New York: Marcel Dekkar 1991: 523-42.
11. Chen H. and Kuo C. Relationship between respiratory muscle function and age, sex and other factors. *Jour Appl Physiol.* 1989, 64: 943-48.
12. Wright B.M. and Mckerrow C.B., Maximum forced expiratory flow rate as a measure of ventilatory capacity. *Br. Med. J.* 1959,2: 1041.
13. Lockhart W., Smith D.H., Mair A. and Wilson W.A., Practical experience with the peak flow meter. *Br. Med. J.* 1960, 1: 37.
14. Fairbairn A.S., Fletcher C.M., Tinker C.M. and Wood C.H., A comparison of spirometric and peak expiratory flow measurements in men with and without chronic bronchitis. *Thorax* 1962, 17: 168.
15. Malik S.K. and Wahi P.L., Prevalence of chronic bronchitis in a group of north Indian adults. *J. Indian Med., Assoc.* 1978, 70: 6.
16. Gregg I. and Nunn A.J., Peak expiratory flow in normal subjects. *Br. Med. J.* 1973, 3: 282.
17. Malik S.K., Jindal S.K., Banga N. *et al.* Peak expiratory flow rate of healthy north Indian teachers, *Ind. J. Med. Res.* 1980,71: 322-24.
18. Malik S.K., Jindal S.K., Jindal Y. and Bansal S., Peak expiratory flow rate in healthy adults. *Indian J. Chest Dis.* 1975, 17: 166.
19. Shah J.R. and Mehta R.H., Peak flow rate as a measure of pulmonary ventilatory capacity. *Indian J. Surg.* 1961,23:397.
20. Singh H.D., Peak flow rate in Indians. *Indian J. Physiol. Pharmacol* 1967,11: 129.
21. Kamat S.R.,Thiruvengadam K.Y. and Rao T.L., A study of pulmonary function among Indians and assessment of the Wright peak flow meter in relation to spirometry for field use. *Am. Rev. Resp. Dis.* 1967,96: 707.
22. Natarajan S. and Radha K., Peak expiratory flow rate in normal south Indians. *Indian J. Chest Dis. Allied Sci.* 1978,20:178.
23. Malik S.K., Jindal S.K., Sharda P.K. and Banga N., Peak expiratory flow rate of healthy school boys from Punjab. *Ind. Paed* 1981, 18,517.
24. Padmavati S. and Arora R., Sex differences in chronic cor pulmonale in Delhi. *Brit. Jour. Dis. Chest.* 1976, 70: 251.
25. Malik S.K., Jindal S.K. and Banga N. Differences in ventilatory capacity of rural and urban adult women from northern India, *Ann Natl. Acad. Med. Sci.* 1982, 18, 51-55.
26. Kamat S.R., *Chronic obstructive pulmonary disease—An Indian perspective. In: Lung disease in the tropics,* O.P. Sharma, Ed. (Marcel Dekker Inc., NewYork); 1991, p.399.
27. Malik S.K., Chronic bronchitis in north India. *Chest* 1977, 72, 800.
28. Malik S.K., Profile of chronic bronchitis in north India—The PGI experience (1972-1985). *Lung India* 1986, 4, 89.
29. Jindal S.K. and Malik S.K., *Tobacco smoking and non-neoplastic respiratory disease. In: Tobacco and health; the Indian scene,* L.D. Sanghvi and P. Notani, Eds. (UICC Workshop, Tata Memorial Centre, Bombay) 1983; p.30.
30. Malik S.K., Behera D. and Jindal S.K., Reverse smoking and chronic obstructive lung disease. *Br. J. Dis. Chest* 1983, 77, 199.
31. Wig. K.L., Guleria J.S., Bhasin R.C., Holmes Jr. E., Vasudeva Y.L. and Singh H., Certain clinical and epidemiological aspects of chronic bronchitis as seen in northern India. *Indian J. Chest.Dis.* 1964,6, 183.
32. Viswanathan R., Chronic bronchitis emphysema syndrome, incidence, aetiology and natural history. *Indian J. Chest Dis.* 1964, 6, 171.
33. Joshi R.C., Madan R.N. and Brash A.A., Prevalence of chronic bronchitis in an industrial population in north India *Thorax* 1975, 30, 61.
34. Viswanathan R., Prasad M., Thakur A.K., Prasad S.S., Sinha S.P., Prasad S.N., Prakash N, Modi R.K. and Singh T.R.B.P.N. Epidemiology of chronic bronchitis: Morbidity survey in Patna urban area. *Indian J. Med. Res.* 1966,54, 105.
35. Fletcher C.M., Peto R., Tinker C. and Speizer F.E., *The natural history of chronic bronchitis and emphysema* (Oxford University Press, London) 1976; p. 122.
36. Postma D.S., Burema J., Gimeno F., May J.F., Smit J.M., Steenhuis E.J., Weele L. TH VD and Sluiter R.J., Prognosis in severe chronic obstructive pulmonary disease, *Am. Rev. Respir. Dis.* 1979,119: 357.
37. Burrows B. and Earle R.H., Course and prognosis of chronic obstructive lung disease. A prospective study of 200 patients. *N. Engl. J. Med.* 1969,280: 397.
38. Diener C.F. and Burrows B., Further observations on the course and prognosis of chronic obstructive lung disease. *Am. Rev. Respir. Dis.* 1975,111: 719.
39. Woolcock A.J., Epidemiology of chronic airways disease. *Chest* 1989, 96 (Suppl 3): 302S.
40. Crofton J. and Masironi R., Chronic airways disease the smoking component. *Chest.* 1989, 96 (suppl 3): 349S.
41. Hodgkin J.E., Prognosis in chronic obstructive pulmonary disease. *Clinics Chest. Med.* 1990,11: 555.
42. Jindal S.K., A field study on follow up at 10 years of prevalence of chronic obstructive pulmonary disease and peak expiratory flow rate, *Ind. J. Med. Res.* 1993, 98: 20-26.
43. Bhatia R.S. *et al.* COPD and kitchen education; Paper selected for award session by ICS; 1995.
44. Behera D. and Jindal S.K., Respiratory symptoms in Indian women using domestic cooking fuels. *Chest.* 1991, 100,385.
45. Cotes J.E., *Lung function assessment and application in medicine,* 3rd ed. (Blackwell Scientific Publications, Oxford) 1974, p. 340.

46. Burrows B., Cline M.G., Knudson R.J., Taussig L.M. and Lebowitz M.D., A descriptive analysis of the growth and decline of the FVC and FEV_1. *Chest* 1983, 83: 717.
47. Malik S.K. and Jindal S.K., Normal values of peak expiratory flow rate in healthy north Indian adults—Revision of prediction formulae. *Indian J. Chest. Dis. Allied. Sci.* 1985, 27: 50.
48. Jindal S.K. and Wahi P.L., *Pulmonary junction laboratory in the tropics; needs, problems and solutions. In: lung disease in the tropics,* O.P. Sharma, Ed. (Marcel Dekker Inc., New York) 1991; p.523.
49. Tiwary R.S., Pruthi H.S., Lakhera S.C, *et al.* Pulmonary functions in ulcerative colitis, *JAPI* 1989, 37: 773-74.
50. Greenstein A., Janowitz H. and Sachar D., The extra intestinal complications of Crohn's disease and ulcerative colitis, a study of 700 patients. *Medicine* 1976, 55: 401-408.
51. Wright R., Lumsden K., Luntz M.H. and Sevel D., Abnormalities of the sacroiliac joints and uveitis in ulcerative colitis. *Q.J. Med.* 1965,34: 229-36.
52. Thornton J.R., Teague R.H., Low-Beer T.S. and Read A.E., Pyodermagangrenosum and ulcerative colitis. *Gut* 1980,21: 247-55.
53. Johnson M.L. and Wilson T.H., Skin lesions in ulcerative colitis. *Gut* 1969, 10: 255-59.
54. Krisner J.B. and Shorter R.H., *Inflammatory disease,* 2nd Ed. Philadelphia, Lea and Febiger 1975, 142-43.
55. Isenberg J.I., Goldstein H., Korn A.R., Ozerman R.S. and Rosen V., Pulmonary vasculities: An uncommon complication of ulcerative colitis. *N. Engl. J. Med.* 1968,279: 1376-77.
56. Eade O.E., Smith C.L. and Whorwel P.J., Pulmonary function in patients with inflammatory bowel diseases. *Gut.* 1977,18: A 432.
57. Sharma M.P. and Kar P., Pulmonary functions in ulcerative colitis. *J. Assoc. Physicians India* 1985,33:613-14.
58. Jones G.R. and Malone D.N.S., Sulphasalazine induced lung disease. *Thorax* 1972, 27: 713-16.
59. Udwadia F.E., Tropical Eosinophilia—A correlation of clinical histopathologic and lung function studies. *Diseases of Chest* 1967,52: 53 1-38.
60. Nesarajah M.S., Pulmonary functions in tropical eosinophilia before and after treatment with diethyl carbamazine. *Thorax* 1975, 30:574-77.
61. Kamat S.R., Pimparker B.D., Store S.D., Warrier N.V.U. and Fakey Y.C., Study of clinical, radiological and pulmonary function patterns of response to treatment in pulmonary eosinophilia *Ind. J. Chest. Dis.* 1970, 12: 91-110.
62. Abdullah A.K., Siddiqui M.A., Qureshi M.U. and Aziz Khan, Ventilatory impairment in tropical eosinophilia and its comparison with asthma. *Indian J. Chest Dis. Allied. Sci.* 1977, 19: 82-87.
63. Singh R.P., Narang R.K., Bihari K. *et al.* Ventilatory functions in TPE, *JAPI,* 1989,37: 775-77.
64. Narang R.K. and Jain S.C., Oral diethycarbamazine in tropical pulmonary eosinophilia. *Brit. J. Chest. Dis.* 1966, 60: 93-100.
65. Irfan M., *et al.,* Pulmonary functions in patients with diabetes mellitus; Lung India 2011; 28: 89-92.

PULMONARY FUNCTIONS TESTING; INTENSIVE PULMONARY CARE UNITS; PULMONARY PHYSIOTHERAPY

Introduction[1]

The enormous burden of pulmonary tuberculosis (TB) has masked the equally staggering problem of non-tuberculous pulmonary disease in most tropical countries[1] including India. Although 25-30% of total outpatient attendance at Indian hospitals was attributed to pulmonary diseases,[2] around 65% of the patients attending the chest clinic are diagnosed as having non-tuberculous lung disease.[3] Unfortunately, the development of pulmonary medicine in this country, unlike other tropical countries, has not paralleled the enormity of the problem. Only recently trend has shifted from Govt./Municipal chest clinics to private chest clinics.

Existing Facilities

Testing facilities available in large 500-bedded hospitals in 60 Indian centres showed that although 20% of centres had no pulmonary function test laboratory (PFT) at all, most others were ill-equipped (Table 1.37). Frequently, the laboratory consisted of a spirometer, which was generally under utilized and often non-functional.[3] Pakistan, Nepal and Bangladesh have similar situations.[3]

Table 1.37: Available facilities in 60 PFT labs of Indian medical colleges

Test	*PFT using No.*	*Labs the test %*	*Test per week (cumulative average ± SO)*
Spirometry	48	80	22 ± 15
Blood gas analysis	18	30	38 ± 28
Diffusion test	11	18.3	8±3
Plethysmography	4	6.7	6
Exercise testing	3	5	<1

The need to develop a pulmonary service is now being realized.[4,5] The American model can be considered as an example. Physicians dealing with lung disease generally lack the initiative to enlighten themselves regarding advances in the field of pulmonary medicine.

PFT Laboratory Need, Concept and Equipments

The principal purpose of a clinical laboratory in a hospital is to assist the physician by providing a set of lung function tests to determine the presence and degree of respiratory disease and disability. The tests may also provide objective assessment of type, degree and progress of a disease and monitor therapy. A respiratory laboratory in an industrial or occupational setting has the more specific purpose of establishing the relationship between disease and to a particular exposure agent.

A study spirometer is the most basic requirement. Addition of a few peak flow meters is useful. An arterial blood gas analyzer is optional for small laboratories, but mandatory for larger hospitals and laboratories at the level of state medical colleges.[6] These laboratories would also require facilities for measuring functional residual capacity and diffusion capacity, broncho-provocation, and broncho-reversibility testing.

Referral laboratories should have near-complete facilities, including whole body plethysmography, exercise testing, and mass spectrometry. It is useful to integrate facilities for cardiac catheterization and echocardiography to allow for an overall assessment of cardiopulmonary functions.

Respiratory laboratories play a vital role in monitoring hemodynamic and pulmonary mechanics. Lung mechanics can be assessed with volume, pressure, and flow measurements with the help of volume displacement (e.g., water-seal) spirometers and pneumotachographs. For the assessment of gas exchange, monitoring of inspired, expired, and arterial O_2 and CO_2 is required, necessitating O_2 and CO_2 monitors (preferably a mass spectrometer) and blood gas analyzers. Hemodynamic monitoring in the acute care setting occurs largely at the bedside, with central venous or right heart and pulmonary artery catheterization with flow-directed, double- or triple-lumen catheters. A thermodilution catheter with quadruple lumen has an additional line for computer connection to the thermister for measuring cardiac output.

A field unit is an important component as an *extended mobile laboratory,* for epidemiological purposes, especially for obstructive lung diseases.[1] Specialized laboratories such as those for industry, sports institutes, aviation, diving and high-altitude science have more specific needs. Developing countries, including India, depend heavily on the importation of highly automated and sophisticated respiratory equipment. Lack of trained technologists, rapid changes in model designs, and non-availability of spare parts add to the problems.[1] Financial considerations have a great bearing on establishing and running a laboratory. A strong case can be made for the indigenous development of technology, but accuracy must not be sacrificed.[7] Voltage fluctuations are wide and frequent in developing countries, necessitating built-in-stabilizer designs. Hot and humid climates shorten the life of bags and tubing used for collecting and storing gas mixtures.

Laboratory Management: Staff and Computerisation[1]

The administrator in charge, is usually the departmental head. It is difficult to prescribe definite qualifications, but they are expected to be similar to those recommended in an American hospital: a clinician with an M.D. degree who is authorized to practice medicine with certification (or eligibility for certification) by a subspeciality board of pulmonary diseases.[8,9] A post doctoral physician in pulmonary medicine is ideal to head a department and the laboratory. As an alternative, a postgraduate in medicine or in *tuberculosis and chest diseases* with at least 5 years of clinical and teaching experience on the faculty of a respiratory diseases department may be suitable to run the laboratory.

The laboratory staff may include a technical supervisor and a few assistants, technicians and laboratory attendants. The American Thoracic Society recommends a high school background with strong mathematics training.[8] A 2 years combined degree course in cardiopulmonary laboratory technology can be started at two or three institutes equipped with the requisite resources.[1]

Computer technology invaded in a big way and has tremendous application in pulmonary medicine in India.[10] While the use of computers has increased the speed and accuracy of-tests, it has posed problems of quality assurance and increased investment.[8,11] Moreover, most of the systems use Western values for predictive data to create local hard disc or floppy based databases.[12]

Lung Function Tests: In Children andAdults[1]

There are significant variations in normal lung function values among different populations. These may relate to ethnic groups, environmental factors, altitude, level of habitual physical activity and habits of tobacco smoking.[13] Variations of the order of 25% were found in different ethnic groups quantified on the basis of stature.[14] A difference of 13% for vital capacity (VC) and forced expiratory volume (FEV) has been reported between blacks and whites.[15] Indian, Bantu and Chinese have lower values than Europeans.[13,16-20] These differences are generally attributed to differences in body stature and lung size. True ethnic anthropometric variations may exist when age, body size, environmental, and nutritional status are standardized as far as possible.[21]

A large number of reports on normal spirometric values have been produced in the last decade from several tropical countries of Asia and Africa based on findings in both children and adults.[22-31] Caution must be observed while deriving prediction formulae regarding standardization procedures. Guidelines published by American Thoracic Society including recommendations for spirometry systems are most useful.[31] Volume and speed of spirometer should be regularly calibrated and leaks tested. Careful recording of patients' age, height and weight is important. Methodology should be precise and analysis accurate.

Although the indications for lung function testing in children are similar to those in adults, the technical requirements and other specifications differ.[32-34] Several prediction equations available for white children are nearly identical.[35] These predictions may not be applicable to children of other racial groups.[36] Studies from India and some other tropical countries including Libya and Jordan, have used prediction equations that incorporate coefficients for age and height.[22,27,30] These are likely to vary from place to place. It may not be feasible for each laboratory to have its own standards. However, each laboratory can test a group of normal subjects and compare these with the standards available for the particular racial group prevalent in the region.[1]

Lungs are still growing in children, so no single value can be considered as normal for a particular age group and there is a broad range of normal values. Because age and height are more reliable parameters in children, these are used for prediction.

Respiratory Testing in Paediatric Patients[37]

Lung function tests in the management of children have little to offer as paediatric population in the developing countries.[38] It remains undoubtedly true that, for the majority of children with respiratory problems, the diagnosis is primarily made on the history and clincial findings. However, there are situations in which even very simple lung function tests have a major contribution to make and can prevent the clinician commencing inappropriate and potentially dangerous treatment.[37]

Diagnosis

Lung function tests provide information on the functional rather than the anatomical abnormalities and so can rarely be used to establish a diagnosis on their own. However, they identify whether the problem is airways obstruction, restrictive lung disease (stiff lungs), secondary to neuromuscular problems, or a combination of these. Asthma is perhaps the main exception to this since the demonstration of striking short-term variability in airways obstruction is synonymous with asthma, regardless of the trigger responsible.

Guide to Therapy

Serial lung function tests either in the laboratory, or in the clinic, or at home have an important role in assessing the value of any therapy. These tests allow us to identify children who have very little respiratory reserve and yet complain of few symptoms. Such children, particularly those with severe asthma, are either in or on the verge of respiratory failure and can deteriorate with alarming speed, often in the middle of the night, sometimes with fatal results.

Prognostic Value

Respiratory function tests can also be used to provide evidence on the severity of the lung damage in those with chronic respiratory problems so that appropriate advice can be given on the likely long-term outcome as well as while counselling the growing child and teenager on suitable working environments.

Research

An important role of paediatric respiratory units is undoubtedly the evaluation of current and new forms of treatment, preferably under double-blind conditions. The techniques are also of value in indentifying the effect on the growing lungs of severe lower respiratory tract infections, as well as they will lead to lines of treatment that can limit or prevent these crippling diseases.

School children almost always approach lung function tests with an enthusiasm that makes them excellent subjects. At the other extreme the sleepy newborn baby swallows oesophageal balloons and tolerates face masks and so is almost as easy to study. Those who fall between these groups represent a far greater challenge to the clinician's ingenuity and patience.

Children Over the Age of 5 Years Peak Respiratory Flow Rate

The single most widely used parameter is undoubtedly the peak respiratory flow rate as measured by a Wright peak flow meter or one of the more recent (and cheaper) derivatives, the peak flow gauge and the Wright mini peak flow meter. Children use these devices with ease, although the low range peak flow meter is preferable for those under the age of 6 years.

Many studies have shown that the child's height is the best parameter on which to base normal lung function values. The available data for peak flow and most other lung function tests have been summarized.[39] Although mildly reduced in severe restrictive and neuromuscular diseases, the peak respiratory flow rate is primarily an index of airways obstruction and can be used to assess the degree of airways obstruction as also the degree of airways liability induced by exercise[40] or histamine challenge, or relieved by bronchodilator drugs, allowing the identification of those with childhood asthma.

All children with asthma should atleast have their peak flow rate recorded at each medical attendance. Those who have persistently reduced peak flow rates should be referred to an appropriate specialist clinic to establish whether they have associated irreversible airways obstruction or need additional therapy to improve their reserve.

Vital Capacity and Respiratory Volume Curve

Virtually all those caring for children with respiratory disease have access to a method for measuring the vital capacity, that is the total amount of air the child can expel after maximal inspiration and are able to derive useful information from analysis of the forced expiratory volume (FEV) curve. The vital capacity can be measured using wet or dry spirometers or obtained by electronic integration of the signal from a flow-sensing device, for example a pneumotachograph or hot wire anemometer. Unlike the peak respiratory flow rate, the vital capacity is a relative sensitive index of restrictive lung disease and neuromuscular weakness. However, it is also reduced in the presence of moderate to severe airways obstruction, particularly if it is measured as part of the FEV assessment. A significant increase in vital capacity on a slower and more controlled expiratory manoeuvre confirms that significant airways obstruction is present.

Analysis of the FEV curve is primarily used to identify airways obstruction. The most common measurement is the volume of air expelled in the first 0.75 or one second, the $FEV_{0.75}$ and the FEV_1, respectively. For children under the age of 12 years the $FEV_{0.75}$ is more sensitive because many young children can blow out their full vital capacity (FVC) in little more than one second and have an FEV_1/FVC ratio approaching unity, compared with that of 75 per cent in the adolescent and adult. The FEV/FVC ratio is sometimes used to define the degree of airways obstruction. This is not always helpful in view of the fact that the FVC may be reduced to less than half in severe airways obstruction, thus reducing the sensitivity of the ratio. Some favour the maximum mid-expiratory flow rate, the mean of the flow from 25-75 per cent of vital capacity, obtained by drawing straight line through these points on the FEV curve and calculating the mean flow rate from the slope. Although more sensitive, the reproducibility is less satisfactory and the range of normal data is wide.

The expiratory volume manoeuvre can also be used to provide more detailed information by constructing flow volume loops. These can be achieved by feeding the readings of the pneumotachograph or hot wire anemometer onto the vertical axis of a rapidly responding X-Y plotter or storage oscilloscope, and the intergrated volume signal onto the horizontal axis.

Alternatively, differentiators are available that can derive flow from the volume signal of a spirometer. In addition to recording the peak expiratory flow rate the trace can be used to measure flow rate at 25 per cent and 50 per cent of vital capacity, V_{25} and V_{50} respectively. A striking fall in V_{25} suggests that the obstruction is primary in the small airways. Additional information can be achieved if the child rebreathes a gas mixture containing 80 per cent helium and 20 per cent oxygen immediately prior to a repeat flow volume manoeuvre. When the flow limitation is in the large airways, that is, where the flow is relatively high and turbulent, the helium mixture produces a striking improvement in the flow due to helium's low density. When the restriction is in the small airways and the flow is laminar little alteration is seen because the viscosity of helium is close to that of air. Comparison of flow volume curves on breathing helium and air can therefore be used to identify early changes in small airways obstruction. All these parameters can be displayed and calculated for various values using microprocessors, in pre-programmed computers.

Lung Function Measurement[1]

The devices discussed so far fail to measure the amount of gas remaining in the lungs at the end of full expiration, the residual volume. This volume is increased in airways obstruction but reduced in the presence of restrictive lung disease. There is usually little change in neuromuscular disease.

The easiest and cheapest method of obtaining this volume is to connect the child to a closed circuit, including a spirometer, containing a known volume of a marker gas, usually helium. The child rebreathes from the circuit for 3-4 minutes to allow equal distribution of the helium in his lungs, while the carbon dioxide expired is absorbed and replaced by oxygen. The volume of gas in the lungs at the point, the child was connected to the circuit, usually the functional residual capacity, can be calculated from the percentage change in helium concentration and the initial volume of the circuit. If the child combines the procedure with a forced vital capacity manoeuvre, the total lung capacity and the residual volume can also be calculated.[37] These measurements can be helpful in assessing children with severe scoliosis but underestimate the true residual volume and functional residual capacity in the presence of severe airways obstruction and air trapping.

These volumes can more accurately be recorded by measurements using a total body plethysmograph. In this technique the child sits in an airtight chamber, preferably with Perspex walls. Once pressure stabilization has occurred the child breathes through a shutter/pneumotachograph system. The shutter is closed at the end tidal point for three to four breaths while the child continues to make respiratory efforts. The resulting thoracic volume change produces alterations in the pressure within the chamber which can be monitored and calibrated against a syringe. The pressure changes within the lungs can be recorded by a second pressure transducer which leads to the mouth-piece proximal to the shutter. From these measurements the total volume of air in the lungs at the point of shutter closure can be calculated. When combined with a forced vital capacity manoeuvre it is again possible to measure the other lung volumes.

Most children over the age of 6 years tolerate this procedure after a short training period, but inevitably this is a technique that is limited to specialized centres. Most applications are research, but the technique can be useful in children with undiagnosed lung disease by identifying those with irreversible airways obstructions, particularly if repeated after 7-14 days on systemic steroids.

The total body plethysmograph can also measure the degree of airways obstruction directly, as airways resistance. This added facility, although again useful in research, does not help significantly in the management of individual child.

The ability to measure gas transfer, present in most adult respiratory units, is of little benefit in the management of children with respiratory diseases. Equally, the closing volume technique, using either a bolus of radioactive xenon or inhaling nitrogen after a period of oxygen breathing, has also proved to be difficult and unreliable in children.

Of greater importance has been the introduction of radioactive ventilation-perfusion scans using the gamma camera. The best results in children have been achieved by first giving an intravenous injection of Tc-labelled albumin microspheres which lodge in the pulmonary capillaries and provide information on the distribution of blood to the lungs. The child then inhales^{81} Kr. This has a half-life of only 13 seconds and so repeated measurements can be obtained with the child nursed in different positions. These techniques have been very useful in situations where congenital abnormalities such as lung cysts are suspected, or when the contribution of a lobe to total exchange is under dispute.

There have also been dramatic advances in the techniques available to study cilial function. There is little doubt that cilial function is often depressed in many acute and chronic respiratory problems but that in addition there are children, including those with Kartagener's syndrome, who have a primary defect in cilial structure and function. These can be diagnosed by examining the cilia on nasal or bronchial epithelial biopsies under the light microscope to demonst rate the presence or absence of cilial beating, and under the electronmicroscope for abnormalities of the dynein arms within the cilia. Further functional information can be obtained by measuring the rate at which labelled polystyrene microspheres are cleared from the trachea after inhalation, using the gamma camera.

Measurements of compliance are difficult in all except the most cooperative of children, because reliable results can be obtained after they have swallowed oesophageal balloons by relating transpulmonary pressure to volume changes during slow expiration.

Newborn Baby[37]

Lung function testing in the newborn period presents special problems, but with care, the mechanical characteristics, lung volumes, and control of respiration can be studied in considerable detail. These tests have played little part in the management of individual babies, but have revolutionized our understanding of the changes occurring at birth and the effects of a variety of lung problems on the function and subsequent development of the lung.

Noninvasive Monitoring Systems[37]

The main role of noninvasive systems has been to evaluate the normal spontaneous respiratory pattern, its chemoreceptor control mechanisms, and how it changes with sleep, age and disease.

Trunk Plethysmograph

The first relatively noninvasive system developed was trunk plethysmograph. This consists of an airtight box which contains the child's body and seals around the child's face. This system undoubtedly provides useful information on the spontaneous breathing patterns and the responses to a variety of stimuli. Attempts have been made to use this technique to study lung mechanics by simultaneously recording the intrathoracic pressure, but problems arise due to phase shifts introduced by alveolar compression and expansion which results in low compliance and high resistance values.

Impedance

In this technique electrodes are placed on each side of the thorax and a high frequency AC current is generated. The peak voltage is kept constant and the current transmitted across the chest measured, falling by about 5 per cent in inspiration as the ratio between intrathoracic and blood/tissue increases. These signals are undoubtedly obtained noninvasively, but they are affected by movement and produce a signal that cannot be directly calibrated and is out of phase with tidal exchange.

Paired Magnetometers

Paired magnetometers attached to the chest wall have also been used to investigate respiratory patterns. Best results are obtained by also measuring abdominal excursion with a further set of magnetometers and deriving a signal trace from the two signals.

Respitrace

Recently, vests have been produced commercially that incorporate a zigzag copper wire. When appropriately conditioned electronically these act as induction coils with variable output depending on the circumference monitored. Usually two wires are used, one around the thorax and the other on the abdomen. By combining these two signals, trace can be obtained that relates closely to tidal exchange at the mouth. If calibrated against a pneumotachograph, a long-term noninvasive quantitative record can be achieved. The record is also of interest because the phase between the thoracic and abdominal traces can be used to identify sleep states: the traces are approximately 180° out of phase in rapid eye movement sleep but in phase during quiet sleep.

Barometric

A further noninvasive system has been to nurse the baby in an airtight chamber carefully maintained at a constant temperature. The baby's tidal exchange produces pressure changes due to the temperature gradient between the baby's lungs and the air within the chamber.

Nasal Thermistor

Finally, breathing has been monitored by mounting a thermistor at the nares, or by sampling expired gases using a low flow carbon dioxide meter or mass spectrometer. These systems are not helped by the tendency for a baby to breathe predominantly but inconsistently through a single nostril.

Methods Suitable for Short-Term Measurements

Pneumotachograph

The device most commonly used to measure tidal exchange is a pneumotachograph mounted in a face mask. This tends to alter the baby's respiratory pattern to some extent, and a bias flow of air into the face masks is essential to prevent rebreathing. It is also necessary to heat the pneumotachograph to approximately 37°C to prevent condensation, which increases the resistance and alters the calibration. Since the pneumotachograph operates under conditions of laminar flow it is sensitive to changes in viscosity, and hence in both gas composition and gas temperature. Fortunately the changes in temperature and composition between inspiration and expiration largely cancel out.

The pneumotachograph is usually used in conjunction with a method for measuring intrathoracic pressure, in the form of an oesophageal balloon, a water-filled catheter, or a micropressure transducer mounted on a nasogastric tube. The water-filled catheter must be at least 6 FG in diameter for an adequate frequency response and be continuously perfused because bubbles tend to form which damp the response. Positioning in the lower third of the oesophagus provides the most reliable results and is achieved by advancing the tip of the device into the stomach and then withdrawing slightly until the pressure reverses its phase relationship with volume. Once in place the systems can be used to calculate the dynamic compliance, a measure of the stiffness of the lungs by relating the tidal exchange to oesophageal pressure change at points of zero flow. Dynamic compliance is useful measurement in healthy babies but tends to overestimate the stiffness of the lungs when the babies are breathing rapidly or have associated airways obstruction. Similarly, the degree of airways obstruction can be calculated by relating the flow trace and the oesophageal pressure at the midvolume points.

Alternatively, pressure volume loops can be constructed and the work of breathing needed to overcome elastic recoil and airways resistance calculated separately, either manually or with the help of a micropressure.

Spirometer

The volume trace can also be obtained by connecting face mask to a suitably designed and rapidly responding water-filled spirometer which has a capacitor or microtorque transducer mounted on the spindle to provide a calibrated electronic signal.

Reverse Plethysmograph

Alternatively, the face mask can be connected to a rigid 100-litre container and the pressure changes developed in the system monitored by a sensitive pressure transducer. Both the reverse plethysmograph and spirometer systems can be used in conjunction with intrathoracic pressure signals to calculate lung mechanics and work of breathing.

Total Body Plethysmograph

Infants are relatively easy to study in suitably constructed total body plethysmographs[3] and there is currently a commercial available model. In the first few days of life, results can be achieved in quiet sleep after a feed. Subsequently, sedation is usually required. A seal at the face is achieved either with soft flanged face mask or by creating ring of silicone putty that gently adheres to the face. Most home-made systems incorporate facilities for measuring intrathoracic pressure so that lung mechanics can be simultaneously calculated.

Problems arise if the plethysmograph is also used to measure airways resistance, due to the relatively low breathing rate that produces significant pressure changes (see above). These can be overcome by arranging for the baby to rebreathe into a bag mounted in the chamber and by ensuring that the expired gases are fully humidified and maintained at 37°C.

Gas dilution techniques are also applicable to babies but tend to underestimate lung volumes in the presence of air trapping. Additional functional information can be obtained using the ventilation perfusion techniques discussed above.

Infants and Preschool Children

These children have largely been ignored as being too difficult to study. However, they are a very important group as they suffer most frequently from respiratory problems. Between the ages of 2 years 9 months and 5 years it is usually possible to obtain information on airways obstruction, using the following two techniques.

Peak Flow Rate

Most young children enjoy breathing into the low range peak flow meter and, with practice, reasonably reproducible results are forthcoming, allowing response to exercise, histamine, and bronchodilator drugs to be assessed. Interpretation can be difficult and it is preferable to have a second independent system.

Forced Oscillation Technique

This method has proved invaluable in young children. In this procedure, a child breathes quietly through a pneumotachograph that is connected to a box. The box has a loudspeaker mounted in its wall. This loudspeaker is driven by a sine-wave generator set at 6 cycle/s. Since this is the natural resonance frequency of the healthy respiratory system, any pressure generated at the child's mouth by the superimposed sine-wave flow is due to airways obstruction rather than compliance or inertia. These measurements can be obtained with a minimum of cooperation. Unfortunately this attractive theory breaks down in severe lung disease, but studies have nevertheless shown that the device continues to detect change reproducibly.

Children under the Age of 3 Years

Between the newborn period and 3 years of age children require sedation, usually commencing with 80 mg/kg body weight of chloral.

Total Body Plethysmograph

Often sufficient information can be obtained by measuring thoracic gas volume and airways resistance as in the neonatal period, using a child total body plethysmograph with a volume of approximately 250 litres.

Forced Oscillation Technique

This technique can also be used, substituting a mouthpiece for a face mask. As before, repeated measurements allow the detection of response to therapy. If more information is required for diagnostic purposes, mouth volume and intrathoracic pressure can be measured, again as in the neonatal period. However, the passage of oesophageal balloons and catheters becomes progressively more difficult and distressing to the child, even after sedation.

Respiratory Jacket

This technique seems to be particularly useful in the first few years of life. It consists of a thin-walled rubber inflatable jacket which encompasses the baby's chest wall and abdomen. When the jacket is inflated to a pressure of 3-4 cm H_2O, respiratory exchange produces pressures within it of approximately 1 mm H_2O which can be relayed via a pressure transducer to a suitable recorder. Calibration is achieved by injecting and withdrawing a known volume of air from the jacket and measuring the change in the end-tidal baseline. This system has been used in two ways.

Measurement of Breathing

The jacket has allowed the assessment of lung function in critically ill babies too sick to tolerate sedation. The babies are nursed in the jacket. A nasogastric feeding tube is then perfused with water and withdrawn so that the tip lies in the lower oesophagus. From the two signals, thoracic volume change and intrathoracic pressure, pressure volume loops can be constructed with the help of a desk-top computer so that virtually instantaneous readings of lung mechanics and work of breathing can be obtained. With this method it is possible to follow the natural history and assess the response to a variety of therapies.

Static Compliance

The jacket has also been used to measure the change in thoracic volume produced by raising the pressure at the sedated child's mouth during spontaneous breathing. This is achieved either by connecting a child's face mask intermittently to a pre-pressurized container or by using a pressure-limited ventilator in the continuous positive airway pressure mode. By relating inflation pressure to the end-tidal volume, static compliance can be measured.

Finally, again ventilation-perfusion studies are entirely applicable to this group and are helpful if localized lung disease is suspected. Lung function tests on children under the age of 3 years should be reserved for those who have chronic respiratory problems, proving difficult to diagnose and for research investigations.

There is a general lowering of lung function as one moves towards the equator. While North African adults have values similar to those of Europeans and Americans, these values are lower in persons living further south.[13,14,19,21-23,41] On the Indian subcontinent, Pakistanis and North Indians have higher values than those of South Indians.[24,25,28,33] Highlanders are an exception, such as the natives of Nepal, Bhutan, Ladakh, New Guinea and Peru, who have larger lung volume.[13,14,42,43]

The "best fit" equation is chosen. The "best fit" equations are those with height, age and age squared as coefficients (Table 1.38). The predictions using these equations are compared for standardized height. Current values are similar to the Western values reported earlier.[44,45]

Measurement and Normal Values

The range of spirometric values in a normal population is rather broad and it is useful to define the *lower limit of normal* expressed as the lower 95th percentile, provided that the distribution of the data is Gaussian.[46] The lower 95th percentile is the value above which 95% of the normal subjects fall. The 5% of the population whose percentage predicted values fall below this normal 95th percentile are thus considered abnormal. This increases the sensitivity of prediction.[1] Lung function may change due to factors other than disease, which are often dismissed as *noise* by clinicians.[47] Although the technical factors may relate to the instrument and the procedure, the biological factors may vary with the subject and the environment. A well-judged and balanced measurement is therefore essential while interpreting these tests (Tables 1.39 to 1.42).

Peak Expiratory Flow Rate

Peak expiratory now rate (PEFR) remains an important test for both epidemiological and clinical purposes.[48,49] This is especially true for tropical countries, because it is cheaper and easier to perform. The values are closely correlated with estimation of FEV_1 and of airway resistance.[50,51] The PEFR is quite satisfactory. On the other hand, high sensitivity of electronic meters may introduce too many false-positive results.[1] Similar criteria apply to PEFR as to spirometry. Curvilinear equations based on height and age are most suitable.[49,52,53]

Table 1.38: Regression coefficients for prediction equations for healthy North Indian adults

Function	*K*	*Age (yrs)* (b_1)	*Age*^{2} *(yrs)* (b_2)	*Ht. (cm)* (b_3)	*Lower limit of normal*
Men					
FVC(L)	–3.44	–0.013	–0.00005	0.048	2.75
FEV_1(L)	–1.9	0.025	0.00006	0.036	2.13
$FEF_{25-75\%}$ (L/M)	59	–2.6	0.007	1.5	87
Women					
FVC(L)	–2.05	–0.014	–0.00004	0.035	1.81
FEV_1(L)	–1.07	–0.03	0.00013	0.027	1.53
$FEF_{25-75\%}$ (L/M)	23	–2.6	0.01	1.5	79

Table 1.39: Distinguishing features of obstructive pattern

	FEV$_1$	*FVC*	*FEV*$_1$*/FVC*	*Response to bronchodilation*	*Lung volume*	*DLCO*
COPD chronic bronchitis	↓,	↓,	↓,	NC	↑	NL
Emphysema	↓,	↓,	↓,	NC	↑	↓
Asthma	↓,	↓,	↓,	↑	↑	NL
Upper airway obstruction	↓,	↓,	↓,	NC	NL	NL

↓ =Reduced, NC =No change, ↑ Increased, NL =Normal

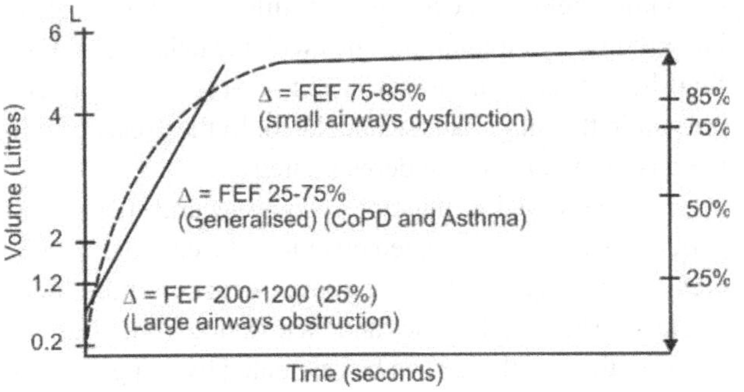

Fig. 1.2: Interpretation of spirometry

Table 1.40: To assess severity obstructive lung disease

Category	*Absolute FEV_1/FVC%*
Normal	≥ 74
Mild obstructive	65-74
Moderate obstructive	45-64
Severe obstructive	<45

Table 1.41: Distinguishing features of restrictive pattern

	Airflow FEV_1/FVC	*Lung volumes*	*DLCO*
Interstitial lungs	↔ or ↑	↓	↓
Neuromascular disease	↔	↓	↔
Pleural disease	↔	↓	↔
Surgical resection	↔	↓	↓

↑ = Increased, ↔ = No change or Normal, ↓ = Decreased

Table 1.42: Severity of restriction

Category	*% Predicted*	
	VC%	*TLC %*
Normal	≥ 81	≥ 81
Mild restriction	60-80	66-80
Moderate restriction	51-65	51-65
Severe restriction	< 50	< 50

Blood Gases Analysis and Pulmonary Diffusion Capacity[1]

Determination of arterial gas pressures and pH has a great significance in patient management. This facility is generally required round the clock for most of the clinical departments of a large hospital. It is difficult to specify absolute quality control requirements because of the differences in analyzers and quality control procedures. Accuracy and precision are the minimum requirements.

The clinical usefulness of diffusion capacity is doubtful, but the applications include diagnosis of diffuse interstitial pulmonary diseases and suspected emphysema. Standard technique should be followed to minimize the variation.[54] With the recent availability of computerized, electronic equipment, it has become easier to measure diffusion capacity. Reports on normal subjects from India have been scanty.[55,56] In a recent study on normal subjects from Bombay, diffusion capacity was found to be lower among Indians.[23]

Clinical Applications: Diagnostic and Therapeutic[1]

Caution is necessary regarding diagnosis by over-interpretation of lung function test results.[57,58] Abnormal lung function indicates respiratory defect. The defect may relate to ventilation (obstructive or restrictive), perfusion, or gas exchange. Obstructive diseases such as bronchial asthma, chronic bronchitis, and emphysema are the common diseases that require PFT laboratory assistance for diagnosis. Pulmonary parenchymal involvement, both primary and secondary to systemic diseases, also shows characteristic findings on lung function assessment. Some of these problems, such as tropical eosinophilia and schistosomiasis, are characteristically seen in tropical countries.

Around 50% of pulmonary function tests are done in India, for preoperative assessment, similar to the Western experience.[59-61]

The role of lung function assessment in both determining treatment and following the response to therapy for diseases of airways, as well as those of lung parenchyma, is well established. In tropical countries, most clinicians in the past used to have generally relied on clinical judgement. This is no longer true. With the routine availability of peak flow meters and cheaper office spirometers, ventilatory monitoring has become easier regular in use and more practical procedure these days. This is especially important for asthma, in which fluctuations in airway obstruction are wide and clinical assessment can be misleading.[1]

Abnormal spirometry may serve as a screening tool only.

Respiratory Equipment: Precaution Against Infections

With advancing science, the number and quality of diagnostic and therapeutic equipment are increasing. Use of spirometer in the pulmonary laboratory is no exception.[62] There are some reports on transmission of nosocomial infection by use of equipment during administration of aerosols by nebulizers.[63-64] Bacterial contamination has been found in one third of the home nebulizers. Both gram positive and gram negative bacteria have been isolated.[65]

Transmission of respiratory pathogens by a spirometer is not a fully established fact though some workers have cultured microorganisms from spirometers in regular use.[66-69] With the availability of compact electronic spirometers, spirometry has become more popular in India in the last decade. But disinfection procedures for spirometers have never been taken seriously. The prevalence of infective respiratory diseases is much higher in India. A theoretical risk of nosocomial infection to subsequent users does exist. Houston *et al.*[67] cultured many non-pathogenic organisms from their spirometer tubing, but organisms like Aspergillus and acid fast bacillus have also been reported.[70]

Pathogenic bacteria, AFB and Aspergillus are isolated from tubings of spirometer, not considering viruses which form the largest factor in respiratory infections. Patients of COPD are more prone to infections.[71] Aspergillus may cause bronchospasm by immune response in susceptible individual,[72] although use of spirometer doesn't have any risk of additional cross infection but it has been suggested to prevent transmission of such infections.[73] Outbreaks of infection have been noted which could be traced to the source, but in majority of instances it may not be possible. Hence precautions are definitely advisable.[74]

Change of mouthpiece alone may not be sufficient. All the tubings and connectors should be cleaned with detergent, rinsed and dried following each use. As the above measures appear inconvenient, the use of *low impedance bacterial barrier system,* essentially a disposable bag in box, is available as an alternative. The box opens into the spirometer and the mouthpiece is attached to the open end of the disposable bag. This prevents the contamination of the spirometer by exhaled air which goes into the disposable bag.[74] A segregation chamber is economical and handy and could prove useful as well as cost affective alternative.[70] The risk of infection during the use of diagnostic equipment is as high as during the use of therapeutic equipment for respiratory conditions.[63-65,71,72] Respiratory diseases account for second largest cause of death in rural India.[74] The advancement of technology should be a mode of service and not doing any sin.

With the help of PFT laboratories diseases such as fibrosing alveolitis, sarcoidosis and others, hitherto considered *extremely rare* in these countries, have been recognized and treated with increasing frequency.[75-77]

A Brief Description of Lung Function Tests[78-81]

Ventilatory Functions

These include lung volumes under static conditions and forced expiratory flow rates under dynamic states. Vital capacity (VC), expiratory reserve volume (ERV) and inspiratory capacity are measured by breathing into and out of a spirometer. Reserve volume (RV), functional residual capacity (FRC) and (TLC) total lung capacity are measured either by helium dilution or by body plethysmography.

Repeatedly breathing in and out of a known volume reservoir containing helium, the helium gets diluted and is not absorbed into pulmonary circulation. Thus with the help of previous and final helium concentrations in the reservoir, the gas volume present in the lungs can be calculated. In the presence of bulk, the gas in the lungs is underestimated.

Here body plethysmograph gives an accurate reading, where patient breathes into a sealed box via a closed mouthpiece. The pressure changes within the thorax cause compression and rarefaction both in the lungs and plethysmograph. Thus volume of gas within the thorax can be calculated by using Boyle's law by measuring pressure changes both at the mouthpiece and in the plethysmograph.

Lung volumes need to be cautiously interpreted keeping in mind the age, sex, height etc. and therefore values between 80 and 120 are generally considered to be normal values. MMFR, a sensitive measurement, needs to be cautiously interpreted with abnormal small lungs (with low TLC and VC).

Three types of abnormal pattern have been observed. In obstructive pattern, expiratory flow rates are decreased. When the disease is fully established, MMFR as well as FEV_1/FVC ratio are decreased, although FEV_1/FVC may be normal in initial stage of obstructive lung disease. TLC may be increased or normal. Residual volume is elevated. RV/TLC is increased. VC is decreased, possibly because of elevated RV.

In restrictive pattern, both VC and TLC are decreased. In parenchymal restrictive disease, RV is decreased without affecting FE flow rates. In extrapulmonary restrictive pattern, TLC is decreased. RV and expiratory flow rates are preserved.

In mixed pattern, there is an overlapping. However, when the predicted values differ by more than 15%, the more severe abnormal one indicates predominance of obstruction or restriction. And if a smaller difference is present, it indicates a mixed pattern and may require other tests to correlate.

Lung function tests provide adequate information in diagnosis and differential diagnosis as well as therapeutic evaluation of pulmonary disorder but lung disease may be present in the absence of abnormal ventilatory functions.

Reversibility Test

It is performed in doubtful cases of bronchial asthma and chronic bronchitis, chronic bronchodilator therapy is stopped, an aerosol bronchodilator is administered, followed by LFTs. Less than 25% increase in values shows slight reversibility, upto 50% moderate and more than 50% shows marked reversibility.

Provocation Test[82,83]

A variety of provocation tests are performed to diagnose causes of cough, bronchial asthma and follow-up of therapy of bronchial asthma. Both specific and non-specific allergen challenger can be used to establish the proof of sensitivity in the allergic alveolitis and occupational asthma of those specific agents. Nevertheless, several unresolved aspects of bronchial provocation tests need to be reviewed, such as:

a. Cut-off between normal and abnormal is not defined.
b. Comparison with reported studies become difficult with differing laboratory techniques.
c. There is subject variability to provoking agents (cold air, hypertonic aerosols, exercise, histamine, methacholine).
d. There are perhaps different mechanisms producing episodic airflow obstruction.

Exercise Test[84,85]

This is used to assess any symptoms of cardiopulmonary systems and also to demonstrate abnormal function, if any; complications may occur to the tune of 0.01% where ventricular arrhythmia is the most common one, followed by precipitation of ischemic heart disease and exertional hypotension. Caution is also to be observed in patients with pulmonary hypertension.

Pulmonary Circulatory Function Tests

These include measurement of pulmonary vascular pressure and cardiac output, involving invasive cardiac catheterisation, recording pulmonary arterial and capillary wedge pressures, using thermodilution method respectively. Using the following equation, pulmonary vascular resistance which is normally 50 to 150 (dynes)/cm^5 can be calculated:

PVR = SO (PAP—Pcw)/CO.

PVR = Pulmonary vascular resistance.

PAP = Pulmonary artery pressure (mean immunity).

PcW = Pulmonary capillary wedge pressure immunity, and

CO = Cardiac output in (L/min).

Pulmonary arterial pressure rises in response to increased vascular resistance. Pulmonary vascular resistance increases in pulmonary thrombosis, in response to alveolar hypoxia causing vasoconstriction and in case of destruction of pulmonary vessels.

If pulmonary vascular resistance increases due to pulmonary vessel diseases, like recurrent pulmonary emboli intraluminal thrombotic disorder, secondary pulmonary vessels involvement in systemic disease scleroderma, the hypoxemia doesn't have significant role. Otherwise it plays a major role in chronic obstructive and interstitial lung diseases as well as chest wall and sleep apnoea syndrome. In fact, pulmonary vascular resistance occurs as result of stimulation due to hypoxemia which is feature of all the diseases of respiratory system. Pulmonary hypertension generally develops if the resistance is prolonged and significant.

Gas Exchange Disturbances

Gas exchange which depends upon alveolar ventilation, rather than total minute ventilation is given as:

$$PaCO_2 = 0.863 \times VC\,O_2 / VA$$

immunity L/min L/min

If VCO_2 is fixed, increase in alveolar ventilation would decrease $PaCO_2$ and vice versa.

The diffusion process of both O_2 and CO_2 through alveolar wall and pulmonary capillaries endothelium is quite rapid, taking l/3rd of the transit time of the erythrocytes through the capillary bed of the lungs and is not much seriously affected during disease state. During exercise the erythrocyte transit time in the lung circulation is shortened, the diffusion is impaired, contributing to hypoxaemia. Such an impaired diffusion produced by exercise, can be measured as diffusing capacity. The partial pressure of the arterial gases, i.e., of O_2 and CO_2 as PaO_2 and $PaCO_2$ are the driving gas pressures rather than exact quantity. The actual amount depends upon the binding capacity of the blood in the form of oxygenated haemoglobin, depending on the concentration of Hb in the blood and PO_2, where PO_2 determines the Hb percentage saturated with O_2.

O_2 Content = 1.34 × Hb × saturation + 0.0031 × PO_2 in normal blood.

The capability of each gram of saturated Hb is to carry 1.34 ml of O_2. Thus PO_2 gives measurement of oxygenation of arterial blood, which can be measured by oximetry.

Another important assessment is alveolar-arterial O_2 gradient called A-a gradiant, which during hyperventilation will rise because of low PCO_2 and vice versa. This can be calculated as follows:

$PAP_2 = FIO_2 \times (PB{-}PH_2O){-}PaCO_2/R$

FIO_2= Fractional concentration of inspired O_2 (breathing at room air level).

PB = Barometric pressure (at sea level 760 immunity).

PH_2O = Water vapour pressure (saturated air at 37°Cg 47 immunity).

R = Respiratory quotient (ratio of CO_2 production to O_2 consumption and is usually 0.8).

In a healthy person, PAO_2-PaO_2 is normally less than 15 and may increase with age upto 30 in the elderly.

CO_2 elimination can be measured by partial pressure of CO_2 in arterial blood, i.e., $PaCO_2$which is independent of pH bicarbonate status of the blood. Diffusing capacity is assessed by diffusing capacity of the lungs for CO in (DLCO). This depends on alveolar capillary surface area, pulmonary capillary blood volume, ventilation perfusion (V/Q) mismatching and Hb of the patient. This is useful test to pin point disease afflicting alveolar-capillary bed, but abnormal DLCO doesn't necessarily mean that diffusion limitation is responsible for hypoxemia of patient. Three main diseases like interstitial lung disease, emphysema and pulmonary vascular disease in which DLCO is diminished.

Diffusing capacity is impaired due to congestive cardiac failure and alveolar haemorrhage as in Goodpasture's syndrome.

Arterial Blood Gases

Clinical utility realised especially during hypoxemia, when exposed, PO_2 contributes to it. It can occur at high altitude or during anaesthesia or during smoke inhalation. Such type of hypoxemia is seen in cyanotic congenital heart disease, pulmonary odema and pneumonia. Less commonly it is seen in hereditary hemorrhagic telangiectasis (Oster-Rendu-Weber Syndrome) and pulmonary vascular malformation in liver cirrhosis.

Ventilation perfusion as a cause of hypoxemia is seen in asthma, chronic obstructive lung disease, and pneumonia and interstitial lung diseases.

ABG Analysis[86] Is Done to Assess

- O_2 status.
- Ventilatory status.
- Acid-base status.

PaO_2 (Partial pressure of O_2 in arterial blood) usually in an adult is 90-100 mm of Hg. Given to breathe O_2, PaO_2 increases proportionately to inspired traction of O_2 (FiO_2).

Expected PaO_2 of normal person is estimated by using a formula. Expected $PaO_2 = FiO_2\% \times 5$. E.g. a person in 40% or will have expected $PaO_2 = 40 \times 5 = 200$ mm Hg.

In diseased lungs, PaO_2 will not rise at the same rate as in a normal person; leading to shunt traction because of ventilation perfusion mismatch with rise in shunt traction.

Rate of rise in PaO_2 with increase in FiO_2, completely stops further any rise in PaO_2 after shunt traction exceeds 40-50%.

PaO_2/FiO_2	*Status of O_2 nation*
500	Good
250-500	Acceptable
100-250	Poor
<100	Critical

Ventilation

Normal $PaCO_2$ is 35-45 mm Hg and is always related to alveolar ventilation of a patient.

Minute volume of healthy adult is 100 ml/kg/minute. 60% actually ventilates; 40% is dead space ventilation.

- ↓Alveolar ventilation would ↑ $PaCO_2$ (Arterial).
- With normal $PaCO_2$ (Arterial); if minute volume is increased.
- With normal $PaCO_2$ (Arterial); don't assume patient to be normal.
- Patient in distress can't sustain increased levels of ventilation for a prolonged period, may get exhausted and many require ventilatory support.

Acid-Base Status

	Respiratory acidosis	*Respiratory alkalosis*
Acute	10: 1	10:2
Chronic	10: 3	10: 4
Directly proportional	For every 10 mm Hg rise in $PaCO_2$ Bicarbonates HCO^-_3 rises by 1 or 3 mm Hg	For every 10 mm Hg fall in $PaCO_2$ HCO_3 concentration falls by 2 or 4 mm Hg

PH*: N 7.35-7.45; Acidosis <7.35; Alkalosis >7.45.

* Not true when patient is on mechanical ventilation.

$PaCO_2$

N–35-45 mm Hg. Abnormal PH with N-$PaCO_2$ = Metabolic disorder. Abnormal PH with abnormal $PaCO_2$ in opposite direction = respiratory disorder.

HCO^-_3 Level

N-22-26 mmol/L. N HCO^-_3 with abnormal PH = respiratory disorder, Abnormal PH and abnormal HCO^-_3 in the same direction = Metabolic disorder.

For accuracy: Quantitate the change in PH with a change in $PaCO_2$.

Respiratory Disorder

In Acute: PH changes by 0.008.
In Chronic: PH change by 0.003.
E.g. If $PaCO_2$ is 60 mm Hg, if it were acute respiratory acidosis (7.1), expected ↓ in PH would be 60 (Observed $PaCO_2$) –40 (Normal $PaCO_2$) = 20×0.008 = 0.16.

So, calculated PH would be (N) 7.4-0.16 = 7.24. Now, if measured (observed) PH is 7.1 which is lower than expected value (7.24), there is associated metabolic acidosis.

Prediction with HCO^-_3

In Metabolic Acidosis
Expected $PaCO_2 = 1.5 \times HCO^-_3 + 8 \pm 2$
In Metabolic Alkalosis
Expected $PaCO_2 = 0.7 \times HCO^-_3 + 21 \pm 2$
Anion Gap = $(N^+ + K^+) - (HCO^-_3 + Cl^-)$
Normal value = 3-11 mmol/L
In Metabolic Acidosis

- ↑ed in diabetic ketoacidosis.
- Normal in renal tubular acidosis, saline infusion.

GAP-GAP Ratio

$$\frac{\text{(AG) Anion gap excess}}{HCO^-_3 \text{ deficit}} = \frac{\text{(Measured AG-12)}}{24\text{-}HCO^-_3 \text{ (measured)}}$$

If ratio is <1, measures anion gap acidosis exists along with metabolic acidosis. If ratio is >1, metabolic alkalosis coexists.

Strong Ion Difference (SID)

Anion Gap (AG)

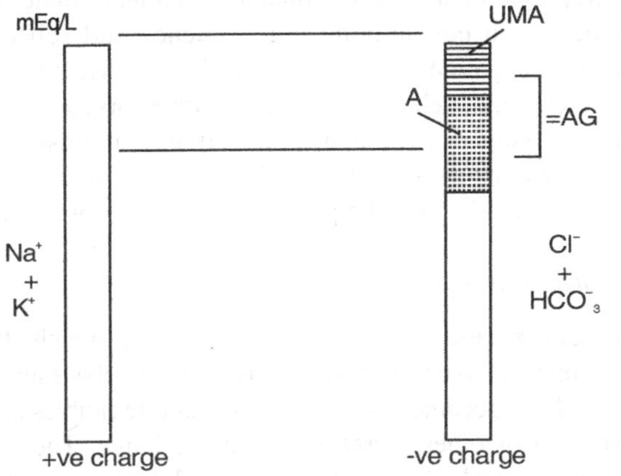

$(Na^+ + K^+) - (HCO_3^- + Cl^-) = AG$

Strong Ion Gap (SIG)

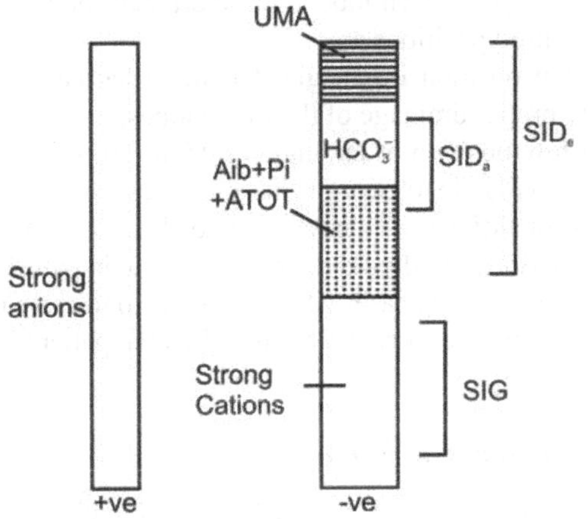

$SID_a = (Na^+ + K^+ + Mg^{++} + Ca)^{+++} - (Cl^- + Lactate^-)$

SID_a -

SID_e* = SIG

SID_e e.g. is normally – 40 mEq/L

- UMA – Unmeasured anions
- A^- – Weak acids
- Albumin and phosphates and strong anions (UMA) such as lactates.

Stewart's approach explains fluid induced acid-base phenomena and also provides a framework for designing fluids for specific acid-base effects.

The concept of intensive pulmonary care units was conceived as early as 1952, but the recognition came as a national team work under a pulmonologist only in USA.

The respiratory emergencies which are nearly cent per cent fatal need immediate transfer and management of these patients in an intensive pulmonary care unit. The staff under the leadership of pulmonologist, well equipped with haemodynamic and cardiopulmonary monitoring, blood gas analyser etc. should be available to take care of acute respiratory failure due to pulmonary disease like massive pneumonia with septicemia COAD, or acute respiratory failure due to single vital organ damage or multi-organ failure. All poisoning cases should be straight forward and the intensive pulmonary care unit should have close team work association with other medical specialists to monitor and manage associated disease (if any) like hypertension, diabetes mellitus, ischemic heart disease and anaemia with or without hypoproteinemia which is quite common in set up like ours.

No doubt the equipment and their maintenance increase the cost and hence their existence has been questioned[87,88] but the overall survival does improve with these services. 5% of beds in any hospital should be reserved for an organised unit[89,90] and pulmonary problems being a major cause of death in any critical set up, intensive pulmonary care services need to be given priority. A 15-20 bedded intensive pulmonary unit may provide satisfactory services to 1lac population and should be considered at least in the hospitals attached to medical colleges under the guidance of a pulmonologist, which, apart from community services, shall impart training to the undergraduates and working staff as well, since medicine department has many sub-specialities and pneumology is a coming up, and expanding field in our tropic. As more and more post doctoral pulmonologists are coming on Indian medical arena, the need for intensive pulmonary care unit becomes the prime need of the present medical care. It is the services in pulmonology which need to be updated with the available resources and not pressurised by sale campaign of westernised business which treats health care as a marketable commodity. The improvement in chest care management should never mean to add services of CAT scans, magnetic resonance imaging, linear accelerators etc. A pulmonologist will not only use an appropriate drug for the disease but also recognise the drug induced pulmonary disease, thereby removing the offending agent and instituting the necessary therapy.[91,92] The high-tech services for intensive care units should not only have impressive symbol value as opposed to use value,[93] rather it should mean to bridge a gap between a chest physician and a patient with chest disease, giving him the best pulmonary care during respiratory emergency.

Therapeutic fiberoptic bronchoscopy has given favourable results in critically ill patients of retained airways secretions, impacted mucus plugs with lobular or lobar collapse.[94] Tracheostomy has been of help[95] although increased incidence of infections has been suggested by others.[96,97] However, aseptic precautions, regular microbiological surveillance, selective decontamination of digestive tract, use of sucralfate instead of H_2 receptor inhibitors or antacids and effective implementation of FOB under the supervision of a pulmonologist could achieve infection control and healthy pneumology.[98-101]

A medical consultant will be able to serve an ailing chest in judicious way no doubt, but a trained chest specialist will provide a pulmonary care in a motherly way and we feel that such patient will be safer in such hands. We are not against these services. But we must be rational and selective.[102] If finances allow, diagnostic aids like ECG, X-ray, arterial blood gas analysis, isotope lung scanning, pulmonary arteriography with a further updated support from echocardiography, digital substraction pulmonary angiography, computed tomography, magnetic resonance imaging, radioisotope imaging, fibreoptic angioscopy can be added to such units. At the same time, leaving aside the overdiagnosis and underdiagnosis in pulmonary emergencies, pulmonary embolism is among the most misdiagnosed and mistreated conditions encountered in hospital practice. Many a times, the investigations may not be useful as the yield is generally non-specific. Even the gold standard investigations to reach a conclusive diagnosis may require a trained pulmonologist. There is a failure to make a clinician's knowledge operational in routine clinical settings especially because of a typical or subtle features of presentation of pulmonary emergencies, deficiencies in the physical examination, inherent limitations of conventional diagnostic measures and some time confusion introduced by co-existing disorders. There lies the need for a pulmonologist manned intensive pulmonary care unit to have a well timed diagnosis as well as treating approach, rendering a service to community as well as training the future chest physicians in emergency chest management. Critical care pulmonology definitely signifies its important role.[103] Opinions may vary and statistics too vary in different reports, but action has to be taken keeping in view the overwhelming problem, despite such a varying concern.[104] It is the delayed referrals to the hospital and admission of neurologically dead patients on ventilator in the intensive respiratory care which increases the cost of the treatment and apparently reduce the effectiveness.[104-108]

Pulmonary Physiotherapy

Pulmonary physiotherapy is an individualised treatment programme. The pulmonologist prescribes and guides and physiotherapists apply these guidelines in patients of chest ailments.

Aims of Physiotherapy

1. To assist in the removal of excess bronchial secretions.
2. To ensure adequate ventilation of all areas of the lungs and to help prevent atelectasis and/or consolidation.
3. To maintain mobility and blood circulation by free active exercise.
4. To ensure the maintenance of a good posture by accurate positioning and advice.
5. To help rehabilitate the patient to a full and independent life as possible by always considering the overall team approach to his management.

The physiotherapist working in a hospital has an important role to play both as an individual and as a team-mate. He is a key person in encouraging independence and self-care, in teaching the patient and his relatives how to use and care for equipment (e.g., nebulisers and air compressors) and to ensure that his living environment is as suitable as possible. The physiotherapist does not treat a diagnosis per se, but uses the techniques available to help solve the patient's problems.

Postural Drainage

Postural drainage is used to treat disorders in which stagnant secretions due to chronic bronchitis, bronchiectasis and cystic fibrosis have become infected. This technique enables drainage of sputum or other secretions from the lungs. The affected person lies on a bed and each lobe of the lung is drained in turn by the adaptation of different postures.

Depending on which lobe is to be drained the three most commonly used positions are:

1. Head low position at an angle of 45 to 60 degrees. This will ensure proper drainage of the lower lobes.
2. Head low position at an angle of 15 to 30 degrees. This posture will help to clear the middle lobes.
3. Supine or sitting position will help to clear the upper lobes.

Postural drainage should not be carried out in patients with cardiac problems or in cases who are unable to tolerate it. This technique should be carried out only when the patient is on an empty stomach.

Postural Drainage at Home

Postural drainage can also be carried out effectively at home. A forced expiration is also very useful. Those who are more disabled may need percussion or shaking from an assistant. Most patients can clear their secretions effectively with a correct huffing technique.

In most cases treatment will be required for at least 15 to 20 minutes twice daily. A useful method is to place a 15 cm pile of newspapers or magazines tied tightly together, in the centre of the bed with pillows on top. The patient can lie over this in various positions to drain several areas of the lung.

Percussion

Percussion should always be applied over a blanket or towel. The mechanical effect of percussion is to loosen secretions from the bronchial walls. In the presence of rib fractures or surgical incisions, percussion is avoided. Other contraindications include haemoptysis, acute pleuritic pain, osteoporosis or metastatic deposits in the ribs or spine and active pulmonary tuberculosis. Possible adverse effects of chest percussion include the onset of cardiac arrhythmias.

Shaking and Vibrations

Chest shaking is most commonly employed in the treatment of a ventilated patient. The physiotherapist should place his hands on the chest wall with the elbows slightly bent, but with his body well positioned over the patient. As the patient pauses at maximum inspiration the physiotherapist should vigorously shake the chest through the expiration. On inspiration the physiotherapist should relax and repeat the manoeuvre through each expiration.

Coarse, vigorous shakings may be used to dislodge very thick tenacious secretions unless the condition of the patient dictates otherwise. The patient's condition determines how vigorously the technique is to be applied. Factors such as pain, and frailty and size of the patient should be taken into account and the technique moderated accordingly. Contraindications include osteoporosis or metastases in the ribs and spine, haemoptysis and acute pleuritic pain.

Since vibrations have a finer action they are used when other techniques are contraindicated. Though not as effective as coarse shakings, in some patients with fractured ribs or a painful surgical incision they may be the only procedure tolerated.

Breathing Exercises

The term *breathing exercises* is often misleading as it implies that the patient is physically exerting himself. Many patients suffering from respiratory disease already expending far too much effort on respiration and need breathing guidance to have a more relaxed and economical pattern of breathing.

Diaphragmatic Breathing

In this method, effort is put on forward movement of the whole abdominal wall. The physiotherapist places both hands over the abdomen. The patient gently breathes in, allowing the abdominal wall to swell. On breathing out the abdomen slowly sinks back to rest. The upper chest and shoulders should remain relaxed throughout. The emphasis should be on gentle breathing with the minimum of effort. It is vital to remember that the expiratory phase is completely passive; any forced or prolonged expiration may increase airways obstruction. In normal expiration the airways shorten and become narrower, so if the airways are already partly obstructed and the patient forces expiration the flow of air will be further reduced.

Segmental Breathing

Localised breathing exercises are useful for assisting in the removal of secretions and improving movement of the thoracic cage. It is unlikely that individual lobes of the lung are ventilated by these exercises.

The physiotherapist should place the palm of his hand in the mild-axillary line over the 7th and 8th ribs. His fingers should be relaxed and well round the posterior aspect of the thorax. The patient is instructed to relax and breathe out, allowing the lower ribs to sink down and in this, movement must not be forced. At the end of expiration the physiotherapist should apply firm pressure against the chest and instruct the patient to expand the lower ribs during inspiration against his hand. This is referred to as rib-spinging. Pressure should be released at the end of inspiration and the weight of the hands follow the chest back to rest. Pressure is reapplied when the patient is ready to breathe in again.

When the aim of the treatment is to expand collapsed lung tissue, the emphasis should be on holding the maximum inspiration for three seconds and then *sniff* in a little more air. Where there is a region of lung which has partially obstructed airways or decreased compliance, the alveoli will fill at a slower rate than the unaffected areas. Lung areas with airways disease or scattered areas of atelectasis need more time to expand than unaffected areas, therefore, slow deep breathing with a hold on inspiration allows them more chance of gaining ventilation. Once the patient has learned the correct technique, he is taught to give pressure himself.

Humidification

In this process, the air inspired by the patient is humidified by minute particles of water (or normal saline). By increasing the amount of humidification in the inspired air, there is deposition of these airborne water particles onto the mucous membranes of the bronchial tree. This helps to decrease the viscosity of bronchial secretions thus aiding in postural drainage. The inspired air can be humidified by plain steam inhalation or by mechanical humidification. This is achieved by passing compressed air or ultrasound waves through a chamber containing water.

Cough/Snuff

The optimum method of clearing bronchial secretions from the lungs is a cough followed by expectoration. Coughing and snuffing are forced expiratory manoeuvres which, by producing a rapid flow of air combined with a narrowing of the airways, dislodge secretion and move them towards the pharynx. Snuffing is less strenuous than coughing.

Suction

Airway suction is frequently required in order to facilitate the removal of bronchial secretions. Suction is given in the following cases:

1. Whenever secretions can be heard in an intubated tracheostomy patient.

2. For retained secretions in the patient who is unable to cough and expectorate efficiently due to confusion, pain or fear.
3. It is also useful in unconscious patients where respiratory muscles are paralysed due to disease or drugs.
4. Before and during the release of the cuff on a tracheostomy tube.

The frequency of treatment will be determined by the assessment and it may be as little as once or twice a day or as frequently as at 2-hourly intervals. Occasionally a patient will require treatment at intervals throughout the night.

As a team member the physiotherapist has to liase with other disciplines and continual consideration of the overall management of the patient is vital. Each patient is a separate individual and even though *conditions* may be the same, the treatment programme must be planned differently for each person.

REFERENCES

1. Jindal S.K. and Wahi P.L., *Pulmonary function laboratory in the tropics; Needs, problems, solutions.* IN: Sharma O.P. (ED); Lung disease in the tropics; Marcel Dekker Inc. N-York; 1990.
2. Rao K.N., Epidemiology of chest diseases. *Indian J. Chest Dis.* 1971, 13: 17-24.
3. Jindal S.K., Bhaskar V.B. and Behera D., Respiratory disease pattern in a large referral hospital in India. *Lung India* 1989, 7: 119-121.
4. Jain S.K., Is teaching and respiratory medicine keeping pace with the clinical needs? *Ind.J Chest. Dis. Allied Sci* 1988, 30: 1-4.
5. Malik S.K., Developing pulmonary medicine (pulmonology) in India—A viewpoint. *Indian J. Chest Dis. Allied Sci* 1985, 27: 254-56.
6. Malik S.K., Setting up pulmonary laboratories in India. *Indian J. Chest Dis. Allied Sci* 1986, 28: 257-262.
7. Bhatia R.S., Role of accurate testing in clinical diagnosis; *J. Med. Surg.* 1987, 27: 14.
8. Gardner R.M., Clausen J.L., Epler G., Hankinson J.L., Permutt S. and Pulmmer A.L., Pulmonary function laboratory personnel qualifications. *Am. Rev. Respir Dis.* 1986a, 134: 623-624.
9. Abramson J.F. and Van Kessel A.L., *Laboratory management; qualifications of personnel. In Pulmonary Function Testing Guidelines and Controversies.* Edited by J.L. Clausen, New York, Academic Press 1982.
10. Jindal S.K. and Jindal U.N., *Computer use in medical field. In Hospital Administration and Management,* Vol. 1. Edited by S.L. Goel and R. Kumar, New Delhi, Deep and Deep Publ., 1988; pp. 213-229.
11. Crapo R.O., Gardner R.M., Berlin S.L. and Morris A.H., Automation of pulmonary function equipment user beware *Chest* 1986, 90: 1-2.
12. Bhatia R.S. Effective medical communication; JAPI 1992, 40: 483-84.
13. Woolcock A.M., Colman M.H. and Blackburn C.R.B., Factors affecting normal values for ventilatory lung function. *Am. Rev. Respir. Dis.* 1972, 106: 692-709.
14. Cotes J.E., *Lung Function.* Oxford, Blackwell Scientific Publishers 1979; 329-387.
15. Rossiter C.E. and Weil H., Ethnic difference in lung function: Evidence for proportional differences, *Int. J. Epidemiol* 1974, 3: 55-56.
16. Jain S.K. and Gupta C.K., Lung function studies in healthy men and women over forty. *Indian J. Med. Res.* 1967, 55: 612-691.
17. Jain S.K. and Ramiah T.J., Spirometric studies in healthy women 15-40 years age. *Indian J. Chest. Dis.* 1967, 9: 1-12.
18. Jain S.K. and Ramiah T.J., Normal standards of pulmonary function tests for healthy men 15-40 years old. Comparison of different regression equations (prediction formulae). *Indian J. Med. Res.* 1969, 57: 1453-66.
19. Johannsen Z.M. and Erasmus L.D., Clinical spirometry in normal Bantu. *Am Rev. Respir. Dis.* 1968, 97: 585-597.
20. Da Costa J.L., Pulmonary function studies in healthy Chinese adults in Singapore. *Am. Rev. Respir. Dis.* 1971, 104: 128-131.
21. Miller G.J., Ashcroft M.T., Swan A.V. and Beadnell, H.M.G.S., Ethnic variation in forced expiratory volume and forced vital capacity of African and Indian adults in Guyana. *Am. Rev. Respir. Dis.* 1970, 102: 979-981.
22. Sliman N.A., Dajani B.M. and Dajani H.M., Ventilatory function test values of healthy adult Jordanians. *Thorax* 1981, 36: 546-549.
23. Udwadia F.E., Sunavala J.D. and Shetye V.M., Lung function studies in healthy Indian subjects. *J. Assoc. Physicians India* 1987, 36: 491-496.
24. Kamat S.R., Tyagi N.K. and Rashid S.S.A., Lung Function in Indian adults subjects. *Lung India* 1982, 1:1-11.
25. Ayub M., Zaidi S.H. and Burki N.K., Spirometry and flow-volume curves in healthy normal Pakistanis. *Br. J. Dis. Chest.* 1987, 81: 35-44.
26. Lam K.K., Pang S.C, Llan W.G.L., Hill L.E., Snell N.J.C., Fayers P.M., Nunn A.J. and Prime F.J., Predictive nomograms for forced expiratory volume, forced vital capacity and peak expiratory flow rate in Chinese adults and children. *Br. J. Dis. Chest.* 1983,77: 391-396.
27. Malik S.K. and Jindal S.K., Pulmonary function tests in healthy children. *Indian Pediatr* 1983, 22: 677-681.
28. Malik S.K., Jindal S.K. and Jindal V.K., Vital capacity and forced expiratory volume, one second (FEV_1) in normal, healthy North Indian adults (I). *Bull. Postgrad. Inst. (Chandigarh);* 1987a, 21: 179-186.
29. Al Fayez S.K., Salieh M., Ardawf M. and Zahran F.M., Effect of sheesha and cigarette smoking on pulmonary function of Saudi males and females. *Trap. Geogr. Med.* 1988, 40: 115-123.
30. Shamassain M.H., Thompson J. and Ogston S.A., Forced expiratory indices in normal Libyan children 6-19 years. *Thorax* 1988, 43: 467-470.
31. AmericanThoracic Society. Standardization of spirometry—1987 update *Am. Rev. Respir. Dis.* 1987a, 136: 1285-1298.
32. Polgar G. and Promadhat V., *Pulmonary Function Testing in Children: Techniques and Standards.* Philadelphia, W.B. Saunders 1971.
33. Taussiq L.M., Chernick V., Wood R., Farrel P. and Mellins R.B., Standardization of lung function testing in Children J. Pediatr 1980,97: 668-678.

34. Lemen J.R., *Pulmonary function testing in the office and clinic. In Disorders of the Respiratory Tract in Children.* Edited by E.L. Kendig and L.C. Chernick. Philadelphia, W.B. Saunders, 1977.
35. Polgar G. and Weng T.R., The functional development of the respiratory system. *Am Rev. Respir. Dis.* 1979, 120: 625-695.
36. Binder R.E., Mitchell C.A., Schoenberg J.B. and Bouhuys A., Lung function among black and white children. *Am Rev. Respir. Dis.* 1976, 114: 955-959.
37. Milner A.B., Respiratory testing in children, *J. Appl. Med.* 1982, 8: 895-901.
38. Bhatia R.S., Public and profession; signs of suspicion and undercare; causes and cure in present paediatric practice; *Curr Med. Pract.* 1991, 35: 9-11.
39. Polgar G., Promadhat V., *Pulmonary function testing in childhood.* Saunders, London, 1971.
40. Godfrey S., *Exercise in Children.* Saunders, London, 1974.
41. Williams D.E., Miller R.D. and Taylor W.F., Pulmonary function studies in healthy Pakistani adults. *Thorax* 1978,33: 243-249.
42. Boyce AJ., Haight J.S., Rimmer D.B. and Harrison G.A., Respiratory function in Peruvian Quechua Indians. *Ann. Hum. Biol* 1974, 1:137-148.
43. Cotes J.E. and Ward M.P., Ventilatory capacity in normal Bhutanese. *J. Physiol* 1966, 186: 88.
44. Godman H.I., Becklake M.R., Respiratory function tests. Normal values at Median altitudes and the prediction of normal results. *Am. Rev. Tuberc.* 1959, 79: 457-467.
45. Ferris B.G., Jr., Anderson D.O. and Zickmantel R., Prediction values for screening tests of pulmonary function. *Am. Rev. Respir. Dis.* 1965, 91: 252-261.
46. Knudson R.J., Slatrin R.E., Lebowitz M.D. and Burrows B., The maximal expiratory flow-volume curve: Normal standards, variability and effects of age. *Am. Rev. Respir. Dis.* 1976, 113: 587-600.
47. Hruby J. and Butler J., Variability of routine pulmonary function tests. *Thorax* 1975, 30: 548-553.
48. Prime F.J., Respiratory function tests for a clinician. *Br. Thorac. Tuberc. Assoc. Rev.* 1973, 3: 1-12.
49. Gregg I. and Nunn A.J., Peak expiratory flow in normal subjects. *Br. Med. J.* 1973, 3: 282-284.
50. Wright B., McKerrow C.G., Maximum forced expiratory flow rate as a measure of ventilatory capacity. *Br. Med. J.* 1959, 2: 1041-1047.
51. Zamel N., Youssef H.H. and Prime F.J., Airway resistance and peak expiratory flow rates in smokers and non-smokers. *Lancet* 1963, 1: 1237-1238.
52. Jindal S.K., Bansal S.K. and Malik S.K., Peak expiratory flow rate in healthy North Indian adults. *Bull. Postgrad. Inst. Chandigarh* 1974, 8: 92-96.
53. Malik S.K. and Jindal S.K., Normal values of PEFR in healthy North Indian adults—Revision of prediction formulae. *Indian J. Chest. Dis. Allied Sci.* 1985, 27: 50-51.
54. American Thoracic Society, Statement, Single breath carbon monoxide diffusing capacity (transfer factor). *Am. Rev. Respir. Dis.* 1987, 136: 1299-1307.
55. Guleria J.S., Pande J.N., Sethi P.K. and Roy S.B., Pulmonary diffusing capacity and high altitudes. *J. Appl. Physiol* 1971, 31: 536-543.
56. Pandel J.N., Gupta S.P. and Guleria J.S.,Clinical significance of the measurement of membrane diffusing capacity and pulmonary capillary blood volume. *Respiration* 1975, 32: 317-324.
57. Butler J., The pulmonary function test–cautious over-interpretation. *Chest* 1981,79: 498-500.
58. Becklake M.R., Concepts of normality applied to the measurement of lung function. *Am. J. Med* 1986, 80: 1158-1164.
59. Malik S.K. and Jindal S.K., Clinical pulmonary function laboratory, fifteen years of assessment. *Lung India* 1988, 6: 59-60.
60. Woolf C.R., Organization of a hospital routine pulmonary function laboratory. *Can. Med. Assoc. J.* 1968, 98: 542-549.
61. Hughes D.T.D. and Empey D.W.,Ten years experience in running a pulmonary function laboratory. *Br. Med. J.* 1972, 4: 470-473.
62. Altose M.D., *Practical aspects of pulmonary function testing:* In: Baum G.L. (ED) Textbook of pulmonary diseases 4th Edition, Boston, Little Brown and Co. 1989; 101.
63. Graven D.E., Lichtenberg D.A., Goularte T.A., *et al.* Contaminated medication in nebulizer's mechanical ventilator circuits: Source of bacterial aerosols. *Am Jour. Med.* 1984, 77: 834-38.
64. Sanders C.V., Luby J.P., Johanson W.G., Serratia marcescens infections from inhalation therapy medications; nosocomial outbreaks. *Ann Intern. Med.* 1970, 73: 15-21.
65. Barnes K.L., Bacterial contamination of home nebulizers: *Br. Med. J.* 1987, 295: 812.
66. Renfrow D.P., Thomann C.A., Rutala W.A., *Infection risks associated with spirometry.* 12th Annual Educational Conference, Association for Practitioners in Infection Control 1985, 12: 161.
67. Houston K, Parry P. and Smith A.D., Have you looked into your spirometer recently: *Breath* 1981,12: 10-12.
68. Isles A., Maclusky I., Corey M., *et al.* Pseudomonas capacia infection in cystic fibrosis; An emerging problem. *J. Pediat* 1984, 104:206-210.
69. Singh Y, Arya A. and Mathur D.S. Bacteriology of spirometer tubing evaluation of methodology to prevent transmission of infection. *JAPI* 1993, 41: 193-94.
70. Johnson W.G., Pierce A.K. and Sanford J.P., Nosocomial respiratory infections with gram negative bacilli. *Ann. Int. Med.* 1972, 77:7101-7106.
71. Pepys J., Clinical and therapeutic significance of patterns of allergic reaction of lungs to extrinsic agents. *Am. Rev. Respir. Dis.* 1977, 116: 573.
72. Gold P.M., Sachweisinger D.W., *Pulmonary Laboratory Infection Control and Safety* in Clausen J.L. (ed). Pulmonary Function Testing, Guidelines and Controversies, New York, Grune and Stratton 1984; 15-18.
73. Oza Y.K., Infections via respiratory equipment; A potential hazard; *JAPI* 1993, 41: 189.
74. Director Gen. of Health Services. Central Bureau of Health Intelligence; *Cause of Death Statistics: Health Information India,* New Delhi, Govt. of India Press 1988; 199.

75. Jindal S.K, Malik S.K, Deodhar S.D. and Sharma B.K., Fibrosing alveolitis: A report of 61 cases seen over the past five years. *Indian J. Chest. Dis. Allied. Sci.* 1979, 21: 174-179.
76. Sharma S.K., Pande J.N. and Guleria J.S., Diffuse interstitial pulmonary fibrosis. *Indian J. Chest. Dis. Allied.* Sci. 1984, 26: 214-219.
77. Bambery P., Behera D., Gupta A.K, Kaur D., Jindal S.K., Deodhar S.D. and Malik S.K., Sarcoidosis in North India: Clinical profile of 40 patients, *Sarcoidosis* 1987, 4: 155-158.
78. Gold W.M. and Boushey H.A., *Pulmonary function testing;* IN Respiratory Medicine; Murry J.F. and Nadel J.A. (ED) Philadelphia, Saunders 1988; 611-82.
79. Weinberger S.E., *Principles of pulmonary medicine,* Philadelphia, Saunders 1986.
80. West J.B., *Pulmonary pathophysiology*—The essentials, 3rd Ed; Batlimore; Williams and Wilkins, 1987.
81. West J.B., *Respiratory physiology—The essentials,* 3rd Ed; Batlimore, Williams and Wilkins 1985.
82. Melillo G. *et. al.*, Guidelines for the standardization of bronchial provocation tests with allergens; Allergy 1991:46:321.
83. Cock Croft D., Berschied B., Standardisation of inhalation provocation tests; Chest 1982;82:572.
84. Jones N.L., Clinical exercise testing; 3rd Ed; Saunders, Philadelphia, 1988.
85. Ries A.L., The role of exercise testing in pulmonary diagnosis; Clin Chest Med. 1987;8:81.
86. Shenoy A., Rapid interpretation of arterial blood gases; J Anaesth Clin Pharmacol 2010; 26(S): 49-53.
87. Bayer R., Callahen D., Fletcher J., *et al.* The care of the terminally ill—Mortality and economics; *N. Eng. J. Med.* 1903, 308: 1490-94.
88. Detsky A.S., Stricker S.C., Mulley A.G. and Thibault G.K., Prognosis, survival and the expenditure of hospital resources for patients in an intensive care unit. *N. Eng. J. Med.* 1981, 305: 667-72.
89. Safar P. and Grenvik A, Critical care medicine; organising and staffing intensive care units; *Chest* 1971,58: 535-37.
90. Petty T.L., Lakshminarayan S., Shah S., *et al.* Intensive Respiratory Care Unit; Review of 10 years experience; *JAMA* 1975,23: 34-37.
91. Copper J.A.D. Jr., White D.A., Mathary G.A., State of the art: Drug induced pulmonary disease: *Amer. Rev. Resp. Dis.* 1986,133: 321-40,498-505.
92. Vijayan V.K., Drug induced respiratory disease; IN: Chandrasekharan S. Ed; Medicine Update: *Assn. Phy. India;* Bombay 1993, 3: 177-186.
93. Attinger E.O., *High technology;* The pendulum must swing back, World Health Forum 1987; 8.
94. Prakash U.V. and Olopade C; Bronchoscopy in critical care unit. Mayo Clin Proc 1989, 64: 1255-63.
95. Abhyankar N.Y., Bhambure N.M., Kasekar S.G., *et al.* Intensive respiratory care service—8 years experience *Ind. J. Chest. Dis. All. Sci.* 1992, 34: 65-72.
96. Marsh H.M., Gillespie D.J. and Baumgartner A.E. Timing of tracheostomy in critically ill patients; *Chest.* 1989, 96: 190-193.
97. Heffner J.E., Medical indications for tracheostomy; *Chest* 1989, 96: 186-90.
98. Ledingham L.M., Alcock S.R., Eastaway A.T., *et al.* Triple regimen of selective decontamination of digestive tract, systemic cefotaxime and microbiological surveillance for prevention of aquired infection in intensive care; *Lancet* 1988, i: 785-90.
99. Tryba M. and May B. Acute treatment of severc haemorrhagic gastritis with high dose sucralfate; *Lancet* 1988, i: 1304.
100. Garvey B.M., Mc Cambley J.A. and Tuxen D.V., Effects of Gastric alkalization on bacterial cotomization in critically ill patients; *Critical Care Medicine* 1989, 17: 211-16.
101. EDITORIAL; Stress ulcer prophylaxis in critically ill patients. *Lancet* 1989, ii: 1255-56.
102. Bhatia R.S. and Batta S., Routine investigations. Let us be selective and rational; *JAPI* 1992, 40: 493.
103. Bhatia R.S. and Sibia S.S., Intensive pulmonary care units: An urgent need: A viewpoint; *Lung India* 1995; 13(2): 75-76.
104. Chang R.W.S., Jacobs S., Lee B; *et al.* Predicting deaths among intensive care unit patients; *Crit. Care. Med.* 1988, 16: 34-42.
105. Fulop M., Adel H.N., Webster A., *et al.* Cost effectiveness of critical care; *Crit. Care. Med.* 1989, 17: 1223-27.
106. King Edward's Hospital Fund: Intensive care services; *Anaesthesia* 1989, 44: 428-31.
107. Purdie J.A.M., Ridley S.A. and Walkce P.E.M., Effective use of regional intensive therapy units; *Brit. Med. J.* 1990, 300: 79-81.
108. Cohen I.L., Lambrinos J. and Fein I.A., Mechanical Ventilation for the elderly patient in intensive care, *JAMA* 1993, 269: 1025-29.

PRACTICAL PROCEDURES IN PULMONARY MEDICINE (THERAPEUTIC AND DIAGNOSTIC)

Lung Biopsy[1]

Biopsy of the lung is considered when serological and other investigations fail to determine the aetiology of pulmonary disease. It may also be carried out to *stage* known disease prior to therapy. All techniques have a morbidity rate and a mortality rate and should be employed only after the patient has been seen by a chest physician. The method used is dictated by the clinical state of the patient, the likely aetiology, and the local expertise. When infection is the probable diagnosis, trials of different antimicrobial therapies may be justified. The patient's clinical state must not be allowed to deteriorate too far before lung biopsy is considered. In immunocompromised patients, many carry out lung biopsy early in view of the wide range of causes of pulmonary disease in these subjects.

Endoscopic Techniques

The low morbidity rate associated with techniques employing a fiberoptic bronchoscope makes it the instrument of choice for biopsy of localized and diffuse pulmonary disease. The bronchial tree can be explored and endobronchial pathology biopsied. If the resting arterial PaO_2 can be raised to 13.3 kPa by giving supplementary oxygen via a single nasopharyngeal catheter, the procedure should be carried out under local anaesthetic; if not, a light intravenous anaesthetic is used and the patient is ventilated with 100 per cent oxygen using a commercial adaptor to allow passage of the bronchoscope without interrupting ventilation. Abnormalities of coagulation must be corrected, by infusion of fresh frozen plasma and/or platelets and so on, before undertaking the procedure. A bronchial biopsy is taken to confirm abnormal haemostasis and in some conditions, for example sarcoidosis and malignancy, this may enable to make a diagnosis that involves the bronchial mucosa as well as the peripheral lung tissue. The required samples are then taken in the following order.

1. Selective Cultures

A sterile double-sheathed brush is passed through the bronchoscope channel and into the bronchial tree. The distal plug is expelled and the sheath is passed into the area for biopsy, under fluoroscopic control, until the end lies 2 cm from the pleura. The central sheath is advanced and the brush is passed into the pulmonary tissue. The steps are then reversed and after withdrawal, the outside sheath is wiped with 70 per cent alcohol and the end is cut off. The central sheath is passed out followed by the brush which is smeared onto a variety of bacteriological plates, and the end is cut off into an anaerobic culture medium.

2. Brush Biopsy

A sterile single-sheathed cytology brush passed as above to within 1 cm of the pleura. The brush is passed in and out of the sheath and when inside the sheath again it is withdrawn. The outside of the sheath is wiped with 70 per cent alcohol and the brush pushed out and smeared into five glass slides, four of which are immediately fixed. These are subsequently examined using Gram's stain, Ziehl-Nielsen stain, haematoxylin and eosin stain, and a silver technique for detecting fungi and pneumocystis carinii. The unfixed slide is stained to pick up lymphoma and leukaemic infiltration.

3. Alveolar Lavage (Small Volume Lung Wash)

The end of the bronchoscope is impacted in a subsegmental bronchus leading to the area to be sampled. Aliquots of sterile saline (50 ml each, containing no preservative and buffered to pH7) are inserted through the central channel of the bronchoscope and recovered with suction trap to which mechanical suction is applied. Upto 300 ml may be used to obtain sufficient material for study. In case of non-infective chronic pulmonary disease the fluid is collected into a siliconized glass bottle in an ice-bath to prevent macrophage adherence. A differential cell count may support the clinical diagnosis and help predict the response to steroids. In other patients analysis of the deposit may allow diagnosis of infection and malignancy.

4. Transbronchial Lung Biopsy

This technique provides small (2 mm) sample of alveolar tissue. Standard biopsy forceps are passed down in the closed position until they lie 1 cm from the pleura. With great experience this position can be judged by *feel.* However, since biopsies taken too distally may cause pneumothorax and those taken too proximally may cause significant haemorrhage, the procedure should be conducted under fluoroscopic control.

During inspiration the forceps are opened and advanced such that they remain 1 cm from the pleura. During expiration they are closed tightly grasping peripheral bronchiolar tissue. The forceps are then withdrawn and the tissue removed by shaking them in the open position in an appropriate fixative (10 per cent formalin for routine histology and glutaraldehyde for electron microscopy). For immunofluorescent microscopy the biopsy material is removed with a fine needle, placed on the wall of a plastic container, and sent in ice for immediate freezing. Four to six biopsies are taken provided that there is no significant bleeding. In view of the risk of pneumothorax, biopsies should be taken from only one lung at a time.

Complications

1. Pneumothorax occurs not that frequently, but it is more common in ventilated patients in whom it may be delayed for several hours.
2. The risk of significant haemorrhage is about 0.3 per cent. It can be controlled by routinely *wedging* the end of the bronchoscope in the segmental bronchus prior to biopsy. If this fails, a no. 4 Fogarty catheter can be passed through the central channel of the bronchoscope and inflated to tamponade the bronchus.

Bronchogenic carcinoma can spread along the mucosal surface, in the submucosal lymphatics, or in peribronchial tissue.[2-6] Mucosal tumour usually presents as an exophytic mass within a bronchus and the diagnostic yield of bronchoscopic forceps biopsy although very high[7-10] is widely variable (71 to 97 per cent). Five biopsy specimens are enough to provide a diagnosis. Insufficient sampling could result in lower diagnostic yields, but needless repetition of endoscopies should be avoided[11] to minimise the complications of the procedure.

A careful biopsy technique to get maximum diagnostic yield includes good visualisation of the tumour mass, accurate placement of the forceps and cleaning the tumour of overlying blood clots.[7]

Two biopsy specimens of an endoscopically visible

bronchigenic carcinoma can provide almost 100 per cent diagnostic yield[12] and the role of bronchoscopist's judgement in placing the biopsy forceps accurately is most important.[13]

Nonendoscopic Techniques (Transthoracic Needle Methods)

1. Fine-needle Aspiration

This provides a small volume of fluid and is likely to give diagnosis by cytology or microbiology. The needle must not cross a fissure as this increases the risk of pneumothorax. A suitable approach is decided from plain radiograph and screening of the chest. The chest wall is infiltrated down to the pleura with local anaesthetic and a thin-walled needle (20 cm × 18 gauge), with a bevelled stylet is passed at the upper margin of a rib into the area for biopsy. If possible the patient should hold his breath in expiration during the procedure. The stylet is removed and while rotating the needle in the lesion a 10 ml syringe is used to aspirate.

Thoracic percutaneous needle aspiration and core biopsy are minimally invasive procedures to sample lesions of lung parenchyma as well as lesions of chest wall, pleura and mediastinum, using image guidance such as CT or ultrasound, using local anaesthesia. A chest X-ray must be obtained to check for pneumothorax as it is common complication in almost 20-25% of cases, in addition to haemoptysis (in 5-15%), pleuritic chest pain without pneumothorax (2-5%) and vasovagal reaction (1%) of cases.

Basic competence is awared after 10 procedures in a supervised setting, requiring 10 procedures to be performed every year to maintain competency.[14]

2. Cutting-Needle Biopsy

The needles used for this are adaptations of a device described by Silverman (1938)[15] and they provide sufficient material for histology. The incidence of haemorrhage, pneumothorax, air embolism, and even death are such that this technique is now rarely used.

3. Trephine (Drill) Biopsy

This provides a core of tissue and is suitable for diffuse lung disease. A hollow needle with a distal cutting edge is driven by a pneumatic drill and the noise generated must be demonstrated to the patient before the procedure is undertaken. In diffuse pulmonary disease a biopsy is taken posteriorly from the right lower lobe. Local anaesthetic is injected down to the pleura in an area chosen by placing markers on the chest wall prior to radiology. A 2 cm incision is made just above a rib and, with the central stylet in place, the trephine is pushed through the parietal pleura. During expiration the stylet is removed and the drill connected. With the trephine rotating at maximum speed it is pushed slowly into the lung for a distance of 3-4 cm. The drill is detached, a 20 ml syringe attached, and while maintaining maximum suction the trephine is withdrawn. The specimen is ejected by flushing the trephine with sterile sodium citrate solution and is divided into sections for the chosen method of examination.

Pneumothorax is more common with trephine biopsy than with transbronchial lung biopsy. The procedure should therefore be reserved for conditions such as cryptogenic fibrosing alveolitis that can neither be diagnosed nor accurately staged from a small sample.

Open-Lung Biopsy

Samples of lung tissue are removed through an 8-10 cm incision under general anaesthesia. The temptation to biopsy the lingula should be resisted because it is often the seat of non-specific inflammatory change. Samples from the obviously abnormal and the minimally involved areas are taken. Each specimen should be divided into sections and processed as follows:

1. Fix one in 10 per cent formalin for routine histology.
2. Freeze one for rapid histology and immunofluorescent studies.
3. Send a small (5 ml) sample in a dry container in ice for electron microscopy.
4. Send an unfixed sample in a sterile container for microbiological examination.
5. If pneumocystis carinii infection is likely, press the cut surface of the lung onto a glass slide and stain this *imprint.*

All lung biopsy techniques have an associated morbidity rate, and should only be employed when the information sought is likely to influence clinical management. Even open-lung biopsy may not reveal diagnosis in all the cases and findings may be non-specific in upto 25 per cent of non-immuno-suppressed patients and in as many as 45 per cent of immuno-suppressed patients.

Pleural Biopsy

Closed pleural biopsy using Abram's punch should form part of the routine investigation of pleural effusion.[16] The common causes of pleural effusion (malignancy and tuberculosis) are infrequently diagnosed from examination of pleural fluid alone.

Pleural biopsy is done by a needle, in which a small piece of pleura is taken for microbiological and histopathological evaluation.[17] It is indicated in all patients with exudative pleural effusion of unknown etiology. Pleural biopsy has its value in establishing the diagnosis of tuberculous pleural effusion.The demonstration of granuloma (even non-caseating) strongly suggests tuberculous etiology in more than 95% of the patients with exudative pleural effusion, while in less than 5% of the patients the aetiology may be rheumatoid arthritis, sarcoidosis or fungal disease. Pleural biopsy has little value (vs. cytologic examination) in the diagnosis of malignant pleural effusion as in approximately 30% of such patients only visceral pleura is involved while parietal pleura is spared.[4]

Indications

1. Exudative pleural effusions of unknown etiology, e.g., tuberculous, malignant etc.
2. Pleural thickening of unknown origin.

Contraindications

1. Local skin disease.
2. Un-cooperative patient.
3. Patients with empyema, because of risk of development of subcutaneous abscess.
4. Patients with respiratory failure as it may get precipitated if complicated by pneumothorax.
5. Patients with bleeding disorders.
6. Patients on anticoagulant therapy.

Material and Procedure

Materials needed for pleural biopsy are:
- Lignocaine 2%.
- Sterile gloves, guaze, cotton and drape.
- Betadine, spirit etc.
- Adhesive tape.
- Disposable syringes and needles: 5 ml, 20 ml.
- Three-way stop-cock.
- Sterile container (vac).
- Autoclaved pleural biopsy needle.
- Sterile surgical blade.
- Plain vials and formalin.

Technique[1]

Premedication with papaveretum 10-15 mg intramuscularly may not always be necessary but is helpful in the majority of patients. The anterior rib which lies at the upper border of the effusion is noted from the posteroanterior radiograph. This rib is found on the patients and a line extended horizontally around the chest with the patient stitting upright. A site is chosen on the interspace below this line and above the level of the other hemidiaphragm, midway between the spine and the posterior axillary line. The percussion note over this site should be confirmed as being dull. After disinfecting the skin, the chest wall is infiltrated down to the pleura with local anaesthetic containing adrenaline (the latter reduces bleeding and allows prolonged anaesthesia). The needle used for local anaesthesia is passed through the pleura to check that the fluid can be aspirated and therefore separates the lung from the chest wall. (If no fluid can be withdrawn, another site is chosen since dry pleural biopsy may require patience.) Then 50 ml of fluid should be withdrawn into a sterile syringe through a 19 gauge needle before making an incision, to avoid traumatic bloodstaining. The fluid is examined conventionally.

A small pointed scalpel is pushed through the anaesthesized area at the upper border of a rib and parallel to it. Abram's punch is connected to a 20 ml glass syringe and pushed through the pleura in the closed position. During this insertion the needle should be *guarded* by holding it 4-5 cms from the tip to prevent entry of its whole length. A knob on the proximal end of the needle indicates the position of the side hole. The needle is opened and the position of the side hole within the pleural space is confirmed by aspirating a little fluid through it. The punch is rotated so that the hole points towards the diaphragm and, while firm pressure is exerted downwards on the needle with the left hand, it is slowly withdrawn.

A common mistake is to wait until the needle *catches* before closing it by clockwise rotation of the syringe. This invariably results in biopsy of intercostal muscle. The punch should be withdrawn gradually and a biopsy attempted every few millimetres; the needle then being pushed a short way into the chest to see if tissue has been caught. If not, the needle is pulled out a little further, until tissue is obtained. Five to seven biopsies are taken, directing the hole inferiorly and laterally but never superiorly (thus avoiding the intercostal nerves and vessels). At the end of the procedure upto one litre of fluid can be withdrawn to make the patient more comfortable if this is needed.

Abram's Needle Parts

1. A large outer trocar.
2. An inner cutting cannula.
3. An inner solid stylet.

The outer trocar is blunt, so a stab incision is required for its insertion into the skin. The inner cutting cannula fits tightly in the outer trocar and it can be locked in two positions—a closed position in which the inner cannula obstructs the notch on the outer trocar to make it airtight; and an open position in which the notch on the outer trocar is open, so that biopsy can be taken.

An indicator knob in the hexagonal grip of outer trocar indicates the position of the notch, when it is in the pleural space.

For insertion of Abram's needle—the stylet is placed inside cannula which is placed inside the trocar (in closed position) and the needle is inserted by to and fro motion till it reaches the pleural space. Once the pleural space is reached, the stylet is removed and a 20 ml syringe is attached to the cannula and then cannula is placed in open position (by rotating it anticlockwise to open the notch on the outer trocar) and fluid is aspirated to ensure that notch is inside the pleural space. The pleural biopsy needle is slowly withdrawn until it hooks the parietal pleura. Then, the cannula is rotated in a clockwise manner to cut the parietal pleura.

Once the biopsy sample is obtained, the needle should be withdrawn from the pleural space in closed position. The needle and biopsy specimen should be removed from the needle and preserved in a plain vial with formalin. It is important to note that the moment the needle is removed from the chest, the biopsy hole should be immediately occluded with a finger to prevent suction pneumothorax.

The procedure should be repeated and at least three biopsy specimens from different quadrants (viz. 3,6,9 O'clock positions) should be obtained. One specimen should be sent for culture for mycobacterium, or other micro-organisms and the rest should be processed for histopathology.

At the end, the biopsy tract should be sealed by placing a sterile guaze with adhesive tape to make it airtight.

Cope's Needle Parts

1. A large outer cannula with a sharp end.
2. Inner biopsy trocar—hollow blunt tipped and hooked.
3. Inner needle—hollow/bevelled.
4. Stylet.

Initially the stylet with inner needle is inserted in the large outer cannula and then inserted into the pleural space after local anaesthesia. Inner stylet is removed with bevelled needle from outer cannula while patient is holding breath at the end of normal expiration and immediately the hooked biopsy trocar (to which 20 ml syringe is attached) is inserted into the outer cannula. A small projection on the proximal end of biopsy trocar indicates the position of the biopsy hook. Withdraw the hooked trocar with outer cannula till parietal pleura gets hinged into the hook, then push the outer cannula over the inner hooked trocar by rotating clockwise till it cuts the hinged parietal pleura. Remove the Cope's biopsy needle from the chest wall and preserve the biopsy specimen and repeat the same procedure as above to get at least 3 specimens of parietal pleura. After the biopsy procedure a chest radiograph should always be taken to rule out any pneumothorax.

Percutaneous pleural biopsy does not differ much from a standard thoracentesis. Initial vital signs are obtained but continuous monitoring is not required. Site of biopsy can be selected with the use of CT or ultrasound. Diagnostic yield is increased with multiple passes. Pleural brushing can also be obtained through the pleural needle. Uncontrolled coagulopathy is a contraindication. Absence of free-flowing pleural fluid increases the risk of pneumothorax. Complications in less than 1% of cases have been reported in the form of pneumo/haemothorax, diaphragm-lacerations, lacerations of lung, liver and spleen and even tumour seeding along the needle-tract. Five procedures in a supervised setting establish basic competence which is required to be maintained by performing five procedures per year.[18]

Complications

1. Pneumothorax: More frequent with Cope's needle than with Abram's needle.
2. Bleeding: Haemothorax may result.

When two operators have failed to obtain diagnostic tissue on one occasion each and it is considered justifiable to pursue the diagnosis, the next procedure is usually an open pleural biopsy through a small incision under general anaesthesia. In some centres pleuroscopy under local or general anaesthesia is employed using either a rigid instrument or a flexible fibreoptic bronchoscope.

Inserting a Chest Drain[19]

The insertion of an intercostal catheter (chest drain) should be a simple, painless, sterile and safe procedure which may in certain situations be life-saving.

The overriding indication for the insertion of all chest drains is to enable a collapsed or partially collapsed lung to be re-expanded, thereby improving pulmonary function. The underlying reasons for the deflated lung may be manifold but include trapped intrathoracic air (pneumothorax). This condition can be unilateral, bilateral, recurrent, or tension in type, and can be spontaneous or follow either injury or rupture of a lung, a compound fracture of the chest, or rupture of a viscus of the mediastinum or abdomen. Fluid may also embarrass the re-expansion of a lung. This may consist of blood (haemothorax), pus (pyothorax or empyema) from a lung infection, chyle (chylothorax), or oesophageal contents resulting from rupture of mediastinal viscus.

Equipment

Most chest drains are inserted electively with the patient in bed or sitting by his bed. The basic kit for insertion of a chest drain should comprise:

1. A gown, a mask and gloves for the operator.
2. Adequate sterile linen or disposable towels.
3. A razor.
4. A bacterial cleansing solution (Iodine, Betadine, Hibitane, or Catevlon).
5. A 10 ml syringe and needles.

6. One per cent plain lignocaine 10 ml.
7. A scalpel and blade.
8. An atraumatic needle with nylon, linen, or silk and a needle holder.
9. A pair of forceps and at least one arterial clip.
10. A pair of scissors.
11. A drain clamp, a chest catheter (see Table 1.43 for sizes) and a trocar and cannula.
12. Approximately 1 m of red connecting tubing and associated connections.
13. An underwater seal bottle, filled with sterile water to a known volume which should be marked.
14. A well briefed nurse or assistant.

The Tudor-Edwards empyema trocar and cannula is preferred by thoracic surgeons because it is sharp and flanged and allows easy access of an intercostal catheter. There are two adult sizes: 8 mm (medium) accepting a 22F catheter and 9.5 mm (large) accepting a 26F catheter.

Table 1.43: Recommended drain sizes

Neonates	10-16 F
Infants	12-20 F
Children	20 F
Adults	26 F

The Argyle-type thoracic catheters are packaged with an introducer which is less sharp than the Tudor-Edwards' trocar and is more difficult to insert between the ribs. It may also plunge deep into the chest as soon as the pleural space is entered and is documented as having frequently entered lung tissue, the spleen, the liver, all structures of the mediastinum, and in particular the heart. The catheters which are available in packaging separate from the introducer are made from plastic, silicone, or silastic materials and all contain radio-opaque markers and side holes as well as an end hole. They constitute good catheters to insert through the preferred Tudor-Edwards empyema trocar and cannula.

A Malecot catheter made of soft rubber is more gentle and comfortable for the patient and can be located close to the chest wall. It will similarly pass through a trocar and cannula, or can be inserted under direct vision.

Red rubber tubing supplied in numerous diameters makes an excellent chest drain and is more suitable for use in the operating theatre than at the bedside. It is more difficult to manipulate into a suitable position within the thorax than plastic or silicone catheters and easily kinks unless the introductory hole is made adequate.

Site of Insertion

The site of insertion of the chest drain depends on the nature of the material to be removed. Except in the emergency situation of a tension pneumothorax, the site of drainage should be checked with reference to the clinical localizing signs and X-ray appearances. Air (the principal nitrogen component of which is poorly reabsorbed) rises to the top of the chest while fluids accumulate at the base. Either air or fluid may loculate, becoming trapped between lobes or between the lung and the mediastinum. If both air and fluid are to be removed from the chest, it is more prudent to insert two appropriately sited drains than a compromise single drain that is not ideal for either the apical air or a basal fluid collection.

1. Posterior to the pectoralis major muscle in the anterior axillary line through the fifth interspace—This commonly chosen site is appropriate in that there is no major muscle through which drain must be inserted except for the intercostals. A drain at this site is easy to insert and angles well towards the apex of the thoracic cavity. Its disadvantages are that the skin site is potentially infected with large quantities of skin flora and is difficult to clean before insertion. The axillary contents, the artery, the vein, and the branchial plexus are at risk, particularly when attempting to insert Argyle-type catheters since in trying to angulate the drain to the apex the thoracic cavity may be missed and the drain inserted extrathoracically into the axilla. A drain inserted through these intercostal spaces can cause subcostal neuropraxia if left in the chest for an inappropriately long time due to pressure on the intercostal bundle of the interspace. Should the patient require thoracotomy, for example, a pleurectomy, the drain willl lie in the line of the incision and the drain site will undoubtedly be discharging pus thereby rendering a *clean* operation *dirty*.
2. Anteriorly in the midclavicular line through the second intercostal space—This is one of the easier sites for access but has the disadvantage of traversing the pectoral muscle. Since this muscle is effectively transfixed, it limits the amount of possible movement of the arm because of the pain and makes it difficult for the patient to cooperate with the physiotherapist. Neuropraxia of the subcostal nerve similarly occurs if the drain is left in position for an inappropriate length of time. It is, however, difficult to ensure that a drain introduced with a trocar angulates to the apex of the pleural cavity and does not take a downward course within the chest.
3. Posteriorly through the first intercostal space—This position is preferred by thoracic surgeons for pneumothoraces. The surface marking is midway along a line linking the vertebral prominence and the medial border of the spine of the scapula. This is the least intrathoracic course for the drain which lies at the most appropriate place for pockets of air that accumulate at the apex. There is no

possibility of neuropraxia of a subcostal nerve in the first interspace as there is no subcostal groove. This permits the drain to be left in-situ indefinitely if necessary. Also the nursing care of a posterior drain is most easily managed and the patient has full mobility of both arms and pectoral muscles thus allowing better cooperation with his physiotherapist. Furthermore, there is a psychological advantages in view of the vicious nature of the equipment in having the patient facing away from the operator. The patient sits on a chair at his bedside and leans on the bed, or may sit on his bed with his arms resting on pillows on a bed-table.

Drains should be held in the chest by the retaining suture. A small dressing is applied around the drain site and an erect chest X-ray taken to verify the correct positioning of the tube and degree of expansion of the lung. The underwater seal bottle must be kept on the floor at all times and the drainage tube connections made firm. If the lung fails to expand, it may be aided by application of a vacuum pump (sucker) to the short limb of the underwater seal bottle. The low volume sucker may impede the release of air from the chest which then tracks into the tissues producing surgical emphysema. This complication also arises from the use of too small a drain or from a side hole of the drain being in the subcutaneous tissue. The nursing staff should be instructed to check the pressure on the sucker and that there are no leaks within the tubing system. They should also record every 4 hours whether the drain is bubbling, singing, or static and the volume and nature of fluid drained. Patients with intercostal drains should be X-rayed daily to verify the drain position, the degree of expansion of the lung, and the extent of the pneumothorax or effusion. Chest drains are removed once the lung has re-expanded and the pleural drainage ceases (all chest drains produce an obligatory serious drainage of about 50 ml a day from irritation of the pleura and lung). It is customary before removing a drain to clamp it overnight and review the absence of pneumothorax on the morning X-ray. Should this have recurred, it is easier to release the clamp than to reinsert the tube.

Possible causes of persistent bubbling from a chest drain or inability to expand the lung are:

1. Leak in tube.
2. Side hole out of the chest.
3. Too small a sucker.
4. Too large a leak.
5. Bronchopleural fistula.
6. Drain in a bullous cyst.

Should the lung leak fail to stop always think of:

1. Tuberculosis.
2. Malignancy.
3. Steroids.

Pericardial Aspiration[20]

Pericardial aspiration may be a diagnostic or a therapeutic procedure.[20] When performed as a diagnostic manoeuvre its purpose is to obtain pericardial fluid for analysis, microscopy, and culture as safely and atraumatically as possible. In most centres it is more reliable and profitable to obtain pericardial fluid for diagnostic purposes while performing open pericardial biopsy through a limited thoracotomy, a procedure that carries a relatively low risk in experienced hands and a much greater chance of yielding a diagnosis.

When pericardial aspiration is to be performed to relieve life-threatening cardiac tamponade it should be done expeditiously (although not usually *within minutes*. However, it is ever unusual for the patient's deterioration to be so rapid and profound that a more complete and controlled aspiration is impossible).

Where the aetiology of the effusion is known before pericardial tapping (elective procedure) a decision should be made as to whether any therapeutic agent is to be introduced into the pericardial space. For example, the cytotoxic agent thiotepa is used in some cases of neoplastic effusion. Two routes can be recommended: the xiphisternal and via the apical region. It is useful to be familiar with both.

Anatomy of the Xiphisternal Region

When viewed in the sagittal section, the xiphisternum articulates with the body of the sternum slightly posteriorly and is often difficult to palpate accurately. The costal margin is easily palpable and the position of the xiphisternum can be predicted. Deep palpation in this area may be curiously uncomfortable particularly when there is hepatomegaly, and with a reasonable comprehension of the anatomy of the region there should be no need to discover everything anew through the skin. In the routine that the aspirating needle takes when inserted xiphisternally, the anterior pericardium is reflected at a more or less acute angle and becomes the diaphragmatic pericardium. In this angle lies the *acute margin* of the heart which is the free border of the rather triangular right ventricle. Along it runs the acute marginal artery. Both this artery and the relatively thin-walled right ventricle are at risk.

Anatomy of the Apical Region

When approached from the apex, the left pleural space and lingula are closely related and care must be taken that a concomitant pleural effusion is not tapped. At the apex of the heart the coronary vessels are smaller than elsewhere and in less danger, although they are by no means invulnerable. If the exploring needle penetrates the heart in this region it is likely to enter the thick-walled left ventricle, which can be entered with relative impunity compared with the thinner-walled right ventricle or worse still the atrium. For these reasons the apical route is strongly recommended by some physicians.

A 5-inch or 6-inch needle covered by a plastic cannula is best used for the aspiration, although a standard intracardiac needle can be employed. A suitable needle is the BD Longdwell Teflon needle (no. 6734,16 gauge × 6 inches) which is designed for direct left ventricular puncture but well suited to pericardial aspiration.[21] Alternatively a 5-1/4 inch Angiocath can be used.

Whenever possible the needle should be attached to an ECG for continuous monitoring. If an Angiocath is to be used the distal centimetre of the cannula needs to be cut off so that the plastic hub of the cannula can be slid along the needle to expose the proximal centimetre of the metal barrel for the attachment of the ECG. A sterilized lead with a crocodile clip at each end is then clipped onto the needle. The other end is clipped onto the precordial lead of an ECG machine, with the limb leads attached to the patient in the usual way.

If the machine is set for recording V leads then complexes approximately equivalent to lead V_2 are obtained as the needle enters the skin. If the needle touches the surface of the ventricle the complex changes abruptly with marked ST-segment elevation or ventricular ectopic beats. If the atrium is touched the P-wave morphology alters, often with atrial ectopic beats. If such changes occur, the needle should be withdrawn a little.

Although ECG monitoring increases the safety of the procedure, it must be recognized that it is not foolproof and it should only be used with equipment that is electrically fully isolated.

Technique for Performing Pericardial Aspiration

Whenever possible, before embarking on pericardial aspiration, echo cardiography should be performed to confirm the diagnosis and estimate the depth of the pericardium at the aspiration site. If cardiac or thoracic surgeons are not carrying out the aspiration, they should be informed about the procedure in case their services are later required to manage unexpected complications. In addition blood is sent to the labroatory for grouping. The procedure is performed with the patient in bed or on a couch, preferably in the ICU. The patient should be recumbent with the thorax inclined (head up) at an angle of 45°. A defibrillator must be ready for use at the bedside.

An aseptic technique is used. The patient's skin is prepared using an antiseptic skin preparation and towels are positioned. A solution of one percent plain lignocaine (without adrenaline) is injected into the skin with the smallest available needle (usually 25 gauge). When the skin is infiltrated the needle is changed to the larger 21 gauge and the subcutaneous tissues in the anticipated route of the pericardiocentesis needle are infiltrated. The pericardium is extremely sensitive, when the needle touches the pericardium the operator realizes it because the patient gives a start. This should also be infiltrated. As with all injections of local anaesthetic agents, the syringe should always be aspirated slightly before injecting. If the pericardium is encountered in this way the inexperienced operator is reassured that he is in the correct area.

A 1 cm skin incision is made and a three-way tap and 20 ml syringe are attached to the needle. If the xiphisternal approach is used the needle is inserted into the angle between the xiphisternum and the left costal margin at about 45° to the anatomical transverse plain, and directed a little towards the patient's left. If the diagnosis of pericardial effusion is correct there should be reasonable depth of fluid before the heart is encountered and if the needle is advanced slowly and aspirated continuously the procedure should be quite safe. When the needle is clearly withdrawing pericardial fluid the plastic cannula should be advanced over it and the needle withdrawn.

If the apical route is to be used the needle is inserted 1 cm outside the apex beat and in the intercostal space below it, but always within the area of cardiac dullness. The needle should then be directed towards the right shoulder tip. If the apex is impalpable the needle should be inserted just inside the area of cardiac dullness.

Specimens should routinely be sent for culture and a heparinized sample sent for cytology. If the fluid is blood stained it is probably wise not to insert air for the purpose of post aspiration contrast radiography. If recurrence of the pericardial tamponade occurs then clearly a more definitive surgical procedure should be considered.

Modified Seldinger Technique

If X-ray screening facilities are available in the ICU, a modified Seldinger technique may be used. A guide wire is first introduced into the pericardial space via the large needle inserted as described above. When the guide wire is in-situ a plastic annual or catheter can be threaded along it. This technique is valuable for long-term drainage of purulent or carcinomatous effusion and for the instillation over periods of several days of antibiotics or antimitotic agents. However, screening facilities are desirable.

To sum up, pericardial aspiration is a life-saving technique which can be relatively, although not absolutely, safely performed by any well trained doctor. It should certainly be in the therapeutic armamentarium of all hospital-based junior physicians and surgeons, particularly those involved in accident and emergency departments.

Galen[22] gave the first postmortom description of pericardial effusion in a monkey and later successfully trephined the sternum of a young man to relieve his pericardial effusion. Larrey (1829),[23] Napoleon's surgeon, inserted a catheter into a pericardial wound and removed 7 beakers of wine-coloured fluid which resulted in the remarkable recovery of his patient. Pericardiocentesis has been used in medical practice since

1940.[24] Using a trochar, Franz Schuh[25] in 1940, did the first *blind* pericardiocentesis in a 24-year-old woman. Billroth (1875)[26] later commented on this technique that *Paracentesis of the pericardium is an operation which in my opinion, approaches very closely (what) some surgeons would term as prostitution of the surgical art and others madness... Perhaps a later generation will think otherwise.* With this prophesy, pericardiocentesis by needle aspiration became a widely accepted technique for the relief of pericardial effusion and tamponade.[27]

The human pericardium normally contains upto 50 ml of clear fluid. When measured with a fluid-filled or transducer-tipped catheter, pericardial pressure is nearly equal to intra-pleural pressure and varies from -5 to +5 cms of water during the respiratory cycle.[28] The transmural distending pressure of either ventricle is the difference between intracardiac and intrapericardial pressures.[29] Hence, any increase of pericardial pressure will result in a decrease of ventricular filling. Three phases of haemodynamic alterations with pericardial effusion and increasing pericardial pressure, have been recognized.[30]

Phase I: Pericardial effusion is small and is detected only by echocardiography. Significant physical signs are absent. Pericardial as well as right and left ventricular diastolic pressures are higher than normal, but they do not equilibrate. Cardiac output may be less than normal. Inspiratory fall in arterial systolic pressure may be exaggerated but is not diagnostic of pulsus paradoxus.

Phase II: Pericardial pressure is elevated and equilibrates with right ventricular diastolic pressure, both being higher than normal, but less than left ventricular diastolic pressure. Cardiac filling is impaired reducing the cardiac output. In many (both not in all) the inspiratory fall in arterial systolic blood pressure is more than 10 mm Hg, diagnostic of pulses paradoxus.

Phase III: Pericardial pressure is markedly elevated and has equilibrated with both right and left ventricular diastolic pressures. Cardiac output is markedly reduced with prominent pulsus paradoxus in all patients.

Intravenous infusion of fluids to increase the filling pressure can temporarily alleviate the manifestations of cardiac tamponade. Conversely, reduction of filling pressure by diuresis, blood loss or inadvertant administration of preload reducing agents could result in precipitous fall in stroke volume and cardiac output. Thus, hypovolaemia and low ventricular filling pressures could easily cause *low pressure tamponade* in patients with pericardial effusion.[30]

Removal of pericardial fluid using subxiphoid[31,32] approach should reverse the haemodynamic changes triggered by the effusion, if the pericardium is normal. However, in some patients with chronic pericardial effusion, even after complete aspiration of fluid and restoration of fluid and restoration of pericardial pressure to normal, the right atrial/jugular venous pressure may remain high.[29] This indicates visceral pericardial constriction, diagnostic of effusive restrictive pericarditis. Under such circumstances, pericardiectomy alone can restore the altered haemodynamics.[28,31]

Haemodynamic measurements during pericardiocentesis are quite useful.[33] Simultaneous measurement of intrapericardial and right heart pressures have helped to identify (25%) patients with effusive constrictive pericarditis early in the natural history of the disease. Fluid can be removed when a catheter is percutanously introduced into the pericardial cavity.[33] The technique is safe and simple. Moreover, the same catherer could be used to measure the pericardial pressure which could be compared with right atrial pressures. The catheter could easily drain thick pericardial exudates and could be left in the pericardial cavity for 24 hours or more. The technique could be undertaken in any intensive cardiac care room which has a fluroscopy machine and facility for pressure monitoring. Haemodynamic studies in pericardial disease is incomplete without measurement of both right and left ventricular diastolic pressures. Equalisation of right and left ventricular diastolic pressures is an important criterion for the diagnosis of both tamponade as well as constriction. Measurement of pulmonary capillary wedge pressure by a balloon catheter in the intensive care room, or retrograde or transeptal left ventricular catheterisation in a catheterization laboratory is essential, if one is attempting to delineate the full haemodynamic spectrum of pericardial disease. Such elaborate measurement protocols are not warranted in the routine management of patients with pericardial disease.

The highly sensitive technique of echocardiography could easily diagnose even the smallest of pericardial effusions. For periodic assessment of severity of effusion, echocardigraphy is the safest, simplest and most reliable of all techniques available. However, in spite of the beautiful and vivid description of many M-mode, 2-dimensional and Doppler echocardiographic signs of pericardial effusion and tamponade, cardiac tamponade continues to be a clinical diagnosis. The triad of physical signs viz. decreasing arterial pressure, increasing jugular venous pressure and quiet precordium identifies patients with clinical cardiac tamponade. Levine *et al.* (1991)[34] tested the hypothesis that right atrial and/or ventricular diastolic collapse in M-mode and two-dimensional echocardiography may indicate early pericardial tamponade. Of the 54 patients in whom they detected echocardiographic signs of tamponade, 94% had systolic blood pressure more than 100 mm of Hg and 58% had cardiac index more than 2.32L/Min/m^2.[23] Pericardiocentesis resulted in haemodynamic improvement but dyspnoea and tachycardia were seldom alleviated. They felt that even though invasive catheter pericardiocentesis could be undertaken with few complications, the natural history and optimal management strategy of patients with pericardial effusion and minimal signs of pericardial fluid on echocardiography should not tempt us to proceed with pericardiocentesis in all patients.

The Barcelona experience has taught us that *diagnostic pericardiocentesis* is of limited value due to high incidence of false positive and false negative findings except in suspected purulent pericarditis.[35] The technique of pericardiocentesis and haemodynamic measurements may appear to be simple, but there are potential risks particularly in the hands of inexperienced operators.

Complications of pericardial tapping include ventricular arrhythmias, ventricular puncture, perforation and even death.[36,37] Even pleural contamination, coronary arteries laceration, subepicardial haematoma, trauma to stomach, pneumothorax and venti-fibrillation have been described.[38] Ventricular laceration can be decreased by using a figtail catheter in children.[39] Moderate and severe cardiac tamponade must be treated by drainage of pericardial fluid, but pericardial effusions even with mild tamponade may under many circumstances be safely managed expectantly.[40] Clinical and echocardiographic evaluation may suffice to identify this subgroup of patients.

An Emergency Tracheostomy[41]

Of the many dramatic life-saving operations, emergency tracheostomy must be one of the most effective-potentially hazardous, yet dramatically rewarding. A patient presenting with a rapid respiratory obstruction arising in the upper air and food passages as a result of tumour, burns, injury, or other lesion, which prevents oral tracheal intubation in the manner of an anaesthetic procedure, provides the indications for the type of emergency tracheostomy described below. The tracheostomies carried out for a respiratory obstruction that allows time for the patient to be taken to the operating theatre, anaesthetized, and possibly intubated—but atleast able to lie still in proper surgical surroundings—form an intermediate group.

The Indications

When the patient is suffused and struggling, purple-faced with a neck lesion all too evident, and sometimes comatose, for example lying in a road traffic accident with stridor. Similarly, sufferers with a rapid increase in size of a tumour of the pharynx or the larynx (sometimes while under radiotherapy) present an alarming but obvious surgical target.

Whether still, struggling, or suffering from fits the patient is best managed, preferable with the aid of an assistant, while lying supine with a cushion or coat under the shoulders and with the neck hyperextended. In these circumstances impaired consciousness is often a blessing. Indeed fully conscious patients resist any such manipulation and may lapse into coma due to asphyxia.

With the head and neck held straight and the chin well up a horizontal incision is made across the neck, having located the thyroid and cricoid cartilages, if possible, by palpation. Vertical incisions, starting at the readily identifiable thyroid cartilage and leading downwards, served well for those suffering from Ludwig's angina in the past but are not so appropriate in the road traffic accident era. A transverse incision gives access to a trachea that is well deviated from the midline and is also useful in those with such smashed larynxes where landmarks are lost. Tissues are then spread horizontally in the midline to reveal the strap muscles and vertically in the midline between them when the forefinger is plunged into the wound to seek a palpable trachea.

Haematoma or major injury may cause the trachea to be far displaced from the midline. It is advisable to insert both forefingers into the wound and spread them laterally in an attempt to find the trachea. Engorged veins, normally trivial, constitute major bleeding hazards as of course does the isthmus of the thyroid gland. Haemostasis is permissible at this stage, by means of the crude application of artery forceps to the more obvious ones (avoiding the laterally placed vessels in the carotid sheath). Once located, the stabilization of the trachea is invaluable and a hook under the cricoid ring, drawing the trachea upwards and forwards, is of great help.

Under these circumstances a vertical midline slit, preferably through the second, third, and fourth rings of the trachea, gives access to the airway. A tiny nick in the trachea of pinpoint dimension is worthwhile in the first instance, air and blood frothing from it reassure the operator that it is correctly located. A pair of forceps spread into the incised trachea may well be accompanied by a rewarding air exchange there and then. If this does not occur artificial respiration should ensure that it does.

Intubation of the trachea with a tracheostomy tube is a rapid necessity and is best done with a metal tube with an introducer and tapes knotted around the neck if these are available. Worse are a plastic tube with an introducer, a plastic tube without an introducer, and an anaesthetic endotracheal tube introduced by being compressed between the jaws of a pair of artery forceps.

Suction if available is of massive benefit. Applied orally by the operator via a length of tubing it is satisfactory in the short term and in any event is one of the first aids to be sought since blood and secretions may block the lower airway even when the tracheostomy has been well established. Artificial respiration should be begun as soon as the tracheostomy is established if no respiratory movements are made by the patient. Once respiratory excursions do start it is worthwhile maintaining the patient in the lateral position with the head down. The emergency is over when the patient, with a clear dry airway, is restored to consciousness and becomes biddable, the tracheostomy is secure, and humidified oxygen can be presented to the tracheostome in a proper post operative environment.

Removing a Foreign Body from the Trachea and Bronchial Tree[42]

The father of all bronchoscopists, was undoubtedly Chevalier Jackson.[43] A foreign body in the aerodigestive tract is an important cause of morbidity and mortality in the two extremes of life. Chocking is the leading cause of accidental death in infants, under 12 months of age.[44]

Foreign bodies in tracheobronchial tree have always been of interest to the endoscopists and radiologists, as well as to the otolaryngologists. All types of bizarre foreign bodies[45-49] have been described in air passages such as seeds, clips, pins, safety-pins, buttons, mutton pieces, bones, coins, dentures, nose rings and still the list is incomplete.[50] Most of the reports on foreign bodies are concerned with either the type of foreign bodies or the technique of anaesthesia and/or endoscopic removal of foreign bodies.[45,46,48,50-54]

Entry of the foreign body in the air passage is more common in the right main bronchus in comparison to left and in most of the reported series, foreign bodies have not been reported in peripheral bronchi. This is because of the anatomical shape and configuration of the tracheobronchial tree, since the right main bronchus is wider and more in line with trachea than left main bronchus which is narrower and forms a sharp angle with the trachea.[55] Isolated reports of unusual foreign body in air passage also belong to foreign bodies of main bronchus or lower bronchi.[46,48,50,56]

Commonly the patients with foreign bodies present with history of cough, gagging or spasmodic chocking, audible wheeze and increasing dyspnoea. Often the characteristic wheeze can be appreciated by listening to the breath sounds with the unaided ear held against the chest or in front of the open lips and on skiagram there is evidence of obstructive emphysema or collapse of lung.[55] Foreign body also deserves consideration in differential diagnosis of an upper zone opacity.

Aetiological Factors

A few foreign bodies are due to occupational hazards (for example in professional tailors, and carpet layers). Other causes are epileptic fits (causing broken dentures) and dental extraction. Some objects are inhaled when they are used in games, for instance peashooting or throwing nuts up and catching them in the open mouth. However, the majority of inhaled bodies occur in children (80 per cent; Table 1.44).

A lot of the blame must lie with parents who are careless allowing children to play or move about while eating, giving small children or infants food that they cannot chew and which therefore tends to remain in their mouths or to be swallowed whole, permitting small children to have chewing gum, allowing children to play with small objects, and leaving small objects lying about (pins, nails, screws, tacks, drawing pins etc.) which they can easily inhale.

Falling, tripping, receiving a sudden push in the back, fighting, running, jumping, laughing, crying and vomiting (especially when triggered by small food particles, saliva, or water) are followed by deep inspiration. The foreign body is sucked in through the widely opened glottis, during these situations.

Any object, edible or inedible, that finds its way into the mouth might be inhaled. Some foreign bodies are universally found (for instance screws, nails, pins, peanuts, teeth, bones and dentures) while others are more common in certain countries. In India peanuts, beetle nuts, beads and tamarind seeds are frequent, whereas in the Middle East salted watermelon, melon and marrow seeds (sold in comer shops), peanuts, pistachio nuts, beans, chick peas, and beads are usual. Even within the same country there are regional and seasonal variations.

80 per cent of the patients are children. The foreign body is found mostly in the right side (73.5 per cent) and rarely in the upper lobes (in our series only one was found in the right upper lobe). The foreign body removed most frequently is a peanut (38 per cent) and plastic objects as offenders (20 per cent) are on the increase as more and more plastic products are coming around in life.

Foreign bodies come in all shapes and sizes. In general, the smaller and smoother they are, the more easily they are tolerated.

1. Of the minerals, metallic objects produce the least reaction (iron and steel even less than the other metals) glass produces very little reaction.
2. Animal substances set up more extensive reactions than minerals, but less than vegetable substances.
3. Plastic substances produce a severe reaction.

Table 1.44: Characteristics of laser[70-72]

Laser	*Wavelength (Manometer)*	*Colour*	*Transmission*	*Photo-coagulation*	*Smallest spot size (at 200 mm)*	*Eye protection*
1. Carbon dioxide laser	10,600	Invisible	Rigid	No	0.2 mm	Clear glass
2. Argon laser	458-475	Visible blue green	Fiberoptic	Yes	0.15 mm	Amber lens
3. Nd: YAG laser	1,060	Invisible infra-red	Fiberoptic	Yes	0.03 mm	Light green glass
4. KTP-532 laser	532	Visible light	Fiberoptic	Yes	0.00002 mm	–

4. Vegetable substances cause the most severe reactions of all. Peanuts are particularly irritant. Beans by absorbing moisture, swell and cause complete obstruction of the bronchus.

Mobile foreign bodies can cause increasing damage, especially if they are sharp and irregular. The damage begins at initial impact on inhalation. The subglottic areolar tissue in children under 2 years swells very quickly, rapidly producing severe laryngeal and subglottic oedema. The bronchus becomes inflamed and bleeding occurs easily to the touch. Later on, granulation tissue develops and might completely cover the foreign body. In atelectatic lungs, infection easily develops (pneumonitis, lung abscess, or empyema). In long-standing cases, bronchiectasis might become irreversible and necessitate lung resection.

It may be mentioned that heavy-handed bronchoscopy can cause more damage than the foreign body itself.

The parents or relatives must be interviewed to find the cause of choking. In the vast majority of cases they provide a clear history of choking, while some are doubtful. Therefore, always believe the parents even if sometimes they might confuse the issue by saying that the child has *swallowed something,* and secondly, if in doubt, act—even if the bronchoscopy proves negative.

Symptoms and Signs

Occasionally the patient is symptomless. If the foreign body is large and lying in the trachea or at the bifurcation or is bilateral, the patient is often extremely distressed, has stridor and rib recession, and might die of suffocation within a few minutes.

A cough is the most frequent symptom. It is more troublesome and irritating when the foreign body is free and moving in the trachea (a tracheal tap may be felt and heard on coughing).

A wheeze, when present, is due to partial obstruction of the bronchus. It may confuse the diagnosis and the patient may mistakenly be treated for asthma. The wheeze is usually unilateral.

Dyspnoea is present when there is atelectasis or obstructive emphysema. In old or neglected cases, infection may supervene and the patient presents with lung abscess, consolidation, bronchiectasis or empyema.

Posteroanterior and lateral radiographs of the chest are essential in suspected cases. The diagnosis is simple enough when the foreign body is radio-opaque, although even then it might be partially hidden by the shadowing due to infection or atelectasis of the lung. When the foreign body is non-opaque, there are usually changes which suggest its presence, atelectasis of a lobe, or lung if there is complete obstruction of the bronchus, or hyperinflation (obstructive emphysema; with the foreign body acting as a ball valve. At times the latter can simulate atelectasis of the opposite lung (hence the importance of inspection of all orifices at bronchoscopy).

However, the X-ray is sometimes completely normal (may be 15 per cent of cases) and may give rise to the erroneous conclusion that there is no foreign body. Bronchoscopy must be performed if there is a history suggesting inhalation.

Treatment

Bronchoscopic removal should be carried out in a theatre capable of undertaking a thoracotomy, and should only be performed by a skilful operator, aided by an experienced anaesthetist. Some patients should be X-rayed just before transfer to theatre, in case the foreign body has moved.

Preparation

Checking and careful selection of equipment are essential. The flexible bronchoscope is of no use for a removal procedure.There are six Negus bronchoscopes to chose from for adult, adult-small, adolescent, child, infant and suckling. The choice is difficult when the patient is a child under 2 years. The bronchoscope must be small enough to pass the vocal cords and reach the lower lobe bronchi. If it is too big, not only can it traumatize the vocal cords and subglottic area but also cannot be passed far enough down the bronchial tree.

Secondly, select suitable suckers and grasping forceps.This is very important especially in the case of an infant and suckling bronchoscope. The surgeon must do it himself. Check that at least two suckers can go through the chosen bronchoscope and are patent. From a variety of grasping forceps, select those that can be passed through the appropriate bronchoscope and check that they are in working order and that the jaws are in good condition.

Thirdly, check the lights (batteries and bulbs). A fibro light source is better and more reliable but a spare bulb should always be available.

Fourthly, allow a period of adaptation in the darkened room and practise looking through the chosen bronchoscope to become familiar with the small visual field.

Finally, pass the open forceps through the bronchoscope a few times. As the jaws come out of the tip of the bronchoscope, they spring in to a wide open position. There is a special feel to it. They are then ready to grasp the foreign body.

Anaesthesia

General anaesthesia by an experienced anaesthetist are essential. Anaesthesia has been made less hazardous for the patient and easier for the anaesthetist since the introduction of Sander's injectors.[57] These use the Venturi principle for ventilating the patient via the bronchoscope without obstructing surgeon's view. Because ventilation is achieved by using a pressurized supply of oxygen at 60 psi and entraining air, some other means are required to keep the patient unconscious and relaxed. These involve the injection of intermittent doses of induction agents and muscle relaxants intravenously, and this in turn means establishing an intravenous route. This is used throughout in adults but in children, a *gas induction* may be necessary with the intravenous cannula being inserted when the patient is unconscious. Anaesthesia is then maintained by intermittent doses of intravenous agents as in adults.

The advantage of this technique is that relaxation and adequate ventilation of patient can be maintained throughout what may be a lengthy procedure, giving the operator (especially the less experienced) more time for the removal of the foreign body.

Bronchoscopic Procedure

The patient is positioned on the operating table (or special trolley) in such a way that the head and neck are resting on the small upper flap. Initially the neck is slightly flexed and the head slightly extended. The head must be straight. The left middle finger is placed on the upper jaw and pulls it back. The thumb and index finger retract the lips and direct the tip of the bronchoscope. The search for the foreign body starts at this point since it might have been coughed up and by lying in the larynx or pharynx. The lubricated bronchoscope is passed behind the tongue, in the midline, and the tip gradually moved toward until the epiglottis is visualized. The tip of the bronchoscope is passed behind it and the epiglottis is lifted forwards. (The bronchoscope should not be pushed down at this stage, the inexperienced do this very often and the result is to enter the oesophagus). Immediately the arytenoids and vocal cords come into view. As the patient is paralysed, the cords are in the open position. The bronchoscope is rotated 90° and passed between the cords. The head of the table is extended gradually and is required for the rest of the procedure.

The trachea is recognized as a widely open tube with cartilaginous rings. A systematic search is carried out. If the foreign body is in the trachea, it is usually quite easy to grasp, but can also as easily slip down into one of the bronchi. Every part of the trachea and bronchial orifices must be recognized and inspected. Particular care should, of course, be given to the probable site of the foreign body since it may be completely obscured by secretions or granulation tissue.

Principles for Removal of the Foreign Body

The end of the bronchoscope is brought as near to the foreign body as possible. Its axis must be in alignment with bronchus and the foreign body in full view in the middle of the bronchoscopic field. This ideal position for grasping is maintained by fixing the bronchoscope to the upper jaw with the fingers of the left hand. If the foreign body is hard (for example bone, metal or denture) then strong forceps are required otherwise it may slip. If the foreign body is soft (for example a peanut) then special delicate forceps should be chosen otherwise it might be crushed.

The chosen forward-grasping forceps are passed with the jaws open through the shaft of the bronchoscope. When they come out of its lower end, they spring open even more and pass on either side of the foreign body. This seems to be the best way of preventing a downward drift of the object. The forceps are closed and the foreign body is pulled back to the tip of the bronchoscope, using the right index finger to prevent bending of the forceps. The fingers of the left hand fix the forceps shaft rigidly to the bronchoscope. They are then brought out in one piece in such a way that the biggest diameter of the foreign body passes through the anteroposterior (wider) opening of the glottis. If the foreign body has sharp points (for example a pin, safety pin, or drawing pin) or irregular sharp edges (like a denture, piece of metal, or piece of bone) then it must be manipulated and rotated in such a way that the point of sharp edge is drawn into the safety of the bronchoscope or trails behind. If the point of the pin is engaged in the bronchial wall, then it must be disengaged by pushing the pin further down and then grasping the point and pulling it into the bronchoscope. There are special side-grasping forceps for closing safety pins and soft staples. If the foreign body slips off the jaws, it is usually because it was caught in the glottis, it was not pulled firmly enough against the tip of the bronchoscope, or the wrong forceps were used.

The following rules help:

1. Always rebronchoscope the patient even if the foreign body has been successfully removed, for three reasons: to find out if there is another one present (especially in the case of peanuts), to suck out sputum or pus that has accumulated behind the foreign body, and to see if there has been any damage to the mucosa.
2. If resistance is encountered on traction, stop immediately to prevent damage to the bronchus and find out the cause: the forceps' jaws might have grasped a carina between segmental bronchi or the foreign body might have caught on the bronchial mucosa.
3. If the foreign body cannot be removed safely, abandon the procedure and resort to thoracotomy. It is better to admit failure, than to have a successful removal of the foreign body, and produce severe or even fatal damage.

Complications

1. *Laryngeal Oedema:* Always be on the look out for this, especially in children and if the procedure was a lengthy one. It should be treated using an oxygen tent with humidification, antibiotics and hydrocortisone. Also, an endotracheal tube might be required for 24-48 hours. Tracheostomy should be carried out if the above measures fail.
2. *Surgical Emphysema and Pneumothorax:* These may occur as a result of bronchial damage. They necessitate intercostal intubation or urgent operation and might be fatal.

3. *Bleeding:* Bleeding caused by the tearing of a vessel or rough handling, might also be fatal.

Thoracotomy and Removal of the Foreign Body[42]

The foreign body is felt and located. If possible it is brought up in a larger bronchus which is exposed, opened, and carefully resutured after its removal.

Late Operations

Abscess or repeated bronchiectasis may require late thoracotomy or lobotomy.

Lasers in Respiratory Medicine—Clinical Application

The use of laser energy in medicine is still in its infancy, but its role has been well established.[58] The application of laser technology for the diagnosis and treatment of congenital, benign and malignant respiratory diseases has added exciting dimensions for physicians. Laser is an acronym for *light amplification by the stimulated emission of radiation.* The principles upon which lasers are based was put forth by Einstein in 1917.[59] In 1960 it was Maiman who first discovered the laser using a ruby crystal. Polanyi and associates performed first tracheobronchial surgery using carbon-dioxide (CO_2) laser, which was coupled with modified rigid bronchoscope.[60,61] Since then various permutations and combinations were made for effective, controlled delivery of laser energy through bronchoscope for palliation of obstructing, congenital, benign and malignant diseases of tracheobronchial tree. Limitations associated with rigid bronchoscopic system, prompted the development of a flexible (fiberoptic) bronchoscopic system. Further technological advancement and development of newer lasers have further improved the techniques.[62,63]

Photodynamic therapy for treatment of malignant tumours uses certain porphyrins as relatively tumour selective photosensitizers. A wide variety of tumours take up and retain these materials, which results in complete eradication of the local tumour. This therapy appears to be particularly applicable to treatment of early stage lung cancer and can be palliative for several other more advanced cancers.[64-67]

To treat respiratory diseases, some of the features of laser energy-tissue interaction are:[58]

i. An inherent haemostatic effect.
ii. Minimal production of edema in tissues post application.
iii. Rapid healing due to minimal peripheral tissue damage.
iv. Minimal tissue scarring.

These features have proved laser to be the best surgical-knife. Basic differences between the various types of laser are (i) wavelength (ii) beam spot size (iii) exposure time to tissues (iv) temporal behaviour of laser, i.e., whether continuous or pulsed. These factors determine the (i) cutting, (ii) vapourization, and (iii) coagulation effects of lasers on tissues.[68,69]

Types of Laser used in Respiratory Medicine

i. Carbon dioxide laser.
ii. Neodymium: yttrium aluminium-garnet (Nd:YAG) laser (diagram).
iii. Argon laser.
iv. Potassium titanyl phosphate (KTP-532) laser.

CO_2 laser is the most widely used laser. The surgical superiority of this laser is because of (i) predictable laser-tissue interaction, (ii) clearly visible operating field, (iii) the capacity to control coagulation and vapourization of the tissues, (iv) less need for tissue manipulation, and (v) less post application edema. The CO_2 laser has proved beneficial for the treatment of many diseases of the respiratory system. These diseases include recurrent respiratory papillomatosis, stenosis, granulation tissue, adenoma, webs and palliation for obstructing carcinoma.[73]

The Nd:YAG laser energy is absorbed by dark colours, such as haemoglobin and melanin and transmitted clear liquids, with little loss of energy. The hallmark of the Nd:YAG laser and tissue interaction is scattering of the laser energy within the tissue. The ability of the laser to produce deep tissue coagulation makes it ideal for vascular tumours of the airway.[74-76]

The Argon laser is capable of delivery via a fiberoptic system with beam size as small as 0.15 mm and has been utilised for selected small tumours, like haemorrhagic nodules, polyps and vascular granulomas. The Argon laser colour absorption for red makes it more suitable for photocoagulation of blood vessels than for tissue ablation. Most recently Argon laser has been used for photodynamic therapy.[77]

The KTP-532 laser possesses the advantage of having a very small spot size (200 μm) and delivery via fiberoptic system. It has sharp edge of the aim beam; it has been successfully used in papillomas, carcinomas and photosurgical procedures.[78,79]

Complications[58]

i. *Bleeding:* Generally diffuse, oozing and small haemorrhages may occur in tumours. Major bleeding may occur if the tumour has invaded the artery and become centrally necrotic. If such tumour is lasered upto the necrotic area, bleeding may occur which can only be controlled by thorocotomy and ligating the vessels.[80]

(ii) *Perforations:* When using the lasers, there is always danger of perforation. The anatomy is frequently severely distorted by maligant tumours, greatly increasing the possibility of inadvertent tracheal or bronchial perforations and subsequent pneumothorax, fistula formation or exsanguinating haemorrhage. Intratracheal or intrabronchial haemorrhage is a complication that may be very poorly controlled through the bronchoscope and may require open thoracotomy.

(iii) *Development of Smoke:* When the irradiated tissues evaporate, smoke develops which is ventilated into periphery of the lungs. The biological effects of the smoke are known to cause detrimental effects on pulmonary airway resistance, gas exchange and mucociliary functions.[81]

(iv) *Fibrinous Plaques:* Laser irradiation causes a partially carbonized defect which is frequently covered by tenacious rubber-like plaques within a day. Since the bronchial clearance is partially blocked by this defect, materials from periphery collects there, forming an amorphous mass. It cannot be coagulated out by laser and practically not possible to aspirate them endosurgically. These plaques can be removed by forceps with rigid bronchoscopy.

Clinical Applications

(i) *Tracheal Stenosis:* It is characterised by granulation tissue in acute phase, and later on by scarring. Some tracheal collapse may occur due to loss of tracheal cartilage from tracheostomy. The carbon dioxide laser can be used to treat certain types of tracheal stenosis with high rate of success. It is the granulation phase which responds well to CO_2 laser vapourization. The tracheal stenosis that has a non-circumferential fibrotic scar without tracheomalacia, responds to CO_2 laser management. CO_2 laser is used to make radial incision and subsequent dilatation of the trachea.[82]

(ii) *Recurrent Respiratory Papillomatosis:* The laser excision of paryngeal papillomas is an easy and efficient method. Broncho laser helps in clearing obstruction, broncho-tracheal pathology and save from imminent asphyxia as well as cure those affected with stenosis or obstruction due to benign tumour.[83] The laser excision does not reduce the incidence of recurrent disease, requiring repeated treatment. The future therapy for the papillomatosis would require laser therapy with adjuvant medical therapy such as interferon or photodynamic therapy.[84]

(iii) *Malignant Neoplasms and Its Cytoreduction:* The management of patients with obstructing neoplasms of the tracheobronchial tree is difficult. Pre-operative evaluation of patient is necessary to assess cardiovascular status, coagulation function, and degree of tumour involvement of trachea. Laser treatment in carcinoma of bronchus is essentially palliative and is suitable for only a few patients.[85] Subjects selected for laser treatment must have predominently endobronchial growth with normal bronchial anatomy still identifiable. CO_2 laser, and Nd: YAG laser are used. Good palliation is obtained in just over half the cases of partial obstruction of trachea or main bronchus, but best results are obtained in lesions of main carina. Re-expansion of collapsed lung is achieved in some cases with risks of pneumonia and massive haemoptysis.[86-89] Some patients may require stents in-situ after laser therapy.

In some instances cytoreduction (debulking) of large upper airway carcinomas has been accomplished prior to definitive radiation therapy. Laser treatment has the advantage of having no toxicity or dose limit and may be used in cases of poor respiratory functions. It is better tolerated than radiation or chemotherapy.[90,91]

Photodynamic Therapy of Tumours

The history of photodynamic therapy dates back to more than thirty centuries to India and China, where plant extracts containing psoralens were applied to skin and exposed to sunlight to darken areas of skin of individuals suffering from vitiligo and leucoderma. The photochemical basis for photodynamic therapy is the sensitized photo-oxidation of biomolecules. Clinical photodynamic therapy to date has utilized hematoporphyrin derivatives (HpD) dihematoporphyrin ester (DHE) and Rhodamine-123 as photosensitizing agent.

Photodynamic therapy involves the systemic administrations to living tissues of a photosensitizing agent, which is then activated by a specific laser wavelength, causing destruction of target tissue, due to development of concentration gradient within the tumour cells having higher amount of drug than the surrounding normal tissues leading to cytodestructive release of high energy oxygen radicals.[92]

The major advantages of photodynamic therapy are, the possible early diagnosis of malignancy and the proven ability to destroy malignant tissues with preservation of surrounding normal tissue.[93,94]

Laser has thus, multiple uses in bronchotracheal pathology for emergency removal of obstruction, palliative airway restoration and sometimes a curative resection.[95-97]

The laser used is YAG-Neodymium, and the power ranges from about 40 to 90 watts, in a continuous or pulsatile beam. The intervention is carried out under general anesthesia and curarization. Use of a rigid bronchoscope is compulsory for operative security. As compared to other fiberscopes, it has a better visual field, attributable to the optics with which it is equipped, and is easier to clean. As it can be firmly wedged in the bronchotracheal tree, accurate beam transmission is ensured. Further, it enables continuous aspiration of secretions and hemorrhage by using a large-caliber aspirator, and also easy extraction of large tumour fragments.

Participation of trained anesthetists is of prime importance during the intervention, which is often long (1 or 1-1/2 hours) and not devoid of functional risks or hemorrhagic complications. The patient is supervised by the same team during the following 12 hours in a resuscitative room.

REFERENCES

1. Knight R.K., How to biopsy the lung and pleura? J. Appl. Med 1982, 8: 71-73.
2. Kramer R. and Som M.L., Bronchoscopic study of carcinoma of the lung, Arch, Otolaryngol 1936, 23: 526-43.
3. Rabinovitch J., Hochberg L.A. and Lederer M., Primary (Bronchogenic) carcinoma of the lung with histopathologic study of forty necropsies. J. Thorac. Surg 1940,9:332-45.
4. Griess D.F., Mc Donald J.R. and Clagett O.T., The proximal extension of carcinoma of the lung in the bronchial wall. J. Thorac Surg 1945, 14: 362-68.
5. Cotton R.E., The bronchial spread of lung cancer Brit. J. Dis. Chest 1959, 53: 142-50.
6. Seppala A.J., Endoscopic aspects of bronchogenic carcinoma, A Study of 815 cases, Acta Otolaryngol 1958, 59:81-86.
7. Sarkar S.K., Joshi Narayani, Purohit S.D., Gupta A, Sexena A., Bhatnagar M., Madan A. and Sharma T.N., Diagnosis of endoscopically visible bronchogenic carcinoma by using different tissue sampling techniques, *Lung India* 1988,3: 149-51.
8. Zavala D.C., Diagnostic fiberoptic bronchoscopy, Techniques and results of biopsy in 600 patients, Chest 1975,68: 12-19.
9. Kvale P.A., Dode F.R. and Kini S., Diagnostic accuracy in lung cancer: Comparison of techniques used in association with flexible fiberoptic bronchoscopy, Chest 1976, 69: 752-757.
10. Martini N. and Mc Cormack P.M., Assessment of end-oscopically visible bronchial carcinoma, Chest 1978, 73: 718-720.
11. Pande J.N., Sharma S.K., Tandon M., Verma K. and Guleria J.S., Fibreoptic bronchoscopy in the diagnosis of malignant lesions of lung—a three-year experience, Indian J. Chest. Dis. and Allied Sci 1982, 24: 244-50.
12. Popovich J., Kvale P.A., Eichenhom M.S., Radke J.R., Ohorodnik J.M. and Fine G., Diagnostic accuracy of multiple biopsies from flexible fiberoptic bronchoscopy—A comparison of central versus peripheral sarcoma, Am. Rev. Respir. Dis 1982, 125: 521-23.
13. Sarkar S.K., Mali Ram, Khandelwal P.P., *et al.* Bronchogenic carcinoma—optimal number of biopsy specimens required for diagnosis; *Lung India* 1990,8: 153-55.
14. Dennie C.J., *et al.,* Transthoracic needle biopsy of lung–results of early discharge in 506 patients, Radiology 2001, 219: 247-51.
15. Silverman I., A new biopsy needle, American Journal of Surgery 1938, 40: 671.
16. Abrams L.D., A pleural-biopsy punch. Lancet 1958, i: 30.
17. Mittal V., Pleural biopsy, Medinews 1993, p. 23.
18. Screaton N.J., Flower C.D., Percutaneous needle biopsy of pleura; Radiolo Clin North Amer 2000, 38: 293-301.
19. Walesby R.K., How to insert a chest drain and aspirate a pleural effusion. J. App., Med 1981, 7: 587-90.
20. Treasure T. and Cotter L., How to aspirate the pericardium, J. Appl. Med 1981, 7: 335-36.
21. Glancy D.L. and Richter M.A., Catheterisation and Cardiovascular Diagnosis 1975, 1:311.
22. Galen C. *DeAffectionibus Localis.* Book V and Book VIII.
23. Larrey DJ., Clin. Cardiol. (Paris) 1829, 2: 291.
24. Kilpatri Z.M. and Chapman C.B. On pericardiocentesis Amer. J. Cardiol 1965, 16: 722-28.
25. Spodick D.H., Medical History of Pericardium, Amer. J. Cardiol 1970, 26: 447.
26. Rondelet G., Cited by Beck C.S. and Moore R.L., The significance of the pericardium in relation to Surgery of the pericardium in relation to Surgery of the Heart. Arch. Surg. (Chicago) 1925, 11: 550.
27. Vijayaraghavan G., Pericardiocentesis; Need for haemodynamic monitoring, JAPI 1992, 40:652-53.
28. Morgan B.C., Guntheroth W.C. and Dillard D.H., The relationship of pericardial to pleural pressure during quiet respiration and cardiac tamponade, Cir. Res 1965, 16: 493.
29. Lorell B.H. and Braunwald E., *Pericardial disease 'Heart Disease.* Ed. Braunwald E. 8th Edn. WB Saunders Co. Philadelphia, P. 1485.
30. Reddy P.S. and Curties E.I., Cardiactamponade, Cardiology Clinics1990, 8:627.
31. Santos G.H. and Frater R.W.M., The subxiphoid approach in the treatment of pericardial effusion. Ann Thorac Surg 1977, 23: 467-70.
32. Friedrikson R.T., Cohen L.S. and Mullins C.B. Pericardial windows for pericardiocentesis, Am. Heart. J 1971, 82L: 158-62.
33. Kulkarni S.M.,Sundaram U., Desai D.M. *et al.* Value of haemodynamic studies during pericardiocentesis in a cardiac catheterisation laboratory, JAPI 1992,40: 655-57.
34. Levine M.J., Lorell B.H., Diver D.I. and Come P.J., Implications of echocardiographically assisted diagnosis of pericardial tamponade in contemporary medical patients: Detection before hemodynamic embarrassment, JACC 1991, 17: 59.
35. Soler-Soler J., Permanyer-Miralda G. and Sagrista-Sauleda J., A systemetic diagnostic approach to primary acute pericardial disease. The Barcelona Experience, Cardiology Clinics 1990, 8: 609.
36. Krikorian J.G. and Hancock E.W., Pericardiocentesis. Am. J. Med.1978, 65:808-14.
37. Wong B., Murphy J. and Chang E., The risk of pericardiocentesis, Am. J. Cardiol 1979, 44:1110-14.
38. Kotte J.H. and McGuire J., Pericardial paracentesis, Mod Concepts Cardiovasc Dis 1951, 20:102-103.
39. Hock J.E., Bass J.L. and Kulik T.J., Chronic percutaneous pericardial drainage with modified pigtail catheter in children, Am. J. Cardiol 1984, 53: 1179-82.
40. Shabetai R., The effects of pericardial effusion on respiratory variation in haemodynamics and ventricular function, JACC 1991, 17: 249.

41. McKelvie P., How to do an emergency tracheostomy? J. Appl. Med 1981, 7: 766-67.
42. Henri Moussalli, How to remove a foreign body from the trachea and bronchial tree? J. Appl. Med 1981,7: 497-503.
43. Jackson C., *Disease of the Air and Food Passages of Foreign Body Origin.* Saunders, London 1936.
44. Eller C.W. and Haugen R.K., Food asphyxiation, New Engl. J. Med 1973, 289:81-82.
45. Harboyan G. and Nassif R., Tracheo-bronchial foreign bodies—A review of 14 years experience, J. Laryngol Otol 1970, 84: 403-09.
46. Kaker P.K. and Saharia P.S., As unusual foreign body in tracheobronchial tree, J. Laryngol Otol 1972, 86: 1155-57.
47. Pande G., Iron nails in the tracheobronchial tree, Ind. J. Otolaryngol 1976, 28: 192-193.
48. Maru Y.K., Puri N.D. and Majid A., An unusual foreign body in tracheobronchial tree, J. Laryngol Otol 1978, 11: 1045-48.
49. Chawla R.K., Sachdeva O.P., Yadav S.P.S., Kaushal A.N., Chawla K. and Raj Baldev, Unusual presentation of foreign bodies in bronchus, Ind. J. Chest. Dis 1988, 30:231-33.
50. Mohan V., Bushan B., Kumar A. and Gupta S.D., An unusual foreign body in the bronchial tree—Case Report Ind. J. Chest. Dis 1983, 25: 149-51.
51. Sambamurthy V., Ramanjaneyulu P. and Ramachary V., Foreign body in food and air passages, Ind. J. Otolaryngol 1971, 23: 84-87.
52. Heimlich M.J., A life saving manoeuvre to prevent food choking, J. Am. Med. Ass 1975, 234: 298-401.
53. Black RE., Choi K.J., Syme W.C., Johnson D.G. and Matlak M.E., Bronchoscopic removal of aspirated foreign bodies in children, Am. J. Sur 1984,148(6):778-81.
54. Laurence A.S. and Burton A., Removal of inhaled peanut using a fiberoptic bronchoscope, Anaesthesia 1986, 41 (12): 1271-72.
55. Jain N.K., Garg V.K., Sharma V.K. *et al.* An upper lobe tracheo bronchial foreign body; *Lung India* 1990, 8: 203-205.
56. Gupta R.L., Foreign bodies in food and air passages, Ind. J. Otolaryngol 1964, 16:35-44.
57. Sanders RD., Delaware Medical Journal 1967, 39: 170.
58. Shukla A.K., Garg M. and Bhasin R.C, Clinical application of lasers in respiratory medicine, *Lung India*, 1992, 10: 41-44.
59. Schawlwo A.L. and Townder CH., Infrared and optical lasers, Phys. Rev., HZ 1958, 112: 1940-49.
60. Malman T.H., Stimulated optical radiation in ruby, Nature 1960, 187:493-494.
61. Polanyi T.B., Bredemeier H.C. and Davis T.N. Jr., A CO_2 laser for surgical research, Med. Biol. Eng. Comput 1970, 8: 541-48.
62. Hopkins H.H., *Physics of the fibreoptic endoscope* in Gerci G. (ed): Endoscopy, New York Appleton Centrury Crofts, 1976.
63. Cortese D.A., Kinsey J.H., Woolner L.B., Payne W.S. Sanderson D.R. and Fontana R.S., Clinical application of a new endoscopic technique for detection of in-situ bronchial carcinoma, Mayo Clin. Proc 1979,54:635-42.
64. Balchum O.J., Doiron D.R., Profio A.E. and Huth G.C, Fluorescence bronchoscopy for localising easily bronchial cancer and carcinoma in situ. Recent Results, Cancer Res 1982, 82:97-120.
65. Doiron D.R., Profio E., Vincent R.G. and Dougherty T.J., Fluorescence bronchoscopy for detection of lung cancer, Chest 1979, 76: 27-32.
66. Cortese D.A. and Kinsey J.H., Hematoporphyrin derivative phototherapy in the treatment of bronchogenic carcinoma, Chest 1984, 86: 8-13.
67. Dougherty J.J., Kaufman J.E., Goldfarb A., Weishaupt K.R., Boyle D. and Mittleman A., Photoradiation therapy for the treatment of malignant tumour, Cancer. Res 1978, 38: 2628-35.
68. David H. and Sliney M.S., Laser-tissue interactions Clinics in Chest Medicine 1985, 6(2): 203-208.
69. Goldman L. and Rockwell R.J., *Lasers in medicine* New York, Gordon and Breach 1971.
70. Polanyi T.G., Physics, Physics of surgery with lasers, Clinics in Chest Med 1986, 6:179-202.
71. Crockett D.M. and Reynolds B.N., Laryngeal laser surgery, Otol.Clin.North. Am 1990; 23(1):49-66.
72. Shapshay S.M. and Simpson G.T., Lasers in bronchology, Otol. Clin. North Am 1983, 16(4):879-86.
73. McElvein R.B. and Zorn G., Indications, results and complications of bronchoscopic carbon dioxide laser therapy, Ann. Surg 1984, 199: 522-25.
74. Unger M. and Atkinson G.W., *Nd-YAG laser applications in pulmonary and endobronchial lesions.* In Joffee S.N. (ed) Neodymium-YAG laser in Medicine and Surgery, New York, Elsevier Pulb. Co 1983, 72-81.
75. Toty L., Personne C, Colcehn A. and Vourchs G., Bronchoscopic management of tracheal lesions using the neodymium yttrium aluminum garnet laser, Thorax 1981,36: 175-78.
76. Dumon J.P., Bourcerau J., Meric B., Rebound E. and Garbe L. *Report of 1000 YAG laser endobronchial resections.* In Joffee S.N. (ed). Neodymium YAG laser in Medicine and Surgery. New York, Elsevier Publ. Co. 1983: 60-69.
77. Gillis T.M., Strong M.S., Shapshay S.M., Incze J. and Simpson G., Argon laser and soft tissue interaction, Otolaryngol Head Neck Surg 1984, 92: 7-12.
78. Atiyah R.A., *The KTP-532 laser in laryngeal surgery* KTP/532 Clinical Update No. 21, Sept. 1988.
79. Fried M.P., *The KTP/532 laser in head and neck surgery,* KTP/532 Clinical Update No. 16 April 1988.
80. Mallow A. and Chabot L., *Laser safety handbook,* New York. Van Nostrand Reinhold Company, 1980.
81. Freitag L., Champman G.A., Siekczak M., Ahmed A. and Russin D., Laser smoke effect on the bronchial system. Lasers Surg. Med 1987, 7(3): 283-88.

82. Shapshay S.M., Beamis J.F., Hybels R.L. and Bohigian R.K., Endoscopic treatment of subglottic and tracheal stenosis by radial laser incision and dilation, Ann Oto Rhino Laryngol 1987, 96: 661-64.
83. Steiberg B.N., Too W.L., Schneider P.S. and Abramson A.L., Laryngeal papilloma virus infection during clinical remission, New Engl. J. Med 1983, 308: 1261-64.
84. Toty L., Laser in Bronchopneumology, La Med. En Fra 1987, p.37-42.
85. Gell A.F. and Epstein J.D., Laser in treatment of Lung Cancer, Chest 1984, 86(5): 622-66.
86. Hetyel M.R., Millard F.J.C., Rayesh Bridges C.E., Nanson E.M., Swain C.P. and William I.P., Laser treatment for carcinoma of the bronchus. Br. Med. J 1983, 286: 12-18.
87. Unger M., Bronchoscopic utilization of the Nd: YAG laser for obstructing lesions of the trachea and bronchi, Surg. Clin. North. Am 1984, 64(5): 931-38.
88. Strong M.S., Vaughan C.W., Polanyi I.B. and Wallace R., Bronchoscopic carbon dioxide laser surgery, Ann. Otol 1974, 83: 769-76.
89. McElvein R.B. and Zorn G., Indications, results and complications of bronchoscopic carbon dioxide laser therapy. Ann Surg 1984, 199: 522-25.
90. MacElvein R.B. and Zorn G., Carbon dioxide laser therapy. Clin. In Chest. Med 1985, 6: 291-95.
91. Dougherty T.J.,Photodynamic therapy, Clinics in Chest Med 1985, 6(2): 219-36.
92. King E.G., Doiron D., Man G., Profo A.E. and Huth G., Hemaroporpyrin derivations as a tumour makrer in the detection and localisation of pulmonary malignancy. Recent Results Cancer Res 1982, 89:90-96.
93. Hayata Y., Kato H., Konaka C, Matsushima Y. and Nishimiya K., Fiberoptic bronchoscopic laser photoradiation for tumour localisation in lung cancer. Chest 1982, 82: 10-18.
94. Kensey J.H., Cortex D.A.I., and Sanderson D.R., Detection of hematoporphyr in fluorescence during fiberoptic bronchoscopy to localise early bronchogenic carcinoma. Mayo Clin. Proc 1978, 53: 594-600.
95. Toty L., Personne C.L., Colchen A. and Vourch G., *Tracheal surgery under Nd-YAG. Necessity of using a modified rigid bronchoscope.* Laser Tokyo 81. The 4th Congress of the International Society for Laser Surgery, Tokyo, Japan 23-27 Nov 1981; 20-24.
96. Toty L., Personne C.L., Colchen A., Leroy M. and Vourch G., Indications and results of the use of YAG laser in bronchology. Apropos 89 cases, Rev. Fr. Mal. Resp 1980, 8: 201-210.
97. Toty L., Personne CL., Colchen A. and Yourc H.G. Broncho-scopic management of tracheal lesions using the Neodymium Ytrium Aluminium Garnet laser. Thorax 1981, 36: 175-178.

PREOPERATIVE PULMONARY ASSESSMENT

It is well known that subjects with pulmonary disability due to variety of causes are at increased risk to develop postoperative morbidity.[1] Physicians and pulmonogists are often called upon to evaluate such patients in the preoperative period. Pulmonary complications are the most frequent causes of postoperative morbidity and mortality. Advances in surgical and anaesthetic techniques have markedly reduced the incidence of bronchoaspiration, atelectasis and infections. But a significant number of patients continue to develop postoperative bronchospasm, pulmonary embolism, pulmonary oedema and acute respiratory failure even in the best of centres.[2] In these situations it is important to employ a systematic strategy in order to detect, categorise and quantitate the respiratory disability. This would be an essential prerequisite to ensure vigilant pre-intra and postoperative attention from the pulmonary viewpoint. Further, such a strategy would allow institution of measures to correct reversible aspects of lung compromise in an attempt to reduce morbidity after the surgical procedure.

Both preoperative pulmonary evaluation for surgery and prediction of postoperative lung function is possible, largely with the help of pulmonary function tests (PFT), in addition to chest radiography and other investigations. While all patients should undergo preoperative check up from the pulmonary standpoint, certain categories should receive particular attention. These include elderly subjects, those with past or current chest diseases, obese individuals, smokers and those with chest wall or spinal deformities. In practice, subjects with chronic obstructive pulmonary disease form the bulk of subjects, who need special attention and evaluation. Subjects with chronic airflow limitation invariably have varying degrees of ventilation perfusion inhomogeneity. This is in turn due to airway smooth muscle spasm, fixed airway narrowing, airway collapse (as in emphysema) and intraluminal secretions.

Pulmonary function testing is helpful mostly in patients with presence of one or more risk determinants.[3] These include all patients schedule for thoracic or upper abdominal surgery and with underlying chronic lung disease. Other risk factors are: history of smoking and/or sputum production, severe obesity and age over 70 years. Type of surgery is more important than type of anaesthesia. The gas exchange abnormality is further aggravated by factors related to surgery such as supine posture, atropine administration, preoperative sedation, narcotic analgesia, pain, depressed cough reflex, inadequate expectoration and lack of hydration. Retained secreations may lead to areas of atelectasis.

Patients with restrictive deficit are also subject to hightened risk of post operative complications, though perhaps not to the same extent as those with diffuse airways obstruction. Pulmonary fibrosis of a diffuse nature (due to many causes), post-tubercular scarring, pleural thickening and calcification, spinal deformities and obesity are some of the common situations encountered. Post operative complications like atelectasis are related, to some extent, to the site of surgery. For instance, thoracic operations as well as cardiac surgeries are very often complicated by basal atelectasis. Surgical procedures with subcostal or upper abdominal incisions are more often followed by lung events than lower abdominal or inguinal incisions. Obesity, particularly when gross, adds to the risk of post operative atelectasis.[4] Whenever elective surgery is planned it is very desirable to have comprehensive evaluation of patients including their chest.

An adequate history and physical examination with focus on detection of possible lung compromise, supported by standard skiagrams are of central importance. Identified as at hightened risk, these subjects are then referred to the chest service, for detailed assessment. Such referrals, at a preliminary stage, serve two important functions. Firstly, these patients can be assessed as outpatients. The assessment should be on OPD basis, saving considerable hospital costs for the patient. Laboratory diagnosis and clinical assessment (diagnosis) go hand in hand.[5] But unnecessary investigations, the exact number of which one cannot precisely say, is unethical and unfair. Even routine urine analysis may not give new diagnosis of 0.5% and 0.83 to 7.04%.[5] This has to be strengthened with improved quality testing.[6]

Simple spirometry, with measurement of forced vital capacity, forced expiratory volume in 1 second, the ratio thereof and peak expiratory flow rate are invaluable tools in the assessment of the type and magnitude of pulmonary impairment. In cases of obstructive deficit, the degree of bronchodilator response has to be assessed. A rapid appreciation of the nature of the impairment in terms of obstructive, restrictive or mixed types can be obtained by using a simple monogram. This is of particular use to non-pulmonologists and anaesthetists. The vital capacity as percentage of predicted is plotted on the horizontal axis and the FEV/FVC on the vertical axis. When a given patient's values are plotted, a glance will convey the risk stratification. In most cases, spirometry including forced expiratory graph is adequate.[7,8] Spirometry is readily available, inexpensive and easy to use. A simple graph gives information on vital capacity (VC), forced vital capacity (FVC), timed forced expiratory volumes (such as FEV_1) and forced expiratory flows such as mild expiratory flow rates (FEF 200-1200 and FEF 25%-75%). The FEV_1/FVC ratio shall help in defining airway obstruction. Spirometric indices depend upon age, sex and height, differently in different ethnic groups. Therefore, there are no single values which can be suggested as normal and abnormal. Maximal voluntary ventilation (MVV) is helpful, though often tiresome, in a sick patient. It is done by asking the patient to breathe in and out as fastly and deeply as possible for 10-15 seconds.

Detailed assessment of lung function is required in only a fraction of cases such as those undergoing lung resection or with significant cardiopulmonary disease. This may include measurement of total lung capacity (TLC) and residual volume (RV), diffusion capacity (DLco) and arterial blood gas analysis. Regional lung function can be assessed with the ventilation and perfusion scans. Balloon occlusion of the pulmonary artery in conjunction with right heart catheterization is done to evaluate operatability such as pneumonectomy.[2] PFT criteria indicating high operative risk are listed in Table 1.45.

Table 1.45: Accepted PFT criteria that indicate high operative risk

Spirometry		
FVC	$\leq$	50% predicted
FEV_1	<	2.0 L
MVV	$\leq$	50% predicted
DLco	$\leq$	40% predicted
Art. blood gases $PaCO_2$	>	45 mm
Hypoxaemia		Not reliable

Functional status of pulmonary vasculature is assessed by temporary balloon occlusion of right or left main pulmonary artery. An increase of pulmonary arterial pressure by over 30 mmHg indicates non-operatability. Specialized studies, besides spirometry are needed on patients undergoing lung resection to evaluate the suitability of anticipated resection and prediction of adequacy of post resection function.[8] These are shown in Table 1.46.

Table 1.46: Sophisticated tests

1. Spirometry
2. Bronchospirometry (differential spirometry)
3. Lung scanning
4. Ventilation and perfusion studies.

Simple and easy method such as exercise testing is yet another important method of assessment.[8] Simple tests such as climbing one flight upstairs of six minute exercise tolerance, gives a good clinical indication of cardiopulmonary status. Evaluation of peak oxygen uptake (VO_2) and ventilation (V_e) is helpful but not the main criteria to determine operatability. Another simple approach is the assessment of ventilated part of the lung likely to be resected.[9] This is based on careful analysis of radiological and bronchoscopic studies. Predicted post operative test such as FEV_1 is equal to:

$$\text{Measured preoperative } FEV_1 \times \frac{\text{Number of Segments to remain Postoperatively}}{\text{20 Minus the Number of Non Ventilated Segments}}$$

(20 is the total number of segments, 10 in each lung, drawn as equal divisions on a plain chest roentgenogram by horizontal lines).

The use of PFT in patients undergoing open heart surgery or coronary artery bypass grafting has been proved beyond doubt. Patients staying in I.C.U. for shorter periods had better preoperative FVC, FEV_1 and FEF 25%-75%, Elevated $PaCO_2$ (> 45 mm Hg) is also associated with higher mortality. Patients undergoing coronary artery bypass with a graft from left internal mammary artery may have temporary left diaphragmatic dysfunction, causing difficult weaning from the ventilator. It is therefore, advisable to evaluate the respiratory function of such patients preoperatively.

The measurement of arterial blood gases and pH, if available, adds an important dimension to the understanding of the impact of the disability on gas exchange and pH homostasis, and help in more accurately assessing the risk of untoward postsurgical events.[10,11] Clearly, patients with mild to moderate hypoxemia alone can be more easily managed with supplemented oxygen; those with pre-existing resting hypercapnia are far more likely to dramatically worsen in the postoperative situation and may need ventilatory support till the stress period is tided over. The interaction between the surgeon, physician and the anaesthetist would evolve the measures to improve lung function, choice of premedication and nature of anaesthesia, to suit individual patient's needs. Subjects with chronic airflow limitation can very often benefit by cessation of smoking, bronchodilators, antibiotics and chest physiotherapy. Asthmatics have to be given careful preoperative treatment including parenteral hydrocortisone as well as bronchodilators in an optimal fashion. These patients often may not only develop profound worsening of asthma in the post surgical period, but are at great risk of adrenal crisis.[12]

Close monitoring with PFT is required for pulmonary complications in high risk patients, those with cardiopulmonary disease, multiple trauma, burns, septicemia and those undergoing lung resection. Serial blood gas determinations and chest radiographs are helpful for early detection of a serious complication of adult respiratory distress syndrome (ARDS) in postoperative periods. These tests may also help to diagnose pulmonary thromboembolism. Serial spirometric evaluation is required in patients of bronchial asthma, chronic obstructive or other lung diseases for adequate control and detection of deterioration.[13] In patients undergoing resectional lung surgery, lung function testing is essential for making assessment of residual function and respiratory disability.[2] Table 1.47 gives a precise picture of drugs commonly used in respiratory ailments.

Table 1.47: Classification of drugs used in respiratory diseases

1. *Drugs Used in the Therapy of Cough*		
A. Antitussives	B. Expectorants	
a. Opiates codeine, noscapine, dextromethorphan.	a. Direct stimulants effective orally: Oil of eucalyptus, anise oil, lemon oil, cedar wood oil and alcohol.	
b. Antihistaminics: Diphenhydramine, chlorcyclizine, demethoxanate.	b. Reflex stimulants: Potassium iodide, potassium citrate, ammonium chloride, ammonium carbonate, ipecacuanha, extract of adhatoda.	
c. Miscellaneous: Benzonatate, ethyl dibunate, pepridone, pimetine.		
2. *Bronchodilators*		
A. Adrenergic drugs a. Non-selective adrenergic agonists Adrenaline, ephedrine. b. Beta adrenergic drugs: Isopernaline, salbutamol, terbutaline.	B. Methylxanthines Theophylline aminophylline	C. Anti cholinergic drugs Etofylline
3. *Immunomodulators*		
A. Corticosteroids a. Systemic hydrocortisone, prednisone, prednisolone, betamethasone dipropionate.	B. Disodium cromoglycate	C. Ketotifen
4. *Mucolytics* Acetylcysteine, bromhexine, guaifenesin, pancreatic dornase.		
5. *Therapeutic Agents*		
A. Systemically used agents	B. Locally used drugs (inhalational agents): Antibiotics: Gentamicin Antiparasitic Agents: Pentamidine	

REFERENCES

1. Ford G.T. and Guenter C.A., Toward prevention of post operative pulmonary complications Amer. Rev. Resp. Dis 1984, 130: 4-5.
2. Jindal S.K., *Perioperative pulmonary function testing;* IN: Shankar P.S., ED: Med Update. API Bombay 1995, 5: 434-37.
3. Zibrak J.D. and O' Donnell C.R., Indicating for preoperative pulmonary function testing, Clin in Chest. Med 1993, 14: 227.
4. Pasulka P.S., Bistrain B.R., Benotti P.N. and Blackburn G.L., The risk of surgery in obese subjects; Ann. Int. Med 1986, 104: 540-46.
5. Broughton P.M.G., The cost of unnecessary test by day and night, Brit. Med. Jour 1987, 294: 1530-34.
6. Bhatia R.S., Should we subject every OPD patient to routine urine testing? J. Assn Phys. India 1993, 41: 57.
7. Hayhurst M.D., Preoperative pulmonary function testing, Resr. Med 1993, 87: 161.
8. Celli B.R., What is the value of preoperative pulmonary function testing? Med. Clin. North Amer 1993, 77: 309.
9. Egeblad K., Aunsholt N.A., Funder V. Nielson P.H., A simple method for predicting pulmonary function after lung resection, Scand J. Thorac Cardiovas Surg 1986,20: 103.
10. Schoonover G.A. and Olson G.N., Pulmonary function testing in preoperative period, A review of literature, J. Clin. Surg 1982, 1: 125-37.
11. Tisi G.M., Preoperative identification and evaluation of the patient with lung disease, Med. Clin. North Amer 1987, 71: 399-412.
12. Bhatia R.S., Preoperative pulmonary assessment, Curr, Med. Prac 1993, 37: 140-42.
13. Bhatia R.S., Sibia S.S., Intensive pulmonary care units, An urgent need, A viewpoint, *Lung India* 1995, 13(2):75-76.

Congenital Conditions

2

These are described in two groups: (A) Congenital abnormalities of upper respiratory system; and (B) Congenital abnormalities of lower respiratory system.

GROUP A

Congenital Laryngeal Stridor[1,2]

Noisy breathing or hoarseness or aphonia with dyspnoea and inspiratory retraction of intercostal and supraclavicular spaces in the newborn is generally referred to as congenital laryngeal stridor. Differential diagnosis include laryngeal spasm of tetany, laryngeal odema due to trauma or aspiration. These patients are undernourished, as they have difficulty in nursing. There is dyspnoea, especially during feeding. Cyanosis is rarely seen.

Stridor after four days of neonatal life, is due to congenital anomaly of epiglottis or laryngomalacia. Laryngeal anomalies include malformation of laryngeal cartilages, intraluminal webs and duplication or malformation of vocal cords. Other causes of stridor include generalised chondromalacia of trachea and hairy fibroma of larynx (congenital tumor), retension cyst, bronchial left cyst and thyroglobal duct remnants.

Extra laryngeal causes include birth trauma, hypoplasia of mandible, macroglossia, haemangioma, lymphangioma or cyst, enlarged thymus, congenital vascular anomalies, goitre (congenital) and Pierre-Robin syndrome (Mandible hypoplasia, pseudomacroglossia and glossoptosis). Laryngoscopy, general physical examination and fluoroscopic observations (for vascular abnormalities) help in pinpointing the diagnosis.

Management

Laryngomalacia does not require any treatment. Symptoms gradually and spontaneously clear over a period of one year. Cysts, webs, tumors and laryngeal malformations require excision, dilatation, laryngoplasty or tracheostomy. Forward pulling of the tongue and mandible relieve stridor associated with macroglossia and mandible hypoplasia.

These infants need careful nursing and slow feeding to avoid aspiration and need to be protected from chest infections.

CONGENITAL WEB[1,2]

Tracheal stenosis may be seen as congenital web, absent or deformed tracheal cartilages. The condition is not common but needs an emergency measure to diagnose and treat, especially if the web is complete because in such situations, neonate shall get quickly asphyxiated. Stridor and dyspnoea occurs when the web is not complete. Anophthalmia and laryngeal atresia may coexist. Tracheal stenosis may be diffuse, segmental or funnel like. Last variety may be associated with left pulmonary anomalies.[3-5]

Laryngoscopy is both diagnostic and curative. Anterior division of the web, followed by retension of a non-irrigating metal or silicone keel until epithelialisation occurs, is the real treatment. Direct laryngoscopic incision or excision of web does reunite and has always proved unsuccessful. Tracheostomy is rarely required in cases where serial dilatation is to be performed.

TRACHEO ESOPHAGEAL FISTULA[6-9]

The most common congenital anomalies tracheal agenesis and atresia are quite rare and communicate as a fistula with the esophagus and may be due to a deviation of the septum between the esophagus and trachea or to an altered growth along the septum, where absence of growth results in a fistula and deficient growth results in atresia. Clinically, there are five types, most common being where an upper blind segment ending in a pouch above the tracheal bifurcation and a lower segment from the stomach connecting the trachea with a small fistulous tract.

The first one or two fluid or feed are followed by sudden return either by mouth or nose. The child coughs, struggles and may become cyanotic. Although no feed goes into the trachea but the bile and gastric secretions regurgitate via the fistula into the trachea. Pneumonia is a serious problem in these infants.

The symptoms in the 2nd type are similar to the previous one but the X-ray shows an opaque abdomen devoid of gas in the stomach and intestines. The lower esophageal segment is rudimentary and the pulmonary symptoms are only due to overflow or aspiration of feed.

The H-type tracheoesophageal fistula without atresia is suspected in children or infants who give an abnormal response to cough, choking and respiratory embarrassment to fluids as compared to solid food. Repeated pneumonias are common.

The last types include upper segment of trachea connected with the trachea, with or without the connection of the lower segment. First feed of the infant may prove drowning, leading to cough and cyanosis.

X-rays are quite helpful. Radio opaque will not pass through into the stomach in oesophageal atresia and contrast media like iodised ointment (in place of barium), just one ml, would reveal blind end of esophagus at the tracheal bifurcation.

The H-type fistula casually requires lateral and oblique cinefluoroscopy.

Management

Surgical management, the early, the best, before dehydration and pneumonia occurs, is the choice. Gastrostomy may be required if the neonate is underweight.

Adequate antibiotic cover, aseptic incubator, delicate nursing care under a team work look-after by surgeon and pulmonologist, upright position and nutrition via intravenous line along with bronchoscopic aspiration to prevent infections. and atelectasis are useful measures. After, 2-3 days post operatively, first feed of 0.5% saline, followed by 5% glucose if tolerated, should be followed by diluted milk. Tracheobronchomegaly is another congenital condition, where trachea is unusually dilated. Symptoms may be assent, or appear in adulthood, as wheeze, dyspnoea, respiratory distress stridor, cyanosis and apnoea. It is an autosomal recessive trait defect that produces this condition. Treatment is symptomatic, mainly for the recurrent infections.[10]

GROUP B

Dysmorphic Lung

A complex bronchovascular malformation of the lung is called dysmorphic lung. It involves right lung more frequently than the left and is associated with lung hypoplasia (disordered growth), pulmonary vascular anomalies of arterial collaterals, vascular abnormality, pulmonary artery atresia or even absence of the pulmonary artery (aplasia) etc. There is evidence of disordered growth of the lung (hypoplasia, sequestration) and vascular abnormality consisting of systemic arterial collaterals or anomalous venous return of all or most of the lung or abnormal anatomy of the pulmonary artery (atresia or absence).[11] The right lung is involved far more frequently than the left.

Pulmonary Agenesis

Agenesis of the Lung

Agenesis of the lung is a very rare congenital anomaly. It reflects an arrest in embryonic development, exhibiting failure of development of the primitive lung bud. It is obviously not compatible with life. There can be complete absence (agenesia), rudimentary bronchus without lung parenchyma (aplasia) or disordered growth of bronchovascular and lung parenchyma (hypoplasia).[12] Lober agenesia is rarely reported. Pulmonary hypoplasia is commonly seen in association with anomalies which compete with the lungs for space, such as diaphragmatic hernia. A case of aplasia of left lung has recently been reported in Indian literature.[13]

Lung agenesia is responsible for recurrent pulmonary infection during infancy. Coexisting congenital anomalies of other systems like gastrointestinal, genitourinary, skeletal and cardiovascular are common feature.

Nearly in 50% of cases survival is low even with unilateral pulmonary agenesia, which is otherwise compatible with life and occurs as an isolated lesion. It involves both sides and almost equally both the sexes and comes to light in infancy or childhood only when complicated with bronchopulmonary complication.[14-16] Ipsilateral facial anomalies may occur with unilateral agenesis.[17]

Radiologically it demonstrates a homogeneous opacity of the hemithorax with a shift of the mediastinum to the affected side. Differential diagnosis includes pneumonia, empyema, and atelectasis.[18] CT scan reveals smaller hemithorax with hyperinflated other lung, mediastinal shift to the affected side and other associated rudimentary or absence of carive, bronchial, tracheal bifurcation or pulmonary vessels.[19,20] Bronchoscopy reveals an abrupt ending of the main bronchus and bronchography reveals rudimentary bronchus, often ending in a blind pouch. Angiocardiography is rarely required.[18] Prognosis depends on the functional capacity of the remaining lung. Recurrent respiratory infections need therapy with antibiotics.

Azygos Lobe

Azygos lobe is actually a part of right upper lobe. Normally the embryonic right lung bud grows cephalad, lateral to azygos vein. During foetal development, the azygosvein normally shifts medially into the mediastinum and onto the vertebral column. Occasionally (0.1 percent) such a migration fails to occur and a portion of the bud passes medial to azygos vein resulting in an invagination of the visceral pleural as the lung bud grows cephalad.[21] The so-called azygos lobe hardly has any physiological or pathological significance. There is no abnormality of the bronchial tree. Radiologically the pleural line extends as a smooth concave from the lung apex to the take-off of the upper lobe bronchus. The vein appears as an ovoid density of the caudal end of the pleural line giving an appearance of an inverted comma with a long tail.[22]

Cystic Adenomatoid Malformation[23]

It is associated with other congenital anomalies. Even prematurity and still births are also commonly associated.

The condition has predilection for lower lobes. The condition may be responsible for acute respiratory distress in newborn, but may be detected in about 50% of cases in early childhood, presenting with chronic recurrent chest infections. Dextrocardia is an associated anomaly, with congenital bronchiectasis. Differential diagnosis includes sequestration, infected congenital cysts and bronchiectasis.

This rare developmental anomaly of terminal respiratory structures, having incidence of 1 in 10,000-35,000 births, occurs in 4-7th week of fetal life.

Common features and complications include:

- Cough > 85%.
- Sucking difficulty > 70%.
- Breathing difficulty > 70%.
- Fever 60%.
- Recurrent pneumonia > 25%.
- ARDS 40%.
- Other complications > 10%.

Chest X-ray shows a multicystic *swiss cheese* configuration with over-expanded affected region, and mediastinum is shifted towards normal side.

Thoracotomy reveals partially aerated dense mass studded with cysts. Histopathology shows respiratory tissue and irregular tubules lined with disorganised respiratory epithelium that resembles an adenoma.

Early surgery is the treatment of choice and has good prognosis. Lobectomy is the choice although pneumonectomy may become necessary in certain cases.

Diverticula[24]

These congenital anomalies generally exist as asymptomatic malformations. These may be communicating freely with the airways, generally in the distal part of the trachea.

Accessory Lung[24]

It is a rare congenital anomaly which is invariably situated at the lung base, mostly on the left side. The accessory lung has no communications with tracheo-bronchial tree. It has systemic supply, rather than pulmonary. Histopathology may reveal varying appearance from normal lung parenchyma to that of cystic space with bronchial element and with or without alveoli.

Bronchial Cysts

These arise during embryonic development of the tracheobronchial tree. These occur at tracheal carina and are mostly asymptomatic. Cystic structures lined with bronchial epithelium may evolve during development, which do not have any communication with the airways and are located in the pulmonary parenchyma at the periphery, especially of the lower lobes. These are called bronchial cysts. They may be solitary or multiple.[22] They may expand rapidly during neonatal period to cause cardiorespiratory embarrassment. These are more common in males. The cysts are filled with mucus, which may get infected in later life and enlarge in size or develop communication with the bronchial tree, and may get partially air-filled and infected.[25] Even bleeding may occur into the cyst. When enlarged, compressive symptoms and even severe respiratory distress may occur. Antibiotics form mainstay in medical treatment and surgical management can be done by incomplete cystectomy.[26] Surgery is indicated for large or chronically infected cysts.[27-30] Sequestration must be ruled out with preoperative evaluation with arteriography and bronchoscopy.

Bronchopulmonary Sequestration[17,22,25,31-34]

Bronchopulmonary sequestration mostly congenital refers to an area of the non-functioning abnormal lung tissue isolated during development from the rest of the lung having a systemic blood supply from an aberrant branch of aorta instead of pulmonary artery. Characteristically it has no connection with the tracheobronchial tree. In case communication exists, it gives a cystic appearance. In about 70 per cent of reported cases the condition is intralobar, wherein the abnormal lung tissue is located within the visceral pleura of a pulmonary lobe and does not have its useful pleural covering. In extralobar sequestration, the lung tissue is separated completely like an accessory lobe having its own visceral pleura in the inferoposterior mediastinum adjacent to lung and esophagus, generally on the left side. Extralobar type is seen in the lower lung zone mostly in the left hemithorax. It has an arterial blood supply from the aorta and venous drainage occurs into the azygos vein. Other congenital anomalies may accompany in 50% of cases. Tracheobronchial communication is not seen but oesophageal communication may occasionally be present. This type is generally detected in the childhood, as an unexplained dense triangular mass in the posterior lower lung field on chest X-ray.

Intralobar variety, unlike extralobar, do not have accompanying anomalies, therefore, patient presents late in life. It is located above the diaphragm and always in the lower lung zones, posterior basal segment being its most common site. There is a persistence of a branch from primitive dorsal aorta. Normally these branches disappear with the development of a pulmonary artery. In this condition there is insufficient pulmonary arterial vascularization during foetal lung development. The aberrant artery may arise from descending thoracic aorta or from intercostal artery or from branch of abdominal aorta. The sequestrated lung receives anomalous branch from thoracic aorta in 70% and rest of the cases from abdominal aorta. The vessel reaches by passing through inferior pulmonary ligament. There is pulmonary hypoplasia along with cystic degeneration and fibrosis. The condition may in some cases be acquired after birth due to vasoconstriction in the regions of bronchial obstruction. There is no effective anastomosis between pulmonary and systemic arteries. The venous drainage occurs into the pulmonary venous system.

The sequestrated area may consist of large bronchial walls, thin-walled cysts, polycystic areas with an irregular intermingling of cysts and alveolar parenchyma or alveolar structures. The bronchial branchings do not communicate with those of the normal lung. An accessory lobe can be differentiated from sequestration by presence of its communication with the trachea or one of the major bronchi, generally on the left side, and has a supply either from pulmonary or systemic circulation. The condition often presents recurrent episodes of infection in young adults especially in intralobar type which remains asymptomatic until young adulthood. The infection can reach the sequestrated lung by contiguity or through haematogenous or lymphatic spread.

Chest X-ray shows an opacity in the posterior mediastinum with a fluid level in the posterior basal segment, not distinguishable from other congenital cystic malformations. Bronchoscopy does not outline any bronchial tree or bronchial connection with the cystic-cavitary structures with displaced airways in the neighbourhood. The chest CT demonstrates multiple cystic cavities and reveals a systemic feeding artery from the descending aorta. Arteriogram should be done in both the types. The arterial phase film from an aortogram reveals a systemic feeding artery, and venous phase shows the venous drainage into the pulmonary vein. Barium esophagogram will rule out any communication to esophagus. Rarely it presents as homogenous opacity or multiple cystic areas. Recurrent pneumonia and focal bronchiectasis may result due to repeated infections.

Risk of abscess formation in the sequestrated lung due to poor bronchial drainage can't be ruled out. Surgical management includes resection of mass, taking care of the origin of aberrant vessel especially from the abdominal aorta to avoid disastrous bleeding. Lobectomy for intralobar type and resection for the extralobar type is the treatment of choice.

Lobar Emphysema[35-40]

Congenital Obstructive Lobar Emphysema

Lobar emphysema clinically presents with massive distention of lung lobe or segment which causes a mediastinal shift and contralateral lung is compressed. Apart from sequestration, cystic adenomatoid malformation and bronchogenic cyst, it is one of the four structural lesions responsible for respiratory distress in newborn. It may have associated cardiovascular, malformations, in about 40% of cases. A part of the lobe, usually the right middle or left upper lobe, is affected.

There is a check valve type of obstruction, possibly due to defective cartilage in the bronchi (25% cases), mucosal fold, bronchial stenosis and external compression by aberrant vessels, tumors etc. Cause of obstruction may not be identified in 50% of cases.

Respiratory distress may occur within 4 days to 4 months. In 50% of cases, it has occurred within first 4 weeks of neonatal life. Lungs may be hyper-resonant. Breath sounds are decreased. X-ray chest shows hyperlucent lungs and pneumothorax needs to be differentiated. Congenital lobar emphysema presenting in late childhood or adulthood for the first time offers diagnostic challenge and should be kept in mind to avoid unnecessary intervention for pneumothorax. Compressed lung can be differentiated from atelectasis by chest radiograph where diaphragm is depressed on both sides with lobar emphysema compared to normal or elevated in the side of primary atelectasis. A varying degree of lobar emphysema due to aspiration of mucus or aminiotic fluid or by acute bronchiolitis may occur but resolves with medical therapy. Surgery is indicated in progressive respiratory distress. Lobectomy is the choice, as mortality rate is 50% with surgical intervention.

Scimitar Syndrome

Also known as hypogenetic lung syndrome or mirror image lung syndrome. It is a rare complex spectrum of congenital malformation of the right lung (Hypoplasia) and of the right pulmonary artery, a systemic arterial supply from the abdominal aorta by an aberrant pulmonary artery to the hypoplastic right lung base, and partial anomalous pulmonary venous return from the right lung to the inferior vena cava.[41] More.in females, the condition may remain asymptomatic.[42] In older children and adults, the syndrome may present with recurrent pulmonary infections, fatigue and dyspnoea. Hemoptysis and pulmonary artery hypertension, both are uncommon presenting complaints beyond infancy.[43] Abnormal tortuous pulmonary vein as cause of cough and chest pain in an adult is called pseudosimitar syndrome.[44]

The volume of right hemithorax is diminished due to hypoplasia of the right lung. Anomalies include errors of segmentation and lobation, pulmonary arterial hypoplasia, right bronchus hypoplasia, and rightward displacement of the heart. Coexisting congenital heart diseases and frequently secondum atrial septal defect is present in the 1/4th of cases. Pulmonary arterial hypertension is commonly seen.[44]

Chest X-ray shows a diminished volume of right hemithorax, rightward displacement of the mediastinum, small right pulmonary artery, absence of one or both fissures and increased perfusion of the left lung. The right heart border is indistinct. An abnormal vein draining from the right lung in the form of a curved scimitar (Turkish sword) to the subdiaphragmatic inferior vena cava or to the right atrium is the characteristic feature. It is visible as a broad curved or thin straight band parallel to the right heart border which disappears at the diaphragm. There may be eventration of the right hemidiaphragm.[22]

Bronchography reveals dilatation of trachea, tracheal or bronchial diverticula, abnormal distribution of the right bronchi, absence of upper lobe bronchus and sometimes bronchiectasis. Angiogram demonstrates anomalous venous drainage, a diminished size of the right pulmonary artery and branches of abdominal aorta penetrating the diaphragm to supply the right lung. Computed tomography demonstrates the indistinct right heart border[45] and retrosternal opacity noticed on chest X-ray to be due to mediastinal shift.[46] Vascular anomaly can be visualized non-invasively by MR technology.[47]

Recurrent lung infections may require pneumonectomy and a significant left-to-right shunt, anastomosing Scimitar veins to the left atrium.[22] Hemoptysis occurs due to rupture of hypertrophied systemic pulmonary anastomoses or bleeding from bronchiectatic segment in hypoplastic lung.

'Horse Shoe' Lung

It is a rare congenital anomaly where posterobasal segments of the right and the left lungs are fused by an isthmus of pulmonary parenchyma behind the pericardial sac. The condition, may occur in association with anomalies typical of *Scimitar* syndrome[48] in many patients. The isthmus has branches from the right pulmonary artery and the right bronchus. It shows female predominance and many present with pulmonary manifestations in the first few years of their lives. Chest X-ray reveals multiple thin walled retro cardiac cystic lesion in addition to the features of *Scimitar* syndrome. Computed tomography (CT) of thorax shows the two lungs are not separated by pleura unlike Scimitar syndrome.[22] Surgical resection of hypoplastic lung and isthmus is the treatment.[49]

Primary Ciliary Dyskinesia

It is also known as immotile cilia syndrome or ciliary dyskinesis syndrome (CDS). Originally documented by Siewart in 1904,[50] it was Kartagener who described it in detail in 1933.[51]

Defects in the ultrastructure of the cilia and of the sperm[52] may affect their motility and function. It is referred as immotile cilia syndrome. As the cilia do not function normally,[53] the term primary ciliary dyskinesia is often preferred since some cilia may exhibit very slow and uncoordinated motility. Genetic lack of dynein arms in the cilia of the bronchial mucosa and nasal mucosa and absence of outer hook-like configuration in the dynein arms in the cilia of the middle ear in such patients has been documented. The condition may also develop from lack of radial spokes, clumping of fibrils, absence of central singlets, transposition of a peripheral doublet, microtubular disorganisation and axonemal defects.[54-56] There is loss of orientation and these respiratory cilia are unable to beat in a coherent way.[57] The sperm tails stand straight and stiff without exhibiting any motility. They cause male infertility. The situs inversus appears to develop from malrotation of the embryonic gut[58] when it is not guided by ciliary movements during the early part of gestation.

A classic example of immotile cilia syndrome, where apart from a generalised ciliary defect, situs invertus, recurrent infections in the form of chronic sinusitis, otitis media and bronchiectasis are also present. It develops as a congenital abnormality and is inherited as an autosomal recessive condition.[22]

Complete expression of Kartagener's syndrome is less frequently seen than partial expression. Men suffering from such syndrome are sterile. Complete situs invertus may be seen only in 50% of cases, with dextrocardia.[59] A genetic disorder of primary ciliary dyskinesia which is characterized by the triad of sinusitis, bronchiectasis and situs inversus (dextrocardia, left hepatic flexure and right descending colon with sigmoid colon). Polydactyly and clubbing are also seen.[59] Prevalence of triad of least agenesis 1:20,000to 40,000 and of ciliary dyskinesia syndrome without situs inverstus is 1:10,000 of population.[60]

Impaired mucociliary clearance causes stasis of airway mucus as a consequence of abnormal ciliary ultrastructure.[61] There is an obstructive ventilatory defect with greatly reduced FEV_1. Fertility, congenital heart defect and pectum excavatum are also rarely associated with this syndrome.[62] Timely treatment for infertility should be offered and unnecessary evaluation of symptoms is avoided.[63] The congenital ciliary abnormality has chronic lung diseases affecting the mucociliary mechanism as important differential diagnosis, where non-specific structural changes occur in cilia. The saccharin test is helpful to measure nasal mucociliary clearance.[64] All cases with bronchiectasis should be investigated for CDS but all cases of dextrocardia with respiratory symptoms may not be the cases of CDS.[65] A case of primary ciliary dyskinesia with pulmonary arterial hypertension responding to oral sildenafil has recently been documented.[66]

Diaphragmatic Hernia[22]

The herniation of diaphragm may occur through a triangular space at the posterolateral rib cage called Foramen of Bochdalek and this occurs more frequently on the left side. Hypoplasia of the lung along with decreased number of alveoli is an associated feature. Patient comes with features of aspiration pneumonia and of malnutrition. Chest X-ray shows signet radiolucencies from air filled loops of bowel in the chest. Respiratory distress due to lung compression from distended bowel may occur and can be deflated by passing nasogastric tube.

Minor defects can be medically managed by frequently seen small feeds, continuous upright posture and anti spasmodics. Surgical closure may be necessary for major defects. Similar herniation, though rarely, may occur anteriorly through Foramen of Morgagni. It is generally on the right side and may contain omentum and transverse colon. Patient may present with cough, dyspnoea or constipation. Chest radiogram reveals an opacity in the anterior mediastinum. Transverse colon can be confirmed by barium enema. Surgical correction may be required. Diaphragmatic hernia with intrathoracic kidney has been documented.[67]

Congenital Eventration of the Diaphragm[22]

Maldeveloped diaphragm may cause eventration of part or whole of the diaphragm on one or both sides. In that case, diaphragm is thin and fibrous. It is raised to bring peritoneum in close contact with pleura. Mediastinal shift occurs to the opposite side. Child may present with symptoms of respiratory distress. Chest radiogram and fluoroscopy reveal elevated diaphragm. Marked eventration requires surgical application.

REFERENCES

1. Ferguson C.F. and Kendig E.L., *Pediatric Otolaryngology* W.B. Saunders Co., Philadelphia, 1972.
2. Vaughan V.C., KaMes McKay Rs. and Nelson W.E., *Nelson Textbook of Pediatrics,* 10th Ed, 1975 W.B. Saunders Co., Philadelphia, 1975.
3. Altman R.P. *et al.*, Tracheal agenesis, Recognition and management, J. Paed. Surg 1972; 7: 112.
4. Hophinson J.M., Congenital absence of trachea; J. Path 1972; 107:63.
5. Contrell J.R., Guild H.G., Congenital stenosis of trachea; Amer J. Surg 1964; 108: 297.
6. Herweg J.C. and Ogura J.H., Congenital tracheo esophageal fistula with esophageal atresia, J. Pediat 1955,47: 293.
7. Holder T.M., Cloud T.C., Lewis J.E. In *et al.,* Esophageal atresia and tracheoesophageal fistula; Pediat 1964,34: 542.
8. Holinger P.H., Johnston K.C. and Potts W.J., Congenital anomalies of the oesophagus, Acta Oto Cary (Suppl) 1952, 100.
9. Ghai O.P.; *Essential pediatrics,* 2nd Ed; Interprint, N. Delhi; 1990.
10. Al-Mallal Z, Ouantok O.P., Tracheo-bronchomegaly, Thorax 1968; 23: 320.
11. Portridge J.B., Oaborne J.M. and Slaughter R.E., Clin. Radiol 1988, 11-19.
12. Boyden E.A., Development anomalies of the lung. Amer. J. Surg 1995, 89; 79.
13. Bedi R.S.; Unilateral total homogeneous opacity of left hemithorax; Curr Med Journ 1996; 2(1): 58.
14. Singh N.P., Rohtagi R.; Unilateral agenesis of the lung; JAPI 1996; 44(10): 723-24.
15. Singh R.P., *et al.*, Agenesis of lung, JAPI 1987; 35(3): 235-36.
16. Banerjee A. *et al.*, Agenesis of the lung; Ind J Chest Dis and All Sci 1990; 32(4): 229-32.
17. Schwartz Seymour I, Shires G. Tom, Spencer Frank C and Husser W.C., *Schwartz's principles of surgery;* 6th Ed. McGraw Hill; New York, 1994.
18. Sokos C.G., M.C. Millan I.K.R., Agenesis of the lung, Brist J Dis Chest 1977; 71: 183-97.
19. Argent A.C., Cremin B.J., CT in agenesis of lung in infants; Brist J Radiol 1992; 65: 221-24.
20. Mendelson D.S. *et al.*, Hypoplasia of the lung; CT appearance; Mount Sinai J Med 1986; 53: 297-98.
21. Boyden E.A., *Segmental Anatomy of the Lungs,* McGraw Hill, New York, 1955.
22. Shanker P.S., Chest Medicine; 4th Ed. Oxford and IBH Pub. Co., New Delhi, 1994.
23. Craig J.K., Kirkpatrick J. and Neuhanger E.B.D., Congenital cystic adenomatoid malformation of the lung in infants, Amer. J. Roentg 1956, 76: 516.
24. Wexler H.A., Valdes-Depena M., Congenital cystic adenomatoid malformation: A report of three unusual cases; Radiology 1980; 126: 737.
25. Uanghan III V.C., James Mckay R. and Nelson W.E., Nelson's Text Book of Paediatrics, 10th Ed, WB Saunders Co., Philadelphia, 1975.
26. Wesley J.R., Heidelberger K.P., *et al.* Diagnosis and management of congenital cystic disease of the lung in children, J. Pediat. Surg 1986, 21: 202.
27. Kergin F.G., Congenital cystic disease of lung tissue associated with anomalous arteries, J. Thorac. Surg 1952; 23: 55.
28. Gallagher H.S., Cytomegalic inclusion disease of infancy, Report of case associated with cysts of lung with recovery following lobectomy, Amer. J. Clin. Path 1952,22: 147.
29. Anonymous, Bronchogenic cyst; BMJ 1973; 2: 501.
30. Huchin P., Congenital cystic disease of the lung; Rev. Surg 1971; 28: 79.
31. Sperling D.R. and Finck E.J., Intralobar bronchopulmonary sequestration. Amer. J. Dis. Child 1968, 115: 362.
32. Rana S; *et al.,* Congenital anomaly of the lung; Lung India; 2014; 31: 182-83.
33. Willians A.O., Enumal F.I., Extralobar pulmonary sequestration; Thorax 1968; 23: 200.
34. Clements B.S., Warner J.O., Pulmonary sequestration and related congenital bronchopulmonary vascular malformations, nomenclature and classification based on anatomical and embryological considerations; Thorax 1987; 42: 401.
35. Campbell P.E.,Congenital lobar emphysema; Aust. Paed. J 1969,5:226.
36. Browder J.A. and Billingsley J.G., Regional obstructive lung disease in children, Amer. J. Dis. Child 1970, 119:322.
37. Gruenfield G.E. and Gray S,H., Malformations of the lung, Arch. Path 1941, 31: 392.

38. Santra A; *et al* Congenital lobar emphysema presenting late childhood; Lung India; 2014;31:302-04
39. Ceran S; *et al.* Congenital lobar emphysema-Is surgery routinely necessary? Afr. J Pediatric Surg; 2010;7:36-37
40. Abushalin AM; *et al.,* Bilateral congenital lobar emphysema– a rare cause for respiratory distress in infancy; Anu Thor Med; 2012;7:250-52
41. Khan A., *et al.,* Scimitar syndrome: PG Med J 2005;8:216.
42. Mordue B.C., A case series of five infants with scimitar syndrome: Adv Neonatal care 2003: 3: 121-32.
43. Reddy R., *et al.,* Scimitar syndrome—A rare cause of hemoptysis; Eur J Cardiothoracic Surg 2002; 22: 821.
44. Vyas S., *et al.,* Pseudo-Scimitar syndrome; Lung India 2012;29:363-65.
45. Bhupali A.K., *et al.,* Use of 64 slice CT in scimitar syndrome; JAPI 2010; 58: 698-700.
46. Wang C.C., *et al.,* Scimitar syndrome—incidence, treatment and prognosis; Eur J Pediat 2008;167:155-60.
47. Sinha R, *et al.,* Scimitar syndrome—Imaging by M.R. angiography and doppler echocardiography: Ind J Chest Dis All Sci 2004; 46; 283-86.
48. Fredman R.M., Burrows P.E. and Moes C.P.F., Amer. Jour. Roentgenol 1986,146:211-15.
49. Crotfon and Douglas' Respiratory Diseases; Seaton A., Seaton D. and Gordon Leitch A., Ed, 4th Ed; 1989; Oxford University Press, Delhi.
50. Siewart A.K., Berlin Munchen Tieraerztl Wochenschr 1904;2: 139-41.
51. Kartagener M., Beitr Klin Tuberk 1933;83:489-501.
52. Afzelius B.A., A human syndrome caused by immotile cilia; Science 1976;193:317-19.
53. Gmner P., *et al.,* Evidence for congenitally non-functioning cilia in the tracheo-bronchial tract in two subjects; Amer Rev Resp Dis 1975; 112: 807-809.
54. Rossman C.M., *et al.,* The dyskinetic cilia syndrome; Chest 1980;78:580-82.
55. Lie H, Ferkol T., Primary ciliary dyskinesia–recent advances in pathogenesis, diagnosis and treatment; Drugs 2007; 67: 1883-92.
56. Gary A., *et al.,* Primary ciliary dyskinesia–An underdiagnosed entity; JAPI 2010; 58: 704-06.
57. Rutland J. and Cole P.J., Non-invasive sampling of nasal cilia for measurement of beat frequency and study of ultra structure; Lancet 1980; 2: 564-65.
58. Sturgess I.J., *et al.,* Transposition of ciliary microtubules; New Eng J. Med 1980; 303: 318.
59. Cole P.J., *et al.,* Cilia in local host defence; Eurp J.Resp Dis 1983 (suppl); 126:64,31.
60. Kapur V., *et al,* Kartagener's Syndrome; Lancet 2009;373:1973.
61. Eavey R.D., *et al.,* Kartagener's syndrome:A blinded controlled study of cilia ultrastructure;Arch Otolaryngol 1986;112: 646-50.
62. Shukla V., *et al.,* An unusual presentation of kartagener's syndrome; JAPI 2011; 59: 266-67.
63. Mishra M., Kartagener's syndrome–A case series; Lung India 2012;29:366-69.
64. Stanley P., *et al.,* Etticacy of a Sachharin test for screening to detect abnormal mucociliary clearance;Brit J.Dis Chest 1984; 78:62.
65. Joshi J.M., Kamble R.T., Clinical spectrum of DCS; JAPI 1997;45:699-700.
66. Dutta G., *et al.,* A case of primary ciliary dyskinesia with pulmonary arterial hypertension responding to oral sildenafil; JAPI 2011; 59:738-40.
67. Shah A.D., *et al.,* Bochdalek hernia with intrathoracic kidney; Lung India 2012;29:273-75.

CYSTIC FIBROSIS (CF)

Introduction

Cystic fibrosis is a severe, autosomal recessive disease affecting one in 2500 live births in the British population. The clinical expression of cystic fibrosis is variable, although most patients show progressive pulmonary disease and pancreatic insufficiency with malabsorption. The average life expectancy for people with cystic fibrosis is 20 years, but these data relate to patients who were first treated more than 20 years ago and there have been considerable advances in treatment since then.[1] The carrier frequency in the British population is approximately one in 25; as for all autosomal recessive disorders, most infants with cystic fibrosis are born into families with no previous history of the disorder. The gene mutated in cystic fibrosis has been shown to code for the cystic firbosis transmembrane regulator.[2-4] A three base pair deletion at position 508 of the protein accounts for about 78% of cystic fibrosis mutations in the British population.[5] Two point mutations, G551D and R553X,[6] account for a further 4% of cystic fibrosis mutations. These three mutations can be detected simultaneously by using the polymerase chain reaction, which will identify approximately 82% of carriers in the population. A simple mouthwash test serves as a reliable method of obtaining DNA for such an analysis.

Cystic fibrosis is the most frequent lethal genetic syndrome amongst White children and now it is not so rare among Indians. The occurrence has been estimated at 1:600 in Namibian Dutch Africaaners, 1:15 in Italians, 1:2000 in Caucasians, 1:17,000 in American Blacks, and 1:90,000 in Orientals.[7] An autosomal recessive inherited generalised systemic disorder, cystic fibrosis has no link with the blood groups of HLA antigens. It consists of a triad of chronic pulmonary diseases, pancreatic insufficiency and increased electrolytes in the sweat.[8] It occurs in 25% of siblings of an index case. It is not uncommon in India and cases are being regularly diagnosed in centres where physician's awareness to this diagnosis is higher. Possible reasons for underdiagnosis of this disorder in developing nations are varied clinical spectrum of the disorder, and lack of facilities such as sweat chloride estimation and molecular diagnosis kits. In the Madras series the youngest was aged two years and six months while the oldest was 48 years. In heterozygous carrier parents, children have 1:4 chances of being homozygous for cystic fibrosis.[7]

Next to asthma, CF is the most common cause of obstructive airways in youngsters. The carrier rate of the CF gene among European Caucasions is 1:25. In the United States approximately 5% of the population (10 million) are carriers. The exact incidence in India is not known, though few report in Indian literature confirm that it is not as rare a disease as believed.[9-10] Recently, first report of cystic fibrosis multiplex occurring in the same family is reported.[11]

Antimicrobials should be started early when cough develops into nocturnal or productive cough and lung symptoms and signs increase despite normothermia. The most troublesome bacteria in CF is Pseudomonas aeruginosa, occurring in 6-10% of normal population and 80-90% of patients at CF centres. For biliary diseases ursodeoxycholic acid, 15-25 mg/kg/day has been found useful. Variceal bleeding is controlled with somatostatin and octreotide. Vasopressin is also effective in this condition.

For lungs destroyed by cystic fibrosis, lung, heart lung and double lung transplants have been tried. The major complications have included acute rejection, opportunistic lung infections and obliterative bronchiolitis.

Aetiology and Pathology[12]

This common genetic disorder of childhood respiratory system is transmitted as an autosomal recessive trait and usually manifests its symptomatology in homozygous persons at an early age. There is widespread involvement of exocrine glands leading to thickened secretions whose basic defect is not known exactly. However, it is known to result in alterations of cellular chloride transport and measureable potential differences across the membranes of affected cells.

Eosinophilic solidified secretions block the intralobular pancreatic ducts leading to cystic dilation of ducts, atrophy of acini and diffuse fibrosis. Similar changes may occur in intra-hepatic biliary ducts and gallbladder. The exocrine defect also affects reproductive system and sweat glands.

In the respiratory tract and alimentary tract the mucous secreting glands may be distended with hypersecretion. At birth the lungs are normal, Later there is hypertrophy of mucous glands and goblet cells. The viscid mucous secretion with greatly elevated flow viscosity causes partial or complete obstruction of smaller bronchi and bronchioles. It results in impaired ventilation, air trapping and impaired ciliary clearance machanism. The stagnant secretion with *p*-hydroxy phenyl acetic acid provides a good *nidus* for growth of bacteria especially Staphylococcus aureus and Pseudomonas aeruginosa. They cause a low grade, persistent infection and enhance the secretion and mucosal oedema, thus accentuating the obstruction. Such recumbent episodes destory the cilia and cause squamous metaplasia. The wall of the bronchioles and bronchi are weakened leading to bronchiolectasis and bronchiectasis. Aspergillus fumigatus can invade the damaged bronchial passages and induce hypersensitivity.

Clinical Features

The clinical features in cystic fibrosis are due to two basic abnormalities,[7] production and physiochemical behaviour of mucous causing obstruction of ducts in various organs[9] and increased secretions of chloride, sodium and potassium (to some extent) from the sweat glands, possibly due to reduced reabsorption by duct cells.[13]

The pulmonary manifestations appear in infancy following a respiratory infection, presenting with persistent cough, expectoration of purulent viscid sputum, tachypnoea,[14] wheeze (shortness of breath), haemoptysis and pneumothorax. The episodes are recurrent. Staphylococcus aureus and Pseudomonas aeruginosa are the dominant organisms in cystic fibrosis.[15]

Nasal sinuses are frequently involved. Even nasal polypi develop in 10 per cent of the cases. Pancreatic insufficiency presenting malabsorption, weight loss, stunted growth, protuberant abdomen and steatorrhoea may be associated. Non-pulmonary changes are slow dark adaptation of the pupil, biliary cirrhosis or fatty changes in the liver, the circulatory collapse, male infertility (absence of spermatozoa in 80-90% cases) and fertility in females is markedly reduced but those reaching adulthood are fertile.[16] The physical signs include cyanosis, clubbed digits a barrel shaped chest and signs of consolidation or collapse and crepitations. Differential diagnosis include ciliary dyskinesis syndrome. Impaired mucociliary transport in cystic fibrosis is essentially due to thick and viscid secretion. It is not associated with ultrastructural defects in ciliated cells.[12] Some cases of cystic fibrosis mutations may have milder clinical course.[17] Its diagnosis should be considered in an adult with bronchiectasis or a child with asthma as differential diagnosis and should be looked for high levels of sweat chloride. 94% of Indian patients have respiratory dysfunction. Knowledge about all mutations, molecular screening and subsequent genetic counseling shall be a right step forward.

Investigations

Chest X-ray shows collapse or consolidation with peripheral mottling. Widespread bronchiectasis may be present (Table 2.1). Pulmonary functions show increased airflow resistance, in the form of obstructive pattern with reduced flow rates and deceased compliance. Hypoxaemia present may be disproportionate to the lung destruction.

Table 2.1: X-rays finding in cystic fibrosis

1. Small ill-defined consolidation, maximal in the upper zones with or without cavitation.
2. Bronchial wall thickening and the signs of bronchiectasis both usually maximal in the upper zones.
3. Evidence of airway obstruction.

The sheet anchor for diagnosis is sweat chloride estimation. It is carried out with pilocarpine or urocholine to stimulate the cholinergic sweat glands. Although simple, the test is subject to many possible errors. A laboratory with experience of doing the test frequently is the ideal choice, as very careful control of technique is essential. A flame photometer is used to estimate the Na levels and titrimetry for chloride levels. Chloride is a more reliable indicator, and has a better discriminatory capacity between CF and non-CF conditions.

A false positive sweat test could be due to number of reasons, including laboratory error, untreated adrenal insufficiency, ectodermal dysplasia, saccharoidosis and malnutrition. False negative results can occur in oedema. While doing the test it is important to ensure that evaporation does not decrease the sample size of the sweat. Sweat Na and Cl levels do not correlate with the severity of disease. Levels of 40-60 mmol/L are usually diagnostic in young children.

Definitive diagnosis is clinched when sweat chloride exceeds 60 mmol/L in a patient with (i) chronic obstructive pulmonary disease or (ii) exocrine pancreatic insufficiency or (iii) family history of cystic fibrosis. DNA methods provide absolute diagnostic proof, if two mutations are identified. In Caucasians about 70% of subjects with CF have the delta 508 deletion, compared to more than 50% of subjects in India.[18] A 30 mutations screening programme has recently been launched. DNA technology also offer prenatal diagnosis of the disorder, currently revised diagnostic criteria for CF include; presence of typical clinical features (respiratory, gastrointestinal or genitourinary) or a history of CF in a sibling, or a positive newborn screening test (Immunoreactive trypsinogen) plus two elevated sweat chloride levels obtained on separate days or identification of two CF mutations or an abnormal potential difference measurement.

There is high fecal content of free fatty acids and tyramine. The rectal suction biopsy shows widely dilated crypts filled with mucous.

The condition may progress leading to corpulmonale and respiratory failure. Early recognition and treatment prevents early occurrence of respiratory disability. The carrier of the gene can be recognised by culture of skin fibroblasts as they show metachromatic inclusions in the cells.[12]

The treatment includes towards improvement of general health, control of infections and maintenance of clear airways. The diet should have high protein, high calorie and low fat with supplemental fat soluble vitamins, pancreatic enzymes and additional salt during hot weather. The removal of viscid secretions from the airways has to be facilitated by regular chest physiotherapy involving postural drainage, clapping and aerosol inhalations. To clear the viscid secretions, antibiotics and aerosols containing mucolytic agents may be beneficial. Table 2.2 shows clinical signs, investigations and differential diagnoses.

Table 2.2: Cystic fibrosis (Fibrocystic disease)

Transmitted as an autosomal recessive trait, clinically characterized by fibrosis and cyst formation in pancrease and lungs.

- **Investigations:**
  Sweat chloride: High
  Faecal fat: High
  Serum pancreatic enzymes and B.immunoreactive trypsin: Low
- **Clinical signs:**
  Clubbing of fingers
  Salty taste to skin
  Haemoptysis
- **DO:**
  Chronic bronchitis
  Cirrhosis
  Malnutrition: Malabsorption syndrome

Antibiotics for Acute Infection

While there is general agreement that antibiotics should be used in high dosage and for adequate periods in the treatment of active infection, there are differing views on their use in the prevention of infection, some favouring continuous, others intermittent therapy.

Management of cystic fibrosis essentially includes antibiotic therapy, proper hydration, chest physiotherapy, postural drainage and management of obstructive lung disease.[19]

In the absence of Ps. aeruginosa, chest physiotherapy should be given frequently, and clearing of secretions may be aided by inhalation of saline given by aerosol. The choice of antibiotic should be related to the sensitivity of the pathogen isolated from the respiratory tract. Flucloxacillin, 12.5 mg/kg body weight given orally upto 1 g daily will be indicated in the majority of patients. If there is no clinical response lincomycin 50 mg/kg body weight upto 1 g daily, or sodium fusidate 20 mg/kg body weight per day in three divided doses may be substituted. Very rarely chloramphenicol 50 mg/kg weight upto 1 g daily if the paitent is gravely ill and not responding to other agents may be given for two to three weeks monitoring the total cell count in blood.

When the patient is vomiting or severely ill, antibiotics may be given intravenously. Treatment should be continued for a month after the pulmonary infection is considered to have cleared. To avoid the emergence of resistant strains of staphylococcus, it is recommended that sodium fusidate should always be used in combination with another anti-staphylococcal drug.

When sputum culture is positive for Ps. aeruginosa, some of these patients respond to frequent intensive physiotherapy but if they are acutely ill, intravenous gentamicin 6-8 mg/kg body weight daily in three divided doses alone or combined with carbenicillin 200-400 mg/kg body weight in six divided daily doses should be given.

When these antibiotics are given together, their effect appears to be additive. Gentamicin dosage should be adjusted. Blood urea should be checked before starting therapy. Probenecid 0.5-1 g daily will delay renal excretion of carbenicillin and so raise blood levels. Gentamicin and carbenicillin should not be mixed together for administration. Both antibiotics should be given by separate injection slowly over 15-20 minutes.

In certain advanced centres, especially in the States, gene therapy for cystic fibrosis has been attempted. This has followed identification of the CF gene, in the long arm of chromosome 7 band q-31. The most common mutation is F508 (phenyl alamine deleted in the 508th position). It is found in upto 75% of affected individuals in some ethnic European populations. Others have various sub sets, such as, CF-PS, indicating sufficient functioning of the pancrease, and CF-Pl when there is pancreatic insufficiency. Table 2.3 gives brief information.

Table 2.3: Gene therapy for cystic fibrosis

Gene therapy is a new modality for cystic fibrosis (CF) and is to be widely tested in clinical trials all over the UK in the next three years.
The treatment advised for some cases of CF is DNase therapy, with the use of human DNase enzyme to clear the large quantities of DNA found in the lungs of patients with CF. The DNA accumulates in the lungs following destruction of inflammatory cells. It increases the mucosal viscosity and inhibits antibiotics from acting effectively. It has shown promising results in a study at the National Heart and Lung Institute, London, UK. However, researchers feel that gene therapy is not a magic wand; it may be ineffective in major manifestations of cystic fibrosis including male infertility and gastrointestinal disorders. Alternative and complementary therapies must also be developed.

Ref.: Bio Med; 1994; 2(1): 11.

The nutrition balance is often disturbed in CF. This is caused by malabsorption due to obstruction in the pancreatic duct and absence of enzymes in the gut lumen, as well as reduced intake due to anorexia, abdominal symptoms and depression and increased energy expenditure due to advanced lung disease.

To correct the nutritional balance, dietary intake upto 150% of the caloric requirement, by elemental, semi-elemental or poly food products increase may be required. Permanent feeding by gastrotomy is rarely required.

Cystic Fibrosis and Gene Therapy: Viewpoint

Patients suffering from cystic fibrosis have a defective copy of the gene that normally enables cells to construct the channel by which chloride can pass in and out of cells. As a result, salt accumulates in the cells lining the lungs and digestive tissues, turning the surrounding mucus into a sticky suffocating paste. Therapy available today includes antibiotics which help to control the respiratory infections. Slapping and pounding can also help to dislodge some mucus from the blocked airways. But the destruction continues.

Splicing the normal gene into the cold viruses caused the gene to become active, thus preventing build up of mucus. The cells that acquire the new gene would start manufacturing their own chloride channels and start excreting normally. Gene therapy shall transform life forever. In cystic fibrosis, respiratory epithelium is being targeted via liposome and adenovirus for transmembrane regulatory enzyme replacement.

Prophylaxis

Antibiotics prescribed for prophylaxis should be given in the full therapeutic dose. In the first year of life continuous antibiotic therapy is recommended even in the absence of overt symptoms, and because, *Staph. aureus* appears to have a predilection for the lungs of children with cystic fibrosis, an antibiotic effective against this pathogen must be given. Erythromycin when given for prolonged periods has the advantage of being palatable and of causing less gastrointestinal upset in infants than flucloxacillin. It is also effective against H. influenzae which may be present.

Flucloxacillin is the antibiotic of choice when staphylococcus has been shown to be resistant to erythromycin. All antibiotics may cause diarrhoea but erythromycin less frequently than flucloxacillin. The estolate preparation causes jaundice and should be avoided.

After the age of one year continuous antibiotic, therapy may be discontinued if the patient has no persistent cough, his chest radiograph is clear with no pathogens grown from a cough swab, and is thriving. The patient should be reviewed about every two months. Erythromycin or flucloxacillin should be started at the onset of any kind of respiratory tract infections and given for at least one week, or longer if symptoms persist or signs develop in the lower respiratory tract.When there is evidence of chronic infection and productive cough and/or changes on chest radiograph, continuous antibiotic therapy should be given and continued into the pre-school and early school years.

In later school life (after about eight years of age) continuous therapy may be discontinued. Should there be an increase in cough or volume of sputum and/or a poor weight gain, a return to continuous therapy may be necessary.

Aerosols

Some clinicians consider that certain aerosols play a part in the treatment of the respiratory symptoms.

Aerosols may be used to administer:

(i) *Moisture:* This helps loosen secretions. For this purpose normal saline is nebulized and inhaled for 10 minutes (2 ml approx) before physiotherapy.

(ii) *Bronchodilators:* For this an equal quantity of saline and salbutamol 0.5 per cent solution (1-3 ml) is given, but it should only be used when there is evidence of reversible airways obstruction.

(iii) *Antibiotics:* Cloxacillin 125 mg in 3 ml of saline or gentamicin sulphate 40-80 mg diluted to 3 ml is administered with water. Neomycin sulphate 250-500 mg in 3 ml of normal saline may be given twice daily after physiotherapy. Neomycin is active against both staphylococci and some Gram negative organism, but it is ototoxic and high tone deafness occurs with prolonged use. Therefore, hearing should be tested at two to three monthly intervals during treatment.

(iv) *Mucolytic agents:* N-acetylcysteine-2 ml of a 10 per cent solution, may be given before physiotherapy. It can be irritating and has an unpleasant smell. Mucolytic agents such as bromhexine hydrochloride or carboxymethyl cyste in have not been proved to have any long-term value in cystic fibrosis.

Pancreatic Enzymes and Vitamin Supplements

These should not be given unless there is pancreatic dysfunction. Extra salt is only indicated if there is excessive sweating, as occurs in febrile illness or during a prolonged heat wave.

Fat soluble Vitamin A 5000-10000 units and Vitamin D 500-1000 units (twice the usually recommended dose according to age), should be given daily. Vitamin K may be given if the prothrombin time is prolonged. Blood levels of Vitamin E are frequently low but the clinical significance is unknown.

Immunization

Immunization against diphtheria, pertussis, tetanus, and poliomyelitis should be performed at the appropriate ages and with the usual exceptions and precautions.

Live measles vaccination is strongly advised as pulmonary complications following measles may be serious. It should be given at one year of age. Prior to vaccination a patient in contact with measles should be given protective gammaglobulin.

Influenza vaccination is recommended if the particular virus responsible for an epidemic is identified and an appropriate vaccine is available. Respiratory viruses, particularly influenza viruses, cause infective respiratory exacerbations and deterioration of pulmonary function in patient with cystic fibrosis.[21] Moreover, these patients have an increased risk of dying from influenza or its complications.[22] The vaccine is well tolerated. The most common side effect in the patients can be pain at the injection site. No infective pulmonary exacerbation has been recorded. An active annual influenza vaccination programme is suggested.

The uptake of cystic fibrosis carrier testing in the community is high through general practices (66%) or family planning clinics (87)%. Screening by inivitation letter achieves a much lower uptake (10%). This is in line with findings from other screening programmes.[23]

Knowledge of cystic fibrosis in the community is limited, as the previous studies have shown.[24,25] Good educational material on genetics in general and cystic fibrosis in particular is lacking. The main aim or cystic fibrosis screening is to allow couples to make fully informed reproductive choices. These could include choice of partner, whether or not to have children, egg or sperm donation, adoption, antenatal diagnosis with or without termination of affected pregnancies, or choosing to have children without using the information. Couples may opt not to have children. A prenatal test to determine whether or not the foetus was affected can be done.

Screening programmes have the potential to do more harm than good if those who test positive either do not receive adequate counselling or remain anxious or distressed.[26,27] Therefore, a small proportion of carriers whose needs are not met by the combination of education and counselling offered at present, new areas need be explored.

With the discovery of cystic fibrosis gene,[28,29] prenatal screening for CF is now possible with restriction fragment length polymorphism. Screening the population for the CF gene has also become feasible. The ultimate solution is to inform all concerned, educate all concerned, counsel prospective couples, support the family and consider all the ethical issues. Early detection and management results in longer survival.

Lung transplantation in cystic fibrosis gives a short-term survival rate of 70% in the experienced centres.[30,31]

Most important aspect of cystic fibrosis includes to suspect the disease in a red scaly infant who fails to thrive, anemic, odematous and hypoproteinemic.[32] Recognition of rash as a sign of cystic fibrosis complicated by protein energy malnutrition (PEM) will allow an early diagnosis, treatment and subsequently improve the outcome in such patients. PEM is reported to be upto 13% of infants with cystic fibrosis, especially in early 6 months of life, and is associated with high morbidity and mortality.[32-37] It has, therefore, been proposed to include cystic fibrosis among the differential diagnosis of nutritional dermatoses of infancy, especially when there is a failure to thrive, odema and hypoproteinemia are also present.[38]

REFERENCES

1. Royal College of Physicians. *Cystic fibrosis in adults.* RCP, London; 1990.
2. Rommens J.M., Iannuzi M.C., Kerem B.S., *et al.*, Identification of the cystic fibrosis gene: Chromosome walking and jumping, Science 1989;245:1059-65.
3. Riordan J.R., Rommens J.M., Kere m B.S., *et al.* Identification of the cystic fibrosis gene: cloning and characterisation of complementary DNA, Science 1989; 245: 1066-72.
4. Kerem B.S., Rommens J.M., Buchanan J.A., *et al.* Identification of the cystic fibrosis gene: genetic analysis, Science 1989, 245: 1073-80.
5. Watson E.K., Mayal E.S., Simova L, *et al.* The incidence of Delta F 508 CF mutation and associated haplotypes in a sample of English families, Hum Genes 1990; 85: 435-36.
6. Cutting G.R., Kasch L.M., Rosenstein B.J., *et al.* A cluster of cystic fibrosis mutations in the first nucleotide binding fold of the cystic fibrosis conductance regulator protein, Nature 1990,346:366-69.
7. Scanlin T.F., Cystic fibrosis in pulmonary diseases and disorders, Fishman A.P., (ED), McGraw-Hill Book Co. 2nd Ed 1988, 2: 1273.
8. Mahashur A.A., Cystic Fibrosis (Editorial), JAPI 1993, 41: 71-72.
9. Deivanayagam C.N. *et al.* A clinical profile of cystic fibrosis in South India; *Lung India* 1990; 8: 167-72.
10. Reddy C.R.R.M., *et al.*, Cystic fibrosis of pancrease in India, J Peditr 1969, 75.
11. Narsingan S.N. *et al.* Two cases of cystic fibrosis in one family, JAPI 1993, 41:111-12.
12. Shankar P.S., Chest medicine, 4th Ed., Oxford and IBH Pub. Co., New Delhi 1994.
13. Schultz I.J., Micropuncture studies of sweat formation in cystic fibrosis patients, J Clin Invest 1969, 48: 1470-77.
14. Browning Gilbert E. and Tobin M., Importance of respiratory rate as an indicator of respiratory dysfunction in patients with cystic fibrosis, Chest 1990, 97: 1317-21.
15. Hoiby N. and Kock C., Pseudomonas aeruginosa infection in cystic fibrosis and its management, Thorax 1990, 45:881-84.
16. Kerem *et al.* and Lynch A., Screening for cystic fibrosis, ethical and social issues, Amer Rev Resp Disease 1991, 143: 457-60.
17. Santra G, Banergee S., Adult cystic fibrosis—A rare diagnosis from India; JAPI 2012;60:45-47.
18. Ashavaid T.F., *et al.*, Cystic fibrosis in India—A systemic review; JAPI 2012; 60: 39-41.
19. Prayor J.A. *et al.*, Effect of chest physiotherapy in oxygen saturation in patients with cystic fibrosis, Thorax 1990, 45: 77.
20. Misra S., Human gene therapy—A brief overview of the genetic revolution; JAPI 2013;61:41-47.
21. Ong E.L.C., Ellis M.E., Webb A.K., Neal K.R., Dodd M., Caul E.L., *et al.* Infective respiratory exacerbations in young adults with cystic fibrosis, role of viruses and atypical microorganisms, Thorax 1989,44: 739-42.
22. Eickhoff T.C., Sherman I.L. and Serfling R.E., Observations on excess mortality associated with epidemic influenza, JAMA 1961, 176: 776-82.
23. Thompson T.C., Inviting infrequent attenders to attend for a health check: Costs and benefits, Br. J. Gen. Pract 1990;40.
24. Williamson R., Allison M., Bently T., *et al.*, Community attitudes to cystic fibrosis carrier testing in England: A pilot study, Prenatal Diagnosis 1989; 9: 727-34.
25. Watson E.K., Silliamson R. and Chapple J. Attitudes to carrier screening for cystic fibrosis, Br. J. Gen. Pract 1991, 41: 237-40.
26. Skrabanek P., Preventive medicine and mortality. Lancet 1986, i: 143-44.
27. Mant D. and Fowler G., Mass screening: Theory and ethics. BMJ 1990, 300: 916-18.
28. Rommeno J.M., *et al.*, Identification of the cystic fibrosis gene: Chromosome. Walking and jumping, Science 1989, 245: 1059-65.
29. B. Nadler H.L., *et al.*, Prenatal detection of cystic fibrosis, Lancet 1981,2: 122-26.
30. Geddes G.M. and Hodsen M.E., The role of heart and lung transplantation in the treatment of lung cystic fibrosis, J Roy Soc Med 1989, 82 (Suppl), 16: 49-53.
31. Scott J., *et al.*, Heart lung transplantation for cystic fibrosis, Lancet 1988, 2: 192-94.
32. Abdman S.H., Accurso F.J., Bowman C.M., Persistent morbidity and mortality of protein calorie malnutrition in young infants with cystic fibrosis. J. Pediatr. Gastroenterol Nutr 1986, 5: 393-396.
33. Fleischer D.S., DiGeorge A.M., Barness L.A. and Cornfeld D., Hypoproteinemia and edema in infants with cystic fibrosis of the pancreas, J. Pediatr 1964, 64: 341-348.
34. Lee P.A., Roloff D.W. and Howatt W.F., Hypoproteinemia and anemia in infants with cystic fibrosis. JAMA 1974, 228: 585-588.
35. Lloyd-Still J.D., Khaw K.T. and Schwachman H., Severe respiratory distress in infants with cystic fibrosis. Pediatrics 1974,53:678-682.
36. Abman S.H., Reardon M.C., Accurso F.J., Hammond K.B. and Sokol R.J., Hypoalbuminemia at diagnosis as a marker for severe respiratory course in infants with cystic fibrosis identified by newborn screening. J. Pediatr 1985,107: 933-935.
37. Abman S.H., Accurso F.J. and Sokol R.J., Hypoalbuminemia in young infants with cystic fibrosis. J. Pediatr 1990,116: 840-841.

38. Darmstadt G.L, Schmidt C.P., Wechsler D.S., *et al.*, Dermatitis as a presenting sign of cystic fibrosis, JAMA India 1993, 13: 107-116.

PULMONARY ARTERIOVENOUS FISTULA[1-6]

Fistulous vascular pulmonary communication may be large and multiple or localized or scattered and small. Associated with angiomas in the liver, gastrointestinal tract including buccal mucosa and nasal mucosa, these may form part of hereditary hemorrhagic telangiectasia (Rendu-Osler-Weber syndrome) which accounts for half of the cases reported. Diagnosis is easy in 20% of cases presenting clinically with dyspnoea (in 31-67% of cases), cyanosis, polycythemia and clubbing, especially seen with large fistulae. 50% of patients may have features of Rendu-Osler-Weber syndrome with recurrent epistaxis, gastro-intestinal bleeding, dizziness, diplopia, aphasia, convulsions etc. Rarely a massive haemoptysis may occur. Complications occur at least in 25% of all patients, locally as haemothorax and cerebral thrombosis as a consequence of polycythemia. Condition is slightly more in females, usually single, and the malformation is closely related to the pleura, oftenly involving the lower lobes. Chest X-ray shows opacities due to large fistulae. Small fistulae can be visualized as abnormal pulsations by fluoroscopy or tomography. The site, size, extent and distribution of the fistulae can be demonstrated by bilateral pulmonary angiography which remains gold standard investigation. Non-surgical methods include embolization or occlusion procedures, using balloons and steel coils. This embolotherapy has 'easy to repeat' advantage over surgery and achieves goals of therapy in improving dyspnoea, preventing lung haemorrhage and preventing neurological sequelae. Complications of embolotherapy include self-limiting pleurisy, air embolism and paradoxical embolisation of the device. Surgical excision of solitary localised lesion by lobectomy or wedge resection is useful. But postoperative reappearance of small fistulae occurs even after extensive pulmonary resection. Cyanotic patients with multiple fistulae are inoperable.

REFERENCES

1. Khurshid I., Downie G.H., PA malformation; PG Med J 2002; 78: 191-97.
2. Montani D., *et al.,* Fatal rupture of pulmonary arteriovenous malformation in hereditary haemorrhagic telangiectasis and severe PAH; Eurp Respir Rev 2009; 18:42-46.
3. Brown S.E., Wright P.W., *et al.,* Staged bilateral thoracotomies for multiple pulmonary AV malformation complicating hereditary hemorrhagic telangiectasis J. Thorac. Cardiovasc. Surg 1982, 83: 285.
4. White R.J. Jr *et al.* PA malformations: Diagnosis and trans catheter embolotherapy; J Vas Interv Radio 1996; 7: 787-804.
5. Kundu S., Life threatening haemothorax–A rare presentation of pulmonary arteriovenous malformation; JAPI 2010; 58: 695-98.
6. Saxena S., *et al.*, PA malformation treated with embolotherapy: JAPI 2003; 51; 398-400.

PRIMARY PULMONARY HYPERTENSION

This is a disease of unknown origin where hypertension of lesser circulation along with right sided heart failure occurs.[1] Disease is rare in childhood but can be seen at any age.

Atherosclerotic changes and thickened antrima of pulmonary arterioles and arteries with hyperplasia of muscular and elastic tissues, causing pre-capillary obstruction of the pulmonary vascular bed and leading to pulmonary hypertension.

There is no evidence of emphysema, pancreatic fibrosis and hyposcoliosis, neither any cause of chronic corpulmonale can be detected. Recurrent pulmonary emboli and extreme obesity (Praeder-Willi syndrome) in adults and gross tonsillar and adenoidal hypertrophy and ventriculojugular shunt tube inserted for treating the hydrocephalus can also produce pulmonary hypertension, should be kept in mind.

Right sided heart failure with or without tricuspid insufficiency is the ultimate aftermath. The chain of changes include pulmonary artery aneurysmal dilatation and right ventricle resultant dilatation and hypertrophy respectively. There is hoarseness of voice from 2-70% of cases due to compression of left recurrent laryngeal nerve by the triangle formed by aorta, pulmonary artery and ligamentum arteriosum.[2-6]

Clincially

Clinical features include chest heaviness with or without pain, dizziness, with or without syncope and early fatigability. Peripheral extremities are cold and cyanotic. Jugular venous pressure is raised, hepatomegaly and odema follows as right sided heart failure develops. Heart is moderately enlarged with right apical tap. Thrills are absent and murmurs are insignificant. Soft systolic murmurs can be heard. First heart sound is ventricular apical followed by pulmonary ejection click. A presystolic gallop may be audible. Chest X-ray reveals prominent hilar pulmonary vascular markings compared to peripheral clear lung folds and right ventricle and pulmonary artery are also quite prominent (Table 2.4).

Table 2.4: X-ray findings in primary pulmonary hypertension

1. Right ventricle is enlarged.
2. The apex of the heart is lifted off the diaphragm.
3. Lateral view shows an all anterior enlargement without any displacement of lower oesophagus.
4. Features of pulmonary arterial hypertension are present like enlargement of pulmonary artery and hilar arteries with normal vessels within the lungs.

Diagnosis

Cardiac catheterisation is confirmatory. Right ventricular and pulmonary hypertension with normal pulmonary wedge pressure is demonstrated. Cardiac output is low and arterial oxygen saturation is normal. Eisenmenger's syndrome can be differentiated with cardiac catheterisation which demonstrates site, size and direction of the shunt. If reversed, intra-atrial shunt through foramen ovale is coexisting with primary pulmonary hypertension, the clinical picture of primary pulmonary hypertension shall simulate the Eisenmenger's syndrome. Pulmonary hypertension in SLE also simulate primary pulmonary hypertension[7,8] but it has a higher amount of antiphospholipid antibodies.[9-10] Pulmonary venous hypertension and left sided lesions with raised pulmonary venous hypertension can be differentiated as pulmonary wedge pressure is elevated significantly in these conditions.

Treatment and Outcome

The results of treatment are disappointing as the disease is progressive. Management of congestive cardiac failure gives relief.

REFERENCES

1. Wood P., Pulmonary hypertension. Med. Clin Cardiovas. Dis 1959;28:513.
2. Rich S., Primary pulmonary hypertension; Proc. Cardiovas. Dis 1988; 31:205-238.
3. Abraham M.T., Cherian G., Primary pulmonary hypertension in India; Ind. Heart Journ 1981;33:5-15.
4. Kinare S.G., Deshpande J., Primary pulmonary hypertension in India; Indian Heart Journ 1987;39:9-18.
5. Rajsekhar D., *et al.*, Primary pulmonary hypertension; Natural history and prognostic factors; Ind. Heart Journ 1994; 46: 165-170.
6. Shah K.D., Hoarseness of voice: A manifestation of primary pulmonary hypertension; JAPI 1997; 45: 629-630.
7. Asherson R.A. and Okley C.M., Pulmonary hypertension and SLE, J. Rheumatol 1986, 13: 1-3.
8. Asherson R.A., *et al.*, Immunological studies in primary idiopathic pulmonary hypertension. Eur. J. Rheum. Inflamm. 1984,7:75.
9. Mackworth Young Charles, Antiphospholipid antibodies, More than just a disease marker?Imm. Today 1990, 11:60-65.
10. Saluja S., Pulmonary hypertension, JAPI 1990,38: 878.

POLAND SYNDROME

It is characterized by unilateral chest wall hypoplasia and ipsilateral hand abnormalities having ipsilateral renal hypoplasia has been documented.[1]

REFERNECE

1. Gude D. *et al.*, Poland syndrome with a rare association; JAPI 2012;60;56-57.

PULMONARY ARTERY HYPOPLASIA[1,2]

It is a congenital abnormality of pulmonary artery, with compensatory hyperinflammation secondary to atelectasis, bronchial obstruction and unilateral acquired bronchiolitis (Swer-James-Macleod syndrome) or hypoplastic pulmonary artery with recurrent chest infections (Swer-James syndrome).

REFERNECES

1. Harkel A., Isolated unilateral absence of a pulmonary artery; Chest 2002; 122: 1471-77.
2. Sunavala A. J., *et al.*, Left pulmonary artery hypoplasia presenting with unilateral hyperluscent lung; JAPI 2011; 59: 179-81.

ALCAPA (Abnormal Left Coronary Artery Arising from Pulmonary Artery

Rarely seen in adults and adolescents; 1 in 3 lac births, where 90% of patients die in first year of life. Survival happens because of collaterals between left and right coronary system. Cardiomyopathy, ventricular arrythmia and death may occur. 10% only survive upto 2 decades of life. ECG shows inverted T in L_1, AVL and ST squaring in V_4-V_6. Surgical closure of coronary ostium from pulmonary artery help in improving survival.

HEMANGIOMA

Constitute 0.5% of all mediastinal tumours, originating from vascular endothelium, representing developmental malformations, rather than true tumours. No gender preponderance, 75% appear before the age of 35 years. 68% are located in anterior mediastinum. Surgical removal is preferred treatment modality.[1,2]

REFERNECES

1. Agarwal PP *et al.*, Case 130– Media stinal hemangioma; Radiology 2008;246;634-37.
2. Das A; *et al.*, Hemangioma in the posterior mediastinum; Lung India 2014;31:186-88.

Immunological Disorders

3

Immunological lung diseases involve immune effector mechanisms. These include bronchial asthma, hypersensitive pneumonitis, iatrogenic immunologic lung disease related to organ transplantation, following immunosuppressive therapy and those associated with AIDS. This also includes bronchogenic carcinoma and cystic fibrosis where degree of tissue destruction, and even survival are determined by immune response.

Immunological Lung Diseases

Gell and Coombs classification in brief is given below:

A. Hypersensitivity Reaction (HR) Type I—Immediate or anaphylaxis reaction within 10-30 minutes. IgE plays an important role, e.g., Asthma.
B. HR Type II—Cytotoxic tissue specific antibody IgG or IgM react with antigen using complement, presenting with symptoms of haemoptysis and rapidly progressing renal failure, e.g., Goodpasture's syndrome.
C. HR Type III—Due to immune complex formation both IgG and IgM involved. Smaller complexes, e.g., uremia, septicemia complexes contain complements, vasculitis and granuloma formation, e.g., Extrinsic allergic alveolitis, fibrosing alveolitis, connective tissue disease and polyarteritus.
D. HR Type IV—Reaction within 24-72 hours after exposure to antigen such as virus (varicella, mumps), bacteria (Mycobacteria-cum-tuberculosis), fungi and parasites. Tuberculin test is classic type IV reaction. Sarcoidosis graft-rejection and tumour immunity are other examples.

Immunological lung diseases that do not fit into a single Gell and Coombs category are as follows:

1. ABPA-Combine type I, III and IV reactions.
2. Chronic hypersensitivity pneumonitis-combine type III and IV.
3. HIV infection, organ transplant and lymphocytic interstitial lung diseases have some immunologic basis.
4. Local immune reactions in interstitial fibrosis.
5. Asthma is more than simply an IgE triggered anaphylaxis.

EXTRINSIC ALLERGIC ALVEOLITIS[1-5]

Hypersensitivity Pneumonitis

This is a kind of hypersensitivity alveolar reaction at the lung periphery that occurs in response to exposure to varied variety of organic dust particles. Often history of exposure to allergic agents like spores of fungi, vegetable material like barley, bagasse, hay etc. and animal proteins like avian, bovine and insect material is present.

Aetiology

The hypersensitivity reaction occurs in pre-sensitised persons on exposure to the antigen. The repeated exposures sensitises the nonatopic persons who are predominantly affected. The disease adopts a chronic course if the repeated exposures are containing high concentration of the antigen. Farmer's lung is the classical example which is described separately under occupational diseases. Other diseases of this kind include bagassosis and mushroom picker's lung (actinomycetes-M. faeni), malt worker's disease, cheese worker' s lung and coffee worker's lung (asperagillus clavatus P. casie and dust of coffee beans), sequoiosis (red wood saw dust), suberosis (coak dust), pituitary snuff taker's lung (bovine posterior pituitary extract), pigeon fancier's lung (pigeon and budgerigar droppings), etc. Improperly maintained air conditioners allow growth of thermophilic actinomycetes and other fungi causing humidifier pneumonitis which is described in Chapter 3.2.

Pathogenesis

A sequence of complex immunologic events occur due to sensitisation from a previous exposure to the antigen. An intense re-exposure causes an interaction between the antigen and the memory system. Precipitins and compliment fixing antibodies are formed which in turn lead to formation of immune complex aggregates of antigen and antibody, that are responsible for both pulmonary and systemic reactions. The symptoms appear only 3-8 hours after the exposure. Precipitins against the thermophilic actinomycetes are present in the serum. This suggests that the reactions are the result of an immune mediated Arthus reaction. Not that all those exposed to antigen developing antibodies would suffer, it is only a small number of persons who develop symptoms, depending upon the concentration of the antigen inhaled as well as host susceptability. The immune complexes are not present in the alveolar septa or in the granuloma. Possibly a mononuclear leucocyte mediated component plays a role in its pathogenesis.

A delayed type of hypersensitivity reaction also plays a role in the development of chronic disease, which is further supported by the presense of large number of lymphocytes in the BAL fluid. This stresses the role of local sensitivity in the development of the disease.

Pathology

There is inflammatory reaction in the walls of alveoli and the pulmonary interstitium, in the form of odema, transudation and exudation as well as leucocytic infiltration, followed by polymorphs and plasma cells. Later on non-caseating granulomas are formed because of interstitial and intra alveolar inflammation with mononuclear cells infiltration. Granulomas which are seen in the alveolar spaces and intra alveolar septa comprise macrophages, monocytes, lymphocytes and plasma cells. Where intense mononuclear activity is considered to be diagnostic, few foam cells and giant cells are also seen. The functional defect due to involvement of bronchioles and histological changes in the alveoli causing obstruction is sometimes referred as bronchiolo-alveolitis. Prolonged exposure may lead to diffuse interstitial fibrosis due to cellular infiltration of alveolar septa. An increased deposits of reticulin and collagen may convert granulomas into spherical scars. The process may end up into a **honeycomb lung** with cystic spaces surrounded by fibrous tissue and development of pulmonary hypertension and cor pulmonale due to obliteration of pulmonary arterioles.

Clinical Presentation

Clinically both systemic and pulmonary features are encountered. The systemic reactions appear within 3-4 hours of exposure and are similar to those infections. They include fever, chills, generalised pains and aches, headache, anorexia etc. Pulmonary symptoms include dyspnoea and chest tightness. Generally symptoms subside within 24 hours but persist if there is continued exposure to the antigen. There is history of rapid weight loss. Clinically there is irritating cough with progressive dyspnoea without wheeze. On examination, inspiratory basal crepts are present. The clinical manifestations directly depend upon the degree of intensity and frequency of exposure. Many a times patient is able to explain this symptom to be connected with dust exposure. Further stopping of exposure to the dust definitely cuts down serious disability of pulmonary illness. In case the exposure continues, the features of irreversible lung changes with fibrosis may develop without any features of acute illness. Ultimately features of right sided heart failure supervene.

Investigations

Positive skin reaction to relevant antigen is exhibited because of precipitins in the serum. The skin test may not be positive even in the presence of precipitins in the serum as in case of Farmer's lung. There is neutrophilic leucocytosis without eosinophilia. Serum IgG level is raised. Nevertheless a negative serologic and skin tests do not necessarily exclude the diagnosis of extrinsic allergic alveolitis.

BAL fluid analysis gives information regarding inflammatory events occurring in the interstitium of the lung in the form of increased lymphocytes with T suppressor cells. T/B cell ratio is also increased. IgG and IgM levels are also raised.

Two patterns are commonly seen on chest X-ray. Diffuse mottling (nodular shadows) affecting mid-zones and sparing both apices and bases, occurs in acute disease. Hilar nodes and pleura are not affected and unlike miliary tuberculosis, nodules do not have sharp and distinct borders. Lung volume is almost diminished in case of continued exposure but nodular shadows clear up if the exposure is stopped. Honeycomb changes are seen in advanced cases only. In case of budgerigar's lung, fibrosis occurs in the upper part of the lung, simulating chronic fibrosis of tuberculosis.

Lung biopsy shows infiltration of alveolar septa with lymphocytes, plasma cells and histiocytes. Pulmonary function tests in an acute disease, there is no airways obstruction and lung volumes FEV I, FVC and TLC are reduced. In chronic disease there is reduction in diffusion capacity to carbon monoxide (DLco). PaO_2 tension is low which decreases further on exercise. Alveolar-arterial oxygen gradient is lowered. $PaCO_2$ is normal or low. There is high minute ventilation at rest and on exercise.

Prevention and Treatment

These conditions are essentially preventable by avoiding exposure to inciting antigens. The acute episodes are self-terminating on stopping exposure to antigens. Continued exposure to antigen for a prolonged period leads to a progressive functional deterioration because of the development of structural pulmonary changes. A short course of corticosteroids give for

2-4 weeks and then gradually tapered off, hastens recovery but further stoppage of exposure to dust in early stages is the main stay in reverting to the original condition. In budgerigar's disease steroids are of no use. Even the withdrawal from contact with budgerigars brings limited improvement. However, the removal of contaminated humidifier or airconditioner does help in preventing humidifier lung disease. Differences from bronchial asthma are listed in Table 3.1.

Table 3.1: Distinguishing features

Bronchial Asthma	**Extrinsic Allergic Alveolitis**
1. Pulmonary involvement only	1. Pulmonary and severe systenic upsets
2. Rhonchi +++	2. Crepts +++
3. **Lung Function Test** Reversible air ways obstruction	3. **Lung Function Test** Restrictive pattern

REFERENCES

1. Shankar P.S., Extrinsic allergic alveolitis, IN, Chest Medicine, 4th ed, Oxford and IBH Publ. Co., N-Delhi, 1994.
2. Leatherman J.W., Michael A.F., Schwartz B.A. and Hoidal J.R., Lung cells in hypersensitivity pneumonitis; Ann Inter Med 1994; 100: 390.
3. Grant I.W.B., IN; *Current perspectives in the immunology of respiratory diseases,* Kay A.B. and Geotzl E.J. (ED) Churchill Livingstone, London, 1985.
4. Crofton and Douglas Resp. Diseases Seaton A, Seaton D and Gordon Leitch A; ED: 4th ed; 1989; Oxford University Press; Delhi.
5. Haslam P.L. *et al.*, Mast cells atypical lymphocytes and neutrophills in BAL in extrinsic energic alveolitis: Comparison with other interstitial lung diseases; Amer Rev Resp Dis 1987; 135: 35-47.

HUMIDIFIER DISEASE

Introduction

Humidifier disease is a lesser known clinical respiratory disease. There is fever with respiratory symptoms caused by contaminated water of humidifier system by certain algae, bacteria, fungi, etc. Humidifier disease was first described by Pestalozzi in 1959.[1] The common features are fever, cough, breathlessness and tiredness starting 4-12 hours after the beginning of exposure. The symptoms resolve spontaneously in one or two days. Patient is febrile and respiratory disease is attributable to humidification system contaminated with algae and bacteria as was reported in 1969 by Her Majesty's Inspector of Factories.[2]

There have been precipitating outbreaks of asthmatic attacks, Legionnaire's disease, etc. Humidification units may cause disease entity quite different from the classical extrinsic allergic alveolitis, known as humidifier disease, humidifier fever or humidifier lung. The vast use of desert cooler khas screens, etc. in our country is a potential source for such epidemics during summers. However, Indian reports in this context are conspicuously absent, probably due to lack of awareness rather than non-occurrence.

Clinical Features

The clinical features of humidifier disease are very similar to extrinsic allergic alveolitis. The incubation period of the disease is 4 to 8 hours after the exposure.

Symptoms include fever, cough, breathlessness, tight chest and discomfort, headache, and pain in joints. Fatigue and polyuria have also been reported by some investigators.[3] In occupational settings, the symptoms are generally reported on the first working day of the week. Diagnostic plan is shown in Table 3.2.

Table 3.2: Diagnosis of humidifier disease

1. Positive history of exposure	3. *Clinical Signs:* Inspiratory crepts
2. *Symptoms:*	4. *On Investigation:*
a. *Common* Malaise, Fever, Cough, Breathlessness	No-X-ray findings Polymorphonuclear leucocytosis PFT: Decreased lung diffusion
b. *Variable* Chest pain, Joint pain, Polyuria	

Chest examination reveals inspiratory crepts present at the bases of the lungs in acute episodes.

Investigations

Unlike extrinsic allergic alveolitis, radiographic abnormalities are generally absent in cases of humidifier disease. Polymorphonuclear leucocytosis is often detected on a peripheral blood smear examination.

History is most important. Suspected cases should be routinely investigated for history of exposure to humidified environment at home or at work. Lung diffusion capacities which may be reduced and may evince a restrictive pattern during an acute episode.

Inhalation provocation test and immunological investigation have been tried to demonstrate the aetiology and to isolate the responsible organism in outbreaks affecting many individuals. Bronchial provocation tests are carried out using water of the humidifiers or a freeze dried extract of the humidifier saline. Pickering *et al.*[4] carried out provocation tests using organism isolated from the humidified environment. However, these failed to elicit any response.

Demonstration of precipitating antibodies against micro-organisms found in humidifier water or in the environment confirm the exposure and although not diagnostic, yet it is a supportive evidence. Nordman[5] compared the prevalence of antibodies and symptoms in six outbreaks and found that precipitins could be found in 82-100 per cent of the affected subjects.

Conflicting reports exist about the usefulness of skin pricks test. Friend *et al.*[6] observed a positive reaction with freeze dried extract of humidifier water in 9 of the 15 exposed subjects and no reaction in 30 unexposed controls. However, other investigators were unable to elicit such reactions.[4,7]

Aetiology

A large variety of micro-organisms have been isolated from water in the humidifier and from surrounding environment, however causal relationship with majority of these could not be proved. Five organisms have been isolated during various outbreaks (Table 3.3). It has been suggested that the febrile illness might be caused by bacterial endotoxins or the soluble antigens might produce soluble aggregates and resultant complement consumption; whereas relatively insoluble antigens remain in the gas exchange region of the lungs and cause a granulomatous reaction. The pyrexial episodes of humidifier disease might represent the first stage in a sequence of events which ends in a full attack of extrinsic allergic alveolitis (Table 3.4). On the other hand a mechanism other than immune complex complement activation may be involved possibly via the alternate pathway.[8-12]

The fact that tolerance to endotoxins occurs during continued exposure and the tolerance is rapidly lost when the exposure is discontinued supports the endotoxin theory. The hypothesis was further supported by the findings of a well established epidemic of humidifier disease in Finland.[13] The role of fungal toxins in production of the disease has not been thoroughly investigated and needs to be examined in greater detail because in humid situations where organic matter is stored or handled, the growth of different fungi cannot be controlled.

The Occupational Factor

Outbreaks of this disease have been reported from printing presses, stationery and textile manufacturing units. Chances of outbreaks are more in industries where carefully controlled humidity is required. In the western countries, majority of the outbreaks have been reported to occur during winter months probably because of greater recirculation of heated air. However, in tropical countries the seasonality of the disease occurrence may vary in relation to climatic conditions and subsequent use of humidifiers.

Workers in certain industries in India where organic material is handled and also has high levels of environmental humidity, specially during particular seasons, are also at a high risk. In fact diseases with similar symptomatology have been reported by Clerk and Gupta[14] in small flour mills and in hemp processing units.[15] In workers of small flour mills the symptoms observed were cough, dyspnoea, chest discomfort with minimal clinical signs and no changes in X-ray picture. The authors attributed the disease to high levels of fungi and spores in the environment. Different species of Aspergillus and Rhizopus were detected in the ambient environment.[16]

In the hemp processing industry, hemp material and associated bacteria have been increminated. Vaccines prepared from these antigenic materials when used for immunotherapy resulted in a significant improvement of symptoms in the affected workers.[17] Further a number of outbreaks of humidifier disease have been reported from textile mills. The features of this disease are quite similar to mill fever reported among textile workers and therefore, an investigation of the relationship

Table 3.4: Differential diagnosis: Extrinsic allergic alveolitis

Humidifier disease differs from classical extrinsic allergic alveolitis in following ways:

1. The development of tolerance after continuous exposure and its loss following cessation of exposure is seen only in humidifier disease.
2. Radiographic changes are not seen in humidifier disease.
3. Occurrence of pulmonary fibrosis has not been demonstrated.
4. Humidifier disease may be triggered off by very small concentrations of the antigen.

Table 3.3: Organisms commonly found

Organism	*Source of infection*	*Reference*	
Protozoa	Humidifier water	Edwards	1980[3]
Pullularia	Water in home sauna	Metzger *et al.*	1976[9]
Flavobacterium	Humidifier water	Rylander *et al.*	1978[8]
Cephalosporium	Sewage flooding	Patterson *et al.*	1981[10]
	Humidifier water	Patterson *et al.*	1981[11]
Bacillus Subtillis	Water in printing factory	Parrot and Blyth	1980[12]

between humidifier disease and mill fever should also be investigated and a study of the prevalence of humidifier disease in other small high risk units.

Clinical Management

What mind does not know, eyes don't see. The clinician must be aware of this disorder and of the many different forms it may take. Though usually the disease resolves in 24 hours through development of tolerance, it may be a starting point for chronic respiratory disease and as such the patient needs to be properly monitored.

In the acute stage the patient should be given symptomatic treatment schedule. The treatment should be individualised so as to prevent complications or exacerbations of previously existing lung conditions.[18]

Prevention

Pulmonologists and industrial physicians can collaborate in this field.[19] Control of growth of organisms in humidifier systems is the sheet anchor of the preventive programme. The growth of the organisms can be suppressed or prevented by input water filters or by steam injection of water which avoids recirculation and cooling. Frequent cleaning of storage tanks may reduce but do not eliminate the growth of organisms. Disinfectants are contraindicated as they encourage the growth of some species of bacteria and are themselves likely to be inhaled.

Other measures can be periodic monitoring for microbial content of the environment in high risk industries and situations. Special precautions are required for control of bacterial growth in environments with humidity control and where large quantities of organic materials are stored or used.

REFERENCES

1. Pestalozzi C. Febrile Group erkrankungen in einer Mod ellschreinerei durch Inhalation von mit Schimmelpilzen kon taminiertem Befeuchterwkasser (Befeucherfieber). Schweiz. Med. Wochenschr 1959, 89:710-713.
2. HM Chief Inspector of Factories, Annual Report, London 1969.
3. Edward J.H., Microbial and immunological investigations and remedial action after an outbreak of humidifier fever. Br. J. Indu. Med 1980, 37: 55-62.
4. Pickering C.A.C., Moore W.K.S. Lacey J. Holford Streven Strevens V.C. and Pepys, J. Investigations of a respiratory disease associated with an air conditioning system, Clin. Allergy 1976, 6: 109-118.
5. Nordman H., Humidifier syndrome in occupational lung disease (ed Bernard J *et al.* Reven Press, New York 1984, 97-107.
6. Friend. J.A.R. Gaddie. J. Palmer, K.N.V., Pickering C.A.C. and Pepys, J., Extrinsic allergic alveolitis and contaminated cooling-water in a factory machine, Lancet 1977, 1: 297-303.
7. Newman-Taylor A. Pickering, CAL Turnerwarwick M. and Pepys J., Respiratory allergy to a factory humidifier contaminant presenting as pyrexia of undetermined origin, Br Med J 1978, 2:94-95.
8. Rylander R., Haglind P., Lundholm M., Mattsby L. and Stengist K., Humidifier fever and endotoxin exposure, Clin Allergy 1978, 8:511-516.
9. Metzger W.J., Patterson R., Fink J., Semerdjian R. and Roberts M. Hypersensitivity penumonitis due to contaminated water in a home sauna, J Am Med Ass 1976, 236 : 2209-2211.
10. Pattern R. Fink, J.N. Roberts, M. Kelly J.F. and Sommers H.M., Antibody activities in sera of patients with humidifier fever, J Allergy Clin Immunol 1978, 62: 103-108.
11. Patterson R., Fink J.N., Miles W.B., Kelly J.F., Schleuter D.B., Tinkelman D.G. and Roberts M., Hypersensitivity lung disease presumptively due to cephalosporium in homes contaminated by sewage flooding or by humidifier water, J Allergy Clin Immunol 1981, 68: 128-132.
12. Parrot W.F. and Blyth W. An other casual factor in the production of humidifier fever, J Soc Occup Med 1980, 30: 63-65.
13. Muittari A., Rylander R. and Salminoja-Sloanen, M., Endotoxins and bath-water fever, Lancet 1980, 2: 89.
14. Clerk S.H., Gupta B.N. Flour mill workers disease, ITRC Bull 1982, 3: 2-3.
15. Cislerk S.H., Gupta B.N. Mehrotra N.K. and Zaidi S.H., Hemp workers disease, Proceedings of the International Symposium on Industrial Toxicology, Lucknow Nov 4-7, 1975.
16. Gupta B.N. and Singh K.P., Mycological studies in small flour mills, Bio Mem 1983,8: 95-102.
17. Gupta B.M., Mehrotra N.K., Clerk S.H., Saxena A.K, George P.A., Chadra H. and Mahendra P.N., Immunotherapy in hemp workers having respiratory complaints. Ind J Med Sci 1980; 34: 72-85.
18. Srivastava A.K., Gupta B.N., Humidifier disease, A lesser known clinical entity, Ind J Clin Pract 1992, 2: 25-27, 50.
19. Bhatia R.S., Humidifier disease (Humidifier lung and humidifier fever); *Lung India* 1994, 12 (4): 198-200.

GOODPASTURE'S SYNDROME[1-6]

Introduction

Syndrome is characterised by recurrent episodes of pulmonary haemorrhage occurring rarely in association with or followed by development of glomerulonephritis, as mediated by antibody to basement membrane antigen. As such pulmonary haemorrhages can occur in glomerular diseases like Wegener's granulomatosis, systemic necrotizing vasculitis, SLE, cryoimmunoglobulinemia, Henoch-Schönlein purpura and in certain non-glomerular diseases like legionella infection (Table 3.5). The condition has been observed predominantly in young men.

Aetiology and Pathology

In 80 per cent of patients, a cytotoxic type II reaction mediated by antibodies reacting with basement membrane of the glomeruli

Table 3.5: Goodpasture's syndrome

Definition: Syndrome of pulmonary haemorrhages and renal failure due to damaged basement membranes in the kidney and lungs.
DD: Differential diagnosis
Bronchitis
Glomerulonephritis
Pneumonitis
Tuberculosis

and alveoli appear to be responsible for the condition and the capillary disruption which leads to haemorrhage, In a small number of patients immune complex disease may provoke the disorder.

Clinical Features and Investigations

The presenting symptoms is haemapyts's, and rapidly progressing renal failure. The condition presents with mild dyspnoea, cough and haemoptysis. Renal involvement consists of a rapidly progressive glomerulonephritis. There is evidence of microcytic hypochromic anaemia.

Hilar pulmonary infiltrates seen on chest X-ray predominantly in the lower lobes, though simulate the radiological appearance of idiopathic pulmonary haemosiderosis, are labile due to a rapid course of the disease. The diagnosis is established following needle biopsy of the kidney or transbronchial biopsy via a flexible fiberoptic bronchoscope. There may be a normal or focal proliferative and necrotizing glomerulonephritis. Extensive extracapillary proliferation (Crescents) is frequently seen.

This is a type II hypersensitivity reaction where there is an interaction with the basement membrane of the alveoli and that of the glomeruli of the kidney. Immunofluorescent staining demonstrates a linear pattern of deposits of antibasement membrane antibody immunoglobulin IgG and complement C_3 along the glomerular and alveolar basement membrane. The diagnosis is confirmed by radioimmunoassay which demonstrates that the antibodies eluted from involved tissues are specific for solubilised basement membrane from the lung and kidney. This is not demonstrable in those patients in whom immune complexes are playing a role in the pathogenesis. Electron-microscopic studies don't show electron dense deposits. Bronchoalveolar lavage shows haemosiderin-laden macrophages as a non-specific finding.

Prognosis

The course in variable, patient may have initial haemoptysis and a long-term remission or recurrent haemoptysis may occur and the glomerular disease may not progress, But in most of the cases, it is the progressive renal disease which becomes fulminant, leading to oliguric renal failure. The prognosis is grave with a life expectancy of less than two years if untreated.

Treatment

Treatment is essentially supportive that includes dialysis for renal failure, and oxygen and assisted ventilation for respiratory failure. Corticosteroids are given to control pulmonary haemorrhage. A combination of immunosuppressive agents and intensive plasma exchange (plasmapheresis) appear to be beneficial. The former eliminates or diminishes the production of cytotoxic antibodies and the latter helps in the removal of circulating antibody or immune complexes. In refractory cases with life threatening pulmonary haemorrhage, nephrectomy may benefit. Patient can best be managed with haemodialysis or/ and transplantation. Renal transplantation is considered when the level of circulating anti-basement membrane antibodies have vanished or decreased to undetectable levels.

REFERENCES

1. Salent D., Immunopathogenesis of crescentic glomerulonephritis and lung purpura, Kid Inter 1987,32:408.
2. Shankar P.S., *Goodpasture's Syndrome* , IN, Chest Medicine; Oxford and IBH Pub. Co. (P) Ltd, New Delhi, 1994, 4th ed.
3. Brenner B.M. and Rector F.C., Fd; Kidney; 3rd ed; Philadelphia; Saunders 1986; 1014-83.
4. Reynolds H.Y., Immunologic lung disease (Part I and II); Chest 1982; 81:626 and 745.
5. Harman E.M., Immunologic lung disease; Med Clin North Amer 1985; 69: 705.
6. Curtis J.L., Warnock M.L., New Concepts in the pathogenesis of immune lung injury; Sem Resp Med 1991; 12:156.

Respiratory Infections

4

VIRAL INFECTIONS OF RESPIRATORY SYSTEM

Viral infection of the respiratory tract is commonly encountered in all age groups the world over. Though the majority of these are benign and self-limiting, they are still responsible for greater mortality and morbidity in children, elderly persons and in patients with chronic diseases. The respiratory viruses produce a wide range of clinical responses and different clinical syndromes. The type of respiratory illness depends on the type of the cells affected in the respiratory tract. The involvement may be confined to the upper or lower respiratory tract or both. The important clinical syndromes in the upper respiratory passages are common cold, febrile cold, sore throat (pharyngitis, laryngitis), influenza, flu-like illness, tracheobronchitis and otitis media. The affections in the lower respiratory tract are croup, bronchiolitis, bronchitis and pneumonia.[1]

Viruses enter through the oronasal passages where they multiply and cause local inflammatory changes associated with oedema, secretion of mucous and necrosis of the cellular epithelium. There is involvement of the lymphadenoid tissue as well. The infection is of a temporary nature as it involves the surface except the adenoviral infections where the virus persists for some time in the deeper tissues.[2]

The existence of virus in the respiratory tract is pathological. The secretion of interferon in the nasal mucosa curtails the multiplication and spread of virus only to a certain extent as its effect is inhibited by oxygen. Most of viral infections show seasonal variance as they occur in the winter season, often assuming an epidemic form. Coxsackie and ECHO infections occur during summer. The infection from rhinoviruses is prevalent throughout the year. The viral infections invite the development of secondary bacterial infections.

Viral infections stimulate production of circulating IgG antibody and local IgA antibody, which are responsible for preventing reinfection as a blessing in disguise.[3] However, viral infections reccur frequently due to a decline in circulating antibody (IgG) level, variation in the antigenic configuration of viruses, existence of multiple serotypes, and low level of secretory antibodies (IgA) in the respiratory secretions during the subsequent infection from para-influenza and respiratory syncitial viruses, as there is no constant relationship between their levels in the serum and secretions. A majority of viral respiratory infections have no specific treatment.

The acute respiratory illnesses produced by respiratory viruses are shown in the Table 4.1.

Common Cold

Coryza[2,5-11]

An acute illness of short duration presents as an acute inflammation of the upper respiratory passages. The condition is frequently due to rhinoviruses. There are nearly 100 serologically distinct antigenic strains of the virus, hence there is life long susceptibility of man to the infection. They do not possess a common antigen. They grow in the presence of low temperature, acidic pH and oxygen, which are provided in the nasal mucosa. Other viruses like para-influenza, respiratory syncytical, ECHO 28 coronavirus and coxsackie A 21 are capable of producing similar illness.

The virus invades the nasal mucosa causing oedema and desquamation of epithelium. The sub-mucosa shows infiltration with polymorphs and lymphocytes. It spreads especially in an overcrowded atmosphere. The airbrone virus spreads through infected droplets.

Symptoms of nasal irritation, nasal stuffiness, sneezing, sore throat, the conjunctival irritation and watery nasal discharge occur after an incubation period of 48 to 72 hours. Later it becomes thick and mucopurulent. An irritant dry cough, husky voice, retrosternal discomfort and aches in the limbs occur, although condition is usually afebrile.

Table 4.1: Common viral respiratory infections [4]

Virus	*Common*	*Occasional*	*Infrequent*
Rhinovirus	Common cold	Bronchitis and asthma	Bronchopneumonia (in children)
Coronavirus	Common cold	Bronchitis and asthma	Bronchiolitis and pneumonitis
Respiratory syncytial virus	Bronchiotitis and pneumonitis (in children)	Common cold (in adults)	Pneumonitis (in elderly)
Parainfluenza viruses	Croup (in young children)	Common cold and pharyngitis	Bronchitis (in adults)
Adenoviruses	Common cold and pharyngitis (in children)	ARD	Pneumonia in children and immuno-suppressed patients
Influenza A	Flu like illness	Pneumonia	Pneumonia } synonymous
Influenza B	Flu like illness	Rhinitis and pharyngitis	Pneumonia } synonymous
Enterovirus	Non-specific febric illness	Rhinitis and pharyngitis	Pneumonia } synonymous
Herpes simplex virus	Gingiostomatitis (in children) and pharyngotonsilitis (in adults)	Pneumonitis	Disseminated infection (in immunocompromised patients)

Nasopharynx, sinuses, middle ear and the lower respiratory tract are affected. The role of corona viruses in lower respiratory tract infection is unclear. The infected mucosa is susceptible to secondary bacterial invasion. Routine laboratory tests are non-contributory.

The treatment is symptomatic. No specific antiviral treatment is available. The prophylactic vaccine offers little protection, rather its role has been questioned, due to multiplicity of antigenic strains. The secondary bacterial infection may require small doses of antibiotics. Intranasal spray of interferons is useful.

Feverish Cold[2,5,12,13]

Fever is not a feature in common colds and may be associated in some without severe nasal manifestations. It causes a great deal of weakness and prostration confining the patient to bed. It is more incapacitating than the common cold. The rhinoviruses, adenoviruses and influenza viruses are responsible for feverish cold.

Influenza[2,4,13-16]

Influenza is a highly infectious disease prevalent the world over, and causes great morbidity and high mortality.

Aetiology

Three antigenically distinct types of influenza group of myxoviruses are: A, B and C. The virus is antigenically unstable. The A strain is the usual cause of extensive outbreaks and is responsible for epidemics and pandemics, especially between months of October and April. The B strain causes small outbreaks in localised areas and it has no distinct seasonal pattern. There is no cross immunity between infections from A and B strains. The C strain occasionaly produces common cold and *does not affect the lower* respiratory tract.

It spreads through infected droplets. It involves predominantly the respiratory epithelium including nasopharynx, trachea and bronchi. Viral infection initially involves the ciliated columner epithelial cells, followed by alveolar cells, mucous gland cells and macrophages. There is oedema, hyperaemia and hypersecretion of the mucosa of the upper respiratory tract. There is also desquamation of the mucosa, ciliary damage of the trachea and bronchi, which predispose to the secondary bacterial infection and result in pneumonia. Degenerative changes can be seen histopathologically in the form of granulation, vacuolization, swelling and pyknotic nucleus, columner epithelium is replaced by flat and metaplastic epithelial cells. Primary viral infection itself may be responsible for occasional pneumonia. The severe constitutional symptoms appear to be due to viraemia. The exact pathogenesis of systemic symptoms remain unknown.

The diagnosis of the condition is easy during an epidemic. It spreads rapidly to all members of the family. After a short incubation period of one to two days the condition manifests as abrupt onset of fever, chills, malaise, headache, myalgia and anorexia. The fever may be associated with rhinitis and mild conjunctivitis, followed by a non-productive cough. The condition may progress to bronchitis and pneumonia. Fine crepitations are audible on auscultation of the chest. There is leucopaenia. In such cases complications like respiratory distress, cyanosis and death may supervene from peripheral circulatory failure or heart failure. High mortality is noted in middle-aged and elderly persons and those with cardio-respiratory diseases. The damage to the respiratory tract epithelium and defective clearance mechanism may lead to secondary pneumonia particularly with Streptococcus pneumoniae and Staphylococcus aureus, and may terminate fatally.

A four-fold rise in titre of complement fixing antibodies from acute to convalescent serum indicates recent influenza infection. Serum antibodies can be measured in the second week by haemaglutination inhibition neutralisation test, ELISA and anti-neuraminidase antibody assays also. There is no specific therapy and symptomatic treatment is given to relieve headache and body ache, cough and insomnia. Uncomplicated cases resolve within 2-5 days, with a post-influenzal asthenia in few patients. Even pulmonary function abnormality may persist. Antibiotics are given to counteract the secondary bacterial infections. Steroids are helpful in the treatment of shock and adrenal crisis but their use in routine is responsible for many complications.

Complications occur as a result of bacterial infections. Fibrin thrombi in alveolar capillaries along with haemorrhages and necrosis have been documented.[4] Eosinophilic hyaline membranes may also be found lining in alveolar ducts. Primary influenza has a predilection for those with mitral stenosis and with chronic pulmonary disorders. Rey's syndrome, having an afebrile onset with nausea and vomiting followed by jaundice, hypoglycemia and encephalopathy, is seen in 1 per cent of cases. Cerebral odema and anoxic changes in the neurons have been documented. The correlation between aspirin, influenza infection and Rey's syndrome has also been noted. Occasionally myositis, rhabdomyolysis and myoglobinuria may occur. Uncommon complications include myocarditis, pericarditis, encephalitis, transverse myelitis and Guillain-Barré syndrome.

A polyvalent vaccine elicits a wide immunological response. 50-80 percent protection is obtained. 5 percent of patients experience low grade fever and systemic symptoms 24 hours after vaccination. The administration of 1-adamantanamine hydrochloride (amatadine) 200 mg orally daily for 10 days as a prophylactic drug to the household contacts appears to protect against influenza A infection. 5-10 per cent of persons will experience mild CNS side effects like anxiety, insomonia etc. Rimantidine, closely reltated structurally to amantidine, is also effective in the prevention and treatment of influenza A infection and it is less toxic. 70-100 per cent effectiveness as prophylaxis of these drugs has been documented. Vitamin E has been used to increase platelet count. A combination of nitazoxanide, chloroquine, orettamivir and montelukast has shown to have good result in (HINI virus) swine flue,[17] chikengunia and seasonal influenza.

Flue-Like Illness[12,18]

Afebrile illness simulating influenza occurs due to infection from adenoviruses, para-influenza and enteroviruses. High grade fever may be present in severe cases and there may be relative bradycardia. Type 3 and 7 of adenovirus is responsible for this fever.

Sore Throat[4,12,19]

Acute Pharyngitis

Second to beta haemolytic streptococcus, adenovirus is the frequent non-bacterial cause of sore throat, tonsilitis and pharyngitis. Influenza and enteroviruses may also cause it. Pharynx and tonsils are inflamed and may be covered with exudate. It is difficult to distinguish clinically between viral and streptococcal sore throat. Baterial culture of throat swab is important.

Adenoviruses are an important aetiological agents in acute respiratory illness in all age groups. The virus size is 70 to 90 millimicrons. They have a group specific antigen demonstrable by compliment fixation test and there is no type specific antigen. There are 31 antigenic types. The infection produces a catarrhal inflammation of mucosa of the respiratory tract and of eyes. The type of illness depends on the age group. Types 3, 4, 7, 14 and 21 commonly involve the respiratory tract. Types 4 and 7 cause ARD (acute respiratory distress).

Pharynx is inflamed with patchy exudation over tonsils. It is associated with fever, malaise, cough and sore throat with difficulty to swallow. There may be cervical lymphadenopathy. Routine laboratory tests are non-contributory. Febrile catarrh, acute pharyngitis, pharyngoconjunctival fever, kerato-conjunctivitis, pharyngolaryngotracheitis and pneumonia in children may be other associated syndromes in adenoviral infection. Infection is generally mild and self limiting. Specific antiviral therapy is not available. Utility of Live Vaccine has been utilised only in types 4 and 7 infections.

Herpangina[2,20,21]

Coxsackie A 1-25 serotypes, cause afebrile illness with sore throat. It is seen in children. There is pharyngeal conjestion. Multiple vesicles appear on pharynx, fauces, soft palate and tonsils and they ulcerate rapidly. The virus is associated with malaise, sore throat, fever and headache.

Bornholm's Disease[2]

The infection with coxsackie 1 to 6 types, is associated with fever, cough, headache, muscular pain in the lower part of thorax and upper part of the abdomen. Pleural rub may be audible (pleurodynia). The illness is self-limiting and treatment is symptomatic only.

Croup[2,22,23]

This is generally caused by para-influenza I, although para-influenza virus has five different antigenic types. It causes illness especially in children between ages of three months and three years. Respiratory syncytial virus, coheno and roheno viruses have been incriminated. The manifestions vary from mild upper respiratory illness to flu-like illness in adults. The antigenic type II strain of the virus is associated with croup, and obstructive laryngotracheobronchitis.

Manifestations include hoarseness, suprasternal, intercostal and sternal retractions, cough, inspiratory stridor, dyspnoea and cyanosis. As the obstruction increases, breath sounds may become inaudible and strider may apparently decrease, and, infact, unfortunately misinterpreted as a clinical improvement. Generally preceding it, there is mild cold, rhinorrhoea and low grade fever, later on there is brassy cough with mild inspiratory strider. Differential diagnosis includes laryngeal diphtheria and oedema of epiglottis. The latter is associated with septicemia and there is no hoarseness of voice as the larynx is not affected.

Humidified oxygen is useful in relieving the laryngeal spasm. Secondary bacterial infection is treated with antibiotics. Periodic inhalation of a racemic adrenaline may help in rapid resolution. Tracheostomy may be required in some cases.

Bronchiolitis[4,12,24-29]

It is caused by one serological type of the virus called respiratory syncytial virus (RSV). It forms an important cause of acute lower respiratory tract infection in infancy and childhood. Peak incidence is at 6 months. Severe bronchiolitis may be associated with para-influenza virus types I and III, enterovirus, influenza virus and adenovirus. RSV infection causes febrile lower respiratory tract disease in adults including severe pneumonia in the elderly. Children who are immunocompromised appear to be more susceptible to RSV infection. There is inflammation of lower respiratory passages with severe obstruction at the level of bronchioles. The infection is associated with necrosis of respiratory epithelium, submucosal oedema, and peribronchial lymphocytic infiltrates to result in tracheobronchitis, obstructive brochiolitis and even pneumonia.

The narrow bronchial lumen is further reduced due to bronchiolar spasm, causing airway resistance. The airflow is reduced and there is increased airflow resistance both during inspiration and expiration. Alveolar air trapping occurs, causing emphysematous changes. If obstruction is complete, atelectasis occurs as the trapped air is absorbed.

Hypoxemia occurs due to diminished ventilation and diffusion, retaining the CO_2 which leads to respiratory acidosis. Wheezing may occur if the child has been earlier senitized by the same viral infection. In such cases, eosinophils may be present in the respiratory secretions. It is highly infectious and tends to occur in epidemics. The infection involves the whole of the respiratory tract, resulting in hypoxaemia and hypercarbia. It causes mild upper respiratory tract infection in adults.

RSV causes bronchiolitis in infants, with symptoms of rhinorrhoea, anorexia and listlessness. The internal antibody does not appear to have a protective effect. Later on it is associated wih cough, fever, severe dyspnoea, retractions, wheeze, cyanosis, over inflated chest and bronchi. In severe cases, respiratory sounds may be inaudible. Respiratory distress can be out of proportion to the extent of the physical pulmonary signs. There is severe airways obstruction. Patients with respiratory allergy and asthma may present with a syndrome indistinguishable from bronchiolitis. Chest X-ray reveals hyperinflation and perihilar infiltrates. Lateral views are more informative. Diaphragm may be pushed down. Total leucocytic count may be slightly increased or normal.

Ribovirin aerosols reduce the severity of the illness. Antibiotics are unnecessary and antihistaminics are not indicated. Bronchodilators may be judiciously used. The disease may settle spontaneously within four to seven days. 10% mortality has been reported. Bronchial asthma has been observed to occur in 25% cases of acute bronchiolitis. Assisted ventilation is needed in severe cases only. 40% oxygen concentration is adequate.

Bronchitis[1,4,5,8,9]

Bronchitis may develop as a complication of upper respiratory tract infection. It presents with cough, mucopurulent expectoration and wheeze. Fever is not a constant feature and dyspnoea is not severe. It may precipitate an attack of chronic bronchitis.

Viral Pneumonia[2,4,9,28,30]

Pneumonia can occur as a primary viral infection in infants ('respiratory syncytial virus and para-influenza virus in the elderly and, debilitated individuals from adenoviruses and influenza viruses. Often secondary infections cause trouble. Fever may or may not be the presenting feature.

Viral pneumonias are responsible for one fourth cases of total pneumonic infections. There may be fever, dyspnoea and increasing respiratory rate. Secondary bacterial infections complicate, especially the pneumococcal infection which invades the respiratory mucosa damaged by viral infection, commonly in infants under one year of age. Adenoviruses have been associated with disseminated disease and pneumonias in immunosuppressed patients including patients with AIDS.

Investigations

The diagnosis of viral infection is based on demonstration of virus and four-fold rise in specific antibody titre during convalescence. This is not a routine practice in the tropics.

Isolation of the virus can be done by the use of tissue culture techiques in the first week of infection. There are different cultures to isolate different viruses. Immunofluorescence and electron microsopy techniques are also utilised to demonstrate viruses quickly.

A four-fold or greater increase in the antibody tire in the serum *can be demonstrated* by the complement fixation test. Serological test for rhinovirus and echovirus are not done routinely because of the numerous serotypes.

Giant Cell Pneumonia[31-34]

This is one of the rare pulmonary involvements by Rubeola virus, especially in children suffering from systemic illnesses like congenital or aquired immunodeficiency leukemia, malnutrition etc. Measles, usually a self limiting infection, may involve respiratory tract leading to croup, bronchitis, and bronchiolitis.

The giant cell pneumonia may occur in the absence of typical measles infection. Clinically patient may have moderate respiratory distress, manifesting as tachypnoea and dyspnoea. Chest examination reveals both inspiratory and expiratory rales. There is pulmonary infiltration with multinucleated giant cells in the lung parenchyma. Proliferation of alveolar lining and metaplasia of bronchiolar epithelium may occur. The giant cell formation seen in Hecht's pneumonia and in cystic fibrosis is not a histological feature of pneumonia in measles infection. Chest X-ray shows generalised patchy infiltrates with areas of overinflation. It is the secondary bacterial infection by pneumococci and straphylococci which is quite common and leads to formation of empyema and lung abscess.

No specific treatment is available. Appropriate antibiotics for secondary infections should be used. Prophylactic dose of gammaglobulins does not alter frequency or severity of the superadded bacterial infections. Inactivated vaccine is not indicated because of the development of atypical measles. Live attenuated vaccine is recommended for measles, which apart from pregnant women, cannot be given to immunocompromised and leukemic children who are more prone to this pneumonitis. However, there have been vaccine failures.

Cytomegaloviral Pneumonia[35-44]

This is one of the opportunistic infections seen in 15-20% of bone marrow transplant patients. Peak risk period is 5-13 weeks after transplant. Risk factors include old age, immuno-suppression, viremia, acute graft-versus-host disease and granulocyte transfusion. Cytomegaloviral syndrome in AIDS patients presents with fever, malaise, fatigue, myalgia, loss of appetite and night sweats.

There is unproductive cough, hypoxia and trachypnoea. Chest X-ray shows bilateral interstitial or retin to nodular infiltrates, involving the periphery of lower lobes, spreading centrally. Since high antibody titre does not serve the diagnositc purpose, lung biopsy is indicated. Differential diagnosis include pulmonary haemorrhage, other bacterial or viral infections. Prophylaxis is important, especially in high risk patients. CMV immunoglobulin reduces the CMV associated syndromes in sero negative renal transplant recipients. Ganciclovir alone is less effective but in combination with CMV immunoglobulin, the response rate is enhanced to 50-70 per cent in CMV pneumonitis.

BACTERIAL PULMONARY INFECTIONS

Pneumonia

Pneumonia continues to be a leading cause of mortality in USA.[4] Pneumonia is an infection localised to the gas exchanging units of the lung, characterised by consolidation of a part or whole of the lung from an acute inflammatory exudate into the alveolar spaces. The alveoli are involved in bacterial infections and the interstitium in non-bacterial pneumonia. The microbial invasion of the bronchioles and alveolar units elicits an inflammatory response.[2] In bronchopneumonia, there is a patchy and diffuse involvement but without consolidation.[19]

Pneumonia may be classified on anatomical or on aetiological basis. In the former it is referred to as lobar, segmental and lobular (bronchopneumonia when bilateral pneumonia). Clinically pneumonia can be community aquired, nosocomial, aspiration pneumonia and pneumonia in immuno-compromised host. So, varies their pathogenesis, diagnosis, treatment and prognosis.

Aetiology wise; the infective agents such as bacteria (Streptococcus pneumoniae, Staphylococcus aureus, Streptococcus pyogenes, Klebsiella pneumoniae, H. influenzae, My. tuberculosis and Legionella pneumoniae), virus (influenza, respiratory syncytial virus in infants), Chlamydia, rickettsia (R.burnetti), microbiological agent (mycoplasma), protozoa (Pneumocystis carinii) and fungus (Aspergillus and dimorphic fungus) are recognised as causative agents in most cases. Other causative agents are chemical (irritant gases, lipoid, beryllium) and physical (radiation injury) agents, hypersensitivity (eosinophilic pneumonia) and collagen diseases (non-eosinophilic infiltrates). Pathologically, five distinct histological types such as lobar pneumonia, bronchopneumonia, tuberculous pneumonia, bacterial superadded infection and necrotizing pneumonia may occur.

An increasing number of immunocompromised patients develop pneumonia. The infants and children become frequent victims because of poorly developed immune response and relatively narrow airways, so are the elderly persons, who are suffering from chronic disease. Tables 4.2 and 4.3 detail about pneumonia and their classification.

Table 4.2: Pneumonitis

Tests:	Total count is raised Sputum culture +ve
Presentation:	
Signs:	Bronchial breathing: Dull percussion note: Crepitations: Pericardial friction rub: Whispering pectoriloquy: Vocal fremitus: Hypoventilation
DD: (Differential diagnosis)	Other Pneumonias: Pulmonary infarction: Atelectasis: Subphrenic abscess: Bronchitis: Bronchogenic carcinoma

Predisposing Conditions[2,46]

Any interference with the defence mechanisms of the respiratory tract (impaired consciousness, depressed cough reflex, and regurgitation of gastric contents) may lead to inhalation of foreign material and infected secretions providing basics for the development of pneumonia. Viral infections of the respiratory tract, especially influenza, causes damage to its epithelium and predisposes to bacterial pneumonia. Pneumonia often complicates in patients suffering from chronic bronchitis, bronchiectasis and cystic fibrosis because of inadequate drainage of bronchial secretions and retained secretions from bronchogenic carcinoma may lead to pneumonia.

Patients on immunosuppressive therapy are frequently susceptible to infections. Patients with immune deficiency (AIDS) have an increased risk of infection by pneumocystis carinii and cytomegalovirus. Immunologic disorders like leukaemia, lymphoma and multiple myeloma and hypo-gammaglobulin-aemia predispose to pneumonia. Anaerobic cause pneumonia may occur in debilitated patients. Factors which may precipitate pulmonary infections are listed in Table 4.4.

Host Defence[4,47-50]

In the upper respiratory tract and large airways, mechanical mechanisms which exclude particulate material, are: (i) anatomic barriers, such as the epiglottis and tight apical cellular junctions

Table 4.3: Pneumonia's classification[45]

I. Bacterial infections	*II. Viral or probable viral infections*	*III. Other infections*	*IV. Mycotic infections*	*V. Aspiration of amniotic contents (fetal anoxia)*	*VI. Loffler's syndrome*	*VII. Hypostatic pneumonia*
• Pneumococcus • Streptococcus • Staphylococcus • H. influenza • Friendlander's bacillus • Tubercle bacillus • Treponema pallidum	• Bronchiolitis and interstitial pneumonitis • Giant cell pneumonia • Influenza	• *Pneumocystis carinii pneumonia* *Q fever* • *Mycoplasma pneumoniae pneumonia*	• Coccidioidomycosis • Histoplasmosis • Blastomycosis • Cryptococcosis • Mucormycosis • Nocardiosis • Sporotrichosis thrush	• Food • Foreign bodies • Zinc stearate • Dust • Kerosene • Lipoid substances		

Table 4.4: Factors that precipitate or promote pulmonary infection

Defence barrier	*Factor interfering with defence*	*Disturbed mechanism*
1. Alveolar macrophage	Inspiration of silica/asbestos particles	Destroyed macrophages
2. Cough reflex	Pain	Reduction in forceful expiration
	Sedatives and narcotics	Inhibition of cough reflex
3. Ciliary action	Atmospheric pollution and cigarette smoking	Depressed ciliary activity
	Chronic bronchitis	Overproduction of mucus rendering Ciliary activity ineffective
	Anesthetics	Depressed ciliary activity
4. Mucus secretion	Dehydration	Fluid deficit due to production of scant and viscous mucus
	Inspiration of dry air	Production of viscous mucus
	Anesthetics	Depressed mucus production

between epithelial lining cells of the mucosa; (ii) reflex closure of the glottis, (iii) frequent branching of the pulmonary tree which leads to aerodynamic filtering of inspired air, (iv) mucociliary clearance of particulates that impact on the mucosa, and (v) the cough response. The infectious agents, bacteria in particular, after crossing these defences are deposited in the alveoli, another group of host factors comes into action. The terminal units (alveolar ducts and alveoli) do not contain ciliated epithelium and mucus-secreting cells (goblet cells and mucous glands) and coughing does not effectively clear material from the alveoli. Clearance is dependent on phagocytic cells and humoral factors.

Opsonins[4]

When bacteria or particles reach the alveolar surface, alveolar macrophages rapidly phagocytose some inert particles but the viable bacteria is more slowly ingested. Coating or opsonizing the organisms will enhance phagocytosis approximately by ten fold. Non-immune opsonins are found in the film of fluid on the alveolar surface (lipoprotein surfactant from type II pneumocytes and large fragments of the glycoprotein, fibronectin, produced locally by alveolar macrophages or delivered from intravascular sources). Immune opsonins include IgG antibody and a complement factor. C3b enhance attachment to specific plasma membrane receptors. These opsonins may be locally produced or are developed as part of systemic humoral immunity.

The complement system in the airways is activated along the alternative pathway, can lead to lysis of a succeptible organism and generation of opsonic C3b. Phagocytosis is followed by intracellular killing, but at a slower rate than in polymorphonuclear leukocytes (PMNs) and by less well-defined mechanisms involving both oxygen dependent and independent pathways. In contrast to PMNs, macrophages usually lack cycloperoxidase; but production of superoxide and H_2O_2 are enhanced by macrophages activation. *Pathogenesis* of respiratory tract infection involve immune defenses both humoral in the form of B lymphocytes augmenting phagocytic defence mechanism that initiate acute inflammatory response, and cell mediated immunity in the form of T lymphocytes and biological activity both by lymphokine directed delayed hypersensitivity reaction as well as T cell cytotoxicity. This cell-mediated microbial and cytotoxic activity initiates subacute, chronic and granulomatous responses.

In addition to phagocytosis, subsequent containment and destruction of microbes hinge on the effectiveness of the macrophages to kill the organisms and the development of an inflammatory reaction. Phagocytosis and macrophageal killing of organisms lead to an inflammatory reaction. Alveolar macrophages can survive months to years and are capable of handling repeated microbial offence. Being motile cells, they can migrate quickly to other alveoli through the pores of Kohn or move to more proximal areas of the respiratory tract. Macrophages are instrumental in degrading antigenic material and presenting it to appropriate alveolar lymphocytes which in turn may initiate specific immune responses. Macrophages may gain entry into lung lymphatics in respiratory bronchioles also and are transported to regional lymph nodes—the site of humoral and cellular immune responses for the lung. Many secretory products of macrophages are essential participants in the immune effector system and thus contribute to chronic inflammation and to fibrogenesis or granuloma formation. All this is regulated by lymphocytes which control the lung macrophage functions related to cellular activation and inflammation. They are also directly involved in the formation and regulation of antibody responses and activation of dormant cytotoxic lymphocytes.

Lymphocytes retrieved from normal alveoli account for about 10 per cent of airway cells. Seventy per cent of these are T-lymphocytes and proportions of the major subpopulations are similar to those in peripheral blood. Among the helper T-cells is a small percentage of HLA-DR-positive lymphocytes (7 per cent) that secrete in major amount of interleukin 2. Killer T cells may be dormant but can be activated by Y-interferon. Several important cytokines produced by T-lymphocytes activate alveolar macrophages and include Y-interferon and macrophage-inhibitory factor. Acquired cell-mediated immunity (CMI) is necessary if the macrophage population is to contain or kill certain intercellular microbes.

PMNs are usually separated from alveolar spaces by three planes, tissue-capillary endothelium, interstitial space, and alveolar epithelium. PMN movement into the alveoli is on orderly chemotactic reaction initiated from the alveolar side. Pathways involved include macrophages that help promote the acute inflammatory response, including chemotaxis. Production of chemotactic factors, particularly leukotriene B4, from macrophages can attract PMNs from pulmonary capillaries and venules and alter pulmonary capillary permeability. Other chemotactic and capillary permeability-altering factors include C3a and C5a and components of the kinin systems. The combined action of these agents promotes the accumulation of PMNs, fluid and other humoral substances in alveoli.

Clinical illness usually occurs in response with the appearance of an inflammatory chest roentgenogram that reveals an infiltrate. The systemic effects of pneumonia—such as chills and fever, malaise and myalgias are due to production of certain interleukin I (ILI) and tumor necrotic factors by alveolar macrophages.

Ultimately the lung tissues may become consolidated. Release of proteolytic enzymes (e.g., PMN-derived clastase) can contribute to lung injury. Their neutralization by several inhibitor proteins, alpha-antiprotea and possibly alpha-macroglobulin can minimize destruction of lung tissue. Successful control of the infection brings complete resolution and healing, but little is known about the processes that halt the acute inflammatory reaction in pneumonia and initiate recovery.

Laboratory Tests

Typically there is leukocytosis with a high percentage of polymorpho nuclear cells and with a *left shift,* whereas changes in leukocyte counts may be minimal in viral and other pneumonias. The white blood count becomes under the effect of coexisting hepatorenal disorders, alcoholism, accompanying cytotoxic therapy etc.

Microscopic examination and culture of respiratory secretions are essential for the treatment of pneumonia. Blood cultures reveal the aetiologic agent and, if positive, can affect the prognosis and is potential for metastatic infection. A freshly obtained specimen of expectorated sputum should be prepared for a gram's stain and culture. If the patient is not producing sputum, an attempt is made to induce secretions. P. carinii can be identified in the induced sputum of about 80 per cent of the patients with this pneumonia who have AIDS and in a smaller percentage of patients with non-HIV disease. If it is impossible to induce an adequate respiratory sample, more invasive measures like transtracheal aspiration, fiberoptic bronchoscopy, percutaneous transthoracic needle aspiration, thoracentesis, or open-lung biopsy, can be considered.

Percutaneous transtracheal aspiration is a direct approach that eliminates much of the contaminating oral microbial flora, but it carries a risk to the patient and is now rarely employed in most centers.

Fiberoptic bronchoscopy with BAL and a protected brush catheter provides another diagnostic aid. The risk of bronchoscopy is small, even in patients with extensive pneumonia. Administration of supplemental oxygen is carried during the procedure and Oximetry is used to monitor its effect. Platelet transfusions to correct thrombocytopenia are usually recommended. A direct view of the affected lung anatomy may disclose an endobronchial obstruction. Removal of secretions or a mucus plug could make the procedure of therapeutic as well as diagnostic value. Usually the lavage fluid or catheter brush culture will contain the offending pathogen. However, microbial cultures from the bronchoscopy specimens also contain contaminating flora from the nasopharynx and interpretation can be confusing.

Transbronchial biopsy provides lung tissue for culture and histology. Multiple biopsies of pieces 2 to 3 mm in size are usually obtained from at least two segments of a lobe if a diffuse lesion is present. A specific aetiologic diagnosis in 50 to 95 per cent of cases can be made.

Complication arising from bronchoscopy include hemorrhage and/or pneumothorax in about 5 per cent of cases. Occasionally, a chest tube will be needed to treat the pneumothorax. About 25 per cent of patients develop a postbronchoscopy fever about 4 to 8 hours after the procedure, usually lasting less than 24 hours.

Percutaneous transthoracic needle aspiration—a diagnostic modality—is sometimes helpful in pneumonia, although needle aspiration guided by computed tomography (CT) is performed more frequently to diagnose discrete lung lesions. Spread of micro organisms along the needle track and pneumothorax are common complications.

Small size pleural effusions can occur with Mycoplasma and Legionella infection as well, and pleural tuberculosis characteristically causes effusions. A diagnostic thoracentesis is indicated to determine whether the fluid contains organisms and/or has the characteristics of an empyema. Cellular analysis and certain chemical tests (pH, lactic dehydrogenase, glucose, and total protein) will identify pleural fluid to be a transudate or exudate. Empyema can develop with pneumonitis or lung abscess in adjacent lung tissue; the fluid is exudative and like pus. Micro organisms may be seen on stained smear and usually grow from cultures. Repeated thoracentesis to drain the fluid or use of an indwelling chest tube to effect continuous drainage is usually necessary in an empyema to hasten healing and to prevent or minimize future complications like pleural adhesions.

If a parapneumonic effusion develops in the course of pneumonia, thoracentesis is indicated if:

i. Fever has persisted for 72 hours after beginning the treatment with appropriate antibiotics.
ii. A large effusion develops that is contributing to discomfort and impaired breathing or is increasing in size; and
iii. There is evidence that once freely movable fluid has become loculated.

Diagnostic Open Lung Biopsy[4]

This is often necessary in the immunocompromised patient with an advancing, pulmonary infiltrate, especially, when the bronchoscope is noncontributory. Severe hypoxemia or other complications make the risk excessive. A properly performed and handled open-lung biopsy will reveal a specific aetiology for pulmonary infiltrates in over 90 per cent of patients.

Treatment entails appropriate support with fluids, antipyretic drugs, oxygen, airway suction or gravity (postural) drainage, and broncho-dilator drugs if brnchospasm is present. Antibiotic therapy remains the cornerstone of medical management (Tables 4.5 to 4.7).

Three principles of antimicrobial therapy deserve emphasis, (i) all necessary specimens for appropriate bacteriologic cultures should be obtained before therapy is initiated so that there is a reasonable chance to recover the

Table 4.5: Treatment: Factors to be considered before starting empirical therapy in respiratory infections

1. History of allergy
2. Age of the patient
3. Pregnancy
4. Renal and hepatic functions
5. Genetic factors

Ref: Mahashur AA and Chaudhuri RA; Current therapy in common bacterial respiratories I J C P 1993: sp issue; P 17-22.

Table 4.6: Treatment of respiratory infections

Site	*Drug of choice*	*Dose*
URTI		
Sinusitis and tonsillitis	Ampicillin, amoxycillin, cephlexin,	250-500 mg QDS
	cotrimoxazole	(800 + 160) BD
Pharyngitis	Roxythromycin	80 mg bd
Common cold	Symptomatic treatment: Antihistaminics, steam inhalation	
LRTI		
(Pneumonitis) community acquired	Erythromycin, ampicillin, cephlexin	250-500 mg qds 6-24 million units/day
Nosocomial	Ciprofloxacin or cefotaxime	200 mg IV bd 8 mg IV tds
	+ Amikacin	5 mg/kg IV tds
Aspiration pneumonia	Ampicillin	4 gm/kg/ddIV
	Gentamycin	3 mg/day/dd IV
	Meteronidazole	500 mg IV/6 hrly
Immunocompromised host	Antimicrobials given according to causative organism	
	Carbenicillin	300 mg/day/ddIV
	Aminoglycoside	3-5 mg/kg/day/ddIV

Table 4.7: Microbes and microbials (Specific and senisitive)

Organism	*Drug of choice*	*Dose*
Pseudomonas	Carbenicillin	30 mg/day IV
	Gentamycin or Tobramycin	3·5 mg/kg/day IV
Klebsiella	Gentamycin or Tobramycin	3-5 mg/kg/day IV
	Cephalothin	1-12 gm/day IV
Proteus	Ampicillin	10-12 gm/day IV
	Aminoglycoside	3-5 mg/kg/day IV
Staphylococcus aureus	Cloxacillin	4 gm/day IV
	Cephalothin	1-12 gm/day IV
	Vancomycin	15 mg/kg/12 hrly IV
Fungal	Amphotericin B	0.4-0.6 mg/kg/d ay IV
Pneumocystis	Cotrimoxazole	20 mg/kg/day TMP or 160 mg/kg/day
Carinii	Pentamidin or isetheonate	4 mg/kg/day IV
Mycoplasma pneumonia	Erythromycin	500 mg, 6 hrly
Legionellosis	Erythromycin	500 mg, 6 hrly
Viral pneumonia	Amantidine hydrochloride	4-8 mg/kg/day
Streptococci	Ampicillin	500 mg qds
E. coli	Aminoglycoside +Cephalosporine	As above
H. influenza	Ampicillin	4-6 gm/day

organism; (ii) initial drug therapy should be as specific as the evidence pointing to the aetiologic agent allows, yet sufficiently broad to cover the common micro organisms; and (iii) a few days of broad-spectrum antimicrobial treatment usually will not cause superinfection or selection of drug-resistant bacteria. At the same time, the choice of antimicrobial should be made depending on clinical setting in which pneumonia is diagnosed, its severity and host characteristics. However, microbiological confirmation is feasible in 1/3rd of cases only, even in developed countries.

Gram Positive Pneumonias

Pneumococcal Pneumonia[2]

Pneumococcal pneumonia is a disease of considerable uniformity. This is the most common type of bacterial pneumonia encountered accounting for 40 to 50 per cent of all pneumonias in India. It is due to an infection by streptococcus pneumoniae. It is characterised by chills, fever, chest pain, cough and rusty sputum.

Aetiology

Streptococcus pneumoniae is a gram positive, lancet shaped organism. It occurs in pairs. There are 86 different serotypes, of which, 1, 2, 3, 6, 7, 14 and 19 strains have been recognised as infective types responsible for pneumonia in previously healthy individuals.[51] Type 3 pneumococcal pneumonia usually has poor prognosis, probably because type 3 infections occur frequently in the aged and in patients with immunodeficiency states and other debilitating diseases, such as diabetes and congestive heart failure.[52] The usual lesion in adults is segmental or lobar in distribution, but in children and the aged, bronchopneumonia characterized by patchy involvement, is frequent.

This is commonly seen during winter and early spring following a viral infection of the respiratory tract. The infective type may remain in the nasopharynx sometimes and the carriers play an important role in the spread of the disease. The exposure to cold, fatigue, debility, alcoholic intoxication, effects of anaesthesia, viral infections, and inhalation of irritant gases lower the resistance and make the lungs susceptible to infection. Conditions like congestive heart failure, and chronic bronchitis may also predispose to pneumococcal pneumonia.

Pathology

The organisms normally present in the upper respiratory tract are aspirated into the alveoli of the dependent lung segments where they multiply. An immediate inflammatory reaction with chemotaxis of neutrophilic leucocytes and outpouring of oedema fluid into the alveoli occurs, as the pneumococci are powerful stimulants for oedema fluid. The large amount of oedema fluid carries the pneumococci through the pores of Kohn into contiguous lung segments.[2]

Four stages of the pneumococcal consolidation are, congestion, red hepatisation, grey hepatisation and resolution. Initially the capillaries are markedly congested along with exudation of fluid into the alveoli, with the result the lung becomes airless and firm, having a liver like consistency (red hepatisation). The alveoli are filled with red blood cells, few polymorphs and fibrin. The capillaries are intensely compressed. The inflammatory process extends to the pleura, probably from a lymphatic spread. The pleural surface is covered by a fibrinous exudate. In grey hepatisation, the capillaries are markedly compressed and present a greyish yellow appearance. The alveoli are filled with a large number of pneumococci and a few red blood cells. This involves either a lobe or a segment and the spread is limited by the pleural boundaries of the lobe. As the resolution starts, the alveoli are invaded by macrophages, which engulf the leucocytes and digest the cellular debris. The proteolytic enzymes of disintegrating leucocytes liquefy the material which is either absorbed or expectorated. There is no necrosis of the alveolar walls as the inflammatory process is superficial and the exudate is intra alveolar. The deeper tissues remain unaffected. Hence, it clears up completely without causing any lung damage. As the resolution occurs, the small amount of pleural fluid collected during acute process gets absorbed. When there is improper bronchial drainage, as in chronic bronchitis, a delayed resolution may occur.

Clinical Features

Often pneumonia is noted in previously healthy young adult males, following a history of cold or upper respiratory infections. There is a sudden shaking chill in more than 80 per cent of the cases and a rapid rise in temperature, with corresponding tachycardia and an increase in respiratory rate (tachypnea).

About 75 per cent of patients develop severe pleuritic pain and cough, productive of pinkish or *'rusty'* mucoid sputum within a few hours. The chest pain is agonizing, and respiration becomes rapid shallow and grunting. Many patients are mildly cyanotic as a result of hypoxia caused by altered V/Q (ventilation-perfusion ratio), because of passage of blood via poorly ventilated alveoli. Patients appear acutely ill; but nausea, headache and malaise are not prominent, and most individuals are alert. Pleuritic pain and dyspnoea are the dominant complaints.[53] With crisis, the elevated temperature falls rapidly along with profuse sweating.

On clinical examination, the patient is acutely ill and presents flushed face and warm body. Cyanosis may be present. There is tachypnoea with shallow rapid respiration. Vesicles of herpes over the lips (Herpes labialis) is a common complication.[2]

In cases which terminate fatally, there is usually extensive pulmonary involvement, and dyspnoea, cyanosis, and tachycardia are prominent. Circulatory collapse or a picture resembling adult respiratory distress syndrome has been observed.[54] Unilateral pulmonary edema can mimic as pneumonia.[55] Death in a few patients is associated with empyema or some other suppurative complications such as meningitis or endocarditis.

The movements are restricted on the affected side of the chest. A friction fremitus may be felt. It is dull to percussion with increased vocal fremitus and vocal resonance. A typical tubular breathing is heard from consolidation of the underlying lobe. Crackles (fine crepitations) are heard at the end of inspiration due to separation of the alveolar walls. Pleural rub may be audible in few cases. Whispering pectoriloquy is characteristically heard. The signs of consolidation are confined to the involved lobe. With improvement, the breath sounds alter their character and crepitations disappear gradually.

Deviation of the trachea away from the affected lung suggests pleural effusion or empyema. The occurrence of pleural effusion may mask the features of consolidation. A stoney dull note with absence of breath sounds is noted.

Investigations

There is polymorphonuclear leucocytosis and the ESR is raised. The sputum examination with Gram's stain is vital to demonstrate Gram positive, lancet shaped diplococci in association with polymorphs. X-ray of the chest reveals a homogeneous opacity confined to the lobe or even a segment. A typical pattern of consolidation may be seen in patients with underlying pulmonary disease. The costophrenic angle is obliterated in cases of pleural effusion and the opacity reaches a high level towards the chest wall. Pneumococcal capsular antigen can be demonstrated in sputum or blood by countercurrent immunoelectrophoresis. Hypoxaemia, hypocapnia and respiratory alkalosis have also been documented.

Complications

Complications like delayed resolution, fibrosis, peripheral vascular collapse in early phase and lung abscess, or empyema may occur as rare complications. Other systemic complications such as pericarditis, endocarditis, arthritis and meningitis, or non-specific complications, such as, actute dilatation of stomach or ileus and impairment of liver functions, may occur rarely.

Management

The treatment should be started immediately. The sputum culture results are obtained in 24 hours and it may necessitate change in the antibiotic in other types of pneumonia. Streptococcus pneumoniae are sensitive to penicillin. Management modalities have been tabulated in Table 4.8.

Table 4.8: Bacterial pneumonia: Management

1. Appropriate antibiotics.
2. Physiotherapy for segmental drainage.
3. Oxygen if there is distress or cyanosis.
4. Treatment of intercurrent cardiac failure.
5. Maintenance of nutrition, fluid and electrolyte balance.
6. Diazepam rarely in cases of delirium.
7. Vaccination against pneumococcal pneumonia for highly vulnerable patients.

In the absence of resistance or of hypersensitivity to it, penicillin G (benzylpenicillin) is the drug of choice for all manifestations of pneumococcal infections. Strains of pneumococcus manifesting increased resistance to penicillin have been recovered infrequently from humans; and although the level of such resistance does not often preclude treatment with this antibiotic, awareness of the phenomenon is necessary.[56,57]

Crystalline penicillin is administered in doses of I mega unit intramuscularly every six hours. Response to penicillin is dramatic and it causes rapid defervescence and subsidence of symptoms in a majority of patients. The treatment should be continued with procaine penicillin until the temperature has been normal for 72 hours or is maintained for a minimal period of one week to prevent relapses. Ampicillin in a daily dose of I to 2 gm is also beneficial.

Cephalosporins in parenteral doses of 1 to 2 g daily are effective in pneumococcal pneumonia but must be administered with caution to those hypersensitive to penicillin. The tetracycline in doses of 1 to 2 g daily, erythromycin doses of 1.6 g daily, or clindamycin in doses of 1.2 g daily are efffective treatment for pneumococcal pneumonia if it is caused by a sensitive strain, but they are recommended only for patients who have had untoward reactions to penicillins or cephalosporins. Erythromycin or amoxycilin can be used in ambulatory patients also. Aminoglycoside such as gentamicin, tobramycin, and amikacin should not be employed to treat pneumococcal infection.

In case of a failure or delay in the response, other causes must be looked for such as, pulmonary infarction, Klebsiella pneumonia, pulmonary tuberculosis or complications like empyema, lung abscess, or bronchial obstruction hindering the drainage as seen in the bronchogenic carcinoma or foreign body aspiration.[2]

Empyema should be detected and treated as early as possible. When an effusion is found, fluid should be removed and examined for bacteria, leukocytes, glucose concentration and pH. The presence of bacteria, pus, a pH below 7.0 and/or pleural fluid glucose below 2.2 mmol/L (40 mg/dL) are indications for institution of closed-chest tube drainage. Failure to cure empyema early may be followed by pleural fibrosis and may necessitate subsequent surgical decortication of the lung to restore pulmonary function.

The sputum should be examined for the presence of AFB and malignant cells. Other types of organisms may be revealed by culture and sensitivity tests. Pulmonary infarction has sudden onset of pain in the chest and haemoptysis. It may be recurrent with involvement of different parts of the lung. Bronchoscopy may be necessary to exclude the presence of bronchial obstruction.[58]

The oxygen administration is necessary to counteract hypoxaemia. The pleuritic chest pain is relieved by local application of heat or by administration of salicylates or paracetamol. Sometimes when the pain is severe, pethidine 50 mg intramuscularly may be necessary. Rarely intercostal nerve block with 1-2% procaine may be required when pain is severe.

Prognosis and Prevention[59-63]

The fatality rate in patients over the age of 12 years with bacterimic pneumococcal pneumonia treated with an antibiotic is 18 per cent, and in patients over the age of 50 and in those with underlying systemic illness, it is significantly higher. Resistant streptococcal pneumonia C are increasingly being reported and require close scrutini and changes in the recommendation of treatment.[62]

Signs of poor prognosis include leucopenia, bacteremia, multilobar involvement, any extrapulmonary focus of pneumococcal infection, presence of pre-existing systemic disease, circulatory collapse, and occurrence of the infection in the first year of life or after the age of 55. Infection with pneumococcus type has a higher mortality rate. Persons of all ages with sickle cell disease have an increased risk of developing pneumococcal infection, and the vaccine is recommended for those with this disorders over the age of 2 years. Since anatomic or functional asplenia is associated with fluminant overwhelming pneumococcal septicemia with disseminated intravascular coagulation, giving rise to a clinical picture resembling that of the Waterhouse Friderichesen syndrome, such individuals should also be immunized. However, the vaccine dose not contain the antigens of all pneumococcal types, and infection caused by non-included types may occur occasionally in immunized subjects.

Reactions to the vaccine are usually absent or mild, such as local pain, erythema, and elevation of temperature. Because of the persistence of pneumococcal antibodies after a single injection of vaccine, reimmunization is not necessary. The aggregate efficacy of the vaccine in preventing bacterimic infection is 65 to 70 percent in immunocompetent adults. Currently, vaccines of capsular saccharide conjugated to proteins such as diphtheria toxoid which are antigenic in infancy, are under development for pediatric populations. Pneumococcal vaccine may be administered concomitantly with influenza viral vaccine, provided each vaccine is injected from a separate syringe at a separate site. Vaccination of elderly patients who have been discharged from the hospital, after successful treatment, has been suggested, to prevent recurrent hospital admissions because of pneumonitis.[63]

Staphylococcal Pneumonia

Staphylococcal pneumonia (S. aureus) causes approximately 1 per cent of community-acquired bacterial pneumonias. It affects infants and children commonly, 3/4th of the patients are below 1 year of age. It can be primary parenchymal infection but most frequently occurs as a complication of measles, cystic fibrosis[19] influenza and upper respiratory infections. It may occur as a complication in the compromised hosts among adult population and in debilitated and ill patients.[61] It may occur in hospitalised patients recovering from surgery or being treated with corticosteroids or multiple antibiotics.

Primary staphylococcal pneumonia in infants and children frequently presents with high fever and non-productive cough. Multiple thin-walled abscesses, or pneumatoceles, are present on the chest roentgenogram. Empyema formation is common. In older children and healthy adults staphylococcal pneumonia is generally preceded by an influenza-like respiratory infection (influenza, measles, or other viruses). Onset is abrupt, with chills, high fever, progressive dyspnoea, cyanosis, cough and pleural pain. The sputum may be bloody or frankly purulent.[64-67] Lungs show impaired percussion note, crepitations and pleural rub. The signs of consolidation are rare.

There is leucocytosis. Blood culture is positive only in 20-30 per cent of cases. X-ray chest shows bilateral patchy opacities and small multiple lung abscesses which may develop into thin-walled cavities. Huge pneumatoceles may be noted in infants. The condition may lead to pleural effusion, empyema, pulmonary fibrosis and bronchiectasis is common in adults. Plenty of polymorphs and gram positive cocci within the leucocytes are present in the sputum.

Staphylococcal pneumonia must be differentiated from other pneumonias. The preceding influenza-like illness, rapid onset of pleural pain, cyanosis, and prostration out of proportion to physical findings should suggest primary staphylococcal pneumonia.

Penicillin may be given in doses of 1 mega unit every six hours.[68] But erythromycin 500 mg six hours or cloxacillin 500 mg six hourly are to be given.[69] Cephlosporin is effective against staphylococci and is resistant to penicillinase. Cephalexin and cephradine can be given orally in doses of 250 to 500 mg six hourly or cephalothin and cephaloridine in similar dosage parenterally.[70] Two weeks treatment is usually sufficient. The circulatory collapse is controlled by administration of hydrocortisone hemisuccinate 200 to 300 mg in the form of continuous intravenous infusion for 24 hours. The mechanical block created by secretions necessitates suction or aspiration through bronchoscope. Hypoxaemia is corrected by administration of oxygen.[2]

Empyema usually necessitates chest tube drainage and may be complicated by the formation of loculations or bronchopleural fistulas. Ultrasound or computed tomography scan may be required to identify loculated collections of pus for drainage.[4]

Streptococcal Pneumonia

It occurs as a complication of viral infections (Streptococcus pyogenes) or following secondary invasion during lowered internal resistance (Streptococcus viridans).

There is a patchy haemorrhagic consolidation. The distribution is diffuse involving many lobules. There is inflammation of the bronchial walls and alveoli. The alveoli are filled with inflammatory exudate. Both radiologically and pathologically it is usually a bronchopneumonia.[19]

There is an abrupt onset of fever chills, myalgia, dyspnoea, cough, pleuritic chest pain and hemoptysis. Patients are severely ill and often cyanotic.[71-73] A characteristic feature of streptococcal pneumonia is the early and rapid accumulation of copious amounts of serosanguinous empyema fluid.

Often there is preceding acute pharyngitis due to streptococcal infection. The condition may make an insidious onset in debilitated patients with fever, cough, tachycardia, tachypnoea, bloody or purulent sputum. The pleura is involved early in the course of the disease with production of this turbid effusion. The features are essentially of bronchopneumonia and clinical signs of consolidation are uncommon. Fever comes down by lysis. Bacteremia occurs in 10 to 15 per cent of the cases. Potential complications include mediastinitis, purulent pericarditis, pneumothorax and bronchiectasis.[4] Therapy consists of at least 4 to 6 million units of parenteral penicillin daily in the form of aqueous procaine penicillin G, given every 6 to 12 hours intramuscularly, or intravenous aqueous crystalline penicillin G.

The resolution is delayed and occurs with fibrosis. Empyema is frequent and requires usually chest tube insertion for adequate drainage. Total leucocytic count is raised.

The organism can be demonstrated in the sputum, and serum ASO titre is raised during the illness due to beta haemolytic streptococci.[2]

Gram Negative Pneumonia

When there is a poor resistance to infections (chronic alcoholism and debilitating conditions) and altered defence mechanisms (recent surgery, multiple antibiotic therapy, corticosteroid therapy or tracheostomy), there is a chance of infection from aerobic gram negative organisms (Klebsiella, Enterobacter and Serratia).[74]

Klebsiella is being frequently isolated among individuals suffering from pneumonia.[75,76]

Klebsiella Pneumonia

It accounts for less than 1 per cent of all cases of pneumonia.[77] The infection from Klebsiella pneumoniae, an encapsulated Gram negative bacillus first described by Friedlander in 1882[77] is associated with rapidly progressive pneumonia with necrotic lesions.

It is noted more frequently in debilitated individuals, alcoholics, diabetics and malnourished people.[78] It is common in middle aged and elderly men. Infection is unusual in children but nursery epidemics have rarely been reported. At the same time, it accounts for 18-64 per cent of community acquired and 30 per cent of nosocomial gram negative pneumonias.[79]

The upper lobe is more frequently affected and later it may spread to other lobes. The condition is rapidly progressive with tissue necrosis resulting in thin-walled abscess cavities. A fibrinous exudates covers the pleural surface, and adhesions develop early. Empyema develops frequently. 25 per cent cases have bacteremia[80] and abscess formation occurs in more than 25 per cent of cases.[81,82]

There is a sudden onset of high fever, chills, pain in the chest, dyspnoea and cough. Cough is associated with jelly-like blood stained sputum. The patient is acutely ill with fever, cyanosis and tachycardia. There will be signs of consolidation. The signs of pleural effusion or cavitation may supervene. Even a case of myocarditis has been reported.[83]

X-ray chest shows dense opacity and the interlobar fissure is often bulged outwards due to volume expansion of the involved lobe. The occurrence of multiple small thin-walled or large abscess cavities is frequent. The sputum smear shows sheets of short encapsulated gram negative bacilli by Gram's stain and culture of the sputum.[84-86] The leucocytosis is not marked.

Untreated cases carry a high mortality which may be as high as 50 per cent in sporadic cases but lower during epidemics. The recovery is slow and often it leaves behind parenchymal damage with residual fibrosis. Resolution is the feature in subacute form of the disease.[87] There is no response to penicillin. Treatment should be initiated immediately with aminoglycosides. Gentamycin is to be given in a dose of 80 mg intramuscularly eight hourly, or streptomycin 1 gm twice daily for five days along with chloramphenicol 0.5 gm six hourly for five to ten days. The organism is sensitive to cephalosporins but develops resistance rapidly. The maintenance of fluid and electrolyte balance, oxygen and clear airways are essential during treatment. Surgical intervention may be required to drain empyema or abscess. Endotoxic shock and intravascular coagulation are serious complications in untreated cases.[88]

The infection from enterobacter and serratia occurs in debilitated persons who are hospitalised. Though clinically the features simulate that of Klebsiella infection, the chances of abscess formation are less. They all are resistant to cephalosporins.[2]

Haemophilus Influenza Pneumonia

This is an aerobic gram negative bacteria present in the upper respiratory tract of normal individuals, only capsulated strains are pathogenic to produce bronchopneumonia. It is a second common cause of community acquired pneumonias and is responsible for 1/3rd of cases of bacterial pneumonitis, between 4 months to 4 years of age.[89-91] Nearly 50 per cent cases show positive culture growth. Streptococcal pneumonia poses a difficult differential diagnosis.

Additional symptomological associations include sinusitis, otitis media and exacerbation of chronic bronchitis. Infection is common in cases with asplenia, sickle cell disease and immunocompromised patients. Patient may have fever, dyspnoea, or cough. Chest X-ray may show bronchopneumonia as well as segmental pneumonia. Infrequently pneumatocele may occur. Pleural effusion and empyema are quite common.

Treatment

Ampicillin, amoxycillin are the commonly used drugs. Steroids are only indicated in cases of acute affection of epiglottis.[92, 93]

Prevention

Rifampicin 20 mg/kg/day should be given as a single dose for 4 days to all the household contacts.[94] Immunisation of children at 18 months with an injection of conjugate vaccine is recommended.[95]

Whooping Cough

It is caused by gram negative bacillus Bordetella pertussis. The infection is highly communicable, 70-100 of cases occurring due to household contacts and 25-50 of cases occurring in school contacts. Children are affected as early 4 years of age in developing countries. 50 per cent of cases are infants and 15 per cent under the age of 15 years in USA4.[1] The route of transmission is by droplet infection from infected persons.

Incubation period is 7-10 days. Non-specific catarrhal stage is followed by proxysmal stage wherein sneezing, eye bulging, vomiting, fever and proxysmal cough are disturbing features for 2-4 weeks. Reappearance of fever indicates suppurative complication. Convalescent phase may last upto a month or so. 45 percent of patients are hospitalised, 75 per cent being below the age of 6 months. Pneumonitis occurs in 12-20 per cent of cases below one year of age, either as interstitial pneumonitis or as bronchopneumonia. It may be suspected as a cause of persistent cough in adults.[96]

Pulmonary complications are pneumothorax, atelectasis, bronchiectasis, diaphragmatic hernia and activation of tuberculosis. Extrapulmonary complications are CNS involvement in 1.7 per cent; encephalitis in 0.5 percent cases, otitis media, umbilical hernia and hemorrhages.

Total leucocytic count may be increased from 20,000 to 50,000/cumm with 60 percent lymphocytosis. Direct examination of specimen and positive culture may be diagnostic in 15-20 percent. Organism can be cultured on Regan-Lowe, Bordet-Gengon or modified Stainer-Schote agar. Direct fluorescent antibody test has variable sensitivity and ELISA is not of much help.[97] Differential diagnoses have been tabulated in Table 4.9.

Table 4.9: Whooping cough: DD
Allergic bronchitis
Coryza
Cystic fibrosis
Foreign body aspiration
Pneumonia
Tracheobronchitis

Treatment

Antibiotics are not indicated. Erythromycin is useful in 40 mg/kg/day in 2 divided doses for 2 weeks. Relapse occurs in 10 per cent of cases.

Prevention

Erythromycin should be given to all contacts of the patients. Immunised persons should get booster of DPT. Efficacy of whole cell and a cellular type of vaccines is effective in 80-90 per cent of cases and if suffer, the attack is very mild.[98]

Pneumatocele[99]

It occurs commonly in children, rare in adults, in association mostly with staph pneumonia.

Chest X-ray: Multiple air fluid levels with collapse lung at places.

Differential Diagnosis include:

- Bulla
- Lung abscess
- Herniated bowel in hemithorax.

Proposed by Conway in 1951, Boisset in 1972 concluded that bronchial inflammation which ruptures the bronchiolar walls, causing formation of air passage, where air dissects the passage to the pleura, thus forming pneumatocele, through a bursting lesion of the lung.

Absence of Kohn's pores in newborn, the infectious etiology in the presence of obstruction, pneumatocele occurs as the air continues to enter with no way out of segment due to absence of Kohn's pores. Rare occurrence of pneumatocele in adults signifies the value of Kohn's pores.

Undernutrition and hyper IgE syndrome often predispose in younger age, whereas infections (See the following box), trauma, pollutant (hydrocarbon ingestion) and positive pressure ventilation precipitate pneumatocele.

Infections :

- Staph aureus
- Strep pneumoniae
- Haem influenza
- Kleb pneumoniae
- S. marcescens
- E coli
- Group A streptococci
- Myco tuberculosis
- Pseudomonas aeruginosa
- Adenovirus

Management

- Antimicrobial treatment of pneumonia.
- Close watch.
- Rarely surgical intervention required.
- Large pneumatocele may burst causing tension pneumothorax.
- A tense pneumatocele may deviate mediastinum to contralateral side, requiring surgical drainage.[99]

Tularemia (Rabbit Fever) (Dear Fly Fever)

It is caused by gram negative aerobic coccobacilli called Francisella tularensis, found in animals and transmitted to human beings either by direct contact through ingestion or by inhalation. 200 cases have been reported of this arthropod borne disease in USA.[4]

Pulmonary involvement occurs in 10-15 per cent of cases. There is history of non-productive cough, with or without dyspnoea and pleuritic chest pain.

Pathogenesis

There is an inflammatory reaction with foci of alveolar necrosis with polymorphic activity initially, followed by mononuclear cells infiltration, leading to granuloma formation. Cervical and mediastinal lymphadenopathy occurs, followed by abscess formation and rupture.

Healing occurs with fibrosis and calcification of granuloma. Chest X-ray shows bilateral patchy infiltration in the form of ovoid densities. Lobar pneumonia and pleural effusion may occur. Pericarditis, endocarditis, osteomyelitis and meningitis may occur.[100-103]

Differential diagnosis includes mycoplasmal pneumonia. History is suggestive in 40 per cent of cases towards diagnosis. Blood culture is negative. Differential diagnoses are shown in Table 4.10.

Table 4.10: Tularaemia: Differential diagnoses

1. Cat-scratch disease
2. Rickettsial infection
3. Infectious mononucleosis
4. Fungaemia
5. Meningococcal infection

ELISA may be of help in first week, agglutinins level rises in 1-2 weeks. A delayed type of skin test is positive during first week of infection. Streptomycin 7.5-10 mg/kg 12 hourly is effective. Gentamicin can also be used. Relapse rate is 20 per cent when treated with tetracyclines and chloramphenicol.

Prevention

To avoid skinning with animals especially the rabbits. Multipuncture intradermal vaccine made from F. tularensis, recommended by CDC, is affective.

Prognosis

Life-long immunity is achieved following infection with F. tularensis.[104] Mortality is 8 per cent. Mortality of 1-3 per cent even with the treatment may occur.[105]

Other Gram Negative Pneumonias

Escherichia coli, Bacillus proteus and Pseudomonas aeruginosa occasionally produce pneumonia in compromised hosts with malignant disorders, cystic fibrosis or prolonged antimicrobial therapy. Often, they are demonstrable but assume significance as aetiological agents if isolated repeatedly in heavy growth. The clinical features are similar to other Gram negative infections. Proteus pneumonia, however makes a more insidious onset. The condition needs therapy with gentamicin, carbenicillin or ticarcillin.[2]

Legionnaire's Disease (Pontiac Fever)

Legionnaire's disease is a multi-system disorder affecting the lung, kidney, alimentary tract and central nervous system.[106] It is second most common cause of severe community acquired pneumonia requiring intermittant positive pressure ventilation. It occurs in middle-aged or elderly persons, frequently among males who are 3 times more affected than females. Infection is uncommon in children. It spreads by airborne route and it has been noted to occur frequently in hotel or hospital surroundings. Infection is responsible for 1-3 per cent cases of community acquired pneumonias, 10 per cent nosocomial pneumonias and 30 per cent hospital infections.[4] Person-to-person transmission does not take place. A higher incidence is noted in patients with some underlying disease or in those receiving immuno-suppressive therapy. Even alcohol and smoking are considered precipitating factors.

It is caused by Gram negative, aerobic, coccobacillus-Legionella pneumophila, and other Legionel-la-like organisms.[107] Legionellosis consists of a spectrum of diseases, one Pontiac fever is a flu like self-limiting syndrome, seen in immunocompromised patients. Legionella pneumophila serotype (type-1) accounts for 50 per cent of human infection, out of 34 species and 50 distinct serogroups. Biochemical analysis, autofluorescence, immunofluorescence, staining and gas liquid chromatography are used to characterise these strains and subtypes.[108,109] These organisms are present in soil excavations and in air conditioning cooling towers and evaporative condensers. The organism has an affinity for water, particularly if blue-green algae are present.

There is an incubation period of two to ten days. Infection spreads through endobronchial, hematogenous and lymphatic routes.[110] The pathologic changes are essentially alveolitis with bronchiolitis and hence confined to the lungs where it produces an acute fibrinopurulent patchy bronchopneumonia and the alveolli are filled with polymorphs admixed with macrophages and a large amount of fibrin. Multilobar consolidation may occur. Abscess formation, with a central necrosis is seen in 25 per cent of fatal cases. Pleural effusion may occur but empyema is not seen. The toxins of the bacteria may cause an acute necrosis and encephalopathy.[2] Bacteremia occurs in 1/3rd of cases, causing extrapulmonary infection.

Onset is acute, with prodromal features consisting of malaise, muscle ache, slight headache and anorexia. It is followed by fever, chills, non-productive cough, dyspnoea and prostration. There can be vomiting, abdominal pain, diarrhoea, oliguria, disorientation, confusion and delirium. These symptoms are due to toxic encephalopathy. Rarely cranial or peripheral nerves are involved. Purulent expectoration may occur in 50 per cent of cases and haemoptysis occurs in 1/3rd of cases. Chest examination shows the presence of crackles and later signs of consolidation.

Moderate polymorphonuclear leucocytosis is seen in 10 to 20 per cent of cases. Chest X-ray shows patchy infiltrates, which later progress to lobar shadows either unilaterally or bilaterally. Gram stain of sputum shows few polymorphs without any bacteria. There is marked hypoxaemia, proteinuria and elevated liver enzymes. Often there is hyponatraemia in 50-70 per cent of cases and hypophosphatemia. There is absence of bacterial pathogens on Gram's staining. The causative agent may be demonstrated by direct immunofluorescence of the transtracheal or percutaneous lung aspirate using Gimenez stain or Dieterle's silver impregnation stain and cultured on charcoal yeast extract agar in two to four days. A four-fold rise in fluorescent antibody titres against L. Pneumophila develop after three weeks of infection.[2]

The disease may pursue a mild to fatal course. Pulmonary complications are empyema (rarely), lung abscess, respiratory failure and systemic ones include hypotension, DIC, ITP, renal failure. Other complications include prosthetic valve endo-carditis, pericarditis, myocarditis, pancreatitis, pyelonephritis, liver abscess, etc.[108,111,112] Death occurs from respiratory failure, shock, hypotension and acute renal failure. The condition is treated with erythromycin 0.5 gm six hourly orally or intravenously in critically ill patients over a period of three weeks. Rifamycin may be used in those who are severely ill and in those showing poor response to erythromycin. The condition needs supportive therapy with oxygen, mechanical ventilators, volume replacement, vasoactive agents and dialysis,[113] important features are shown in the Table 4.11.

Table 4.11: Legionnaire's disease

Investigations:
Total cell count and ESR are high, U protein +ve
Indirect fluorescent antibodies +ve
DD:
Bronchitis
Influenza
Pneumonia
Renal failure
Treatment:
Erythromycin is affective
Rifamycin may be used

Prognosis and Prevention

Mortality is 15 per cent. It has decreased from 80 per cent to 25 per cent with the use of erythromycin in immunocompromised patients. However, postinfection residual pulmonary fibrosis has been reported. *Rifamycin* has been recommended as an additional agent though clinical experience has not been reported. Jaundice is likely to be more common in such patients.

Proper surveillance of water systems and amplifiers and regular cleansing and sterilization should be done.

Bronchopneumonia

Bronchopneumonia is a combination of bronchiolitis and pneumonia. There is a patchy involvement. The inflammatory process spreads downwards along the airways to a number of terminal bronchioles and respiratory bronchioles and alveoli.

It is noted when there is damage to the normal defence mechanism of the lower respiratory tract with depression of cough and paralysis of ciliary clearance mechanism. It facilitates retention of bronchial secretions. In such situations the region is invaded by the commensal organisms present in the upper respiratory tract.

Bronchopneumonia is seen in young children during or after measles and whooping cough, aged persons, debilitated individuals and post-operative conditions.[2] There is no specific pathogen, however, staphylococcus, streptococcus, streptococcus pneumoniae, and H. influenzae are incriminated as causative agents. There is bilateral patchy inflammation with inflammation crossing anatomic divisions between lobes. The bronchioles are infiltrated by lymphocytes. The alveolar *exudate* shows polymorphs and fibrin. There may be destruction of bronchioles and interstitial tissue leading to fibrosis and bronchiectasis. The resolution is incomplete.[2]

It has a gradual onset, with fever, cough and dyspnoea, the sputum is viscid. Often it causes obstruction to the bronchioles leading to collapse. The temperature and pulse are increased. There is tachypnoea. Bronchial breathing is heard in different regions and there may be diminished breath sounds in some areas. Crepitations and ronchi are audible either in bases or throughout the lung.

X-ray chest shows scattered areas of ill-defined opacities especially in the basal regions. The response to the antibiotics is poor.

It is treated with crytalline pencillin 1 mega unit, along with streptomycin sulphate 1gm intramuscularly daily.

Non-bacterial Pneumonias[2]

Unlike bacterial pneumonias, these pneumonias are associated with systemic manifestations such as headache, pain, mild fever and relatively few respiratory symptoms. They have interstitial exudate unlike alveolar exudate of bacterial pneumonia. The sputum is rarely present and pleural effusion is uncommon. Radiologically the shadows are more florid than the clinical signs. Peripheral leucocyte count is within normal limits.[114]

Rickettsial Pneumonia

Q fever (Queensland Fever) is caused by Coxiella burnetti first described in 1935 from Australia, and later on from the U.S.A. and the U.K. A history of contact with cattle or sheep is present. The process is patchy, consisting of microscopic areas of conjestion and odema.[4] Pulmonary involvement varies from 0-90%.

An eosinophilic exudate is present in the alveolar spaces with desquamation of epithelial cells, and infiltrations of the alveolar walls with lymphocytes, plasma cells, erythrocytes, and a large macrophages but there are very few polymorphs. After an incubation period of one to two weeks, the condition develops insidiously with systemic manifestations and minimal respiratory symptoms. There is persistent low grade fever, severe headache, malaise and loss of weight. Cough and dyspnoea may be present. Occasionally crepitations are heard. There is bradycardia.[2] Chest pain is not a feature.

X-ray chest shows patchy opacities. WBC count may be normal. The complement fixation test shows a raising antibody titre. Rickettsias can rarely be seen microscopically in the tissue section. They can be readily identified by immunofluorescent technique. Failure to demonstrate them has no diagnostic significance.[115] The condition may be complicated by endocarditis. The daily administration of tetracycline in 2 to 4 gm dose improves the condition, but doesn't have rickettsiocidal property. Chloramphenicol is *also effective*. Supportive treatment for hypotension and dialysis for acute renal failure is indicated.

Chlamydial Pneumonia

Psittacosis (Ormithosis)

Psittacosis is an uncommon acute systemic infection due to Chlamydia transmitted by infected psittacine birds (Parrots and Parakeets) and fowl (pigeons, turkeys and ducks)[27,116] and can result in pulmonary manifestations, such as pneumonia.

Aetiology and Pathology

It is caused by C psittaci, a gram negative obligate intracellular bacteria 90 species of which have been documented. It enters the body through the respiratory passages by inhalation while a person is handling infected birds. There is an incubation period of 7-15 days. There is a hematogenous systemic spread with the organisms localising in the liver, spleen, lung, kidney, central nervous system and cardia. There is an inflammatory reaction both in the interstitial as well as respiratory surfaces of alveoli and also in the perivascular spaces. Both alveolar walls and interstitial lung tissue are thickened; odema, necrosis and hemorrhage may occur.[117] Histologically, the filled fluid may show lymphocytes, erythrocytes and pathognomic macrophages containing cytoplasmic inclusion on bodies called LCL.[4] The respiratory epithelium of bronchi and bronchioles remains intact.

Clinical Features

These may vary from a *transient viral like* illness to severe fatal pneumonia.[118] The incubation period is one to two weeks. The onset may be acute or insidious. The initial symptoms are high fever, severe headache, myalgia, photophobia and non-productive cough. Later cough becomes productive of scanty mucoid expectoration. Chest pain due to pleurisy may occur though pelural effusion is rarely seen. Respiratory rate may be increased, dyspnoea with cyanosis may occur in extensive psittacasial involvement. Epistaxis may occur in 25 per cent of cases in early course of the disease. Photophobia, pericarditis and myocarditis have also been reported.[4] Haemoptysis may occur.

A macular rash (Horden's spot) may occur over the face. There can be gastrointestinal symptoms and deteriorating mental status. Clinical examination may reveal crackles over the lung bases. Splenomegaly, erythema nodosum and relative bradycardia are other systemic findings. Immunity to reinfection is probably permanent.

Investigations

No specific laboratory or radiological signs are *present.* The chest X-ray shows patchy opacities often with segmental distribution. The white cell count and ESR are normal. The condition mimics non-bacterial pneumonia. A four-fold rise in complement fixation antibody titre in the sera drawn during the acute and convalescent stages is diagnostic.[2]

Treatment

Chlamydial infection responds to the administration of tetracycline, and it has to be given in a dose of 500 mg orally four times a day for a week. In severe cases, hospitalisation with intensive pulmonary care may be indicated.

Chlamydia Pneumoniae Pneumonia

This is a recent infection described by Grayston J.T., *et al.*[119,120] 50 isolates have been obtained from patients world-wide. The clinical spectrum includes acute upper respiratory tract symptoms like pharyngitis, sinusitis, followed by bronchitis and pneumonitis, especially in young males. The pneumonia resembles that caused by Mycoplasma pneumoniae.

Symptoms include fever, non-productive cough, and upper respiratory tract symptoms. Chest examination is minimal contributory. There is no leucocytosis. Chest X-ray shows small segmental infiltrates. Pneumonitis may be severe and necessitates hospitalisation, in the elderly patient, requiring respiratory support.

Retrospective diagnosis can be made by chlamydial complement fixation. Cell culture techniques can be routinely applied for diagnosis. C. pneumoniae has shown sensitivity to erythromycin and tetracyclines in vitro studies.

Mycoplasmal Pneumonia

Upper respiratory tract infection to pneumonia can be caused by Mycoplasma pneumoniae, earlier recognised as Eaton Agent.[2] Although affects mouth organ systems, the Mycoplasma pneumoniae infection has protean clinical manifestations.

Mycoplasma are the smallest free living micro organisms. Mycoplasma pneumoniae are not present in healthy people. They are noted in the oropharynx during infection and convalescence.

The condition manifests as rhinitis, pharyngitis, tracheobronchitis, pneumonia or may cause acute exacerbations of chronic bronchitis after an incubation period of one to two weeks. The classical clinical syndrome consists of acute or subacute tracheobronchitis.[121] The infection is common in adolescents and young adults. It spreads by infected respiratory secretions. With infiltration of large round cells and mononuclear cells, the alveoli are filled with oedema fluid, red cells and macrophages.

The onset is acute with constitutional symptoms like fever, chills, headache, malaise, arthralgia, myalgia, rash and anorexia. The respiratory manifestations are absent initially. In one to five days a scratchy sore throat is followed by cough which initially is dry and irritating, later becoming productive of mucoid or mucopurulent expectoration. Often cough is paroxysmal becoming worse at night. There may be retrosternal soreness and dyspnoea. The infection often precipitates wheezing episodes in bronchial asthmatics and may exacerbate COPD. Physical examination of the chest reveals relatively few signs and basal crepitations are audible most often.

The chest *X-ray* reveals reticular interstitial infiltrates initially and air space pneumonia develops later on. The infiltrates are generally segmental or lobar in their distribution. Patchy areas of bronchopneumonias, especially of the lower lobes is common in more than 3/4th of cases. Areas of subsegmental atelectasis may appear. Small pleural effusions may develop in some cases. ESR is elevated moderately, with leucocytosis seen only in 25% of cases. Though sputum shows polymorphonuclear leucocytes, it is negative for bacteria. The mycoplasma can be isolated from sputum or throat swab but it is very slow to grow. These have also been isolated in cases of children with lower respiratory tract infectionl.[122] The sera from acute and convalescent phase obtained nearly three weeks apart shows a four-fold rise in the antibody titre demonstrable by the complement fixation and indirect fluorescent antibody techniques. These tests have value in confirming the diagnosis retrospectively. User friendly, sensitive, specific, rapid and low cost serological or amplified/non-amplified methods of detection of mycoplasma/its nucleic acid are the need of the hour for management of mycoplasma pneumoniae infection.[123]

The disease is benign and self-limited. The course is prolonged with low mortality.[124] The disease settles within 2-4 weeks, without any treatment.[4] Some cases may progress to respiratory syndromes including ARDS. Occasionally complications like otitis media, bullous meningitis, coagulopathies, non-cardiogenic pulmonary odema, haemolytic anaemia, thrombocytopaenic purpura and Stevens-Johnson syndrome may occur. Rarely life threatening or fatal episodes may occur. Arthritis, myocarditis and pericarditis may also be seen.[12]

The condition is treated with tetracycline or erythromycin, 500 mg orally four times a day for one week.[125,126] The radiologic shadow makes rapid clearing.

Radiation Pneumonia

Radiation exposure may cause radiation cancers, genetic mutations and radiation pneumonia apart from effect on stem, bones growth, teeth, lung etc.[127,128] Radiation pneumonia is an inflammatory condition of the lung caused by irradiation during radiotherapy. Therapeutic irradiation undertaken for the treatment of cancer of breast, oesophagus, lungs and lymphomas and use of radioactive isotopes in thyroid disorders are likely to result in radiation pneumonia.[2]

The alveolar lining cell becomes swollen with a lymphocytic cellular infiltration of alveolar walls. The alveoli are filled with an exudate containing desquamated alveolar cells and macrophages. The bronchioles show destruction of surface epithelium and there is excessive secretion of mucous. Pneumonitis is progressive with a tendency to develop diffuse fibrosis[129] yet little lung damage following nearly lethal amounts of whole body irradiation exposure has been documented.[4]

Clinically, there is a rapidly increasing dyspnoea, dry cough and pain in the chest. The latter may occur due to rib fracture following radiation injury. Initially, there is dysphagia of short duration from radiation oesophagitis. There is no fever. The breath sounds are diminished and crepitations are audible.

Hb may be low, ESR is elevated. X-ray chest reveals opacity around the hilum and mid-zones simulating pulmonary oedema. It may progress to fibrosis. The lung damage is limited to the area of irradiation and shows some improvement in the course of a few weeks. There is a restrictive ventilatory abnormality. The diffusing capacity is reduced.[2]

In the acute stages for relief of symptoms and to halt the inflammatory process, corticosteroids are useful. They inhibit its progress to fibrosis. Prednisolone is given 40 mg reduced to a maintenance dose of 10 mg and is administered for three to six months. Oxygen administration is necessary to correct hypoxaemia.[2] Antibiotics are often indicated to prevent bacterial infection. There are known forms of therapy for prevention of late effects of radiation exposure.

Lipoid Pneumonia

The pulmonary inhalation of oil is likely to result in diffuse pneumonia or fibrotic granuloma. The inert mineral oil liquid paraffin, used as laxative or used as nasal drops may be inhaled by elderly people with neurological disturbances.[2] The malnourished young children may inhale milk or cod liver oil, which undergoes hydrolysis liberating fatty acids. This may happen as a part of aspiration of mild or oily preparation, in case of forced feeding or improper positioning (horizontal) during feeding or presence of cleft palate.[130]

There is a proliferative interstitial inflammation. Around the oil, a polymorphonuclear reaction occurs in the alveoli followed by macrophages and giant cells forming an intra-alveolar exudate. The severity of pulmonary reaction depends upon the type of oil inhaled, vegetable oil being less irritating than animal oil, because of high fatty acid content, which is most damaging.[131] The alveolar walls get thickened infiltered of lymphocytes and plasma cells, leading to fibrosis of the alveolar walls with the destruction of alveoli and obliteration of blood vessels.[132]

Clinically, there can be cough with mucoid expectoration and dyspnoea may be present. There may be signs of consolidation and crepitations may be audible. X-ray chest shows reticular or nodular shadows. The sputum may show macrophages filled with fat droplets (on staining with Sudan III). The sputum is obtained for examination on fat free diet for one week. The lung functions show a restrictive defect without airways obstruction.[133] Prognosis is guarded because of secondary bronchopneumonic infections which are quite common.[131]

There is no specific treatment. Infant's position should be changed frequently to avoid development of hypostatic pneumonia. Prevention lies in stopping the use of oily nasal drops or laxatives in those with danger of aspiration.

An endogenous lipoid pneumonia as a localised lesion can appear in chronic respiratory diseases like lung abscess, bronchiectasis and may even complicate carcinoma. The degenerating lung tissue results in deposition of cholesterol esters and is taken up by macrophages in the alveoli and alveolar walls.[2]

Chickenpox (Varicella) Pneumonia

Chickenpox infection is a universal mild form of infection in the childhood. In 1/3rd of cases during the course of chicken-pox, lungs may get involved especially in young adults and in 20 per cent cases of middle aged individuals. The pneumonic symptoms develop three to five days after the appearance of the rash and may deteriorate. It is manifested by pleuritic pain, cough, blood stained sputum and dyspnoea. It may be associated with shock, hypotension and cyanosis. Lungs show crepitations bilaterally.[2] Secondary bacterial infections are quite common.

There are patchy areas of haemorrhagic consolidation and focal necrosis in the lungs. The alveolar walls are congested and there is infiltration of macrophages, lymphocytes and polymorphs.[2]

Chest X-ray reveals nodular infiltrates with interstitial pneumonitis. There are bilateral opacities of variable size in both lung fields, being marked in the mid and lower zones. Lab tests include Fluorescent Antibody to Membrane Antigen

(FAMA) and ELISA which are quite sensitive.[4] Immune prophylaxis includes Varicella-Zoster immunoglobulin (VZIG)[134,135] intravenously within 72 hours of infection, although its effectiveness in adults and pregnant women is questioned. Alive attenuated vaccine, VZV (Varicella-Zoster vaccine) has been proposed for normal and immunocompromised host for prevention.[136]

Treatment is mainly supportive. Mortality is as high as 20% in acutely ill patients. Pneumonia resolves slowly in two to three weeks almost parallel to resolution of skin lesions. Steroids better be avoided because the condition may even be fatal. Acyclovir may be of use in severely ill patients. In few cases small soft nodular opacities persist indicating a fibrotic process, which later undergo calcification over a period of years. It appears that the people, on retrospective analysis, who were not severely ill during acute infection are likely to have calcification.[137] Differential diagnosis includes tuberculosis and histoplasmosis. Systemic complications of chickenpox include myocarditis, nephritis, arthritis, hepatitis glomerulonephrits etc. Immunocompromised patients should be protected from exposure, since the disease is contageous.

Pulmonary Meliodosis

An acute respiratory infection can occur from Pseudomonas Pseudomallei Whitmore's Bacillus[138] an aerobic Gram-negative becillus closely related to the causative agent of glanders, presenting with fever, productive cough, pleuritic chest pain, weight loss and haemoptysis.[2] The condition may be a primary pneumonia following inhalation or by a hematogenous spread.[139] Tachypnoea may be out of proportion to fever. Chest examination may reveal few rales. Liver and spleen are not palpable in undisseminated cases. The disease may have a varying clinical course from simple bronchitis to fulminant necrotising pneumonia. Multiple hepatosplenic and cutaneous abscesses with a fulminant respiratory failure and radiologically mimicking tuberculosis can be the presentation in melioidoses.[140] There can be disseminated abscesses following septicemic episodes and present as pneumonia, arthritis, hepatitis, meningitis or osteomyelitis, uncommonly pleural effusion and bilateral hilar lymphadenopathy may occur.[141]

Primary focus of infection may be skin, subcutaneous tissue and lungs. Diabetes, renal disease, immunosuppression, alcohol, pregnancy and drug abuse act as precipitating factors. Mortality is high, 80-90% in case of disseminated sepsis.[142] There is leucocytosis with normocytic normochronic anemia. The radiological picture simulates pulmonary tuberculosis with nodular infiltration or abscess formation in chronic cases giving rise to thin-walled cavities in the upper lobes which are usually involved. The growth of the organism on culture of sputum or of skin pustules can be obtained and an elevated titre of haemagglutinins and complement-fixing antibodies are diagnostic. A negative complement fixation test does not exclude disease as it is seen in l/3rd of cases. At the same time, serological positivity indicating subclinical infection is quite common as compared to clinical human melioidosis which is rare.

Tetracyclines alone or in combination with chloramphenicol, in doses of 2 to 3 gm are effective. The treatment has to be prolonged with a minimum period of eight weeks to prevent recurrence. Ciprofloxacin is not effective against P. pseudomallei.[143] In case of multiple resistance strains trimethaprim-sulfamethoxazole combination has been recommended for 60-150 days. Patients allergic to sulphonamides, can be treated with ceftazodime and cefotaxime. Carbapenem helps in rapid cure. Even multiple drug regimen is suggested for acutely pneumonitic patients, using levaimisole 150 mg twice a week as adjuvant therapy.[144,145] Mortality is 100% in untreated cases and more than 50% in cases with septicemia despite antibiotics therapy. There is no active immunisation.[4] Recently, two cases of this imported infection are reported in Indian patients.[146,147]

Glanders

Glanders is a generalised infection in man by nonmotile, aerobic, gram negative organism called Pseudomonas mallei occurring from horses and donkeys. In inhaled form, nasal ulceration, pneumonia, lung abscess and empyema are common. Pneumonia may also be seen in septicemic form. Diagnosis is made either by culture or four-fold rise in complement fixing antibody titre after 2-4 weeks of infection. Sulfadiazine is the drug of choice given for 3-4 weeks.

Hypostatic Pneumonia[131]

This occurs as a complication in patients who are kept lying in one position for quite a long time. This can be seen in elderly patients also who are debilitated and bed ridden.

The clinical symptomatology is not characteristic. There is no pyrexia or dyspnoea unless there is some other underlying cardiopulmonary disorder. Physical examination of chest is not much contributory. Respiration sounds are feeble with few fine crackles. Pathologically, there is dependent conjestion, odema and pneumonitis.

Management includes treatment of primary cause. Prophylaxis is important in the form of advice to frequently changing the positions of patient, especially the elderly, immobile due to any cause.

Community Acquired Pneumonia

Pneumonia is the most common fatal community acquired infection. Guidelines on management of community acquired pneumonia have been laid down by Infectious Diseases Society of America.[148]

Most cases of community acquired pneumonia requiring hospital admission are caused by Streptococcus pneumoniae (34%); Mycoplasma pneumoniae is the next and most frequent cause (18%); legionnaires' disease as a sporadic condition is uncommon (2%); and the combination of influenza and Staphylococcus aureus is rare but disastrous. The most valuable of the widely available and rapid aetiological investigations are Gram's stain of sputum (insensitive but with a high positive predictive value in pneumococcal infection), blood culture, sputum culture, and cold agglutinin detection (present in 56% of mycoplasma infections with a specificity of 96%).

A fatal outcome was associated with hypotension and tachypnoea and with a rise of the blood urea concentration in hospitalised patients. The overall mortality was almost 6 per cent. Of those who had been treated, only a fifth had pneumococcal penumonia compared with almost half of those who had not received antibiotics. The survey emphasises that these infections must be taken seriously.[148]

The British Thoracic Society recommends that the management of patients with community acquired pneumonia can be improved. As soon as clinical features of pneumonia are evident in an adult treatment with an antibiotic effective against S. pneumoniae should be started and if Mycoplasma infections are prevalent at the time, or there are other suggestive clinical features, erythromycin or tertracycline should also be given. During influenza outbreaks at least one (and, in view of the lethal effect of staphylococcal superinfection, perhaps two) anti-staphylococcal antibiotics should be prescribed. Patients should be referred to hospital if they fail to improve with treatment at home, if their diastolic blood pressure is less than 60 mm Hg, if their respiratory rate is over 30 per minute, or if they are confused or elderly. If the patient is critically ill or if epidemiological evidence suggests legionella infection, treatment for that condition should be added. Thus, though we may rightly condemn the indiscriminate prescription of antibiotics, their timely and informed use in patients with pneumonia is vital and rewarding.[149] Although rapid antibiotic delivery is expected in the lungs because of their being highly vascular organs, yet several factors may interfere with antibiotic access and action in the lungs.[150] The therapy should be initiated as early as possible.

Desquamative Interstitial Pneumonia

Desquamative Interstitial Pneumonia (DIP) is a chronic lung disease of unknown cause characterized by a heavy accumulation of mononuclear cells, mostly macrophages, in the distal air spaces of lungs. It was first described by Liebow in 1962 and later additional 18 cases were reported in 1965 by Liebow, Steer and Billingsley.[151]

Interstitial pneumonitis has been classified into six variants:[152]

1. Usual interstitial pneumonitis.
2. Desquamative interstitial pneumonitis.
3. Giant cell interstitial pneumonitis.
4. Lymphoid interstitial pneumonitis.
5. Bronchiolitis obliterans with interstitial penumonitis.
6. Plasma cell interstitial pneumonitis.

DIP usually is a disease of adults, although Tal *et al.*[153] have reported three siblings who developed/DIP during early infancy. About 60 per cent of the reported cases have been in males. Clinically, symptoms consist of dyspnoea, non-productive cough, and weight loss. Arthralgia and myalgia may be present. Physical findings may be absent or may be limited to basal rales, with or without clubbing. Triangular opacities consising of confirmed reticulonodular and acinar patterns extending into both lung bases from the hila, loss of lung volume and hilar lymphadenopathy are seen on chest X-ray. Spontaneous pneumothorax has been described in three of the 12 cases.[154]

Aetiology

The cause of DIP is unknown. It is not certain whether it represents a foreign body type reaction, sequelae of infection or an autoimmune phenomenon. Rheumatoid factor, anti-nuclear factor and the lupus erythematosus phenomenon have been reported in DIP.[155,156]

Pathology

As a result of loss of type I alveolar epithelial cells and proliferation of type II cells, the alveolar spaces are filled with large mononuclear cells that were originally believed to be desquamated type II cells.[157]

Corticosteroids are recognised as the treatment of choice in DIP.[155] However, spontaneous remissions have been described. Immunotherapy (cyclophosphamide) is indicated in those patients who do not respond to steroids. Failure to respond to steroids could be because of coexisting interstitial fibrosis or advanced disease. Chloroquine has also been suggested in the treatment of DIP. Both antemortem and postmortem cases have been reported.[158,159]

Nosocomial Pneumonia

Introduction

Pneumonias can be classified, from the clinical stand point, into the community acquired and the hospital acquired (nosocomial).[160] The former has been separately described. Nosocomial pneumonias pose a particular problem in post-operative patients[161] and in-patients in intensive care units despite an advancement in diagnostic techniques and use of potent blood spectrum antimicrobials. These pneumonias are important because:

a. The microbiology distinctly differs from the community acquired pneumonias.
b. They constitute a leading cause of mortality from hospital acquired infections.

c. There is a steady rise in number.
d. Nearly 1 per cent of hospitalised and 60 per cent of intensive care unit patients develop pneumonia.
e. Fatality occurs in 1/3rd of cases.
f. Presentation is quite vague, therefore delayed diagnosis.
g. Early recognition and bacterial diagnosis does improve chances of survival.

Risk Factors

1. Residence in intensive care unit.
2. Ineffective cough reflex.
3. Elderly patients, above 60 years of age.
4. Depressed alertness due to age, disease or recent surgery.
5. Indwelling catherter, nasogastric tube or endotracheal intubation done.
6. Arteriovenous shunt or fistula.
7. Accompanying diseases like diabetes mellitus or congestive heart failure.
8. Impaired mucocilliary mechanism due to underlying chronic lung disease.

Epidemiology

Nearly 80 per cent of nosocomial pneumonias are caused by gram negative bacilli like Pseudomonas aerugenosa, Klebsiella pneumoniae, E. coli and Proteus species.[162,163] Pseudomonas aerugenosa accounts for 15-20 per cent of cases while E.coli, Enterobacter, Klebsiella and Proteus species are responsible for 30-40 per cent of cases. Other gram negative aerobic bacilli like Serratia, Citrobacter and H. influenzae may be responsible for 1-4 per cent of nosocomial pneumonias. Gram positive aerobic organisms like Staphylococci and Streptococci account for 15-20 per cent of cases, while 10-20 per cent cases are polymicrobial. 2-5 per cent cases may be due to anerobic organisms.

The spectrum and sensitivity pattern to microbial agents, of these organisms may vary from hospital to hospital inflenced by infection control measures in an institution as well as by the use of antibiotics both for community as well as hospital infections.

Pathogenesis

Lack of host resistance and easy access of the organism to the lower respiratory tract is responsible for nosocomial pneumonia. Risk factors include immunodeficiency status, haematologic factors, malignancy and immunosuppressive therapy. Gram negative as well as other opportunistic pathogens gain access to the alveoli either through subclinical aspiration of naso-pharyngeal secretions, facilitated by gastric acid aspirations causing chemical injury to pulmonary tissue. Haematogenous spread from extrapulmonary areas like skin and urinary tract may also occur. Even contaminated ventilation system tubing and inhalor therapy equipment have been implicated. Gastric colonization with gram negative bacilli may play a casual role in developing nosocomial pneumonia in-patients in the intensive care units.[164] Therefore, the protective role of drugs enhancing gastric motility, acidifying the enteral feed (ph 3.5), and antacids as well as protective role of prophylactic broad spectrum antimicrobials, have been questioned?

Diagnosis

Diagnostic criteria include identification of the organisms, and effect on lung functions, apart from clinical features like pyrexia, leukocytosis, purulent secretions and of course radiological shadows. Total count is not helpful, neither purulent secretion with fever is specific for nosocomial pneumonia. Radiological differential diagnoses include pulmonary emboli, ARDS, atelectasis and fluid overload. Similarly, bacteriological diagnosis poses a lot of difficulties. Culture from sputum, secretions or tracheal aspirate may be fruitful but does not differentiate between infection and colonization. BAL gives a better profile but again the results are equivocal. The protected brush specimen (PBS), with the fiberoptic bronchoscope is considered to be quite reliable in diagnosing bacteriologically.

Management

It includes prompt recognition and elimination of risk factors. Positioning of obtunded patient in a swimmer's position and isolation as early as possible. Empirical therapy should be started. Antimicrobials can be used as given below:

a. Penicillinase resistant penicillins like naficillin, oxacillin against Staphylococcal infection.
b. Extended penicillins like piperacillin, mezlocillin, azocillin and ticarcillin for gram negative infections including pseudomonas.
c. Betalactams, aztreonam and imipenem in immuno-compromised patients.
d. Cephalosporins like cefotaxime and ceftazidine in pseudomonas infection where group (c) agents are ineffective. Empiric therapy is instituted before the culture reports are received. This may be a combination of beta lactam broad spectrum antibiotic with an aminoglycoside or double beta lactam therapy is started. Alternative regimens may include fluoroquinolones like ofloxacin and aztreonam in combination with vancomycin, clindamycin or metronidazole or a beta lactam, vancomycin combined with an aminoglycoside; a fluoroquinolone combined with metronidazole or clindamycin.

Strict infection control measures, judicious prescribing of antimicrobials, antibiotics resistance surveillance programme and antibiotic cycling should be adopted to control infections due to these MDR resistant bacteria in hospitalized (ICU) patients.[165]

Pneumonia in Immunocompromised Patient

Immunity is compromised in AIDS patients, the modern plague engulfing the world. Use of corticosteroids and other immunosuppressive drugs in connective tissues disorders and auto immune diseases, application of chemotherapy in various malignant disorders and organ transplantation-surgeries also leads to alteration in immunity of these patients. This results in infections, lungs being the most common site and ultimately proves fatal. Out of various opportunistic infections in immuno suppressed patients which are listed in Table 4.12 pneumocystic carinii pneumonia, tuberculosis and pyogenic bacterial pneumonia are HIV related pulmonary disorders which are effectively treatable.

Table 4.12: Pulmonary infections in HIV disease/AIDS

HIV related
Tuberculosis
Nocardiosis
Possibly HIV related
Pyogenic bacterial pneumonias
Non-infectious lymphoid interstitial pneumonitis
Opportunistic infections
Pneumocystic carinii pneumonia
Pulmonary toxoplasmosis
Pulmonary cryptococcosis
Pulmonary strongyloidosis
Disseminated histoplasmosis
Disseminated MAC infection
Cytomegalovirus and Herpes simplex pneumonias

Immunodeficiency Pneumonia[166-167]

IgA immumnodeficiency is more common than selective IGM deficiency, which has 0.03% community incidence. This state of dysgammaglu bulinemia, often has other immunoglobulins normal except raised IgE levels. Earlier thought to be occurring in childhood, is now recognized first time in adulthood with recurrent chest infections including pneumonia.

Preventive vacination against capsulated organisms and viruses have yield no benefit as there is failure of even IgG responses to capsular organisms despite normal IgG levels.

REFERENCES

1. Medical Research Council. Brit. Med. Jour 1965, 2: 319.
2. Shankar P.S., Chest Medicine, Oxford and IBH Publ Co. (P) Ltd. N. Delhi 1994, 4th ed.
3. Report of the MRC Working Party. Brit Med. Jour 1965, 2: 211.
4. *Harrison's Principles of Internal Medicine.*, Wilson J.D., Braunwald E., Isselbacher K.J., *et al.*, 12th ed., Vol 1, McGraw Hill, N.York 1991.
5. Gwaltney J.W., *Rhinoviruses, IN: Viral Infections of Humans,* Evans A.S. (Ed), New York, Plenum 1982.
6. Rossman M.G., *et al.*, Structure of a human common cold virus and functional relationships to other picornaviruses, Nature 1985, 317: 145.
7. Tyrrell D.A.J., Common colds, Inter Virology 1986, 25: 177.
8. McIntokn K., *Coronaviruses, IN, Virology,* 2nd Ed; Fields BN (ed) N. York, Raven 1989.
9. Larson H.E., *et al.*, Isolation of rhinoviruses and coronaviruses from 38 colds in adults, J. Med. Virol 1980, 5:221.
10. D'Alessio D.J., *et al.*, Short duration exposure and the transmission of rhinoviral cold, J Infect. Dis. 1984, 150: 189.
11. Teryar P.J., Report of a workshop on respiratory syncytial virus and parainfluenza viruses, J Infec. Dis 1983; 148: 528.
12. Baum S.G., *Adenoviruses, IN, Principles and practice of 'Infectious diseases,* 3rd (ed); Mandell G., *et al.*, (ed); Wiley; N, York 1990.
13. Murphy B.R. and Webster R.G., *Orthomyxo viruses, IN, Virology,* 2nd ed; Fields B.N.(ed), Raven, N. York 1989.
14. Centres for disease control, Prevention and control of influenza; Morb. Mort, Week Rep 1989, 38; 297.
15. Dolin R., *et al.*, A controlled trial of amantidine and rimantadine in the prophylaxis of influenza A infection, N. Eng. J. Med 1982, 307: 580.
16. LaMontagne J.R., *et al.*, Summary of clinical trials of inactivated influenza vaccines, 1978; Rev. Inf. Dis 1983, 5: 723.
17. Rana H., *et al.*, Epidemiology and clinical outcome of HINI in Gujarat from July 2009 to March 2010; JAPI 2012;60;95-97.
18. Wright P.F., *Parainfluenza viruses, IN, Textbook of human Virology,* Belshe R.B. (ed); Littleton M.A., PSG Publi. 1985.
19. Wigand R., *et al.*, *Adenoviridae,* 2nd Report, Inter Virology; 1982, 18: 169.
20. Ghai O.P., *Essential pediatrics,* 2nd ed, Interprint, N. Delhi, 1990.
21. Kaplan M.H., *et al.*, Group B Coxsackie virus infectious infants younger than three months of age, a serious childhood illness, Rev, Inf. Dis. 1983, 5: 1019.
22. Denny F.W., *et al.*, Croup, An 11-year study in a pediatric practice, Pediat 1983; 71: 871-876.
23. Tooley W.H. and Lipow H.W., *Inspiratory obstruction,* IN; Rudolph A.M., Pediatrics, Connecticut, Prentice Hall, Intemational 1987.
24. Hall C.B., *et al.*, Aerolized ribavirin treatment of infants with respiratory syncytial viral infection: A randomised double blind study, N. Eng. J. Med 1983,308: 1443.
25. Henderson F.W., *et al.*, Respiratory syncytial virus infections, Reinfections and immunity, N. Eng. J. Med 1979, 300: 530.
26. Mufson M.A., *et al.*, Respiratory syncytial virus epidemics; Variable dominance of subgroups A and B strains among children 1981-86, J. Inf. Dis 1988, 1: 143.
27. Glezen W.P., *et al.*, Risk of primary infection and reinfection with respiratory syncytial virus. Amer. J. Dis. Child 1986, 140: 543.
28. Englund J. A., *et al.*, Resp. Syncytial virus infection in immuno-compromised adults, Ann. Int. Med 1988, 109:203.
29. Hall C.B., Powell K.B., Mac-Donald N.E., *el al.*, New Eng. Jour. Med 1986, 315:77-81.
30. Zuhradnik J.M., *et al.*, Adenovirus infection in the immuno-suppressed patients, Amer. J.Med 1980;68:725.
31. CDC, *Measles prevention,* Suppl. statement, Morb. Mort Week Rep 1989; 38: 11.
32. Centres for disease control: *Measles prevention:* Recommendation of the immunization practices Advisory committee; Morb. Mrtt.Week, Rep 1987,36:409.

33. Fulginitsi V.A., Helfer R.E., Atypical measles in adolescent siblings 16 years after killed measles virus vaccine; JAMA 1980; 244: 804.
34. Gustafson T.L., *et al.,* Measles outbreak in a fully immunized secondary school population, N. Eng. J. Med 1987;317:771.
35. Ho M., *Cytomegalovirus, Biology and infection,* Plenum. N. York 1982.
36. Meyers J.D., *et al.,* Risk factors for CMV infection after human marrow transplantation; J. Inf. Dis 1986;153:478.
37. Reed E.C., *et al.,* Treatment of CMV pneumonia with genciclovir and intravenous CMV immunoglobulin in patients with bone marrow transplants; Ann. Int. Med 1988;109:783.
38. Skolnik P.R. and Hirsch M.S., *Therapy and prevention of CMV infections;* In: Declerq E. (ed); Clinical use of antiviral drugs; Bortin; Martinus Nijhoff 1988.
39. Bowden R.A., *et al.,* Cytomagalovirus immune globulin and seronegative blood products to prevent primary cytomegalovirus infection after marrow transplantation, N. Eng. J. Med 1986, 314: 1006.
40. Emmanuel D., *et al.,* Cytomegalovirus pneumonia after bone marrow transplantation successfully treated with the combination of ganciclovir and high dose intravenous immuno-globulin, Ann. Int. Med 1988,109:777.
41. Jacobson M.A. and Mills J., Serious CMV disease in AIDS, Ann.Int.Med 1988; 108: 585.
42. Onorato I.M., *et al.,* Epidemiology of CMV, Recommendations for prevention and control, Rev. Inf. Dis 1985;7:479.
43. Synderman D.R., *et al.,* Use of CMV immunoglobulin to prevent CMV disease in renal transplant recipient, N. Eng. J. Med 1987, 317: 1049.
44. Draw W.L., Diagnosis of Cytomegalovirus infection, Rev. Inf. Dis 1988; 10: 5468.
45. Boat T.F., *Lower respiratory tract, bacterial pneumonias and pneumonias of other causes.* In, Behrman R.E., Vanghan V.C. and Nelson W.E., ed; Textbook of Pediatrics; WB Saunders Co., Philadelphia 1987.
46. Shankar P.S., *Changing Patterns in Pneumonias,* In, Post-graduate Medicine, 2, V. Pasrameshvara (ed) Bombay, Association of Physicians of India 1988, p. 202.
47. Renolds H.Y., Lung inflammation, Normal host defence or a Complication of some diseases, Ann Rev. Med 1987,38: 295.
48. Pennington J.E. (ed). Hospital acquired pneumonias, Semn, Resp, Inf 1987,2: 1.
49. Verghase A. and Birk S.L., Bacterial pneumonia in the elderly, Medicine 1983, 62: 271.
50. Reynolds H.Y., Pulmonary host defence, Chest 1989,95(8): 223.
51. American College of Physicians, Ann. Int, Med 1982,96: 207.
52. Research Committee British Thoracic Society, Community-acquired pneumonia in adults in British Hospitals in 1982-83, A study of aetiology, mortality prognostic factors and outcome. Quart. J. Med 1987, 62: 195.
53. Austrian R., *Life with the Pneumococcus.* Philadelphia, University of Pennsylvania Press 1985.
54. Fruchtman S.M., *et al.,* Adult respiratory distress syndrome as a cause of death in penumococcal pneumonia, Chest 1983,83: 598.
55. Pandya G.J., *et al.,* Unilateral labor pulmonary edema; JAPI 2012;60:60-62.
56. Applebaum P.C., World-wide development of antibiotic resistance in pneumococci, Eur, J, Clin, Microbiol 1987, 6: 367.
57. Kludman K. and Koornh of H.J., Drug resistance patterns and serogroups or serotypes of pneumococcal isolates from cerebrospinal fluid or blood 1979-86, J. Inf. Dis 1988, 158: 956.
58. American Thoracic Society, Amer, Rev, Respir, Dis 1970, 101: 116.
59. Paton J.C., *et al.,* Antibody response to Pneumococcal vaccine in children aged 5 to 15 years Am. J. Dis. Child 1986,140:135.
60. Bolan N., *et al.,* Pneumococcal vaccine efficacy in selected population in the United States, Ann. Inter. Med. 1986, 104: 1.
61. Shapro E.D. and Clemens J.D., A controlled evaluation pneumococcal vaccine for patients at high risk of serious pneumococcal infections, Ann, Intern, Med 1984, 101: 325.
62. Cunha B.A. ed., Antimicrobial therapy, Med Clinic North Amer 1995; 79: 581-97.
63. Bhatia R.S., Pneumonia in the elderly: Role of vaccination; Lung India 1993;11:124.
64. Tooley W.H. and Lipow H.W., *Bacterial pneumonia.* In, Rudolph A.M., Pediatrics, Connecticut, Prentice Hall International 1987.
65. Lefrock J.L., Molavi A., Lentnek A., The pneumonias: In, Clinical approaches to infectious diseases of the lower respiratory tract, ed; Levison M.E. 1984, John Wright, Boston.
66. Pfaller M.A. and Herwaldt L.A., Laboratory, clinical and epidemiological aspects of coagulase-negative staphylococci, Clin Microbiol Rev 1988, 1: 281.
67. Martin M.A., *et al.,* Coagulase-negative staphylococcal bacteremia. Mortality and hospital stay, Ann. Intern. Med. 1989,110:9.
68. Brumfitt W. and Hamilton-Miller J., Methicillin-resistant Staphylococcus aureus, N. Eng. J. Med 1989, 320: 1188.
69. Lacey R.W., Treatment of staphylococcal infection; J Antimicrob Chemotherapy 1983, 11: 03.
70. Grassi C., Recent Advances in Respiratory Medicine 1986, 4;65.
71. Auckenthaler R., *et al.,* Group G. Streptococcal bacteremia: Clinical study and review of the literature., Rev, Infect, Dis 1983; 5: 196.
72. Brennan R.D. and Durack D.T., *The viridans streptococci in perspective, in Current Clinical Topics in Infectious Diseases.* J.S., Remington, M.N., Swartz (eds), New York, McGraw Hill, 1984.
73. Edwards M.S. and Baker C.J., *Streptococcus agalactiae (Group B treptococci), Principles and practices of Infectious Diseases.* 2nd ed. G.L. Mandella, *et al.,* (eds), New York, Wiley 1985, p. 1155.
74. Crane L.R., Lerner A.M., Gram negative bacillary pneumonias, In: Respiratory infections, diagnosis and management; ed; Remington J; Raven Press, N. York 1983.
75. Levison M.E., Kaye D., Pneumonias caused by gram negative bacilli:An overview; Rev, Infect Dis, 1985 (Suppl): 7: S656.
76. Mandell G.L. (ed): Principles and Practices of Infectious Diseases, 3rd ed; John Wiley, N York 1990.
77. Majumdar A.K., Klebsiella pneumonia with lung abscess in a male child, JAPI 1992, 40: 767-68.
78. Verghese A., Berk S.L., Bacterial pneumonia in the elderly, Medicine 1983,62: 271.
79. Johnson C.C. and Finegold S.M., *Bacterial Pneumonia.* Lung abscess, Empyema in Murry J.F. and Nadel J.A. Textbook of Respiratory Medicine, Vol I., Philadelphia W.B. Saunders Co 1988,803: 55.

80. Pierce A.K. and Sanford J.P., Aerobic Gram negative bacillary pneumonias, Am. Rev. Respir. Dis 1974, 110:647.
81. Seaton Anthony, *et al., Lung Abscess,* Crofton and Douglas's Respiratory Disease, 4th ed, 1989, p. 359.
82. Bhat K.S., *et al.,* Kleb, Pneumonia with lung abscess, JAPI 1990, 38: 378.
83. Jagdish J.S., *et al.,* Acute myocarditis in association with Kleb. pneumonia, JAPI 1987, 35: 652-54.
84. Arya T.V.S., Arora R.C., Klebsiella pneumonia with lung abscess, JAPI 1989, 37: 549-51.
85. Schaberg D.R. and Turch M., *Diseases caused by Gram negative enteric bacilli.* In Braunwald E., *et al., (eds),* Harrison's Principles of Internal Medicine 1 lth edition, New York, McGraw Hill Book Co 1987, 583-89.
86. Hirschmann J.V. and Murray J.F., *Pneumonia and lung abscess.* In Brounwald E., *et al.,* (eds). Harrison's Principles of Internal Medicine, 11th edition, New York, McGraw Hill Book Co 1987, 1075-82.
87. Hinshaw Corwin H., Murray F, John. *Bacterial Pneumonias: Diseases of Chest:* WB Saunders Co., Philadelphia, 4th Ed. 1980; p.269.
88. Sheagren J.N., Septic shock and corticosteroids, New Eng., J. Medcine 1981,305:456.
89. *American Academy of Pediatrics Committee on Infectious Disease. Haemophilus influenzae infections* In; 1988, Red Book, Petr G., *et al.,* ed., ElK Grone village IL; Amer. Acad. Ped 1988, 204-10.
90. Borenstein D.G. and Simon G.L., *Hemophilus lnfluenzae Septic arthritis in adults,* A report of 4 cases; Medicine 1986, 65,191.
91. Ginsburg C.M., *et al.,* Report of 65 cases of H. Influenzae type B pneumoniae, Paed 1979, 64: 283.
92. Label M.H. *et al.,* Dexametherone therapy in bacterial meningitis; Results of 2 double blind placebo controlled trials; N. Eng. J. Med 1988, 319: 964.
93. Mayo Smith M.F., *et al.,* Acute epiglottis in adults; An eight-year experience in the State of Rhode Island; N. Engl. J. Med 1986, 314: 1133.
94. Murphy T.O., *et al.,* Risk of subsequent disease among day care contacts of patients with systemic H. influenzae type disease, N. Eng, J. Med 1987, 316: 01.
95. Weinberg G.A. and Rrawff D.A., Polysaccharide-protein conjugate vaccines for the prevention of H. influenzae disease, J. Pedia 1988, 113: 62.
96. Robertson P.W., *et al.,* Borde Fena pertussis infection—A case of persistent cough in adults. Med. J. Aust 1987,146: 522.
97. Onorato I.M. and Wassilak S.G.F., Lab diagnosis of pertussis; Ped. Inf. Dis 1987, 6: 145.
98. Blennow M., *et al.,* Primary immunization of infants with a cellular pertussis vaccine in a double blind clinical trial, Pediat 1988, 82: 293.
99. Thukral A., *et al.,* Pneumatocele in an adult; JAPI 2011; 59: 186-87.
100. Kaiser A.B., *et al.,* Tularemia and rhabdomyolysis; JAMA 1985, 250: 241.
101. Evans M.E., *et al.,* Tularemia; A 30 years experience with 88 cases; Medicine 1985, 64: 251.
102. Sanford J.P., Landmark Perspective. Tularemia; JAMA 1985, 250:3225.
103. Harper J.L., *et al.,* Tularemic meningitis in a child with mononuclear leucocytosis, Paedia, Inf. Dis 1986,5: 595.
104. Koskela P. and Salminen A., Humoral immunity against Franciella tulereus is after natural infection, J.Clin. Microbiol 1985, 22: 973.
105. Pann R.L., Kina seuritz G.J., Factor associated with a poor outcome in Tularemia. Arch. Int. Med 1987,147: 265.
106. Crafton and Douglas's Respiratory Diseases; Seaton A, Seaton D and Gordon with A;ED: 4th ed; 1989, Oxford University Press, Delhi.
107. McDade J.E., Shopard C.C. and Frasser D.W., *et al.,* New Engl. J.Med 1977, 297: 1197-1203.
108. Winn W.C., Jr., Legionnaire's disease; Historical perspective, Clin. Micro. Rev 1988, 1: 60.
109. Fang G.D., *et al.,* Diseases due to the Legionellaceae (other than L.Pneumophila): Historical, microbiological, clinical and epidemiologic review; Medicine (Baltimore) 1989, 68: 116.
110. Muder R.R., *et al.,* Mode of transmission of L.pneumophila. A critical review, Arch. Inter. Med 1986,146: 1607.
111. Tompkins L.S., *et al.,* Legionella prosthetic valve endocarditis, N. Eng J. Med 1988, 318: 530.
112. Cunha B.A. (ed) Legionnaire's disease, Sem. Resp. Infact 1987, 2: 189.
113. Hubbard R.B., *et al.,* Severe community acquired pneumonia; Treatment; Complications and outcome: QJM 1993,86: 327-32.
114. Wather C.G. and Sudlow M.F., Postgr. Med. Jour 1986,62: 369-76.
115. Moulton F.R. (ed), *The Rickettsial diseases of man,* Washington D.C., Amer. Assn. for Solvanc of Sci 1948.
116. Stepanek D., *et al.,* Chalaymidosis in cattle and in man; A epidemiologic and serologic study; J. Hyg. Epidem Microbiol Immunol 1983,27: 445.
117. Coults II, *et al.,* Clinical and radiographic features of psittacosis infection, Thorax 1985,40: 530.
118. Coults II, Mackenzie S. and White R.J., Clinical and radiographic features of Psittacosis infection; Thorax 1985, 40: 530.
119. Gorayston J.T., Chlamydia pneumoniae, Strain TWAR; Chest 1989, 95: 664.
120. Grayston J.T., *et al.,* A new chlamydia pneumoniae strain.TWAR; isolated in acute respiratory tract infections; N. Eng. J. Med 1986, 315: 161.
121. Broughton R.A., Infections due to Mycoplasma pneumoniae in childhood, Ped. Inf. Dis. J 1986, 5: 71.
122. Nagayama Y., *et al.,* Isolation of M. pneumoniae from children with lower respiratory tract infections. J. Inf. Dis 1988, 157: 911.
123. Kashyap S., Sarkar M., Mycoplasma pneumoniae–Clinical features and management; Lung India 2010; 27: 75-85.
124. Chanock R.M., Mycoplasma infection of man: New Engl, J. Med 1965, 273: 1199 and 1257.
125. Wilson J.D., *et al.,* ed: Harrison's Principles of International Medicine; 12th ed; Mcflraw Hill, NewYork, 1991.
126. McCracken G.H., Jr. Current status of antibiotic treatment of M. pneumoniae disease, Ped. Inf. Dis. J 1986, 5: 167.

127. Mettler Jr. F.A., Mosiley J.R.D., *Medical effects of radiation;* Orlando, Florida, Grone and Stratton 1985.
128. Committee on the Biological effects of ionising radiation. National research council Health effects of exposure to low levels of ionizing radiation (BEIR V), Washington D.C., National Academy Press, 1990.
129. Felson B: Chest Roentgenology; WB Saunders; Philadelphia, 1973.
130. Bromer R.S. and Wolman I.J., Lipoid pneumonia in infants and children, Radiology 1939,32: 01.
131. Nelson's Text Book of Paediatrics, Vanghan IIIVC; James Mckay R., Nelson W.E. 10th ed, 1975, W.E. Saunders Co.
132. Spencer H., Pathology of lung; Pergamon Press; Oxford 1985.
133. Pinkerton H., The reaction oils and fats in the lung, Arch. Path 1928:5:380.
134. Brunell P.A., *et al.,* Prevention of varicella by zoster immune globulin, N. Eng. J. Med 1969,280: 1192.
135. Zaia J.A., *et al.*, Evaluation of varicella-zoster immunoglobulin. Protection of immunosuppressed children after household exposure to varicella; J. Inf. Dis 1983, 147: 737.
136. Gershon A.A., *et al.,* Live attenuated varicellla vaccine JAMA 1984, 252: 355.
137. Knyvett A.F., The pulmonary lesions of chikcenpox, Quat. J. Med 1966, 35: 1313.
138. Dodin A. and Galimand M. WHITMORE's bacillus, observations in 39 cases, Amer. Rev. Resp. Dis 1975, 112: 331.
139. McCormick J.B., *et al.,* Human to human transmission of P. Pseudomallei, Ann. Int, Med 1975,831: 512.
140. Krishnan P., *et al.,* Malioidosis; JAPI 2008; 56: 636-39.
141. Wanvarie S., Melioidosis certain interesting presentations and treatment, Trop. Med 1984, 36: 165.
142. Ray V., *et al.,* Septicemic melioidosis; JAPI 2009; 57: 598-99.
143. Gillespie S.H., *et al.,* in Vitro susceptibility of P. pseudomallei to DNA Gyrease inhibitors; J., Antimic Chemother 1987, 20: 612.
144. Dance D.A.B., *et al.,* Antibiotic resistance in pseudomonas pseudomallei, Lancet 1988; 1: 1994.
145. McEniry D.W., *et al.,* Susceptability of P. pseudomallei to new betalactam and aminoglycoside antibiotics; J. Antimicro Chemothe 1988, 21: 171.
146. Murli R., *et al.*, Surat '94: Was in meliodosis? Interesting observations from the first case of imported meliodosis in India; JAPI 1996; 44: 218-19.
147. Handa R., Bhatia S., Wali J.P., Meliodosis: A rare but not forgotten case of ever of unknown origin; Brit. J. Clin. Pract 1996;50:116-17.
148. Mandell L.A., *et al.*, Inf. Disease Soc of America/American Thor. Soc. Consensus guidelines in the management of community acquired pneumonia in adults; Clinical Infectious Diseases 2007;44:527-72.
149. Innes J.A., Community acquired pneumonia, BMJ 1987, 295: 1083-84.
150. Lonks J.R., Medeiros J.A., The growing treat of antibiotic resistant strept pneumoniae; IN; Cunha B.A., E.D., Antimicrobial therapy; Med Clinic North Amer 1995; 79: 523-35.
151. Liebow A.A., Steer A. and Billingsley J.C., Desquamative interstitial pneumonia. Am. J. Med 1965,39: 369.
152. Liebow A.A., Definition and classification of interstitial pneumonias in human pathology; Alveolar, interstitium of lung. International Symposium, Paris 1974, Prog., Respir, Res 1975, 8: 1.
153. Tal A., Maor E., Bari-Ziv J. and Gorodischer R., Fatal desquamative interstitial pneumonia in three infant siblings, J, Pediatrics 1984, 873-876.
154. Gaensler E.A., Goff A.M. and Prowse C.M., Desquamative interstitial pneumonia, N.Eng J. Med 1966, 274: 113.
155. Hilman B.C., Interstitial and hypersensitivity interstitial pneumonitis and their variants. Pediatr. Rev 1980, 1: 229.
156. Schatz M., Patterson R. and Fingk J., Immunologic lung disease, N.Engl. J.Med 1979, 300: 1310.
157. Gaensler E.A., Carrington C.B. and Coutu R.E., Chronic interstitial pneumonia Clin. Notes. Respir, Dis 1972,10:3.
158. Chaudhary P.K., *et al.,* Desquamative interstitial pneumonia, JAPI 1993, 41: 303-305.
159. Broor S.L., Upeet Kaur, Dutta B.N. and Sapru R.P., Desquamative Interstitial pneumonia. Indian J. Chest Dis, and Allied Sciences 1977, XIX (2) 96.
160. Jain S.K, Acute chest infections, nosocomial pneumonia: An overview: IJCP 1993,4: 13-14.
161. Garibaldi R.A., *et al.,* Risk factors for post operative pneumonia; Amer. J. Med 1921, 70: 677.
162. Lynch J.P., Nosocomial pneumonia, J. Resp. Dis 1992,13: 1015.
163. Jay S.J., Nosocomial infections, Med Clin North Amer 1983, 67: 1251.
164. Heyland D., Lionel A.M., Gastric colonization by gram negative bacilli and nosocomial pneumonia in the intensive care unit patients, Chest 1992, 101: 187.
165. Shete U.B., *et al.,* MDR Acinobacter ventilator-associated pneumonia; Lung India 2010; 27: 217-20.
166. Yel L; *et al*; Clinical and immunological features in IgM deficiency; Int. Arch Allergy Immunol; 2009; 150:291-98
167. Dhir V; *et al.,* An unsure cause of recurrent pneumonia in adults; Lung India; 2014;31;296-98.

SUPPURATION

Lung Abscess

Lung abscess is a localised collection of pus in the parenchyma of the lung as a result of suppuration and necrosis from a pyogenic infection or from necrosis in a neoplasm, when the purulent material cannot be drained because of partial or complete bronchial obstruction. Abscess means, therefore, collection of necrotic material with inflammation and infection and should be preferred over the term cavity which is usually a radiological description.[1]

Aetiology and Pathology

The condition is secondary to some antecedent cause in a majority of cases. Still a significant number of cases are present as (simple) primary lung abscess.[2] The abscess can develop following inhalation of infected material, following bronchial obstruction, embolism or pneumonia or from spread of infection from neighbouring structures. The abscess may be single or multiple.[3] Various causes have been tabulated in Table 4.13.

Table 4.13: Common causes of lung abscess (Aetiological classification)

1. Primary necrotizing pneumonia
   a. Aerobic: Staphylococcal, Klebsiella, Streptococcal, Tubercular, Legionellar
   b. Anaerobic: Bacteroides, Actinomycosis, Nocardiosis
   c. Parasitic: Amoebic, Lung flukes (ectinococcal)
   d. Fungal: Aspergillosis, Histoplasmosis, Coccidioidosis.
2. Aspiration pneumonia.
3. Bronchial obstruction: Foreign body, Tumor—Bronchogenic Metastasis (Rarely).
4. Systemic sepsis: Septic pulmonary emboli
   Vasculitis (Wegener's disease)
   Pulmonary infarction.
5. Pulmonary trauma: Penetrating injury, foreign body, haematoma.
6. Direct extension from extra parenchymal affection: Pleural empyema, hepatic, mediastinal or subphrenic abscess.
7. Miscellaneous: Infected cyst, Silicosis, Coal miner's pneumoconiosis.

Inhalational abscess is the most common mode of development. The septic material from naso-oropharyngeal regions may be aspirated into the bronchioles. The gravity and posture determine the localisation. The posterior segment of the upper lobe and the superior segment of the lower lobe form the common sites for inhalational abscesses,[4] more frequently on the right side because of the existence of the right bronchus in direct continuation of the trachea.

The infection in the upper respiratory passages including gingivodental sepsis can be aspirated following tonsillectomy or dental extraction. The septic material can be inhaled during comatose conditions, under the effects of anaesthesia, alcoholic stupor, epilepsy, drowning, electroconvulsive therapy, tracheostomy and post-operative states. The diseases of oesophagus, such as achalasia and carcinoma of the upper third of the oesophagus may predispose to the development of abscess. It can develop following inhalation of a foreign body or in the obstructed lung segments secondary to bronchostenosis or bronchial adenoma or bronchogenic carcinoma. In children, abscess develops as a complication of staphylococcal or Klebsiellar pneumonias.[5, 6] Also it may develop in sequestration of lung or in association with bronchial cyst, stenosis or foreign body.[7]

The aspirated infective material may obstructs the smaller air passages and causes collapse.[8] Often the aspiration is difficult to prove. The infection spreads to that area resulting in the development of a mass of inflammatory tissue. It undergoes necrosis with formation of cavity. The wall of the cavity is irregular initially and consists of granulation tissue. The blood vessels get thrombosed. The bronchi get eroded and the communication enables the expectoration of the necrotic tissue. The infection spreads to the surrounding areas. The drainage into the bronchus may help in spontaneous recovery in some cases. The abscess heals with complete evacuation of contents and collapse of the wall of the cavity. There may be some residual scarring. The abscess may become persistent due to continued presence of infection or FB and partial evacuation of its contents.

Generally the infection is mixed, and may showing growth of Streptococcus pyogenes, Staphylococcus aureus, Streptococcus pneumoniae, Klebsiella pneumoniae and Pseudomonas aeruginosa. Rarely Proteus and H. influenzae cause necrosis. Anaerobic streptococci, bacteroides, clostridia, fusobacterium, and spirochaets may develop in such devitalized tissue and are common in inhalational abscess.

Pyaemia or septic embolisation from the veins of the pelvis or lower limbs or from the right side of endocarditis lead to multiple lung abscesses. Such haematogenous spread of Staphylococcal infection results in suppuration with formation of small abscesses. They are located essentially in the periphery in the subpleural areas. It may rupture into pleural space causing pneumothorax or pyopneumothorax. Aseptic emboli may get infected by mixed bacterial flora. Abscess may develop from vasculitis as seen in Wegener's granulomatosis.[3]

Pneumonitis from Staphylococcal infection leads to the development of multiple acute lung abscesses involving both lungs. The abscess often enlarges progressively as pneumotocele, due to valvular obstruction of the bronchial communication that allows entry of air into the cavity on inspiration and prevents its exit during expiration. Klebsiella pneumoniae causes a necrotising pneumonia leading to the development of lung abscess. It involves the upper lobes commonly. Rarely Pneumococcal pneumonia causes lung abscess as a complication. Though the advent of antibiotics has reduced the incidence the condition is still encountered due to improper management of pneumonias.[3]

Spread of infection from neighbouring organs and structures below the diaphragm may result in abscess formation or may follow perforating injuries. Large areas of inflamed fibrotic lung tissue coalesce, with added vascular insufficiency, to form a cavity, as in advanced cases of silicosis.

Clinical Features and Physical Signs

Regardless of aetiology the clinical manifestations of lung abscess are uniform.[1] In addition to the features of predisposing condition, the development of the lung abscess manifests with acute onset of symptoms. In some, the condition may develop insidiously. Often the typical presentation of the abscess is altered due to the use of antibiotics in the treatment of infective conditions at an early opportunity. Patient has a febrile onset with chills and cough. It is associated with diffuse pain over the chest, which sometimes may have pleuritic character. Dry initially, cough is soon associated with expectoration. It is profuse and purulent, often, with definite postural relationship. It may be foetid in anaerobic lung abscess. The production of sputum may not be evident in septic pulmonary emboli. There may be haemoptysis, often massive from erosion of blood vessels. The patient becomes acutely ill with loss of appetite and loss of weight. In contrast to pneumonia, dyspnoea is not a prominent feature.[9]

The physical chest signs depend on the site and contents of the cavity whether full or empty. There may be bronchial sounds with rales as in consolidation or dull, cavernous or emphoric breath sound.[10] Majority of patients show signs of consolidation. The signs of cavitation are rarely encountered and are found when the cavity is superficial and partially empty. The deep seated abscess may not reveal any signs. Even with an established pneumonia, it becomes difficult to distinguish between a lung abscess and pleural effusion and empyema, because the spread to the pleura may mask the picture. A chronic lung abscess presents with a classical productive, foul smelling cough, intermittent fever, dyspnoea, weight loss and loss of appetite. Clubbing may occur in few weeks.

Investigations

Lung abscess is associated with polymorphonuclear leucocytosis and anaemia of infection. The sputum shows pus cells and elastic tissue. The elastic tissue is demonstrated after treating the sputum smear with sodium hydroxide as it dissolves mucous elements. The sputum can be examined for the existence of acid fast bacilli and malignant cells. The culture shows the growth of mixed bacterial flora. Anaerobic cultures from the sputum obtained following transtracheal aspiration may show growth of anaerobic streptococci. The pathogens may not be isolated in those who have received antibiotics already.

Chest X-ray may reveal a homogeneous opacity initially. There is radiolucent area, later indicating its opening into the bronchus. It will then have a fluid level.The outline of the abscess wall is shaggy initially and becomes well formed later. Multiple thin-walled cavities are noted when there is septic pulmonary emboli. Blood cultures are positive.[3]

CT scanning may be of help in differentiating parenchymal abscess, an empyema, a bronchopleural fistula creating an empyema, an infected cyst or an emphysematous bulla with fluid levels. CT view of the lung can demonstrate even a cavity within the pneumonic area more evidently.

Bronchoscopy should be cautiously performed in cases of cavities with large amount of fluid as sudden fluid discharge into the airways may prove hazardous.

Complications have been significantly reduced by early recognition of the condition and treatment; however, empyema, pyopneumothorax, cerebral abscess, amyloidosis and arthritis may occur occasionally.

Differential Diagnosis

Important differential diagnosis includes cavitated bronchogenic carcinoma. The squamous cell carcinoma exhibits such a tendency. The walls of the cavity are thick and irregular. Often it causes haemoptysis. It may even exist with out symptoms. The retained secretion secondary to the obstruction from bronchial neoplasm may get infected, and result in an abscess. Though the infective element clears with treatment, the investigations for existence of neoplasm has to be carried out in all persons over the age of 40 years and in smokers. Bronchiectasis is another differential diagnosis, where chronic suppurative copious mucous production is characteristic compared to carcinoma and lung abscess. Acute febrile illness is feature of lung abscess, especially in necrotising pneuomonitis, although bronchiectasis and carcinoma may have febrile illness due to exacerbation of inflammatory process. Bronchography rules out bronchiectasis while bronchoscopy and biopsy of the lung are essential for diagnosis of carcinoma of the lung.[11]

The examination of sputum for tubercle bacilli should exclude tuberculosis where there will be a history of cough, weight loss and chronic ill health. Tuberculous cavities are often multiple and without any fluid levels. Infection from dimorphic fungi may lead to lung abscess. Nocardial asteroides may invade the infected areas. The emphysematous bullae may get infected and appear as an apparent cavity with a fluid level and they do not show much evidence of consolidation in the surrounding area. Colonies of aspergillus may grow in the devitalised tissue of the lung abscess. Hiatus hernia may demonstrate fluid level behind the heart simulating a lung abscess but without producing any respiratory symptoms.[8]

Prognosis

The early and effective use of antibiotics and postural drainage, the lung abscess can be cured without resorting to surgery. Mortality has been significantly reduced following the introduction of antibiotics in the management. The lung abscess secondary to bronchogenic carcinoma has a poor prognosis. Prognosis is also poor in cases of large abscess cavity, more than 6 cm diameter of more than 8 weeks duration, multiple abscesses of necrotizing pneumonia, abscess with bronchial obstruction (secondary abscess) and in elderly people.[11-17]

Treatment

Inhalation abscess can be prevented by pre-operative treatment of foci of infection with antibiotics. The removal of foreign body by bronchoscopy halts its progress into an abscess. Majority of lung abscesses make good recovery with medical treatment using antibiotics and postural drainage.

Bed rest and a high protein nutritious diet are important. Antibiotic therapy has to be instituted with crystalline penicillin in doses of 1 to 2 mega units intramuscularly every 12 hours. Streptomycin sulphate 1 gm I.M. daily may be added during the initial period for 15 days to make the therapy effective. Tuberculosis must be excluded before its addition to the therapy.

Further line of treatment is guided by the bacteriological sensitivity. Majority of organisms—both aerobic and anaerobic—are sensitive to the above antibiotics. Even in the absence of growth of any organisms, penicillin is the drug of choice. Klebsiella lung abscess is treated with gentamycin and chloramphenicol. The treatment with procain penicillin is continued in other cases till complete disappearance of the radiologic shadows. The clinical response is assessed by noting a decrease in the quantity of the sputum, absence of pyrexial episodes, disappearance of an offensive smell of sputum, gain in weight, general sense of well-being and disappearance of lung signs. The antibiotic therapy has to be continued till the closure of the abscess cavity even when the patient has become asymptomatic. Generally it has to be given for at least six weeks.[3] Promotion of good drainage of secretions enhances recovery.[9]

Postural drainage by gravity facilitates the evacuation of the content of the abscess cavity. The position adapted depends on the location of abscess.[3] Percussion and clapping the area of abscess during physiotherapy assists in the expectoration of the contents and hastens its resolution. Drainage of pleural space may be indicated for loculated fluid and empyema, if they are complicating lung abscess.

Diagnostic and therapeutic usefulness of bronchoscopy in the management of lung abscess cannot be underweighed. It helps in the exclusion of an underlying neoplastic condition and in the removal of foreign body if there is a history of aspiration. The tenacious exudate can be aspirated and the material can be studied for bacteriological identity and sensitivity to various antibiotics. The location of draining bronchus helps in guiding postural drainage.[18]

Refractory cases after six weeks with rigorous medical management are considered chronic. The inadequate medical treatment predisposes to its chronicity apart from other underlying primary diseases. Pneumonotomy—a percutaneous insertion of drainage tube or pneumonostomy—an open drainage procedure can be performed.[19-23] However, in a majority of cases penicillin and postural drainage are sufficient to achieve complete cure. The antibiotics have to be continued even after that period, if the patient is producing sputum, but surgical intervention may be deferred. The chronic cases with sepsis haemorrhage and destruction of the lung or bronchial carcinoma need pulmonary resection, performing either segmental resection or lobectomy. Intraoperative bronchoscopy adds safety as well as provide accurate irrigation and aspiration of the airways.[1] It is also useful in massive haemorrhage.

Rarely bronchial artery embolisation is required because of presence of rich collateral circulation in the lung. The coexisting disease has to be treated. Similarly. surgical intervention may be required for complications like empyema and bronchopleural fistula.[3]

REFERENCES

1. *Schwartz's Principles of surgery;* 6th ed., McGraw Hill, New York, 1994.
2. Schweppe H.E., Knowles J.H. and Kane L., New Engl Jour. Med 1961,265:1039.
3. Shankar P.S., *Suppuration, Chest Medicine,* 4th ed, Oxford and IBH Publ. Co. N. Delhi, 1994.
4. Brock R.C., *The Anatomy of the Bronchial Tree.* London Oxford University Press 1946.
5. Ramani A., Kundaje G.N., Staphylococcal lung abscess, J. Assn. Phys. India 1989, 37: 715-16.
6. Majumdar A.K., Klebsiella pneumonia with lung abscess in a male child, J. Assn. Phys. India 1992,40:767-68.
7. Ghai O.P., *Essentials of Paediatrics,* 2nd ed; Interprint, N. Delhi, 1991.
8. Johnson W.G., *et al.,* Aspiration pneumonia, anaerobic infections and lung abscess, Med. Clin. North Amer 1980, 64: 385.
9. *Harrison's Principles of Internal Medicine,* Wilson J.D., Braunwald E., Isselbacher K.J., *et al.,* Ed. 12th ed., Vol 2; McGraw Hill, New York, 1991.
10. Bhatia R.S., Pulmonary sounds in common lung diseases; Lung India 1994; 12: 89-92.
11. Schacter E.N., Suppurative lung disease, Old problems revisited, Clin. Chest. Med 1981, 2:41.
12. Mahler D.A., D'Esopo N.D., Peri-emphysematous lung infection, Clin. Chest. Med 1981, 2: 51.
13. Alexander J.C. and Wolfe W.G., Lung abscess and empyema of the thorax, Surg. Clin. North Amer 1980, 60:835.
14. IeRoux B.T., Mohlata M.L., *et al.,* Suppurative diseases of the lung and pleural space, Curr. Probl. Surg 1986, 23: 1.
15. Pohlson E.C., McNamara J.J., *et al.,* Lung abscess; A changing pattern of the disease, Amer. J. Surg 1985, 150: 97.
16. Scaton A., *et al., Lung abscess;* in: Crofton and Douglas's Resp. Diseases, 4th ed, Oxford Blackwell Sci. Publ 1989.
17. Johnson C.C., and Finegold S.M., *Bacterial pneumonias, lung abscess, empyema.* in; Murry J.F., Nadel J.A. (ed). Textbook of Resp. Medicine; VoL (1) WB Saunders Co., Philadelphia, 1988.

18. Bhatia R.S. and Sibia S.S. Therapeutic uses of FOB; Lung India 1994; 12: 138-39.
19. Yellin A., Yellin E.O., *et al.* Percutaneous tube drainage. The treatment of choice for refractory lung abscess, Amer. Thorac. Surg 1985, 39: 266.
20. Lacey S.R. and Kosloske A.M., Pneumonostomy in the management of paediatric lung abscess, J. Ped. Surg 1983, 18: 625.
21. Kosloske A.M., Ball W.S., *et al.* Drainage of pediatric lung abscess by cough, catheter, or complete resection, J. Ped. Surg 1986, 21: 596.
22. Lacey S.R. and Kosloske A.M., Pneumonostomy in the management of paediatric lung abscess, J. Ped. Surg 1983, 18:625.
23. Weigssberg D. Percutaneous drainage of lung abscess, J.Thorac. Cardio. Vas. Surg 1984, 87:308.

ENTERIC LUNG ABSCESS

Before discussing enteric lung abscess, typhoid fever is required to be briefly discussed.

Epidemiology

The worldwide incidence of typhoid is approximately 12.5 million cases annually with more than 62 per cent of the cases occurring in India and other Asian countries[1] and 35 per cent in the African continent.[2] Typhoid has been a bane of nations and almost every nation in the world has paid a price because of this disease.[3] But progressive improvement in sanitation, water supply and environmental hygiene has resulted in decrease in the annual incidence of reported cases of typhoid in European countries and the USA. In the U.K. typhoid fever has been almost eradicated with approximately one case per 1,000,000 population which is perhaps the lowest in the world.[3,4]

Epidemiological studies all over the world have been rather few. In a study[5] from Delhi an incidence of 110 among males and 75 among females per 100,000 population in Delhi was reported. A limited study in an urban slum showed 1 per cent of children upto 17 years age to suffer from typhoid fever every year. It is difficult to really get the true incidence of the disease. In developing countries as there is an initial fall but, again there is a spurt in the incidence and morbidity of typhoid, for which a number of factors ranging from poor sanitation and hygiene, improper water supply, emergence of drug resistant strains are apparently contributory.

Pulmonary enteric affection is very common and generally has a hematogenous spread as pyemia occurs. Infection by intravenous route during platelet transfusion may occur. There has been a changing trend in the clinical presentation of typhoid fever[1] in the recent years. Almost half the number of cases are showing a typical symptomatology, with a variable onset. Early diagnosis is important to guide the patient for proper and prompt management, thus, avoiding complications of enteric fever. Apart from metabolic derangements, other complications like glomerulonephritis, nephritis, orchitis, parotitis, myocarditis, cholecystitis, hepatitis, appendicitis, enteric pneumonia, hemiparesis, encephalopathy, intestinal haemorrhage, perforation, circulatory failure etc. are variously encountered because of endotoxaemia[2-9] that occurs during bacteremic phase of the disease which gives rise to abscess formation.[10] Pre-existence of a cavity may precipitate enteric lung infection and ultimately the lung abscess. But in that case, it cannot be called as true abscess.[11]

Routine blood tests, widal test and blood culture are sufficient investigations in clinching the diagnosis, although many other tests like bone marrow culture, ELISA for detecting salmonella antigen with monoclonal antibodies,[12] increased values of adenosine deaminase activity in enteric fever[13] are available. At the same time, doubts about the reliability of widal tests[14] and utilisation of absence of eosinophils in the peripheral blood smear for the diagnosis of typhoid fever have been suggested. Again neutropenic lymphocytosis may be responsible for absence of eosinophils but absence of eosinophils in leucocytosis cannot be explained, in case of enteric fever of less than a week's duration.[15] Normal WBC, raised eosinophils and raised level of SGPT have also been suggested.

Management of uncomplicated cases is not difficult. Multidrug resistant strains of salmonella typhi have been reported to be endemic in some parts of the world including India. Chest X-ray shows a cavity with watery fluid levels. Cavity wall may show fibrotic changes in case the abscess is of longer duration or it is pre-existing due to other pulmonary pathological disorders including tuberculosis.[11] Fibreoptic bronchoscopy may not reveal any intrabronchial pathology. Mucosa may be inflammed, smeared with blood and streaky clots with or without secretions. The bronchial brush from the affected lobe is positive for S. typhi. Sputum culture is positive for S. typhi.

Management

Medical management includes treatment with chloramphenicol which remained the drug of choice and the gold standard treatment available since decades, although various recent reports have shown resistance to this drug in vitro. The reason for chloramphenicol resistance in S. typhi can be explained either due to mutation or aquisition of a transferable extra chromosomal resistance factor. The indiscriminate use of chloramphenicol in various other infections, in subtherapeutic dosages and for a subtherapeutic period[16] along with recurrent exposure of the drug in the same fashion is an important factor in the causation of chloramphenicol resistance.[16,17]

The use of other drugs, individually or in combination have been tried, these include cotrimoxazole, cotrimoxazine, ampicillin, amoxycillin, gentamycin, cephalosporins and quinolones. Cotrimoxazole is effective, cotrimoxazine is a better combination. Amoxycillin is better than ampicillin which is even inferior to cotrimoxazole and diarrhoea with ampicillin are other factors restricting their use. Gentamicin can be added[18] but is not without adverse effects.[19] The quinolones and cephalosporins are other potent effective drugs, but adverse reactions to ciprofloxacin are not that uncommon.[20,21] Even sporadic cases of resistance to these drugs are also seen in clinical practice.[22] Newer combinations of azithromycin and cefixime are also being used. Resistance probably results from either a mutation in gene controlling DNA gyrase or a permeability barrier to ciprofloxacin in the cell envelope.[23] Therefore, it is better to keep these potent currently available effective tools as reserve therapy.[24] Surgical management includes lobectomy[11] in case the cavity is not closing, infection is recurring or haemoptysis, especially when we are aware of emergence of chloramphenicol resistant salmonella typhi strains. Steroids are only indicated in high doses in typhoid fever with delirium, stupor, coma or shock.

Prevention

It can broadly be discussed under, (1) Control of infection, (2) Environmental sanitation, and (3) Immunisation. Where it is high time to correctly diagnose at an early phase a case of enteric fever, there the use of chloramphenicol and quinolones in proper dosage, for proper period is most essential. This avoids emergence of resistant strains as well prevent enteric complications including pulmonary complications like abscess, consolidation etc. which may take 3-4 weeks to develop. Where preventive measures for disease like HIV infection need be effectively pursued, these infectious disease like enteric fever, which causes more of morbidity especially in developing countries, need necessary preventive measures to be supplemented in this direction. Here lies the role of vaccination. Unfortunately the parenteral typhoid vaccination programme does not match with the rest of vaccinations.[1] At the same time, none of the three vaccines (parental and oral)[25-28] has proven capability of giving full protection.[29,30,31]

REFERENCES

1. Bhatia R.S., Typhoid—Changing trends in presentation and treatment, Curr. Med. Pract 1992; 36: 109.
2. Bhatia R.S. and Batta S., Enteric Orchitis—A rejoinder, J. Assn. Phys. India 1990; 38:809.
3. Khosla S.N., Heart in enteric, J. Trap.Med.Hyg 1981, 84:125-131.
4. Bhatia R.S., Enteric glomerulonephritis, Antiseptic 1989; 86:330.
5. Bhatia R.S., Hemiparesis in typhoid fever, Curr Med Pract 1994; 38: 19-20.
6. Beryl E., Wilde L. and Stanley, Salmonella typhi in sputum. Medical J. Australia 1997;126:307.
7. Kundu A.K., Typhoid hepatitis; JAPI 2002; 50: 719-20.
8. T. Hayness Harvill, Typhoid Pulmonary Abscess, J. Am. Med. Assoc 1942; 119:494-496.
9. *Harrison's Principles of Internal Medicine,* Wilson J.D. *et al.*, Ed., Salmonella Infections, 11th Ed 1987; 596-97. McGraw Hill Book Company.
10. Kenneth M.A., Perry Thomas and Holmes Sellors, *Pneumonia in Salmonella Infections. In Chest Diseases* 1963. 2nd Ed. chapter 3, Butterworth and Co.
11. Swarnkar J.S., WakodkarTB., Kirolikar S. *et al.,* Salmonella typhi lung abscess with mycetoma—A case report, Lung India 1990; 8: 149-52.
12. Cherkasov V.I., Rubistov I.V., Erovichen Kov. A.A., *et al.,* Diagnostic significance of various methods for detection of infections anti-genemia in patients with typhoid fever and paratyphoid fever A and B. Terap. Arth 1988; 60:33-34.
13. Galanti B., Nardie I.B.S., Russo M. *et al.,* Increased lymphocyte adenosine deaminase in typhoid fever, Scand J. Infect. Dis 1981; 13: 47-50.
14. Bhatia R.S. Serodiagnosis of typhoid fever, Curr. Med. Pract 1991; 35:332.
15. Bhatia R.S., Eosinophils in PB smear in typhoid, value in diagnosing and therapy evaluation. A short study, Currr. Med. Pract 1993.
16. Bhatia R.S., Changing trends in presentations and treatment of enteric fever, J. Assn. Phys. India 1992; 40: 283-84.
17. Khub Chandani R.P., Sainani G.S., Mahajan M.N., Drug resistant enteric fever, J.Appl.Med 1990;16:735-37.
18. Bhatia R.S., Author's reply, J. Assn. Phys. India 1993.41:182.
19. Singhal K.C., Verma K., Kumar P., Bhatia R.S. Adverse reaction to gentamicin, Ind. Journ. Pharm 1991; 23:64-68.
20. Bhatia R.S. Adverse reactions to ciprofloxacin, J. Assn. Phys. India 1991; 39:972.
21. Bhatia R.S. SJS following a single dose of ciprofloxacin, JAPI 1994; 42:344.
22. Bhatia R.S. Typhoid fever not responding to ciprofloxacin therapy, J. Assn. Phys. India 1992; 40:705-06.
23. Lewin C.S., Allen R.A., Aymes S.G.B. Potential mechanism of resistance of the modern fluorinated 4 quinolones, J. Med. Microbiol 1990; 31: 153-62.
24. Bhatia R.S. and Batta S. Routine use of ciprofloxacin JAPI,1992; 40: 417.
25. Hejfec L.B., Results of the study of typhoid vaccine in four controlled field trials in USSR, Bull.WHO 1965; 32:1-14.
26. Hornick R.B., Cireisman S.E., Woodward T.E. *et al.*, Typhoid fever, pathogenesis and immunology control, Part (2):N. Eng. J. Med 1970; 283: 739-746.
27. Simanjuntak C.H., Paleologo F.P., Punjabi N.H. *et al.*, Oral immunisation against typhoid fever in Indonesia with TY 2L a vaccine, Lancet 1991; 338: 1055-59.
28. Bhatia R.S. Live oral TY 2L a vaccine, J. Assn. Phys. India 1992; 40:492.
29. Bhatia R.S., Typhoid vaccinations: Should it be left to the traveller's to choose? Med. Pulse 1998; 5: 16-17.

30. Schwartz E. Shlim D.R., Eaton M., *et al.*, The effect of oral and parenteral typhoid vaccination on the rate of infection with S. typhi and S. para typhi. among foreigners in Nepal Arch. Intern. Med 1990; 150:349-51.
31. Bhatia R.S., Sibia S.S. Immunization against typhoid: A short review; JAPI 1994; 42:424.

BRONCHIECTASIS

Bronchiectasis is characterised by its chronic course[1] and is defined on anatomical basis as a condition characterised by abnormal and permanent distortion and dilation of the sub-segmental airways.[2] The disabling disease has recurrent acute pulmonary infections over a chronic mucopurulent expectoration.

Aetiology

Obstruction, infection, immunodeficiency and congenital anomalies are few precipitating factors, predisposing to bronchiectasis. It is generally initiated in childhood. The infective fevers of childhood like measles and whooping cough and the secondary bacterial infections associated with thick viscid sputum are likely to cause obstruction of multiple small bronchi and destruction of its components. Often there is previous history of recurrent viral infections as bronchitis or bronchopneumonia. Primary tuberculosis with compression of the bronchus by the lymph nodes, bronchostenosis, foreign body inhalation, aspiration of infected material, unresolved pneumonia, bronchial adenoma and neoplastic growth can lead to the occurrence of bronchiectasis.

Diffuse bronchiectasis occurs in congenital conditions like ciliary dyskinesis syndrome, cystic fibrosis, alpha 1 antitrypsin deficiency, Young's syndrome, bronchomalacia (Williams-Campbell syndrome) and panhypogammaglobulinaemia.[5-7] Allergic bronchopulmonary aspergillosis may cause bronchiectasis of medium sized bronchi. Diffuse bronchiectasis may occur by repeated aspirations due to nasogastric intubation, unconscious state, neuromuscular impairment of cough or swallowing and incompetence of gastroesophageal sphincter.[8] Focal bronchiectasis is often limited to a segment or lobe. Localised bronchiectasis may result from foreign body, tuberculosis, pressing hilar node or metastasis or a congenital anomaly. Second to fourth order segmental bronchi in the basal segments of lower lobes, the right middle lobe and the lingula are the most frequently involved. Isolated upper lobe may, rarely, be involved in case of tuberculosis. Nearly one third of cases are unilateral bilobar, one third being unilobar and one third are bilateral.[9-11] It occurs from foreign body aspiration, benign lung tumours and inflamed lymph nodes compressing the orifice of bronchus, thus allowing poor bronchial drainage and enhancing susceptibility to repeated infections.[10]

Pathogenesis[2]

Two important factors infection and collapse are responsible to a variable extent in the production of bronchiectasis, may be alone or two together contribute in the pathogenesis of bronchiectasis. Bronchiectasis may be focal, localised to a segment or lobe or diffuse. Weakening of the bronchial walls due to infection can lead to bronchiectasis without collapse or obstruction in case of tuberculosis.

During acute infections, the aspirated infected material may block the lumen of small bronchi and bronchioles. The infection causes ulcers of the walls leading to endobronchial abscess. The obstruction of the segmental bronchus does not lead to collapse as the aeration is still maintained by collateral air drift (bronchiolitis obliterans) resulting in the interruption of the free communication of the bronchial tree upwards and cause bronchial dilatation in the abscence of obstruction.

An obstruction of the large airways from foreign body or adenoma may cause collapse beyond the obstruction and secretions accumulate distally and get infected if they are not promptly relieved. Inflammation of the bronchial wall will cause destruction of the elastic muscular tissue, thus, its weakening and eventual dilatation. Primary tuberculosis produces a similar effect. The obstruction in the lumen of the medium and small sized bronchi leads to collapse and shrinkage of the lung. It generates sufficient intrapleural negative pressure to stretch and distend the unobliterated parts of the peripheral airways. It causes reversible bronchiectasis in the early stages. However it becomes irreversible with time when collapse has stayed long enough and is super-added with infection. The parenchymal damage and fibrosis exert traction on the bronchial wall to cause dilatation. The infection from staphylococcus, streptococcus and H. influenza causes damage to the wall, thus preventing it to go back to the original size. It loses the ability to contract on expiration and the secretions accumulate, thus the secondary infections persist. Micro organisms release various inflammatory products and also attract neutrophils which often release various proteolytic enzymes, including neutrophil elastase, at the site of inflammation, which are in turn responsible for various pathologic feature in bronchiectasis such as epithelial damage, bronchial gland hyperplasia and connective tissue damage regulating in bronchial distoration.

Pathology[2]

The components of the bronchial wall are destroyed. The elastic tissue, muscle, cartilage, glands and lymphoid tissue undergo complete destruction and are replaced by fibrous tissue. The normal size and shape is not maintained and the subsegmental airways become tortuous and dilated. The changes may vary from mild tubular dilatation to cystic or saccular changes with almost grossly deranged unrecognisable architecture. The peribronchial fibrosis exerts traction from outside. Many of the small bronchi and bronchioles are completely destroyed by the inflammatory process. The epithelium exhibits squamous metaplasia and there is infiltration with chronic inflammatory cells in the submucosal region. The increased intrabronchial pressure during inspiration distends the weakened wall containing fibrous remnants. There is vascular occlusion, and the dilated bronchi terminate abruptly. The cilia are damaged and paralysed, thus affecting the removal of the secretions. The excess mucous production and its stagnation facilitates the growth of organisms and persistence of infection. The viscid or purulent exudates obstruct the airways partially and lead to poor aeration of the lung. There is intense neovascularisation of bronchial arteries. There occurs hypertrophy of bronchial arteries as a part of inflammatory process, creating a local extensive pre-capillary shunt from left to right into the pulmonary venous system, thus laying the substrate for haemorrhage and hemoptysis.[1-5]

Bronchiectasis has predilection for lower lobes, on the sides, left side is commonly involved. The basal segments of the lower lobe, apical segment of the lower lobe, lingula or middle lobe and posterior segment of the upper lobe are the common sites of affection. The condition is bilateral in one-third of the cases. However, it may be limited to one lobe or segment. The clinical manifestations are noted more frequently among three to four decades of male population.[2]

Clinical Features

Patient may not have any symptom in mild bronchiectasis, and diagnosis is made on bronchography (Dry bronchiectasis). The clinical features develop insidiously and the symptoms are noted when there is infection leading to collection of secretions in moderately severe bronchiectasis.

The patient has a raspy, frequent, paroxysmal cough. It is productive of mucopurulent or purulent expectoration in varying amounts. The sputum becomes foetid when the tissues are invaded by anaerobic streptococci, fusiform bacilli, bacteroids, and gram negative organisms. Due to paroxysmal character of cough, the patient may bring out large amounts of expectoration with a definite postural relationship. It is noted on rising in the morning or on lying down at night indicating to be due to a drainage of secretions from a major bronchus.[1] A history of persistent cough and purulent sputum since childhood is diagnostic of bronchiectasis. Haemoptysis is another feature but it generally stops without treatment.[1] Sometimes hyperaemic walls and granulation tissue[11] may lead to life threatening haemoptysis.

During infection i.e. bronchitis and bronchopneumonia) fever and rigor may be present, pleuritic chest pain may be noted due to spread of infection to pleura. Breathlessness on exertion occurs with progress of the disease and depends on the extent of lung involvement and presence and absence of acute infection. In fact, recurrent pneumonia should lead to suspicion of bronchiectasis in an isolated lung segment involvement. The persistence of the disease leads to general ill health, loss of appetite and loss of weight.[2]

The clinical signs have a basal distribution with diminution of movement, impairment of percussion note and sticky coarse crepitations. The crepitations are persistent. The signs of collapse or fibrosis may be present. Cyanosis may be evident. Clubbing of both of fingers and toes is common. The upper lobe bronchiectasis may be secondary to tuberculosis. Signs of secondary pulmonary hypertension and cor pulmonale usually develop with the end stage bronchiectasis. Various signs and differential diagnoses have been shown in Table 4.14.

Table 4.14: Bronchiectasis

Signs: Cavernous breathing
Clubbing of fingers
Crepitations
Hypoventilation
DD: Amyloidosis, bronchitis, lung cancer, pneumonia, tuberculosis

Investigation[2]

Chest X-ray shows areas of collapse and ring shadows. Vascular markings are often increased and may be crowded together. There may be displacement of the fissure or of the mediastinum from the collapsed lobe. If sinusitis is accompanying, sinus X-ray may reveal sinus thickening, opacity or air fluid levels. Bronchoscopy may demonstrate strictures, growth and foreign bodies. It is not recommended otherwise to visualize bronchiectatic areas. Bronchography is the definite diagnostic test, especially when the resection is contemplated, to define the anatomy (Table 4.15). These days it is rarely indicated, as lung CT scanning is a sensitive and convenient way to detect bronchiectasis. Only recently bronchoscopic shuttle, where flexible fiberoptic bronchoscope has been used to carry the catheter for bronchography.[3,4]

Table 4.15: Bronchographic changes in bronchiectasis

1. Cystic:	When the dilatation is like a bunch of grapes (70%).
2. Fusiform:	When the dilatation is spindle shaped (5%)
3. Cylindrical:	When the dilatation is uniform like a cylinder (20%)

The sputum should be examined for the volume, frequency and colour for pyogenic bacteria and tubercle bacilli. The culture reveals mixed flora. ESR is elevated. There may be leucocytosis in the presence of active infection. The transcricoid instillation of radio-opaque iodized oil (lipiodol) allows anatomical localisation of bronchiectatic airways. The absence of peripheral filling indicates its inability to conduct. There is pooling of contrast medium in the dilated and distorted bronchial passages. The bronchial dilatations are distinguished as saccular, fusiform and cylindrical types and they may coexist in the same individual. The smaller bronchioles of the airways are not seen. The normal tapering of the bronchioles is absent and they appear dilated.

Lung function are altered depending on the regions involved in the process. Spirometry reveals an obstructive defect in diffuse bronchiectasis in initial stage and it may be combined with a restrictive defect in the presence of parenchymal destruction in the advanced stage of the disease. The area affected by bronchiectasis show reduction in ventilation, decreased V/Q ratio and diminished perfusion. Arterial blood gas values reveal hypoxemia and respiratory alkalosis. The level of immunoglobulins must be measured in suspected cases of immunodeficiency. Nasal mucosal biopsy to define ciliary ultrastructure under electron microscope, assessment of sperm motility, and electrolytes analysis of sweat are useful screening test for bronchiectasis in dyskinetic cilia syndrome, young's syndrome and cystic fibrosis.

Complications

Complications may be local or systemic: local complications can be recurrent pneumonias, haemoptysis, pleurisy, empyema and lung abscess, cerebral abscess; systemic ones include hypoproteinemia, septicemia, arthritis and secondary amyloidosis. Progressive respiratory failure and corpulmonale occur in severe cases, when ventilation is compromised.

Management[1-5]

The institution of antibiotics at the early stages of respiratory infection in childhood prevents the development of bronchiectasis. Evacuation of the secretions by postural drainage and control of infection with antibiotics form the main line of treatment. The posture adopted depends on the lobe or segment affected. There is good drainage from the upper lobes during an upright position, from the middle lobe in a recumbent position with the normal side up and from the lower lobes while the patient is lying face downward at the elevated foot-end of the bed. It reduces the amount of pus and toxaemia secondary to it. Percussion tappings help in bringing out the secretions easily.

The antibiotics help in controlling the infection. However, the relapses are frequent on cessation of administration of the antibiotics. Prolonged antibiotic therapy in severe cases of bronchiectasis with tetracycline or penicillin reduces the sputum volume and purulence rapidly and reduces the disability.

Favourable response is considered only when there is decrease and thinning of sputum along with resolution of systemic symptoms, which may take upto a week. Associated pneumonitis may get radiological clearing in few weeks, so much time bronchiectasis may require for clinical recovery. Antibiotics should be reserved only for acute exacerbations since prolonged prophylactic use may not be of value; rather it might create development of resistant strains. Beneficial effects of mucolytics and expectorants and of oral theophylline through improved ciliary activity is not proved. Complete cessation of smoking is essential.[1] Management modalities have been shown in Table 4.16.

Lobectomy or segmental surgical resection enables to get rid of the damaged lung. Before undertaking the resection, the pulmonary function studies and bronchography on the healthy side have to be carried out to find the efficiency of the lung. Majority of patients do not require surgery. Surgery is indicated only when the disease is localised with possibility of complete excision.[12,13] In dry bronchiectasis with marked recurrent haemoptysis, the affected segments may be removed. Surgical intervention may be necessary in some cases when there is difficulty to control the infection with postural drainage and in the absence of response to medical therapy. However, the necessity of surgery has markedly declined in the recent years.[2]

Table 4.16: Bronchiectasis: Management

1. Stop smoking
2. Specific antibiotics
3. Taking care of acute exacerbations
4. Postural drainage
5. Bronchodilators
6. Surgical resection of chronically infected lobe-
7. Prognosis can be good with proper care
8. Precautions: Beware of amyloidosis and cor pulmonale

Even bronchial haemorrhage can well be controlled by bronchial artery embolization rather than surgery. In case there is an extensive pulmonary involvement with destruction, lung transplantation is the choice.

Prevention

Cessation of smoking, chest exercises with deep breathing, nutritious diet and prompt treatment of infections during acute exacerbations. Annual vaccination against influenza and pneumococcal infections along with immunisation against measles and pertussis should be done.[1]

REFERENCES

1. *Harrisons' Principles of internal medicine:* Wilson J.D.; Braunwald E., Isselbacher K.J., *et al.*, (ED); 12th Ed, Vol. 2, McGraw Hill, New York 1991.
2. Shankar P.S., *Chest Medicine,* Oxford and IBH Publ. Co. N. Delhi, 4th ed., 1994.
3. Haruno M.M., Williams Jr. JH; The flexible fiberoptic bronchoscope shuttle, Chest 1992; 102: 914-45.
4. Hira H.S., FFB as a carrier of catheter for bronchography; JAPI 1997; 45: 763-65.
5. Crofton and Douglas's Respiratory Diseases, Seaton A, Seaton D and Gordonleitch A, ed., 4th ed., 1989; Oxford University Press, Delhi.
6. Sturgers J.M. and Turner J.A.P., Recurrent illness due to immotile cilia syndrome J. Resp. Dis 1982; 3:48.
7. Reynolds H.Y., Host defence impairment that lead to respiratory infections; Clin. Ches. Med 1987; 8:339.
8. Iokara T., *Lung infections and diffuse interstitial diseases of the lungs,* In; Sabiston D.C., Spender F.C. (ed), Gibbon's Surgery of the Chest; 4th ed, Saunders, Philadelphia, 1983.
9. Swartz M.N., *Bronchiectasis, In, Pulmonary diseases* and *disorders,* 2nd ed; Fishman A.P., ed., McGraw Hill, New York; 1988.
10. Barker A.F. and Bardara E.J., Bronchiectasis: Update of an orphan disease, Amer. Rev. Resp. Dis 1988,137:969.
11. Schwartz Seymour I., *et al.*, Schwartz's Principles of Surgery, 6th ed; McGraw Hill Inc, N. York 1994.
12. Wilson J.F. and Decker A.M., The surgical management of childhood bronchiectasis; A review of 96 consecutive pulmonary resection in children with non-tuberculous bronchiectasis, Ann. Surg 1982; 195: 354.
13. Tokaro T., Sethi G., *et al., Thoracic surgical infections,* In: Simons R.L., Howard R.J. (ed); Surgical infectious diseases. Appleton Century Crofts; N. York 1982.

ANAEROBIC BACTERIAL INFECTIONS

The normal anaerobic flora of oropharynx or of gastrointestinal tract may enter into the lower respiratory passages, producing pathological changes of pleuropulmonary regions, presenting as aspiration pneumonia, necrotizing pneumonia, lung abscess and empyema.[1]

Aetiology

The anaerobes are non-sporulating Gram positive microaerophilic streptococci (peptostreptococci) and Gram negative rods (Bacteroides melaninogeniscus, Bacteroides fragilis, B intermedius or Fusobacterium nucleatum). The aspiration of oropharyngeal secretions or of gastrointestinal contents that have been regurgitated during the course of some other diseases is common in patients with compromised consciousness (chronic alcoholism, general anaesthesia, cerebrovascular accident or narcotic addiction), convulsions, periodontal diseases, immunosuppression or dysphagia.[2] The gravitational flow facilitates occurrence of infection in the posterior segments of the upper lobes or superior segments of the lower lobes in recumbancy or basal segments of the lower lobes in upright or semirecumbant positions. Haematogenous dissemination of pelvic or abdominal abscesses or direct extension of subphrenic abscess[3] can also lead to anaerobic infection.

Pathology

There is development of air space (pneumonic) consolidation initially which soon undergoes necrosis and liquefaction resulting in an abscess in one to two weeks. The infection may spread to the pleura leading to the occurrence of empyema. In an overwhelming infection, development of multiple small abscesses may prove fulminant.[3]

Anaerobic infections of the chest include[4-8] the following:

Anaerobic Aspiration Pneumonitis

It needs to be differentiated from two other aspiration pneumonias:

i. Pneumonitis due to aspiration of solid or food. In these cases, major airways are obstructed resulting into atelectasis, with non-specific inflammation. Removal of foreign body is the treatment.
ii. Mendelson's syndrome—results from regurgitation of gastric contents containing chemical material, resulting into odema of alveolar lining with transudation of the alveolar spaces. This develops within hours of aspiration, especially following anaesthesia. Patients become febrile, hypoxic and tachypnoic. Sputum production is minimum. Respiratory failure may develop. Total leucocytic count increases and chest X-ray shows complete whiteout bilaterally.
   Antibiotics are given only when secondary bacterial infections occur, featured by persistance of fever, increased sputum, leucocytosis etc.
iii. Bacterial aspiration pneumonitis—develops quickly, especially in hospitalised patients or alcoholics. Such patients have low grade fever, malaise, increased sputum production with mixed flora. Chest X-ray shows segmental consolidation.

Necrotizing Pneumonia

These are numerous small abscesses scattered over many lung segments. It is less common than aspiration pneumonia and lung abscess and may have indolent or fulminant course.

Anaerobic Lung Abscess

It is the result of a subacute anaerobic respiratory infection. Patient has fever with chills, malaise and foul smelling sputum for the last few weeks. Abscess may be single or multiple, but present in the dependent lung segments. Differential diagnosis includes lung abscess, tuberculosis and carcinoma.

Bronchoscopy doesn't enhance drainage and surgery is never indicated because of fear of spilling the abscess contents into the normal lung segment.

Empyema

A long standing an aerobic lung infection results into empyema, the clinical presentation of which is similar to other anaerobic chest infections. Extension from subdiaphragmatic infection or infective pulmonary emboli from intra-abdominal or genital organs[9] in case of females, can also result in anaerobic pneumonitis and empyema. There is foul smell in the expectorations. Pleuritic chest pain is present.

A pneumonia patient with foul smelling sputum and persistence of fever, receiving antibiotics, should be suspected of loculated empyema that can be confirmed with ultrasound, and needs drainage.

REFERENCES

1. Barlett J.G., Gorbach S.L. and Finegold S.M., Amer. Jour. Med 1974; 56:1202.
2. Barlett J.G. and Gorbach S.L., Jour. Amer. Med. Assn 1975; 234:935.
3. Shankar P.S., Anaerobic bacterial infections; Chest Medicine, Oxford and IBH Publ. Co. (P) Ltd., New Delhi, 1994; 4th ed.
4. Wilson J.D., Braunwald E., Isrelbacher K.J., *et al.*, ED. Harrison's principles of internal medicine 12th ed. McGraw Hill, New York, 1991.
5. Gorbach S.C. and Bartlett J.G., Anaerobic infections N. Eng. J. Med 1974; 290:1177.
6. Girbach S.C., Anaerobic bacteria; IN, Principles and practices of infectious diseases, 3rd ed; Mandell G.L., *et al.*, ed, Wiley, N. York 1990.
7. Finegold S., ED, Anaerobic infections in humans, Academic, Orlando F.L. 1989.
8. Finegold S.M., Anaerobic bacteria in human disease; Academic, N. York, 1977.
9. Gibbs R.S., Microbiology of the female genital tract, Amer J. Obs. Gynae 1987; 156:491.

ACUTE RESPIRATORY INFECTIONS (ARI) IN CHILDREN

Acute respiratory infections (ARI) in children form a major cause of paediatric illness in the world and a persistence source of childhood mortality in many developing countries.[1-3] The incidence of respiratory tract infections is parallel to sudden death syndrome in infants in pediatric community.[4] Acute respiratory infections which occur as one case out of five cases of upper respiratory infections,[5,6] though being effectively tackled under an approved comprehensive ARI control programme of service and research by WHO[2] yet require to be handled as an integral part of primary health care so as to achieve the goal of health for all by 2,000 A.D.[7]

ARI have been rated among the principal causes of paediatric morbidity and mortality in developing countries, a part from malnutrition and diarrhoeal diseases[8-10] where the risk is 30-70 times higher as compared to developed nations.[1] The epidemiological profile of ARI in India conforms to that of most developing countries.[2,11] 80 per cent having a mild course of the disease, i.e., not having fast breathing, chest indrawing or drinking trouble because of breathing difficulty, causing 14.3 per cent of an infant and 15.9 per cent of preschool mortality.[12] Recently lower respiratory infections accounting for 20-24 per cent of childhood deaths have been reported.[13]

Virus has been isolated in 25 per cent cases of pneumonia in developing countries.[14] In a study on preschool children with pneumonia, on culturing lung aspirates, were found to have 50 per cent of cases with bacterial pathogens, 30 per cent with virus and no agents recovered in rest of the cases. Half of those with viral infection, also had bacterial invasion, therefore, accounting for 2/3rd as bacterial aetiology, either primary or in combination with virus.[14] In another study on severe acute lower respiratory infections, bacterial aetiology was confirmed in 70 per cent of all cases, caused by streptococcus pneumoniae, haemophilus influenzae and staphylococcus aureus.[2] This provides a scientific basis for routine administration of antibiotics in managing moderate to severe ARI within the community.[2] The drug of choice being cotrimoxazole but ampicillin/amoxycillin proved to be a better alternative except for side effects like diarrhoea and rash and also cost factor can be considerable. Precipitating factors for chest infections in children are shown in Table 4.17.

Table 4.17: Chest infection: Precipitating factors in children

1. Defective defensive mechanism (Agammaglobulinemia).
2. Cystic fibrosis.
3. Congenital anomalies like cleft palate, congenital bronchiectasis, tracheoesopageal fistula, etc.
4. Vascular defects like abnormal polymorphs, neutropenia, increased pulmonary blood flow.
5. Deficient gag reflex.

Fast breathing is the best sign that a child has pneumonia[1,14] requiring prompt management rather than clinical differentiation of viral or bacterial origin[7] although these chest sounds can be differentiated clinically, yet are not very reliable.[14]

A short study reveals lack of knowledge to the attending mothers. No casualty occurred in group (a) and (b). 2/8 died in group (c) and 3/6 readmitted, 1/3 expired and 2/4 were malnourished out of those who died. Male predominance may not be seen owing to a trend toward a smaller family[15] where the female child does get her due care.[7] The ARI attack rate as well as duration of the attack is similar for both normal birth weight and low birth weight, although mortality is higher in the latter. Fever is important since it compels the parents to rush to their doctors[16] but 20 per cent of the parents are not aware of the grave consequence of the disease their child is suffering from. Deep tracheal aspiration has proved to be a good specimen for lab evaluation.[18]

Thus ARI control can be achieved not only by case management but also by immunisation and health education.[2] As suggested by WHO/UNICEF, stress should be laid on:

i. Educating the mothers regarding dietary habits, improving hygiene and general resistance of the children through nutritional measures.
ii. Proper vaccination for vaccine preventable serious ARI such as diphtheria, pertussis and measles, protein polysaccharide conjugates of endemic serotypes of H. influenzae and S. pneumoniae and use of purified protein components or attenuated live virus with syncytial and paramyovirus vaccines.
iii. Priority to breast feeding.
iv. Minimising air pollution by banning parental smoking.
v. Helping parents to learn to dispense simple supportive measures and differentiating the gravity of disease, deciding in time to seek medical help.

These disease preventive and health promotive measures would yield a healthy paediatric existence in the society, reducing both disease and death in child population, thus indirectly raising the health index of community.[19,20] The decline in mortality rate is however much slower, compared to developed countries where ARI mortality has rapidly declined.[17] A suitably geared up national programme of the country for ARI control is the need of the present time.

REFERENCES

1. A Joint WHO/UNICEF Statement; Basic principles for control of acute respiratory infections in children in developing countries 1986, 7-17.
2. Kumar Y., Practical aspects of the WHO Programme on acute respiratory infection and health systems research in India; Tuberculosis and respiratory diseases.
3. Forsyth K.D., *et al.,* Lung immunoglobulins in the sudden infant death syndrome, BMJ 1989; 298:23-26.
4. Proceedings of 26th World Conference of IUATLD, Nov. 1986.
5. Bhatia R.S., Public and profession—Causes and cure in present paediatric practices, CMP 1991; 35:09-11.
6. Monto A.S., *et al.,* Acute respiratory illness in an American community, JAMA 1974; 227:2:164-68.
7. Bhatia R.S., *Acute respiratory infections in children—Present trend, future course;* Paper accepted for 15th International Conference of Eastern region of IUATLD, Dec. 1987.
8. Pio A., Leowski J. and Ten Dam H.G., The magnitude of problem of acute respiratory infections. In: Dougles RM; Kerby-Eaton E.;Eds. Acute respiratory infections in children; Proceedings of an International Workshop, Adelaide; Dept. of Community Medicine, University of Adelaide 1985.
9. Railey I.D., The epidemiology, aetiology and management of acute respiratory infections. In: Tuberculosis and respiratory diseases, Proceedings of 26th World Conference of IUAT Nov. 1986.
10. Shann Frank, Treating pneumonia in children, ARI News 1985; 1:6.
11. Kumar V., Personal Communication, March1988.
12. Registrar General of India, Survey on infant and child mortality 1979, Ministry of Home Affairs, N. Delhi 1983.
13. Cherian T., *et al.,* Lower respiratory infection can be diagnosed by simple clinical signs, Medical Times 1988; 18:1.
14. Shann Frank, Reader's views, ARI News 1985; 3:8.
15. Bhatia R.S. and Sibia S.S., ARI in children in private practice at Ludhiana, Punjab, Lung India 1992:10:161-164.
16. Bhatia R.S., Over-prescribing and under-reporting, ARI News, London 1987; 8:8.
17. WHO, Case management of acute respiratory infections in children in developing countries; report of a working group meeting. Geneva.;WHO:1985;WHO/RSD/85:15.
18. Rathi S., *et al.,* Our experience of clinical profile of ARI in children; 4th National Pulmonary Update,1996, Coimbatore.
19. Bhatia R.S., ARI in paediatric practice; Curr Med Journ 1996; 2(1):59.
20. Bhatia R.S., ARI in children: Our experience; Update Med and Surg; RCPS, Glasglow, ed, Jagdesan K, *et al.,* 1988:162-68.

OESOPHAGEAL ACHALASIA AND CHEST INFECTIONS

Recurrent chest infection can be sole manifestation of oesophageal achalasia in child. Oesophageal achalasia is quite uncommon in children.[1] Classically, dysphagia, regurgitation and retrosternal pain are cardinal symptoms.[2] Rarely, cases with achalasia may be first recognised because of pulmonary manifestations alone.[3]

Achalasia under 4 years of age constitutes less than 5 per cent of all patients.[4,5] However, in two recent paediatric series totalling 37 cases, nearly 25 per cent cases were under 5 years and 4 were below 2 years of age.[1]

Regurgitation occurs in about 70 per cent of cases and may be positional.[3] Regurgitation at night may go unnoticed but can lead to pulmonary aspiration. Respiratory manifestations are irritative recurrent pneumonitis, lung suppuration and even bronchiectasis.[2] In 20 children with achalasia, 25 per cent had associated respiratory symptoms.[4]

Early recognition and awareness about this rare presentation of achalasia is important as timely surgical management can save the child from prolonged morbidity and permanent lung damage.[6] Careful history and barium swallow lead to diagnosis. Absence of gastric air bubble, uniform, oesophageal dilatation with an air filled fluid level and tapered 'bird-beak' deformity at lower oesophageal sphincter because of failure of relaxation are radiographic features. Treatment consists of oesophageal dilatation and stenting. Repeated balloon dilatation if fails, cardiomyotomy is considered.

REFERENCES

1. Silverman A. and Roy C.C., Pediatric Clinical Gastroenterology, London C.V. Mosby Co 1983; 158-6l.
2. Bedi R.S., Recurrent chest infection—sole manifestation oesophageal achalasia in a child, JAP1 1993, 41:230-31.
3. Berk J.E., Bockus Gatroenterology, Vol. 2, Philadelphia W.B. Saunders Co 1985; 4584-87.
4. Azizkhan R.G., Tapper D. and Eraklis A., Achalasia in childhood: 20 years experience, J. Pediat, Surg 1980; 15: 452-56.
5. Elder T.B., Achalasia of cardia in childhood, Digestion 1970; 3:90-96.
6. Menzies Gow N., Gummer J.W.P. and Edwards A.M., Results of Heller's operation for achalasia of the cardia. Br. J. Surg 1978; 65; 483-85.

PULMONARY TUBERCULOSIS

Introduction

Tuberculosis is a disease of great antiquity and man has lived with it for many centuries.[1] A major health problem in most of the developing countries, tuberculosis continues to challenge medical practitioners and health professionals. Nearly one and a half million new cases of tuberculosis are being discovered every year in India, of whom one fifth are sputum positive. Robert Koch (1882) was the first to establish the causative organism—tubercle bacilli.[2] The disease originates from the person infected with pulmonary tuberculosis, expectorating tubercle bacilli. The development of infection is affected by socio-economic factors, living and dietary status and degree of exposure and immunisation status of the population. Clinical and radiological examination, confirmed by sputum smear examination clinches the diagnosis. Identification of infectious cases and their adequate treatment is necessary to break the chain of further transmission of tubercle bacilli. Chemotherapy is a powerful therapeutic tool against tuberculosis if used sensibly. Used in a right combination, with proper dosage and for proper duration, chemotherapy effectively arrests and cures the disease. Nevertheless, successful chemotherapy faces practical limitations due to inadequate dosage and inadequate drug regimens, irregular drug intake with frequent interruptions and early discontinuation of drugs, drug toxicity, drug resistance etc. Possibly innocence, ignorance and illiteracy play a significant role, especially in countries like India.[3] Improvement in socio-economic infrastructure of the population along with accurate diagnosis and adequate treatment of case is likely to play a vital role.

Aetiology

Mycobacterium (Myco.) tuberculosis (Table 4.18) is the causative organism, which is rod shaped, straight or slightly curved organism, measuring 1-4 microns by 0.3-0.6 micron, with rounded ends, occurring singly, rarely in clumps. It is non-motile, an acapsular and strictly aerobic organism, susceptible to sunlight. Cell wall of the organism appears to be a filamentous, consisting of glycolipid, peptidoglycan and mycolic acids, as revealed under electron microscope.[4] It is quite thick and lipophilic and is responsible for acid fastness, resistance to various anti-microbials, lytic enzymes and even certain nutrients. Cytoplasm of the cell is quite thin, containing mesosomes, ribosomes and vacuoles in its central core. Mycobacteria can exist in human and bovine (mammalian), avian, piscine and marine forms. Myco. tuberculosis var. hominis and Mycobact. Tuberculosis africans are responsible for tuberculosis in human beings. It is called acid fast bacillus (AFB) due to its distinct tinctorial property of acid-fastness. The organism is stained by using carbolfuchsin or carbolauramine and resists decolorization by acid and alcohol.[5] It gives a brilliant red appearance when stained with fuchsin by Ziehl-Neelsen method. It fluoresces golden yellow when examined under ultraviolet light following staining with carbolauramine.

Table 4.18: Mycobacterium tuberculosis: Salient features

1. An aerobic organism.
2. Grows best at pH 7.4 and PO_2 of 100-140 mm of Hg.
3. Divides every 16-20 hours.
4. Cavity lesion may contain 100 million or more.
5. In a virgin population of mycobacterium tuberculosis, there may be 1: 100,000 or more of single drug resistant mutants.
6. Many more secondary resistant mutants may be present in those patients who receive inadequate therapy.
7. In a tubercular patient, four types of populations may be present:
   - Extracellular in cavities
   - Extracellular-closed caseous lesions
   - Intracellular (within macrophages)
   - Dormant bacilli

The organism is susceptible to sunlight and heat, but survives in the dark, and resists freezing and drying. It can be killed on exposure to 1-2 per cent phenol, 80 per cent ethyl alcohol and 40 per cent formalin. It resists action of sodium hydroxide, HCL and sulphuric acid. It is non-chromogenic, and does not produce any acid with glucose. It produces nicotinic acid, peroxidase and catalase as it grows and causes reduction of nitrates to nitrites. Bovine strains do not reduce nitrates and are weakly niacin positive.

The organism grows very slowly in culture and multiplies by binary fission. These can be grown both on solid and liquid media. Growth requires pH of 6.8-7.0, temperature 37°C and both oxygen and carbon dioxide. The colonies grown over Lowenstein-Jensen (LJ) medium are dry, friable and rough with spreading edges. Human strain may have variable virulence for different laboratory animals.[6] Only recently, a new method of culture and sensitivity for Myco. tuberculosis has been tested, giving results in four days, compared to standard LJ medium, which gives results usually in 4-6 weeks to 2-3 months.[7]

As tubercle bacilli do not seem to produce any toxins or extracellular enzymes, these cause disease by multiplying within the phagocytic cells, withstanding thereby the host defence and intracellular enzymatic digestion. It has complex antigenic nature, its proteins elicit both humoral as well as cellular immune response, while carbohydrates elicit primarily humoral response.

Transmission of Infection

Tuberculosis originates in a patient whose sputum forms the source of infection. The contacts of smear positive cases run a greater risk of getting infection and disease, whereas patients negative by smear microscopy and positive only by culture are less dangerous to the community than those positive by smear.[8] Entrance of organism (infection) occurs by inhalation of airborne droplet nuclei. The bacilli are discharged from a pulmonary focus in the form of tiny droplets of mucus as the patient coughs, spits, talks, sneezes etc., which get dried and become droplet nuclei. It is estimated that a smear positive case of primary tuberculosis infects almost 10 persons during one year.[9]

There is a marked disparity in getting infection and occurrence of clinical disease by Myco. tuberculosis. The host tissue reacts to the infection and may mount an immune response to effectively control the infection. But if the infection is overwhelming or the host resistance is poor, the disease develops, of course, affected by other factors like genetic, immunologic, environmental etc. People at the extreme of age are more susceptible. Malnutrition and undernutrition, occupational exposure to silica dust, alcohlism, smoking and diabetes mellitus increase the susceptibility to develop tuberculosis. Partial gastrectomy, large dose of steroids, and infections like measles, whooping cough and influenza may enhance the susceptibility to developing tuberculosis.[1]

The infectiousness of the tuberculous patient declines rapidly as soon as the therapy is commenced, making the index case much less infectious to the contacts. The number of bacilli also start falling within few days of starting the treatment, decreasing the infective potential of the patient as well in a few weeks.

Tuberculous infection may occur by ingestion of raw milk from tuberculous cows—Bovine tuberculosis. Such an infection is quite uncommon in India as milk is traditionally boiled before its consumption.

Immunology

There is an increased resistance (tuberculo-immunity) to re-infection in persons infected with tubercle bacilli. Infection can be natural or artificial following vaccination. In addition, those infected develop a delayed hypersensitivity to tuberculoprotein. These changes are cell-mediated and are specific immunologic reactions.

Acquired Immunity

Tuberculo-immunity is a cellular type immunity, and tubercle bacilli are facultative intracellular organisms. Although there is production of antibodies, they play a little role in the defence against the disease. The acquired immunity in tubercle bacilli is specific. T-lymphocytes derived from thymus play a significant role. Alveolar macrophages recognise the entry of tubercle bacilli and present the antigen to T-lymphocytes. They produce an extracellular substance—Lymphokine, which activates the macrophages, which in turn trap tubercle bacilli in the centre of granuloma and bring about intracellular inhibition of multiplication of the organisms.[10] A variety of antigens in the cell wall and cytoplasm of the mycobacterium are responsible for granuloma formation, macrophage activation, host toxicity and adjuvanticity.[1]

Delayed Hypersensitivity

An altered state of host tissue reactivity, which exists following tubercular infection, can be detected by introducing tuberculin (tuberculoprotein) into the skin, which gives a delayed type of acute inflammatory response (reaction), that develops fully by 72 hours. Initial response of capillaries, dilatation and neutrophilic exudation, is followed by an induration consisting of macrophages and lymphocytes. The reaction is mediated by T-lymphocytes, involving accumulation of circulating sensitised lymphocytes in response to the specific antigen. Both these reactions are different and exist separately in the body. Degree of tuberculin hypersensitivity is inversely related to degree of acquired resistance. Those exhibiting marked degree of tuberculin hypersensitivity, possess greater susceptibility to active progressive disease. Once infected, animals show greater degree of resistance to re-infection. Similarly, human beings vaccinated with BCG develop an ability to resist further infection.

The number of circulating T-lymphocytes in the blood determines the cell-mediated immunity. It gets depressed in the active phase of the tuberculosis, as is reflected by a significant fall in the level of T-cell count.[11] T-cell count can serve as a marker of immunocompetency and an indicator of clinical severity of pulmonary tuberculosis, while B-lymphocytes count remain normal.[12] The cellular immune response improves with chemotherapy. Antibodies to proteins, glycolipids and polysaccharides components of tubercle bacilli can be demonstrated both in active and inactive tuberculosis. Role of antibodies produced by B-cells in the pathogenesis of tuberculosis is not clear.[1]

Pathogenesis

Tuberculosis is a chronic intracellular infection due to Myco. tuberculosis, having a complex pathogenesis. Infection can develop in two types of patients; those who had no previous infection and those who had previous infection with Myco. tuberculosis. The latter receive infection either from virulent strains of tubercle bacilli or from living attenuated bovine strains of mycobacteria in the form of BCG vaccine. They differ from those who had no previous infection of mycobacteria in demonstrating tuberculin in hypersensitivity and acquired immunity to infection.

Tuberculosis occurs in the form of primary tuberculosis and non-(post) primary tuberculosis. The latter term is applied when the disease occurs in persons with remote primary infection.[14] Primary tuberculosis develops after the first infection with Myco. tuberculosis. The organism enter the respiratory tract by inhalation and the lesion develops in the well ventilated mid or lower lung zones. In majority of cases, healing occurs with or without calcification. In some the lesion gets encapsulated with collagenous tissue and remains viable for many years. Haematogenous spread to remote areas like lung apices, brain, kidney, intestines, bone and spleen may occur. In few cases, primary infection may progress into an active disease, especially in those who have not developed acquired cellular immunity against tuberculosis.

Post primary tuberculosis develops either from reactivation of a quiescent endogenous primary lesion or as an exogenous infection from an active case. This activation of primary focus may occur in later life due to decreased resistance of the individual. Post-primary tuberculosis is characterised by localised lesion with necrosis, that pursues a chronic course.[1]

Primary Tuberculosis

The infection (disease) is referred to in those who have never had a previous infection with tubercle bacilli. It is commonly seen in childhood and adolescence.

Pathology

The organism enters the lungs by inhalation and reach the alveoli, where these are rapidly phagocytosed by polymorphs. This is followed by replacement of these cells by macrophages (epitheloid cells), within which the tubercle bacilli remain viable and continue to multiply slowly at a rate of one multiplication every 24 hours, giving a pneumonia picture with an inflammatory cellular reaction with serofibrinous exudation. Unhindered multiplication of mycobacteria goes on since no resistance has developed in the body. Rupture of macrophages release the bacilli, which spread by way of lymphatics, involving the hilar and paratracheal lymph nodes. The lung lesion which is generally sub-pleural, the draining lymphatics and together with regional lymph nodes constitutes the primary (Ghon's) complex. Entry to blood stream and dissemination to systemic organs may occur before the arrival of T-lymphocytes in sufficient number to control the infection. Macrophages have to be activated before they can destroy the tubercle bacilli. In majority of cases, after a period of few days or weeks, as the acquired immunity develops, this leads to marked reduction in the multiplication of the bacilli, resulting into resolution of pneumonic process. Further dissemination of tubercle bacilli stops and the condition resolves without any residual evidence of tuberculous infection. This is accompanied with development of cutaneous hypersensitivity to tuberculoprotein. Alternatively, some of the epitheloid cells become multinucleated giant (Langhans) cells and collection of large number of macrophages produce a granuloma, which gets encased in collagen fibres, followed by lymphocytic accumulation at the periphery.

In majority of the cases, the lesions get arrested and calcification occurs. In small number of cases, progression of the lesions continue and cellular immunity is unable to prevent its progress. There occurs cellular destruction, forming an amorphous cheesy mass called caseation which results in cavitation. Lymph nodes get enlarged in the hilum. The body is sensitised to tuberculoprotein by the time the infection reaches the lymph nodes. They press and compress the bronchi, causing collapse of the lung lobe, which either re-expands if the inflammation subsides (epituberculosis) or leads to subsequent bronchiectasis.[1]

Clinical Presentation

In majority of cases primary complex goes unnoticed as there are no signs and symptoms. Tuberculin skin test becomes positive within 6 weeks of infection. Chest skiagram shows presence of calcification in later years of life as the hallmark of having had tuberculosis. Some patients may have a short febrile episode, malaise and dry cough, which is often ascribed to an influenza-like illness. Loss of appetite, loss of weight and generalised ill-health may be seen in very few cases. Cough with low grade fever, stridor, wheeze simulating asthma or paroxysmal cough simulating whooping cough may be present in few cases due to pressure effect of enlarged lymph glands on trachea and bronchus. Chest examination is also non-contributory except in few cases where local dullness, absent breath sounds, localised crepitations or wheeze due to pressure effect may be heard.

Diagnosis

Diagnosis of primary tuberculosis becomes difficult due to vague symptomtology. History of contact with a patient of tuberculosis, in an unhealthy child may make clinical suspicion, a reality. Chest X-ray may show unilateral parenchymal lymph node complex. Initially it is quite small, involving the mid or lower zones. Enlarged lymph nodes may be found compressing the middle lobe to cause atelectasis, that appears as a homogenous opacity. Tuberculin test is positive with 5 TU within 6 weeks of infection, but negative test does rule out the possibility of tuberculosis.

Tuberculin Test

Robert Koch's extensive search to find cure of tuberculosis ended in discovering tuberculin test which is being used even today for epidermiological tool in surveillance of tuberculosis and even used in diagnosing tuberculosis. However, predictive value and specificity of the test greatly varies with host and environmental factors. Listeria type of reaction is demonstrable after 10 days of infection and the skin test reactivity is evident at 18-24 hours of inoculation of tuberculin. Unlike destructive type of Koch's reaction, this is non-specific, non-necrotic and protective type of reaction. Mycobacteium vaccae and BCG exclusively induce Listeria type of reaction, whereas Myco. Kansasii, Myco. avium, Myco. scrofulaceium and Myco. tuberculosis induce Koch's type of reaction. Tuberculin test makes use of Koch's type of reaction that is demonstrable after 4-6 weeks of primary infection, at 48-72 hours of skin testing.

Following infection with Myco. tuberculosis, person becomes hypersensitive to its santigenic protein. The bacillary antigen comes in contact with T-lymphocytes and specific antibodies are formed on their surface. When tuberculoprotein is introduced into the skin of an infected person (for testing purposes), the lymphocytes combine with the antigen and release lymphokinines to produce a delayed hypersensitivity reaction (type IV), in the form of inflammatory reaction with exudation of fluid and accumulation of macrophages. This generally takes some time as the sensitised circulating lymphocytes must reach a sufficient number to initiate the inflammatory reaction at the site of infection. Erythema and induration occur in response to cell mediated response.

A positive reaction indicates an infection of Myco. tuberculosis. The person is either suffering from active tuberculosis or has suffered from it in the past. The reaction is positive strongly, even with a very little dose in patients with active disease. Purified protein derivative (PPD) is available in India. Mantoux test, Heaf multipuncture method and Tine test are commonly used methods for tuberculin test. In India Mantoux test is commonly employed while Tine test is almost obsolete. Multipuncture is popular in U.K.

On the flexor surface of forearm a bleb is raised with 0.1 ml of PPD-T/RT23 equivalent to 5TU injected intradermally and reading is taken after 48-72 hours. Erythema and induration indicate positive reaction. Induration is measured transversely in the long axis of forearm and more than 10 mm in diameter is considered positive. A negative reaction is observed in pre-allergic period. Reversion of tuberculin sensitivity may occur in advanced stage tuberculosis, and miliary tuberculosis. The sensitivity is depressed in viral infections (influenza, measles, infectious mononucleosis), mycoplasmal pneumonia, sarcoidosis, renal failure, AIDS, lympho-reticular malignancy, drugs (steroids anti-histaminics, immunosuppressive drugs), pregnancy and in old age.[1]

Prognosis

The acquired cellular immunity, virulence of the organism and its dose determine the course of the primary tuberculosis. It is a benign form and systemic disturbances are almost absent in majority of the cases. Some patients may show hypersensitivity manifestations like pleurisy and effusion, phlyctenular conjunctivitis or erythema nodosum (not common in India). Progressive lesions are seen especially in those with close contact with infected person, massive or recurrent exposure, malnourished persons, lack of immunity or intercurrent infections. Risk of haematogenous spread causing miliary or meningeal tuberculosis is high in these cases. Primary complex does not require any treatment, however, close observations of the child regarding development of clinical disease is essential in these cases. Such cases should be immediately treated on minimal radiological evidence of the disease as there are greater chances of development of complications by dissemination or of progressive disease.

Miliary Tuberculosis[1]

Haematogenous dissemination of tuberculous bacilli causing widespread systemic lesions of tuberculosis is referred to as miliary tuberculosis.

Pathology

Depending upon poor host resistance or overwhelming infection, miliary tuberculosis frequently develops in children after primary infection in populations with widespread tuberculosis. The spread is localised to the lungs only if the focus erodes into pulmonary artery, but becomes systemic when the pulmonary vein is eroded. A granulomatous reaction, producing small foci of the size of millet seed is elicited by the bacilli wherever they are deposited. These may become cellular with collection of epitheloid cells, with minimal caseation (hard tubercles) or caseation with exudation and a large number of bacilli (soft tubercle).

Clinical Presentation

Clinically, patient may have a sudden onset of fever, bodyache, malaise, headache and prostration. Cough is a late feature. Tuberculous meningitis may be associated feature. Both heart and respiratory rate are increased. However, chest examination is non-contributory. It is only in the late stage, fine crepitations may become audible. There may be hepatosplenomegaly. Meningeal signs may appear early or during the illness, associated with funduscopic evidence of choroidal tubercles.

Investigations

Radiological findings are evident only when miliary shadows are of 1-2 mm in diameter, presenting as a *snow storm,* where small miliary shadows are distributed in both the lungs, from apices to bases. Lesions being predominantly interstitial, there are less chances of demonstration of tubercle bacilli in the sputum smear. Tuberculin test may be negative or weakly positive. Total count may show leucopenia or leucocytosis. Liver or bone marrow biopsy may show tubercles but it is trans-bronchial biopsy which demonstrate the typical lesions. Rapid on-site evaluation (ROSE) can improve diagnostic rapidness and accuracy of TBNAand adequacy of sample for molecular studies.[13]

Diagnosis, Course and Prognosis

Presence of miliary shadows on chest skiagram in an acutely ill child with fever clinches the diagnosis. History of contact, enlarged spleen and choroidal tubercles further confirms the diagnosis. The condition is fatal, if not treated energetically.

Non-Primary Tuberculosis

This refers to all types of tuberculosis that occur after the first few weeks of primary infection when immunity to the mycobacteria has developed. Its source of infection can be either endogenous reactivation or exogenous reinfection. Tubercle bacilli acquired by primary infection remain viable but *dormant* in the tubercles of lung or lymph nodes. Reactivation of these occurs if there is reduction of local immunity. Re-infection can occur from virulent tubercle bacilli. TB might induce glucose intolerance and worsen glycemic control in diabetics. Duration of illness and host immune status influence radiologic manifestation of TB. Lower lung involvement is common in diabetics compared to upper lobe infiltrates in non-diabetics, many a times misdiagnosed as cancer or community acquired pneumonia. TB patients who donot have upper lobe involvement are less likely to have positive sputum smear and cultures for AFB.[14]

Pathology

Interaction between the host immunologic response and the infecting tubercle bacilli, where a local breakdown of resistance enables the organism to grow, leads to various pathological changes. There is a necrotising hypersensitivity reaction, resulting localised or extensive lesions. These lesions exhibit different stages of necrosis, and repair, caseation, cavitation and fibrosis. Tubercle is a primary lesion in tuberculosis, due to predominance of macrophages, it is called a granuloma. As they reach the alveoli, tubercle bacilli elicit an acute inflammatory reaction, with exudation of fluid, containing polymorphs, which are replaced by' macrophages within 24 hours. They phagocytose both polymorphs as well as the bacilli. Phosphatides in the bacilli gets spread in the cytoplasm and converts the macrophages into epitheloid cells. Many of these fuse to form giant cells. Later, invasion by mononuclear cells occurs and get altered into epitheloid cells. This causes enlargement of the nodule, which becomes globular in shape; however, their size and number may vary.

Reticulin fibrils and lymphocytes enter between these epitheloid cells surrounded by a large number of lymphocyctes, mostly T-suppressor cells. This gets enveloped by a fibrous cap. Lymph nodes involvement is conspicuously absent.[15] Unhindered growth and multiplication of tubercle bacilli goes on due to local breakdown in cellular immunity. A necrotising hypersensitivity to a large amount of tuberculo protein accumulated at the site leads to coagulative necrosis in the centre of the tubercle. Cellular outline as well as the nuclei of the inflammatory cells disappear and the whole area is changed into a structureless and homogenous cheesy mass. This process is known as caseation. Softening of caseous material occurs because of imbalance in antigen-antibody or changing local concentration of enzyme inhibitors.[16] The area is avascular and all the lymphocytes as well as macrophages have been destroyed. Dying macrophages liberate hydrolytic enzymes like proteinases, lipases and nucleases, which create a dangerous situation by liquefying the caseous material, thus making the disease progressive, because the liquefied material is rich in nutrients and form a good culture medium for growth and multiplication of the bacilli. Also the liquid material moves along the bronchi spreading to other pulmonary areas. The coughed out material contains plenty of tubercle bacilli, hence becomes a transmitting continuous source of infection. Cavity left behind in place of liquid material, offers a good culture medium for the multiplication of the organism. A cavity of the size of 2 cm may contain 100 million tubercle bacilli.

Bronchial mucosal tuberculous inflammation may behave as a check valve, allowing air entry during inspiration and not allowing its exit during expiration. This may cause distension and rupture of the cavity into the pleura, resulting in pneumothorax or hydro/(pyo) pneumothorax. If the bronchus gets blocked by the necrotic material, it may facilitate absorption of the cavity, otherwise a patent bronchus make the cavity chronic. Haemorrhage may occur as the blood vessels and their aneurysmal dilatation running across the cavity get ruptured.[1]

The cellular immunity prevents multiplication of the bacilli and their further dissemination. Fibroblasts lay down fibrous tissue to localise the lesion. Healing may occur with residual fibrous nodules containing viable bacilli (Simon foci or nodule),[17] i.e., regression occurs replacing caseous tissue by fibrosis. Marked destruction of lung parenchyma along with irregular fibrosis is seen in chronic pulmonary disease.

Classification (Post Primary Tuberculosis)

Tuberculosis has been classified into five classes by CDC and The American Thoracic Society: (1) Tuberculosis exposure without evidence of any infection or positive tuberculin test; (2) Tuberculous infection without disease with positive tuberculin skin test without any evidence of clinical, radiographic or bacteriologic evidence of tuberculosis; (3) Tuberculous infection with clinically active disease having clinical or radiographic evidence of current tuberculosis, with conclusive isolation of Mycobacterium tuberculosis. This group is further defined by following features: location of disease, bacteriological status and chemotherapy status; (4) Tuberculosis not clinically active, wherein there is a history of previous episode of tuberculosis or abnormal stable radiographic finding in a person with a positive reaction to tuberculin skin test, negative bacteriologic studies and no clinical and/or radiographic evidence of current disease; and (5) Tuberculosis suspect includes persons wherein diagnosis of tuberculosis is considered. Chemotherapy status are included in class 4 and 5. Class (0) refers to no exposure to tuberculosis and a negative reaction skin test and person is not infected.[18]

Clinical Presentation

Pulmonary tuberculosis has protean manifestations. The onset is gradual, with symptoms of cough, expectoration, fever, loss of weight and haemoptysis. Tuberculous pneumonia, however, may have acute onset with high grade fever, cough and weight loss. At the same time, there can be an active disease without any clinical features and diagnosed only by a radiographic abnormality on chest X-ray. Constitutional symptoms are attributed to nosogenic substances released by the organism into the circulation. These include fever with night sweats, lassitude, loss of weight and appetite. Fever is an important feature and may be irregular often with an evening rise. Probably tumor necrotic factor (TNF) and interleukin-I released by the bacilli act as pyrogens.[19,20]

Temperature is generally normal in tuberculous pneumonia but hectic fever is noted in cavitation. Cough may be mild but persistent and productive as the disease advances, thus drawing attention of the patient as well as the physician. The sputum is mucoid, mucopurulent or blood-tinged sometimes, the amount of which increases with the cavity form-ation. It is not foul smelling. The severety of cough and extent of disease, however, are not related. Haemoptysis may be a first or presenting symptom in pulmonary tuberculosis, especially in young adults. Otherwise, it is a feature of advanced stage of the disease. Amount of bleeding may vary from blood-tinged sputum to expectoration of large amount of fresh and frank blood. Cause of bleeding is the breakdown of a focus in initial stage and erosion of an artery in a necrotic arc or cavity wall, in later stage of the disease. Chest pain or discomfort is another important feature, which may be due to recurrent cough or pleurisy. Breathlessness is a feature with extensive disease. Dyspnoea may occur with the development of massive pleural effusion, pneumothorax or fibrosis. Clubbing may be seen in long standing case of tuberculosis.[21] Involvement of the larynx leads to hoarseness of voice. Loss of weight occurs due to anorexia, toxaemia, increased metabolism, increased protein and lipid turnover by suppressed activity of lipoprotein lipase.[22]

There can be a family history of tuberculosis or history of contact with a sputum positive case. In all these cases, family history of 2/3rd of cases is present.[23,24] History of direct or indirect contact is present in half of the cases.[25] One third to half of the cases belong to 5-10 years of age group.[26] Most of the children have lowering of body resistance due to infectious diseases like whooping cough or measles and pulmonary involvement may be followed by meningial spread.[27,28]

Clinical examination may reveal pallor, pyrexia, tachycardia and sometime tachypnoea. There may not be any abnormality despite relatively advanced disease in some cases. Post-tussive apical crepitations has long been considered an early abnormality. Breath sounds may be feeble, harsh or cog-wheel type. Signs of consolidation may be present. Chest may be asymmetrical in fibrotic lesions, with a mediastinal shift towards the affected side. Dullness, bronchial breathing and crepitations may be present in cases of cavitation and consolidation. Cavernous breathing and post-tussive suction are present in cavitory lesions. There can be signs of pleural effusion, pneumothorax or hydropneumothorax. Unlike leprosy, polar lesions are less frequent.[29] All types except childhood tuberculosis are showing declining trends.[30]

Investigations

The diagnosis is essentially clinical and supported by smear examination of the sputum and chest X-ray. Radiological abnormalities are noted in the chest X-ray film in the presence of symptoms. Tubercular radiological shadows must be proved by sputum examination. The shadows are generally in the upper zone in the form of nodular or patchy shadows, cavity or cavities and calcification.

Initial lesions are exudative, with ill-defined oval or round shadow in the upper zone which may progress to form a density or a homogenous density in the later stages or may regress and get calcified. Shadows are soft, confluent, may be puffy and ill-defined. Initially cavity has a thick wall, which becomes thin in the later stage of the disease, surrounded by punctate or nodular densities. Mediastinum may be distorted due to fibrotic lesions which exhibit linear or dense shadows. There can be crowding of the ribs, mediastinal shift to the affected side and pulled up diaphragm. There can be shadow of cavity filled with caseous material, homogenous shadow of tuberculoma, obliteration of costophrenic angle due to coexisting pleural effusion if small and as a uniform dense shadow with its concavity towards hilum and a mediastinal shift to the opposite side when large and miliary shadows scattered bilaterally from apices to bases. Hyperlucency without any lung markings is seen in pneumothorax and a horizontal fluid level makes its presence in hydro-pneumothorax. Small effusions can be detected by lateral decubitus film. CT helps in recognition of calcification. Ultrasound can also identify minimum pleural effusion.

Bacteriological confirmation is made by demonstrating acid fast bacilli (AFB) by staining in a sputum smear. If sputum continues to remain positive despite chemotherapy for 3-6 months, drug resistance should be suspected since number of organisms come down quickly following adequate chemotherapy. Sputum examination should be done for three consecutive days. The number of bacilli present in the smear is generally related to concentration of bacilli in the sputum. Morning sample, on an empty stomach, preferably secretions from the lower respiratory tract, is collected in a clean container, from which a smear is subjected to staining by Ziehl-Neelsen (ZN) method to see tubercle bacilli under microscope as pink rods against a light blue background. Cold staining using Gabett's methylene blue is a good alternative to ZN procedure.[31,32] Techniques sparing the use of alcohol have been tried but technical superiority of ZN method appears well founded.[3] Since the incidence of disease caused by non-tubercular mycobacterium (NTM) is on a constant increase,[33-36] and its high incidence being in AIDS patients,[36] protein finger printing[37] and immunoblotting identification for NTM have been described.[38]

Sputum culture provides a definite identification of tubercle bacilli. Unlike the smear procedure, in culture, the size of inoculum is 0.1ml and the colonies are visible without any difficulty. CO_2 increases the mycobacteria yield in primary culture in 10% concentration, while 40% CO_2 is lethal.[39] Laryngeal swab, fasting gastric aspirate or bronchial lavage specimens can be used both for smear and culture tests. The smear examination is simple, easy to perform and less expensive unlike culture which is a definite identifying technique. Causes of false negative results in smear examination are given in Table 4.19. Culture is much more sensitive than microscopy and provides precise species identification. Most popular egg-based media are Lowenstein-Jensen buffered egg-potato medium and American Trudeau Society egg-yolk-potato flour medium. Agar-based media such as Middlebrook 7H-10, Middlebrook 7H-11 and Dubos oleic-albumin agar are also important. Metabolic tests like niacin accumulation, catalase production and nitrate reduction are used to identify various mycobacteria. Drug sensitivity tests for M. tuberculosis are helpful to find most effective anti TB drugs as well as appraisal of patients' response to anti TB chemotherapy.

Table 4.19: False –ve results in sputum smear examination: Causes

1. Improper or unsuitable sputum collection
2. Defective slide preparation or faulty slide fixation
3. Slide material is washed away
4. Under or over staining
5. Inadequate slide examination

Bronchoscopy is a useful diagnostic and therapeutic tool.[40] Fiberoptic bronchoscopy establishes aetiological diagnosis in 66 per cent of cases,[41] and aetiology of haemoptysis can be established in 33 per cent of cases, but reactivation of tuberculous lesion[42] and spread of tuberculosis following bronchoscopy has been reported.[43-45] In case sputum is not available, washings from the affected lobe have been found serving the purpose.[46,47] Haematological investigations include total leucocytic count, which is not much altered, peripheral film may show hypochromic microcytic anaemia, ESR may or may not be elevated.

Tuberculin test positivity increases as the length of the time between vaccination and tuberculin testing increases.[48] Complex antigenicity of mycobacterial cell wall or cytoplasm gives rise to various antibodies (antipolysaccharide, antiprotein and antiphosphatides), that can be revealed by haemagglutination, gel diffusion and compliment fixation tests, but these tests are neither specific nor sufficiently sensitive to detect active disease. High levels of adenosine deaminase (ADA) activity have been corelated with tuberculous infection. However, higher levels of activity are also found in enteric fever, bronchogenic carcinoma, and infectious mononucleosis.[49] Higher levels may also be present in pleural tuberculosis.[50] More sensitive methods like enzyme linked immunosorbent assay (ELISA) and radio immuno assay (RIA) are being used to detect and quantify the bacillary antigen in the circulation. ELISA and SAFA (soluble antigen fluorescent antibody) are used for serodiagnosis of tuberculosis, having more sensitivity and specificity, especially the SAFA.[51] A-60 ELISA shows 90-95 per cent diagnostic sensitivity and specificity but not an absolute diagnostic test.[52] ESAT-6 antigen is the most important virulent factor of MTB but may, be seen in some species of NTM as well.[53]

Diagnosis and Differential Diagnosis

Asthma, pneumonitis, lung abscess, bronchiectasis, tropical eosinophilia and bronchogenic carcinoma need to be differentially diagnosed as they simulate tuberculosis in its different stages. Many patients in India are found taking treatment for tuberculosis and ultimately diagnosed having late stage of bronchogenic carcinoma. Table 4.20 lists differential diagnosis.

Table 4.20: Pulmonary tuberculosis: Differential diagnosis

1. Lung cancer
2. Sarcoidosis
3. Other pulmonary disease (since TB can mimic most of the pulmonary disorders)

Complications

Long standing pyrexia: Tuberculosis is an important cause of long standing fever in 2/3rd of cases.[54,55] Being common manifestation of tuberculosis, sometimes, it becomes the only complication in patient having long standing pyrexia not responding to any other treatment.

Pleurisy and pleural effusion: An acute fibrinous pleurisy may develop in pulmonary tuberculosis. There may be fever, cough and pleuritic chest pain progressing to cause exudative, thick, straw coloured effusion. The protein contents are more than 3 gm/dl, specific gravity more than 1.015, pleural fluid to serum protein ratio is more than 0.5, LDH is more than 200IU, pleural fluid to serum LDH ratio is more than 0.6, glucose contents are 60 mg/dl and ADA, which is an enzyme of T-lymphocytes, is markedly elevated.[56] The lymphocytes are increased. Sputum test for AFB in diagnosing tuberculous pleural effusion has very low sensitivity and often result in underdiagnosis.[57] This test if combined with N-PcR definitely improves the diagnosis of pleural tuberculosis.[58]

Empyema

The pleural fluid may get infected, containing large number of polymorphs. Sometimes, it may get encapsulated. Recently a case of tuberculous pyopneumothorax necessitans has been reported.[59]

Atelectasis

Due to pressure over the bronchus by an enlarged lymph node in tuberculosis has been documented. Erosion by the lymph node, followed by bronchial mucosal odema, causing bronchial obstruction appears to be the possible mechanism.[60]

Pneumothorax

Rupture of a subpleural tuberculous focus or cavity results in spontaneous pneumothorax. There is sudden onset of dyspnoea and chest pain or tightness. Those with valvular type may have respiratory distress, tachycardia and cyanosis.

Bronchiectasis

It may develop secondary to bronchial compression by enlarged lymph node or primary complex or granulation tissue or bronchostenosis. This is generally seen in the upper lung lobe and there may be dilatation of the bronchi beyond the obstruction.

Laryngeal Involvement

Tuberculous laryngitis occurs in extensive disease. Patient manifests with soreness of throat, dry hacking cough, and hoarseness of voice. Oedema, ulcer, granuloma or paralysis of vocal cords may occur.

Aspergilloma

Aspergillus fumigatus may grow on the walls of healed open tuberculous cavity, which ultimately gets detached and remains like a free ball within the cavity, producing recurrent episodes of haemoptysis.

Cor Pulmonale

Destruction of pulmonary tissue and vasculature, endarteritis and vasoconstriction are responsible for cor pulmonale. In other words it occurs as a result of extensive chronic fibrocaseous tuberculosis. It manifests with dyspnoea, cyanosis and right sides heart failure. Incidence of pulmonary hypertension has dramatically reduced due to early diagnosis and management with chemotherapy.[61]

Bronchial Carcinoma

Bronchial carcinoma may originate from scars of old tuberculosis. Tuberculosis and lung cancer, carcinoma of tongue, skin, breast and parotid[62] are reported to co-occur.

Cutaneous manifestation of systemic disease and occurrence in an unusual presentation of lupus vulgaris in a case of pleural effusion has been reported.[63] Mediastinal lymphadenopathy in a patient with malignancy may not be always metastatic disease. EBUS guided TBNA if show granulomatous pathology may tilt the diagnosis towards TB.[64]

Other Organs

Pulmonary tuberculosis may be accompanied with tuberculosis of other organs. Involvement of tongue, oral mucosa, middle ear and mastoid, temporal bone, tubercular dysphagia, mediastinal lymph nodes communicating with oesophagus, pancreas and epiglottis with tuberculous infection has been reported.[65-70] Immune thrombocytopenia (ITP) may rarely be associated with lymph node tuberculosis or disseminated TB. In addition to corticosteroids, anti-D immunoglobulin and oral Eltrombopag (aTPO agonist to increase platelet production along with anti koch's treatment cured ITP.

Tuberculosis and AIDS

India has the largest HIV-infected population in the world. Those infected with Mycobacterium tuberculosis add to the gravity of the situation enhancing both morbidity and mortality in these dually infected patients. It is wise to exploit the situation with utilization of tuberculin test with a different cut off criterion for the early diagnosis of mycobacterial infection amongst HIV positive population. HIV/TB coinfection is more common during heterosexual HIV transfer sufferers. Positivity of sputum for AFB and Mantoux test is low. Disseminated TB is common in these patients of dual infection. Almost one third of cases have mediastinal lymphadenopathy.[72]

Introduction

An ancient (Tuberculosis) and a modern pandemic (HIV/AIDS) grew into each other in a decade and became a joint pandemic in the 1990s.

Tuberculosis is responsible for maximum morbidity and mortality in HIV infected patients. In India the HIV seropositivity in TB patients ranges from 0.4-4.9% with a rising trend.[73,74] Those with dual infection are 25-30 times at higher risk of developing active tuberculous disease than those with M. tuberculosis infection alone. Out of 300 million people infected with M. tuberculosis in India, 12 million are supposed to be of active tuberculosis, where only 25% of these cases have positive sputum test for AFB. Prevalence of TB is 50% in the age group of 15-50 years whereas prevalence of HIV infection is 0.5%. In a recent survey, a rising trend has been recorded in Punjab as well. Difficulty in diagnosis of TB in HIV disease occurs because of the following features:

1. Extrapulmonary disease.
2. AFB negativity.
3. Tuberculin test negativity or weak response.
4. Lower and middle zone involvement.

Due to constraints of laboratory facilities[75] in India, tuberculin test positivity with cut off criterion of 2 mm can be ultilized in early detection of mycobacterial infection amongst HIV positive individuals, especially when CD4 count is not possible.[76] The positive tuberculin reaction when stratified by induration measured reveals positivity of test (2 mm induration) in HIV +ve cases in 80% as compared to 24% in HIV –ve cases.

Clinical Picture

Clinical features are most atypical, where lungs are less affected and the disease is more disseminated to other organs. Sputum smear and stool smear are positive for AFB hardly in 40% of cases. This necessitates the need for more sensitive and rapid diagnostic tests. The dual infection has pulmonary involvement in 74-100% of cases and physical findings are indistinguishable between those with and those without HIV infection, posing a lot of difficulty in differential diagnosis. In early stage with CD4 count >200 cells/mm,[3] pulmonary involvement occurs in upper lobe in 70-90% of cases with fever, chill, weight loss. In later stage, CD4 count < 200 cells/mm^3, pulmonary TB is atypical, involving middle and lower lobes, miliary and extrapulmonary in 40-80% of cases. Extrapulmonary involvement in the form of lymphadenitis, miliary or disseminated tuberculosis, has been included as AIDS indicator disease in the Indian context. Features of TB and HIV in early and late phase are shown in the Table 4.21. Spontaneous pneumopericardium in TB and HIV disease is a very rare entity. Usually it is self limiting; a large symptomatic pneumopericardium may need needle aspiration or tube decompensation. High concentration O_2 therapy may also help in absorption of air.[77]

HIV disease with tuberculosis often presents with chronic meningitis, presenting with headache and altered sensorium. Fever and signs of meningial irritation are less common.

Diagnosis

Diagnosis is difficult in AIDS since TB has unusual presentation and lack of simultaneous histologic reaction in some cases due to depressed cell-mediated immunity. Those with relatively well preserved cell immunity (manifested by positive tuberculin test and lack of other HIV associated infections), chest findings are similar to those of reactivation TB in immunocompetent patients, including cavitation and upper lobe infiltration. In contrast, those with immunosuppression due to HIV infection have chest findings that are typical of primary TB in immunocompetent patients such as hilar lymphadenopathy; miliary TB and pleural effusion. Sputum smear positivity for AFB may vary from 31-82%. All types of pleural involvement may occur. Those with isolated unilateral involvement may have better prognosis.[78] Multi-drug resistant TB (MDR-TB) is caused by a strain of Mycobacterium tuberculosis that is resistant to or more antitubercular drugs, usually isonized and rifampicin. It is

Table 4.21: TB and HIV disease

	Early phase	*Late phase*
Clinical features		
Site	Upper lobe	Middle and lower lobes
Pattern	Infiltration, cavitation, focal	Infiltration, miliary, diffuse
Pleural effusion	—	+
Hilar lymph nodes	—	+
Extrapulmonary TB	+	+++
	—	(Abdominal, lymph nodal,
	—	CNS involvement)
Investigations	—	
Sputum	+	+
Blood culture	—	+
Stool culture	—	+
Biopsy	+	—
Granuloma with giant cells and	+	—
AFB	—	++
Tuberculin test	+	—
CD4 cells count	> 200 cells/mm^3	< 200 cells/mm^3

a serious problem and case fatality in HIV with MDR-TB patients is 70% in 4-6 weeks as compared to non-HIV with MDR-TB where it is 25%. It is being labelled as 'The third epidemic', as most malignant opportunistic infection, i.e., MDR-TB and yet associated with HIV infection.

Primary resistance in developing countries like India is 15%. Acquired resistance from initial resistance is constantly increasing and this resistance problem shall further worsen with HIV endemic. In MDR-TB risk factors include inadequate treatment or non-compliance, especially in lower socio-economic patients, or with cavitory lesions or HIV infection, I/V drug users or following anti-cancer therapy or organ transplant.

Mechanism of development of resistance includes:

a. Natural resistance due to spontaneous mutation.
b. Primary resistance by developing tuberculosis from a patient who is infected with resistant microorganisms.
c. Acquired resistance in those having inadequate therapy and thus produce strongest predictors for MDR-TB.
d. Initially resistance may be seen in those who have taken the chemotherapy intentionally or unintentionally.

Pathology

In early stage of HIV infection, if CD4 cell count is more than 200 cell/mm^3, microscopic findings include central caseation with granulomas, giant cells and few AFB. In late stage with CD4 cell count < 200 cells/mm^3, central necrosis is seen with absence of giant cells, lymphocytes and granulomas and abundant AFB.

Immunology

It is considered if more than 5 mm in HIV positive patients. A positive test increases the likelihood of TB whereas a negative test does not exclude TB. Also HIV induces spectrum of immune abnormalities in the host by binding to CD4 molecules and chemokine receptors. Anergy apoptosis and immune activation are diverse immunological changes that are observed in the host. Chemokines block the entry of a retroviral strain, which exhibits tropism for the given receptor and may thus open new therapeutic options to treat HIV infected patients in future.

Pathogenesis

In an immunocompetent person, on infection with M. tuberculosis, the organism is presented in the macrophage through ingestion; thereafter the processed mycobacterial antigens are presented to T cells CD4 cells secrete lymphokines that enhance the capacity of macrophage to ingest and kill the mycobacteria. In majority of the people the infection is contained and TB does not develop, although a number of format bacilli remain in the body. Only 10% of cases develop clinical TB, soon after primary infection or years later as reactivation TB. The consequences in the HIV positive background are possibly due to defects in T cells and/or macrophages functions.[79]

Progressive depletion and dysfunction of CD4 cells, coupled with defects in macrophage and monocyte function, forms the hallmark of HIV infection. An epidemiological evidence favours that HIV infection increases the risk of reactivation of latest TB and also the risk of progressive disease from new infection.[80]

Treatment

Effective treatment of HIV infection can be achieved by using highly active anti-retroviral therapy (HAART) that improves immunologic functions and reduce incidence of infection and death by suppressing HIV replication.

Infection with HIV during pregnancy can increase the risk of:

- Spontaneous abortion.
- Preterm labor.
- Premature membrane rupture.
- Abruptio placenta.
- Low birth weight baby.
- Still birth.
- Ectopic pregnancy.

And also, there is an increased risk of UTI and bacterial pneumonia.

Risk of transmission of HIV to baby is:

1. 30-40% Transplacental
2. 50% During labor/delivery
3. 10-20% Breast feeding.

Effective treatment of tuberculosis with four drugs (rifampicin, isoniazid, ethambutol and pyrazinamide) for two months, followed by three drugs for seven months gives 80% conversion after three months of treatment. However, relapses have been reported, but mortality, if occurs, is due to other opportunistic infections. Adverse reactions to drugs are more frequent in these cases, 90% of these occur in the first two months. Rifampicin should not be given to those patients who are being treated with protease inhibitor. Rifabutin can be used in place of rifampicin with protease inhibitors—indinavir or nelfinavir, since these inhibit metabolism of rifabutin and increase the risk of uveitis; but to be avoided with saquanavir (since it reduces levels of saquanavir 45%) and sitonavir as well as not to be used with non-nucleoside reverse transcriptase inhibitor (NNRTI). In treating MDR-TB, a 5 drug regimen has been suggested, while treating MDR-TB in HIV patients, six drugs have been suggested to be used. There is a need to add two new drugs instead of one. Rifampicin results in anti-fungal treatment failure in AIDS patients who are in ketaconazole and itraconazole.

A case control study in a large New York City Hospital that included MDR-TB cases with and without HIV revealed that 5 or 6 drugs combination that was used included either of the following additional drugs:

1. Capreomycin plus ciprofloxacin.
2. Capreomycin plus cycloserine.
3. Ciprofloxacin + cycloserine + capreomycin.

In meningial tubercular involvement in HIV disease, in areas where initial resistance is less than 4%, three to four drugs combination for minimum of 12 months but 50% of patients may need longer treatment is adequate because of concurrent HIV disease. In case of infection with MDR-TB, more than four drugs including ciprofloxacin, clofazimine, clarithromycin or cyclosporine should be dispensed. It has to be differentiated from M. avium intracellulare infection, typically presenting as mass lesions such as tuberculoma, cerebreal or spinal cord abscess. Prevention of these infections, both TB and AIDS—the ancient and modern plagues—to raise their ugly heads, can only be done through public awareness and education regarding correct behaviour, and code of conduct in their sexual needs. While treating the patients with HIV disease, the aim is maximal suppression of HIV replication for as long as possible. Three-drug combination of two nucleoside analogues with a protease inhibitor, initiated early in the course of HIV infection forms the current standard care of HIV patients.[81] Patients of organ transplant recipients should be carefully given rifampicin as problem of hepatic damage increases in the presence of various immunosuppressive drugs and antifungal drugs who is suspected of having tuberculosis.

Chemoprophylaxis

HIV patients with positive tuberculin test have a 10% risk per year of developing TB compared to a 1% per year or a 10% lifetime risk among HIV negative individuals. Public education regarding correct sexual behaviour forms the cornerstone, in preventing this dual infection. Chemoprophylaxis of healthy contacts is highly important. Chemoprophylaxis with isoniazid alone may not look to be a prudent step. 5 mm induration instead of 10 mm should be the criterion for positive tuberculin test. So, criteria for isoniazid chemoprophylaxis has been suggested to be either tuberculin test of more than 5 mm induration with 51U or CD4 cell count below 200/cw mm, and prophylaxis is recommended for 12 months for any person of any age. CDC and American Thoracic Society have recommended preventive therapy especially in patients exposed to ciprofloxacin 750 mg BD or ofloxacin 400 mg or pyrazinamide 25 mg/kg/day for contacts deemed likely to be newly infected with MDR-TB and at high risk for active disease.

ART prophylaxis[82] includes:

a. Antepartum AZT daily.
b. Nevirapine at onset of labor.
c. AZT+3TC during delivery.
d. (AZT+3TC) Twice daily × 7 days postpartum.

- AZT–Azidothymidine.
- 3 TC–Lamivudine.

BCG is beneficial in HIV infection in preventing the TB infection and putting aside the theoretical fear of disseminating BCG infection in HIV infected infants. BCG vaccination should be given to all infants even when the mother is a known or suspected case of HIV infection, however, BCG should be withheld from patients with symptomatic HIV infection. In case of dissemination of infection, successful treatment can be done with isoniazid and rifampicin. Pyrazinamide is not effective as original strain of BCG showed resistance to pyrazinamide.

AIDS vaccine trials and their evaluation have been entrusted to NARI of ICMR. There are certain difficulties such as maintenance of high level immune response and variability of virus. Ideal HIV vaccine would be that which works against all the major five subtypes of the virus.[83] Trials have been started recently. We have to wait for 3-5 years for their results.

Comments

Deficient cell-mediated immunity is the common denominator, both for tuberculosis and HIV disease. More than 50% of AIDS cases suffer from tuberculosis in India. Radiological and other effects of this dual infection are shown in Tables 4.22 and 4.23. Reactivation of tuberculosis is common in early HIV disease. Clinical presentation and response to anti-tubercular therapy is similar to non-HIV tubercular disease. Progressive HIV disease with severe immunodeficiency leads to extrapulmonary and disseminated tuberculosis requiring aggressive and prolonged treatment. Incidence of multi-drug resistant tuberculosis has increased. MAC infection is often a late opportunistic infection. Six or more drugs combination including fluoroquines is recommended for combating MDR-tuberculosis. Sparfloxacin, although, has shown dose related activity both in vivo and vitro, a caution has been given to use in MDR-TB,[84] only after extended human studies are undertaken. Prevention of MDR-TB is more important than treating MDR-TB.

Table 4.22: Chest X-ray findings in pulmonary TB in association with HIV infection

Hilar lymphadenopathy	42%
Pleural effusion	29%
Upper lobe infiltrates	25%
Miliary pattern	13%
Cavitation	06%

Table 4.23: TB and HIV infection

1. Reactivation common
2. Difficult diagnosis
3. Poor prognosis
4. Extrapulmonary lesions of TB
5. MDR-TB

Management

Currently, chemotherapy has proved to be a strong weapon against tuberculosis and chemotherapeutic regimens have revolutionised the management of tuberculosis. Anti-tuberculosis drugs are either natural antibiotics or synthetic preparations, having bacteriostatic or bactericidal properties. Isoniazid and rifampicin are potent bactericidal drugs. Isoniazid has sterilizing activity.[85] Rifampicin and pyrazinamide are the most potent sterilizing agents. Streptomycin and pyrazinamide are less potent bactericidal drugs. They kill the bacilli in a semi dormant stage. Rifampicin kills bacilli in dormant stage as well as when they exhibit short periods of active metabolism in suitable environment. Pyrazinamide kills bacilli in the areas of inflammation, within the macrophages as well as inhibit/their growth in an acid environment. Rifampicin and isoniazid can effectively prevent emergence of resistance to other drugs. Such an activity is lesser with streptomycin, ethambutol, pyrazinamide, PAS and thiocetazone, in a descending order. Crippling eye complications and sequelae have occurred with thiocetazone, therefore deleting this drug from Indian pharmacopia has been suggested.[86]

The drugs for short course chemotherapy regimens should have ability to prevent resistance as well as possess sterilizing activity. Drugs for intermittent regimens, should have long half life, potent bactericidal activity, capability to kill large number of bacilli by a single dose, and a long lag phase after exposure to the drug before growth restarts. The treatment aims at controlling the active disease, sterilizing the lesion, rendering the patient non-contagious and preventing both complications as well as relapse. Various anti-tuberculosis drugs and their site of action have been tabulated in Tables 4.24 and 4.25.

Immune reconstitution inflammatory syndrome (IRIS) occurs due to rapid immune reconstitution as a consequence of successful ART, TB-IRIS occuring in 11-45% of cases in dual infection, and 3.5% cases of HIV+ non tuberculous mycobacterial IRIS. Pulmonary TB-IRIS manifestations include:

- Progressive pulmonary infiltrates
- Pleural effusion
- Lymph node compression of airways.

IRIS occurs when ART is initiated easy enough.[87]

Intermittent chemotherapy: Using three or four drugs an initial intensive therapy, following which two drugs are administered twice a week at a higher dose, that may be sufficient to prevent multiplication as bacilli take several days after exposure to anti-tuberculosis durgs (a lag period of 3-7 days in their growth), during which if drugs are given, the growth and multiplication of bacilli can be effectively checked. Apart from ethambutol and intermittent rifampicin therapy, isoniazid induced flu-like syndrome has also been documented as a rare side effect.[88]

In pregnancy, 4 drug first line ATT can safely be given; Aminoglycosides be avoided, so are PAS, fluoroquinolnes, cyclocer and ethionamide.

Streptomycin, fluoroquinolones, ethambutol and less hepatotoxic isoniazid can be given in liver dysfunction.

In renal disease, haemodialysis and post renal transplant, drug to drug interaction must be taken care of. In HIV and TB dual infection, if ATT and ART are considered together, complete revision of treatment is required.[89]

Short Course Chemotherapy in Tuberculosis (TB)

Prolonged therapy in tuberculosis has problems due to time factor in the form of irregular drug intake, emergence of resistance and high rate of treatment defaulters. This has led to popularity of short course drug regimens, which have proved to be highly effective. These are acceptable in all age groups.[90] A 9 months regimen with initial 2 months 4 drug regimen has been advocated.[91] However, effectivity of pyrazinamide after one month did not offer any additional benefit, in retreatment cases, with primary treatment failure.[92] Streptomycin and pyrazinamide are contraindicated in pregnancy.[93] Individualised care of geriatric patients has been suggested especially in developing countries like India, where old age pension (stipend) is not available.[94]

Streptomycin and rifampicin in combination with isoniazid are capable of destroying actively growing extracellular living bacilli at a neutral pH in the cavity wall. Rifampicin has an

Table 4.24: Anti-tuberculosis drugs

Drug	*Dose*	*mg/kg*	*Major toxicity of drug*
Isoniazid	300 mg	5-6	Hepatitis, drug fever, peripheral neuropathy
Rifampicin	450/600	10-12	Hepatitis, influenza-like syndrome, thrombocytopenia
Streptomycin	0.75-1.0 gm	15-20	Renal and vestibular toxicity
Pyrazinamide	1.5-2.0 gm	35	Hyperuricemia, hepatitis
Ethambutol	600-800 mg	25/15	Optic neuritis
PAS	12-15 gm	240	Diarrhoea, hepatitis
Ethionamide and Prothionamide	0.5-1 gm	10-15	Hypersensitivity reactions
Cycloserine	0.5-1 gm	10-15	Depression, psychosis, convulsion
Kanamycin, Viomycin and Capreomycin	0.75-1.0 gm	15-20	Vestibular and renal toxicity

Table 4.25: Site of action of commonly used drugs in tuberculosis (TB)

Isoniazid:	Active on organisms which are extracellular both in cavities and in the macrophages (Intracellular).
Streptomycin:	Active on organisms both in the cavities and in closed lesions (Extracellularly).
Rifampicin:	Active on extracellular (both in cavities and in closed caseous lesions) and on intracellular (within the macrophages).
Pyrazinamide:	Active on intracelluar-acid medium .
Ethambutol:	In high doses it is bactericidal on all the four types of bacterial population *i.e.* extracellular (in cavities and in the closed caseous lesions), intracellular (within the macrophages) and the dormant bacilli. In normal dose it is bacteriostatic.

additional potent power of eliminating the persisters, which multiply slowly or intermittently. Rifampicin and isoniazid are effective against intracellular bacilli as well as those in a closed granuloma with a neutral pH. Intracellular organisms present in an acidic enviornment of macrophages in a near resting stage are acted upon by pyrazinamide. The relapses occur because of dormant bacilli and intracellular bacilli as they remain viable in host tissue and start multiplying when the resistance declines. Rifampicin and pyrazinamide in high doses can sterilize the lesion and prevent relapse. Isoniazid and rifampicin form the best 2-drug combination. On adding pyrazinamide the three form most effective agents in short course chemotherapyin terms of sterilizing activity and prevention of emergence of drug resistance in chemotherapy. Ethambutol is effective in preventing failure due to initial drug resistance but lacks sterilizing activity.

A high success rate is seen with short-course chemotherapy with triple drug regimens. Patient's compliance is required for only a relatively short period to cure a disease. East African studies have shown a very high sputum conversion with therapy for six months using streptomycin (1 g), isoniazid (300 mg) and rifampicin (450 to 600 mg). There were relapses in 3 per cent (5 of cases) in two years follow-up and in majority of them occurred within 6 months after stopping the treatment. The organisms, however, were drug sensitive and showed response to retreatment.[95] A study at Singapore has shown a good response with six months regimen while using streptomycin, isoniazid, rifampicin and pyrazinamide for two months followed by continuous treatment with rifampicin, isoniazid and pyrazinamide.[96] A good response was noted in a study conducted in the United Kingdom using isoniazid (300 mg) and rifampicin (450 to 600 mg) for a period of nine months with an initial supplement of ethambutol (50 mg/kg) for two months.[97] A United Kingdom study showed that the six months regimen to be as effective as the nine months treatment.[98] Even six months short course daily with two months initial intensive therapy followed by intermittent regimen has been reported to be successful.[98] Streptomycin is given parenterally. Other drugs such as isoniazid, rifampicin, pyrazinamide and ethambutol are administered orally. Streptomycin, isoniazid are generally given at prefixed doses of 0.75-1 gram and 300 mg respectively to all patients irrespective of their body weight. The dose of ethambutol is 25 mg/kg. For rifampicin the patients are subdivided into two body weight classes. The daily doses 450 mg for those weighing less than 50 kg and 600 mg for those weighing more than 50 kg. Pyrazinamide is given in a daily dose of 1.5, 2.0 and 2.5 g respectively for patients weighing less than 50 kg, between 50 and 74 kg and more than 74 kg.[99]

Different regimens of short course chemotherapy have in common isoniazid and rifampicin in the continuation phase. The six months treatment is advised as the standard regimen for all newly diagnosed cases. The treatment may be daily throughout or daily initially and intermittent in continuation or intermittent throughout. In the continuation phase isoniazid and rifampicin may be administered thrice or twice a week.[100] Various combinations for daily and intermittent regimens have been suggested.[101,102] A well-organised and well supervised six months regimen will cure practically all patients and retreatment may be necessary for only one or two percent who relapse bacteriologically.[103] Short course chemotherapy requires a lesser quantity of drugs. The risk of toxicity is low. The cost is also low. It has the advantage of better co-operation from the patients. It has rapid sterilizing effect on the lesions. But it appears T.B, is going to remain a significant health problem for many more decades.[104] Hepatotoxicity is common with anti T.B. drugs except streptomycin.[105,106] Beneficial effects of indigenous adjuvants have been documented.[107] Hypersensitivity reactions are quite often in first four to six weeks of treatment.[108,109] Routine sensitivity test on pretreatment culture is not recommended.[110] Modified slide culture and sensitivity using bright field microscope provides quick drug sensitivity in a week's time and hence is a safe and rapid alternative.[111] In a quite sick patient two drugs minimum are to be continued.[112] Chemotherapy of TB remains an active and changing field which continues to stimulate interest and research.[113] No modification in the chemotherapy regimen is necessary because of diabetes.[112]

Drug resistant tuberculosis: Treatment in patients whose organisms are resistant to standard anti-tuberculosis drugs poses many difficulties. The organisms remain viable and multiply. The drug resistance may be primary (natural) or acquired. Initial drug resistance on previously untreated patients demonstrates drug resistance of organisms presumably being infected from another patient who has acquired resistance and occasionally from natural resistant wild strains. Acquired drug resistance refers to a situation where the patient who had drug sensitive bacilli initially which later became resistant due to inadequate or inappropriate or irregular treatment. The drug resistant organisms result from mutation. In India the primary drug resistance for isoniazid or streptomycin either alone or in combination respond favourably to short course chemotherapy consisting of rifampicin, isoniazid, pyrazinamide and ethambutol or streptomycin either alone or in combination for two months followed by rifampicin and isoniazid for another four months. Poor bacteriological conversion and radiologic deterioration while on chemotherapy indicates emergence of acquired drug resistance. It is necessary to undertake drug sensitivity tests. The management poses many problems. The patients should be retreated for atleast 12 months from the time the sputum smears become negative. It is preferable to have the drugs which the patient had not received earlier and which do not show cross resistance. Rifampicin, ethambutol and pyrazinamide are highly effective and well tolerated. Prothionamide, cycloserine and one of the aminoglycosides (Kanamycin, viomycin or capreomycin) may be added.[114]

Rifabutin and refapentine have shown sensitivity in rifampicin resistance strains,[115,116] in combination with thioridazine and clofazimine[117] in experimental MDR-TB models and in Myco. intercellular infection in patients with AIDS.[118] Refapentine has less stationary phase bactericidal activity than F(22).[119] Ofloxacin, in cases resistant to isoniazid has shown to decrease the number of viable mycobacterium tuberculosis,[120] which has been found susceptible to betalactam antibiotic and augmentin (amoxicillin and clavulanic acid).[121] Many effective alternative medicines including cycloserine[122] are available. Ofloxacin, ciprofloxacin and ansamycin are effective in resistant cases.[123,124]

Newer Drugs

- Nitro-dihydroimidazo oxazole derivative-delamanid.
- Diaryl quinolone bedaquiline.
- Nitro imidazole-oxazine.
- Oxazolidinones.
- Ethambutol analogues are giving promising results.

Newer modalities of drug delivery, especially nanotechnology, to enhance patient adherence, reduce pill burden and shorten treatment duration are being looked for their potential.[115] Role of physicians and medical staff is important to ensure patient compliance.[125] Immunomodulators such as levamisole, reimun, immuvac, immunoglobulin (I/V), cytokines are suggested to reduce the pool of infection as they increase host immunity.[126]

Use of systemic corticosteroids significantly increase the incidence of tuberculosis, especially in high prevalent areas by facilitating or reactivating earlier infection because of general decrease in host defenses.[127] ZN staining rapid culture and sensitivity are cornerstone in management of TB. Resection surgery, and treatment for 2-3 years with the use of molecular diagnostics and culture sensitivity offers correct treatment lines.[128] Role of surgery and surgical procedures are shown in Tables 4.26 and 4.27.

Table 4.26: Indication of surgery in pulmonary tuberculosis

Tubercular empyema (Collapsed lung)
Cavitary lesions
Coin lesions
Bronchiectasis
Posterior mediastinal mass
Massive haemoptysis

Table 4.27: Surgical procedures done in pulmonary tuberculosis

Decortication
Lobectomy
Pneumonectomy
Pleuropneumonectomy
Thoracoplasty
Rib resection and drainage
Exploratory thoracotomy

Residual radiologic outcome in TB after ATT shows:

Residual pulmonary lesions	45%
Pleural	34%
Mediastinal	31%

DOTS—THE PRESENT DAY TREATMENT OF TUBERCULOSIS[129]

Introduction

WHO declares tuberculosis as a global emergency, requiring an urgent action against the increasing number of TB cases as well as multi-drug resistant cases. Inadequate treatment either as underdose treatment or adding single drug to a failing regimen (addition syndrome) allows the growth of drug resistant mutants, thus resulting in development of acquired drug resistance. An increasing concern regarding high relapse rate requires timely intervention to address optimal duration of supervised intensive phase and operational difficulties in implementing daily supervised treatment.[129]

Disease and the Drug

Number of drugs available for chemotherapy are although limited, yet sufficient to tackle the problem when given in combination regimens. The most effective regimen today is short course chemotherapy for a fresh case comprising 2 RHEZ (daily), 4 HR (daily or intermittently). Hong Kong trials have proved that intermittent therapy is at least as effective as daily therapy. Optimum compliance is important for the outcome. Resistance can best be prevented by using 4 drugs regimen. Compliance problem is related to patient himself, the drug bioavailability and socio-economic factors. WHO has recommended intermittent chemotherapy given as short course, fully supervised plan to be implemented in India. This has been included under revised National TB Control Programme. Non DOTS treatment regimen under RNTCP where patient shows ADRS to rifampicin and/or pyrazinamide i.e. 2 months of SHE and 10 months of HE.[130]

DOTS

Concept of directly observed therapy is not new. What has been advocated by WHO now is to be higher dose intermittent therapy 2 (EHRZ) 3, 4 (HR) 3 i.e. short course chemotherapy given thrice a week in higher doses. This is called DOTS (Directly Observed Therapy Short-course) Table 4.28. The drugs are taken by the patient under the supervision of a health worker. This also ensures regularity in drug consumption Drug dosage and typical regimens are shown in Tables 4.29 and 4.30.

Table 4.28: Components of DOTS

1. Diagnosis is primarily by sputum microscopy
2. Regular and uninterrupted supply of drugs
3. Directly observed treatment is given by health workers
4. Systemic evaluation and monitoring is done and cure rates are main indicators of the programme success
5. Political commitment

Table 4.29: Dosage of anti-TB drugs

Drug	*Daily (mg/kg)*	*Intermittent (mg/kg)*
Rifampicin	10	10
INH	5	10
Ethambutol	15	30
Pyrazinamide	25	35
Streptomycin	15	15

Table 4.30: Current RNTCP regime for treating MDR-TB (Drugs)

1. • Pyrazinamide
   • Levofloxacin
   • Ethionamide
   • Ethambutol
   • Kanalmycin
   • Cycloserine
2. Susceptibility pattern (indurdua lised) as per DST (Drug sensitivity testing)
3. PAS clofazimine Inclusion makes superior option
4. Apply only weight-based regime and restrict fluoroquicolone overuse.

Ref: RNTCP-DOTS plus guidelines; Available at www.tbindia. Accessed Jan 31, 2014.

Directly observed therapy may not be possible, especially in rural population because of lack of infrastructure. In urban areas, lack of cooperation by the people especially during maintenance phase; when the patient becomes active, may create defaulters. Benefit of intermittent therapy are as follows. Lesser drug toxicity and minimum complications thereof; because lesser drugs are consumed that improves patient's compliance; and lesser drugs means more of economy, hence minimising lesser chances of dropouts, in between the treatment.

Prevention of MDR-TB is more important than treating MDR-TB. 2nd line treatment is expensive and also drugs are irregularly available. DOTS with four drugs is probably the best option in countries where levels of MDR-TB both primary and acquired are very high. What is most important is strict supervision for administering the drugs under intermittent therapy. Diagnosis must be made on firm footing, quality medicines are ensured through out the treatment and periodic assessment monitoring must be given the utmost importance. We should join hands to completely eradicate this ancient plague through strictly applying DOTS therapy in treating tuberculosis. Let the last train not be missed.

Prevention and Control

Detection of all bacillary positive cases and their effective treatment to make them non-infectious forms the basis of prevention of tuberculosis in a community. Transmission of infection is kept maintained by sputum positive cases. Adequate treatment of infective cases need be efficiently done. Otherwise, they form other group to spread the disease to susceptible persons of all ages in the community. Improvement in environmental hygiene and health education at all levels of society may help in reducing the spread of the disease. Chemotherapy should be organised in a proper manner right from the beginning of the treatment. Family members' co-operation, health orientation and education, and explaining to all the family members is very important as they help in encouraging, motivating and supervising the patient's. treatment. Social factors, public awareness and role of voluntary organizations have been listed in Tables 4.31 to 4.33. Nevertheless, discrimination, stigmatization and denial remain problems in many areas.

Table 4.31: Role of voluntary organization
They have following contributions: 1. Social awakening and community participation 2. Health education through posters and films 3. Case detection has increased by arranging camps for symptomatics 4. Financial contribution

Table 4.32: Social factors accountable in the treatment of tuberculosis
1. Working ability of the patient
2. Earning capacity
3. Maintaining the family
4. Personal and social status
5. Contributing to community health status
6. Securing future for self and the family

Table 4.33: Public awareness regarding tuberculosis
1. Tuberculosis is curable
2. Facilities should reach the masses
3. People must be made to understand the effects of smoking, unhygienic conditions, polluted water, insanitation and unhealthy homes and community environments in contributing towards the disease.

Active and passive approaches are applied for case finding. In active approach, cases of tuberculosis are detected out of general population or from a specific group of persons at risk, by using screening methods like mass miniatures radiography, mass tuberculin testing, contact examination etc. In passive approach, those who are reporting with symptoms are subjected to be diagnosed and treated. Active case finding and effective treatment brings about clinical and community health benefits.[130,131] Therefore, case finding and treatment of all these cases must be integral part of control programme of tuberculosis.[132] As tuberculosis advances rapidly in a patient to become smear positive,[133] which is potentially dangerous to the community, methods of prevention should be given due importance.

Vaccination prevents occurrence of cases of active disease, following infection with tubercle bacili.[134,135] Also, the risk of serious complications of primary tuberculosis in children is reduced by immunization with BCG (Bacillii de Calmette et Guerin) vaccination.[136] The benefit is great in communities where tuberculous infection and disease are high. Controlled trials in tuberculin negative persons receiving BCG vaccination have shown the development of protection against the disease ranging from 14 per cent to 80%.[137] BCG lowers the risk of complications in children of primary disease;[138] however, this was shown to be of disputed value by a recent trial in a community around Madras, in India.[139] Global experience show similar results regarding BCG's efficacy due to variation in susceptibility or exposure to infection. The vaccine has been incorporated in the expanded programme of immunization (EPI) in India and is administered to infants or young children.[140] The success of vaccination is exhibited by tuberculin conversion. An accelerated reaction with rapid conversion is seen in persons after revaccination (Willi's phenomenon). Though it induces a satisfactory reaction initially, the sensitivity wanes in subsequent years. The fading away of scar BCG of 8 per cent in ten to fourteen years age group, creates problem in interpretation, while indices of tuberculosis are being computed.[141] BCG is must for children with negative tuberculin test, at a high risk rate of new infection.[142] BCG shows protection against both high and low virulent challenges.[143]

Tuberculosis continues to be a major public health problem in developing countries despite efforts to control it. About 2 per cent of our population is suffering from the disease, out of which about 1/5th is continuously excreting tubercle bacilli in the environment through sputum and expectoration. The limitation of use of X-ray and culture examination as case-finding measures, inadequate and improper chemotherapy, limitations in medical care and malnutrition in community play an important role in the persistence of tuberculosis in the country. Since TB is a socio-economic problem, recently efforts have been put to involve community into the control programme at Bombay in India.[144] Role of television is commendable in creating awareness against preventable infectious diseases including tuberculosis.[145] It is stressed that rather than changing the strategy at this juncture, it is required to reactivate and strengthen the existing programme.[146] NTP has assessed that short course chemotherapy is quite satisfactory at peripheral level.[147] What is vital is to diagnose and institute adequate chemotherapy[148] and guide the patients regarding drug, diet and disease to improve compliance.[149] But higher percentage (54.5%) of patients showing resistance to one or more drugs suspects short course chemotherapy becoming fruitless.[150] Only recently, rifampicin resistant tuberculosis following rifabutin prophylaxis has been reported in New Eng. J. of Medicine. First case of M. Monalense, which is a potential human pathogen associated with pulmonary disease has also been reported from India.[151]

Man-made disorder of totally drug resistant TB should not be allowed to occur at any cost, because Indian health economy may not be able to tackle the same.[152] Drug resistance pattern studies may help in further planning long term studies.[153-155] Out of 9 million people around the world suffering, only 10,528 people suffered in US from TB in 2011. And FDA approved new anti TB drug, after four decades, as a part of combination therapy against MDR-TB, i.e., sirturo (bedaquiline).

REFERENCES

1. Shankar P.S., Pulmonary tuberculosis, Quat. Med. Review 1991; 42:1-23.
2. Koch R., Die Aetiologieder Tuberkulose. Berlin, Klin. Wochensch 1982; 19: 221.
3. Bhatia R.S., TB and AIDS—Update article; JAPI 2000; 48: 613-16.
4. Barksdale L., Kim K.S., Mycobacterium Bacteriol 1977, Rev. 41:217.
5. Kanai K., The staining properties of isolated Mycobacterial cellular components as revealed by the Zihel-Neelsen procedure; Amer. Rev. Respir. Dis 1962, 85:442.
6. Grosset J., Tuberculosis, Bacterial and immunology; In IB and Respiratory disease 1987, PPS International 150-52.
7. Mitchison D.A.,The virulence of tubercle bacilli from patients with pulmonary tuberculosis in India and other countries, Bull. Int. Un. Tuberc 1964; 35: 287.
8. Raj Narain, Subbarao M.S., Chandrasekhar P., Pyaralal, Microscopy positive and microscopy negative cases of pulmonary tuberclulosis, Amer. Rev. Respir. Dis 1971; 103:761.
9. Styblo K. Recent advances in epidemiological research in tuberculosis. Advances in Tuberculosis Research 1980, 20:1-63.
10. Chaparas S.D., Immunity in tuberculosis 1982, Bull WHO 60:447.
11. Baganha F., Lina A., Garcao F. and Cardeiro R. Pulmonary tuberculosis and immunological changes; Bull. Int. Un. Tuberc 1993; 58:252.
12. Shimao T. Tuberculosis epidemiology and control programme, In: TB. and respiratory diseases 1984, International 153-55.
13. Gasparini S, Banifazi M; ROSE of transbronchial aspiration; why not; Lung India 2014; 31:203-04
14. Patel A.K., *et al.,* Radiological presentation of patients of pulmonary TB with diabetes; Lung India 2011; 28:70.
15. Van den Oord J.J., de Wolf-Pestem C, Pachett F. and Desmet, V.J. Cellular composition of hypersensitivity type granuloma, Immunohistochemical analysis of tuberculosis and sarcoidal lymphadenitis, Hum. Pathol 1984;15:559-65.
16. Styblo K. The relationship between the risk of TB infection and the risk of developing infectious TB, Bull IUAT 1985; 60:03.
17. Stead W.W. Tuberculosis among elderly people, An outbreak in nursing home; Ann. Inten. Med 1981; 94: 606-10.
18. Diagnostic standards and classification of tuberculosis; Amer Rev Res Dis 1990; 142: 725-35.
19. Dinarello C.A., Cannon J.C., Wolff S.M., *et al:* TUMOR necrosis factor as 2 factors (cachectin) is an endogenous pyrogen and induces production of interieukin-1; Jour. Exp. Med 1986; 163:1433-50.
20. Wallia R.S., Fuilware H. and Ellmer J.J., Direct stimulation of monocyte release interleukin-l by mycobacterial protein antigens, Jour. Immunol 1996; 136:193-96.
21. Rao Sukesh, Rau P.V.P., Sahoo R.C., Clubbing in pulmonary tuberculosis—A clinical radiological correlation, Lung India 1992, 10:69-70.
22. Bhandari B., Mandoruare S.L., A study of tuberculosis in BCG vaccinated children, Ind. Ped 1982; 19:865.
23. Kakrari V.A. and Pratinidhi A.K., A study of childhood tuberculosis, Ind. J. Tuber 1992; 39:177-80.
24. Padma Ramachandran, Duriapandian M. and Nagarajan M. TB research centre (ICMR). Chemotherapeutic studies of TBM in children; Tubercle 1986; 67:17.
25. Parthasarthy A., Narmada R. and Krishnamoorti K.A., Tuberculosis in BCG vaccinated children, Ind. Ped 1982; 19:785.
26. Rao K.N. Textbook of tuberculosis, Ind. Ed., Bombay 1982.
27. Rao S.P., Bhasambe M.S., Vaccine preventable diseases in Eastern Maharashtra: A Hospital based analysis, Ind. Ped 1991; 28:629.
28. Lucas S.B., Histopathology of leprosy and tuberculosis: An overview, Brit. Med. Bull 1988; 48: 584-99.
29. Target diseases included in UIP; Monograph on intregrated training on National Programme for mother and child development 1990; 111.
30. Gokhale S., Qadir S., Nagra J.S. and Chakraborty A.K., Efficiency of cold staining method of AFB in Sputum. A comparison with ZN method under field conditions, Ind. J. Tuber 1990; 37: 135.
31. Vasantha Kumari R., Jagannath K. and Rajsekhran S., Cold Staining method for AFB, Bull. WHO 1986; 64:741.
32. Sujatha Chandrasekaran, Sreenivas T.R. and Chaudhuri K., Modified sputum microscopy techniques sparing use of alchohol for field application, Ind. J. Tuber 1991; 38:87-90.
33. Gorse C.J., Fairshter R.D., Friedly, *et al.,* Non-tuberculosis mycobacterial disease. Experience in Southern California Hospital, Arch. Intern. Med 1980; 43: 225.
34. Shankar S.V.R., Jain N.K., Chandrasekhar S. and Singh M.M. Prevalence of atypical Mycobacteria in sputum of patients undergoing treatment at a T.B. clinic, Ind. J. Chest. Dis. All. Sci 1989; 31.
35. Wolinsky E. Non-Tuberculous mycobacteria and associated diseases Amer. Rev. Res. Dis 1990; 119:107.
36. Harries A.D. Tuberculosis and HIV infection in developing countries, Lancet 1990; 335:387.
37. Jain N.K., Kachroo B.B., Parsad G., *et al.,* Identification and characterization of mycobacteria other than TB by protein fingerprinting Ind. J. Tuber 1991; 38:91-94.
38. Chauhan M.M., Sreenivas T.R. and Chaudhuri K., Effect of CO_2 on the primary isolation of mycobacteria, Ind. J. Tuberc 1991; 38:81-85.
39. Bhatia R.S. and Sibia S.S., Bronchoscopy: Therapeutic indications, Lung India 1994; 12: 138-139.
40. Seaton A., Seaton D., Leitch Agin, Crofton and Douglas. *Resp. Diseases,* Oxford University Press, Delhi, 4th Ed., 1989.
41. Jain S.K. and Agarwal R.L., Reactivation of a tuberculous lesion following bronchoscopy, Tubercle 1980; 61: 105.
42. Sesma P., Sanchez E., Deben F.M. and Sambede D.S., Tuberculosis pneumonia—A complication of bronchoscopy, Reb. Clin. Espan 1984; 173:185.

43. Rimmer J., Gibson P. and Bryant D.H., Extension of pulmonary tuberculosis after fiberoptic bronchoscopy, Tubercle 1988; 69:57.
44. Agarwal R.L., Manju Agarwal and Agarwal D.K. Spread of pulmonary tuberculosis following bronchoscopy, Ind.J. Tuberc 1992; 39:47-48.
45. Sarkar S.K., Sharma C.S., Gupta P.R. and Sharma R.K., Fiberoptic bronchoscopy in the diagnosis of pulmonary TB, Tubercle 1980; 61-97.
46. S.O.S.Y., Lam W.R. Rapid diagnosis of suspected pulmonary tuberculosis by fiberoptic bronchoscopy, Tubercle 1982; 63:195.
47. Snider D.E. Jr., Bacille Calmette-Guerin vaccination and tuberculin skin test, Jour. Amer. Med., Assn 1985; 253: 438-439.
48. Agarwal M.K., Nath J., Mukerji P.K. and Srivastva V.M.L., A study of serum ADA activity in sputum negative patients of pulmonary tuberculosis, Ind. J. Tuberc 1991; 38:139-41.
49. Maartens G. and Bateman E.D. Tubercular pleural effusions; Increased culture yield with bedside in occulation of pleural fluid and poor diagnostic value of ADA, Thorax 1991; 46:96-99.
50. Kiran U., Shriniwas Kumar R. and Sharma A. Efficacy of three mycobacterial antigens in the serodiagnosis of tuberculosis, Eur. J. Respir. Dis 1985; 66:187.
51. Bhatia R.S. and Batta S. Routine investigations. Let us be selective and rational, J. Assn. Phys. India 1992; 40:493.
52. Coleym K.C., Singh H.P., Karnani I. and Rao M.K.K., Bone marrow in the diagnosis of PUO: A report of five cases; Ind. J. Tuber 1991; 38:163-65.
53. Van Ingen I; *et al.*, Region of difference in non tuberculous my cobecterium speieces adds a phylogenetic and taxonomical character. J. Bateriol; 2009;191: 5865-67
54. Bhatia R.S. Respiratory disease pattern in a private clinic in Ludhiana; Lung India 1995; 13: 125-26.
55. Epstein D.M., Kline L.R., Albeda S.M. and Miller W.T., Tuberculosis pleural effusion,Chest 1987; 91:106-09.
56. Bhatia R.S., *et al.*, Diagnostic value of ELISA and ADA in TB: Need for more specific tests; JAPI 1998; 46:574.
57. Chaudhuri A.D., *et al.*, Role of sputum examination for AFB in tuberculous pleural effusion; Lung India 2011; 28:21-24.
58. Kumar P., *et al.*, Assessment of N-PCR assay in diagnosis of pleural tuberculosis; Detection of M. tuberculosis in pleural fluid and sputum collected in tandem; PLOS One 2010: 5:10220.
59. Singh R.P. and Katiyar S.K. Acute massive atelectasis in pulmonary tuberculosis, Ind. J. Tuber 1992; 39:49-51.
60. Bhatia R.S., Pulmonary tuberculosis—An update; Curr. Med. Journ 1997; 3:50-52.
61. Bhatia R.S. Pulmonary hypertention in pulmonary tuberculosis (Abst); National conference of tuberculosis and chest diseases, Pakistan, 1989.
62. Mathur K.C. Association of malignancy of other organs in case of pulmonary tuberculosis, Ind. J. Tuber 1977; 24(4):167-68.
63. Mukta V., Jayachandran K., Lung and lupus vulgaris; Lung India 2011; 28:127-29.
64. Subramanian S; *et al.*, Meditational lymphadenopathy in malignancy-metastatic or grahulomatous? JAPI; 2014; 62: 78-80.
65. Chakravarti A., Chaturvedi V.N., Samal W. and Narang P. Tuberculosis of the tongue—A case report, Ind. J. Tuber 1992; 39:45-56.
66. Malik M.K., Pratap V.K., Kumar A. and Bhatia S. Tuberculosis of temporal bone, Ind. J. Tuber 1992,39:243-245.
67. Cahan A., *et al.*, TB of oral mucosa; J Craniofoc Surg 2002; 23:533-37.
68. Kumar N; et al., Isolated media stinal TB-a rare entity; JAPI; 2013;61:202-03.
69. Gupta M.M., Wig J.G. and Suri S. Tuberculosis of pancrease—A case report Ind. J. Tuber 1992; 39: 247-49.
70. Rao Sukesh and Rau P.V.P., TB epiglottis—A case report; Lung India 1992; 10: 15-16.
71. Surana AP; *et al.*, ITP-A rare association of lymphnode TB; JAPI 2014;62:74-76
72. Patel A.K., *et al.*, Clinical and laboratory profile of patients with TB/HIV coinfections–A case series of 50 patients; Lung India 2011; 28: 93-96.
73. Vasadevaiah V. HIV infection among tuberculosis patients; Ind. J. Tub 1997:1997; 44: 97-98.
74. Gupta P.R., *et al.*, TB in HIV seropositives in Rajasthan; Lung India 1998; 16: 147-49.
75. Kate S.K. *et al.* Association of HIV infection and pulmonary TB; The Ind. Pract 1998;51: 352-56.
76. Girija Singh Pais, Tuberculin sensitivity in HIV seropositives with TB compared to seronegatives; JAPI 1998; 46: 1029-30.
77. Chopra U; *et al.*, spontaneous pneumo pericardium-can complication in a patient of HIV and pulmonary TB; Lung India; 2013; 30: 148-50.
78. Gupta K.B. *et al.* Pleural involvement in patients coinfected with HIV and M. tuberculosis: Clinico radiological profile: Lung India 1999; 17(2): 65-67.
79. Hedge H.R. Anergy and chemokine receptors; JAPI 2002; 50: 816-18.
80. Bhatia R.S., Bedi P.S., Sibia H.K. HIV infection and TB, TB Update 1997; 1: 14-16.
81. Vajpayee M., Dar L. Anti-retroviral drugs in HIV infection; Ind J Pharm 1999; 31(2): 96-103.
82. Agarwal PK, Parmar V; HIV and pregnancy; IN; A. Muruganathan; Ed; Med update, API 2013:23:67-68.
83. Bhatia R.S., HIV and TB: The ominous connection; In: P.C. Manoria, Ed, PG Med API, Mumbai 1998; 12(III): 104-107.
84. Bhatia R.S., Sibia S.S., Treatment of tuberculosis; Role of sparfloxacin; JAPI 1999; 47:750.
85. Mitchison D.A., Ellard G.A. and Grosset J., New anti-bacterial drugs for the treatment of mycobacterial diseases in man, Brit. Med. Bull 1988; 44:757-774.
86. Deivanyagam C.N. Pulmonary tuberculosis, book review, Lung India 1991;9:38.
87. Shah A; IRIS; IN; SR Joshi; Ed; Med. update, API 2014;24: 432-42.
88. Pandit S. *et al.*, Isoniazid-induced flu like syndrome; a rare side effect; Lung India J, 2013; 30:61-63.
89. Parker JD; TB in special situations; In; SR Joshi; ED; Med update API 2014; 24; 287-96.

90. Soider D.E. Jr, Cohn D.L., Davidson P.T., *et al.* Standard therapy for tuberculosis, Chest 87 (Supp.) 1985, 117S-124S.
91. National Consensus Conference on Tuberculosis, Chest (supp) 1985, 87, Vol. II/suppl.
92. Raja Sekaran S., *et al.,* Value of PZA initial intensive phase of long-term treatment for pulmonary tuberculosis with primary treatment failure, Lung India 1993; 11: 33-36.
93. Citron K.M., Control and prevention of tuberculosis in Britain, Brit. Med. Bull 1988; 44:704-16.
94. Bhatia R.S., Geriatric tuberculosis—An individualized care suggested, J. Assn. Phys. India 1990; 38:253-54.
95. Third East Africa/British Medical Council Research Study: Controlled clinical trial of four short course regimens of chemotherapy for two durations in the treatment of pulmonary tuberculosis, Second Report, Tubercle, Lond 1980; 61:59.
96. Fox W. The modern management of therapy of pulmonary tuberculosis, Proc. Roy. Soc. Med 1977, 70:44.
97. British Thoracic Society: Short course chemotherapy in pulmonary tuberculosis, Third Report, Lancet 1980; 1:1182-83.
98. British Thoracic Society: A controlled trial of 6 months chemotherapy in pulmonary tuberculosis: Results during the 36 months after the end of chemotherapy and beyond, Brit. Jour. Dis. Chest 1984, 78:330-36.
99. Ramkrishnan C.V. Rifampicin—A look back, Lung India 1987, 5:19-28.
100. Medical Research Council's Tuberculosis and Chest Diseases, Unit, Treatment of pulmonary tuberculosis in patients notified in England and Wales in 1978/79, Chemotherapy and hospital admissions, Thorax 1985, 40:113-30.
101. Fox W. Tuberculosis case finding and treatment programmes in the developing countries, Brit. Med., Bull 1988; 44: 717-37.
102. Bhatia S. Update management of pulmonary tuberculosis, Ind. Pract 1991; 44:527-32.
103. Bhatia R.S., Nigam P., Update management of pulmonary tuberculosis CMT 1989; 4:4-27-32.
104. Fox W. Short course chemotherapy for pulmonary tuberculosis and some problems of its programme application with particular reference to India, Lung India 1984; 2:167-74.
105. Bhatia R.S., Tuberculosis—Present approach in management, Curr. Med. Pract 1992; 36:168-70.
106. Bhatia R.S., Comparative study hepatic toxicity of two regimens with and without pyrazinamide, J. Med. Surg 1987; 27:13-15.
107. Bhatia R.S. and Singhal K.C. Hepatitis in patients on anti-tubercular drugs, Ind. J. Bio 1990; 13:15-18.
108. Bhatia R.S., Complimentary role of tefroli with anti-tuberculosis therapy, Ind. Med. Gaz 1989; 123: 292-94.
109. Bhatia R.S. and Sibia S.S. Anti-tubercular drugs—adverse reactions; Curr. Med. Jour 1996; 2 (2): 24-26.
110. Bhatia R.S. Anti-tubercular drugs—adverse reactions, Paper accepted in National Conference on TB and Chest Disease, Pakistan 1989. Reproduced in J. Challenge, Pakistan.
111. Shimao T. Drug resistance in tuberculosis control, Tubercle, Lond 1987; 68 Supp: 5-16.
112. Gupta P.R., Singhal B. Sharma T.N. and Gupta R.B. A modified slide culture technique for quick drug sensitivity testing of M. tuberculosis, Ind. J. Tuber 1992, 39:113-116.
113. Recommendations from committee on treatment of tuberculosis. International Union Against Tuberculosis and Lung Diseases, anti-tuberculosis regimens of chemotherapy; Ind. J. Chest. Dis 1988, 69:5-14.
114. Shankar P.S. Chest medicine, 4th ed., New Delhi, Oxford and IBH Publishers; 1994.
115. Mohan A; *et al.,* newer anti-TB drugs and drug delivery systems; IN; A. Muruganathan; Ed; Med update, API; 2013; 23:388-92.
116. O'Brien R.J., Lyle M.A. and Snider D.E. Refabutin (ansamycin L.M. 427)—A new refampicin S derivative for the treatment of mycobacterial diseases; Rev. Infect. Dis 1987; 519-30.
117. Perumal V.K., Gangadharam P.R.J. Neifets L.B. and Iseman M.D. Dynamic aspects of *in vitro* chemotherapeutic activity of ansamycin on mycobacterium intracellulare Amer. Rev. Resp. Dis 1985; 132: 278-80.
118. Gangadharam P.R.J., Perumal V.K., Jairam B.T., *et al.,* Activity of rifabutin alone or in combination with clofazimine or ethambutol or both against acute and chronic experimental mycobacterium intracellulare infections, Amer. Rev. Resp. Dis 1987; 136:329-333.
119. O'Brien R.S., LYLE M.A., Johnson M.W. and Shider D.A. Ansamycin (LM 427) therapy in AIDS patients with mycobacterium avium (mai) complex infection. A preliminary report (abstract) Atlanta; Proceedings of the International Conference on AIDS 1985; 47.
120. Dickinson J.M. and Mitchison D.A. *In vitro* observations on suitability of new rifampicins for the intermittent: Chemotherapy of tuberculosis, Tubercle, London 1987, 68: 183-193.
121. Sukumara M., Nakamura E., Yoshii S. and Amano H. Theraputic effect of a new antibacterial substance ofloxacin (DL8280) on pulmonary tuberculosis, Am. Rev. Resp. Dis 1985; 131: 352-56.
122. Casal M., Rodrigues F., Benavente M. and Luna M., In vitro susceptibility of mycobacterium tuberculosis, mycobacterium fortuitum and mycobacterium, Chelonel to augmentin; Eur., J. Clin. Microbiol 1986; 5:43, 453-55.
123. Babu Swai, O., Aluoch J.A., Cithui W.A. *et al.* Controlled clinical trial of regimen of two durations for the treatment of isoniazid resistant pulmonary tuberculosis, Tubercle, London 1988; 69:5-14.
124. Crofton J. The prevention and management of drug resistant tuberculosis, Bull. Int. Union Against Tubers 1987; 62:6-11.
125. Jain J.K., Chopra K.K. and Prasad C.P. Initial and acquired isoniazid and rifampicin resistance to myco. tuberculosis and its implication for treatment; Ind. J. Tuber 1992; 39:121-24.
126. Mohanty KC, Vaidya SB; Role of immune modulators in management of drug resistant TB; IN; SR Joshi; ed; Med update API; 2014; 24:297-311
127. Agarwal P.N., Gupta D., Aggarwal A.N. *et al.* Incidence of TB among patients receiving treatment with oral corticosteroids; JAPI 2000; 48: 881-84.
128. Prabhudesai PP, Shah RP; MDR-TB–the present scenario; IN; SR Joshi; ed; Med update, API 2014; 24:318-29

129. Sajal De; High relapse rate in RNTCP; An increasing concern and time to intervene; Lung India 2013; 30:85-86.
130. Sachdeva KS; Management of TB: Indian guide lines; IN; A. Muruganathan; ED: Med update, API 2013; 23;479-83.
131. American Thoracic Society; CDC Control of tuberculosis; Amer Rev. Resp. Dis 1983; 128:336-42.
132. Shankar P.S. Prevention and Control; IN: Pulmonary Tuberculosis, Oxford and IBH Publ. Co., N. New Delhi, 2nd ed 1990; 128-43.
133. Home N.W. Tuberculosis Control, Bull Inter Union Tuberc 1985; 59:107-209.
134. Tuberculosis Prevention Trial Madras: Trial of BCG vaccines in South India for tuberculosis prevention, Ind. J. Med. Res 1980; 72:51.
135. Guidelines for T.B. control programmes in developing countries an Oxfam memorandum Shears P. Oxfam health unit K. Oxfam 1985.
136. Padungehan S., Konjanart S, Kassiratta S., *et al.* The effectiveness of BCG vaccination of the newborn against childhood tuberculosis in Bangkok; Bull WHO 1986; 64:247.
137. Hart P.D. Efficacy and applicability of mass BCG vaccination in tuberculosis control, BMJ 1984; 1:587.
138. T.B. control as an integral part of primary care, General, WHO 1988.
139. Tripathy S.P. Fifteen years follow-up of the Indian BCG prevention trial. In: Proceedings of the XXV IUAT World Conference on Tuberculosis and Lung Diseases, Singapore; Japan Professional Post Graduate Series. International 1987; 69-72.
140. Ten Dam M.G. Research on BCG vaccination; Adv. Tuberc. Res 1984; 21:79.
141. National Tuberculosis Institute, Bangalore: Report: Tuberculin testing in a partly vaccinated population; Ind. J. Tuber 1992; 39:149-158.
142. Leads from the morbidity and mortality weekly report: Use of BCG vaccines in the control of tuberculosis; A joint statement by the ACCP and the Advisory ACCP committee for elimination of tuberculosis; J. Amer. Med. Assn 1988; 260:2983-91.
143. Challu V.K., Chandrasekharan S., Sreenivas, T.R. *et al.* Role of non-tuberculous infection in immunisation against tuberculosis, Ind. J. Tuber 1992; 39:165-70.
144. Desai V.P. and Khergaonkar K.N. Urban TB programme; The Greater Bombay setup; Ind. J. Tuber 1991; 38:235-37.
145. Bhatia R.S. and Batra S., Forum; Ind J. Tuber 1991; 38:239.
146. Chaudhuri K., Tuberculosis programme: Meeting the demand for its review; Ind., J. Tuber 1991,38:189-90.
147. Sreenivas T.R. Shymasundra C.V. and Chaudhuri K. Impact of short course chemotherapy in the operational efficiency of National Tuberculosis Programme, Ind. J. Tuber 1992, 39:107=VII.
148. Mohanty K.C., Rationale of current anti-tuberculosis chemotherapy; IJCP 1993; 3(11):31-37.
149. Bhatia R.S. Adverse reactions to rifampicin; IJCP 1994; 4(9): 67-69.
150. Vasantha Kumari R. *et al.* Bacteriological status and prevalence of drug resistance in district tuberculosis centres in Tamil Nadu; Lung India 1993; 11:27-31.
151. Lily Therese K., *et al.*, First report of isolation of M. Monalense from sputum specimen in India; Lung India 2011; 28:124-26.
152. Udwadia Z.F., *et al.*, Totally drug resistant TB in India; Clin. Infect Dis 2012; 54:579-81.
153. Menon S., *et al.*, Drug resistance profiles of Mycobacteriom tuberculosis isolates to first line anti-TB drugs—A five year study; Lung India 2012; 29:227-31.
154. Soman R; *et al.*, Successful management of highly drug resistant TB with individualised drug susceptibility testing; JAPI; 2014; 62:567-70.
155. Ginsburg AS; fluoroguinolone, TB, and resistance; Lancet Inf. Dis; 2013; 3:432-42.

MAC DISEASE[1-3] (MYCOBACTERIUM AVIUM COMPLEX)

Introduction

Infections by mycobacteria other than M. tuberculosis and M. leprae are increasingly being reported from all over the globe.

Although a number of mycobacteria have been identified causing human disease, MAC is the one of the most frequently isolated respiratory infections, next, of course, to M. tuberculosis. Several other mycobacteria have been held responsible for human infection, M. kansansil and M. fortuitum being reported more frequently. In India, one established case of MAC has recently been reported.

Prevalence

Infection by MAC has an increasing frequency. In a San Francisco Hospital, the percentage of isolates of MAC from patients with respiratory mycobacterial disease has risen from 0.3 per cent to 8.8 per cent over the last 8 years. Similarly, in Japan the prevalence rate of MAC respiratory disease has risen from 0.82 per million population in 1971 to 2.08 in 1987, as compared to M. tuberculosis which has fallen from 133 per million to 42.6 over the same period. Similar trends are reported from African countries too.

Characteristics and Identification

MAC literally means Mycobacterium Avium Complex comprising Mycobacterium avium and M. intercellulare. MAC strains grow slowly in culture. They are comparatively resistant (compared with M. tuberculosis) to most anti-tuberculosis drugs, each of the species constituting the complex. M. avium can grow at 45°C, while M. intracellulare cannot. Both species show resistance to rifampicin, streptomycin, ethambutol, kanamycin, isoniazid and other anti-tuberculosis drugs, highly so in M. avium. However, M. avium shows a rather low level of resistance to quinolones like ofloxacin and ciprofloxacin.

MAC are normally virulent for human beings, and person to person infection does occur. Identification is costly and cumbersome. Of various methods being tried out in distinguishing MAC from M. tuberculosis, *Gen-Probe* using nucleic acids, and DNA probes using DNA strands isolated by enzymatic activity and matching them against the suspect organisms, have shown potential for rapid identification. However, newer techniques with multiple DNA probes have been described and show promising potential. In clinical situations, it may be practicable to investigate patients, diagnosed as positive tuberculosis, who do not respond to standard chemotherapeutic regimes, for atypical mycobacterial diseases, specially MAC disease.

M. avium was classified as one of the members of the tuberculosis family, along with hominis, bovis etc. Recently, however, MAC has been taken out of the M. tuberculosis complex, and is included among the non-tuberculosis mycobacteria. The justification for this reclassification is not exactly clear.

Clinical Features, Pathology and Diagonsis

MAC disease frequently occurs as an opportunistic infection in those already having active or healed organs, especially the lungs. There may be a background of treated pulmonary tuberculosis, pleurisy, chronic bronchitis or any chronic respiratory infection, emphysema, pneumoconiosis, etc. The respiratory disease is like pulmonary tuberculosis in almost all respects, including radiological appearances. Other organs that are affected are lymph nodes, skin, bones and joints. Disseminated MAC disease may also occur, specially in immunocompromised individuals like patients of AIDS, severe diabetics, those on steroids and other immunosuppressive drugs, and may simulate a comparatively indolent miliary tuberculosis.

A diffuse patchy infiltration or pneumonic shadow with or without mediastinal lymph node involvement can be seen on X-ray of the chest. Cavitation is uncommon and, when present, cavity walls tend to be thin. Miliary shadows are rare, but nodular shadows may be seen. The radiological appearances may be entirely those of the previous disease. In pulmonary disease, sputum smears are usually positive for AFB. Especially in immunocompromised persons, one is likely to find hepatosplenomegaly, large retroperitoneal and mesenteric glands and diffuse jejunal wall thickening, on CT scan of the abdomen.

Pathological appearances are like tuberculosis except that the granuloma is not so well defined. Typical granulomata with lymphocytic infiltration, epitheloid and Langhans giant cells and caseation are seen only in a minority of cases. However, in those with AIDS and MAC disease, it is more likely to be an ill-defined granuloma consisting of histiocytes filled with acid fast bacilli, which are seen as unstained striations in H.E. stains but can be demonstrated by Z.N. staining (A newer technique has been described wherein simultaneous H.E. and Z.N. staining has been achieved in histopathological specimens). In immunocomprŏmised individuals bacteraemia and even septicemia are quite likely, the favoured sites of dissemination being lymphatic tissue, meninges and bone marrow.

Diagnosis of MAC disease can be established only through specific culture material. It is not possible to distinguish the infecting mycobacterium from M. tuberculosis (or others) by smear alone, and even routine culture. Subsequently, a DNA probe or other technique is necessary to identify the bacillus.

Management

Various chemotherapy regimes have been suggested. It is seen that combined drug therapy is synergistic so that combinations including some of the known anti-tuberculosis drugs with aminoglycosides such as amikacin and quinolones like ofloxacin, ciprofloxacin are advocated. A new quinolone, sporfloxacin has been found to be effective against M. avium in experimental animals. Clofazimine has been particularly effective against M. intracellulare in vitro, and this bacterium is less resistant to most of standard anti-tubercular drugs than M. avium.

There is no standard regimen for MAC disease. Various combinations suggested and tried are: (i) Kanamycin 1/2 g daily for 2 months, followed by 1g 2-3 times a week, + Rifampicin 450 mg, and ethambutol and isoniazid to be given indefinitely. Cycloserine could replace one of the the oral drugs and streptomycin could replace kanamycin (ii) rifampicin, ethambutol, clofazimine and ciprofloxacin with amikacin in the initial three months. However, as testing and identification take some time, it is better to add isoniazid till MAC is definitely established.

Chemotherapy has to continue for at least 18 months or even indefinitely, in case of those with HIV infection. Reduction of excreted bacillary load can be regarded as partial success and chemotherapy persisted with, may be by adding cycloserine or ethionamide or changing the rifamycin derivative (e.g. Rifabutin).

Surgery is indicated in patients with high bacillary content or in those with persistent positive sputum and resectable lesions. Associated HIV infection should always be kept in mind. Conversely, MAC disease should be strongly suspected in AIDS patients, even in smear negative individuals, and culture of secretion, biopsy material etc. freely resorted to.

Facilities for testing mycobacteria need to be developed, at least on a regional basis. Till that time, it may be wise to consider every case with resistant tuberculosis to be a potential case of MAC.

REFERENCES

1. Kapoor S.R. MAC Disease, Ind. J. Tuber 1992; 39:193-94.
2. Bhatia R.S. HIV and TB: The ominous connection; Manoria P.C. (ed) P.G. Med; API; Mumbai 1998; 12: 104-07.
3. Guha SK; Atypical mycobacterial infection; IN; SR Joshi; ed; Med update; API 2014;24;313-18.

PARASITIC PULMONARY DISEASES

Parasitic diseases are quite common in tropical and subtropical countries. Actually these diseases have plagued man and his domestic animals since the beginning of recorded history. Many of the developed nations in the world have been able to control, if not completely overcome these diseases, at least within their own borders, but the parasites continue to have their heavy toll among the developing countries. Lungs, pleura and chest wall may be affected by a variety of parasites. The parasites are Protozoa (Entamoeba histolytica, Plasmodium falciparum, Toxoplasma gondii and Pneumocystis carinii) or Metazoa (round worms, flat worms and flukes). Nemathelminths (Ascaris lumbricoides, Ankylostoma duodenale, Strongyloides stercoralis, Toxocara canis and catis, Trichinella spiralis, Wuchereria bancrofti, and Dirofilaria immitis), Platyhelminths such as cestodes (Echinococcus granulosus) and trematodes (Paragonimus and Schistosoma) are the examples of metazoa.[1,2]

Clinically they can present features of involvement of intercostal muscles (Trichinosis), diffuse parenchymal infiltrations (migratory phase of nematodes, visceral larva migrans, Schistosomiasis, Paragonimiasis, Toxoplasmosis, and Pneumocystosis), pleuropulmonary manifestations (amoebiasis, hydatid disease, Paragonimiasis), pulmonary hypertension (Schistosomiasis) or tropical pulmonary eosinophilia. Commonly encountered parasitic pulmonary diseases have been described. Recently, interest has been renewed in parasitic lung diseases as opportunistic infections in patients of AIDS.[3]

Pulmonary Amoebiasis

The pulmonary amoebiasis is relatively infrequent though intestinal amoebiasis is quite commonly encountered in India. However, the lung forms the second most common site of extra-intestinal amoebiasis, the most common being hepatic involvement.[1] 10% of world population has amoebic infection.[4] In present times, pathogenic strains of Entamoeba histolytica can be distinguished from non-pathogenic by isoenzyme analysis.[5]

Pathogenesis

Entamoeba histolytica is transmitted by faeco-oral route. Pulmonary amoebiasis is always secondary to hepatic involvement. Therefore, it can be termed as hepato pulmonary amoebiasis. Since both pleura and lungs are involved, it can be termed as pleuro pulmonary amoebiasis. Malnutrition and alcoholism often predispose. The infection may spread by a direct communication from an erosion or rupture through the diaphragm, or through transdiaphragmatic lymphatic channels.[1,2] It occurs in 5 to 30 per cent of patients with liver involvement. Rarely the lungs may be affected through haematogenous spread without involving the liver.

The genesis of primary amoebic lung abscess is thought to be due to the entry of E. histolytica into tributaries of hepatic veins.[6] The venoarterial shunting from the right side of the heart through the pulmonary arteries and its branches into the lungs causes primary pulmonary amoebiasis. Some suggest that dissemination occurs because trophozoites in the intestinal wall burrow into branches of the haemorrhoidal veins instead of the portal vein or because organisms in the liver penetrate hepatic veins.[7]

Primary pulmonary amoebic abscess is a rare condition.[8] Only few cases have been reported.[9-11] Primary form of pulmonary amoebiasis caused by amoeba reaching the respiratory tract by direct embolism from the intestine has not been reported commonly.[8] The pulmonary infection may result from an occult E-histolytica infection of the colon bypassing the liver. Increased incidence of extra intestinal amoebiasis as asymptomatic infection of the colon than symptomatic individuals is well documented.[12]

Similar cases of primary amoebic lung abscess without hepatic involvement have been reported.[10,13,14] Primary amoebic abscess may affect any part of the lung whereas secondary lesions affect the right lower lobe due to direct extension from the underlying liver.[15]

The spread of infection through the diaphragm causes fibrinous pleurisy, pleural effusion, basal pneumonia and lung abscess. The occurrence of pulmonary disease in relation to the right diaphragm is frequent because 75 per cent amoebic liver abscesses are present in the right lobe of the liver.[16] Invasion of lung parenchyma results in interstitial pneumonitis. Inflammatory exudation, and migration of Ent. histolytica is soon followed by consolidation.[17,18] Pleural effusion may develop as a reaction to the amoebic liver abscess or to subdiaphragmatic abscess. There can also be development of amoebic empyema by a spread of infection to the pleural space. A liver abscess can rupture into the pleural cavity or into the lung through the adhesions that have occurred from inflammation. Pleuro-pulmonary amoebiasis is commonly seen with an abscess located in the upper and middle third of the liver and it is less commonly seen on the left side. Empyema can open into a bronchus (bronchopleural fistula).

There are adhesions between the liver and the diaphragm, and between the parietal and visceral pleura that may cause rupture of liver abscess into the lung and a communication may be established with the bronchus (hepatobronchial fistula). Lung abscess consists of dark brown liquid resembling chocolate sauce. Initially the necrotic area is surrounded by an inflammatory exudate consisting of polymorphs to be replaced later by lymphocytes and histiocytes. The margins of the abscess[2] are rich in E. histolytica.

Clinical Features

It is seen frequently in the age group of 20 to 40 years and is common in men. The presentation is insidiously with systemic manifestations of fever, chills, sweating, weakness, loss of appetite and loss of weight. There may be previous history of dysentery in nearly half of the patients.[19] Incidence of pleuropulmonary amoebiasis in relation to primary amoebic infection of the colon varies from 5 to 15 per cent and can present with pleural effusion, consolidation, abscesses, empyema or hepatobronchial fistula.[4]

Pain in the right upper abdomen and sometimes over the right shoulder is quite common. Initially there is dry cough, later it is associated with expectoration of the chocolate sauce sputum. Those in whom a direct communication has been established with the liver may feel a bitter taste of sputum from the presence of bile. Secondary infection may result in production of large amount of purulent sputum. Haemoptysis is rarely encountered.

Clinical examination may reveal wasting and an enlarged tender liver. However pleuro pulmonary manifestations may exist without any enlarged tender liver. The physical in the chest are essentially confined to the basal regions of the right side. There may be tenderness in the lower intercostal spaces and right hypochondrium. The signs of pleurisy and effusion or of consolidation may be elicited. Clubbing and the mediastinal shift absent seen in amoebic empyema.[2,7]

Investigation

X-ray chest reveals an elevated right dome of the diaphragm and its restricted movement. A hump-like localised elevation of the diaphragm is best seen in the lateral view. Right costophrenic angle can be obliterated by a reactionary serous effusion. On screening the diaphragm shows restricted movement. There can be radiological evidence of pleural effusion or ill defined or well encapsulated homogeneous opacity due to consolidation. Radiological abnormalities have been tabulated in Table 4.34.

Table 4.34: Radiological abnormalities

1. Pulmonary	a. Pneumonitis
	b. Lung abscess
2. Pleural	a. Pleuropulmonary lesions
	b. Isolated pleural effusion
3. Diaphragmatic	a. Restricted movements
	b. (R) hemidiaphragm elevated
	c. Pneumoperitoneal adhesions

Amoebic trophozoites or cysts can be present in the stool. There is moderate polymorphonuclear leucocytosis, anaemia and raised ESR. Liver function tests like alkaline phosphatase and serum transaminases may be mild to moderately increased. There is no eosinophilia. Examination of the sputum and of the pleural fluid may reveal the presence of trophozoites of E. histolytica. The pleural fluid may be clear and sterile on culture or it may appear like chocolate coloured sauce.[2] Haemagglutination test may be positive in 80-90 per cent of cases. However, there is evidence of a significantly high background positivity of these tests in endemic areas, as antibodies remain high for a long period following infection. Apart from indirect haemagglutination test which is commonly used, ELISA (enzyme linked immunosorbent assays) are being quite widely used, as these seem to be more specific and sensitive. Never-theless, these tests don't help in establishing the diagnosis.[12] Careful examination of the sputum is always rewarding.[9]

Treatment

Pleuropulmonary amoebiasis responds dramatically to dihydroemetine subcutaneously in a dose of 60 mg daily for 10 days. Quicker and better results can be obtained with a combination of dehydroemetine with metronidazole.[20] This provides the rapid amoebicidal action of emetine[21] and superiority over metronidazole alone.[22] EKG changes have been less pronounced on dehydroemetine therapy as compared to emetine.[23] Since dehydroemetine is excreated thrice as rapidly from the body than emetine, it disappears much earlier from the heart than from the liver, thereby causing transient electrocardiographic changes. Metronidazole in a dose of 400 mg thrice a day orally for 10 days is as effective in the management with lower incidence of side effects, but combination with dehydroemetine gives the best results in hepatopulmonary amoebiasis.[20] Treatment response is similar in case of amoebic liver abcess in patients with HIV disease with low cell count.[23]

The co-existing hepatitis responds to the administration of chloroquin 250 mg twice a day for three weeks. The pleural effusion or empyema has to be aspirated periodically or drained with intercostal drainage. Ultrasonography helps not only in localising the hepatic abscess, but also has a bearing on selection of treatment regimen as well as the time taken for the abscess to resolve.[24] Indications for needle aspiration of the abscess have been more clearly defined. Since medical therapy is effective, needle aspiration is only required[16,25-30] when the abscess is large or those with impending rupture; because complete resolution of the abscess cavity takes a long time and large abscess may even take several years to resolve.[20] Liver abscess needs aspiration with a widebore needle, or either drainage under ultrasound guide which is safe as well as reduces the period of morbidity considerably.

REFERENCES

1. Wilmot A.J. Amoebiasis, In: Woodruff A.W., Ed, Medicine in the tropics. Edinburgh, London: Churchill Livingstone 1974; 111-24.
2. Shankar P.S. Parasitic pulmonary diseases, In: Chest Medicine; Published Oxford and IBH Publ. Co. (P) Ltd., New Delhi 1994; 4th ed.
3. Vijayan V.K. Parasitic lung diseases; Lung India 1997; 15: 49-53.
4. Reed R.L. Amoebiasis: An update; Clin Inf. Dis 1992;14: 385-93.
5. Revdin J.I. Amoebiasis: Clin Inf. Dis 1995; 20:14-66.
6. Chakravarty A., Pulmonary Amoebiasis, J. Indian Med. Assoc 1951; 20:399-402.
7. Hinshaw C.H. and Murray J.F., Parasitic Diseases of the Lung and Thorax. In: Diseases of the Chest, 4th Ed., Philadelphia: WB Saunders Company 1980; 418.
8. Verner H.D. Pulmonary amoebiasis due to hematogenous spread. Report of a case, Bull. Charfotte Mem. Hosp. Charlotte NC 1948; 3:3-6.
9. Ghose A.K. Paul K., Panja M., *et al.,* Primary amoebic lung abscess, J. Assn. Phys. India 1992; 40:200-01.
10. Chaudhury R.N. and Chaudhury M.N.R. Pulmonary amoebiasis. Ind. Med. Gaz 1946; 81:66-68.
11. Gupta S., Minocha S.K. and Singh B. Primary amoebic lung abscess, J. Assn. Phys. India 1992; 40:707.
12. Plorde J.J., Amebiasis. In: Braunwald E., Isselbacher K.G., Petersdorf R.A., Wilson J.D., Martin J.B., Fauci A.S., Ads. Harrison's Principles of Internal Medicine, 11th ed., NewYork: McGraw-Hill 1987,773-76.
13. Webster B.H. Pleuropulmonary amoebiasis a review with analysis of ten cases, Am. Rev. Respir. Dis 1960; 81:683-88.
14. Ochsner A. and Debakey M., Pleuropulmonary complications of amoebiasis, J. Thoracic Surg 1936; 5:225-28.
15. Chatterjee K.D. Parasitology, 11th ed., Calcutta: Chatterjee Medical Publishers 1976; 29-33.
16. Naik S.R., Koshy A. and Nayak N.C. Tropical liver disease, Medicine India 1991; 3:3449-50.
17. Gaude G.S., *et al.,* The lungs in liver disorders; Medicine II Update 1995;3:(1)143-50.
18. Gaude G.S., *et al.,* Lung involvement in amoebiasis; Lung India 1997; 15: 72-77.
19. Bhatia R.S. and Chawla A.S. Tinidazole in amoebiasis and giardiasis, J. Med and Surg 1990; 30: 15-16.
20. Jain N.K., Madan A., Sharma T.N., Sharma D.K. and Mandhana R.G., Hepatopulmonary amoebiasis: Efficacy of various treatment regimens containing dehydroemetine and/or metronidazole, J. Assoc. Physicians India 1990, 38: 269-71.
21. Marcial-Rojas R.A. and Ramiraz-Ronda C.H. *Parasitic diseases of the liver,* In: Diseases of the liver, 5th ed, Schiff L., Schiff E.R.; Eds, Philadelphia, Toronto: Lippincott J.B. 1982; 1165-69.
22. Wilmot A.J., Powell S.J. and Adams E.B., Chloroquine compared with chloroquine and emetine combined in amoebic liver abscess, Am. J. Trop. Med. Hyg 1959; 9: 623-24.
23. Hamide A., *et al.,* Amoebic liver abscess in a patient with HIV infection; JAPI 2002; 50: 832-33.
24. Srivastava S.C., Hepatopulmonary amoebiasis, J. Assn. Phys. India 1991; 39:725.
25. Gibney E.J. Amoebic liver abscess Br. J. Surg 1990;77: 483-84.
26. Sharma M.P., Rai R.R., Acharya S.K., Samant Ray, J.C. and Tandon B.N. Needle aspiration of amoebic liver abscess. Br. Med. J 1989; 299: 1308-09.
27. Dela Rey Nel J., Simjee A.E. and Patel A. Indications for aspiration of amoebic liver abscess. S. Afr. Med. J 1989; 75: 373-76.
28. Maharaj B., Bhoora I.G., Patel A. and Maharajh J. Ultrasonography and scintigraphy in liver disease in developing countries. A retrospective study, Lancet 1989; ii: 853-856.
29. Singh J.P. and Kashyap A. A comparative evaluation percutaneous catheter drainage for resistant amoebic liver abscesses, Am. J. Surg 1989;158: 58-62.
30. Ahmed J., Salama Z.A., Rooby A.E. and Strickland G.T. Ultrasonographic resolution time for amoebic liver abscess. Am. J. Trop. Med. Hyg 1989; 41: 406-10.

PULMONARY MALARIAL DISEASE (PULMONARY MALARIA)

Malarial presentation may have protean clinical manifestation,[1] with fever of short duration with rigors and chills.[2] Apart from afebrile malaria,[3] cerebral malaria,[4] gastrointestinal involvement,[5] anemia,[6] circulatory failure[5,7] urticaria,[8] autonomic neuropathy, Guillain-Barr 'e syndrome,[9] tubular necrosis and proliferative glomerulonephritis,[5] pulmonary involvement with P. falciparum may occur in 3-10% of patients.

There can be obstruction to the flow of blood in the capillaries of the lung following agglutination of red blood cells containing malarial parasites. It produces features of pulmonary oedema with cough, blood tinged sputum and crepitations.[10] The sputum examination may show presence of red blood cells containing malarial parasites. The examination of peripheral blood for presence of the parasites is essential. The condition is treated with chloroquine, oxygen and diuretics. Chloroquine phosphate is given in a loading dose of 1 gm (600 mg base) to be followed by 500 mg in six hours. Then it is continued in a daily dose of 500 mg for the subsequent two days.

Malarial lung involvement may lead to adult respiratory distress syndrome. The condition manifests marked dyspnoea, progressive hypoxaemia, reduced pulmonary compliance, diffuse alveolar infiltrates and marked impairment in oxygen transport despite ventilatory assistance.[11]

People in this part of tropics are suffering from many diseases but one that plagues mankind more dangerously is malaria, possibly because of neglect in prophylaxis and increased labour influx especially in this region.[12] Milder course of pulmonary malaria has also been occasionally experienced.

Diseased red cell corpuscles disturb the pulmonary microcirculations which disturbs oxidative metabolism causing pulmonary venular spasm or microthrombus formation with inappropriate antidiuretic hormone release and fluid overload have been experimentally suggested possible mechanisms, secondary to which hypothalamic dysfunctions occur centrally. And peripherally, elevated pulmonary venous pressure secondary to venous and lymphatic obstruction have been proposed as to be the cause of pleural effusion and pulmonary odema in pulmonary malaria. There is also evidence of immune complexes causing alveolar change. Parasitemia causes generalised vasodilatation, leading to decreased effective circulating blood volume. All these factors increase the permeability of alveolar capillary membrane, leading in turn to interstitial odema, alveolar haemorrhage and other changes of ARDS.[11,13]

Patient comes with high grade fever, cough, usually dry, recurrent and hoarseness. Clinical examination reveals tachypnoea and tachycardia with or without pre-systolic murmur. Occasional crepts may be heard on chest examination. Chest X-ray reveals hazziness with pleural effusion. There is interstitial and alveolar odema with normal size heart.[14] Fluid is sterile and shows eosinophils on Leishman's staining. Peripheral smear is positive for M.P. (malarial parasite).

Milder course of complications may partly be because of use of sub-therapeutic dosage of anti-malarial drug. Full therapeutic dose of antimalarials to a clinically diagnosed case of malaria even if the PBS for MP is negative has been suggested and such diagnostic probabilities must be kept in endemic areas; otherwise this global problem[15] will not hesitate in presenting with different complication.[16] Progressive respiratory failure and hypoxemia may require mechanical ventilation with PEEP. However, mortality is as high as 50% of cases, despite aggressive treatment in complicated cases of pulmonary malaria. To counter the oxidative stress in ARDS, role of antioxidants has been advocated.[14]

REFERENCES

1. Chander Vipan, Mehta S.R., Sharma P.D., Sarkar P.K. and Sharma B.R. Falciparum malaria, Indian J Peed 1989; 56: 365-69.
2. Deb T., Mohanty R.K., Raviok, *et al.,* Atypical presentations of falciparum malaria, J Assn Phys India 1992; 40: 381-84.
3. Bhatia R.S., Afebrile malaria; Ind. J. Clin. Pract 1994, 5(4): 97.
4. Kochar D.K., *et al.*, Cerebral malaria in Indian adults; JAPI 2002; 50: 234-42.
5. Edington G.M. and Gilles H.M., Pathology in the Tropics, 2nd ed., London: Edward Arnold 1976; 17-18, 463.
6. Fleming A.F. Haematological manifestations of malaria and other parasitic infectious diseases, Clin. Haematol 1981; 10: 983-1011.
7. Murphy P.A. Physiological changes in Infected Patients. In: Weatherall D.J., Ledingham, J.G.G., Warell D.A., Eds. Oxford Textbook of Medicine Vol. 2nd ed. Oxford University Press, Oxford 1987; 5.25.
8. Bhatia R.S. Malarial urticaria, Antiseptic 1990, 87: 70.
9. Drago S.D., *et al.*, Guillain-Barr'e syndrome in a case of falciparum malaria; Journ Assn Phys India 1997; 45:161.
10. Shankar P.S. Malarial lung disease; In: Chest Medicine, Oxford and IBH Publ. C. (P) Ltd., New Delhi 1994, 4th ed.
11. Shankar P.S. Adult Respiratory Distress Syndrome, Quart. Med. Rev. 1978; 29: 1.
12. Chawla L.S., Sidhu G., Sabharwal B.D., Bhatia K.L. and Sood A. Jaundice in plasmodium falciparum; 1. Assn. Phys. India 1989; 37: 390-91.
13. Vas C.R., Goyle S. ARDS precipitated by falciparum malaria: A case report; J Diab Assn India 1997; 37: 19-24.
14. Johnson S. *et al.* Acute tropical infections and lungs; Thorax 1994; 49: 714-18.
15. Bhatia R.S. Role of pantothenic in cutaneous reactions to chloroquin: J. Therap and Drugs 1988; 5: 50.
16. Bhatia R.S. Malarial epididymo-orchitis: A case report, Antiseptic 1990; 87(10): 526.

PULMONARY HYDATID DISEASE (PULMONARY ECHINOCOCCOSIS)

Hydatid disease is caused by the cestode (tapeworm), Echinococcus granulosus. This extremely small tapeworm of 3 to 6 mm in length, has the dog as a definitive host and mammals such as sheep, cattle and pig as intermediate hosts. Man in an accidental intermediate host.[2] The disease is seen throughout the world but is often encountered in cattle and sheep-rearing countries such as, Australia, New Zealand, Middle-East, South America[1] and India.[3] Hydatid disease was known to Hippocrates.[4] Hunter (1835) described several cases and was the first to postulate that pelvic hydatid cysts were secondary to rupture of a visceral cyst.[5] Only 2 out of 12 species of

Ecchinococcus granulosis and Ec multilocularis are known to affect man. More serious multilocular or alveolar form has a more restricted distribution, affecting Middle and Eastern Europe, Japan and Alaska.

Life Cycle

The infection is acquired from handling dogs and fecal-oral contamination allows entry of ova containing infective embryo. The protective coat of the ova is digested in the intestine and hexacanth embryo (30 microns in length) is liberated. It pierces the duodenal wall from where it has its access to the portal blood stream and reaches the liver, after crossing the first filter—the liver—it sometimes reaches the lungs. The larva may gain entry into systemic circulation and reaches spleen, kidney, bone and brain. It gets impacted in the capillary bed of the tissues, where it develops slowly over a period of years to cause hydatid (Gk. drops of water) disease.[6]

Pathology

Hydatid disease, as it affects man, is the cystic stage of E. granulosus. Usually the parasite arrests at the liver where it may either be killed by the host or develop into a hepatic hydatid cyst. Hydatid cysts of the liver account for around 60 per cent of all cases.[7] It has been reported that they are usually single and more commonly affect the right lobe. In the remaining 40 per cent of cases hydatid cysts of the lung account for 20 per cent[8] and cysts of bone, soft tissues, spleen, kidney, brain, and heart make up the rest. The cyst develops as a spherical or oval mass predominantly in the lung parenchyma. There is hardly any hindrance to the growth of the cyst in the lung. The cyst elicits little response from the host and causes compression and collapse of the adjacent lung as it enlarges. It may gradually grow to a very large size. A thin layer comprising host tissue, granulation tissue and fibrous tissue of the host surrounds it as pericyst (pseudocyst).

Hydatid cyst consists of two layers—a chitinous laminated non-nucleated hyaline outer layer (ectocyst, exocyst) and a thin syncytial nucleated inner layer (endocyst). The latter acts as a germinal layer and forms small sacs (brood capsules). Daughter cysts with scolex and miniature worm (100 microns in length) develop from the germinal layer and from brood capsules towards the crystal clear fluid-filled cyst cavity (uhilocular cyst). A cyst may contain nearly100 daughter cysts. However the production of daughter cysts is less frequent in the lung than in the liver.[6] The scolices may get separated from the capsule and float inside or may gravitate and form hydatid sand at the bottom of the cyst.[7] The fluid in the cyst is under high tension. Ectocyst and endocyst in spite of being in close contact, they are not linked with each other.

The pulmonary hydatid cysts are classified as simple or complicated. A simple cyst has intact membranes with live parasites inside. The cyst may be single or multiple (20 per cent), unilateral or bilateral (20 to 30 per cent).[3] It may co-exist with hepatic cysts (10 per cent).[9] It grows at a variable rate and later it may rupture into the bronchus or get infected or both and is referred to as complicated cyst.

A small volume of air can enter into the space between ectocyst and pericyst following slight erosion of the ectocyst. Air may get absorbed if the erosion is small and it does not recur. In many instances the ectocyst ruptures into surrounding bronchi causing collapse and fragmentation of the endocyst. It allows expectoration of the fragments of the membrane and hydatid fluid and is replaced with air. Often it becomes the seat of secondary infection.[6]

Clinical Presentation

Patient may be asymptomatic with a small or moderate-sized hydatid cyst. It may be detected accidentally on radiologic examination. The symptoms are noted only when it causes pressure changes in the surrounding lung, pleura or mediastinum. Dyspnoea and discomfort in the chest may occur from a large sized cyst. Haemoptysis occurs at the time of rupture of the cyst. Pulmonary hydatid cysts are more prone to complications, possibly because of lack of support by the rather flimsy lung tissue.[6] Often it is associated with an irritating cough. There can be hypersensitivity reaction with urticaria, rashes and pruritis. The rupture of the cyst is associated with cough and expectoration of watery fluid with salty taste. A massive rupture is associated with leakage of a large amount of hydatid fluid and severe cough. The sputum or pleural fluid may show fragments of hydatid membrane resembling white of a hard-boiled egg of grape-peel like material or white plaques, with hydatid scolex and hooklets. Rarely hepatic hydatid cysts may rupture through the diaphragm and establish a bronchial communication (hepatobronchial fistula) and the sputum is stained with bile.[6]

A dull note on percussion and diminished breath sounds are the features of a large cyst. Pleural spread of the hydatid disease gives rise to signs of pleural effusion. Rarely if the bronchial communication is large, complete evacuation of the contents of the cysts and ultimate obliteration of the cavity may occur. Generally infection develops in the cyst and the cavity becomes filled with disintegrating membrane and pus. The hydatid fluid is clear, colourless and highly antigenic. The cyst may rupture into the pleural cavity and result in the development of secondary cysts and destruction of hemithorax. Histopathological findings include, identification of cyst wall, membranous layer and scolices with hooklets. The outer wall is infiltrated with eosinophils, fibroblasts, giant cells and few lymphocytes.[10]

Investigations

X-ray chest may show a solitary, well circumscribed homogeneous, oval or circular mass with a clear-cut border, varying from 1 to 10 cm in diameter surrounded by a normal lung. The cysts may be multiple, unilateral or bilateral. It may co-exist with a hepatic cyst which is revealed by an elevated diaphragm. The cysts are more commonly found in the lower lobes, often posteriorly on the right side and may give an appearance of a rising sun over the horizon of the diaphragm. Often the dense shadow of hydatid cyst may be mistaken for a tumour or encysted effusion. Very rarely the cysts are irregular and indented. Those cysts in close proximity to the diagphragm, chest wall or mediastinum may be flat on one side. On fluoroscopy, round density becomes oval on deep inspiration, as[6] the shadow alters in shape during forced inspiration and expiration.

When air enters between pericyst and ectocyst it results in accumulation of a thin crescent of air around the periphery of the cyst (perivascular pneumocyst, pericystic emphysema, miniscus sign, pneumopericyst, single crescent sign, *halo* transradiancy). The position of air alters with the posture of the patient. Crescent shaped transradiancy is not characteristic of hydatid cyst alone. It can be noted in aspergillosis, a breaking down carcinoma, or a pulmonary infarct. There can be a communication of endocyst with a bronchial passage and it allows expulsion of cyst contents or allows development of secondary infection to result in an air-fluid level. The broken laminated membranes shrink and the folded up membrane contrasts against the surrounding air which has replaced the fluid, gives an appearance like a crumbled handkerchief or a water-lily within the cyst (water lily sign, lily-pad sign, sign of the Camelot). This sign is not commonly seen because of either complete expulsion of cysts or secondary infection. There can be air-fluid level within the cyst and a crescent sign around the periphery (double arch sign, double dome arch sign, Cumbo's sign, moon sign).[6] At the same time, absence of typical radiological signs like air crescent, water lily sign does not exclude hydatid disease.[11] Even classical signs are radiologically seen only in a small percentage of cases.[12]

Commonly seen findings are listed below:

a. Chest X-ray — Multiloculated cystic lesions
b. U.sonography— Gross fluid in cavity contrast enhanced.
c. CT scan of chest — Fluid and multiloculated non-enhancing fluid density lesions
d. 2D-Echo — Globular echolucent structure

Sometimes, as the contents evacuate, the cavity may distend with air by the hydatid membrane obstructing the draining bronchus at the bottom of the cavity (tension pneumocyst). The cyst may rupture into the pleural space to result in pneumothorax, hydropneumothorax or pyopneumothorax. Pulmonary hydatidosis may have unusual presentations like tension pneumothorax[13,14] spontaneous pneumothorax,[15] pleural effusion,[16] and massive pleural effusion.[17] Horner's syndrome,[18,19] not-resolving and recurrent consolidation,[20] lung abscess,[21] and bilateral consolidation.[22] Calcification of the cyst is extremely rare.

Bronchoscopy is not advocated. It is dangerous to attempt aspiration of the cysts or biopsy of the cyst. It causes rupture and leakage of hydatid fluid that causes anaphylaxis. Also there is long term risk of development of secondary hydatidosis which is possibly the most feared complication of hydatid disease.[7] Ultrasonography is helpful in recognition of the cyst and it exhibits regular walls and an absence of echoes. Ultrasound characteristics of hydatid cyst include an echoic cyst, cyst with internal echoes, cyst with air fluid levels (infected cyst), cyst with thick wal l and lifting of membrane.[11,23] Distal acoustic enhancement is usual,[24-26] ultrasonographic diagnosis appears to be accurate,[27,28] Radioisotope scanning is effective in demonstrating hydatid cyst as cold and nodular but this cannot be differentiated from carcinomatous metastasis. C.T. scan clearly and precisely demonstrates the existence, number and size of both pulmonary and hepatic hydatid cysts. Also they can be differentiated from tumour metastasis and abscess.[7] CT can demonstrate both intact and ruptured cysts.[29] While selective angiography carries a definite risk, needle biopsy is better avoided for fear of anaphylaxis or hydatidosis.[30]

A normal eosinophil count may show an increase during an active growth and following rupture of the cyst. An intradermal injection of 0.5 ml sterile hydatid fluid induces a large wheal with surrounding erythema within 30 minutes and it is later replaced by an area of induration lasting for one to two days (Casoni's test). The test is likely to be positive in 60 to 80 per cent of the cases. A positive Casoni's test has diagnostic importance; but a negative Casoni's test has no significance in the differential diagnosis.[6] The test is very sensitive but not very specific and is now not used in U.K.

Complement fixation test may be positive in 80 per cent of cases of hydatid disease. Antibody titre of one in four to one in eight are often found in people working in farms. A titre of more than one in eight is suspicious of infection. Haemagglutination test is both sensitive and specific. Hydatid antigen is absorbed into tanned erythrocytes which agglutinate with specific antibody upon coming in contact. Latex agglutination and many immuno diagnostic tests[31] are being used to detect hydatid disease. Diagnostic significance of elevated hydatid specific IgE, against hydatid specific IgG, ELISA and Casoni's intradermal test in surgical proven cases have been evaluated,[32] without any correlation and with false positivity in 57.14 per cent of cases.

High levels of IgE in some patients with malignancy have been reported. In endemic care as in our country, where previous exposure to Echinococcus granulosus ova is high, specific IgG rather than IgE may prove more reliable for detection of hydatid disease.[33] However, in Casoni's positive patients, in whom cancer is suspected and they do with high levels of total IgE. In differential diagnosis pulmonary, hydatid cyst should be considered in tropical region in young persons without having conventional risk factors of atherosclerosis.[34] On MRI imaging, cyst shows low signal intensity on T 1-weighted images and high signal intensity on T2-weighted images.[35] Double arch sign or combo sign in diagnostic of ruptured hydatid cyst, represented as air tubble on chest CT and have 85% sensitivity and 96% specificity.[36]

Treatment

Management of disseminated and recurrent hydatid cyst is a much greater problem. Hydropneumothorax has been documented as secondary pleural hydatidosis occurring as complication of ruptured intrapulmonary echinococcosis.[37] Surgery is usually successful in the recurrence of uncomplicated primary cyst.[38]

The surgical treatment consists of enucleation of the cyst. Rapid growth of the cyst and complicated cyst needs pulmonary resection. Hydatid cysts are not commonly located in the upper lobe posterior segment,[30] but no lung anatomical location is exempted. Cysts are to be removed without contaminating the surrounding pleura or lungs and they have to be removed completely without getting ruptured. Rupture of the cyst during surgery or puncture of the cysts by introducing a needle may allow leakage of the contents. It causes implantation of the daughter cysts and severe anaphylactic reaction. High doses of corticosteroids in such situations protect against anaphylaxis. Hydatid cysts have shown total regression following prolonged treatment with mebendazole in a dose of 400 mg daily over a period of three months.[6]

Poor absorption of mebendazole has limited its use. Albendazole is another benzimidazole compound with a much better response[22,39-41] in a dose of 10 mg/kg body weight for 4-6 weeks[37] has been recommended by WHO.[42]

REFERENCES

1. LeRoux B.T. Pulmonary hydatid disease. Thorax 1972; 27: 365.
2. Maniar D.R. *et al.*, Pulmonary hydatidosis; Medical and surgical management JAPI 1996; 44: 63-64.
3. Kulpati D.D.S. Pulmonary hydatid disease. In: Progress in clinical medicine (Series III) Ahuja, MMS (ed) Arnold Heinman, New Delhi 1982; 453-58.
4. Adams F. The Genuine Work of Hippocrates No. 55, Bailliere Tindall and Cox, London 1939; 327.
5. Hunter J. The works of John Hunter, Vol 1 (edited by Palmer, J.F.), Longman, London 1825, 572.
6. Shankar P.S., Pulmonary echinoccosis, In: Chest Medicine Oxford and IBH Publ Co.(P) Ltd., New Delhi 1994, 4th ed.
7. Morris D.L., Management of hydatid disease, J.Appl. Med 1985; 723-730.
8. Roy S.C., Chakravarthy M., Das M.M. and Chatterjee B.P., World incidence of hydatid disease in general and pulmonary disease in particular with special reference to India, J. Ind. Med. Assoc 1970; 55: 212.
9. Bekhti A., Schaaps J.P., Capron M., Dissaint J.P., Santoto F. and Capron A. Treatment of hepatic hydatid disease with mebendazole, preliminary results in four cases, Br. Med. J 1977; 11: 1047-1051.
10. Chakrapani B.S., Vidyasagar B. and Yeli S.M., Solve a problem, Lung India 1991; 9: 68-69.
11. Saidi Farook, Surgery of hydatid diseases, W.B. Saunders Company, Philadelphia, Edn 1976, 268: 81.
12. Crofton J. and Douglas A., Respiratory Diseases, 3rd edition, P.G. Publishing Ltd., Singapore 1983; 439-41.
13. Beker P. and Al Omari M.M. Echinococcal tension pneumothorax, Thorax 1981; 24: 547.
14. Comollam S.J., Jowath A.W. and Wilson R.S.E. Hydatid disease presenting as tension pneumothorax, Dis, Chest 1979, 73: 405.
15. Vidyasagar B., Subbarao H.L. and Babu C.L. Spontaneous pneumothorax caused by tuptured pulmonary hydatid cyst—A case report, Lung India 1988; 6: 79-80.
16. Imari A.J. Pulmonary hydatid disease in Iraq. Am. J. Trap, Med 1962 II: 481-490.
17. Thippanna G. and Vidyasagar C. Pulmonary hydatid cyst presenting as a massive effusion—A case report, Lung India 1987; 5: 74-76.
18. Ramesh Kumar, Gupta K.L., Sakhuja V. and Chugh K.S. Horner's syndrome due to pulmonary hydatid disease. L Assn Physician Ind 1990; 38: 584.
19. Singh R.P., Saxena S., Navrang R.K. and Katiyar S.K. Horner's syndrome in hydatid cyst of lung. Ind. J, Chest. Dis. All. Sci 1984; 26: 119-22.
20. Kaul S., Kaul B.L., Kawusa M.Y., *et al.*, Recurrent pneumonitis from hydatid cyst—A case report; Lung India 1991; 9: 27-28.
21. Dhar S.N. and Kaul B. Hydatid disease of lungs, Seminars in Resp. Medicine 1988; 9: 4.
22. Guleria P., Dhaliwal R.S. and Malik S.K., Pulmonary hydatid disease presenting as non-resolving bilateral consolidation, Ind. J. Chest. Dis. All. Sci 1989, 3,2, 129-131.
23. Hadidi A., Sonography of hepatic echinococcal cyst, Gastro, Radiol 1982; 7: 349.
24. Itzchak V.Y., Rubinstein Z., Heyman Z. and Gerzof S., Role of ultrasound in the diagnosis of abdominal hydatid disease, J. Clin. Ultrasound 1980; 8: 341.

25. Gharbi H.A., Hassin W., Braumer M.W. and Dupuch K., Ultrasound examination of the hydatid liver, Radiology 1981; 139: 444.
26. Choliz J.D.E.D., Olaverri F.U.L., Cases T.F. and Zubieta S.D., Computed tomography in hepatic echinococcosis, Am. J. Radiol 1982; 139: 699-02.
27. Beggs I., The radiological appearance of hydatid disease of the liver. Clin Radiol 1983; 34: 555-63.
28. Pant C.S. and Gupta R.K., Diagnostic value of ultrasonography in hydatid disease in abdomen and chest, Acta Radiologica 1987, 28; 743-45.
29. Gouliamos A.D., *et al.*, CT appearance of pulmonary hydatid disease; Chest 1991; 100:1578-81.
30. Vidyasagar B. and Nagaraja Shetty K.L., Pulmonary hydatidosis in Davangere, Lung India 1987; 5: 70-73.
31. Alkarnai M.A., *et al.*, Advances in diagnosis and management of hydatid disease; Hepatogastroenterology 1990; 37: 327-31.
32. Wattal C., *et al.*, Evaluation of specific immunoglobulin E by ELISA in hydatid disease, Int. Arch. Allerg. Immunol 1988; 87: 98-100.
33. Ray D., *et al.*, Total immunoglobulins in patients with positive Casoni's test, Lung India 1993; 11: 64-66.
34. Kalpna SR; *et al.*, flydatid cyst of lung-an uncommon cause of chest pain in young; Lung India; 2014;31:262-63.
35. Singh S, Gibikote SV; MRI signal characteristics in hydatid cyst; Australia's Radio;2001;45:128-33.
36. Sarkar A; *et al.*, Double-arch sign and air bubble sign-two radiological signs of ruptured lydatid cyst in lung; JAPI; 2014; 62:705-706
37. Walid F; et al., Secondary pleural lydatidosis-complication of intra pulmonary echinococcosis, Lung India, 2014;31:270-73
38. Sajir F; *et al.*, Our eight year surgical experience in patients with pulmonary cyst hydatid; Int. J Chin Exp Med; 2012;51:64-71.
39. Morris D.L., Dykes P.W., Dickson B., Barrines S.E., Bogan J. and Brown F.G.O., Albendazole in hydatid disease, Br. Med. J 1983; 268: 103-104.
40. Morris D.L., Dykes P.W., Dickson B., Barrines S.E., Bogan J., Brown F.G.O. and Smith H., Albendazole, objective evidence of response in human hydatid disease, J. Am. Med. Ass 1985; 253: 2053-57.
41. Officer Brown F.G., Surgical pathology of hydatid cysts of the lung, Postgrad. Med. J 1958; 34: 195.
42. Kumar A., Chattopadhyay T.K. Management of hydatid disease of the liver; Post Grad Med Jour 1992; 68:853-56.

TROPICAL EOSINOPHILIA

Introduction

Tropical Eosinophilia (TE) or tropical pulmonary eosinophilia TPE is a clinical syndrome, prevalent throughout the tropical world,[1] with its characteristic features like hyper eosinophilia, paroxysmal cough, scanty sputum, wheeze and non-descript pulmonary markings in chest X-ray.[2-7] The syndrome is an exaggerated immune response to Wuchereria bancrofti and malayi.[1,3]

Tropical eosinophilia (TE), one of the main causes of pulmonary eosinophilia in tropical countries, is prevalent in filarial endemic regions of the world especially South-East Asia.[8] Even though tropical eosinophilia as a clinical entity was described only in 1940s, the earliest report that conformed to the clinical picture of TE was published in 1916 by Low[9] in a 30-year-old male. Subsequently, Roy and Bose[10] noticed marked leucocytosis and eosinophilia in a group of *asthmatic* subjects who responded to subcutaneous or intramuscular injections of soamin. Frimodt-Moller and Barton[11] in 1940 described a group of sanatorium patients in Madanappalle who had extensive bilateral, evenly distributed miliary mottling in chest X-rays resembling miliary tuberculosis, and blood eosinophilia. They termed this condition as *a pseudotuberculosis condition associated with eosinophilia.* The name *Tropical eosinophilia* was coined in 1943 by Weingarten[12] who accidentally observed that these patients could be treated with neoarsphenamine, as one of his patients with concurrent syphilis was cured of his TE on being given neoarsphenamine for syphilis.

Filarial infection is the cause of TE[13,14] as it is most frequently encountered in those regions where filariasis is endemic.[8,15] A positive filarial complement fixation test (FCFT) and intradermal skin tests using D. immitis antigen is a diagnostic test for TE.[16] Webb *et al.*[17] in 1960 demonstrated microfilariae in the lungs, liver and lymph nodes of patients with TE. Udwadia[15] also had demonstrated microfilarial (indistinguishable from Brugia malayi) in open lung biopsy specimens from TE patients. Elevated concentrations of filarial-specific IgE have also been reported in TE.[18] The observation that diethylcarbamazine (DEC), an antifilarial drug, is useful in the treatment[19,20] further supports the hypothesis of a filarial aetiology in TE. Experimental studies carried out in human volunteers[21,22] had suggested that TE is due to immunologic hyperresponsiveness to human filariasis. Leucocyte adhesion phenomenon[23] and the demonstration that basophils from patients with TE released greater amounts of histamine when cells were challenged with Brugia or Wuchereria antigens than with Dirofilaria antigens[24] provide further evidence that human forms rather than animal filaria are responsible for TE.

Pathogenesis

Histopathological findings such as widely scattered nodules of varying size (1 to 5 mm) over lung surface were first described by Vishwanathan[25] and Dhanaraj.[26] Detailed histopathological studies demonstrating eosinophilic, histiocytic and mixed cell type infiltrations were documented by Udwadia.[15] Pulmonary fibrosis developed in some patients, particularly in those with a longstanding history.[15,27] Mild to moderate thickening of both pulmonary arteries and veins is seen in a patient with TE. The current concept of the pathogenesis of TE suggests that it begins with a lung parenchymal inflammation in individual, highly sensitized immunologically to filarial parasites.[28] The microfilariae released from lymphatic dwelling adult worm is cleared in the pulmonary circulation and the microfilariae degenerate and release their antigenic constituents which trigger the local inflammatory and immune processes.[17,24,27] Morphologically, it had been shown that there is evidence of degenerating microfilariae and diffuse inflammation in the lung parenchyma.[15,17,29,30] Therefore, it can be reasonably hypothesized that the clinical and pulmonary physiological abnormalitites in TE are at least in part due to accumulation of inflammatory cells in the lung parenchyma.

Bronchoalveolar lavage (BAL) studies had demonstrated that TE is characterized by intense eosinophilic inflammatory process in the lower respiratory tract.[31] The concentration of eosinophils in the epithelial lining fluid (ELF) of the lower respiratory tract is many fold greater than that in the blood, suggesting that eosinophils accumulate selectively in the lung parenchyma. Electron microscopic examinations disclose marked alterations consisting of severe degranulation with loss of both the cores and the peripheral portion of the granules. These findings suggest that eosinophils are in an activated state. The significant negative correlation of lung eosinophils with transfer factor[32] is, therefore, compatible with the hypothesis that the toxic mediators liberated by activated eosinophils are responsible for the injury to the lung parenchyma inTE. Polycolonal IgE and parasite-specific IgG, IgM and IgE antibody levels in epithelial lining fluid (ELF) are significantly higher in TE patients.[33] Treatment with DEC for 6-14 days later shows a dramatic fall in the levels of ELF parasite-specific IgG and IgE antibodies without corresponding changes in either the serum antibody levels of ELF polyclonal immunoglobulin levels. Immunoblot comparison of the antigen recognition pattern of ELF and serum antibodies demonstrate a general similarity in parasite antigen recognised. Thus, a profound antibody response to filarial infection is found in the lungs of patients with TE, suggesting that these filaria-specific antibodies play an important role in the pathogenesis of this disorder.[33]

Clinical Features

TE is predominantly seen in males and between the ages of 15 to 40 years.[8] Udwadia[15] has classified the clinical manifestations into 6 forms. They are respiratory form which is the most common form, alimentary form, general form, lymphatic form, mixed form and asymptomatic form with only peripheral eosinophilia. Respiratory form is characterised by cough, dyspnoea and noctural wheezing, occasionally associated with fever, anorexia and weight loss. Clinical examination may reveal rales and rhonchi. Leucocytosis with an absolute increase in eosinophils in the peripheral blood is the hallmark of TE.[12,13] Microfilariae are rarely seen in the peripheral blood.[15] Sputum shows clumps of eosinophils and Charcot-Leyden crystals.[12] Radiological features in TE include miliary mottling, prominent hila with increased vascular markings. In patients with long-standing history, lung fields may show reticulations and in a few cases honeycombing.[27] Chest X-ray may be normal in 20-30 per cent of patients with TE.[15] Before treatment, the main physiological abnormality in acute TE was reduction in the carbon monoxide transfer factor[28,34] which was found to be due to reduction in membrane diffusing capacity (Dm).[35] Mild to moderate obstructive ventilatory defect was seen in 30 per cent of cases and restrictive defect in 50-70 per cent.[27,36] Arterial hypoxemia ($PaO_2 < 80$ mm Hg) was observed in 42 per cent of acute TE patients, but 36 per cent had only hypoxemia (PaO_2 70-80 mm Hg).[36,37]

Management

The diagnostic criteria of TE, therefore, include history of past or present residence in three endemic areas of filariasis, respiratory symptoms, pulmonary infiltrates, peripheral blood eosinophil Z 2000 cells/mm^3 and high serum antifilarial IgG. Initially, the treatment of TE was with arsenic and was abandoned because of its toxicity.[12] Later on, diethylcarbamazin (DEC), a piperazine derivative with antifilarial activity, was found to be the drug of choice[19,20,38] and it is cheap and least toxic. The recommended schedule of treatment with DEC is 6 mg/kg/body weight for 3 weeks.[39,40] Most individuals with TE respond to DEC within 1 to 3 weeks with a progressive reduction in symptoms, clearing of the chest X-rays, reduction in the blood eosinophils count, and improvement in lung function. Relapses occurred in 20 per cent of patients followed upto 5 years.[15] Earlier workers[41] had shown that steroids were also effective in the treatment of TE. The new antifilarial drug, invermectin given in a dosage of 200 ug/kg/day for 2 days was found to be ineffective in TE.

Course of Disease

It had been shown previously that acute tropical eosinophilia left untreated could develop into chronic interstitial lung disease.[15] Studies conducted to know the fate of those patients who were treated *successfully* with a standard three weeks course of DEC had revealed that most patients had shown a marked symptomatic improvement, but peripheral blood eosinophilia (> 2000 cells/mm^3) persisted in 52 per cent, radiographic abnormalities in 44 per cent, cough in 22 per cent and chest signs in 8 per cent.[36] Significant improvement was noticed in almost all aspects of lung function including blood gases, but the mean values for forced expiratory volume in one second (FEV_1), Transfer Factor (TLCO), transfer coefficient (KCO) and membrane diffusing capacity (Dm) continued to be significantly lower than predicted values.[27,28,36] At one month the obstructive defect was persistent in 14 per cent and the restrictive in 16 per cent. Reduced transfer factor and transfer coefficient persisted in 62 per cent and 54 per cent respectively. There was also a marked decrease of the lung eosinophils[42] following the treatment. However, a mild macrophage-eosinophilic alveolitis was presisting at one month despite treatment.[42] Thus, there was incomplete reversal of clinical, hematological, radiological, physiological and pathological changes in TE one month after starting a 3-week course of diethylcarbamazine.[36,42]

The observation that there is incomplete recovery in TE[36] suggests the possibility that the disease can persist despite DEC therapy and lead to chronic dyspnoea with restrictive functional impairment. Majority of patients evaluated 12±2 months later following a standard 3-week course of DEC for acute TE[43] have mild, persistent symptoms referable to the lung, chest X-ray abnormalities, blood eosinophilia and elevated serum IgE and filarial specific IgG.[43] On the average, lung function is consistent with the presence of chronic mild interstitial lung disease. When the inflammatory cells from the lower respiratory tract are examined, there is a persistent eosinophilic alveolitis.[43] A one year follow-up study of 50 patients has revealed that chronic eosinophilic alveolitis in 35 per cent and diffusion defect in 51 per cent persists at 12 months despite treatment.[44] Evaluation of the lower respiratory tract inflammatory cells recovered from post-DEC-treated individuals demonstrates spontaneous release of exaggerated amounts of O_2 and H_2O_2 compared to normal subjects.[43] Treatment with prednisone significantly reduces the lower respiratory tract eosinophilic inflammation and the release of oxidants,[45] permitting minimum time for eosinophilia to exert damaging influence on pulmonary parenchyma.[14,46]

These findings suggest that standard treatment as practised currently, i.e., one course DEC (6 mg/kg/body weight) for 3 weeks is inadequate for a cure in TE. There has been a distinct group of patients who do not respond to DEC therapy.[18,47] Therefore, other modalities of treatment such as long-term DEC with or without corticosteroids have to be evaluated in a controlled clinical trial.

REFERENCES

1. Panda B.N., Raha B., Bhalla J.S., *et al.,* Short term treatment of tropical eosinophilia with DEC; impact on clinical haematological and micrometeric data, Ind. J. Tuber 1992; 39: 117-20.
2. Viswanathan R. and Jaggi O.P., Progress in clinical medicine in India, 1st ed; N. Delhi, Arnold Heinemann 1976; 75-91.
3. Nava FA. and Offesen E.A. Tropical eosinophilia, N. Eng. J. Med 1978; 298: 1129.
4. Suresh V., Srivastava J.N., Dutta V., *et al.,* A clinical study of tropical eosinophilia, Med. J. Arm Forces India 1986; 207-10.
5. Gopinathan V.P., Tropical eosinophilia, A clinical study, Med. J. Aust 1983; 69.
6. Goyal R., Raghu M., Bhagi R.P., *et al.,* Pulmonary function in tropical pulmonary eosinophilia. Ind. J. Chest Dis. All. Sci 1990; 32:29.
7. Geddes D.M., Pulmonary eosinophilia, J. Royal Coll. Phy. London 1986; 20: 139.
8. Ottesen E.A. and Nutman T.V., Tropical pulmonary eosinophilia, Annu Rev. Med 1992; 43: 417-25.
9. Low G.L., An Interesting case of eosinophilia, Trans. Roy Soc. Trop Med. Hyg 1916; 9: 77-81.
10. Roy N.C. and Bose C.C. Introduction: Effectiveness of soamin in cases of asthma associated with eosinophilia, Calcutta Med J 1918; 12: 268-77.
11. Frimodt Miller C. and Barton R.M. A pseudo tuberculous condition associated with eosinophilia, Ind. Med. Gaz 1940; 75: 607-13.
12. Weingarten R.J., Tropical eosinophilia, Lancet 1943; 1: 103-05.
13. Dhanraj L.T., Deselva J.S. and Schancher J.F. The serological diagnosis of eosinophilic lung (tropical eosinophilia) and its etiological implications, Am. J. Trop. Med. Hyg 1959; 8: 151-59.
14. Neva F.A. and Ottesen E.A. Tropical (filarial) eosinophilia. N Engl J. Med 1978; 298: 1129-31.
15. Udwadia F.E. Tropical eosinophilia (In) Pulmonary eosinophilia—Progress in respiratory research. S Karger, Basel 1975;7: 35-155.
16. Dhanaraj T.J. and Schacher J.R. 1/D tests with dirofilaria immitis extract in eosinophilic lung (tropical eosinophilia) Am J. Trop Med Hyg 1959; 8: 640.
17. Webb J.K.B., Job C.K. and Gault W., Tropical eosinophilia. Demonstration of mcirofilariae in liver, lung and lymph nodes. The Lancet 1960; 1: 835-42.
18. Neva FA., Kaplan A.P., Pacheco G., *et al.,* Tropical eosinophilia. A human model of parasitic immunopathology with observations on serum IgE levels before and after treatment. Ann. Allergy Clin. Immunol 1975; 55: 422-429.
19. Dhanaraj T.J., The treatment of eosinophilic lung (tropical eosinophilia) with diethycarbamazine, Quart J Med 1958, 27: 243-263.
20. Ganatra R.D., Seth U.K. and Lewis R.A., Diethylacarbamazine (Hetrazan) in tropical pulmonary eosinophilia E., Afr. Med. J 1958, 35: 493-500.
21. Buckley J.C., Tropical pulmonary eosinophilia in relation to filarial infections (Wuchereария Sp) of animals, Trans Roy Soc. Med. Hyg 1958; 52: 335-36.
22. Buckler J.C., Occult filarial infections of animal orgin as a cause of tropical pulmonary eosinophilia E Afr. Med. J 1955, 35: 493-510.

23. Viswanathan R., Baghi R.C. and Saran R., Leucocyte adhesion phenomenon in pulmonary eosinophilia (Tropical eosinophilia) Am. Rev. Respir. Dis 1973; 107: 298-300.
24. Ottesen E.A., Neva FA., Parajape R.S., Tripathy S.P., Thiruvengadam D.V. and Beaven M.A., Specific allergic sensitisation to filarial antigens in tropical eosinophilia syndrome. The Lancet 1979; 1: 1159-61.
25. Viswanathan R., Post mortem appearances in tropical eosinophilia. Ind Med Gaz 1947; 82: 49.
26. Dhanaraj T.J., Pathological studies in eosinophilic lung, case report, Arch Path 1959; 67-515.
27. Udwadia E.E., Tropical eosinophilia: A correlation of clinical histopathologic and lung function studies. Dis. Chest 1967; 52: 531-38.
28. Poh S.C., The course of lung function in treated tropical eosinophilia, Thorax 1974; 29: 710-12.
29. Dhanaraj T.J., Pacheco G., Shanmugaratnam K. and Beaven P.S. The aetiology and pathology of eosinophilic lung (Tropical eosinophilia) Am. J. Trop. Med. Hyg 1966; 15: 183-89.
30. Joshi V.V., Udwadia F.E. and Gandil R.K., Etiology of tropical eosinophilia. A study of lung biopsies and review of published reports, Am. J. Trop. Med. Hyg 1969; 18: 231-40.
31. Pinkston P., Vijayan V.K., Nutman T.B., Rom W.M., O'Donnell K.M., Cornelius M.J., Kumarswami V., Ferrans V.J., Takemura T., Ynokida O, Revengadam K.V., Tripathy, S.P., Ottesen F.A. and Crystal K.G., Acute tropical pulmonary eosinophilia. Characterisation of the lower respiratory tract inflammation and its response to therapy, J. Clin. Invest 1967; 80: 216-25.
32. Vijayan V.K., Sankaran K., Venkatesan P. and Kuppurao K.V., Correlation of lower respiratory tract inflammation with changes in lung function and chest roentgenograms in patients with untreated tropical pulmonary eosinophilia, Singapore Med J 1991; 32: 122-25.
33. Nutman T.B., Vijayan V.K., Pinkston P., Kumarswami V., Steel C., Crystal R.G. Diffusing capacity in acute untreated tropical eosinophilia, Ind. J. Chest Dis. and All Sci 1988; 160: 1042-50.
34. Vijayan V.K., Kuppurao V.K., Sankaran K., Venkatesan P. and Prabhakar R., Diffusing capacity in acute untreated tropical eosinophilia, Ind. J. Chest Dis. and All Sci 1988; 30: 71-77.
35. Vijayan V.K., Kuppurao V.K, Sankaran K., Venkatesan P. and Prabhakar R., Pulmonary membrane diffusing capacity and capillary blood volume in tropical eosinophilia, Chest 1990; 97: 1386-89.
36. Vijayan V.K., Kuppurao K.V., Sankaran K., Venkatesan P. and Prabhakar R. Tropical eosinophilia: Clinical and physiological response to diethyl carbamazine, Respiratory Medicine 1991; 85: 17-20.
37. Vijayan V.K., Kuppurao K.V., Venkatesan P. and Prabhakar R. Arterial hypoxemia in acute tropical pulmonary eosinophilia, Lung India 1988, 6: 183-185.
38. Baker S.J., Rajan K.J. and Devadatta S., Treatment of tropical eosinophilia: A controlled trial, Lancet 1959; 11: 144-47.
39. Final report, *Joint WHO/Searo Working group on Brugian Filariasis,* Manila WHO 1979; 1-47.
40. Drugs for parasitic infections. Med lett Drugs Ther 1988; 30: 15-24.
41. Sanjivi K.S., Thiruvengadam K.V. and Friedman H.C., Tropical eosinophilia treated with cortisone, Dis Chest 1955; 28: 88-90.
42. Vijayan K.S., Sankaran K., Venkatesan P. and Prabhakar R., Effect of diethyl carbamazine on the alveolitis of tropical eosinophilia, Respirat 1991; 58: 255-59.
43. Rom W.N., Vijayan V.K., Cornelius M.J., Kumarswami V., Prabhakar R., Ottesen E.A. and Crystal R.G., Persistent lower respiratory tract inflammation associated with interstitial lung disease in patients with tropical pulmonary eosinophilia following conventional treatment with diethylacarbamazine. Am. Rev. Respir. Dis 1990; 142:1088-92.
44. Bhatia R.S., Tropical eosinophilia—Atypical presentations, Curr. Med. Pract 1990; 34: 321-24.
45. Vijayan V.K., Role of Steroids in 'chronic' tropical eosinophilia: A bronchoalveolar lavage study, Ind. J. Chest. Dis. and All Sci 1987; 29: vii.
46. Singh D. Pulmonary eosinophilia, J App. Med 1991, 3: 1135.
47. Udwadia F.E. Pulmonary eosinophilia, J. Assn. Phys. India 1978; 26: 283-93 and 428-37.

SCHISTOSOMIASIS (BILHARZIASIS)

200 million people are infected all over the world.[1] The blood flukes of the class trematoda —Schistosoma haematobium and S. mansoni are endemic in Egypt, East and Central Africa, Middle-East and South America and S. japanicum in the Far East. They affect predominantly genitourinary (S. haematobium) and gastrointestinal (S. mansioni) systems.

Man acquires infection as a definitive host from fresh water containing infective cercaria larvae. They enter through the skin when bathing or the buccal mucosa when drinking infected water and reach the systemic circulation after passing through the lungs very rapidly. They develop into adult worms (1 to 2 cms in length) in the intrahepatic portion of the portal system and migrate within four to six weeks to the mesenteric, bladder and pelvic venules. Host of the infected people have few symptoms and only few sufferers develop significant disease.[2]

Pathology

The ova of the adult worms and sometimes the adult flukes may get disseminated to the pulmonary arterioles which accompany the respiratory bronchioles.

The ova get impacted in a pulmonary arteriole producing a nectrotising arteriolitis. It affects the continuity of the media and allows the ova to penetrate the vessel wall. Initially there is cellular reaction around the ova consisting of eosinophils, histiocytes, multinucleated giant cells and later lumphocytes and it results in the occurrence of *bilharzial tubercle.*[3] Later the cellular reaction subsides to leave behind a nodular scar around a disintegrated or calcified ovum. There is intimal thickening in the damaged arteriole leading to its occlusion, but without any thrombosis. A characteristic feature of bilharzial pulmonary endarteritis, develops as recanalisation of the occluding tissue occurs, later which may extend beyond the limits of the occluded arteriole as there is focal destruction of the media to result in the dilatation lesions *angiomatoids*.

Pulmonary hypertension develops due to oblitration of pulmonary arteritis by granulomatous inflammation induced by shunted and emblished eggs.[4,5] This results in right ventricular hypertrophy and dilatation of pulmonary arterial tree. The adult worm in the pulmonary vessels, after their death produces thrombosis, periarteritis and occlusion of the arterial lumen.

The parenchyma of the lungs is not much affected except from the perivascular bilharzial tubercules and the lesions are essentially arterial. Extrapulmonary features include glomerulonephritis and liver fibrosis which develops after 10-15 years prolonged exposure.[6] Periportal fibrosis is much common as compared to clinical presentation, as demonstrated by ultrasound[7,8] and these patients may not have eggs in the stool. Portal hypertension may occur.

Clinical Features

Pulmonary features in the form of mild bronchitis are seen in 33-65% of cases. Initial symptoms like fever, headache, weakness, dry cough, pain may occur 2-6 weeks after exposure.[6] After a long latent period, the individual may present features of pulmonary hypertension. Since the lesions are widespread in the pulmonary vascular territory, there is marked decrease in the pulmonary vascular bed to result in pulmonary hypertension and cor pulmonale. It causes increasing dyspnoea and non-productive cough. However the occurrence of cyanosis and haemoptysis are infrequent. Clubbing is unusual. The condition ultimately terminates in congestive heart failure which is refractory to treatment. Generally these individuals exhibit extrapulmonary schistosomial involvement either of urinary (dysuria, terminal haematuria) or intestinal (dysentery) bilharziasis. In the latter condition there is usually hepatosplenomegaly. Schistosomial infestation must be considered as the probable cause if there is development of cor pulmonale in an individual residing in an endemic area.[9]

Clinical examination of the lungs may reveal crepitations and rhonchi. The second heart sound in the pulmonary area may be loud. Sometimes the manifestations may instead of being in the form of chronic cor pulmonale, present acute features. The patient has severe dyspnoea, cough with expectoration, haemoptysis and cyanosis, because of intense inflammatory response to a sudden shower of eggs reaching the lungs.[9]

Investigation

Chest X-ray may show miliary mottling or diffuse infiltrates. Pleural effusion does not occur. In established cases of pulmonary hypertension, there is marked dilatation of pulmonary trunk and its hilar branches and the right ventricle is enlarged. There may even be aneurysmal dilatation of the pulmonary artery. The lung fields are relatively clear, while the patient presents with pulmonary hypertension and right ventricular hypertrophy.[9]

Stool, urine and rectal mucosal chips when examined may demonstrate the presence of ova. There is moderate leucocytosis and eosinophilia. Pulmonary function studies show a restrictive and obstructive defect and the diffusion capacity is reduced.[10] Needle biopsy of the lung is helpful in establishing the diagnosis. Electrocardiogram demonstrates right axis deviation, right ventricular hypertrophy and incomplete bundle branch block on development of cor pulmonale.[9] IgM, IgG and IgE are elevated.

Treatment

Anti-schistosomial therapy is useful if ova are demonstrable in the sputum or if the patient has acute pulmonary schistosomiasis. Therapy directed against, schistosomiasis is not effective following appearance of features of cor pulmonale. The urinary and intestinal infestation is treated with niridazole orally 25 mg/kg body weight daily in two divided doses for seven days[9] or with praziquantel[11] as a single dose of 50 mg/kg body weight.[9]

REFERENCES

1. Harrison's principles of interna medicine; Wilson J.D., Branunwald E., Isselbacher K.J., *et al.*, (ed) 12th Ed; McGraw Hill, New York 1991.
2. Jordan P., Webbe G., (ed), Schistosomiasis, Epidemiology, treatment and control, London, Heinemann Medical 1982.
3. Warren K.S., Nature (Parasitol. Suppl) 1978; 273: 609.
4. Hiat R.A., *et al.*, Factors in pathogenesis of acute schistosomiasis mansoni, J. Infect. Dis 1979; 139:659.
5. Cheever A.W. and Andrade Z.A., Pathological lesions associated with S. mansoni infection in man; Trans. Royal Soc. Trop. Med. Hyg 1968; 61: 626.
6. Norsh T.E., *et al.*, Schistosome infection in humans, perspective and recent findings, Ann. Int. Med 1982; 97:740.
7. Homeide M., *et al.*, Morbidity associated with S. mansoni infection determined by ultrasound, Amer. J. Trop. Med. Hyg 1988; 39: 196.
8. Homeide M., Diagnosis of pathologically confirmed symmer's periportal fibrosis by ultrasonography, A perspective bonded study, Amer. J. Trop. Med. Hyg 1988; 39:86.

9. Shankar P.S., Chest Medicine, Oxford and IBH Publ. Co (P) Ltd., New Delhi, 4th ed, 1994.
10. Crofton and Douglas's Resp. Diseases Seaton A., Seaton D and Gordon Leitch A., ED, 4th ed, 1989; Oxford University Press, Delhi.
11. Davis A and Wegner D.H.G., Multicentre trials praziquantel in human schistosomiasis; Design and technique; Bull, WHO 1979; 57:767.

PARAGONIMIASIS [PULMONARY DISTOMIASIS (ENDEMIC HAEMOPTYSIS)]

The infestation with oriental lung fluke, paragonimus westermoni of the class Trematoda can present haemoptysis and is the common cause of human infection, 10 of the 43 species can cause infection in man.[1,2]

Paragonimiasis is common in the Far East, Nigeria, Zaire, Cameroons, Latin and South America. The condition is acquired by eating raw or undercooked fresh water crabs or crayfish parasitised with an immature form of the lung. In addition to man, dog, cat, rat and pig are also definitive hosts. The disease is characterised by migration of juvenile worms to lungs in early stage and cyst formation around the worm.

Pathology

Pulmonary response to the worm is an eosinophilic granulomatous reaction which results in the formation of cystic cavities. The cysts are 1 to 3 cm in diameter and consist of reddish-brown material resembling chocolate sauce and the worm. It is surrounded by fibrosis that occurs due to healing and might have communication with the bronchii. It may get secondary infections.[1]

Clinical Features

Pulmonary infection may be asymptomatic. The respiratory symptoms may develop gradually in the form of pain in the chest, often of pleuritic nature, cough, profuse expectoration, anorexia and weight loss. Initially the symptoms are of bronchitis and the sputum is rusty in colour, later there is frank haemoptysis. It may be severe and recurrent.[3] Digital clubbing is common. The pulmonary signs are minimal and generalised crepitations are audible. The specific signs appear only if there is pneumonia or pleural effusion. However, there is absence of fever. Lung abscess occurs in cases of heavy infection. Chronic cases may be associated with severe bronchiectasis. The sputum becomes chocolate coloured and has a peculiar odour.[3] Extrapulmonary involvements include liver and splenic abscesses, epilepsy, hemianopia, optic atrophy, papilloedema etc. Cerebral calcification is detected in 50 per cent of cases.

Investigations

Chest X-ray shows shadows in the form of one or more soft infiltrates anywhere in the lung except in the apices. These are round nodular shadows, cyst like spaces, coin lesions, cavitation, fibrosis, pleural effusion or pneumothorax. Calcification may occur closely resembling that of tuberculosis and the later condition often co-exists with paragonimiasis. CT reveals round low attenuation cysts filled with gas or fluid, characteristically within the consolidation. CT may demonstrate intracystic worms also.[4,5]

Demonstration of golden-brown ova with their characteristic operculated ends in the sputum, pleural fluid or stool are diagnostic. The ova are not demonstrable in the sputum during the first three months of infestation. Fresh unstained sputum is used and the ova are better visualised by the addition of 3 to 10 per cent sodium or potassium hydroxide or 0.1 per cent sulphuric acid to the preparation. Eosinophilia is frequent and is noted early in the course of the disease.[3]

Ova can be demonstrated in sputum, pleural fluid and tissue in 75-80 per cent cases 3 months after infection. Serological tests like complement fixation, latex agglutination, counter immunoelectrophoresis and ELISA are especially useful for extrapulmonary cases.

Treatment

Praziquantel is useful drug when given in dose of 60-75 mg/kg and it is given in three divided doses in a day for 3 days. Cure is almost 100%. Resolution occurs in 3 months.[6] Bithionol (2, 2-thiobis = 4, 6-dichlorphenol) is also effective in a dose of 30 mg/kg body weight administered orally every other day on 10 to 15 occasions. They help in resolution of pulmonary infiltrates and the symptoms disappear.[3]

REFERENCES

1. Harrison's principles of internal medicine, Wilson J.D., Braunwald E., Isselbacher K.J., *et al.*, Ed, 12th ed, McGraw Hill, New York 1991.
2. Nana A., Bovornkitti; Pleuropulmonary paragonimiasis; Semi. Resp. Med 1991; 12: 46.
3. Shankar P.S., Chest Medicine, Oxford and IBH Publ. Co (P) Ltd., New Delhi, 4th ed, 1994.
4. Singh T.S., *et al.*, Pulmonary paragonimiasis: Trans Roy Soc Trop Med Hyg 1986; 80: 967-70.
5. Im J.G., *et al.*, Pleuropulmonary paragonimiasis; radiological findings in 71 patients; Amer J Roentgenol 1992; 159: 39-43.
6. Johnson R.J., *et al.*, Paragonimiasis, Diagnosis and use of Praziquantel in treatment, Rev Inf. Dis 1985; 7: 200.

TOXOPLASMOSIS

An uncommon disease caused by a protozoan, Toxoplasma gondii, which may be congenital or acquired. Often the condition is noted in compromised host.[1] This term is given to the disease caused by the protozoan T. gondii. Besides this, asymptomatic infection with this organism is quite common.[2] It is a worldwide infection,[3] 3-60% of healthy adults in India, 3-70% in USA and 1.5-50% HIV infected patients suffer from toxoplasmosis.[4,5,6]

Aetiological Agents

This obligate intercellular parasite is found in 3 morphologic forms *viz.* trophozoite, oocyst and cyst. The trophozoite is an oval structure measuring approximately 5 um. During acute infection they may be found in all human tissues except the red blood cells. The oocyst is founded in the mucosa of the intestine of the cat family and is excreted in the faeces. These mature within 2 to 3 days and become infectious to man and all animals. Ingestion of animal tissue by carnivores (especially brain, heart and skeletal muscle where organism most often localize) is an important mode of transmission.

Transmission and Life Cycle

Transmission of the disease to man take place through three routes—oral, transplacental and by transfusion.

Oral transmission can occur chiefly in two ways firstly, ingestion of meat contaminated by cysts and secondly ingestion of material contaminated by cat faeces containing oocysts.

Transplacental transmission results when the mother acquires toxoplasmosis during the pregnancy in question. The mother may be asymptomatic (more often the case) and yet transmit the disease. Congenital form predominantly involves CNS and eyes.

Blood and blood products (particularly leucocytes) may very occasionally transmit disease. Particularly affected are immunodeficient patients or those requiring multiple transfusions.

The most common route of entry is thus the gastrointestinal tract. Cysts or oocysts enter through the mucosa, multiply, disrupt the cells and attack neighbouring cells. These are then carried via the blood stream and the lymphatic system to all the organs of the body. The trophozoites proliferate in various organs and are capable of causing foci of necrosis and intense inflammation. The humoral and cell-mediated immune responses of the patients determines the outcome of this initial acute process. In patients with a normal response, trophozoites disappear from the tissues but cysts generally persist leading to chronic infection. In immunocompromised individuals, the acute infection may result in encephalitis, pneumonitis or myocarditis and thus leads to death.

Pathology

Changes may be seen in various organs, but the lymph nodes, eyes and central nervous system show the maximum changes. The lymph nodes show areas of reactive follicular hyperplasia and clusters of epitheloid histiocytes encroaching on the borders of the highly active germinal centres. Foci of necrosis may be seen and trophozoites are demonstrated on staining with Wright's stain.

When the infection is widespread, organs such as heart, lungs, kidney and skeletal muscle may show similar changes. In the lungs, the organisms invade alveolar cells and endothelial cells and elicit a granulomatous reaction with central necrosis.

Clinical Presentation

In immunocompetent individuals, besides fever, sore throat, malaise and rash, lymphadenopathy is the most common mode of presentation. The infection goes unnoticed in 80-90 of healthy cases both adults and children according to data from serological survey.[7] Nearly 20 per cent of pregnant women become symptomatic although transmission of infection in a placental route is relatively more frequent.

Lymphadenopathy is seen in 20 per cent cases, 1 to 3 weeks after exposure and generalized lymphadenopathy occurs in 30 per cent of symptomatic cases.[8]

Unusual manifestations include refractory fever of prolonged duration retichoroiditis (unilateral), pneumonitis with effusion, pericarditis and myocarditis (Table 4.35). Non-cardiopulmonary involvement includes hepatitis, Guillain-Barré Syndrome, meningoencephalitis, intracerebral lesion etc.

On the other hand, the immunocompromised patient[9] presents most often with central nervous system involvement. Thus in patients with lymphoreticular neoplasms, organ transplants or on immunosuppressive therapy, the onset of symptoms or signs related to the central nervous system warrants a search for toxoplasma as the causative agent as 25-80 per cent of cases of encephalitis or brain abscess in AIDS are caused by T. gondii. Myocarditis and pneumonitis may also be seen in such individuals. There is unproductive cough with dyspnoea. Chest auscultation records crepitations. Lymphadenopathy may not be present. Hepatosplenomegaly, rash, or collitis often occurs in acute form in AIDS patients. In case of reactivated toxoplasmosis, the symptoms depend on the site of cyst breaking, release of trophozoites into the tissue and the resultant inflammatory response. Although various dysfunctions like pneumonitis, retinitis, orchitis occurs, CNS manifestations[10,11] are the frequent presentation of this reactivated toxoplasmosis in AIDS, in almost 30 per cent cases.

Lung involvement is uncommon without CNS involvement. Concomitant infections include pneumocystis carinii and cystomegaloviral infections.[12]

Table 4.35: Toxoplasmosis: Clinical features
1. Fever, sore throat, rash, malaise, headache, unproductive cough and dyspnoea.
2. Conjunctivitis, lymphadenopathy, CN S involvement, pericarditis, myocarditis, pneumonitis with effusion.

Laboratory Diagnosis

Laboratory diagnosis can be made by either of the following methods: There is lymphocytosis and they appear as typical mononuclear cells.

a. Innoculation of leucocytes, body fluids, blood or tissue specimens, subcutaneously or intraperitoneally into mice helps in isolating the organism. The samples should be inoculated immediately without freezing or treatment with formation, both of which destroy the organism. The mice are tested for organisms in their intraperitoneal fluid a week after innoculation or earlier if they die. Mice that survive for 6 weeks should be tested for antibody in the serum or their brain histology should be studied for cysts. As a general rule isolation of T. gondii from body fluids may be interpreted as a sign of acute infection while isolation from tissues obtained by biopsy only reflects the presence of cysts and does not prove that the infection is acute.
b. Examination of tissue sections and smears of body fluids can help to establish a histological diagnosis. Trophozoites require special scans for their demonstration and their presence indicates acute infection. On the other hand, demonstration of tissue cysts does not differentiate between acute and chronic infection. However, in lymphadenitis, the histopathological picture is quite characteristic.[13]
c. Serologic tests are used very often to establish the diagnosis. These tests include the indirect fluorescent antibody test (IFA) (positive within a week of infection) and the indirect fluorescent antibody test Sabin-Feldman dye tests (SFDT) both of which measure IgG antibodies. IgG antibody simply indicates prior infection and does not have any casual relation with the current signs and symptoms of infection. Rising titre during the initial stage of infection of IgM anti-toxoplasma antibody will facilitate the diagnosis of an evolving lesion.[14] Both the latter mentioned tests become positive within 6 to 8 weeks of infection. Even a complement fixation (CF) assay can be performed. IgG fluorescent antibody IgG-IFA assay and more sensitive, double sand with enzyme linked immunosorbent technique (DS-IgM-ELISA) can be used. IFA and IgM-IFA may be falsely positive in the presence of rheumatoid factor or antinuclear antibodies. Computed tomography is quite informative in cases of CNS involvement, especially in encephalitis. But it is occasionally normal in initial stages where MRI can demonstrate the lesion.
d. Radiologically, patchy opacities may be seen.
e. BAL and open lung biopsies are useful in diagnosing toxoplasmosis.[15]

Management

Of the drugs mentioned below, only sulfadiazine may be used in pregnancy since pyrimethamine is teratogenic.

The drugs used are:

a. *Pyrimethamine:* In a dose 2 mg/kg body weight (loading dose) for the first 2 to 3 days followed by 1 mg/kg body weight (maintenance dose). The drug is a folic acid antagonist and prolonged administration may lead to megaloblastic anaemia. Concomitant use of folinic acid or bakers' yeast prevents this side effect. Folic acid should not be used since it interferes with the action of the drug on the parasite.
b. *Sulfadiazine*: In a loading dose of 50-75 mg/kg body weight followed by a total daily dose of 100 mg/kg body weight in four divided doses.
c. Tetracyclines 250 mg 6 hourly are also useful. In congenital toxoplasmosis and in reactivated cases, clindamycin and spiramycin are more beneficial drugs.

Irrespective of presence of signs and symptoms of congenital toxoplasmosis, all infected infants should be treated (for active or subclinical disease) to prevent the likelihood of subsequent manifestations of the symptomatic toxoplasmosis.[15] The therapy with the combination is effective in 70 per cent cases in 4 weeks. Clindamycin is also effective in choroid involvement. In immunodeficient patients,[16] the sulfadiazine and pyrimethamine combination gives complete resolution 60-80 per cent cases but relapse is frequent. The addition of clindamycin or spiramycin and glucocorticoids gives better response but at present, there is insufficient experience to recommend these in routine.

Prevention

Heating of meat or freezing it below 20°C kills cysts. Proper hand washing, boiling of water and observing precautions to prevent contamination of food with cat faeces prevents transmission of oocysts. Ideally, donor blood should be screened for toxoplasma antibodies. It is also reasonable to screen blood and organ donor for antibody to T. gondii in seronegative immunodeficient and transplant recipients.

As yet no vaccine is available.

REFERENCES

1. Shankar P.S., Toxoplasmosis, In: Chest Medicine; Oxford and IBH Pbl. Co (P) Ltd. N. Delhi 1994: 4th ed.
2. Sainani G.S., Rarer parasitic disease, J. App. Med 1983; 9: 759-61.
3. Mandal G.L., *et al.*, ED; Principles and practice of infectious diseases; 4th ed; Churchill Livingstone, Edinburgh 1995; 2455-75.
4. Bhopale G.M., Naik S.R., Toxoplasmosis in India; Practitioner 1992; XLV: 237-44.
5. Luft B.J., Remington J.S., Toxoplasmosis encephalitis in AIDS; Clin Infect. Dis 1992; 15: 211-12.
6. Israelski D., Remington J., Toxoplasmosis in non-AIDS immunocompromised host; IN; Remington J., Schwartz M. ED: Curr Clin Topics in Infect Dis; Blackwell Scient. Publ. Boston 1993; 13: 322-56.
7. Brooks R.G., *et al.*, Role of serology in the diagnosis of toxoplasmic lymphadenopathy, Rev. Infec, Dis 1987; 9: 1055.
8. Mccabe R.E., *et al.*, Clinical spectrum in 107 cases of toxoplasmic lymphadenopathy, Rev. Inf. Dis 1987; 9: 754.
9. Wadia R.S., *et al.*, Neurological manifestations of HIV disease; JAPI 2001; 49: 343-48.
10. Conley F., Remington J.S., An outbreak of CNS toxoplasmosis; in West Europe and North America; Lancet 1983; I:781.
11. Israelski B.M. and Remington J.S., Toxoplasmic encephalitis in patients with AIDS, Inf. Dis. Clin. North Amer 1988; 2:429.
12. Young L.S., Protozoal infections in lungs in immuno suppressed patients; Sem. Resp. Infect 1986; 1: 186.
13. Dorfman R.F., Remington J.S. and Isrrelbecher K.J., *et al.*, Flassion, Principles of informal medicine, 12th ed., Vol. 1: 1991; McGraw Hill, N.York.
14. Sati Adya, *et al.*, Serodiagnosis of toxoplasmosis in Calcutta; JAPI 1997; 45: 376-378.
15. Daffos F., *et al.*, Prenatal management of 746, pregnancies at risk for congenital toxoplasmosis, N. Eng, J. Med 1988; 318:271.
16. Israelski B.M. and Remington J.S., Toxoplasmic encephalitis in patients with AIDS, Inf.Dis. Clin. North Amer 1988; 2: 429.

ASPERGILLOSIS

Among the notable saprophytic and commensal organisms of the human host that have become increasingly pathogenic are the ubiquitous fungi of the genus aspergillus.[1] The members of this genus are widely distributed from temperate regions to tropics. The fungal conidia are found in the soil, water and air. Humans, animals, plants as well as food can be always and continuously exposed to the aspergilli conidia.[2] Aspergillus species may cause superficial infection of skin and mucous membrane, but in the lungs it may manifest as actual inhalational pneumonia, saprophytic colonisation or bronchopulmonary aspergillosis (ABPA) or invasive pulmonary aspergillosis.[3] Recently it has been described that invasive pulmonary aspergillosis can affect the lung without any systemic or local disorder, therefore, termed as primary invasive pulmonary aspergillosis.[4]

The clinical manifestations[5] following inhalation of fungus depends on the immunological reactivity of the individual and present as hypersensitivity reaction (bronchial asthma, allergic bronchopulmonary aspergillosis and extrinsic allergic alveolitis), invasive aspergillosis and saprophytic colonisation (aspergilloma). However, presence of the fungi in the respiratory passages without producing any symptoms especially in bronchitics and asthmatics has been documented and may be detected on routine examination of the sputum.

Hypersensitivity Reaction

Allergic Aspergillic Sinusitis

Inhalation of aspergillic antigen gives rise to sneezing, nasal blockage and watery nasal discharge. On examination, nasal mucosa is erythematous, ulcerated and frontal and maxillary sinuses are hazy.[5]

Bronchial Asthma

The inhaled aspergillus antigen on contact with specific IgE fixed to mast cells within the airways produces allergic bronchial asthma in atopic individuals. There is cough and sputum associated with bronchospasm. The symptoms are worse in autumn and winter when the spores are present in plenty. These individuals demonstrate positive immediate hypersensitivity skin test to aspergillus species and peripheral eosinophilia. Transient shadows are seen on X-ray chest.

Allergic Bronchopulmonary Aspergillosis (ABPA)

Aspergilli can penetrate and colonise in the medium sized bronchi, where their growth results in an increased amount of antigen locally and brings a hypersensitivity reaction mediated through reaginic and precipitin antibodies. The condition is referred to as allergic bronchopulmonary aspergillosis and is noted in atopic asthmatic individuals. There is no tissue invasion.

Pathogenesis[6]

The disease process begins with the inhalation of A. fumigatus spores, which are trapped by secretions in the bronchi. As the fungi germinate and form vegetative elements (hyphae), they continuously shed antigenic material in the respiratory tissues which in turn raises IgE levels. The bronchial wall damage and pulmonary eosinophilic infiltration occurs as a result of a chain of immunological reactions, initiated by the combination of antigens released by the hyphae and the IgE and IgG antibodies. The IgE enhances the tissue damaging effect of IgE precipitating antibody. Presence of mononuclear cells infiltrate, granulomata, multinucleate giant cells, chronic inflammatory cells and prominent eosinophilic material in the lungs further favours that an immunological process is involved in allergic bronchopulmonary aspergillosis (ABPA).[7] It is suggested to consider the possibility of ABPA in patients of cystic fibrosis who develop asthma. Environmental factors play no role in primary pathogenesis in causing ABPA.[8]

Pathology[6]

There are two distinct pathological processes:

1. Dense eosinophilic infiltration of pulmonary parenchyma, which is responsible for the characteristic fleeting peripheral radiographic shadows and
2. The bronchial occlusion by mucus plugs infiltered with aspergillus hyphae, causing distal collapse in the chest X-ray. The size of the impacted bronchus determines the extent of the collapse. Proximal bronchiectasis mainly affecting the upper lobes is a sequelae to immunopathological changes and is the major cause of morbidity in ABPA. Histologically, bronchi contain mucus, fibrin, Curschman's spirals, Charcot-Leyden crystals, eosinophils and mononuclear cells.[9]

Patterson *et al.* recognize five stages of ABPA which also indicate their management.[10,11]

Stage 1: Acute stage characterised by typical radiological manifestations and laboratory evidence of aspergillus sensitivity.

Stage 2: A stage of remission in which corticosteroid therapy results in control of asthma, clearing of the chest X-ray and a decrease in the levels of IgE and eosinophilia.

Stage 3: A stage of exacerbation but may not be symptoms producing; there is a rise in IgE levels and X-ray chest may reveal evidence of mucus plugging.

Stage 4: Stage characterised by corticosteroid dependent asthma, which is controlled, with off and on acute exacerbations of ABPA; there is a rise in precipitins, specific IgE and IgG and in total IgE.

Stage 5: A fibrotic stage due to long standing ABPA; characterised by bronchiectasis, fibrosis and functional airway obstruction, not responding to corticosteroids. The rise in precipitins and IgE occurs only during acute episode of ABPA.[12]

Clinically ABPA is characterised by febrile episodes, paroxysmal attacks of breathlessness, wheeze, cough and expectoration, malaise, anorexia and myalgia. Radiological examination shows rapidly fleeting non-segmental pulmonary infiltrates from probable eosinophilic pneumonia mostly in upper lobes or shadows from collapse-consolidation of segments or lobes from impaction of mucoid plugs in the bronchus. Conventional linear tomography is more sensitive than plain radiograph in detecting ABPA.[13] Computerised tomography is useful in assessing lung damage but bronchography gives better details of distribution of bronchiectasis. However, it is not routinely indicated as is potentially dangerous.[14] Since Bennet's first description of pulmonary aspergillosis in man[15] various manifestations of aspergillus lung have been described.[3,4] Nevertheless, the detection of antibodies remains the only serologic test available for detection of most fungal diseases.[16] Although many tests for serum antibodies are of limited clinical usefulness, those for coccidiodomycosis, aspergilloma and bronchopulmonary aspergillosis are quite reliable. Nevertheless, not a single test is completely specific or sensitive to diagnose ABPA.[17] Since first description ABPA in 1952, certain criteria for diagnosis of ABPA which later modified in 1985,[18] have been laid down i.e. history of asthma, eosinophilia, pulmonary infiltrates, positive serology and central bronchiectasis are quite common. The diagnosis of central bronchiectasis can be made either on plain X-ray or bronchogram occasionally. ABPA is the single largest manifestation of pulmonary aspergillosis. A recent report in Indian literature has suggested that appearance of new shadows in a patient of pulmonary tuberculosis may be due to ABPA.[19] Incidence in India has been reported varying from 5.4%, 8% and 20%.[20-22]

Eosinophilia is noted both in the sputum and in the peripheral blood. The specimens included sputum, bronchial aspirate, lung tissue following biopsy and resection. In case of sputum samples early morning specimens are collected on three consecutive days in sterile wide mouth bottles and examined by an experienced mycologist.[23] All the specimens are subjected to direct microscopic examination (KOH, Gram's and ZN-stain). Subsequently they are cultured on Sabourd's glucose agarslants in duplicate and incubated at room temperature and at 37°C for a maximum period of 10 days with daily observation. The aspergillus isolates are identified at genus and species level according to Raper and Fennel.[24] The double diffusion (DD) and counter immunoelectrophoresis (CIE) tests are performed according to standard methods.[25-27] The bands formed following DD or CIE are counted as these may help to differentiate between

ABPA and aspergilloma.[28] The antigens for the serological tests can be prepared according to Bardana, *et al.,*[25,28] using A. niger, A. fumigatus, A. flavus and A. nidulans isolated from the sputa of patients. The sputum may contain solid, brownish plugs and the aspergillus mycelium may be demonstrated using PAS or silver methenamine stain and cultured.

Allergic bronchopulmonary mycosis (aspergillosis) can well be earlier diagnosed in suspected asthma cases by HRCT scan.[28] Sensitivity and specificity of various tests are shown in the following table.

S.No.	Investigation	Sensitivity	Specificity
1.	Eosinophil count > 350/mm^3	90	26
2.	Serum IgE > 1000 ng/ml	80	96
3.	Chest X-ray infiltrate	100	63
4.	Isolation of fungus	30	80
5.	Central bronchiectasis on CT scan	100	100

There is immediate (within 10 minutes) wheal and flare reaction and six hours later oedematous cutaneous hypersensitivity reaction after challenge with antigen. Non-specific positive reaction may be seen in one third of cases, possibly due to coexisting diseases like tuberculosis, rheumatoid arthritis, bronchogenic carcinoma etc.[16,17] Serum IgE levels both total and specific are increased significantly as has been demonstrated.[29,30] IgE and IgG precipitating antibodies to aspergillus antigen are strikingly elevated.

The condition which is single largest manifestation of pulmonary aspergillosis,[17] recurs periodically with plugs of mucus, mycelium and eosinophil cells obstructing the segmental brochi leading to bronchiectasis and fibrosis with great disability. A central bronchiectasis may be seen in plain X-ray. Bronchogram in such cases shows proximal saccular (central) bronchiectasis with normal peripheral filling.[5] Miliary muttling with peripheral eosinophilia and atypical symptoms can be due to due to ABPA, rather than TB.[31,32] The treatment is aimed at removal of the fungi from the airways and reducing the inflammation. IgE levels are also decreased.[18] Aerosolised antifungal drugs such as nystatin 25,000 units/ml, brilliant green 1/5000, primarcin 1 mg/ml have been tried without much success. Corticosteroids are indicated during severe spasm.Continuation of steroids, delay in treatment and dissemination of infection to central nervous system or subcutaneous tissues may have poor outcome and can be fatal in 13 weeks. Treatment with ketocanazole for one year brings significant improvement in of asthmatic symptoms. For acute phase, corticosteroids for 6-8 weeks, and 200 mg/day itraconazole for 12-16 weeks is recommended.[27]

Extrinsic Allergic Alveolitis

Extrinsic allergic alveolitis due to aspergillus clavatus is noted in brewers as malt worker's lung. There are precipitin antibodies against aspergillus in most of the patients.[5]

Invasive Aspergillosis

Invasive aspergillosis occurs mostly in severely immuno-compromised host.[33-35] There can be blood borne dissemination of the fungus and occurrence of metastatic abscesses throughout the body. Often it occurs as a terminal event. Inhalation of nystatin or systemic amphotericin B in large doses and rifampicin may be used in the management. Recently report on invasive pulmonary aspergillosis in non-immunocompromised patients has appeared.[36]

Indian experience includes aspergillosis as well as nocardiosis in patients on immunosuppressive drugs, the incidence of deaths due to such infections accounting for 40 per cent or more.[37,38] Metastatic as well as cavitatory lung lesions have been reported.[37-39] Clinical presentation includes fever (90 per cent cases), pleuritic chest pain (50 per cent) haemoptysis (30 per cent) cases. Radiologically nodular opacitis of 1-3 cm size, cavitating in 50 per cent of cases within 10-14 days are seen and is of good prognostic value.[40] Radiological findings, thus, range from bilateral diffuse pulmonary opacities to extensive pulmonary cavitation. When radiographic features are non-specific and fungal cultures are negative, CT findings of one or more fluffy, inflammatory masses of nodules are diagnostic of invasive fungal disease. A classical feature of these early lesions is the 'halo sign'.[41,42] Each rounded shadow is surrounded by a discrete zone or halo with attenuation slightly lower than the centre of the mass, but higher than the surrounding uninvolved lung. In fact CT appearance gives picture of the pathophysiology of the aspergillus lung infection. Aspergillus fungus invades pulmonary blood vessels causing hemorrhagic infarction of lung tissue. The 'halo sign' represents the zone of hemorrhage and hemorrhagic infarction surrounding the infection focus. Progress in these changes can be used to monitor therapy.[43]

Profound neutropenia is the most common predisposing feature in invasive aspergillosis.[44] Classically, patients receiving cytotoxic chemotherapy for acute haematological malignancy, recipients of organ transplants, and those on high doses of systemic corticosteroids[45] are mostly at risk. Chronic granulomatous disease, alcoholism, influenza, diabetes, and parenteral antibiotics have also occasionally been implicated as predisposing factor.[46-49] Though corticosteroids enhance tissue damage and invasion,[45] it is unlikely that they predisposed to the disease, though they may have influenced the outcome. The role of inhaled steroids have been shown to increase the incidence of superficial fungal infection and may possibly predispose to invasive disease.

Alcohol abuse is known to be a risk factor[47] presumably by affecting the function of neutrophils[50] and macrophages.[51] There are few published case reports of invasive pulmonary aspergillosis after influenza in patients not receiving immunosuppressive treatment.[48-52] The mechanism by which influenza predisposes to invasive pulmonary aspergillosis is unknown but may involve suppression of cell mediated immunity.[53]

Prolonged use of antibiotics in predisposing to invasive aspergillosis is less clear. The persistence of fever during antibiotic treatment may be a more reliable index of fungal disease than is duration of antibiotic treatment.[54]

An association between building work and outbreaks of invasive aspergillosis is recognised.[55] Isolating filamentous fungi in sputum from non-neutropenic patients is usually to reflect colonisation and not invasion. Chronic lung disease and cigarette smoking have, however, been associated with high colonisation rates,[56] so the presence of aspergillus in the sputum should not be used to diagnose invasive pulmonary aspergillosis but should arouse suspicion in a patient with progressive lung infiltrates. Sputum cultures is positive in 8-34 per cent cases, while BAL increases the yield in 50-60% of cases. Bronchoscopy should be performed as early as possible in immunocompromised patients with pneumonias because early diagnosis paves for effective management. Bronchoalveolar lavage fluid can be a rapid and effective technique for diagnosing invasive pulmonary aspergillosis in immunocompromised patients with new pulmonary infiltrates.[57] This technique, however, may not distinguish colonisation from invasion in non-immunocompromised patients.

There is much controversy about using transbronchial and open lung biopsy in managing patients with pulmonary infiltrates. Biopsy may yield a diagnosis and leads to a change in treatment in upto 45 per cent of patients,[58] but this may not influence clinical outcome.[58-59]

Detecting aspergillus antigen in serum and urine by enzyme linked immunosorbent assay (ELISA) has recently been shown to predict the onset of invasive pulmonary aspergillosis in profoundly neutropenic patients after treatment for leukaemia and bone marrow transplantation with positive and negative predictive values of greater than 95 per cent.[60] At present these assays are not currently used in immunocompetent patients.

Lung biopsy is gold standard test. BAL with bronchoscopy and transbronchial biopsy also offer good diagnostic yield. Genexpert and Bactec Culture for M. tuberculosis, glactomawan assay for aspergillus supp and 1,3 β-D-glucan for pneumocytis jiroveci can help in diagnosing. Early HRCT is a useful adjuvant in diagnosing opportunistic lung infections.[61]

Treatment

Amphotericin B in combination with flucytocine gives good results.[60,62] Amphotericin B is effective against all strains of A. fumigatus but has dose dependent nephrotoxicity. Flucytocine is less effective but has an additive action. Combination is the treatment of choice for disseminated aspergillosis.[61]

Aspergilloma

Aspergillus fumigatus or A. niger can develop as aspergilloma as it grows as a saprophyte in a nidus provided by damaged lung tissue as in old tubercular cavities, emphysematous bullae, lung cyst bronchiectasis, lung abscess, pneumoconiosis, suppurative pneumonia, sarcoidosis, histoplasmosis and ankylosing spondylitis.[63,64] The growth is along the walls of the cavity occupying most of the portions of the cavity and ultimately it gets detached and rolled up into a ball lying free in the cavity. The fungus grows and dies continuously depending on the prevailing conditions. The matted fungal hyphae mass embedded in fibrin is referred to as aspergilloma or mycetoma. Upper lobes of the lungs are commonly affected. The cavity has a thick fibrous wall. The fungal mass is yellow or green in colour, surrounded with fibrous tissue. At the centre, there are debris, fibrin, inflammatory cells and a network of fungal hyphae. Primary aspergilloma is an acute complication of invasive aspergillosis in an immunocompromised patient and may occur following vascular occlusion in an area of aspergillus pneumonia with a distal haemorrhagic infarct and cavitation.[65] On chest X-ray it appears as a dense round shadow in a cavity being separated by a crescentic shadow of air. The unmatched radiological and serological diagnosis has been reported to be in 7.7 per cent cases. X-ray may not be conclusive with positive serological evidence in case of aspergilloma with congenital cystic diseases of lung is reported.[24] Serology is positive in 90 per cent cases, with multiple bands[27] but may be negative.

Due to tissue necrosis, recurrent small haemoptysis may occur as the presenting symptom, otherwise, mycetoma does not produce symptoms. There is no eosinophilia. Aspergillus precipitins are demonstrable in the serum. The dead fungus sometimes may liquefy and get expectorated thus undergoing spontaneous resolution or it may get calcified. CT scan is quite useful. In acute allergic phase, areas of non-segmental consolidation are visible in bronchopulmonary aspergillosis. Serial scans reveal that the consolidation resolves to occur elsewhere. Chronic necrotizing pulmonary aspergillosis—an uncommon pulmonary infection, seen in patients with COPD, bronchiectasis, pneumoconiosis, DM, alcoholism, poor nutrition or low dose corticosteroid therapy. Often diagnosed as a case of pulmonary TB due to radiological presence of a cavity in upper zone, even in the absence of AFB; patient eventually gets diagnosed while on ATT during the course of disease with evolution of fungus ball in the cavity.[65]

Systemic antifungal therapy is not effective as the fungus is colonising an air space and not invading tissue. Aspergilloma does not require any treatment. Surgical removal with lobectomy may be indicated if there is recurrent severe haemoptysis, infection and increasing size. However, there is a risk of development of bronchopleural fistula following an operation. When the hemoptysis is life threatening and surgery is contraindicated, bronchial artery embolisation (BAE) can be useful. Pre-operative embolisation of bronchial artery circulation is recommended.[66] In those with adherent pleura, brilliant green, nystatin or pimaricin in waxy emulsion may be injected directly into the cavity. The patients with residual *open healed cavities* following tuberculosis have high risk of development of mycetoma and need to be kept under constant supervision.

REFERENCES

1. Bradana E.J. Jr., The clinical spectrum of aspergillosis. Part 2: Classification and description of saprophytic, allergic and invasive variations of human disease, Crit. Rev. Clin. Lab Sci 1980; 13: 85-159.
2. AL-Doory Y. and Wagner G.E., Aspergillosis, Illinois, Charis C. Thomas 1985; 8.
3. Tenholder M.P., Themany faces of pulmonary aspergillosis, Primary Care 1985;12:353-68.
4. Spiteri M.A., McCall J and Clarks S.W., Successful management of primary invasive pulmonary aspergillosis, Br. J. Dis. Chest 1986; 80: 297-301.
5. Shankar P.S., *Chest Medicine,* 4th Edition, Oxford and IBH Pub. Co., New Delhi 1994.
6. Rupwate R.U., Patterns of aspergillus lung disease; Lung India 1993; 11: 47-55.
7. Chan-Yenug M., *et al.,* ABPA: Clinical and pathological study of 3 cases, Chest 1971; 59: 33-39.
8. Agarwal R; *et al.,* A questionaire-based study on the role of environmental factors in ABPA; Lung India 2014; 31:232-36.
9. Ricketti A.J., *et al.,* Allergic bronchopulmonary aspergillosis; Chest 1984; 86: 773-78.
10. Patterson R., *et al.,* ABPA, Staging as an aid to management, Ann Inter Med 1982; 96: 286-91.
11. Mendelson E.B., *et al.,* Roentgenographic and clinical staging of ABPA; Chest 1985; 87: 334-39.
12. Lee T.M., *et al.* Stage V(fibrotic) ABPA: A review of 17 cases followed from diagnosis, Arch Intern Med 1987,147: 319-323.
13. Fisher M.R., *et al.,* Use of linear tomography to confirm the diagnosis of ABPA; Chest 1985; 87:499-506.
14. Cooke J.C., *et al.,* Role of computed tomography in diagnosis of bronchiectasis; Thorax 1987; 42:272-77.
15. Bennet J.H. On the parasitic vegetable structures found growing in living animals, Trans. R. Soc. Edinb 1982; 15: 277.
16. Klotz S.A., Penn R.L. and George R.B., Antigen detection in the diagnosis of fungal respiratory infections, Sem In Resp. lnf 1986; 1: 16-21.
17. Sahoo R.C., Rau P.V.P., Shivananda P.Y., *et al.,* A profile of aspergillus in lung diseases, JAPI, 1988.
18. Shankar P.S., ABPA, IN, Munjal V.P., Ed., Medicine Update, API, Bombay 1997; 7: 772-75.
19. Bedi R.S., ABPA with co-existent pulmonary tuberculosis: A case report; Lung India 1995; 13: 27-28.
20. Aggarwal A.K., *et al.,* Skin hypersensitivity and precipitating antibodies against A. fumigatus in bronchial asthma; Lung India 1989;7: 67-69.
21. Pamra S.P., *et al.,* ABPA; Ind. J. Tuber 1972; 19: 61-67.
22. Ali M.M., *et al.,* An experience with ABPA in bronchial asthma in Aligarh; Lung India 1994; 12:140-42.
23. Milne L.J.R., Practical Medical Mycology; Ed. by Collee J.G., *et al.,* In; Fungi, 13th ed. Chruchill Livingstone, Edinburgh 1989.
24. Raper K.B. and Fennell D.I. The Genus Aspergillus, Baltimore, The Williams and Wilkins Co., 1965.
25. Bardana E.J. Jr., MeClatchy J.K., Farr R.S. and Minden P., The primary interactions of antibody to components of aspergilli. II. Antibodies in sera from normal persons and from patients with aspergillosis, J. Allergy Clin. Immunol 1972; 50: 222.
26. Warnock D.W., Detection of aspergillus fungatus precepitins, a comparison of counter imumunoelectrophoresis and double diffusion, J.Clin. Path 1977; 30: 388.
27. Gupta R.K., *et al.,* ABPA: A clinical review, JAPI 2012; 60: 46-51.
28. Sarkar A., *et al.,* Occurrence of allergic bronchopulmonary mycosis in patients with asthma–An Eastern India experience; Lung India 2010; 27: 212-16.
29. Shivananda P.G., Pulmonary aspergillosis and its serologic studies; (Abst) ICMRI Bull 1992; 22:107-108.
30. Talwar P., Pathogenic fungal isolations from respiratory tract of patients with chronic lung disease and malignancies; (Abst); ICMR Bull 1994; 24: 31-32.
31. Aneja P; *et al.,* Miliary nodules–An unusual presentation of ABPA Lung India; 2014;31;285-88.
32. Agarwal R; *et al.,* A rare Cause of miliary modules-ABPA; Br J of Radiol 2009;82:e 151-54.
33. Bhatia R.S., Common pulmonary infections in AIDS; Med Update 1999; 7: 1088-90.
34. Louria D.B., Introduction and epidemiology (symposium on infection complications of neoplastic diseases (part 1) Amer. Med 1984; 76: 414-20.
35. Murray J.F., *et al.,* Pulmonary complications of AIDS, An uppdate, Amer. Rev. Resp. Dis 1987;135: 504-509.
36. Hovenden J.L., Nicklason F. and Barnes R.A., Invasive pulmonary aspergillosis in non-immunocompromised patients; BMJ 1991; 302: 583-84.
37. Varma P.P., Chugh S., Gupta K.C., *et al.,* Invasive pulmonary aspergillosis and nocardiosis in an immunocompromised host; JAPI 1993; 41: 237-38.
38. Soman R.M., Pulmonary infections in the immuno-compromised host, JAPI 1991; 39: 633-36.
39. Rubin R.H., Pneumonia in the immunocompromised host; In; Fishmen A.P., ed; Pulmonary diseases and disorders; New York, McGraw Hill 1988; 1745-1760.
40. Filice G.A. and Armstro S., Actinomycosis, Arachinia and Nocardia; In: Fishman A.P., ed, Pulmonary diseases and disorders; New York; McGraw Hill 1988; 1597-1603.
41. Khulman J.E., *et al.,* Invasive pulmonary aspergillosis in acute leukemia: Characteristic findings CT, the CT halo sign and the role of CT in early diagnosis, Radiology 1985; 157:611-14.
42. Kuhlman J.E., *et al.,* Invasive pulmonary aspergillosis in acute leukemia. The contribution of CT to early diagnosis and aggressive management; Chest 1987; 92: 95-99.

43. Kuhlman J.E., *et al.*, CT of invasive pulmonary aspergillosis: Pictorial assay, Amer J Radiol 1988; 150: 1015-20.
44. Gerson S.L., Tailbot G.H., Hurwitz S., Strom S., Lusk E.J. and Cassileth P.A., Prolonged granulocytopenia, the major risk factor for invasive pulmonary aspergillosis in patients with acute leukemia. Ann. Intern. Med 1984; 100: 345-51.
45. Rinaldi M.G., Invasive aspergillosis, Rev Infect Dis 1983;5: 1061-77.
46. Lazrus G.H. and Neu H.M., Agents responsible for infection in chronic granulomatous disease of childhood. J. Pediatr 1975; 86: 415-17.
47. Karam G.H. and Griffin F.M., Invasive pulmonary aspergillosis in non-immunocompromised, non-neutropenic hosts, Rev. Infect. Dis 1986; 3: 357-63.
48. Horn C.R., Wood N.C. and Hughes J.A., Invasive aspergillosis following post-influenzal pneumonia, British Journal of Diseases of the Chest 1983; 77: 407-10.
49. D'Silva H., Burke J.F. and Cho S.Y., Disseminated aspergillosis in an apparently immunocompetent host. JAMA 1982; 248: 1495-97.
50. Ascah K.J., Hyland R.H., Hytcheon M.A., *et al.*, Invasive aspergillosis in a "healthy" patient, Can. Med. Assoc. J 1984; 131;332-335.
51. Louria D.B., Almy T.O., Susceptibility to infection during experimental alcohol intoxication. Trans. Assoc. Am. Physicians 1963; 76: 102-112.
52. Fischer J.J., Walker D.H., Invasive pulmonary aspergillosis associated with influenza. JAMA 1979; 241:1493-1494.
53. Scheinbherg M.A., Blacklow N.R., Goldstein A.L., Parrino T.A., Rose F.B.,Cathart E.S. Influenza: N. Engl. J. Med 1976; 294: 1208-11.
54. Gerson S.L. Talbot G.H., Luske E., Hurwitz S., Strom B.L., Cassileth P.A. Invasive pulmonary aspergillosis in adult leukemia: Clinical clues to its diagnosis J. Clin. Oncol 1985; 3: 1109-16.
55. Barnes R.A., Rogers T.R.F. Control of an outbreak of nosocomial aspergillosis by laminar air-flow isolation. J. Med. Hosp Inf 1989; 14: 89-94.
56. Yu L., Munder R.R., Poorsattar A., Significance of isolation of aspergillus from the respiratory tract in diagnosis of invasive pulmonary aspergillosis. Results from a three-year prospective study. Am. J. Med 1986; 81: 249-254.
57. Kahn F.W., Jones J.M., England D.M., The role of bronchoalveolar lavage in the diagnosis of invasive pulmonary aspergillosis. Am. J. Clin. Pathol 1986; 86: 518-23.
58. Rossiter S.J., Miller C.M., Churg A.M., Carrington C.B., Mark J.B.D. Open lung biopsy in the immunosuppressed patient. Is it really beneficiary? J. Thorac Cardiovasc Surg 1979; 77: 338-45.
59. McCabe R.E., Brooks R.G., Mark J.B.D., Remington J.S., Open lung biopsy in patients with a acute luekemia. Am.J. Med 1985; 78: 609-16.
60. Rogers T.R., Haynes K.A., Barnes R.A., Value of antigen detection in prediciting invasive pulmonary aspergillosis. Lancet 1990; 336: 1210-13.
61. Sharma SK; Pulmonary opportunistic infections in immune-compromised hosts; IN; SB Gupta; Ed; PG Med API; 2014; 28:525-43.
62. Rodenhuis S., *et al.*, Invasive pulmonary aspergillosis in a non-compromised patient (immunosuppressed patient), successful management with systemic amphotericin and flucytocine and inhaled amphotericin, Thorax 1984; 39:78-79.
63. Macleod D.T., *et al.*, Successful treatment of invasive pulmonary aspergillosis complicating influenza A, Brit. Med. J 1982; 285: 1166-67.
64. Glimp R.A. and Bayer A.S., Pulmonary aspergillosis; Arch Inter Med 1983; 143: 303-308.
65. Prasad R., Garg S.R., Progressive increase in cavitation with evolution of fungus ball–a clue to diagnosis of chronic necrotizing pulmonary aspergillosis; Lung India 2009; 26: 95-97.
66. Hughes C.E., *et al.*, Surgery for pulmonary aspergilloma, Preoperative embolisation of bronchial circulation, Thorax 1986; 41: 324-25.

AIDS AND LUNGS: PULMONARY COMPLICATIONS OF AIDS

Pulmonary involvement in acquired immunodeficiency syndrome (AIDS) is most common,[1,2] possibly because of defect in cell-mediated immunity. In addition, Kaposi's sarcoma may involve the lungs.[3] Most of the cases reported have come from USA, followed by Canada, France, Germany, UK and being reported from developing countries including India. It is a sex-linked disease, where infection spreads through homo or heterosexual contact apart from risk from blood and blood products and in drug-abusers.[3]

Aetiopathology

The human deficiency virus (HIV), previously called AIDS-related retrovirus (ARV), the lymphadenopathy-associated virus (LAV) or human T-cell leukemia virus (HTLV-III) is the causative pathogen.[3] It is composed of a dense icosahedral viral core containing two strands of RNA, surrounded by a membrane from host cells previously infected. The viral envelope protein and normal cell protein interact specifically. Reaching inside the cell, the virus RNA are used as a template for conversion into a double standard DNA, that enters the nucleus and gets integrated into host cell chromosome as pro-virus. It may remain as such or pass to daughter cells or synthesize new RNA particles. Lymphocytes subsets responsible for cell-mediated immunity are affected by HIV as it attaches to the CD_4 + cells. Here it captures the genetic mechanism of CD + lymphocytes that is designed for protection against the microbial invasion.[3]

Alterations brought about by infection lead to ultimate destruction of T-lymphocyte subsets (T_4) by inserting a DNA copy of its genome. Helper cells are also reduced (i.e. T (CD_4) cells) so is the ratio of helper-T to suppresser-T cells. The cell-mediated immune response fails as is evident by cutaneous anergy lymphopenia and absence of granuloma formation by Mycobacterium avium-complex infection in the tissues. B cells functions are affected as their ability to counteract infection is impaired. An overproduction of immunoglobulins may occur, that is responsible for escalated frequency of hypersensitivity drug reactions. The production of lymphokines as well as gamma interferon is impaired.

Clinical Presentations

With the emergence of AIDS/HIV disease, frequent use of immuno suppressants and increasing number of organ transplantations, renewed interest in tropical lung diseases has been observed.[3] Pulmonary Kaposi's sarcoma cannot be distinguished many a times from opportunistic lung infections and is generally associated with sarcomatous cutaneous involvement. Other opportunistic infections include Mycobacterium tuberculosis, Hisplasma capsulatum, Candida albicans, Toxoplasma gondii, Coccidioiodes immitis and Herpes simplex. Even pulmonary strongyloidiasis, MAC and Nocardiosis have all been listed in the table.

Pulm. Oppt Infection	Treatment
– Legionella	Levofloxacin 500 OD/Azithromycin 500 OD
– Nocardia	TMP-SMX 160/800 2 Tab. BD
– Rhodococcus equi	Macrolides, Fluoroquinolones, Rifampicin
– M. Turerculosis	ATT/Rifabutin in place of Rifampicin+ Early ART
– Non Tuberculous Mycobacteria MAC	Macrolides+H+R
M. Kaulasii	H+R+E
– CMV	Ist Ganciclovir
	2nd Forcarnet/Cidofovir
– Pneumocystis jirovecii	TMR SMX 160/800 2 Tab. BD
– Cryptococcus	Fluconazole 200 BD
– Invasive pulmonary aspergillosis	1st Voriconazole 4 mg/kg BD 2nd Amphotericin B
– Mucormycosis	Amphotericin B
– Toxoplasma	1st pyramethamine+sulfadiazine 2nd TMP+SMX
– Strongyloides stercoralis	Ivermectin 200 mg/kg/day

General symptoms like fever, fatigue and weight loss are present. Pulmonary symptoms include exertional dyspnoea and non-productive cough. Clinical look may reveal wasted and tachypnoeic presentation. Examination may reveal diffuse lymphadenopathy. Chest auscultation yields few crepitations but features of consolidation are not encountered.[4]

Investigations

Chest X-ray reveals bilateral, diffuse interstitial infiltration in case of pneumonia with P. carinii. Adenopathy, effusion and interstitial alveolar infiltration are seen in Kaposi's sarcoma. Hilar adenopathy and diffuse parenchymal infiltration are found in Cryptococcus neoformans. Atypical findings like involvement of lower lobes and lack of cavitation are the features of tuberculosis. Thus it becomes difficult to distinguish it from other opportunistic mycobacteria. The cursed duet[4-6] tuberculosis in HIV infection is more often extrapulmonary and disseminated. Therefore, chest skiagraph shows diffuse or miliary type of infiltration rather than focal or cavitational lesions.[3] Fine needle aspiration of lymph node has been suggested to be of value in the diagnosis.[7] Tuberculin skin test is negative in these patients. A positive skin test increases the chances of tuberculosis, a negative test doesn't rule out the diagnosis.[8,9]

Pulmonary functions show restrictive defect, with a decrease in the diffusing capacity for CO. Hypoxaemia and an increased alveolar to arterial oxygen tension gradient are frequent in pneumocystic pneumonia. Typical chest X-ray findings along with positive Western Blot Test have been suggested to be sufficient in making the diagnosis of AIDS, especially in developing countries.[2,10] An increased uptake of gallium-67 during lung scanning is present.[11] Identification of causative organism can be made using touch imprints from bronchoalveolar lavage fluid. Further, it may reveal high percentage of neurophils and lymphocytes in BAL fluid in contrast to decrease in lymphocytes in the blood.[3,12]

Bronchoscopy reveals a raised cherry red lesion suggestive of Kaposi's sarcoma. The lesions are focal and less cellular but more scattered throughout the pulmonary interstitium.[3]

Prognosis

Prognosis is generally grave. The risk of repeated infections, even after recovery from one pulmonary complication is high because of persistent immunodeficiency.

Treatment

Treatment depends on the aetiology. Cotrimoxazole and pentamidine are useful in *Pneumocystis Carinii* pneumonia. Pentamidine is preferred over the cotrimoxazole, keeping in view the higher rate of allergic reactions to the drugs. Rifampicin containing standard anti-tuberculosis treatment is effective in tuberculosis.[13] Amphotericin and flucytocine are affective in cryptococcal infections but sinultaneous rifampicin and isoniazid administration has a complex interaction with antifungal drugs, rendering antifungal therapy ineffective in some patients. Ganciclovir is effective in cytomegalo virus infection. Vinblastin and bleomycin are effective in Kaposi's sarcoma.[3]

Attending persons and nursing staff need wearing gowns, masks and gloves, so is important the cleansing and disinfection of instruments.

REFERENCES

1. Bhatia R.S., HIV infection, where we stand today, The Med and Surg 1990; 30: 10-11.
2. Bhatia R.S. and Deivanayagam C.N., HIV disease, The great waster upon us, (Ed); Lung India 1992; 10: 91-93.
3. Sidhu G; Pulmonary manifestations of tropical parasitic diseases; IN; A, Muruganathan; Ed; Med. update; API; 2013; 23:484-89.
4. Shankar R.S., Pulmonary complications of AIDS: In: Chest Medicine; Oxford and IBH Publ Co (P) Ltd, N. Delhi 4th ed 1994; 115-18.
5. Styblo K. The global aspects of tuberculosis and HIV infection; Bull Int. Union Tuber Lung Dis 1990; 65: 28.
6. Barnes P.F., *et al.*, TB in patients with HIV infection; N. Eng. J. Med 1991; 324: 1644.
7. Bhatia R.S., Fine needle aspiration, Simple method of diagnosing tuberculosis in HIV disease, Lung India 1993; 11: 123-124.
8. Beck J.S., Skin changes in the tuberculin test; Tubercle 1991; 72: 81.
9. Ellner J.J., Regulation of the human counter immune response to M. Tuberculosis—The mechanism of selective depression of the response to PPD; Bull Int. Union Tuber Lung Dis 1991; 66: 129.
10. Bhatia R.S. and Sibia S.S., PCP in a patient of AIDS in India, J Assn Phys India 1994; 42: 87.
11. Jeffery R.B., Current problems in Diagnostic Radiology 1988; 17: 78-89.
12. Bhatia R.S., HIV infection and tuberculosis; Ind, J Clin Pract 1995; 6(6): 57-61.
13. Fitz Gerald J.M., *et al.*, The impact of HIV infection on TB and its control; Chest 1991; 100: 191.

PNEUMOCYSTIS PNEUMONIA (PCP)

Nanek *et al.* who in 1953 recognized this infection in Europe in World War II when infants born prematurely to undernourished mothers revealed a peculiar pneumonia with granular frothy fibrillar material filling the alveoli and heavy infiltrates in the interstitial tissue.[1] As a pathologist, finding a patch of pneumocystis pneumonia (PCP) in an infant at post mortem hardly evoked any curiosity in the pre-AIDS era and nor did the finding in a child dying of cancer, or an adult organ recipient on regular immunosuppression. However, Micheal Gotleib[2] added entirely new dimensions to this infection and unlocked the secret triangle of homosexuality, PCP and Kaposi's sarcoma. Recently it is estimated upto 150,000 episodes of PCP in the USA in the next three years.[3]

First case of AIDS from India was reported in 1986.[4] By October 1989, 1650 persons had been detected to be infected with the human immunodeficiency virus (HIV) in India.[5] Forty of them have been diagnosed to have acquired immunodeficiency syndrome (AIDS), a clinical stage which is often characterized by different types of opportunistic infections and cancers. Pneumocystis carinii infection of the lungs is one of the most common opportunistic infections in these patients all over the world.[6] There could be two reasons; firstly, the disease may be actually very rare in India. Only few cases have been reported from India.[7] Six out of 39 pulmonary infection episodes in renal allograft recipients were diagnosed to be PCP on BAL in an Indian series.[8] Secondly perhaps more importantly, there may be practical problems in demonstrating this pathogen in the sputum. This could be because of scant sputum and/or technical difficulty in its identification.

Aetiology

The children and adults on immunosuppressive therapy and immunodeficiency disorders are susceptible. It occurs as an opportunistic infection in a compromised host and in acquired immunodeficiency syndrome. It is also noted in patients treated with immunosuppressive therapy and radiation for the management of organ transplants and malignancy, respectively.

The organism, Pneumocystis carinii, is round or elongated and measures 2 to 4 microns in length. Whether it is a protozoan or fungus, has been classified, using small sub unit RNA (165 like ERNA) there are now data to suggest a stronger phylogenetic link of pneumocystis with member of fungi rather than protozoal.[9,10] The various predisposing factors to this infection are primary immune defects, severe malnutrition, iatrogenic immune defects as produced by steroids, and heavy doses of either cytotoxic drugs or those used in organ recipients including cyclosporin. Patients infected with HIV-I, HTLV-I are particularly susceptible and high degree of suspicion is mandatory.[11] It is one infection where even serological evidence for HIV can be bypassed provided there is no evidence of a primary, secondary or an iatrogenic immune defect. The mode of transmission and the natural habitat of the organism are not clear. The spread is likely to occur by infected droplets. The infection is limited to the lungs. Pathogenesis of PCP, especially in AIDS is poorly understood. Poor relationship between the organism and the disease exists; specific treatment resolves the disease even though organisms persist. And steroids which trigger the infection, may improve the clinical response and cutdown the mortality rate a the same time.

Pathology

The condition may present in an epidemic or sporadic form. In an epidemic form, the lungs show areas of consolidation with the alveoli filled with a foamy eosinophilic exudate containing spherical thick walled cysts of pneumocystis. The alveolar walls are infiltrated with a large number of lymphocytes and plasma cells. Involvement of the pleura is uncommon and systemic dissemination of the organisms is unusual. In sporadic form the consolidation is focal and alveolar exudate may be absent.[12]

Histopathologically two patterns have been described; infantile form with interstitial plasma cell infiltration and adult form with rare such kind of infiltration. However, in both forms an eosinophilic intra alveolar foamy exudate is present, giving an honey combed pattern.

Diagnosis

It can be rested on a rapid onset of dyspnoea, tachypnoea, cyanosis, the *snow storm* densities on X-ray and dicyclinical signs.[13] The differing clinical presentation of PCP in HIV patient *vis-a-vis,* with malignancies has been suggested where the course is more insidious (few months) in the former.[14]

Clinical Features

There can be a sudden onset in sporadic type accompanied by fever, non-productive cough, increasing dyspnoea, lassitude, restlessness and cyanosis. Occasionally crepitations are heard. In epidemic form the manifestations develop insidiously with dyspnoea, lassitude and restlessness but fever is absent.[12] Pleural effusion and haemophtysis are distinctly uncommon.

Investigations

There are bilateral diffuse alveolar and interstitial infiltrates in mid-zone beginning from hilum. The physical signs in chest are minimal compared to the degree of radiologic shadows. Earliest visible radiological abnormality of peribronchial and perivascular cuffing due to inflammation gives rise to an ill-defined hilum. With the progress of the disease, there occurs diffuse reticular peripheral shadowing, which subsequently coalesce to form diffuse homogenous alveolar pattern extending from hilum but sparing the apices and the bases. This has been suggested sufficiently adequate with confirmatory western blot test in developing countries.[7,15] There is no leucocytosis or eosinophilia. There is severe hypoxaemia. The organism is seldom found in smears of sputum or tracheal aspirates. Percutaneous aspiration, fiberoptic bronchoscopy with lavage, brushing and transbronchial biopsy may help to demonstrate the causative agent. Open lung biopsy may be needed in some cases to confirm the diagnosis.[8,16-18]

In tissue sections they are best stained with Gomori's silver methanamine or sulphated toleudine blue reactions. Monoclonal antibodies ($2G_2$ and $6B_8$) have been generated and are of immense use for immunohistochemical localization of the organisms[19] but are too costly for routine use.[13] In smears, Geimsa stain is adequate. However, when the oral cavity is full of candida, finding PCP in the sputum may be extremely difficult.[13]

Both cysts and trophozoites can readily be harvested from patients by bronchoalveolar lavage (BAL).[20] Till recently in the West, BAL with or without transbronchial biopsy was the method of choice for a definite diagnosis. It has been documented that sputum induced by hypertonic saline nebulization[21] is far superior to unaided sputum and the sensitivity of PCP detection is further increased upto 78 per cent by addition of reducing agents such as dithiothreitol (DTT)[22] and use of monoclonal antibodies to penumocystis carinii increase sensitivity to nearly 90 per cent.[14] Though BAL remains gold standard test, HRCT in early stages has a sensitivity of 100% and specificity of 89%, when patchy or nodular ground-glass (opacity) attenuation of PCP is used to indicate PCP even when the chest radiograph is normal. Other causes of ground glass appearance on HRCT include pulmonary odema, pulmonary hemorrhage, alveolar proteinosis, sarcoidosis, extrinsic allergic alveolitis, desquamative interstitial pneumonitis but these have different clinical features. The alveolar arterial oxygen gradient ($AaPO_2$) of more than 30 mm Hg at the start of therapy is associated with a higher mortality. Elevated lactate dehydrogenase levels have been correlated with this infection.[23] Sophisticated procedures like Gallium (Ga),[11,14] citrate radioisotope scanning may reveal early changes but they are costly, time consuming and results are non-specific; thus limiting their utility in routine use.[24]

Treatment

Mortality is higher and death occurs from respiratory failure. Hypoxaemia has to be corrected by controlled oxygen therapy. Daily administration of pentamidine isethionate in a dose of 4mg/kg body weight dissolved in 2 to 3 ml of water intramuscularly for two weeks shows a beneficial response if started early. Combination of trimethoprim and sulphamethoxazole has been found effective when administered in dose of 20 mg and 100 mg/kg body weight respectively orally or intramuscularly for two weeks. It has a protective effect in low doses in high risk patients.[12] However drug reactions are severe enough to discontinue the treatment.[25] In addition, the therapy which was designed keeping in view that the organism is a protozoan, has been challenged.[26,27]

Atypical Form, Complications and Future Directions

The incidence of PCP is higher in homosexuals with heterosexual contact.[28] Other atypical features included cavitation, pneumothorax, interstitial microcalcification, vascular invasion by pneumocystis, proliferation of type II pneumocytes and of alveolar macropahges.[13]

Estimation of T helper cell pool can reliably predict the onset of infection. In 1989, Public Health Service Task Force of the U.S. confirmed the reliability of CD_4 + cell count as a predictor of PCP and recommended 3 to 6 monthly evaluation of T helper status and start of prophylaxis. When CD-4 cells fell below 200 cells per mm^3 (and/or 20 per cent of total lymphocytes), secondary prophylaxis was recommended.[29] Pneumocystis carinii infection can also extend to extrapulmonary sites and induce a granulomatous reaction. Eye lesions like choroiditis[30] have been documented and lesions are recorded in ear, skin and other freak sites. The practice of doing silver stain on tissues in all suspected cases of AIDS would go a long way in detecting such cases. Aerosolized pentamidine prophylaxis for AIDS[31] could partly be responsible for extrapulmonary manifestations. A joint forum for clinical immunologists, pathologists and radiologists to devise strategies for early detection of pneumocystis infection and offering newer modalities of prophylaxis taking into consideration the dosage of drug,[32] the frequency of administration, the mode of administration, the types of nebulizer etc. as well as combination therapy for acute episodes has been suggested.[33]

REFERENCES

1. Nanek J., Jirovee O. and Lukes J., Interstitial plasma cell pneumonia in infants, Annal. Paed 1953; 180: 1.
2. Gotteib M.S., Schroff R., Schanker H.M., Weisman J.D., Fan P.T., Wolf R.A. and Saxon A., Pneumocystis carinii pneumonia and mucosa candidiasis in previously healthy homosexual men: Evidence of a new acquired cellular immunodeficiency. N.Engl J. Med 1981; 305: 1425-31.
3. Hopewell P.C., Pneumocystis carinii pneumonia, Diagnosis. J. Infect. Dis 1988; 157: 1115-19.
4. HIV infection—ongoing studies and future research plants. ICMR Bulletin 1988; 18: 109-119.
5. HIV infection—ongoing studies and future research plants. ICMR Bulletin (Indian Council of Medical Research Publication) 1989; 19: 118.
6. Kovas J.A., Masur H., Opportunistic infections. In: De Vita VT Jr. Hellman S., Roseberg S.A., Eds. AIDS: Etiology, Diagnosis, Treatment and Prevention, London, JB Lippincott 1989; 203-05.
7. Singh Y.N., Singh S., Rattan A., *et al.*, PCP in patients of AIDS in India, JAPI 1993; 41: 41-42.
8. Jha V., Sakhuja V., Gupta D., *et al.*, Successful management of pulmonary tuberculosis in renal allograft recipients in a single centre; Kid intern 1999; 56: 1944-50.
9. Edman J.C., Kovacs J.A., Masur H., Santi D.V., Elwood H.J. and Sogin M.L., Ribosomal RNA sequence shows pneumocystis carinii to be a member of the fungi, Nature 1988; 334: 519-22.
10. Stringer S.L., Stringer J.R., Blase M.A., Walzer P.D. and Cushion M.T., Pneumocystis carinii, sequence from ribosomal RNA implies a close relationship with fungi. Exp. Parasitolo 1989; 68: 450-61.
11. Davey R.T. and Masur H., Recent advances in the diagnosis, treatment and prevention of pneumocystis carinii pneumonia: Anti-microbial agents; Chemotherapy 1990; 34(4): 499-504.
12. Shankar P.S., Chest Medicine; Oxford and IBH (P) Co. Ltd. N. Delhi 1994; 4th ed.
13. Sehgal S., Pneumocystis pneumonia, A time to shed complacence 1993; JAPI; 41: 5-7.
14. Kovacs J.A., Hiemenz J.W., Macher A.M., Stover D., Murray H.W., Shelhamer J., Lane H.C., Urmacher C., Hing C., Longo D.L., Parker M.M., Natanson C., Parillo J.E., Fauci A.S., Pizzo P.A. and Masue H., Pneumocystis carinii pneumonia: A comparison between patients with the acquired immunodeficiency syndrome and patients with other immunodeficiencies, Ann. Intern. Med 1984; 100: 663-671.
15. Bhatia R.S., Sibia S.S., PCP in a patient of AIDS in India, JAPI 1994; 42: 87.
16. Malviya A.N., Singh R.R., Khare S.D., *et al.*, AIDS screening in North India; Clinical spectrum of HIV infection. J. Assoc. Physicians India 1987; 35: 405-410.
17. Malviya A.N., Seth P., Singh R.R., *et al.*, AIDS and HIV-I screening in India, Natl. Med. J. India 1989; 2: 22-25.
18. Pintozzi R.L., Modified Grocott's methanamine silver nitrate method for quick staining of Pneumocystis carinii, J. Clin. Pathol 1978; 31: 803-05.
19. Kovacs J.A., Ng V.L., Masur H., Leoung G., Hadley W.K., Evans G., Lane H.C., Ognibene F.P., Shelhamer J., Parrillo J.E. and Gill V.J., Diagnosis of pneumocystis carinii pneumonia improved: Detected in sputum with use of monoclonal antibodies, N. Engl. J. Med 1988; 318: 589-93. '
20. Stover D.E., White D.A., Romano P.A., Gellene R.A. and Robseson W.A., Spectrum of pulmonary disease associated with the acquired immune deficiency associated with the acquired immunodeficiency syndrome, Am. J. Med 1985; 78: 429-37.
21. Pitchenik A.E., Ganjei P., Torres A., Evans D.A., Rubin E. and Baier H., Sputum examination for the diagnosis of pneumocystis carinii pneumonia in the acquired immunodeficiency syndrome, Am. Rev. Respir. Dis 1986; 133: 226-29.
22. Zaman M.K., Wooten O.J., Suprahmanya B., Ankobiah W., Finch P.U.P. and Kamholz, S.L., Rapid non-invasive Diagnosis of pneumocystic carinii from induced liquefied sputum. Ann. Intern. Med 1988; 109: 7-10.
23. Kagawa F.T., Kirsch C.M., Yenokida G.G. and Lecine M.L., Serum lactate dehydrogenase activity in patients with AIDS and pneumocystis carinii pneumonia: An adjunct to diagnosis, Chest 1988; 94: 1031-33.
24. Tuazon C.U., Delaney M.D., Simon G.L., Witroschip P. and Verma V.M., Utility of gallium scintigraphy and bronchial washings in the diagnosis and treatment of pneumocystis carinii pneumonia in patients with the acquired immune deficiency syndrome, Am. Rev. Respir, Dis 1985; 132:1078-92.
25. Fischi M.A., Dickinson G.M., Voie L.L., Safety and efficacy of sulfamethoxazole and trimethoprim chemoprophylaxis for pneumocystis carinii pneumonia in AIDS, J. Amer, Med. Assoc 1988; 259: 1185-89.
26. Bernard E.M., *et al.*, Pneunocystosis; Med. Clin. North Amer. 1992; 76: 107-19.
27. Rosha D., Dandona P.K., Pneumatocoeles in PCP of AIDS and low dose trimethoprim sulphamethoxazole therapy, JAPI 1995; 43: 635-37.
28. Travis W.D., Lack E.E., Ognibene F.P., Suffredini A.E. and Shelhamer J.H., Lung biopsy interpretation in the acquired

immunodeficiency syndrome (AIDS), Review of National Institutes of Health, Experience with literature, review, Progress in AIDS Pathology 1989; 1: 51-84.
29. Centre for Disease Control, Guidelines for prophylaxis against pneumocystis carinii pneumonia for persons infected with human immunodeficiency virus. Morbid Mortal, Weekly Rep 1989; 38 (Suppl. 5-5): 1-9.
30. Dugel P.U., Rao N.A., Forster D.J., *et al.*, Pneumocystic carinii choroiditis after long term aerosolized pentamidine therapy, Am. J. Opthalmol 1990; 110(2): 113-117.
31. MC Cabe R., Aerosolized pentamidine prophylaxis; Chest 1991; 1: 186.
32. Armastong D., Gold J.W.N., Dryjansk J., *et al.*, Treatment of infection in patients with AIDS; Ann. Int. Med 1985; 103, 738-43.
33. Bhatia R.S., Common pulmonary infections in AIDS; Med. update 1999; 7(4):1088-90.

NOCARDIOSIS

Nocardial infections are the uncommon opportunistic infections[1] occurring especially in patients with impaired immunity. However, they have also been reported in individuals without any immunological disorders.[2] The primary site of these infections is usually the lungs.[3] Pneumonia often develops, which may be lobar and lobular and is often chronic. The lesion may be solitary lung abscess, acute necrotizing pneumonia, scattered lesions mimicking miliary tuberculosis, pulmonary mycetoma, or progressive fibrosis or extending to pleura or chest wall with penetration simulating actinomycosis. Nocardiasis and actinomycosis coinfection in chronic granulomatous disease has also been documented.[4] Haematogenous spread to other parts of the body has been reported.[4] Nocardiosis—an exogenous infection from a pleomorphic aerobic actionomycete—may cause lung abscess and sometimes brain abscess.

Aetiology

Nocardia are Gram positive relatively acid fast filamentous bacterial organisms with branching at right angles. They are present in the soil. Inhalation of nocardia asteroides results in nocardiosis. It is not a contagious disease and person-to-person transmission of the infection does not occur. Often nocardiosis occurs as an opportunistic infection[1] in patients who have pulmonary alveolar proteinosis and in patients who are on immunosuppressive therapy particularly steroids. Rarely lungs may be secondarily affected following inoculation of N. brasiliensis into the skin (mycetoma, Madura foot).[5]

Pathology

Nocardial lesions show suppuration, multiple abscesses with central necrosis and relatively little surrounding fibrosis.[6] Pulmonary involvement is frequent and it may spread to the brain and subcutaneous tissues by haematogenous dissemination.[4]

Clinical Features

Nocardiosis is a systemic bacterial disease, seen in 30-50 years of age, more so in females, and may have acute, subacute or chronic forms. Acute inflammation is associated with fever, malaise, weightloss, cough and mucopurulant expectoration. Clinical presentation is almost similar to aspergillosis, but generally there is no pleuritic chest pain and haemoptysis.[7] In 60-80 per cent cases, the disease remains confined to lungs and metastatic spread to CNS occurs in 20-40 per cent cases if treatment is delayed. In that case mortality is 80 per cent.[8] Pleural spread is common and empyema occurs in one third of cases. Chronic form persists for a long time with dyspnoea and occasionally haemoptysis. Endobronchial as well as pulmonary cavitary lesions have been described.[8-10] The condition may be mistaken for tuberculosis. There can be dark coloured subcutaneous abscesses.[5] When the infection spreads to the brain,[2,10] headache and focal neurologic deficits are noted.

Diagnosis

X-ray chest shows patchy nodular opacities[8] not clearly confined to specific lobes or segments or large irregular nodules often cavitating.[7] Initial diagnosis other than pneumonia include tuberculosis, carcinoma or lung abscess. Pleural effusion is quite common and the lymph nodes may be enlarged. The causative agent may be demonstrated in the sputum. However, the appearance of the organisms is not unique in direct smear. It can be cultured on blood agar or Sabouraud's agar and the rate of growth is slow. There is no serologic test.[5]

The sputum and pus drained from the chest reveals the presence of plenty of pus cells and many gram positive branching filaments. These are subsequently shown to be acid fast by modified acid-fast staining. Culture of the pus on blood agar and L-J medium grows gram positive branching filamentous bacteria which are identified as Nocardia asteroides by negative casein and xanthine hydrolysis and positive urease test. Bronchoscopy, percutaneous lung aspiration, needle biopsy and open lung biopsy may occasionally be required.

Opportunistic infections account for 40 per cent or more deaths in immunocompromissed patents. Along with aspergillosis nocardiosis is being increasingly encountered infection.[14] Nocardia, pneumocystis and tuberculosis need strong consideration in leucopenic patients after kidney transplantation. Metastasis may occur even before the lung lesions although primary organ of involvement is the lungs. Long-term corticosteroid therapy makes the patient susceptible to the infection and to its widespread haematogenous dissemination in the body, leading to a fatal outcome. It is well-known that nocardiosis can be confused with tuberculosis at all stages of the disease. Other differential diagnosis are actinomycosis and other mycobacterial and fungal infections.

Treatment

Sulphonamides are the drugs of choice if instituted early enough and given over a prolonged period.[2] Other antimicrobial agents like cycloserine, clindamycin, erythromycin, ampicillin and recently aminoglycosides have been reported to give encouraging results.[11]

Treatment may have to be continued for 10-12 weeks in minor infections and for over one year in patients with major and disseminated infections. Success rate of 90-95 percent had been reported[12] but continuation of steroids, delay in institution or early discontinuation of treatment often leads to dissemination of the disease with metastatic abscesses[13-16] and has poor outcome.[7]

REFERENCES

1. Talwar P., Sehgal S.C., Pulmonary nocardiosis: A report of eight cases, Eur. Respir. Dis 1980; 61: 103-07.
2. Curry W.A., Human nocardiosis, A Clinical review with selected case reports, Arch Inter Med 1980; 140: 816-26.
3. Gausey W.A. and Seiger B., Systemic nocardiosis caused by N. brasiliensis, Am Rev. Respir. Dis 1974; 109: 134-37.
4. Soneja M., *et al.*, Actinomycosis and nocardiasis coinfection in chronic granulomatous disease; JAPI 2012; 60:66-68.
5. Shankar P.S., Chest Medicine; Oxford and IBH Publ. Co. (P) Ltd., New Delhi 1994; 4th ed.
6. Mathur S., *et al.*, Cytologic diagnosis of pulmonary nocardiosis—A report of 3 cases; Acta cytol; 2005;49:567-70.
7. Padmaja P., *et al.*, Nocardia asteroides colonizing bronchiectatic cavity; JAPI 2002; 50: 590-91.
8. Minero M.V.M.M., *et al.*, Nocardiasis at the turn of the century; Medicine 2009;88:250-61.
9. Tam W.O., *et al. Endobronchial nocardiasis associated with Broncholithiasis;* Monalidi Arch Chest Dis 2008;69:183-85.
10. Hather B., *et al.*, A Cavitary lesion in the lung crossing the fissure; Lung India 2011;28:222-25.
11. Kulkarni S.A. and Kulkarni A.G., Disseminated nocardiosis, JAPI 1991; 39: 779-80.
12. Soman R.M., Pulmonary infections in the immunocompromised host JAPI 1991; 39: 633-36.
13. Varma P.P., Chugh S. and Gupta K.L., Invasive pulmonary aspergillosis and nocardiosis in an immunocompromised host, JAPI 1993; 41: 237-238.
14. Diamond R.S. The growing problem of mycosis in patients infected with HIV; Rev. Inf. Dis 1991; 13: 480.
15. Jha R., *et al.*, Pulmonary infections after kidney transplantation; JAPI 1998; 47: 779-83.
16. Rubin R.H., *Pneumonia in the immunocompromised host;* In: Fishman A.P., (ed) Pulmonary disease and disorders; N. York, McGraw Hill 1988; 1745-60.

ACTINOMYCOSIS

It is a chronic suppurative and granulomatous infection by actionomyces israelii, ulcerated, cristed skin lesions are common in United States.[1]

Aetiology

The organism—Actinomyces israelii—is a slow growing, gram positive, anaerobic, branching filamentous bacterium. It exists as a normal flora in the oral cavity. The infection is endogenous in origin and tends to invade the tissues when they are damaged.[2] The condition is not contagious. However, it spreads by contiguity and rarely hematogenously.

Pathology

The organisms can invade the lungs, pleura, ileocaecal and pelvic regions and rarely the liver. The face and neck are the common sites of infection.[3] The infection is associated with a firm indurated swelling, followed by necrosis in the later stages. The lymph nodes are not involved.

Lung infection results from inhalation of infected material mostly from poor orodental hygiene or oral trauma, and rarely it spreads by contiguity from other regions.[4] Haematogenous spread occurs from an initial pulmonary lesion following aspiration of mouth contents.[5,6] The lower lobes especially in the periphery are affected and there are dense fibrotic lesions[7] with abscess formation in the centre, containing granulation in abundance. Around the colonies of actinomyces, there is infiltration of polymorphs, lymphocytes and fibroblasts. Later on pleura and the chest wall are affected and results in discharging sinuses with characteristic pus containing sulphur granules,[4] seen in one third of cases and pulmonary parenchymal lesion may mimick bronchogenic carcinoma or tuberculosis.[8]

Clinical Features

The condition is seen in the age group of 20 to 50 years, predominantly in men. The thoracic actinomycosis is seen in 15 per cent of cases compared to 60 per cent cervicofacial cases. The manifestations begin insidiously starting with cough, fever, and weight loss. Since symptoms are non-specific, diagnosis is difficult. With the formation of abscess there is mucopurulent expectoration. Flaemoptysis secondary to actinomycosis has been documented.[9] The spread to the pleura results in empyema and it may discharge pus to the exterior in the form of sinuses.[4]

Investigations

X-ray chest shows irregular opacity in the lower zones with pleural effusion. There can be extensive bilateral patchy pneumonitis[8] as diffuse consolidation or there can be cavitation, empyema or fibrosis on chest film. The condition may be unilateral or bilateral. There is characterisitic periosteal reaction with new bone formation in the under surface of ribs. Sulphur granules may be demonstrated in the pus, and from the sinus, empyema or abscess cavity. Microscopy reveals the presence of radiating filaments from the central part of the granules and their ends are clubbed (ray fungus).[4] Cultures are positive only in 25 per cent of cases. Differential diagnosis include tuberculosis, other causes of empyema and bronchogenic carcinoma.

Treatment

Actinomycosis responds to benzyl penicillin given in a dose of 1 to 2 mega units intravenously daily for a longer period[10] from three to four weeks followed by intramuscular or oral penicillin for another six weeks. Persistent pulmonary shadows must draw differential diagnosis of actinomycosis as is highly treatable with benzyl penicillin, and obviates unnecessary surgery. Tetracycline, erythromycin or clindamycin are also effective. Lung resection is rarely required.

REFERENCES

1. Tight R.R. and Bartleft M.S., Actinomycetomian the United States, Rev. Inf. Dis 1981;3:1139.
2. Benhof D.P., Actinomycosis: Diagnostic and therapeutic considerations and review of 32 cases; Laryngoscope 1984; 94: 1198.
3. Giumma S.A., *et al.*, Mycetoma of the head and neck, Amer. J. Trop. Med Hyg 1986;35:594.
4. Shankar P.S., Chest Medicine; Oxford and IBH Pub. Co (P) Ltd., 4th ed., 1994.
5. Hennrikus EF and Pederson L., Disseminated actinomycosis; West J Med 1987; 147: 201-204.
6. Dontfraid F. and Rampal R., Bilateral pulmonary infiltrates in association with disseminated actinomycosis; Chin. lnf. Dis 1994; 19: 143-45.
7. Filice G.A., Actinomycosis; IN; Sarosi G.A. and Davies S.F., Ed., Raven Press, N. York; 2nd ed. 1993; 181-90.
8. M.K. Goel., *et al.,* A case of disseminated actinomycosis; Lung India 1996; 14(4): 172-74.
9. Chawla RK; *et al.,* Haemophysis secondary to actinomy cosis A rare presentation; Lung India 2014; 31: 168-70.
10. Slade P.R., *et al.,* Thoracic actinomycosis; Thorax 1973; 28:73.

HISTOPLASMOSIS

Histoplasma capsulatum infection of human system produces a wide variety of clinical manifestations from short lived self limiting influenza like illness to fatal disseminated multiple organ infection and a choronic infection often pulmonary and mediastinal which very closely mimicks pulmonary tuberculosis.[1] Rarely an unusual fiberoptic lesion with progression like a mass occurs which is often confused with malignancy. This is termed as Histoplasmoma.[2] While disseminated histoplasma infections are usually reported in immunocompromised individuals, other chronic infections are super imposed over old bullous or cavitary lesions. The exact pathogenesis of histoplasmoma is not so clear except that it is thought to be due to excessive laying down of fibrous tissue and collagen due to continued antigenic stimulation around a central core of fungal lesion.[2]

The organism is a dimorphic fungus that exists in mycelial form in nature and in yeast phase in the body. The infection is acquired from soil in the river basins in temperature zones of the world, with a higher incidence in the central United States. India is a non endemic area for histoplasmosis, prevalence rate of 0-12.3% has been reported from various parts of the country by a histoplasmin skin sensitivity survey. Till 1994, only 37 cases have been documented. Lung infection is produced by inhalation of air-borne spores from the infected soil, often contaminated by bird droppings, bat, fowl and chicken excreta. The oval spores of 1 to 5 microns diameter develop in the monocytes and endothelial cells of reticuloendothelial system and the lesions so produced resemble tuberculosis.[3]

Primary Infection

In a previously non-infected individual, inhalation of H. capsulatum spores elicits a non-specific pulmonary response. The fungus grows in the alveoli and interstitial spaces and then spreads along the lymphatics and blood stream and produces metastatic lesions in the spleen and liver. Majority of people living in highly endemic areas develop a primary infection which is asymptomatic generally and resembles the primary complex of tuberculosis. The lesions develop in the periphery of the lung as focal granuloma and involve hilar lymph nodes. Later they undergo caseous necrosis and heal by fibrosis and calcification. Unlike tuberculosis, the calcification is bigger and more extensive. Calcification may be noted in the spleen and liver. Paratracheal lymph nodes characteristically demonstrate 'mulberry' calcification. In two to three weeks after the infection there is development of positive skin reaction for histoplasmin.[3,7]

Acute Histoplasmosis

An acute histoplasmosis may develop following a heavy inhalation exposure to airborne spores with manifestations like cough, pain in the chest, fever, lassitude and malaise. X-ray chest reveals multiple, soft pneumonic infiltrates which, later clear, leaving behind multiple calcification ('Buckshot' calcification).[3] The condition is self-limited. A compression collapse of the lobe may occur due to hilar adenopathy.

Disseminated Histoplasmosis

In a setting of compromised cellular immunity rarely histoplasmosis may develop as an opportunistic infection. The condition may run an acute fatal course in infants and young children with disseminated lesions involving liver, spleen, bone marrow and adrenals. There is hilar and mediastinal adenopathy with parenchymal infiltrates. It leads to cough, often brassy in character, fever, loss of weight, oropharyngeal ulcers, diarrhoea and vomiting. There is hepatosplenomegaly, leucopenia and anaemia. Asian histoplasmosis is characterized by painful ulceration of mucocutaneous junctions (84%) and liability to acute adrenocortical insufficiency due to bilateral adrenal involvement.[4] Adrenal involvement is also common in immunocompromised patients. FNAC is such cases with special staining may be diagnostic. CT studies add to diagnostic yield.[5,6]

Chronic Pulmonary Histoplasmosis

There may be a reinfection type of lesion in adults which runs a chronic progressive course. They present respiratory symptoms like cough, sputum, loss of weight, deep ache in the chest and malaise. The condition is noted in patients with pre-existing emphysema or necrotic cavities. There is tissue necrosis and cavity formation especially in the upper lobes. WBC count is normal. Sputum shows yeast like fungi on Wright's stain. Culture on Sabouraud's media develops filamentous cotton white colonies. Histoplasmin skin test is positive indicating present or past infection though anergy occurs with advancing age and with disseminated lesions. Complement fixation test[3] is positive, demonstrating antibodies.

Histopathology

Histopathology reveals cellular inflammatory exudate of polymorphs, lymphocytes and plasma cells and a large number of macrophages. Ulceration of bronchial walls may be seen in the affected area. Macrophages are largely vacuolated and contain intra cytoplasmic round 2-4 micron diameter bodies. Intense macrophage infiltration is seen in peri-bronchial alveoli and "round organism" is seen lying free in some alveolar spaces. Alveolar septa are oedematous.

Treatment

Amphotericin B is useful in treating the acute disseminated lesions and progressive cavitary lesions. Ketoconazole can be administered in a dose of 200 to 400 mg once a day by mouth and it has to be taken while the patient is fastin.[3]

Excessive Fibrosis

Discovery of histoplasma infections in human was made in 1905 in Panama by Dr. Samuel Tayor Darling, a US army pathologist. It was in 1941 that chronic pulmonary histoplasma lesions resembling pulmonary tuberculosis were reported in autopsy specimens.[8] In fact, Furcolow and Brasher[9] sought out these cases from inmates of tuberculosis sanatoria and found many. Later classic work of Goodwin[10] showed that chronic pulmonary histoplasmosis may actually represent colonization of pre-existing air spaces like emphysema. It goes to the credit of Goodwin and Snell[2] again, to describe a rare fibroma like mass that develops usually around a healed primary focus of this fungal infection. In these cases a central fungal lesion at times necrotic, gets enveloped by concentric layers of collagen, fibrous tissue and at times calcium. This lesion called a histoplasmoma may usually enlarge slowly at the rate of 1-2 cm per year and a 3-4 cm diameter size mass develops in 10-20 years.[2] An enlarging histoplasmoma with pulmonary tuberculosis has been documented.[11] If bacilli cannot be cultured then it could be the situation of histoplasmosis shedding M. tuberculosis from necrosis of an old focus as was seen in 10 cases out of 43 combined infections described by Goodwin.[1,12]

A slowly enlarging nodular mass simulate that of a neoplasm. The condition is associated with a calcified central core and concentric laminations of calcification. Such a lesion may develop around a healed primary focus in hilar or mediastinal lymph nodes and result in occlusion of vascular and bronchial structures.[3]

Importance of histoplasmoma in lung is that it masquerades a slow growing neoplasm and is surgically resectable,[7] features which differentiate it from a neoplasm are, a very slow growth rate over 5 years or more, central calcification or concentric lamellar calcification.[11] Fibrosing meddiastinitis and lyphomediastinal granuloma with broncholithiasis have also been documented. Skin tests and serological tests are not significantly contributory. Hispathology is diagnostic in fibrosing mediastinitis. Sputum test for histoplasma demonstration and positive culture are diagnostic.[13]

REFERENCES

1. Goodwin R.A. Jr., Snell J.D., Hubbard W.W. and Terry R.T., Relationships in combined pulmonary infections with histoplasma capsulatum and mycobacterium tuberculosis. Am Rev. Resp. Dis 1967; 96: 990-98.
2. Goodwin R.A. Jr. and Snell J.D. Jr., The enlarging histoplasmoma, Am Rev. Resp. Dis 1969; 100:1-12.
3. Shankar P.S., In: *Chest Medicine,* 4th ed., Oxford and IBH Publ. Co (P) Ltd. New Delhi, 1994.
4. Randhawa H.S., Khan Z.U., Histoplasmosis in India; Current status; Ind. J. Chest Dis. All Sci 1994; 36: 193-213.
5. Deodhar S., Supp. M., Diagnosis by FNA biopsy; Diag. Cytopath 1997;17: 42-44.
6. Howard H.J., Cramer H.M., Kho J., *et al.,* FNAC of benign adrenal cortical nodules; Acta Cytol 1998; 42: 1352-58.
7. Goodwin R.A. Jr. and Des Prez R.M., Histoplasmosis (State of Art review). Am. Rev. Resp. Dis 1978; 117: 929-56.
8. Meleney H.E., Pulmonary histoplasmosis, report of 2 cases. Am Rev. Tuberculosis 1941; 44: 240-42.
9. Furcolow M.L. and Brasher C.A., Chronic progressive cavitary histoplasmosis as a problem in tuberculosis sanatoriums. Am Rev. Tuberculosis 1965; 73: 609-16.
10. Goodwin R.A. Jr., Snell J.D., Hubbard W.W. and Terry R.T., Early chronic pulmonary histoplasmosis. Am. Rev. Res. Dis 1966; 93: 47-61.
11. Tewari S.C., Chauhan M.S., Jayaswal R., *et al.,* Enlarging pulmonary histoplasmoma associated with pulmonary tuberculosis; JAPI 1989; 37: 769-71.
12. Goodwin R.A. Jr., Owens F.T., Snell J.D., *et al.,* Chronic pulmonary histoplasmosis. Medicine 1976; 55:413-52.
13. Macher A., Histoplasmosis and blastomycosis; Med Clin North Amer 1980; 64:147.

COCCIDIOIDOMYCOSIS

Valley fever, Desert fever-Coccidioidomycosis is a disease caused by a dimorphic fungus, coccidiodes immitis with lesions evolving like pulmonary tuberculosis. The condition is restricted to the semi-desert areas of the Southwestern U.S.A. Central and South America.[1] The primary pulmonary infection is symptomatic only in 40 per cent cases, with symptoms ranging from mild influenza like illness to severe pneumonitis.[2]

Aetiology and Pathology

A primary infection in early childhood develops immunity in people living in endemic areas. The pulmonary lesions are produced by inhalation of *arthrospores* separated from a mycelial phase of the fungus growing in the soil. They develop in the lungs into thick walled spherical structures filled with endospores-spherule of 10 to 80 microns in diameter. They evoke an inflammatory response with an intra-alveolar exudate of polymorphs and monocytes, which may heal or convert into granuloma with central necrosis and fibrosing chronic inflammation of the periphery forms a cavity.[1]

Clinical Features and Investigations

It may present as primary progressive pulmonary and disseminated coccidioidomycosis as the lung is the primary seat of the disease.

Primary Form: Nearly 2/3rd of exposed persons remain asymptomatic. Others develop flu-like illness within two weeks of exposure and present low grade fever, dry cough, headache, chest pain, body ache and arthralgia. Later hypersensitivity manifestations are erythema multiforme, erythema nodosum, toxic erythema, conjunctivitis, episcleritis, arthralgia, arthritis and pleuritis. Pleural effusion may be the only manifestation of primary infection. Self healing is quite common.[1]

Lab tests show leucocytosis, moderate eosinophilia and raised ESR. Skin test with intradermal injection of 0.1 ml of 1:100 strength coccidioid in or spherulin shows a positive response in three weeks. The test is not used diagnostically since 1/3rd of asymptomatic adults who live in endemic areas exhibit positive reaction to skin test. X-ray chest shows patchy infiltrates mostly in lower zones and lymphadenopathy. They resolve completely in majority and in some they leave behind symptomless thin-walled cavities without any surrounding infiltration or nodular opacity due to granuloma (coccidioidoma),[1] which is a coin like lesion formed at the place of healed area of pneumonitis.

Less commonly, a single cavity may persist as chronic sequela in the area of consolidation as chronic pneumonia or may become progressive fibronodular cavitary disease. In this chronic granulomatous host reaction, caseation necrosis may occur. Both lung and lymph node lesions may show calcification. Both IgM and IgG are induced but none of them is protective.[2]

Progressive Form: Progressive lesions are seen in 0.1 per cent of cases especially in dark skinned races. Either immediately or several months later, there may be miliary spread with high fatality rate especially during pregnancy (AIDS), in immunocompromised host or occurrence of disseminated granulomatous lesions in the lungs, skin, bones, meninges or brain.[2-4] There are non-specific systemic manifestations like anorexia, weight loss, low grade fever, prostration and signs of bronchopneumonia.[1] The spread is haematogenous.

Lungs show segmental or subsegmental infiltrate with or without concomitant hilar lymphadenopathy, thin or thick-walled cavities, or fibro nodular shadows. Miliary shadows are evident in disseminated disease. There is absence of granulomatous calcification.[5] The ribs, vertebrae and small bones of hands and feet may show sharply circumscribed areas of destruction. Examination of the sputum or bronchial washings after 10 per cent KOH application may demonstrate the presence of endospores.[6] Culture of the sputum on Sabouraud's agar may show growth of fluffy cotton white colonies. A rising titre of antibodies can be demonstrated by tube precipitin or complement fixation test. Latex agglutination and Agar Celli diffusion tests are useful.[1] The skin hypersensitivity is lost with disseminated lesions indicating a poor host response to an active infection.[1] Therefore, skin test for diagnosis is not of use although is useful for epidemological studies.[2]

Treatment

Primary coccidioidomycosis requires no active treatment. Progressive symptomatic primary lesion, presence of coccidioidal infection outside the chest and meningeal involvement should be treated with Amphotericin B. But relapse are common both in disseminated and chronic progressive pulmonary lesions.[7] Intravenous miconazole or oral ketoconazole appear to be less toxic compared to Amphotericin B. ketoconazole is ineffective in meningeal coccidioidomycosis. Ketaconazole has to be given for several months. Itraconazole gives excellent response in most of the patients.[8,9] Surgical resection is advised if there is a giant cavity or rapidly enlarging cavity, threatening to rupture into the pleural space, or getting colonised by other fungi.[1] Specific surgical indications in cavity disease include haemoptysis, rupture, secondary infection and progressive enlargement.[10] Also in cases of empyema drainage, repair of fistula or symptomatic mycetoma, surgery is indicated.[11,12]

REFERENCES

1. Shankar P.S., Coccidioipodomycosis, In; Chest Medicine; Oxford and IBH Pub. Co (P) Ltd., New Delhi, 1994; 4th ed,
2. Harrison's principles of internal medicines, Wilson J.D., Braunatd E., Isselbacher K.J., *et al.*, ed., 12th ed., McGraw Hill, New York, 1991.
3. Brouniman D.A., *et al.,* Coccidioidomycosis in AIDS; Ann. Int. Med 1987; 106: 372.
4. Bouza E., *et al.,* Coccidioidal meningitis. An analysis of 31 cases and review of literature, Medicine 1980; 60: 139.
5. Drutz D.J., Catanzaro A., Coccidioidomycosis; Part I and II; Amer Rev Resp Dis 1978; 117:559 and 727.
6. Pappagianis D., In: Coccidioidomycosis; Stevens D.A., Ed: 1980; Plenum Medical Book Co., New York.
7. Drutz D.J., Amphotericin B. in the treatment coccidioido mycosis. Drugs 1983; 26:337.
8. Galgiani J.N., *et al.,* Ketaconazole therapy of progressive coccidioidomycosis, comparison of 400 to 800 mg doses and observations at higher doses; Amer. J. Med 1988; 84:603.
9. Gopalakrishnan R., *et al.,* Histoplasmosis in India—Truly uncommon or uncommonly recognised? JAPI 2012; 60:25-28.
10. Solomone S.W., Osborne R., *et al.,* Surgical manifestations and results of treatment of pulmonary coccidioidomycosis. Ann. Throac. Surg 1980; 30: 433.
11. Catanzaro A., Pulmonary coccidioidomycosis, Med Clinics North Amer 1980; 64:461.
12. Bayer A., Fungal pneumonias, Coccidioidal syndromes; Chest 1981;79:686.

CANDIDIASIS (MONILIASIS)

Candida albicans is a widely distributed yeast like fungus. It forms the normal commensals in the mouth, intestine and vagina. Rarely it produces a widespread visceral infection.[1] The fungus proliferates when the normal bacterial flora is disturbed and in chronic debilitating diseases of respiratory tract, leukaemia, lymphoma, diabetes, therapy with tetracyclines, steroids, betamethasone aerosol and immunosuppressive agents, burns, dialysis, trauma, and following operations. The local infection is endogenous. In infants and neonates the infection of the respiratory tract can occur and is associated with oral or pharyngeal thrush.[2] Predisposing factors can be surgical operations, malnutrition, diabetes, radiation, steroid therapy and immunosuppression. Mucocutaneous candidiasis is seen in AIDS. Females, especially in third trimester of pregnancy, are prone to vulvovaginal thrush.[3]

Clinically the bronchial candidiasis presents features of bronchitis with cough and scanty expectoration.[4,5] In pulmonary form, the spread is usually hematogenous and manifestations are severe with dyspnoea, cough, pyrexia, chest pain and haemoptysis, tachycardia and tachypnoea. Radiologically it shows ill-defined patchy opacities.[6] Multiple abscesses may cause a diffuse, vaguely nodular infilterate. The diagnosis is established by transtracheal aspiration of secretions and demonstration of growth of budding yeast cells and filaments on Sabouraud's medium serological tests are of no value. The treatment has to be directed on predisposing factors, discontinuation of inciting drugs and inhalation of nystatin combined with intravenous amphotericin B 0.5 mg/kg/day for few weeks may be helpful in disseminated conditions.

REFERENCES

1. OODFC; Candida and Candidiasis; Baltimore, Saunders, 1988.
2. Shankar P.S., Candidiasis, In; Chest medicine; Oxford and IBH Pub. Co. (P) Ltd., New Delhi 1994; 4th ed.
3. Harrison's Principles of Internal Medicine; (ed) by Wilson J.D., Braunwald E., Isselbacher K.J., *et al.,* 12th ed., Vol. (i) McGraw Hill, New York, 1991.
4. Mandall G.I., *et al.,* E.D., Principle and practices of infectious diseases, 3rd ed; New York; Churchill Livingstone, 1990.
5. Rose H.D., Sheth N.K., Pulmonary candidiasis; A clinical and pathological correlation; Arch Interm Med 1978; 138: 964.

6. Sarosi G., Management of fungal disease; Amer Rev Resp Dis 1987; 127:250.

CRYPTOCOCCOSIS (TORULOSIS)

Cryptococcus neoformans—an opportunistic fungal pathogen—is ovoid, thick-walled yeast like fungus 4-6 micro meter in diameter. It contains a mucinous capsule, with large amounts of polysaccharide material demonstrable by India ink and exists in a budding form. It has four serotypes, A,B,C and D. Cryptococcus exists in soil and thrives often on pigeon droppings. The infection is thought to be acquired by inhalation. Organism is known for its predilection to involve CNS, can infect other body sites but almost all the human infections are thought to originate with a pulmonary focus.[1] Pulmonary infection may have spontaneous resolution. It can assume a pathogenic role as an opportunistic infection in immuno-compromised patients.[2]

Lung infection is associated with lymphocytic reaction initially and later fibrosis. It forms a localised granuloma and may undergo cavitation. Disease may have acute, subacute or chronic course. It may remain asymptomatic or present with fever, cough, pleuritic chest pain and haemoptysis. Cough is present in 20 per cent of cases and chest pain in 40 per cent of cases.[3] Radiologically it presents round shadows in the periphery of the lung which is often confused with malignant lesion. Cavity lesions, pleural effusions and hilar adenopathy are infrequent. Rarely fibrotic lesion are seen. Calcification is not present. Differential diagnosis includes malignancy. Serum antigen tests are positive only in one third of cases. Biopsy may be required to confirm the diagnosis.[4] Disease that has been termed 'awakening gaint' among mycoses,[5] may run a benign course, remaining stable or slowly resolving,[6] or rarely may prove fatal.[7]

Hematogenous spread the infection to the central nervous system gives rise to meningitis. CNS involvement forms the most common symptomatic manifestation and often co-exists with pulmonary lesion. It is often fatal if patients with AIDS develop cryptococcosis.[8,9] 5 flucytocine (150 mg/kg orally) and a low dose of amphotericin B 0.5 kg/kg/day are useful in the treatment of cryptococcal meningitisl,[10] and the treatment has to be continued for a period of six weeks or more.[2] 50-70 per cent patients are cured and average survival of AIDS patients with cryptococcosis has been about 8 months.[3]

REFERENCES

1. Behsman R.E., *et al.,* Cryptococcal skeletal infections; case report and review; Rev Infect Dis 1990; 12(2): 181-90
2. Shankar P.S., Chest Medicine, Oxford and IBH Publ. Co. (P) Ltd., New Delhi, 4th ed., 1994.
3. Harrison's principles of Internal medicine; (ed) by Wilson J.D., Braunwald E., Isselbacher K.J., *et al.,* 10th ed., Vol. 1, McGraw Hill, N. York, 1991.
4. Wadia R.S., *et al.,* Neurological manifestations of HIV disease; JAPI 2001:49: 343-48.
5. Kaufman L., Blumer S., Cryptococcosis; True awakening giant; Pan Amer Health Org Sci Pub 1977;356: 176-84.
6. Kerkering T.M., *et al.,* The evolution of pulmonary cryptococcosis; Clinical implications from a study of 41 patients with or without compromising host factors; Ann Intern Med 1991;94:611-16.
7. Ramani A., *et al.,* Pulmonary and cerebral Cryptococcosis; JAPI 1994; 42(9):736-39.
8. Gal A.A., *et al.,* The pathology of pulmonary cryptococcal infection in AIDS. Arch Path. Lab. Med 1986,110:502.
9. Dismukes W.K., Cryptococcal meningitis in patients with AIDS; J. Inf. Dis 1988, 157:624.
10. Perfect J.R., Cryptococcosis, Inf Dis Clinics North Amer 1989; 3:77.

BLASTOMYCOSIS[1-5]

Dimorphic fungus, blastomyces dermatitidis produces a systemic mycosis in the U.S.A. and Canada. Pulmonary and disseminated forms of the disease involving principally the skin, bone and genitourinary tract have been described. Male/female ratio is 10:1 and there is no occupational predisposition.

The condition results from inhalation of spores in immunocompetant host. A vast majority have an asymptomatic or subclinical course. Infection is not transmitted from person to person. Initial infection may heal spontanenously or become chronic. Lesions are cavitational but endobronchial lesions may appear in chronic cases. Disease spreads systemically *via* hematogenous route. Immunosuppressive treatment may precipitate this infection. The patients often have cough, sputum, haemoptysis and chest pain. Regional lymphadeno-pathy is minimal. Diagnosis is made by culture of the organisms from infected sites. The inflammatory response includes lymphocytes, neutrophils and giant cells. Cavity formation is unusual. Pseudoepitheliomatous hyperplasia may be mistaken for diagnosis of squamous cell carcinoma. Chest X-ray is abnormal in two third of cases. Calcification, hilar adenopathy and pleural effusions are rare. Diagnosis can be clinched by presence of fungus in the sputum cytology smear by experienced hand. Table 4.36 shows differential diagnosis of blastomycosis.

Table 4.36: DD of blastomycosis
Aspiration pneumonia
Actinomycosis
Carcinoma lung
Histoplasmosis
Tuberculosis

Ketoconazole appears to be successful in treating patients. The side effects are much less serious than Amphotericin B.Initial adult dose of 400 mg can be increased to 600-800 mg/day and can be continued for 6-12 months. Mortality rate in treated cases is 15 per cent.

REFERENCES

1. Campbell G.D. and Chapman S.W., Blastomycosis; Semin Resp. Med 1987; 9:164.
2. Klein B.S., *et al.,* Two outbreaks of blastomycosis along rivers in Wisconsin. Isolation of blastomyces dermatitidis from river back soil and evidence of its transmission along water ways; Amer. Rev. Resp. Dis 1987; 136: 1333.
3. Harrison's principles of internal medicines; Wilson J.D., Braunwald E., Isselbacher K.J., *et al.,* (ed); 12th Ed., Vol. 1, McGraw Hill, New York, 1991.
4. Macher A., Histoplasmosis and blastomycosis; Med Clin North Amer 1980;64:447.
5. Baily G.G., *et al.,* Blastomycosis in Africa; Clinical features diagnosis and treatment; Rev. Inf. Dis 1991; 13: 1,005.

Environmental Lung Diseases and Interstitial Lung Diseases

5

AIR POLLUTION, ENVIRONMENT AND LUNGS

Due to rapid urbanisation and industrialisation, many common diseases of the chest and the prevalence of cancer have increased greatly and the usual causes like tobacco smoking, infections or dietary and constitutional factors are not as important as air pollution[1-3] due to occupational or ambient exposure to chemicals and pollutants including automobile pollutants,[4] although many workers don't consider these effects especially when the effects of smoking are accounted.[5] Clean air basically consists of a mixture of 21% oxygen and 79% nitrogen and any addition of newer constituents could be labelled at contaminants. The air pollution, its effects on general and pulmonary health and measures suggested to prevent are described with a brief classification of hazardous industrial substances in Table 5.1.

Sources and Mode of Action[3]

Some important air pollutants are: SO_2, NO_2, SPM (suspended particulates), CO and POM (Polycyclic organic matter). The sources are industrial automobiles or domestic in complete burning of fuel. The main soil pollutants are bacteria, metals and pesticides. The main water pollutants are chemical oil and pesticides. Among non-industrial pollutants, asbestos exposure in Turkey (Zeolite or tremolite), Western India and the Himalayan region are important; silica dust exposure in the Ladakh desert has been shown to be important in causing silicosis.[6] Silica exposure has been observed in workers engaged in cycle manufacturing and polishing. Excessive and inefficient burning of fuel is leading to global warming which is reflected in excess CO_2, reduced atmospheric O_3 and increased fluctuations in climate.

The first introduction to such episodes resulting in a morbidity were the London fog,[7] methylisocyanate leak at Bhopal and the Chernobyl nuclear disaster in USSR. Chronic exposure can lead to repeated bronchitis, exacerbations in bronchial asthma, recurrent and severe lung infections, frequent upper airway irritation, bronchiolitis and in some cases, centrilobular emphysema with dust deposition.[8]

With burning of poor quality of coal, wood, cowdung and waste products in inferior burners of domestic stoves with poorly ventilated kitchens,[9] and with poor and inefficient combustion of fossil fuel in industrial furnaces, automobiles and power plants lead to large scale liberation of air pollutants[10,11] and is responsible for chronic lung disorders. Environmental lung diseases have been grouped as shown in Table 5.2.

Table 5.1: Hazardous industrial substances: Classification

1. Inorganic	:	Coal, Asbestos, Cement, Gold, Beryllium, Stone, Synthetic Fibre.		
2. Organic	:	Cotton, Synthetic Fibre, Sugarcane, PVC, Polymer.		
3. Chemicals	:	a. Inorganic	:	Hg, pH, NH_3, Cl, CCl_4, CO, CO_2, Cyanide, As, HCl, H_2SO_4, HNO_3 Isocyanates.
		b. Aromatic	:	Benzene, Toluene, Aniline, Acids, Xylene, Drugs, Methane, Aldehydes.
		c. Pesticides	:	DDT, BHC, Malathion, Carbamates (MIC).
		d. Fertilizers	:	Urea, Phosphate, Nitrate, Biologic.
4. Pollutants	:	Air	:	S.P.M., SO_2, SO_3, NO_2, O_3, CO, POM.
	:	Water	:	Chemicals, Bacteria, Oxygen demand.
	:	Soil	:	Pesticides, Chemicals, Salinity, Fluoride, Parasites.

Table 5.2: Respiratory tract irritants

1. Mucosal irritation of nose, throat	: SO_2, NH_3, Cl, Acids, Aldehydes, Isocyanates.
2. Irritation of lower airways	: Phosgene, Cl, NO_2, MIC, Petroleum products.
3. Lungs	: Cl, Pesticides, MIC, NO_2, SO_3.
4. Irritation of G.I. system	
i. Stomach	: Alcohol, Acid, Alkali, Hg.
ii. Intestines	: Toxins, Bacteria, Viruses.
iii. Liver	: CCL_4.
5. Kidney	: Aniline, Phenol, Benzene, POM, Hg.
Mechanism of action	
Through O_2 deficit	: CO, N, CO_2, NO_2, Cyanide, Aniline

General Health Damage

The total daily air pollutants liberated could be 2000 to 2400 metric tons, of which 60 per cent may come from automobiles, 5-10 per cent from domestic fuels and the rest from industry. Higher levels of NO_2 have also been reported. High SPM pollution leads to the development of smog due to photochemical oxidation in the air with NO_2, humidity and sunlight. This leads to poor visibility, and other ill effects.[10]

Common complaints may be headache (NO_2, aldehyde, benzene) eye-irritation (NH_3, aldehyde, NO_2), watery nasal discharge, sneezing and post-nasal discharge (SO_2), irritating cough (SO_2, SPM), choking and chest pain (NO_2), irritability (CO), productive cough (SO_2, SPM) and dyspnoea (SO_2, NO_2). Rising trend in respiratory disorder has been attributed to environmental pollution. A direct linkage between tobacco and causation of lymphomas through genetic mutations has been putforth. Almost 50,000 cases of lymphomas have occurred by the end of 2001, and this does not include HIV-related lymphomas.

On long term exposure there is an increased risk of cancer, which is manifest as leukemia or urogenital cancer, seen more frequently in children born around nuclear power plants.[12]

There has been some dispute over the chronic effect of diesel or gasoline exhaust fumes on health, but recent studies in U.S.A. on animals and cardiac patients have shown that advance E.C.G. and rhythm changes are seen on inhalation of 3-4.5 per cent CO in blood.[13,14]

Specific Respiratory Changes[3]

An excess of irritant symptoms occur in new entrants to cities like the eastern suburbs of Bombay or California due to a short burst of pollutant increase (*e.g.* NO_2, SO_2). Though the irritation might decrease later, the lung function effect (particularly FEV_1 and flow rates) persists.[11,15] There is an excess of prevalence of chest symptoms and upper and lower respiratory tract morbidity with greater severity and duration of symptoms. More morbidity and hospital admission occur in young children and deaths are commoner in elderly (50+) subjects and children below 1 year of age. The use of inferior fuels (liberating large amounts of CO, NO_2, SPM and POM) in cooking stoves, may lead to frequent lung infection, poor growth and diminished lung functions, particularly in girls. There is an urgent need for promoting use of cleaner fuels with more complete combustion.[16]

Punjab Pollution Control Board, Patiala has published a report that speaks of state of cleanliness of air in certain cities of Punjab state as shown in the Table 5.3.[17]

Table 5.3: 13.9.93 to 19.9.93 Micrograms/m³ (Maximum values)

Punjab	*Suspended particulates*	*Sulphur dioxide*	*Nitrogen oxides*
Permissible limits res.	200	80	80
1. Amritsar	502	72	28
2. Jalandhar	289	69	31
3. Ludhiana	893	92	31
4. Gobindgarh	549	72	23
5. Sangrur	313	71	24
6. Nangal	315	67	24
7. Derabassi	286	63	26
8. Bathinda	148	25	03

Keeping in view, the late Chief Minister of Punjab had announced to take necessary measures to cleanse Ludhiana city by 1995. Licenses to new industrial units are to be issued only when they submit a compulsory plan of preventing both water and air pollution through the industrial waste. How far this succeeds, is to be seen in the coming years. For the present, there are 1200 water polluting and 2200 air polluting industrial units in Ludhiana and only 626 units have adopted measures and methods to check and prevent environmental pollution. Recently Deputy Commissioner of the city has announced to start local buses on CNG and has also ordered to gradually remove old three wheeler off the road in a phased manner. This shall cut down the automobile pollution from exhaust. But it is premature to say that the orders take practical shape. The studies done in Mumbai show that chronic exposure to ambient air pollution and particularly to SO_2, SPM, NO_2 and POM leads to major chest morbidity and mortality. There is synergism between the pollutants and undernutrition, smoking and a dusty occupation. In addition, there may be a higher prevalence of dermatitis, diarrhoeas, eye problems and stunted growth. The effects can be seen as acute exacerbation of chronic cough, dyspnoea, excessive sputum and decrease in lung function with fluctuating increase of SO_2 and SPM.[2,18,19] Immunologic studies have revealed reduction of salivary IgA, lysozyme, lymphocyte migration, reduced polymorph and WBC counts and blood IgG, IgA and IgM levels. Diesel exhaust alters airway fluid polymorphs, delays clearance of soot particles and lung collagen.[20,21] Acute inhalation of CO, NO_2, or aldehydes may cause excess cough, reduction in FEV_1, and MEFR. Bronchitis[15] may occur with acute exposure to NO_2 during winter; some may silently die, with an added effect of CO pollution. An increased activity of macrophages in the lungs is also seen on exposure to coal smoke.

Even in normal animals, after chronic diesel exhaust inhalation, progressive focal inflammation, epithelial proliferation and focal fibrosis around soot laden alveolar macrophages are seen. This may result in bronchiolar thickening, emphysema and increase in lung collagen.[15] There is a sub-population of susceptible subjects particularly with chronic bronchitis, who react with reduced lung function during exercise at an exposure to 0.3 PPM NO_2.[22]

After inhalation of staph aureus; its intrapulmonary killing is impaired at 5 PPM NO_2.[23] This effect may be seen even at 2.5 PPM if lung resistance is lowered by, steroid treatment. The effect on lung function of NO_2 is enhanced after such bacterial challenge.[23]

Even a distant community may show significantly high morbidity due to effects attributable to unmeasured pollutants like aromatic chemicals, *e.g.,* benzene, POM, aldehydes or mercaptans from the adjoining vicinity.[15]

SO_2 and NO_2 may increase resistance to bacterial (staph) or viral infections, thereby increasing the severity and duration of illness. SO_2 has been shown to increase airway hyper-reactivity. There has been a strong relationship between the level of fine particulate (less than l0 micron aerodynamic diameter) and mortality rates for cardiorespiratory diseases.[24]

While the worldwide increase in the prevalence of cancer has been considered due to viruses, respiratory tract cancer and COPD may be enhanced by pollutants.[3] Indoor pollutions in the developed, temperate countries cause the sick building syndrome, as new centrally heated buildings get exposed to sealing insulating chemicals for several weeks. Symptoms include dizziness, headache, chest pain, malaise, tiredness, irritating cough and choking. Newer studies have reflected the concept of total daily (outdoor, work and home) human exposure to pollutants, so as to individually correlate symptoms to diseases or their course.[11]

As the lung is contract organ, breathing or inhaling over 10,000 litres of air daily, it is but natural that several problems are increasingly being related to inhalant gases.

Progress, Prevention and Treatments[3]

If uncontrolled chronic exposure to pollutants continues, the clinical syndromes, pathologies or diseases worsen, leading to greater morbidity. Acute episodic exposure (like at Bhopal to MIC) leads to fluctuating interstitial lung disease.

Reduction of occupational or ambient urban exposure may arrest or reverse some of the symptoms or reduce the functional disability. Problem of air pollution requires public education, governmental leadership action and co-operation from industry, so that the target-goals are achieved to improve air quality even if varying degrees of legislative forces are to be used. The programmes should be directed towards reducing in complete fuel burning, quality diesel exhaust emission and developing cleaner modes of transport.

Non-specific manifestations of airway obstruction, if reversible, will respond to beta stimulants or theophylline type of bronchodilators in adequate doses daily (e.g. salbutamol 2-4 mg, terbutalin 2.5-5 mg and theophylline 200 mg). Patients who develop frequent lung inflections may need a course of antibiotics (e.g. ampicillin). Those with cardiac or neoplastic problems will have to be appropriately investigated and treated, depending upon the type and stage of the disease and conditions, status and willingness of the patient.

REFERENCES

1. Kamat S.R., Godkhindi K.D., Shah V.N., *et al.,* Prospective 3-year study of health morbidity in relation to air pollution in Bombay, India. Methodology and early results upto 2 years. Lung India 1984; 2: 1-20.
2. Kamat S.R. and Doshi V.B., Sequential health-study in relation to air pollution in Bombay, India, Europe J. Epidemiol 1987; 3: 265-77.
3. Kamat S.R., Environment pollution and lung; In: Dalal P.M., (ed) Medicine Update, Assn Phys., India, Bombay 1991, 1: 143-46.
4. Kamat S.R., Shah S.V., Rupawate R.U., Kulkarni A.V., Gregart J. and Deshpande J.M., The health effects of automobile exhaust and total ambient pollution in Bombay, Lung India 1989; 7: 15-22.
5. Tollerud D.J., Speizer F.E., Weiss S.T., Elting S. and Ferris B.G., The health effects of automobile exhaust VI; relationship of respiratory symptoms and pulmonary function in tunnel and tumpike workers. Arch Environ Health 1983;38:334-40.
6. Barjiv J. and Goldberg G. Simple silica as pneumoconiosis in Negev Bedouins, Arch Environ. Hlth 1974,29:121-26.
7. Ministry of health, mortality and morbidity during the London Fog of December 1952. Report publication health and medicine subjects No. 95 H.M.S. London, 1954.
8. Kamat S.R., *et al.,* Bombay air pollution Health Study, Secions 1- 13, Lung, India 1984; 2: 1-135.
9. Bhatia R.S., *et al.,* Effect of smoking and kitchen environments; Medical Pulse 1997;4(2):65-66.
10. Smith K.R., Biofuels, air pollution and health. A Global review, New York, Plenum Publishing Co 1987; 452.

11. Smith K.R., Air pollution assessing total exposure in part one, the United States part two, developing countries, Environment 1988; 30: 10-38 and 16-35.
12. Gardner M.J., Snee M.P., Hall A.J., Powell C.A., Downes S. and Terrel J.D., Results of case control study of leukemia and lymphoma among young people near sellafied nuclear plant in West Columbia. Br. Med. J 1990; 300: 423-28.
13. Watson A.Y., Bates R.R., Kennedy D.(eds), Air pollution, the automobile and public health. National Acad. Press 1988.
14. HEI Multicenter CO Study team, Alfred E.N., Bleecker E.R., Chaitman B.R., *et al.,* Acute effects of CO exposure on individuals with coronary artery disease. Health effects Inst 1989; No. 25.
15. Kamat S.R., Patil J.D., Gregart J., *et al.,* Air pollution related respiratory morbidity in central and north-eastern Bombay, JAPI 1992; 40: 588-93.
16. Bhatia R.S., Kitchen ventilation and COPD; paper selected for award by ICS, 1994.
17. Bhatia R.S., Respiratory disease pattern in a private clinic in Ludhiana; Lung India 1995; 13: 125-26.
18. Chapman R.S., Calafiore D.C. and Hasselblad Y., Prevalence of persistent cough and phlegm in young adults in relation to long-term ambient SO_2 exposure, Am. Rev. Resp. Dis 1985;132: 261-67.
19. Dodge R., Soloman P., Meyers J. and Hayes C., A longitudinal study of children expose d to sulphur oxides, Am. J. Epideminol 1985; 121: 720-36.
20. Mauderly J.L., Bice D.E., Carpenter R.L., *et al.,* Effect of inhaled NO_2 and diesel exhaust on developing lung. Health Effect Institute Report 1987; No. 8.
21. Mauderly J.L., Bice D.E., Cheng Y.S., *et al.,* Influence of experimental pulmonary emphysema on the toxicological effects from inhaled NO_2 and diesel exhaust, Health Effect Institute Report 1989.
22. Morrow P.E. and Utell M.J., Responses of susceptible subpopulations to NO_2. Health Effects Institute Report 1989; No. 23.
23. Jakab G.J., Modulation of pulmonary defence mechanisms against viral and bacterial infections by acute exposure to NO_2. Health Effects Institute Report 1989; No. 20.
24. Samet J.M., *et al.,* Fine particulate air pollution and mortality in 20 US cities; NEJM 2000; 343: 1742-49.

OCCUPATIONAL DISEASES OF THE LUNGS[1-7]

Occupational diseases are mostly related to work-related environments. The inhalation of various industrial, automobile dust, gases or fumes over a varying period of time is responsible for the development of occupational pulmonary diseases. The peripheral gas exchanging system of the lung is affected where the airborne dust particles enable upon the quality and quantity as well as the size of the respiratory system involved. In addition, individual's defence mechanism of the respiratory tract also play an important role. Pneumoconiosis form the most common pulmonary dusts that accumulate, creating tissue reaction in the lungs. Different types of tissue reactions are seen in the form of pulmonary fibrosis (silica, talc, coal, asbestos etc.), pneumonitis (beryllium, manganese), extrinsic allergic alveolitis (bagasse, mouldy hay), bronchitis with or without emphysema (cotton, wool), asthma (fur, feather , wool, chemicals, vegetables, grain etc.), pulmonary odema (irritant gases), malignancy (asbestos, arsenic, nickle etc .). Certain other occupational non-fibrosing pulmonary disorders include siderosisn (iron), stannosis (TIN), baritosis (Barium). Unlike true pneumoconiosis, nodular opacities giving mottled appearances in the chest X-ray, disappear if further exposure to the dust is stopped.

Occupational history with thorough details of type, degree and duration of dust exposure and clinical examination with radiological and pulmonary function studies help in clinching the diagnosis.

Preventive measures include reducing dust exposure in the working environments, radiological check up of workers at regular periodic intervals and suggesting occupational change in case abnormal shadows or changes or symptoms appear. Various occupational pulmonary disorders have been listed in Table 5.4.

Table 5.4: Occupational lung diseases

1. Pneumoconiosis:	1. Asbestoses 2. Silicosis 3. Coal workers' pneumoconiosis (CWP) 4. Miscellaneous A. Those implicated in ILD also beryllium, cobalt, zinc, cadmium, manganese, nickel B. Chronic granulomatous inflammation and pulmonary fibrosis of beryllium C. Hypersensitivity pneumonitis and pulmonary fibrosis – Diamond polishers – Grinders – Hard metal workers

Contd.

Contd.

2. Organic dust exposure:	• Byssinosis in cotton industry workers • Hypersensitivity reaction in wool workers • Bagassosis from sugarcane dust (Allergic rhinitis, bronchitis and asthma and interstitial pneumonia with fibrosis) Hypersensitivity pneumonitis, farmer's lung, pigeon-breeder's lung, cheese workers' lung, mushroom pickers' lung
3. Pulmonary injury due to chemical gases and fumes:	a. Local irritation of eyes and nose to pulmonary odema, severe pneumonia, ARDS and other systemic involvement (Bhopal gas tragedy of 1984) b. Bronchitis, bronchiolitis, atelectasis, pneumonia, pulmonary odema, ARDS caused by ammonia, SO_2 chlorine, oxides of nitrogen c. Systemic toxicity of metal oxide fumes causing: • Metal fume fever • Polymer fume fever
4. Occupational asthma:	Due to chemical agents and biological agents

REFERENCES

1. Becklake M.R., *et al.,* The relationship between acute and chronic airway responses to occupational exposures, Curr. Pulmobiol 1988; 9: 25.
2. Guidelines or the use of International Labour Office Classification of Radiographs of Pneumoconiosis. Occupational safety and Health Science. 22 (Revised 1980); Geneva; ILO, 1980.
3. Laurunerys R.R., Occupational Toxicology, In: Casarett and Doull's Toxicology. The basic science of poison, 3rd Ed, CD Kloassen M.D., Anden J Douli (ed), N.York, MacMillan, 1986; Chap. 29.
4. Parker W.R., Occupational lung disorders, 2nd ed, London, Butterworth, 1982.
5. Petor Schneiderman M. (ed), Qualification of occupational cancer, Banbury Report, 9, Cold Spring, Harbor 1981.
6. Rom M.N. (ed), Environmental and Occupational Medicine, Boston, Little, Brown, 1983, Chap 13,20.
7. Weill J., Occupational pulmonary diseases acute and accidental exposures to irritant gases, in Pulmonary Diseases and Disorder, Fishman A.P. (ED), McGraw Hill, New York, 1987; Chap 54.

ASBESTOS RELATED DISEASES

Asbestos—an inorganic dust is the most commonly recognized occupational culprit giving rise to chronic pulmonary diseases. Asbestos fiber is an indestructible fibrous mineral with great tensile strength, flexibility, heat resistance, acid and alkali resistance. It consists of a mixture of silicates or iron, magnesium, chromium, calcium and aluminium which when crushed break into fibers. It is extensively used in the manufacture of heat resistant insulating boards, textiles, brake clutch linings, fire retardant, cement, plaster and paints. It is also used in the manufacture of fire fighting blankets and safety garments.[1] It was initially used in 1940, but replaced by man-made mineral fibers[2] like glass wool, fiberglass or skywood in 1975.[3]

Asbestosis

Pathogenesis and Pathology

Asbestos is inhaled during mining and manufacturing process and during demolition or stripping of asbestos containing buildings and products. The risk is not limited to asbestos-handlers but also to those who have moderate exposure.[4] Asbestos elicits a fibrogenic response in the lung parenchyma and in the pleura. It has carcinogenic effects on the lung, pleura and peritoneum. It causes pleural plaques, pleural thickening, and pleural effusion and pulmonary fibrosis. Increased prevalence of anti-muscular antibodies an shenmatoid factor in these patients of asbestosis suggests possible sole of immunological reactions in its pathogenesis. Asbestos exposure has been associated with an increased incidence of bronchogenic carcinoma and mesothelioma of the pleura and pericardium.[1]

Pulmonary Fibrosis

Asbestosis is a chronic, non-infectious, non-malignant disease.[4] characterised by diffuse interstitial fibrosing pulmonary disease, which is dually related to level of products in degree and intensity of exposure and duration and takes minimum of 10 years before disease manifests. Chrysotile is less fibrogenic, perhaps due to its rapid elimination from the lungs. Crocidolite appears to be potent to produce a fibrotic reaction. Amphibole fibers get deposited more peripherally. Those less than 5 microns are responsible for the pathologic events . The process begins in the region of respiratory or terminal bronchioles and in the alveoli arising from its most proximal alveolar ducts. Exudation of neutrophils and macrophages into the alveolar spaces is an initial reaction to the deposition of asbestos fibers. Several macrophages envelop the fibers and coat them with an acid mucopolysaccharide. The cytoplasmic enzymes and magnesium exuding from the fibers initiate a fibrotic process.[1] Recent studies shows that during phagocytosis of asbestos fibers, the membrane macrophages are damaged and release enzymes containing lysosomes which destroy lung parenchyma.[3] The process affects the lower lobes first and with prolonged or heavy exposure it ascends.[1]

Frequently a combination of diffuse fibrosis and honeycombing is noted.[5] The inhaled asbestos may get coated with a proteinaceous iron staining material to result in asbestos body (ferruginous body). It has a beaded necklace or dumb-bell appearance and its presence is considered a characteristic index of asbestos exposure.[1]

Pleural Lesions

Asbestos is a potent stimulus for the development of pleural abnormalities,[6] like bilateral pleural thickening or plaques, related directly to dose and duration of exposure.

Pleural Plaques

Pleural plaques occur extrapleurally on the posterolateral aspect of the lower parietal pleura or diaphragm along pathways of lymphatic drainage. They are usually absent on visceral pleura, at costophrenic angles or at the apices. They occur as discrete, elevated, whitish-grey, shiny, rounded areas of hyaline fibrosis. They may be diffuse or nodular, distributed in an irregular fashion and do not produce pleural adhesions. Calcified plaques are opaque and discontinuous. Macroscopically plaques appear as laminated, acellular, collagenous connective tissues. Most of the patients are asymptomatic.[1] Pleural plaques are benign and are not the precursors of mesothelioma.[7]

Pleural Thickening

Focal or diffuse thickening of visceral pleura may occur in asbestosis. It may vary from a thin, milky white discolouration to a thick peel, involving midthorax in the middle or lower zones of lungs, sparing costophrenic angles and apices. Calcification may occur.[1]

Pleural Effusion

Asbestos inhalation is commonly associated with asymptomatic pleural effusion. It is usually sterile exudate, containing a high proportion of eosinophils and may be blood stained. Mostly it is unilateral but may occur bilaterally. Often it occurs as an early feature.[1] The effusion remits spontaneously, only to reappear again, may be gradually progressive.[3]

Clinical Features

There is progressive dyspnoea as the initial manifestation followed by dry cough. The symptoms are slowly progressive and there is loss of weight. The breath sounds are normal as there is usually no airways obstruction. Fine basal crackles are audible bilaterally. They are paninspiratory, often accentuated at the end of inspiration. Pleural rub is not heard despite involvement of visceral pleura in pulmonary fibrosis. Digital clubbing is a feature. In advanced fibrosis, there is cyanosis and appearance of signs of cor pulmonale.[1] Reduction in diffusing capacity is an early sign of severe disease.[3]

Investigations

The sputum shows presence of asbestos bodies (take golden brown colour on haemotoxylin eosin stain) and the workers often expectorate them. It indicates vast exposure to asbestos. But it does not signify asbestosis. Chest X-ray shows linear or band-like shadows from pleural thickening along the lower or mid-thoracic walls. A distinct ground glass appearance may be seen in some cases.[3] It is associated with abnormality involving one or both diaphragms as their flattening or elevation, nodular or irregular shadows adjacent to or on its surface, indistinct or shaggy outline or linear calcification adjacent to the diaphragm (pleural plaques). The cardial outline may become shaggy. Lung lesions show an interstitial pattern that is more prominent at the lung bases. Characteristically they are fine, medium or coarse small irregular opacities. CT gives a better picture.[1]

The condition is associated with restrictive ventilatory defect, reduced lung volumes and impaired diffusion. Large airways function (FEV_1/FVC) is generally well preserved. Hypoxaemia may be noted on exertion. Massive inhalation.[1] may cause progressive pulmonary insufficiency. Fasting urinary hydroxyproline has been suggested to be a useful indicator[8] but doesn't seem to have a diagnostic value.

Treatment

Further exposure to the dust should be stopped on diagnosis of asbestosis as there is no specific treatment. The adverse effects are decreased on reducing the exposure. The workers are advised to stop smoking[9] to decrease the risk of carcinoma of the lung,[1] the risk of which increases in these cases of asbestos exposure.

Pleural Malignancy (Malignant Mesothelioma)

The development of pleural or peritoneal mesothelioma, may occur after an exposure to crocidolite and amosite for a long latent period of 20 years or more. Small amount of asbestos is sufficient for the production of this rare tumour. It can occur even in people living in the neighbourhood[10] of asbestos mines, mills and wastage dumps. This has been proved by experimental work.[11] The association varies from 13 to 99 per cent.[12,13] Cigarette smoking does not appear to play a role in its pathogenesis. Disease mostly presents in 4th to 7th decades of life but infrequently reported at younger age.[14]

It is a diffuse malignant tumour arising from mesothelial cells of pleura, peritoneum and pericardium. Pathologically, it is ivory white, gray or yellow, cut surface is gelatinous. Haemorrhage, necrosis, cavity and fibrosis may be present. Microscopically both epithelial and mesenchymal elements are present along with many transitional cells as seen by electron microscope. Four histological types are: tubulo-papillary (most common), sarcomatous type (predominantly mesenchymal), undifferentiated cell type and mixed type. As it arises from pleura, it spreads along the pleural surface. It encases the lung and invades the fissures. There is accumulation of large amounts of haemorrhagic pleural fluid. Effusion may be insidious but clear. Malignant cells may be present but pyogenic and AFB cultures are negative. It results in manifestations such as dull aching, non-pleuritic chest pain, progressive dyspnoea and loss of weight.[12] The tumour occurs even without any evidence of asbestosis.[1] It is diagnosed on open pleural biopsy. Non-invasive CT scan is both diagnostic as well as of prognostic value.[15] The tumour spreads to the mediastinum and surround the vessels and produce thrombosis, or to the liver by eroding through the diaphragm. The growth may put pressure in esophagus and dysphagia may be an early symptom.[16,17] The condition is rapidly progressive and symptomatic benefit can be obtained by limited resection of the pleura together with chemotherapy containing adriomycin and radiotherapy.[1] Survival of less than six months is usually reported.[17] Combination chemotherapy has been preferred.[18-20] Pirarubin—an anti-reacycline derivative has been able to eradicate tumour completely.[21]

Bronchogenic Carcinoma

Blue asbestos exposure especially in textile workers[22,23] may lead to development bronchogenic carcinoma. Cigarette smoking acts as a powerful co-carcinogen in these patients. Tumours generally develop the lung periphery.[3] Adenocarcinoma appears to be the frequent cell type. The condition develops often in patients without any evidence of pulmonary fibrosis, which is otherwise seen in silicosis when associated with tuberculosis of the lung.[24]

REFERENCES

1. Shankar P.S., Chest Medicine, Oxford and IBH Publ. Co. (P) Ltd., N. Delhi, 1994, 4th ed.
2. Simonato L., *et al.,* The man-made mineral fibre, European historical cohort study, Extension of follow-up. Scandi J. Work Env. Health 1986; 12(1): 34.
3. Harrison's principles of internal medicine, Wilson J.D., Braunwald E., Isselbacher K.J., *et al.*, (ed), 12th ed, McGraw Hill New York, 1991.
4. Craighead J.E. and Mossman B.J., The pathogenesis of asbestos associated disease, N. Engl. J. Med 1982; 306: 1446.
5. Coutts II, Gilson J.C., Kerr I.H., *et al.,* Progression of interpulmonary fibrosis caused by asbestos exposure, Thorax 1981; 36: 232.
6. Crofton and Douglas' Resp. Diseases; Sector A; Sector D. and Gordon Kitch A., ed., 4th ed., 1989, Oxford University Press, Delhi.
7. Elmes P.C., Simpson M.J.C., The clinical aspects of mesothelioma, Quat. J.Med 1976; 45: 427.
8. Ng T.P., *et al.,* Fasting urinary hydroxyproline creatinin ratios in silicosis. Ann Acad Med 1989; 18(6): 692-95.
9. U.S. Department of Health and Human Service, Reducing the Health consequences of smoking, 25 years of progress; A Report of the Surgeon General; DHMS (CDC) Publ. No. 89-8411, 1989.
10. Rishikesh K., *et al.,* Malignant pleural mesothelioma; JAPI 2013; 61: 56-59.
11. Wanger J.C., Berry G. and Timberell V., Mesothelioma rates after innoculation with asbestos and other materials, Br. J. Cancer 1973; 28: 173-85.
12. Peterson J.T., Greenberg S.D. and Patrica A.B., Non-asbestos related malignant mesothelioma, Cancer 1984; 54: 951-53.
13. Cochrane J.C. and Webster I., Mesothelioma in relation to asbestos fibre exposure, A review of 70 serial cases, South Afr. Med. Journ 1978; 54: 279-81.
14. Grundy G.W. and Miller R.W., Malignant mesothelioma in childhood—Report of 13 cases. Cancer 1972; 32: 1216-18.
15. Zahid I., *et al.,* What is the best way to diagnose and stage malignant pleural mesothelioma? Interact Cardiovasic Thorac surg 2011; 12:251-59.
16. Maroy B., Peural Mesothelioma with predominant mediastinal involvement unusual presentation with dysphagia and pneumothorax, Ann Radiol. (Paris), English abst (French) 1981; 24: 661-664.
17. Tewari S.C., Kurian G., Jayaswal R., *et al.,* Malignant mesothelioma in the young (with prosthetic aortic valve—An unusual association), J. Assn. Phys. India 1989; 37: 187-89.
18. Butnor K.J., My approach to the diagnosis of mesothelial lesions, J Clin Pathol 2006;59:564-74.
19. Patel J., Sheppard M.N., Primary malignant mesothelioma of the pericardium; Cardiovas Pathol 2011;20:107-09.
20. Fujimoto N., *et al.*, Malignant pericardial mesothelioma with response to chemotherapy; J Thorac Oncol 2009;4:1440-41.
21. Sridhar K.S., Mussain A.M., Teunn L.G., *et al.,* Activity of Pirarubicin in malignant mesothelioma; Cancer 1989, 63: 1084-91.
22. Doll R. Peto: Effects on health of exposure to asbestos; Health and safety commission, HMSO, London, 1985.
23. Ng J.P., *et al.,* Mortality of cohort of men in a silicosis Register, further evidence of an association with lung cancer, Amer. J. Industr. Med 1990; 17: 163-71.
24. Ng T.P. and Chan S.L., Factors associated with massive fibrosis in silicosis, Thorax 1991; 46: 229-32.

SILICOSIS

Silica flour or finely milled crystalline silica obtained from quartzite ore has multitudes of uses because of its abrasive properties in scoring powders, polishes, toothpastes and sand papers. It is also used as filler in paints and filler for cosmetics, and other manufactured items like rubber and plastic.[1,2]

Acute silicosis is highly prevalent in these silica flour workers is due to high concentrations of respirable dust of nearly pure crystalline silica (99%) found in the workplace. The accelerated progression of silicosis in these workers is due to the higher biological reactivity of the freshly crushed silica since newly fractured silica results in a greater respiratory burst as well as release of lysosomal enzymes from alveolar macro- phages than aged silica.[3,4] This form of silica dust exhibits greater cytotoxic effect on alveolar cellular membrane integrity.[5]

Since its first report from India in 1947 from the Kolar Gold Mines (Mysore), its occurrence has been uncovered in various other industries.[6] Mycobacterial infection is a common complication of silicosis.

Even though the diagnosis of active tuberculosis is confirmed by the finding of tubercle bacilli in the sputum, the sputum positivity is often impeded by the anatomical peculiarities of silico tuberculosis such as obturation of bronchi caused by shrinking silicotic nodules and scars, deforming bronchitis and silicotic lymph nodes. The tuberculin test *per se* does not have much importance for the diagnosis of tuberculous activity by the tuberculin conversion in a patient with silicosis. It is an important sign when there are also appropriate radiological signs of tuberculosis. Therefore radiology is the most important method for diagnosing silicosis, tuberculosis and silicotuberculosis.

In pure silicosis, the first change is mostly the accentuation of the basic lung structures (broncho vascular markings) and this is followed by rounded opacities. In pure tuberculosis round opacities appear first and thereafter linear opacities and cord extending to the hila appear. The small opacities of silicosis are localised predominantly in the upper and middle lung fields and have no connection with the hilum whereas tuberculosis nodules seen in the upper lung fields often appear in rows and are associated with cords extending to the hila. Mass shadows caused by progressive massive fibrosis due to silicosis is not limited by interlobar fissure but in case of tuberculosis it is limited by fissures.[7]

Massive silicotic shadows are mostly irregular shaped and have no connection with the hila but not uncommonly their lateral margin can be very smooth creating interface that parallels lateral chest wall. However the unique characteristic feature is the presence of overinflated emphysematous changes between the massive opacities and pleural surface.[1] Prior tuberculous infection of the lung or the pleura of silica worker will lead to a typical asymmetric form of silicosis because of the residual scars of tuberculosis. Egg shell calcification of hilar node is pathognomonic of silicosis even though it may also occur in sarcoidosis but the presence of irregular and asymmetrical calcified opacity should lead to suspicion of tuberculosis. Tuberculous cavity is often round or spherical whereas silicotic cavities are irregularly shaped because of the mechanical effect of shrinking fibrotic masses. Although regular sputum examination in silicotics is the safe method of detecting tuberculosis in silicotics.[8] It is invariably the chest skiagram features which give a key to the diagnosis.[8] In addition, connective tissue disorders like rheumatoid arthrits and SLE might coexist.[6]

Radiological signs that are suggestive of tuberculosis in silicotic lung are (i) new parenchymal shadows especially the soft and asymmetric opacities in the upper zones; (ii) rapid enlargement and growth of few shadows; (iii) rapidly changing lesion particularly if cavitated (especially with an irregularly shaped inner wall[9]); (iv) unexpected radiological shadows; (v) development of parchy opacities; (vi) coalescence of nodules; (vii) progression of lesion out of proportion to the intensity of exposure;[10] (viii) pleural or pericardial effusion; and (ix) bronchial narrowing and stenosis.[1,7-10]

Varieties

Three distinctly different disease patterns of silicosis, namely chronic, acute and accelerated have been described.[1,2,7] Chronic is the most usual form and develops after many years of exposure to relatively low levels of silica dust, radiologically presenting as nodular shadows. It may progress into massive fibrosis in 20-40 years. Risk factors associated with massive fibrosis include relatively higher level of dust exposure, tuberculosis if associated, and increased background profusion of small opacities through secondary localising process.[11,12] Regional lymph nodes become fibrotic; heavy silica exposure leads to interstitial nodules.

Acute form called silica proteinosis, first described by Sand Blasters in 1969[13] may develop rapidly in subjects exposed to very high concentration of crystaline silicon over a period of first few weeks to months. Pneumothorax is its rare complication.[14-16] Classical nodular presentation on roentgenogram is absent and lungs show diffuse ground glass appearance, simulating pulmonary odema.[17] The X-ray evaluation can be done as per the standard radiographic pictures by International Labour Organisation.[18] There is an increased production of surfactant along with deficient clearance, leading to alveolar filling of eosinophilic material, simulating pulmonary alveolar proteinosis. There is marked reduction in lung volume, diffusing capacity and compliance, with progressive hypoxemia, leading to death.

Accelerated silicosis refers to fibrosis of upper zones progressing at an intermediate rate (5-10 years) on heavy exposure and fibrosis progresses even after the stoppage of silica exposure, leading to respiratory failure.

Personal risk factors play a minor role and development of various forms is directly related to the concentration of respirable dust in the surroundings and the percentage of free silica in the dust.[17] Clubbing is not a feature. Clinically patient may not have any symptoms, even in severe forms of pneumoconiosis, if there is no further complication of chronic obstructive lung disease, depending upon degree and duration of exposure.[19] Silicosis is a restrictive lung disease, and most of the silicotics have reduced FVC. The degree of dyspnoea or respiratory symptoms do not correlate closely with the reduced FVC, and may be due to airway obstruction possibly caused by silica or cigarette smoking.[20] Repeated inhalations cause silicosis of various grades.[21-23] Disturbance in lung functions starts mainly when the chronic obstructive disease starts.[24] The induction of airways obstruction is exhibited more significantly in smokers.[25-27] Dietary intake and nutritional status are also clinical determinants in immunocompetence and the production of chronic obstructive pulmonary disease.[28]

Patient may have dyspnoea, weight loss, cough with scanty mucoid sputum for few weeks or months.[29] Generally there is no chest pain, nocturnal wheeze or dyspnoea. Haemoptysis is not a feature, may be present in cases associated with pulmonary tuberculosis. Destructive pulmonary impairment,[24,30] as well as obstructive airway disease[31,32] with ventilatory impariment[25] have been reported in silicosis workers. The suggested threshold limit value (TLV) by American Congress of Government Industrial Hygienists for dust containing free silica content of 50 per cent is 0.19 mg/mm^3) per cent of air.[33] In a state pencil industry the total dust concentration of 24.7 mg/m^3, respirable dust 5.53 mg/m^3 containing 54.6 per cent free silica has been reported.[34] In the initial stages in silicosis, bronchitis like symptoms due to physical and chemical irritation occur, ultimately leading to obstructive pattern which is more common.[25] Further deposition of silica dust, produced mechanical impediment of ventilation. As the parenchymal injury results in fibrosis, restrictive pattern emerges.[19] In complicated silicosis, severe airflow limitation and decreased FRC levels have been documented.[35] Fasting urinary hydroxy proline might be useful as an indicator of disease progression in established silicosis.[36]

Aetiopathogenesis

There is a cellular reaction which follows the inhalation and alveolar deposition of free silica particles.

The particles that reach the alveoli are cleared by phagocytosis. These defences are overcome when deposition of particles within the airspaces is excessive. The precise machanism of toxic effects of crystalline silica remains unexplained.[6]

Interstitial localisation of a particle is related to injury of lining cells and is followed by passage of silica through the lymphatics to lymph nodes where nodules develop. The development of lung disease is dose related. On the other hand, fatal diseases can occur after a few months exposure when dust concentrations are very high.

There is potential danger of developing irreversible acute silicosis in silica powdering industry[37] even after a brief exposure. Silica when mixed with other dusts like coal and haematite produces less severe fibrosis after long incubation period (mixed dust fibrosis in foundry workers and haematite miners).[38] It has been observed that if workers are exposed to quartz, it is possible for them to leave the occupation after five or more years, free of symptoms with normal chest skiagram/lung function tests at that time and yet develop classical silicosis and die of respiratory failure even without further exposure.[39] Risk of lung cancer in silicotics is due to smoking. Nevertheless, possible role of silicosis and tuberculosis as the fibrotic seedbed for the growth of lung cancer has been a matter of controversy in occupational medicine,[40-50] and is strongly supported.[51]

Treatment, Prevention and Rehabilitation

There is no treatment as such and prevention is the best cure. Medical removal of offending material provides relief. The treatment of choice is unilateral lung lavage while contralateral lung is isolated and ventilated by using a double lumen endobronchial tube.[8]

Even though this occupational hazard is well recognized, practising good occupational hygiene including substitution by safer materials, removal of dust at the source, strict dust suppression control measures and clean air supply to the operatives by respirators and air stream helmet and the proper use of disposable filtering face pieces are not practised uniformly in developing countries like India. Neither the flourishing industry can be banned altogether nor the effective respiratory protective measures can be strictly enforced due to negligence of authorities and ignorance of the illiterate workers. It is suggested that no worker is allowed to work for more than three years in such an industry. Arrangements for re-employment of such workers in other places should be taken over on priority by the Government agencies.

Predictors of Mortality[52]

- Mixed pattern in spirometry is suggestive of restrictive and obstructive pathology.
- TB and nutritional status have strong influence on mortality.
- Screening early and managing comorbidities in these agate stone workers can slow down early death.

REFERENCES

1. Robert G., Fraser Peter Pare J.A., Pare P.D., Richard S. Fraser and George P. Genereux. Diagnosis of the diseases of the chest.

Third Ed. Vol. WB Saunders Company, 1990, Philadelphia, 2282-01.

2. Morgan W.K.C. and Seaton A., Occupational lung diseases, 2nd Ed . Silicosis WB Saunders Company, Philadelphia 1984; 250-91.
3. Morgan W.K.C., Seaton A. and Parkes W.R., Lipid peroxidases of cell memberone involving oxygenated free radical and bydrocxyl radical in silicosis. Proceeding of VII international pneumoconiosis conference (Pittsburg 1988) 1990. P Part I. Department of Health and Human Services Publication 90-108.
4. Val Vallyaathan, Xianglin Shi, Nar S. Dalal, William I.R.R. and Vincent Castranova, Generation of free radicals from freshly fractured silica dust, Am. Rev. Respir. Dis 1988; 138: 1213-19.
5. Brown G.P., Monick M. and Hunninghake G.W., Fibroblast proliferation induced by silica-exposed human alveolar macrophages, Am. Rev. Respir. Dis. 1988; 138: 85-89.
6. Sainani G.S., Industrial lung disease; J. App. Med 1984, 10: 43-49.
7. International Labour Office Encyclopaedia of occupational health and safety. Vol. I and II Silicosis and Silicotuberculosis, 3rd Ed., Geneva 1983.
8. Seaton A., Gordon A., Leitch Eds., Crofton and Douglas' Respiratory Diseases, 4th Ed., Delhi, Oxford University Press, Delhi 1989; 350, 1050.
9. Dixil E. Snider, Editorial—The relationship between tuberculosis and silicosis, Am. Rev. Respir. Dis 1978; 118: 455-60.
10. Becklake M.R., Pneunoconiosis In, Murry Nadel Ed. Textbook of Respiratory Medicine, WB Saunders Co., Philadelphia 1988. Vol.11,1567.
11. Ng T.P., Chan S.L., Factors associated with massive fibrosis in silicosis, Thorax 1991; 46: 229-32.
12. Leibowitz M.C., Goldstein B., Some investigations into the nature and cause of massive fibrosis in the lungs of South African gold, coal and asbestos mine workers, Amer J Indust Med 1987;12: 129-43.
13. Buechner H.A, Ansari A., Acute silico proteinosis, Dis chest 1969; 55: 274-84.
14. Suratt P.M., Winn W.C. Jr., Brody A.R., *et al.,* Acute silicosis in Tomstone sand blasters, Amer. Rev. Resp. Dis 1977; 115: 521-29.
15. Bates D.V., Macklem P.T. and Christie R.V., Resp. function in disease, 2nd Ed, Philadelphia, WB Saunders 1971; 376.
16. Arora V.K., Seetharaman M.L., Veliath A.J., Silicotic alveolar proteinosis with bilateral spontaneous pneumothorax., JAPI 1992, 40:760-62.
17. Natrajan A.S., Gajalakshmi L. and Karunakaran S., Accelerated silicosis in a silica flour mill workers, Lung India 1992; 10: 33-37.
18. International Labour Organisation, International Classification of radiographs or pneumoconiosis, I.L.O. Office, Geneva, 1980.
19. Mohan Rao N., Siyed H.N., Kashyap S.K., *et al.,* Airway obstruction in silicosis workers, Lung India 1991; 9 : 126-29.
20. Chan S.L., Silicosis, Personal communication, Aug 25, 1993.
21. Gupta S.P., Garg A.K. and Gupta O.P., Silicosis among stone cutters, J.Asso. Phys. India 1969; 17: 163-69.
22. Saini R.K., Yousuf M., Allakaband G. and Kaul S.N., Silicosis in stone cutters in Kashmir, J. Ind. Med. Assoc 1984; 82: 198-201.
23. Jain S.M., Sepaha G.C., Khare K.C. and Dubey V.S., Silicosis in state pencil workers, Chest 1977; 71: 423-25.
24. Rane M.A., Lung function of refractory workers exposed to silica dust, Ind. Indust. Med 1982; 29: 72-78.
25. Jain S.M., Sepaha G.C., Khare K.C. and Dubey V.S., Ventilatory functions and sputum cytology in slate pencil workers of silicosis, Ind. J. Chest Dis. All Sci 1979; 21: 103-09.
26. Rogan J.M., Altifield M.D., Jacobson M., Raw S., Walker D.D. and Walton W.H., Role of dust in the working environment in the development of chronic bronchitis in British coal mines, Brit. J. Indust. Med 1973; 30: 217-26.
27. Morgan W.K.C., Editorial on dust, disability and death, Am. Rev. Respir Dis 1986; 134: 639-41.
28. Edelman N.H., Rucker R.B. and Peavy H.H., Nutrition and respiratory system, Am. Rev. Resp. Dis 1986; 134:347-52.
29. Schott C.D., Silicosis-clinical symptoms, pulmonary function and prevention (Germ), Atemwegs-Lungen Krankh 1985; 11/6:241-46.
30. Theriault G., Peters J.M. and Silliam M.J., Pulmonary function and roentgenographic changes in granite dust exposure, Arch Environ Health 1974; 28: 23-27.
31. Spacilova M., The development of silicosis in relation to bronchial obstruction (Czech), Prac. Lak 1982; 34(6-7): 219-21.
32. Procose E.M., Aspects of pulmonary function in silicosis in South African gold miners. Pneumoconiosis: Proceedings of the International Conference, Johannesburg 1969,508-511.
33. American Conference of Government Industrial Hygienistis (ACGIH), Threshold Limit Value (TLV) for chemical substances and physical agents in work-room environment with intended changes, Ohio, USA 1977.
34. Saiyed H.N., Parikh D.J., Ghodasara N.B., Sharma Y.K., Patel G.C., Chatterjee S.K. and Chatterjee B.B., Silicosis in slate pencil industry—An environment and medical study, Am. J. Indust. Med 1985; 32: 13-17.
35. Mitsura Munukata, Yukihiko Homma, Michiyuki Matsuzaki, Hideki Ogaswara, Yuishi Sasaki and Yoshikaza Kawakami., Rales in silicosis, A correlation with physiological and radiological abnormalities, Respiration 1985; 48:140-44.
36. Ng T.P., *et al.,* Fasting urinary hydroxyproline, creatinine ratios in silicosis, Ann. Aca. Meds 1989; 18: 629-95.
37. Banks D.E., Morring K.L., Boehlecke A.B., Althouse R.B., and Merchant J.A., Silicosis in silica flour workers, Am Rev. Respir. Dis 1981; 124: 445-50.
38. Cotes J.E. and Steel J., Biological effects of silica in work-related lung disorders, 1st Ed, Oxford Blackwell Scientific Publications 1987; 147-49.
39. Raffle P.A.B., Lee W.R., McCallum R.I. and Murray R. In Hunter's Diseases of Occupations, Inorganic Dusts, 6th Ed., London, Hodder and Stoughton 1987; 647.
40. Goldsmith D.F., *et al.,* Does occupational exposure to silica cause lung cancer? Amer J Indus Med 1982; 3: 423-40.
41. Choudhury N., *et al.,* Comorbidities among silicotics at Shakarpur—A follow up study; Lung India 2012;29:6-10.
42. Schuller G., Ruttner J.R., Silicosis and lung cancer in Switzerland. In Goldsmith D.F., *et al.,* ed, Silica, silicosis and

cancer, Controversy in occupational medicine, Praeger, New York 1986.
43. Forestiere F., *et al.,* Silica, silicosis and lung cancer among ceramic workers, A case referrant study, Amer J Indust Med 1986; 10: 363-70.
44. Gudberfsson H., *et al.,* An association between silicosis and lung cancer, A Registry approach, Proceedings of VIth International conference on Pneumoconiosis, Bochum, Geneva International Labour Office, 1984.
45. Heppleston A.G., Silica, pneumoconiosis and carcinoma of the lung, Amer J Indust Med 1985; 3:423-40.
46. Hessel P.A., *et al.,* Case contolled study of silicosis, silica exposure and lung cancer in white South African gold miners, Treatment Amer J Indust Med 1986; 10: 57-62.
47. Tiwari R., *et al.,* TB among workers exported to free silica dust. Ind. J. Occup Environ Med 2007;11:61-64.
48. International Agency for Research on Cancer, IARC Monograph on the evaluation of the carcinogenic risk of chemicals to human, Silica and some silicates, Lyons, France, IARC 1987, vol 42.
49. Ng T.P., and O'Kelly F.J., Silicosis prevalence in granite quarry and construction workers in Hong Kong, J Hong Kong Med Assoc 1987, 39: 160-62.
50. Ng T.P., *et al.,* Silica hazard of caisson construction on Hong Kong, J. Soc. Occup. Med 1987, 37: 62-25.
51. Ng T.P., *et al.,* Mortality of a Cohort of men in a silicosis register, further evidence of an association with Lung Cancer, Amer J Indust Med 1990; 17: 163-71.
52. Mathur M.L., Pattern and predictors of mortality in sandstone quarry workers, Ind J Occup Environ Med 2005;9:80-85.

TALC-INDUCED PLEURO-PULMONARY DISEASES

When we talk of talc, we usually visualize a white, soothing powder, sprinkled on the buttocks of babies to prevent irritation. Cosmetic uses of talc actually represents a fraction of the practical applications of this mineral substance, of which almost 4 million tons are used annually for industrial purposes. Talcum is used in the manufacture of paper, ceramics, painting, lubrication of rubber products (even in chewing gum!). It is the principal excipient of drugs in tablet form. It is also found in shock-absorbers or dashboards of some cars, and in rice or animal food stuffs. The pleuropulmonary pathology of talc is not very clear.[1]

Talc

The word talc denotes a mineral (a hydrous magnesium silicate, lammelar in structure; a composite rock, and an industrial product. The pure mineral is handled only by mineralogists and rock collectors. Crude talc is contaminated to a greater or lesser extent with other minerals, particularly quartz, asbestiform minerals (tremolite, anthophyllite and chrysolite specially), chlorites or carbonates. Talc is considered *pure* and accepted for cosmetic use of the mineral talc content therein if at least 90 per cent (the remaining 10 per cent sometimes contains quartz and fibres!).[2] Medical classification is given in Table 5.5.

Table 5.5: Medical classification of talcs

1. Talc + quartz (5%)
2. Talc + asbestiform minerals
   - Tremolite
   - Anthophyllite
   - Chrysolite
3. Talc + non-fibrous minerals
   - Chlorites
   - Carbonates (dolomite, magnesite, calcite)
4. Talc + chemical and pharmaceutical products
5. Pure talc

Quartz and/or asbestiform mineral predominate in certain industrial talcs, where the quantum of talc as such is very low, or even absent.[3]

Talc-induced Pneumoconioses

A differentiation of at least three types of pneumoconiosis induced by inhalation of talc is necessary, talc-silicosis, talc-asbestosis and talcosis.[4]

Talc-silicosis

Usually occurs in the talc miners following inhalation of talc dust contaminated with a high content of free silica. Radiocinematography reveals a picture of classical nodular silicosis, with similar prognosis,[4] although talc appears to slow down the process of onset of silicosis.[5]

Talc-asbestosis

This has primarily been observed after inhalation of American talcs, particularly in the state of New York.[6-11] It induces chronic respiratory insufficiency, gradual in evolution, which progresses into chronic cor pulmonale. X-ray shows linear fibrosis due to asbestos is associated with signs of nodular pneumoconiosis and pleural plaques—*talc plaques.* Histopathologic lesions do not differ much from those of asbestosis. Two types of ferruginous bodies are encountered in such lesions: characteristic *asbestos bodies* and *talc bodies.*

Talcosis

Talcosis is often a mixed silicosis considered to be an occupational disease[12] induced by inhalation of talc and chlorites or talc and carbonates. Such was the case in the pneumoconiosis induced by the French talc from Luzenac, which typifies this third group. *Luzenac talc* pneumoconiosis is relatively frequent among exposed workers. There is a high correlation between radiologic signs of pneumoconiosis and the duration and intensity of inhalationl.[12] Mostly, they are cases of asymptomatic micronodular pneumoconiosis. X-ray sometimes shows a striking picture, with confluent opacities, pseudoterminal masses and emphysematous bullae. These extensive forms are generally accompanied by a mixed or limited ventilatory deficiency of average intensity. The histopathology is that of pneumoconiosis with lesions of macrophage alveolitis and dense mineral deposits.[13] The sclerotic lesions are less marked, with areas of alveolar rarefaction, emphysema and endovascular arteriolar changes with hyperplasia of the intimal.[4] Bronchoalveolar lavage reveals a sizeable quantity of *talc bodies* and some asbestos bodies.[1]

Bronchopulmonary Cancer and Mesothelioma

Several publications have recorded the presence of talc in neoplastic tissue; however, no experimental study has been able to demonstrate the carcinogenic risk of talc. In a retrospective study on mortality, Kleinteld has reported a frequency of pleuropulmonary cancer among workers exposed to tremolite talc that was four times higher in comparison with a control group.[14] Progressive reduction of talc dust content was accompanied by a significant fall in the incidence of cancer.[15] High incidence of bronchial cancer in workers exposed to talc contaminated with tremolite and anthophyllites has been reported.[16] Contradictory reports in favour[17] against[18-21] have been reported.

Chronic Obstructive Bronchopneumopathies

The role of inhalation of talc in the genesis of chronic obstructive, bronchopneumopathy (COBP) is, by and large, yet to be demonstrated, because the populations studied were often heavy smokers. The restrictive functional alterations related to pleural pathology are probably attributable to asbestos bodies.[22] Two lines of recommendation emanate from these studies: strict observance of norms pertaining to occupational inhalation of dust and laying down of regulations for periodical routine check-up of retired personnel who were exposed to occupational inhalation of talc.[1]

Massive Inhalation of Talcum Powder

Several cases of massive inhalation of dusting talc by infants playing with a box of cosmetic talc left carelessly within their reach have been published.[23-25] This is followed by a two-phased syndrome of respiratory distress: an initial phase of mechanical obstruction, marked by cough and intense dyspnoea a which evolves favourably after nasopharyngeal aspiration, followed after a lapse of a few hours by a second phase of respiratory distress due to tracheobronchial inflammation. The infant presents intense dyspnoea, fever, rales and bilateral pulmonary infiltrate. Death occurs in about 25 per cent of the cases. Postmortem lung study shows lesions of bronchoalveolitis with areas of atelectasis and obstructive emphysema. Massive corticosteroid therapy, intubation with artificial ventilation and prompt bronchoalveolar lavages may help in saving the life.[25]

Talc-induced Fibrogranulomatosis in DrugAddicts

Krainer was first to publish in 1962 followed by a large number of cases of fibrogranulomatosis following repeated intravenous administration of narcotic tablets crudely crushed and diluted (methylphenidate, methadone, pentazocine), generally in heroin addicts during withdrawal, have been published.[26] The symptoms observed are due principally, if not exclusively, to talc which is the excipient in these tablets.

Two clinical pictures can be differentiated, although one cannot be definitive about their aetiopathogenesis,[12,27,28] pulmonary arterial hypertension following development of intra- and perivascular granulomatosis and microthrombus, or interstitial pneumopathy associated with development of interstitial fibrosis and pulmonary arterial hypertension. These interstitial pneumopathies caused by talc-induced fibro-granulomatosis sometimes present all the active signs of sarcoidosis,[29] with a high angiotensin convertin enzyme level, gallium hyperfixation, and high lymphocytosis on broncho-alveolar lavage. These pneumopathies are sometimes corticosteroid sensitive.[1] Pneumoconiostic changes due to repeated attacks of respiratory system involvement, possibly due to hypersensitivity reaction with decreased ventilatory capacity, are reported to be cause of absentism in a working place.[30,31]

REFERENCES

1. Leophonte P., Delaude A., Talc induced lung disease, La Medicine en France 1988; 37-42.
2. Cralley L.J., Key M.M., Groth D.H. and Lainhart W.Sr., Am. Ind. Hyg. Assoc. J 1968; 29: 350.
3. Parker W.R.,Occupational lung disorders, Vol. I, London Butterworth and Co. ed., 1974.
4. Leophonte P., Fabre J., Pous J., Albarede J.L. and Delaude A., Talc-induced pneumoconiosis, Arch. Mal. Prof 1976; 87: 513.
5. Schepers G.W.H. and Durkan T.M., Effects of inhaled talc mining dust on human lung, Arch. Ind. Health 1955,12:182.
6. Kleinfeld M., Gel C.P., Majeranowski J.F. and Messite J., Talc pneumoconiosis, A report of six patients with postmortem findings, Arch Enviton Health 1963; 7: 101.
7. Kleinfeld M., Messite J., Shapiro J., Kooyman O. and Swencicki R., Lung function in talc workers, A comparative physiologic study of workers exposed to fibrous and granular talc dusts. Arch. Environ. Health 1964; 9:559.

8. Kleinfeld M., Messite J. and Langer A.M., A study of workers exposed to asbestiform minerals in commercial talc manufacture, Environ. Res 1973; 6: 132.
9. Messite J., Reddin G., Kleinfeld M., Pulmonary talcosis, a clinical and environmental study, Arch. Ind. Health 1959; 20: 408.
10. Miller A., Terstein A.S., Bader M.E., Bader R.A. and Selikoff I.J., Talc pneumoconiosis, significance of sunlight microscopic mineral particles, Am J. Med 1971; 50: 395.
11. Siegal E.N., Smith A.R. and Greenburg L., The dust hazard in tremolite talc mining including roentgenological findings in talc workers. Am J. Roentgen 1943; 49: 11.
12. Arnett E.N., Battle W.E., Russo J.V. and Roberts W.C., Intravenous injection of talc–containing drugs intended for oral use, Am. J. Med 1976; 60: 771.
13. Leophonte P., Fernet P., Pincemin J., Mousset J.L., Rellier R. and Delaude A.,Chronic respiratory pathology in talc workers, Rev. Fr. Mal. Resp 1980; 8: 43.
14. Kleinfeld M., Messite J., Kooyman O. and Zaki M.H., Mortality among talc miners and millers in New York State, Arch Environ. Health 1967; 14: 663.
15. Kleinfeld M., Messite J. and Zaki M.H., Mortality experiences among talc workers, a follow-up study, J Occup Med 1974; 16: 345.
16. Brown D.P., Dement J.M. and Wangner J.K., Mortality patterns among miners and millers occupationally exposed to asbestiform talc, Dusts and Disease. Lemen R., Dement J.M., ed., Part Forest South, Pathotox ed 1979; 317.
17. Rubino G.F., Scansetti B., Piolatto G. and Romano C.A., Mortality study of talc miners and millers, J. Occup. Med 1976; 18: 186.
18. Selevan S.G., Dement J.M., Wagoner J.K. and Froines J.R., Mortality patterns among miners and millers of non-asbestiform talc. Preliminary report. Dusts and Disease. Lemen R., Dement J.M., eds., Park Forest South, Pathotox ed 1979; 379.
19. Wagner J.C., Berry G., Cooke J.J., Hill R.J., Pooley F.D. and Skidmoe J.M., Animal experiments with talc. Inhaled particles. Welton W.H. ed., New York Pergamon Press 1977; 647.
20. Katsonelson B.A., Mokronasova K.A., Nonfibrous mineral dusts and malignant tumors. An epidemiological study of mortality, J. Occu. Med 1979; 21:15.
21. Leophonte P. and Basset M.F., Pincemin J., Louisa A, Fernet P., Delaude A., Talc worker mortality in France. Retrospective epidemiologic study, Rev. Fr. Mal. Resp 1983.
22. Gamble J.F., Fellner W. and Dimeo M.J., An epidemiological study of a group of talc workers, Am. Rev. Resp. Dis 1979; 119: 741.
23. Cless D. and Anger R., Asphyxia due to inhalation of children's toilet powder, Kinderaztl Prax 1954; 22: 506.
24. Nelmann N., Vidallhet M., Kiffer B., Crance J.P., Grung G. and Andre J.L., Accidental inhalation of talc among infants, Pediatric 1971; 26: 81.
25. Pfenninger J., d' Appuzzo V., Powder aspiration in children, Arch. Dis. Child 1977; 52: 157.
26. Krainer L., Berman E. and Wishinick S.D., Parenteral talcum granulomatosis, a complication of narcotic addiction Lab. Invest 1962; 11: 671.
27. Pare J.A.P., Fraser R.G., Hogg J.C., Howlett J.G. and Murphy S., Pulmonary "mainline" granulomatosis; talcosis of intravenous methadone abuse. Medicine 1979; 58: 229.
28. Tomashefski J.F. Jr. and Hirsoh C.S., The pulmonary vascular lesions of intravenous drug. Hum Pathol 1980; 11: 133.
29. Farber H.W., Fairman R.P. and Glauser F.L., Talc granulomatosis, laboratory findings similar to sarcoidosis. Am. Rev. Resp. Dis 1982; 125: 258.
30. Damodar B., *et al.*, Ind. J. Chest Dis 1983; 20: 21-30.
31. Damodar B., Aggarwal D., Impact of Talc dust on the respiratory system of working population, J Ind Med Assn 1985; 83:41-43.

COAL WORKERS' PNEUMOCONIOSIS (CWP)

Miners exposed to coal dust for several years develop a most common type of pneumoconiosis called coal workers' pneumoconiosis. Associated development of silicosis and industrial bronchitis is known as coal miners are frequently exposed to silica dust in addition to coal particles.[1] Only 5-15 per cent of coal workers of underground mines suffer from CWP and that too, depending upon the type of coal.[2] Pneumoconiosis is more common in factory and transport workers.

Pathogenesis

Airborne coal mine dust (carbon) of less than 5 microns in diameter on inhalation gets distributed throughout the lungs and is deposited in the gas exchange parts. The coal dust is retained more in the upper and middle lobes than lower. Most of the carbonaceous material is engulfed as the macrophages come into action and is carried to the terminal bronchioles, thus facilitating its removal by the mucociliary escalator. Coal dust is not toxic to macrophages and it is not digested by them. As the dust deposit increases, the clearance becomes incomplete and the dust-laden macrophages remain attached to the alveolar walls and respiratory bronchioles. Lymphatic drainage to the regional lymph nodes also occurs.[1]

Dust-laden macrophages disintegrate and stimulate focal proliferation of reticulin, not collagen, fibres which fix the dust and ultimately lead to the formation of star-shaped coal macule. They gradually increase in size. The amount of fibrosis is minimal. The respiratory bronchioles and alveoli surrounding the fibrotic nodules undergo dilation leading to focal emphysema in the centre of the lobule.[2] These changes are seen in simple pneumoconiosis. Finely reticular nodules are present throughout the lung.

A higher concentration of silica and coal in the inhaled dust leads to the development of progressive massive fibrosis (PMF) that presents as a complicated pneumoconiosis. The disability is greater with it. Chest X-ray may show nodular involvement ranging from one centimeter in diameter to the size of involving the whole lobe. Generally the involvements remain restricted to upper half of the lungs. Exact mechanism is not fully understood why PMF occurs in CWP.[2] Suggested hypotheses include:

a. Presence of free silica in the dust.
b. Incapability of clearance mechanism to get off excessive dust load.
c. Possible interplay between immune mechanism and dust or damaged lung.
d. Atypical reaction to Mycobact. tuberculosis.

Tuberculosis generally described but may not coexist with the condition. Dense circumscribed fibrotic masses are located in the upper lobes. There is likelihood of softening and necrosis leading to cavitation either by ischemic necrosis or by tuberculous infection. The fibrotic lesions involving hypertension and cor pulmonale.[1]

The rheumatoid pneumoconiosis (Caplan syndrome) may occur on the background of pneumoconiosis with an appearance of multiple, clearly defined, round opacities in both lungs especially in its periphery. There is seropositive rheumatoid arthritis with characteristic PMF. The condition may occur along with lesions of rheumatoid arthritis or before or after the appearance of the arthritic manifestations. The nodules demonstrate fibrinoid necrosis.[1] The condition occurs in other pneumoconiosis also. Raised gammaglobulins suggests[2] an immunologic mechanism.

The coal workers exhibit radiological changes with the presence of small circular shadows even before the appearance of symptoms. These are graded according to the size as punctiform, micronodular and nodular opacities.[3] They exist in relation with coal nodules and the iron from disintegrated phagocytes makes the nodules radio-opaque. The distribution may be confined to one zone or lung or both the lung fields. The opacities may be small (round or irregular) or large (well or ill-defined).[4]

The clinical features develop in persons who have been exposed to dust for a long period. Progressively increasing dyspnoea is marked in progressive massive fibrosis. Cough is a late symptom. It may be associated with mucoid or inky black sputum (melanoptysis). Chest pain and haemoptysis may occur. The condition takes 10 to 20 years to produce nodular radiological shadows especially in the underground worker and may not show any disability. Generally patients with simple coal workers' pneumoconiosis hardly show any clinical disability.[1]

In the early stages[5] the functional abnormalities are not seen. There is reduction in FVC, FEV_1, TLC and there is abnormal gas distribution with progressive fibrosis. Often the functional abnormality correlates with the number of years worked underground, resulting in sufficient accumulation of carbon in the lungs to produce PMF. The superimposed chronic bronchitis and emphysema show evidence of airways obstruction. The progress of simple CWP can be stopped if dust exposure is avoided, but PMF becomes progressively worse even after stopping exposure to dust. Therefore great care is necessary in prevention of the condition by employing measures for suppression of dust and periodic radiological examination of workers. Tuberculosis needs specific chemotherapy.[1]

REFERENCES

1. Shanker P.S., Chest Medicine, Oxford and IBH Publ. Co. (P) Ltd., New Delhi 1994; 4th ed.
2. Harrison's Principles of Internal Medicine, 12th ed., Vol. 2, Wilson J.D., Brown Wald E., Isselbacher K.J., *et al.*, McGraw Hill, N.York, 1991.
3. International Labour Office, Occup. Safety Hlth 9, 1, 1959.
4. UICC/Cincinnati classification of the radiographs of pneumoconiosis, Chest 1970; 58: 57.
5. Cochrane A.L., Moore F.A., A 20 years follow-up of men aged 55-64 including coal miners and foundry workers in Savley, Brit. J. Indus. Med 1980; 37: 226.

BERYLLIOSIS

Before 1950, one may not be able to understand the aetiologic relationship of beryllium to this occupational disease. The exposure to metal dust and soluble salts of beryllium occur in people engaged in mining, extraction, smelting and fabrication of beryllium or its alloys. Beryllium is used in aircraft industries, atomic reactors, manufacture of X-ray tubes and in ceramics. Its contact with skin or mucosa may lead to occurrence of ulcers and granulomas.[1]

Pulmonary lesions noted are acute and chronic.[2] In the acute form the inhaled dust induces a generalised acute inflammatory reaction in the alveoli. The alveoli are filled with fibrin, red cells and a few polymorphs and the alveolar walls are infiltrated with lymphocytes and plasma cells. Such a picture of chemical pneumonitis is noted in the early weeks of exposure and to high dose of beryllium. There is dry cough, breathlessness and discomfort in the chest. There is no fever. It may slowly resolve completely or may pursue a fulminant course to have fatal end or may rarely progress to chronic type. Chest X-ray shows diffuse miliary mottling. Berylliosis is treated with high doses of corticosteroids and high concentration of oxygen.[1]

The chronic form produces interstitial pneumonitis following exposure to a low dose over long time. Such type of interstitial pneumonitis may occur with aluminium, powdery cobalt, titanium iodide etc. Sometimes it may develop following a latent period of as long as 10 to 15 years after a brief exposure. An immunologic mechanism despite the fact that beryllium is an inorganic dust plays some role. It produces non-caseating epitheloid granuloma in the pulmonary interstitum along with diffuse interstitial inflammation and fibrosis. Hilar lymphadenopathy may be present.[1] Thus the condition will have many of the characteristics of sarcoidosis. Tissue levels of beryllium are measured[3] to differentiate.

The symptoms develop very gradually with progressively increasing dysponea, weakness, fatigue, loss of weight and cough with mucoid sputum. On physical examination there may be evidence of clubbing and crepitations at the lung bases. Chest X-ray shows a fine micronodular infiltrate initially, which with the progress of the disease shows diffuse linear fibrosis throughout the lung fields. The hilar nodes are enlarged. However, the hilar adenopathy does not occur in the absence of lung changes. Spontaneous pneumothorax may occur. The condition progresses to cor pulmonale and cardiac failure. Pulmonary functions show a restrictive pattern and reduction in the diffusion capacity. Occasionally there is hyperuricemia and hypercalciuria.[1] CD4+T cells are increased in BAL fluid, skin tests and beryllium lymphocyte transfer tests are positive.[4] Using laser microphobe mass spectrometry[5] presence of beryllium can be demonstrated on histological section of granuloma with toluidine blue.

Cutaneous delayed hypersensitivity to a patch test with 1 to 2 per cent beryllium nitrate or suphate can be seen. Danger of a flare-up of the underlying lung lesion following the test cannot be ruled out. Steroid therapy controls the disease progression.[1]

REFERENCES

1. Shankar P.S., Chest Medicine; Oxford and IBH Publ. Co. (P) Ltd, N. Delhi, 1994; 4th, ed.
2. Teppler L.B., Hardy H.L.,Chamberling R.I., Toxicity of Baryllium, A monograph, Elsevier, Amsterdam, 1961.
3. Harrison's principles of internal medicine, (ed) by Wilson J.D., Braunwald E., Isselbacher K.J., *et al.*, 12th Ed., 1991; McGraw Hill, New York.
4. Jones-Williams W. and Williams WR, Thorax 1985; 38:41.
5. Jones-Williams W. and Wallach E.R., Sarcoidosis 1989; 6: 111-17.

BYSSINOSIS

Exposure to cotton dust provokes respiratory effects leading to chronic respiratory ailment known as byssinosis,[1] characterised by cough, phlegm or chest tightness and abnormalities in ventilatory function.[2] Byssinosis is a prograssive disease manifesting as a reversible asthma like reaction to dust on the first day of work week (Gr. I) and then leading to one of irreversible airway obstruction (Gr. II and III). Abnormal lung function in cotton mill workers and an increased dysfunction with higher grades of byssinosis has been noted with regard to indirect maximum breathing capacity[3] and FEV_1.[4] A singnificant fall in ventilatory indices such as FIV_1, $FEV_{25\text{-}70\%}$ is observed during works[5] as well as in asymptomatic byssinotics.[6] Those who have worked for several years (usually about 10 years) in the mill, may notice chest tightness, cough, laboured breathing and wheeze several hours after return to work on Monday following the weekend holiday. The symptoms subside in the evening. This is referred to as the 'Monday fever' or 'Monday feeling'. Later in the week the individual will be symptom free. With passage of time, the condition may persist for a long duration or may begin to appear on all days. Dyspnoea becomes persistent and the features of chronic bronchitis and emphysema are added.[7] The pathogenesis of the condition is not clear. Non-immunologic mechanisms appear to induce the disease. Release of chemical mediators such as histamine, hydroxy tryptamine, chemotoxins thrornboxane (TxA_2),[8] prostaglandins and leukotrienes or endotoxins from cotton dust contaminated with bacteria and fungi appear to cause bronchoconstriction.[9]

The pathophysiological changes in cotton workers suggest that small airways, which are the silent zone of lung,[10] are involved early and gradually the abnormality progresses to the larger airways.[11] Among byssinotics, smoking has an additive effect over dust in inducing a further fall in percentage of predicted value.[12-14] Airway dysfunction in cotton dust exposed workers is thought to be due to the liberation of histamine prostaglandins or leukotrienes from degranulation of mast cells cause the chemically mediated bronchoconstriction.

Pulmonary function studies reveal an airways obstruction. There is reduction in FEV_1 and is noted even in stages of the Monday fever and later in the week when there is no tightness of the chest.[7]

For further assessment, the British Medical Research Council recommendations have been modified for use in India.[15,16] The $FEV_{25\text{-}75\%}$ is derived from the middle half of the FVC curve. A reduction of this value below 80 per cent of predicted value is diagnosed as obstruction in small airways, since the smaller airways are the primary target area for the deposition of industrial dust and air pollutants.[17] Decreased flow rates are common is early diseases. There is evidence that $FEV_{25\text{-}75\%}$ is more reliable than other flow measurements commonly used in assessing obstructive pulmonary impairments.[18] The best FVC curve recorded with vital graph spirometer and the percentage of predicted value is computed by the regression equation developed for Indian non-smoking healthy subjects.[19] The FEV_1 and PEFR are also measured at

BTPS before and after the shift.[20,21] There is a significant reduction in $FEV_{25-75\%}$, which is an indicator of small airway dysfunction in cotton dust exposed workers and the reduction is more in byssinotics than non-byssinotics. This is observed in both acute and chronic changes.[22,23]

Removal of the worker from exposure to high concentration of cotton dust can stop the progress of the disease. Dust control and pre-treatment with disodium cromoglycate decreases bronchospasm. X-ray of the chest is non-informative as there are no specific radiological features.

Mill fever (cotton fever) is seen in few who commence work in cotton mills afresh or after a prolonged absence. It presents with symptoms like fever, chills, nausea, sneezing and cough within six hours of exposure. The symptoms subside gradually in few days and the individual develops tolerance and there are no further attacks. The condition appears to be an allergic response to inhaled dust[7] and histamine may be responsible for acute and chronic $PEF_{25-75\%}$ changes, with an additive effect by smoking.[24]

Other occupational pulmonary diseases include siderosis from iron oxide of welding or silver finishing, stannosis from manufacture of tin, glass or fabric, baritosis from electroplating etc.Similarly, pneumoconiosis due to other minerals/substances being used in industries can also occur, e.g., kaolin, mica, antimony, cement, polyvinyl chloride, aluminium, tungsten carbide, barium etc.

REFERENCES

1. Schilling R.S.F., Hughs J.P.N., Dingwall-Fordyce L and Gilson J.C., An epidemiological study of byssinosis among Lancashire cotton mill workers, Brit. J. Indust Med 1995; 121: 217-27.
2. Schilling R.S.F., Byssinosis in cotton and other textile mills, Amer, Rev. Resp. Dis 1956; 101: 497-503.
3. Lammers S., Schilling R.S. and Walford J., A study of byssinosis, chronic respiratory symptoms and ventilatory capacity in English and Dutch cotton workers with special reference to atomospheric pollution, Brit. J. Indust. Med 1964; 21: 124-34.
4. Scharg P.E. and Gullett A.D., Byssionosis in cotton textile mills, Ame Rev. Resp. Dis 1970; 101: 497-503.
5. Alzuhiar Y.S. and Cinkottai F.F., Ventilatory function in workers exposed to tea and wood dust, Med. Sci. Microbiol 1977, 5: 190-97.
6. Bouhys A., Wolfson R.L., Horner D.W., Birani J.D. and Zuskin E., Byssiosis in cotton workers, Ann. Intern. Med 1969; 71: 257-59.
7. Shankar P.S., *Byssimosis,* In, Chest Medicine, Oxford, IBH Publ. Co (P) Ltd.N.Delhi, 4th Ed., 1994.
8. Mundie T.G. and Ainsworth S.K., Byssinosis and thromboxane release from human platelets by cotton dust and bract extracts, Arch. Env. Hlth 1985; 40: 165-69.
9. Mundie T.G. and Ainsworth S.K., Aetiopathogenic mechanisms of brochoconstriction in Byssinosis, A Review, Amer. Rev. Respi. Dis 1986; 132: 1181-85.
10. Bhatia R.S., Disease of small airways of lung; Jour Ind Acad Clin Med 2001; 2: 222-24.
11. Mead J., The lung's quiet zone, New Eng. J. Med 1972; 23:1318-19.
12. Bouhys A., Byssinosis in textile workers. In: Proceedings the International Conference on Pneumoconiosis, Johnnesburg, Oxford University Press 1970; 350-59.
13. Niswochner D.H., Kleineman J. and Rice D.B., Pathological changes in the peripheral airways obstruction in chronic obstructive lung disease, New Eng. J. Med 1669; 279: 1355-57.
14. Bouhys A., Schoenberg J.S., Beck G.J. and Schilling R.S.F., Epidemiology of chronic lung disease in cotton mill community, Lung 1977; 154: 168-86.
15. Parikh J.R., Venkatakrishna-Bhatt H and Panchal G.M., Blood histamine levels in cotton dust exposed workers in a textile mill of Ahmedabad, Amer. J Indust. Med 1987; 12: 439-43.
16. Parikh J.R., Bhagia L.J., Majumdar S.K., Shah A.R. and Kashyap S.K., Prevalence of Byssinosis in textile mills at Ahmedabad, India. Brit. J. Indus. Med 1989; 46: 787-90.
17. Mohan-Rao N., Respiratory function tests, Theoretical background, Indian J. Indust. Med 1989, 35: 150-157.
18. Greg R., Lung Volume Tests, Ch. 1 in Manual of pulmonary function testing, 2nd Edn., CV Mosby Co St. Louis (USA) 1979.
19. Jain S.K. and Ramaiah T.J., Normal standards of pulmonary function tests in healthy Indian J. Med. Res 1969, 57: 1453-66.
20. Venkatakrishna-Bhatt H., Mohan-Rao N. and Kulkarni PK., Circulating histamine levels and lung function test in cotton mill workers, Arch. Hig. Radatoksikol 1988; 39: 371-379.
21. Malcanker M.G., Panchal G.M., Venkatakrishna-Bhatt H., Mohan-Rao N. and Kulkarni P.K., Peak-expiratory flow rate and blood histamine in textile mill workers, J. Soc. Occu. Med. (Lond) 1986; 36: 107-08.
22. Macfadden M.R. and Luiden D.A., A reduction of maximum mid expiratory flow rate. A spirographic manifestation of small airways disease Amer. J. Med 1972; 52: 725-37.
23. Mohan-Rao N. and Venkatakrishna-Bhatt H., Acute and chronic changes in pulmonary function in relation to blood histamine levels in cotton dust exposed workers. Proc. Asian Conf. Occu. Hlth, 12th Sn., 18-22, October, Bombay (India) 1988.
24. Venkatakrishna Bhatt H., Mohan Rao N., Panchal G.M., Small airways dysfunction in cotton dust exposed workers, Lung India 1990; 7: 129-32.

PULMONARY DISORDERS IN WOOL WORKERS

Wool has been identified as a causative factor for occupational asthma.[1] Wool, although, a commonly used organic fiber, yet little attention of researchers of industrial and respiratory medicine in our country or abroad has been paid barring a few reports.[2,3]

Wool dust consists of wool fibers, silica and other organic particles from sheep's skin, dung etc. Various jobs like sorting, opening and carding are the occupations where the workers are subjected to higher concentration of wool dust while workers doing the jobs like spinning, reeling, washing, dyeing and packing are subjected to comparatively lower concentration of wool dust in the atmosphere.

Wool has been reported as physiologically inactive material producing very little allergic or mechanical reactions in lungs.[4-6] However a higher incidence of chronic non-specific bronchopulmonary diseases are reported among the wool workers.[7] There has been difference between those workers exposed to wool dust for more than 10 years having a higher incidence of chronic respiratory diseases than those exposed for less than 10 years.[2] This is because wool fiber itself, alone or in combination with other components of wool dust, is causing chronic mechanical/allergic inflammation of bronchial mucosa and other parts of lung, leading to thickening of bronchial mucosa, and inflammatory response in alveoli and other parts of respiratory tract. There may be a direct relationship with duration of exposure to wool. Patient may have cough, tight chest, breathlessness but these may not be present in all the cases. Eosinophilia is seen in about 1/4th of cases.

Observance of a higher incidence of elevated eosinophil count indicates an interplay of some allergic phenomenon between wool fibers and repiratory mucosa, although wool fiber was observed to have given negative hypersensitivity test. Impairment in ventilatory functions of obstructive nature may be the result of changes in bronchial mucosa, leading to bronchial narrowing. Whether wool fiber itself is responsible for mechanical or allergic inflammation and other components of wool dust are playing an additive role, or the whole phenomenon is because of the other components of wool dust, one can't precisely say. X-ray is not contributory diagnostically. Pulmonary functions may be abnormal in more subjects with elevated eosinophils as compared in those with normal eosinophil count. Workers having longer duration of exposure to wool show more abnormalities in PFT. This derangement is more in smokers than non-smokers.

Smoking has an established role in causation of respiratory diseases especially bronchial pathology and a higher incidence of smoking in wool workers suggests that it is playing additive role. Many patients are seen in our routine practice here in Ludhiana—The Manchester of India.[8,9] Wool may not be a predisposing factor for tuberculosis, cancer, or fungal infection.[10]

REFERENCES

1. Raffle P.A.B., Lee W.R., McCallum R.L. and Murray R., Hunter's Disease of Occupations London Hodder and Stoughton 1987; 878.
2. Bhatia R.S., Pattern of respiratory diseases from a private clinic in Ludhiana, Lung India 1995; 13: 125-26.
3. Zuskin E., Valic F. and Bouhuys A. Effect of wool dust on respiratory functions. Am. Rev. Respir. Dis 1976,114: 705-09.
4. Maxwell I.N., Cited by Sulemani A.A., Incidence of nasobronchial allergy in Bikaner. Thesis submitted to the University of Rajasthan, Jaipur, 1968.
5. Bay Little, Cited by Mathur K.C., Incidence of pulmonary diseases among wool workers. Thesis submitted to the University of Rajasthan, Jaipur, 1970.
6. Patterson J.E., Industrial health, Prentice Hall Inc New Jersey 1977; 70.
7. Mathur K.C. and Mishra S.N., Incidence of pulmonary diseases among wool workers, Ind. J. Chest. Dis 1972; 14:172-78.
8. Bhatia R.S., The challenge of smokeless tobacco; Pulm and Crit Care Bulln 1995; 1: 26.
9. Bhatia R.S., Smokeless tobacco: Cardiopulmonary effects; IJCP 1995; 6: 82-85.
10. Kumar S., Kochar S.K., Sabir M., *et. al.*, Pulmonary disorders in wool workers of Bikaner, Rajasthan, Lung India 1992; 10: 65-68.

GRAIN DUST EXPOSURE[1]

Grain dust exposed patients especially in flour or feedmills, have classical presentation of cough, mucoid secretions, wheeze and exertional dyspnoea, similar to cigarette smokers. The effect is additive as 50 per cent of such workers are smokers. Both FEV_1 and FEV_1/FVC ratio are reduced. Evidence of obstruction on pulmonary function testing is seen only in smoking workers, which adds to the present knowledge with question mark whether smoking has its etfect or smoking workers are more vulnerable.

FARMER'S LUNG

A hypersensitivity pneumonitis seen in farmers, exposed to mouldy hay containing thermophilic actinomycetes spores. Incidence being 10-50 per 1000 in U.K., the prevalence varies with mouldy and stack hay. There is antigen-antibody reaction in the peripheral gas exchanging parts of the lungs, causing an alveolitis, leading to a diffusion defect. Recurrent exposure leads to progressive fibrosis.

Patient presents with cough, fever, dyspnoea without wheeze, 4-8 hours after exposure. History of exposure rules out other diseases like influenza, pneumonia etc. Recurrent attacks are features in chronic forms and patchy fibrotic lesions need to be differentiated from sarcoidosis. Other organic dust exposure occupational disorders include Malt Workers' disease, Mushroom workers' disease etc. Chest X-ray shows fine, miliary mottling or modular shadows in the lower and mid pulmonary zones. Pulmonary functions tests show a restrictive pattern.

Diffusing capacity is decreased and there is evidence of hypoxaemia. Skin tests are non-contributory. Lung biopsy shows infiltration of alveolar septa with histiocytes, plasma cells and lymphocytes.[2] The disease is preventable and acute manifestations are well managed with corticosteroids.

INTERSTITIAL LUNG DISEASES (ILDs)

These are a heterogeneous group of conditions involving alveolar walls and perialveolar tissue. These are non-infectitious and non-malignant disorders. Both acute and chronic forms are described, latter being the most common.

In acute form there is inflammation of alveolar walls and air spaces leading to acute transluminal and mural alveolitis. In chronic disease, the inflammation spreads to adjacent tissue (interstitium and vasculature), eventually leading to firbosis. The resultant scarring leads to gas exchange derangements and ventilatory dysfunction. Bronchiolitis obliterans may occur as a part of ILD because of inflammatory involvement of conducting airways.

Classification of known causes as well as granuloma formation have been described in Table 5.6.

Lymphangioleiomyomatosis[3]

Immature cells of smooth muscles proliferate in and around lung tissue causing obstruction, creating blockage and may develop into constricting lesions and cysts.

This is commonly seen in females in reproductive age; association with oestrogen has been suggested.

Clinically patient may have cough, dyspnoea, haemptysis and spontaneous pneumothorax which may be recurrent. Chest X-ray shows reticonodular shadows, cystic or honey comb appearance. PFTs are normal or increased.

Table 5.6: Alveolar and interstitial inflammatory lung diseases (ILDs)[1]

Known cause	*Unknown cause*
Asbestos	Idiopathic pulmonary fibrosis
Fumes, gases	Collagen vascular disease
Drugs (antibiotics)	SLE, Rheumatoid arthritis
Chemotherapy drugs	Ankylosing spondylitis
Radiation	Systemic sclerosis
Aspiration pneumonia	
Residual adult respiratory distress syndrome	Sjögren's syndrome Polymyositis dermatomyositis

Lung Response
Alveolitis, interstitial inflammation and fibrosis
Pulmonary haemorrhage syndromes
Goodpasture's syndrome
Idiopathic pulmonary hemosiderosis
Pulmonary alveolar proteinosis
Lymphocytic interstitial pneumonitis
Eosinophillic pneumonias
Lymphangiomyomatosis
Amyloidosis

Inherited diseases
Tuberous sclerosis, neurofibromatosis, Niemann Pick disease, Gaucher's disease, Hermansky-Pudlak Syndrome, Gastrointestinal or liver diseases, Crohn's disease, primary biliary cirrhosis, chronic active hepatitis, ulcerative colitis, Graft vs Host disease, bone marrow transplantation

Lung response
As above but with granuloma

Known cause
Hypersensitivity pneumonitis (organic dust)
Inorganic, beryllium, silica

Unknown cause
Sarcoidosis, Langerhans cell granulomatosis
or (eosinophilic granulomatosis)
or (histocytosis)[2]

Granulomatous vasculitis
Wegener's granulomatosis, allergic granulomatosis of Churg-Strauss, lymyphomatoid granulomatosis, bronchogenic granulomatosis

Progesterone may help, oophrectomy is useful, even lung transplantation can be considered for refractory cases.

Inherited Disorders with ILDs

These include:

Phacomatosis, Tuberous sclerosis, Neurofibromatosis, Niemann-Pick disease, Lysosomal diseases, Gaucher's disease.

Hemansky-Pudlak Syndrome

An autosomal recessive disorder. ILD is associated with granulomatous collitis. There is albinism, bleeding distresses and pulmonary fibrosis like IPF. Alveolar macrophages contain cytoplasmic caroid like inclusions.

Gastrointestinal, Liver Disease and ILD

All the three may coexist, like sarcoidosis, Crohn's disease may have asymptomatic lymphocytic alveolitis.

Eosinophilic Pneumonia[4]

It is a disease in which lung hypersensitivity plays a role, although specific cause may or may not be known, e.g.:

1. Extrinsic asthma to fungal antigen—Allergic broncho-pulmonary mycosis.
2. Filaria—Tropical pulmonary eosinophilia.
3. Drug induced eosinophilic pneumonia.

Chronic eosinophilic pneumonia has distinct features, and can be differentiated from IPF (Idiopathic Pulmonary Fibrosis) by the following:

1. Common in old females, affecting between 20-50 years.
2. Radiologically-peripheral pattern of dense lung infiltration, sparing the central portion.
3. Regression and appearance are common.
4. Response to steroids is dramatic.

Clinically patient may have cough, fever, dyspnoea, weight loss etc.

Lung biopsy is diagnostic, showing eosinophilic inflammation.

Graf vs Host Disease[5] (GVHD)

It is seen in 10 per cent of cases in the chronic phase, presenting with cough and dyspnoea. Chest X-ray shows peribronchiolar infiltrates. PFT demonstrate small airways destruction. Lung biopsy reveals focal areas of infiltration with lymphocytes and PMNS, simulating bronchiolitis but without vasculitis. Condition may be fatal, unless dose of immunosuppressants is increased. Viral infection may complicate.

Bronchogenic Granulomatosis[2]

An angiocentric vasculitis causing granulomatous destruction of bronchioles is seen in this condition. The necrotic granulomatosis involves small bronchioles and tissue adjacent to pulmonary arteries. Associated parenchymal inflammation leads to ILD. Eosinophils may be present if asthma is the feature. Hypersensitivity pneumonitis due to organic dust forms a differential diagnosis. Chest X-ray shows unilateral (initially), predominantly upper lobe involvement: infiltrates, lobar consolidation or atelectasis, and nodular linear shadows are other features.

REFERENCES

1. Schwartz D.A., Grain dust endotoxin and airflow obstruction; Chest 1996; 109:575-635.
2. Carrington C.B., Addinton W.W., Golt A.M., *et al.,* Chronic eosinophilic pneumonia, N. Engl. J. Med 1969; 28: 787.
3. Ademson D., *et al.,* Successful treatment of pulmonary lymphangio-leiomyomatosis with oophrectomy and progesterone: Amer. Rev. Resp. Dis 5, 1985; 132:916.
4. Allen J.N., *et al.,* Acute eosinophilic pneumonia as a reversible cause of non-infectious respiratory failure; N. Eng. J. Med. 1989; 321:569.
5. Chan C.K., *et al.,* Small airways disease in recipients of allogenic bone marrow transplants, Medicine 1987; 66:327.

6 Neoplastic Diseases

MALIGNANT TUMOURS

Bronchogenic Carcinoma (Lung Cancer)

Introduction

Primary pulmonary neoplastic diseases were not commonly known in the world at the beginning of this century.[1] But near the end of this century, these neoplastic conditions have become one of the most common malignant disorders especially in males.[2] Rising incidence of lung cancer forms 29% of total cancers and 21% of all deaths among men in European community.[3] However in the last decade, an increasing incidence in men has levelled off in USA, and in some European countries, the incidence of lung cancer in women continues to rise sharply. And it is now exceeding breast cancer as the most common cause of cancer death in United States.[4] Similarly, a rising trend in lung cancer has been seen in the recent years in the developing countries. The increasing incidence has been recorded for the last 50 years in the Indian patients where it is recognised as one of the important causes of mortality due to malignant diseases in the country.[5] The rise is actual or the rise in incidence is due to availability of better diagnostic facilities, is difficult to say as very little information is available on lung cancer in India.[6] In India annual crude incidence rate of lung cancer is 0.1 per million of urban population. A rising trend towards increase has been shown from the few reports available.[7]

Year	1984	1985	1986	1987	1988
No. of cases	414	501	429	501	658

A rising incidence of carcinoma bronchus from 4.2 to 31 per 10,000 hospital admission and still higher[8] 76/10,000, estimated from patients admitted with chest symptoms has been reported. The higher incidence may be due to patients in a chest ward compared to previous reports from general medical ward as well as due to increased awareness, improved diagnostic techniques and availability of facilities and enhanced accuracy of performing personnel.[8] 3.95 per cent of all hospitalised admissions have been reported due to cancers and lung cancer is the 5th common form of malignancy.[9] However, a lower incidence of less than 1% has been reported from a private clinic, may be, such patients prefer to go directly to the institutions that exist in the same city.[10] The incidence in two sexes varies in different parts of the world ranging from 13.5:1 in Holland to 1:1 in Nigeria.[11] An overall male to female ratio of 4.5:1 has been reported, the ratio varying between different age groups, and according to the smoking status.[12] Male predominance is quite common in general and most of the sufferers are above the age of forty. Again the rising yield is attributed to available advanced diagnostic techniques as well as increased awareness about the disease among physicians.[13]

Few facts about Lung Cancer (Bronchogenic carcinoma) are:

- Lung cancer is most common malignancy world wide.
- 95% are either SCLC or NSCLC.
- 5% are sarcomas or chondromas.
- 2,24000 new cases and 1,59000 deaths in 2014 in US alone have been estimated to have occurred.
- Squamous cell carcinoma is the most common variety of NSCLC.
- In US, incidence of adenocarcinoma has, however, increases.[14]

Aetiology

Cigarette smoking is a causative factor in the production of wide range of chest diseases including carcinoma of the lung and is now thought to be the cause of 86 per cent of all lung cancers. There is a linear association between the number of cigarettes smoked and cancer deaths. The risk of development of cancer is great in heavy smokers. No significant improvement in outcome over the last 20 years has been observed despite continued efforts to improve diagnosis, staging and treatment of lung cancer, since direct link of smoking and incidence of disease has not been significantly targeted, strong global initiative on tobacco needs universal support.

Epidemiologists have recognised a significant correlation between cigarette smoking and the development of lung cancer.[15] It is dose dependent and often the cumulative dose of smoking plays a significant role in the development of neoplastic as well as non-neoplastic respiratory diseases as a major risk factor. Environmental Tobacco Smoke (ETS) has been found to be associated with variety of lung diseases, including lung cancer.[16] The smoking index above 300 is a definite risk factor in causing pulmonary neoplastic diseases.[17] Among persons who smoke 30 cigarettes a day, the risk of dying from lung cancer is 30 times greater than in non-smokers. Efforts applied in increasing advancement in non-invasive tests for early diagnosis and screening of asymptomatic subjects has been put side by promoting primary prevention through preventing cigarette smoking as the ideal strategy for future.

The male to female ratio is high in smokers and almost identical for all cell types (20:1). In non-smokers the ratio differed with the cell type. The smoker to non-smoker ratio differed significantly in the age groups below and above 40. Small cell carcinoma is predominantly seen in those upto the age of 40 years and cell type has no significant association with the smoking habit, while in those above 40 years, squamous cell type is most common in smokers and adenocarcinoma in non-smokers.[18] Interestingly, tobacco causes more damage in peripheral parts of lungs in women (adenocarcinoma) and more damage in central parts of lungs in men (small cell and squamous cell carcinomas). The risk of lung cancer is reported to be higher in bidi smokers compared to cigarette smokers. Higher levels of benzo (a) pyrene (a carcinogen) have been reported in the bidis as compared to Indian cigarettes.[19]

The chance of development of lung cancer after abstinence for five years is much less likely among those who have given up smoking permanently, but higher than those of passive inhalation. An increased risk of lung cancer from passive inhalation of cigarette smoke at home or at work cannot be ruled out. Insignificant role of medical profession regarding tobacco has become a big question mark.[20,21] However, thanks are due to the Supreme Court of India for banning smoking at public places. Prevalence of smoking among medical and non-medical students has been documented.[22] However, implementation of this ban order is very poor.

On 31st May—World No Tobacco Day, the revealing hard facts about tobacco in India, are as following:

- Tobacco causes more than 20 categories of fatal and disabling diseases, including cardiorespiratory and malignant disorders.
- 3 billion smokers globally, 112 million in India.
- 5.4 million deaths in the world/per year and 9 lakh Indians die per year—due to tobacco.
- 2-3% rise in tobacco consumption per year, only 2% successfully quit every year. Nicotine replacement therapy helps in quitting.
- 65% of cancers in male and 33% of cancers in female are attributed to tobacco.
- Higher rates of lung diseases are due to tobacco smoke.

Data Ministry of Health

- Tobacco kills more than one million people every year in India.
- India bears highest burden of mouth cancer in world.
- Smoking in women enhances the rate of spontaneous abortions, still births and low birth weight babies and reduces fertility.
- 1.2 crore women take tobacco, 54 lakh inhale and 65 lakh intake (smokeless).
- Among girls between 13-15 years of age, 8.3% are tobacco users, 2.4% use cigarettes, while 7.2% use other forms of tobacco.

In a recent study, 18% of medical college students were found to be smokers, in comparison to 44% of students from other colleges.[22] Non inhalational oral tobacco use is also becoming popular among young generations.

Tobacco in China, the largest population of Asia show figures of real concern; i.e.

- 350 million smokers exist in China alone.
- One third of cigarettes of world are smoked in China.
- One fourth of world's cigarette smokers reside in China.

Tobacco smoke is potentially carcinogenic and it contains 4000[22] individual constituents and to mention few, it has initiators like polycyclic aromatic hydrocarbons (3:4 benzpyrenes) and promoter substances like phenol, fatty acid esters or free fatty acids. Tobacco smoke condensates are able to induce basal cell hyperplasia, squamous metaplasia or bronchial epithelium and appearance of atypical cells with hyperchromatic nuclei. Genetic susceptibility due to higher aryl-hydrocarbon hydroxylase (AHH) has been suggested. Tobacco industry has shown a pseudo cooperative concern for health by showing a decline in employees working in the industry. However, new machines have been installed to churn 14,000 cigarettes per minute round the clock. This has affected both economy and health. According to ITC annual report, in India, total turnover was Rs. 24,000 crore and during the same period, Rs. 29,500 crore have been spent on treatment and management of tobacco-related problems (ICMR—annual report), depicting the actual loss in economy. 4 million people losing their lives is an additional burden.

The incidence of deaths from carcinoma is higher in urban areas and an *urban factor* is incriminated because of atmospheric pollution of town air with auto exhaust fumes, dust, smoke and smog.[23] Kerosene oil burning may be a contributory factor in causation of adenocarcinoma. There have been some reports to consider the role of diet in the lung cancer.[24] Deficiency of vitamin A affects the initiation and post-initiation phases of benzo (a) pyrene-induced lung carcinogenesis and causes a significant increase in the incidence of lung tumor and tumor burden.[25] Betacarotene supplimentation in smokers, however, has possible carcinogenic influences.[26] Genetic predisposition has been ob-served in laryngeal carcinoma, lymphoma, chronic leukaemia and tumours of head and neck.[27]

Occupational hazards[2] are known to be contributory to neoplastic pulmonary diseases, like mining of radioactive ores (radium, uranium etc), asbestos processing, nickel refining, processing of chromates, chlormethyl ethers, inorganic arsenic, coal tar combustion and distillation, exposure to workers in cake ovens, gas retorts, silica workers etc. The effect has synergistic action with cigarette smoking in developing lung cancer. Previous scar due to old pulmonary infection form a weak point for environmental carcinogens which are retained due to damaged blocked lymphatics. Atypical epithelial proliferation in bronchi in fibrosing alveolitis, scleroderma, asbestosis and interstitial fibrosis act as high risk factors. Heavy smoking enhances the risk in the development of tumours often at the lung periphery.[2] Bronchoalveolar carcinoma often develops from atypical epithelial proliferation in the lung having rigid scar tissue undergoing honeycomb changes.

Statistics of Cancer in India (January 2008)

- 2.5 million people suffer from cancer in India.
- 8,00,000 people get afflicted with malignant disorder every year in India.
- 4,40,000 people die of cancer every year in India.
- Tobacco is linked to 5% of all kinds of cancers in India.

Classification

World Health Organisation has classified lung cancer based on the presumed tissue of origin. They arise from the surface epithelium of the bronchial tree, usually from either basal or mucous cells. The incompletely differentiated cells present in the basement membrane of the mucosa proliferate following a carcinogenic stimulus.[2]

Histologically on light microscopy, malignant tumours are classified as squamous cell (epidermoid) carcinoma, small cell carcinoma (oat cell, intermediate cell and combined oat cell), adenocarcinoma (acinar adenocarcinoma, papillary adenocarcinoma, bronchioalveolar carcinoma and solid carcinoma with mucus), large cell carcinoma (giant cell and clear cell carcinoma), adenosquamous carcinoma, carcinoid tumour, and bronchial gland carcinoma (adenoid cystic and mucoepidermoid).[2] WHO international histology classification 1981 to classify tumours has been quite in use.

Squamous cell carcinoma is the most frequent histopathological form, encountered in patients over the age of 60 years and small cell lung cancer predominates below 40 years. Uttarakhand study[28] reveals tobacco as major risk factor in more than 80% of cases. Histopathogenesis of lung cancer of different varieties as shown in the following table.

1.	Squamous cell Ca	45%
2.	Adenocarcinoma	20%
3.	Small cell lung Ca	17%
4.	Undifferentiated	10%
5.	Large cell lung Ca	8%

(a) If the features are undifferentiated—the tumour is labelled undifferentiated. (b) Bizarre picture with large pleomorphic cells is labelled as anaplastic carcinoma.

Based on differences in their biology and treatment, two types are described, small cell lung carcinoma (SCLC) and non-small cell lung carcinoma (NSCLC). There is controversy about the origin of bronchogenic carcinoma from a common precursor cell. According to the 'unitary theory' of pulmonary carcinogenesis, various forms of bronchogenic carcinoma arise from a common bronchial epithelial cell. The non-unitary theory considers that small cell carcinoma arises from lung endocrine cell, unlike the non-small cell carcinoma arising from non-endocrinal bronchial mucosa cell. The general consensus is for unitary hypothesis.[2]

Pathology

Bronchiogenic carcinoma arises from the epithelium lining of the bronchi or bronchiole or from the mucous glands of the bronchi. The tumours may be located near the hilum (central) or in the periphery near the pleura or in the region between the two in the middle zone. Most of the cancers pass through a preclinical-premalignant-phase when bronchial mucosa is undergoing squamous cell metaplasia-carcinoma in situ, that turns out to be an invasive carcinoma later on.[29]

The squamous cell carcinoma forms the most common variety accounting for 50 per cent of bronchogenic carcinoma. Recent studies from India, however, have shown a declining trend of squamous cell carcinoma, varying from 23 per cent, 27 per cent, 32 per cent[5,6,8] compared to earlier Indian studies, possibly because of significant reduction in the percentage of epidermoid carcinomas. There has been a changing pattern of bronchogenic carcinoma from northern and western parts of India, probably due to rising average age in the country or possibly related to a change in the dietary habits.[5,24] It is seen in elderly persons predominantly in men. Often there is a long history of cigarette smoking although it is difficult to explain the large number of non-smokers with squamous cell carcinoma. Air pollution, passive smoking and chemical carcinogens have been implicated influencing its prevalence. The occupational exposure to carcinogens is also related to this type of cancer. It arises predominantly near the hilum from the surface of the epithelium in the segmental or more proximal bronchi. Still a quarter of the cases arise in the periphery.

The tumour is slow growing. Growth may be seen as a mass or an infilterate into the lumen, causing narrowing of the bronchi and ultimately block the secretions. The retained secretions may get infected causing pneumonitis or lung abscess, distal to the obstruction. Secondary changes like atelectasis, bronchiectasis and abscess formation may greatly alter the gross appearance. Partial obstruction may cause focal emphysema. There may be bleeding in the lumen due to erosion by the growth. Ulcerative bronchitis may occur. Even chemical changes causing necrosis and leading to formation of irregular abscess cavity have been documented.[2] The extrabronchial spread into the lung parenchyma, lymph nodes and mediastinal structures may occur. Hypercalcemia due to a parathormone effect without any metastasis to the bone has been reported with squamous cell carcinoma. Absolute lymphocytopenia is a feature that occurs possibly due to elevated levels of cortisols.[30]

Histological features include squamous keratinisation, intercellular bridges and epithelial cell pearl formation. Life expectancy after resection along with presently available chemotherapy is longer than the other types.[2] Histologically, squamous cell carcinoma shows marked heterogenicity, in different microscopic fields.

Adenocarcinoma is often located in the periphery and accounts for 20 to 25 per cent of the malignancies of the lung.[27] It has steadily become the most frequent histological type in the recent years.[31] The higher rate of 21 per cent and even 35.5 per cent have been reported from Indian studies from the south.[5] However, other Indian studies, especially from northern India have reported low incidence of 13 per cent only.[8] The growth originates from mucous glands of peripheral bronchi. The pattern may be glandular or tabular with well differentiated mucus secreting and non-mucus secreting columnar or cuboidal cells. The cells contain opaque cytoplasm and vascular nuclei in the corner. The growth often comes to light because of its secondary metastasis from a haematogenous spread to distal parts of the body. They may arise in the scars in the lung from previous infection. Adenocarcinoma is associated with hilar and/or mediastinal involvement. Smoking of cigarettes is increasingly incriminated as an important cause of the condition. The tumours are more frequent in advancing age with equal frequency among both sexes.[2] Unlike lung cancer which is a nodule or mass lesion, it may present as airspace filling process with an alveolar pattern on chest X-ray.[32] Poorly differentiated form produces diffuse or multiple masses, bilaterally.[33] Therefore, solitary lesions should be earliest surgically managed to prevent disseminationl.[34]

The undifferentiated or anaplastic type of carcinoma accounts for 20 to 25 per cent of the malignancies of the lung. They include small cell and large cell carcinoma. Often they are noted in middle aged men with a history of heavy smoking of cigarettes. They arise from the surface of the bronchial epithelium. The large cell carcinoma usually originates in the periphery and spreads early by lymphatics and blood vessels. The small cell carcinoma arises more frequently in larger bronchi and are centrally located. They grow rapidly and metastatise early and more widely than other histological types. The highly malignant oat cell carcinoma with its rapid growth forms the predominant type. It is composed of undifferentiated small cells with deep stained nuclei occupying the whole of the cell. The primary is very small and may pose difficulty in its location. It spreads submucosally across the bronchus and causes early hilar and mediastinal adenopathy. It has a grave prognosis. Small cell carcinoma contains neurosecretory granules and often produce endocrine paraneoplastic manifestations due to abnormal secretions of corticotrophin like substance leading to Cushing's syndrome, carcinoid syndrome and hyponatremia respectively.[2]

The rate of growth of the tumour (doubling time) varies from 20 to 450 days. The mean doubling time or small cell carcinoma, squamous cell carcinoma and adeno carcinoma are 29 days, 88 days and 161 days respectively. The growth may be inwards either causing constriction or obstruction of the bronchus or outwards into the lung. Growing into the bronchial lumen, initially it causes a partial obstruction in the airways. The obstruction is greater during expiration. It leads to air trapping with localised emphysema. Later the obstruction becomes complete. Spreading of growth in the wall may constrict and narrow the passage. Both these conditions lead to collapse of the distal portion of the lung. It interferes with oxygenation of the blood and facilitates accumulation of the secretions. The micro-organisms thrive in such area and set up an infective process leading to pneumonia or lung abscess. The mechanical obstruction of great vessels in the chest may lead to superior vena cava syndrome. Pleural effusion may occur due to extension of the carcinoma and involvement of pleura or it may be due to spread of inflammatory process or secondary to infarction or to obstruction of lymphatic flow.[2]

The neoplastic growths especially of the central region may spread by direct infiltration along its surface in the submucosa and through the cartilaginous spaces in the bronchial wall, into parenchyma and extrabronchial lymph nodes. The peripheral tumours invade the pleura, chest wall and vertebrae. By invading the submucousal lymphatics, the central growths often spread to hilar lymph nodes ipsilaterally. Later they involve the paratracheal glands. Through the subcarinal lymph glands, spread occurs to the contralateral side and later to the cervical lymph nodes. The growth which spreads outwards, invades structures in the mediastinum with pressure effects on the vessels, nerves and oesophagus. The growth may erode into the pulmonary vein and get disseminated throughout the body. They metastasise to liver, adrenals, cerebral hemispheres, and skeleton especially ribs and vertebrae.[2] To sum up, the most common lung cancer is the squamous cell carcinoma. The cell type is largely influenced by smoking habits, age and sex. Squamous cell and small cell types are common in smokers, and adenocarcinoma is the commonest cell type in females, possibly because of heavy smoking habit prevalent in males in India. Small cell lung cancers arise more in histologically normal epithelium while non-small cell lung cancers arise more in preexisting dysplastic or *in situ* lesions. Common features, stages, aetiology and associated non-metastatic syndromes of lung carcinoma have been shown in Tables 6.1 to 6.5.

Table 6.1: Stages of carcionoma of the lung

Stage	*Best Treatment*		
Stage I (development)	Prevention	-	Stop smoking
Stage II (growth)	Surgery	-	35 per cent 5-year survival
Stage III (spread)	Palliation	-	Chemotherapy for small cell carcinoma

Table 6.2: Aetiology of carcinoma of the lung

Smoking industrial causes
- Asbestos
- Uranium
- Nickel
- Chromate
- Iron and silica
- Mustard gas
- Coal distillation and
- Air pollution from auto exhaust, incomplete burning, dust etc.

Table 6.3: Initial symptoms of carcinoma of the lung

Symptom	*Incidence (%)*
Cough	Almost 90%
Chest pain	More than 50%
Breathlessness	Almost 70%
Haemoptysis	Almost 70%
Pyrexia	Almost 20%
Hoarseness of voice	Almost 30%
Dysphagia	Almost 20%

Clinical Presentation

Metastasis to various parts of the body occurs from a hematogenous spread and growth often becomes evident because of metastasis. The growth may arise from residual pulmonary scars of previous infections. Generally, hilar or mediastinal involvement is an accompanying feature. Both the sexes are equal sufferers and the prevalence of infection is more in advancing age, especially in smokers.

Cancers and heart disease are the two major killer diseases in the west, compared to infectious diseases like pneumonia and tuberculosis in developing countries. Almost half of the new cancers reported annually occur in developing nations, although the types may vary. In India 3.6 per cent deaths are due to cancer.[35] Lung, oesophageal and stomach cancers account for 31 per cent of all cancer deaths in Indian males, compared to oesophageal cancer found in tobacco chewers, lung cancer is more prevalent among cigarette smokers.[36]

The symptomatology depends upon the site of the growth where it is located, the growth and the mode of the spread. The manifestations are due to obstruction of a major bronchus, systemic effects of malignancy and the effect of humoral substances synthesized within the growth. The presentation is quite variable and the ontset of symptoms is often insidious. The most common presentation is a mass lesion with or without collapse, diagnosed clinically in 68 per cent and radiologically in 70.7 per cent of cases. Cavitating mass in 6 per cent, pleural effusion in 25.1 per cent, superior vena caval obstruction in 16.7 per cent are other common presentations, seen in clinical

Table 6.4: Lung cancer

Features	*Symptoms*
Cachexia	Cough, chest pain, haemoptysis
Clubbing	
Bronchial breathing	Hoarseness, osteoarthropathy
Dull percussion note	Hormonal effects: More in oat cell carcinoma
Ronchi, vocal fremitus	
Laser-Trelat sign	

Table 6.5: Non-metastatic syndromes associated with carcinoma of the lung

Endocrine Syndromes	*Neuromuscular Syndromes*	*Others*
• Cushing's syndrome	• Sensory neuropathy	• Pulmonary hypertrophic osteoarthropathy
• Hyponatraemia	• Proximal nueromyopathy	• Thrombophlebitis
• Hypercalcaemia	• Cerebellar degeneration	
• Carcinoid	• Dementia	
• Thyrotoxicosis	• Myasthenia	
• Hypoglycaemia	• Dermatomyositis	
• Gynaecomastia		

practice. Chronic obstructive pulmonary disease and pulmonary tuberculosis may be associated in 20.2 per cent and 3.7 per cent of cases respectively. Metastatic complications are seen in 51.8 per cent cases while non-metastatic complications are observed in 37.7 per cent of cases, excluding anorexia and asthenia. These include clubbing (28 per cent), hypertrophic osteoarthropathy (3 per cent), neuropathy (0.9 per cent), myopathy (0.7 per cent), thromboembolic complications (0.5 per cent), cerebellar syndromes (0.4 per cent). Galactorrhoea is also observed in a male patient with squamous cell carcinoma.[37]

The condition may manifest with respiratory symptoms or with metastatic or non-metastatic extrapulmonary manifestations directly or indirectly pointing towards its existence in the chest. It may be directed as an abnormal shadow in the radiogram of the chest or it may present general manifestations like weakness, lassitude and loss of appetite and weight loss (90 per cent), whose investigations may reveal an existence of tumour. Generally the symptoms are minimal in early stages and develop gradually. It is worth noting that there is a long asymptomatic period in most cases, the physical examination may be normal in 6.4 per cent of cases,[12] and the disease is sometimes detected at this time through a chance X-ray examination. Rarely there can be a positive cytology for malignant cells with a normal chest X-ray (6.4 per cent). The cell type is generally squamous cell carcinoma in such instances.

The respiratory manifestations are due to the growth and its effect on the bronchus (local) and spread to the mediastinum (regional). The common presenting symptoms include cough (88 per cent), chest pain (52.2 per cent), breathlessness and heamptysis (69.2 per cent). The number of symptoms and Feinstein's index have strong negative association with survival.[38] The duration of development of symptoms may be quite short and many a time the extent of disease is found to be significant at the time of hospital admission. Cough is a presenting symptom in endobronchial (central) lesions. Often it is not noticed because of the history of smoking for a long time. Any alteration in the nature of the cough or its worsening needs further investigation. The growth into the lumen of the bronchus behaves as a foreign body and the host attempts to expel it, leads to the production of cough. Though it is dry initially, later it is associated with mucoid sputum. It may become purulent due to secondary infection. It may ulcerate or erode the vessel wall and cause hemoptysis. Commonly the sputum is streaked with blood. A single massive hemoptysis is rare. Occasionally hemoptysis may be massive when the bronchial veins get eroded, which is frequent in squamous cell carcinoma and uncommon in small cell carcinoma as it grows as a submucosal plaque. Unlike central lesions, tumours located in the periphery may attain a large size without production of cough. Sometimes a poorly located ache is noted on the side of a tumour. Later in the course of the disease, severe pain may occur due to pleural or chest wall extension and from secondary deposits. A sharp pleuritic chest pain may be noted secondary to pneumonia or to neoplastic involvement of the pleura, or intercostal nerves. A persistent deep aching chest pain may occur with the neoplastic invasion of the mediastinum.[2]

There may be a history of pyrexial episodes (19.6 per cent). Fever with general weakness due to influenza forms an important differential diagnosis in the elderly. The infection existing in an area of the lobe, or the segment beyond the bronchial obstruction leads to pneumonic episodes. Recurrence is common because of incomplete clearance of infection after antibiotic treatment. In many instances unexplained fever especially of low grade with or without evening rise, and loss of weight with dyspepsia are the presenting complaints.[2] In India this is mistaken quite often for tuberculosis.

Breathlessness may occur due to collapse of lobe or from pleural effusion. It may occur due to the involvement of the phrenic nerve causing paralysis of the hemidiaphragm, or following lymphatic spread of the disease in the lungs. Partial obstruction in the main bronchus due to growth may be responsible for wheeze in few patients. The local and regional extension of the growth as mediastinal metastasis may be responsible for varied clinical presentations. The patient may have hoarseness of voice (30 per cent) and a bovine cough due to paralysis of left recurrent laryngeal nerve from left sided growths, dysphagia (20.8 per cent) for fluids from oesophageal compression, dyspepsia from invasion of vagus nerve, dyspnoea from phrenic nerve involvement, puffiness of face (19.8 per cent) and oedema of upper limbs due to obstruction of superior vena cava from the right sided growth, arrhythmias from cardiac involvement, and ptosis due to pressure on sympathetic ganglia. The invasion of the lower part of bronchial plexus (C_8, T1 and T_2) results in severe pain in the shoulder and down the inner surface of the arm, weakness of upper extremities, parasthesia and vasomotor symptoms (Pancoast's tumour).[2]

Pancoast tumour is a bronchogenic carcinoma, arising from apical or posterior regimental bronchus of upper lobe of the three varieties viz. squamous cell, oat cell and adenocarcinoma, the latter has a quite low incidence of 6 per cent. It was originally described by Pancoast in 1932. A small homogeneous shadow on chest X-ray, at the extreme apex is termed as superior sulcus tumour[39] which stands only for apical bronchogenic carcinoma involving the brachial plexus and sympathetic cervical chain. Differential diagnosis includes rib pressure syndrome and consolidation. Nevertheless, pain appears quite early in the shoulder and arm in Pancoast syndrome.[39]

Clinically there is wasting and clubbing. Clubbing develops rapidly from an increased peripheral blood flow. It is marked in squamous cell carcinoma. Ptosis is present in 2 per cent of cases associated with miosis, enophthalmos, and anhidrosis (Horner's syndrome).The superior vena caval obstruction manifests facial plethora, non-pulsatile venous engorgement of the neck veins and dilatation of the superficial veins over the chest and abdomen as a means of collateral circulation and oedema of the upper extremities. These patients often complain of early morning headache and drowsiness from increased venous pressure in the upper half of the body. There may be signs of pericardial effusion and cardiac arrhythmia, due to direct extension or retrograde spread through mediastinal and epicardial lymphatics.[2]

Lung cancer may have extrathoracic metastasis, paraneoplastic syndromes including endocrine syndromes and skeletal connective tissue syndromes. Different varieties of lung cancer, signs of central and peripheral tumour and associated syndromes have been shown in Tables 6.6. to 6.9.

Table 6.6: Different types of pulmonary neoplasms

Epidermoid carcinoma	Mucoepidermoid
Large cell carcinoma	Neuroblastoma
Small cell carcinoma	Fibrosarcoma
Adenocarcinoma	Melanoma
Non-Hodgkin lymphoma	Unclassified
Carcinoid	

Table 6.7: Signs of a central tumour

1. Tumour may present as a hilar mass, that is smooth or irregular, narrowing the major bronchus.
2. Obstruction by tumour is a combination of collapse and consolidation.

Localised rhonchi and feeble breath sounds at the site of growth due to partial occlusion of bronchus and emphysema locally may be heard in initial stages. Rhonchi are made more prominent by making the patient to lean on the same side and they do not clear on coughing. Later the signs may be of consolidation or collapse or of pleural effusion. The condition may exist without any signs when it is deep-seated. The signs depend on the size of the growth and its effect on extra-pulmonary structures. The growth in the upper part of the lung especially in the superior pulmonary sulcus in its terminal bronchioles may cause pain, weakness and parasthesia in the arm, wasting of muscles of the hand and unilateral clubbing. Pleural effusion may be due to pleural metastasis, or from pleural infection or infarction.

The extrapulmonary manifestations of bronchogenic carcinoma may be due to secondary metastasis or without obvious metastasis. The common sites for the metastatic spread are cervical and auxillary lymph nodes, bones, liver, brain, spinal cord, stomach, adrenals, subcutaneous tissue and contralateral lung including contralateral hilar lymph nodes.

Malignant cutaneous metastasis is a relatively rare occurrence (1-2.7 per cent). Cutaneous metastasis resembles histopathologically the primary and usually it is adeno-carcinoma. Cutaneous squamous cell carcinoma metastasis can be differentiated from the primary skin cancer by the absence of malignant proliferation in surface epidermis. The secondaries in skin are confined to the skin (regional) of the primary growth. These malignant cells reach the skin by direct, lymphatic or hematogeous route. Cutaneous metastasis indicates progression of disease and early fatal termination. The metastasis to stomach is commonly through blood supply and may cause haematemesis and gastric perforation.[40] Commonly, small cell anaplastic carcinoma metastasizing into the stomach has occurred.

Even before the occurrence of bone metastasis, a localised tenderness may be elicited over the bone. Later there may be evidence of pathologic fracture or collapse of the vertebra. The bony metastasis are osteoclastic and are generally in the region above the knee. The secondary deposits in the cerebral hemisphere may lead to epileptic seizures, hemiplegia, alteration in behaviour, confusion, spatial disorientation, headache and cerebellar symptoms with unsteadiness. The spinal cord is another important site for metastasis and manifests with paraplegia. The supraclavicular and/or retroclavicular lymph nodes become palpable on dissemination of bronchogenic carcinoma and usually it occurs on the side of the lung lesion.

Table 6.8: Signs of a peripheral tumour

1. *May present as a peripheral solitary mass.
2. *Generally a round shadow, with irregular border: lobulation, notching and infiltrating edges are commonly seen.
3. *Cavitation within the mass may be present, especially in peripheral squamous cell carcinomas.
4. *Bronchial carcinomas with cavitation may require tomography.

Table 6.9: Skeletal/connective tissue syndromes associated with lung cancer

Syndrome	*Frequency and Association*
1. Clubbing	30 per cent (usually with non-small cell)
2. Hypertrophic pulmonary osteoarthropathy	1-10 per cent (usually with adenocarcinomas)
3. Neurologic-myopathic syndromes (Eaton-Lambert Syndrome)	1 per cent (small cell carcinoma)
4. Coagulative, thrombotic and haematologic manifestations (Trowsseau's syndrome)	1-8 per cent, 1 per cent
5. Cutaneous manifestations (dermatomyositis and acanthosis nigricans)	1 per cent or less
6. Renal manifestations (glomerulonephritis and nephrotic syndrome)	1 per cent or less

Occasionally there is involvement of the contralateral nodes in the neck. Axillary lymph nodes are palpable if the tumour has invaded the chest wall.

Cardiac and pericardial metastasis has been 1.5-20.6 per cent[41] with bronchogenic carcinoma, malignant melanoma, carcinoma breast, lymphoma leukemias. Mode of spread may be direct extension, lymphatic or haemotogenous spread. Initial neoplastic pericarditis in metastatic lung disease is silent and asymptomatic or cardiac tamponade may be the early manifestation.[42] Carcinoma of bronchus is seen with cardiac metastasis in 15-30 per cent of cases. Patients with pericardial effusion tamponade tachyarrhythmias, AV block and congestive cardiac failure have been reported.[43]

In non-metastatic manifestations of different variety, the symptoms may appear even earlier than that of primary growth in some cases. The abnormalities may be metabolic, vascular, haematologic, neuromuscular, connective tissue and bony abnormalities.

In 1928, Brown reported unexpected adrenal hyperactivity in patients of lung cancer. Endocrine disturbance like Cushing's syndrome, and excess secretion of ADH are outstanding metabolic abnormalities. Carcinoid syndrome may occur. All these disturbances are characteristically associated with oat cell carcinoma. Squamous cell carcinoma may manifest features of hypercalcemia without evidence of bony metastasis. Features of thyrotoxicosis, hyperparathyroidism, hypoglycemia (insulin like activity) and hyperpigmentation (melanocyte stimulating hormone) are noted in association with bronchogenic carcinoma. 60 per cent small cell lung cancers and 4 per cent bronchial carcinoid tumours are associated with Cushing's syndrome.[43] 4% cases of small cell carcinoma have cortisol abnormality. In less than 8% of these cases of small cell carcinomas, ectopic adrenocorticotropic hormone secretion producing a clinical syndrome is also observed.

The tumour may produce an ACTH like substance. Similar secretion may occur with growths arising from thymus, pancreas, ovary, thyroid, prostate and colon. It leads to appearance of Cushing's syndrome with muscle weakness, polyuria, glycosuria, hirsutism, pigmentation of the skin and oedema and may prove fatal if appear all of a sudden. The patient instead of losing weight, as noted commonly in malignant diseases gains weight. There is adrenal hyperplasia. However it is associated with hypokalaemia, and hypochloraemic alkalosis. It differs from hyperaldosteronism in having normal secretion of aldosterone. The secretion is not suppressed by the administration of dexamethasone. However l/3rd cases of carcinoid tumor, urinary cortisol decreases by 5% on administration of dexamethsone. ACTH stimulation test does not increase serum cortisol level.[2]

The ACTH levels are otherwise generally higher in lung cancer patients as compared to those with pituitary dependent disease, as demonstrated by using conventional radio-immunoassay for ACTH. Certain patients may not exhibit any manifestations of Cushing's syndrome despite higher Pro ACTH levels in the plasma. It is not the ACTH, but the higher levels of Pro ACTH as suggested by beta lipotrophic hormone, gamma lipotrophic hormone, beta endorphin and methionine enkephalin, that have been demonstrated.[45]

There may be an inappropriate secretion of an ADH like substance especially in small cell carcinoma of the bronchus in 50-68% of cases. It is associated with loss of sodium leading to hyponatraemia, retention of water and increased plasma volume. The sodium depletion results in personality changes with lethargy, mental confusion, irritability and drowsiness. This is called Schwrtz-Bartter Syndrome. Probably there is an inhibition of sodium reabsorption by the proximal renal tubules. The condition shows some improvement with restriction of water intake. Such patients can be differentiated from that with the syndrome of inappropriate ADH secretion caused by ectopic ADH secretion, using radioimmunoassay.[44] In some patients definite ADH hyperactivity may not be seen. Some of these patients may have abmormalities related to atrial natriuretic factor (ANF). Hypercalcemia occurs in the absence of bony metastasis from ectopic parathormone secretion or from effects of prostaglandin osteoclast activating factors.

Osteoclasts are seen at the bone tumour intersurface but biopsies generally reveal large areas of bone tissue adjacent to cancer tissue without any evidence of osteoclasts, indicating a direct effect of the tumour. Hypercalcemia is found in 8% of cases and occurs even in the absence of direct bone involvement, especially in patients with squamous cell carcinoma. Even parathyroid hormone is unlikely to be the cause, since there is no evidence of raised intestinal absorption of the calcium, as shown by calcium balance studies.[87] Prostaglandin production by the tumour adjacent to the invaded bone has been demonstrated and these are known to cause bone destruction, but are unlikely to do so as the half-life of prostaglandins in circulation is too short. Active products of cyclo oxygenase pathway may be present, having a longer half life.

The condition is associated with low serum phosphorus and normal alkaline phosphatase level. The individual manifests symptoms of calcium intoxication, such as polyuria, polydipsia, muscular weakness, loss of appetite, constipation, drowsiness and abdominal pain. The level of alkaline phosphatase is high with normal liver and bone studies. Sudden elevation of calcium level in the blood may be curtailed by the administration of steroids (Hydrocortisone suppression test) or declomycin.[12]

Among the osseous abnormalities, the occurrence of hypertrophic pulmonary osteoarthropathy (HPOA) is characteristic. It can occur in all lung cancers except the small cell variety. The fullblown picture is characterised by digital clubbing, pain and swelling around the peripheral joints—ankle and wrist—simulating rheumatoid arthritis. Clubbing has been the only predominant extrapulmonary manifestation in most of

Indian studies.[46] Radiogram shows bilateral, symmetrical periosteitis at the distal end of the bones of the forearm and legs, wherein the periosteal new bone stands out separately like candle grease or onion peel.[2]

Bone scan shows an increased isotope uptake and rapid turnover of calcium using calcium isotope is demonstrated. There is no specific hormonal mediator as yet which has been limited with HPOA. Elevated GH concentration has been reported by radioimmunoassay. Acromegaly is commonly found in bronchial carcinoid tumour and HPOA is more frequently seen in squamous cell bronchial carcinoma.[44] Somatostatins are found in all bronchial carcinoids and in 25-40% cases of small cell carcinoma. Human placental lactogen and prolactin are reported in 2-5% of cases of bronchial carcinoid but with no clinical consequences.

There may be autonomic disturbance like flushing and increased sweating. Gynaecomastia may be noted with high uninary oestrogen level. The level of alkaline phosphatase is raised. Severe pain is often relieved by removal of the tumour or by vagotomy or irradiation of primary or even on thoracotomy. The administration of corticosteroids or indomethacin often gives relief.

Dermatomyositis, scleroderma, acanthosis nigricans and erythema gyratum can occur as connective tissue and dermatologic disorders. Dermatomyositis presents as dusky purple to red erythema, violaceous rash on face and arms, pain in the girdle muscles, marked weakness, and intense irritation of skin. Steroids relieve the symptoms. Erythema gyratum may appear as dusky red macular itchy rash over face, trunk and limbs. There can be hyperkeratosis and hyperpigmentation of the palms and soles (tylosis) called acanthosis nigricans. Non-bacterial thrombotic endocarditis is commonly seen in adenocarcinoma and bronchoalveolar carcinoma. Involvement of mitral valve gives rise to embolisation to kidneys, CNS and coronary arteries.

Thrombophlebitis migrans as recurrent peripheral venous thrombosis from increased thromboplastin production is also noted in lung cancer apart from the carcinoma of pancreas. Often an embolic episode from it leads to pulmonary infarction. Due to shortened survival of red cells and depression of bone marrow, anaemia can occur. There can be disseminated intravascular coagulation. Even leukamoid reaction may occur.[2]

The neurological abnormalities though rare, yet most interesting complications where cerebellar dysfunction and cerebellar and associated spinocerebellar tract atrophy occurs. Almost 60 cases have appeared in literature since its description in 1919. These are commonly associated with small cell lung carcinoma.[44] However, it is important to rule out other causes of CNS disturbance associated with deficient nutrition such as Wernicke's encephalopathy. A comprehensive classification of paraneoplastic disorders has been described. Four types of disorders affecting neuromuscular system, encephalomeningitis, cortical cerebellar degeneration and peripheral neuropathy and myopathy have been seen. Even motor neurone disease with a solitary brain metastasis in bronchogenic carcinoma is reported, although multiple metastases are more common.

Other manifestations, include corticocerebellar degeneration (ataxia, vertigo, tremors and dysarthria), encephalopathies (progressive dementia and amnesia) usually purely sensory peripheral neuropathy (numbness, loss of sensation, weakness and wasting of muscles), carcinomaneous neurocytosis, myopathies with involvement of girdle muscles leading to their weakness and wasting, polymyositis and myasthenic syndrome with weakness involving the girdle muscles, without affection of the bulbar and ocular muscles.[2]

Cachexia is another metabolic manifestation of cancer. Weight loss occurs in a high percentage of patients but generally at a stage *with widespread metastasis.* But the characteristic cachexia of lung cancer is seen at an early stage when no distant metastases are found. Weight gain is seen following tumour resection but recurrent cachexia usually antedates inert metastatic disease. The syndrome includes weakness, weight loss, fever, anemia, hypoalbuminemia, hypercalcinemia etc. and almost multifactorial in aetiology in most of the patients. Anorexia can be due to electrolyte disturbance as well as depression and linear or abdominal metastases. Taste is usually impaired, further worsened by chemotherapy. Weight loss is due to anorexia but in some weight loss is inappropriate to their chlorine intake. The cause of anorexia is not known as no changes in the appetite or feeding centre in the hypothalamus have been found. The cause of weight loss has been multifactorial. Even study of mediators did not yield.

Hypoglycemia is occasionally seen in lung carcinoma,[44] probably this arises when the tumour which relies heavily on anaerobic glycolysis, falls short of glucose supply, could turn towards using normal resources. The sera of some patients contains high levels of somatomedin, probably an insulin-like growth factor.

The existence of bronchogenic carcinoma may come to light because of symptoms referrable to the intrapulmonary lesion or from manifestations due to metastatic spread within the thorax or outside or from non-metastatic extrapulmonary manifestations. These act as pointers to existence of tumour in the chest.

Cachexia associated with cancer is a frequent problem, yet in spite of a considerable research effort the basic mechanisms involved have not been fully elucidated. The term cachexia is derived from the Greek kakos (bad) and hexis (condition) and the patient with cachexia is often considered to be the textbook picture of the cancer patient.

Cancer cachexia has been rocognised as a common condition since the first large-scale study by Warren in 1932. Its frequency varies with the tumour type and ranges from 8-73 per cent in the gastrointestinal cancers and lung cancer facing the highest incidences. Although weight loss is only one component of cachexia, it does have considerable prognostic value.

Cancer Cachexia Syndrome[44,45]

Cancer cachexia syndrome is well characterized by anorexia and early satiety, weight loss and marked muscle weakness, anemia of a non-specific type, and altered host metabolism, often associated with a raised basal metabolic rate. Cachexia in cancer patients is not directly correlated with food intake or the stage, histological type, or site of the tumour. It may occur with a very small primary tumour and may antedate the clinical diagnosis. It is not always associated with patients who have very large tumour burdens. The patient with cancer cachexia shows features of both starvation and injury. There is usually deficient food intake but the presence of the tumour means, in addition, that some of the ability to regulate the response to starvation is lost. Cancer cachexia, therefore, may be more akin to the condition produced by a major injury or sepsis than that due to simple starvation. The clinical picture of a patient with cachexia is thus of an individual who looks ill, has lost weight, and has a pale skin, often with oedema of dependent parts, anemia, lethargy and weakness.

The clinical signs of vitamin deficiency may be corroborated by the relevant biochemical investigations and usually show a high incidence of subclincial problems. Anthropometric tests confirm the loss of subcutaneous fat and then body mass. Other biochemical investigations often reveal evidence of metabolic disorders including low serum albumin level, electrolyte abnormalities, and tracemetal deficiencies. The immunological abnormalities are often associated with patients who have cancer cachexia. Delayed hypersensitivity skin testing is frequently abnormal in such patients. The psychological reaction of the patient may manifest as he may become withdrawn and depressed or increasingly frightened and anxious. The significance of these depends on the patient, the tumour site, and the extent of the disease. Pathological features of cachexia have been shown in Table 6.10.

Table 6.10: Pathology of cachexia

1. Deficient food intake	Anorexia
2. Excessive loss of body protein	Ulceration Haemorrhage Diarrhea Vomiting
3. Malabsorption	
4. Increased metabolic rate	
5. • Abnormal metabolism of the host affecting	Protein Carbohydrate Fat Hormones Water Electrolytes
• Effect of tumour products	
• Nitrogen trap by the tumour	

Deficient food intake can also be associated with anorexia, this decrease in appetite may be noted even when the tumour is small suggesting that the tumour, or an abnormal metabolic response of the body, produces substances with an anorectic effect. While this is an attractive hypothesis, no firm data exist to confirm or refute it. The anorexia is often profound and extremely difficult to modify by dietary, pharmacological, or psychological methods. Taste for food is altered and its palatability affected.

Loss of protein from the gastrointestinal tract through vomiting or diarrhoea or the sequestration of protein in pleural or peritoneal cavities may add significantly to the problem. Repeated minor bleeds increase the risk of developing anemia and are associated with loss of plasma proteins.

The development of cachexia is the demonstration of an increased basal metabolic rate. The mechanism behind this rise is likely to be complex and it has not been recorded in all patients. Host metabolism is altered because either the tumour produces excess lactic acid (due to an increase in glycolysis) or the body itself develops an abnormal metabolism in the presence of the tumour. This produces a lactic acidosis and the excess lactate is recycled to glucose by gluconeogenesis in the liver and kidneys. The pathway is referred to as the Cori cycle.

The cycle is inefficient in the use of energy since only 2 moles of ATP are produced by anaerobic glucolysis in the breakdown of glucose to lactate. Gluconeogenesis (the conversion of lactate to glucose) requires 6 moles of ATP. Thus the tumour derives little energy in its resynthesis. These studies may not entirely explain the progressive weight loss associated with cancer but they do suggest that the pathways are likely to be contributory. In relation to carbohydrate metabolism, the secretion of insulin may be modified. Glucose intolerance in malignant cachexia appears to be related to abnormal insulin production and to insulin resistance.

Body fat is rapidly mobilized as the patient develops cachexia and there is a significant increase in the level of unesterified fatty acids in plasma. The loss of lean body mass from skeletal muscle is obvious clinically and hypoalbuminaemia is common. The latter is due not only to the decreased albumin synthesis rate but also to an increased fractional catabolic rate. It has been noted frequently that cancer cachexia is associated with a negative nitrogen balance. Water, electrolyte and mineral metabolism may all be abnormal and related to deficient intake or hormonal imbalance. Hormone secretion may be related to the effects of the tumour or to the synthesis of ectopic hormones. A tumour-derived product is also implicated in the mechanism. These factors are produced in addition to the well recognized hormones and have been given the name *toxohormones.*

Management of Cachexia[44,45]

It should be stated clearly at the outset that the best way of dealing with cancer cachexia is to eradicate the malignant disease. If this can be done successfully then the patient improves, his appetite returns and weighty gain ensues.

Before discussing the methods of support available, two potential disadvantages of feeding such patients should be mentioned. The first concerns the possible increase in tumour growth that might occur when nutrients are supplied to the patient. There is little firm evidence for this although it is theoretically possible. The second problem concerns the potentially harmful effects of hyperalimentation in patients with cancer cachexia. In addition to the technical complications of intravenous hyperalimentation the physiological effects of rapid refeeding may be dangerous.

Several newer agents based on alterations in brain amino-acid levels may be of interest. The psychological component may also require correction.

Dietary Supplementation

The addition to the diet of one of the ever-widening range of products for nutritional support may be of value in those patients who have minimal anorexia. Since the sensation of taste may be altered, the unpalatability of some of these products may inhibit their use. Adequate vitamin supplementation should be supplied.

The introduction of the fine-bore nasogastric tube has made an enormous contribution to our ability to feed cancer patients. The method has been employed in the management of cancer with useful effect.

Intravenous Hyperalimentation

This has been extensively used in the management of cancer both to correct weight loss and to enhance the effect of anti-cancer therapy. It cannot reverse cachexia in all patients.

The removal of plasma from the cancer-bearing patients—plasmapheresis—is a technique that has been in used for many years. Changes in appetite and in pruritis and in the immunological responses have been seen in cancer patients after plasmapheresis.

Investigations

Common investigations in lung cancer have been shown in Table 6.11.

Table 6.11: Carcinoma lung: Helpful investigations
1. Chest X-ray
2. Fibroptic bronchoscopy and BAL analysis
3. Computerised imaging modalities
4. Lymph node biopsy and percutaneous needle biopsy and U.S. scanning
5. Pleural aspirate cytology and pleural biopsy
6. Thoracotomy and open lung biopsy

Radiology[2]

A small growth developing into the bronchial lumen may not be visible. Hence plain X-ray may be normal in early stages of lung cancer. The growth must be at least 1 cm in diameter to be recognised radiologically. Early detection requires either bronchoscopy or study of exfoliative cytology. Comparison with the previous film taken a year or two earlier helps in checking the diagnosis. It enables one to determine whether the lesion is present over a long period or is of recent development as well as activity of lesion. Variety of presentations are seen in later stages. Often a circular coin shadow situated in the periphery poses diagnostic problems. On tomography, a notch may be seen facing bronchovascular bundle as it offers resistance for the growth. It may also reveal multiple streaky shadows radiating in all directions from the circular opacity indicating the spread. The presence of calcification in the coin shadow favours a diagnosis of granulomatous condition rather than malignancy, especially in tropic. When the growth is hidden or overshadowed by hilum or cardia, a lateral tomography is necessary. Similarly A.P. tomography is required to visualise the region behind the first rib and clavicle.

The growth shadow on X-ray may simulate pneumonic consolidation. The inflammation distal to the growth clears up with antibacterial drugs. As the underlying neoplasm grows and recurs with shadow, the X-ray examination has to be repeated after six weeks especially in male past 40 years.

The growth may present as a unilateral dense hilar opacity with irregular margin, which may be due to the tumour or due to hilar lymph node metastasis. There can be a collapse of a lobe or of the lung due to complete occlusion of bronchus, presenting as homogeneous opacity and mediastinal shift. It can present as a neoplastic cavity that has a thick wall with irregular inner lining. The cavity may develop following ischaemic necrosis or from the check valve effect of the growth or from lung abscess distal to the bronchial obstruction.

Neoplasms may grow slowly, others rapidly. The latter may become non-resectable due to metastatic lesions.[4,5] The growth may present with features of pleural effusion but without any shift of mediastinum due to coexisting collapse from bronchial occlusion. Rarely it may manifest pneumothorax or pericardial effusion. It may exist with tuberculosis or develop around an old tuberculous focus. Coexisting emphysema or pulmonary infarction may be seen on chest X-ray.

Chest X-ray may reveal erosion of the ribs or fracture of the ribs due to secondary deposits. There may be widening of the mediastinum from lymph node metastasis or raised hemidiaphragm due to phrenic nerve paralysis. The tumour spread along the lymphatics (lymphangitis carcinomatosis) shows that enlargement of hilar lymph nodes and streaky liner shadows radiating from the hilum either unilaterally or bilaterally. Pulmonary osteoarthropathy with periosteal new bone formation may point towards lung cancer. Common radiological features encountered are tabulated in Table 6.12.

Table 6.12: Common radiological features

1.	Hilar	Hilar/perihilar/mass or prominence
2.	Parenchymal	1. Pneumonitis/collapse (due to bronchial obstruction) 2. Peripheral mass (small/large) 3. Apical mass 4. Cavitation in a mass
3.	Intrathoracic extrabronchial	1. Mediastinal mass or widening 2. Chest wall mass 3. Pleural effusion 4. Diaphragmatic elevations

Chest screening demonstrates a raised hemidiaphragm with paradoxical movement on respiration and on sniffing. It indicates phrenic nerve paralysis and the mediastinal spread of malignancy. Bronchogram may exhibit block or narrowing in the bronchi. Displacement of oesophagus especially when the mediastinal glands are involved, can be demonstrated by barium swallow examination.

Transesophageal endoscopic ultrasound scanning had 60-90% sensitivity and 70-100 specificity in staging lung cancer and is found to be superior and specific as compared to CT, PET, mediastinoscopy as well as transbronchial aspiration. Even it is far more accurate in diagnosing mediastinal lesion of tuberculosis/sarcoidosis in characterisation and obtaining tissue diagnosis, with the use of tru-cut biopsy under real time ultrasound guidance.[46]

Cytodiagnosis[2]

An analysis of exfoliated malignant cells is a very useful diagnostic test, but false positive tests are obtained even in expert hands. The cancer cells may be stained with 1 per cent methylene blue or with heamalum and eosin. The study of cell morphology help in recognising the type of carcinoma in many cases. The cells of small cell carcinoma are distributed in clumps or streaks and contain darkly stained big nucleus with stripped cell carcinoma and a thin rim of cytoplasm. The squamous cell carcinoma is associated with keratinised cells of variable size and shape. They contain irregular dark stained nucleus with coarse chromatin and abundant cytoplasm. The darkly stained cells appear in clumps. Adenocarcinoma is difficult to recognise by cytology.

The early morning fresh sputum preferably blood streaked secured after deep cough should be used for staining. The cytological studies may be diagnostic, even before the presence of radiological changes. Sputum cytology for diagnosing lung cancer is effective and is just a poor man's bronchoscopy.[47] However, it has often been neglected. Thin prep method improves yield of sputum cytology.[48] Low cost and easy availability makes it practically useful in diagnosing lung cancer at tertiary care centres. Caution must be taken as false positive results are often obtained during or immediately following inflammatory conditions of the lungs, asthma and one to two weeks after bronchoscopy. Cellular yield may become indistinguishable from the cells of squamous cell carcinoma in the presence of chronic inflammatory changes in the lung like bronchiectasis and tuberculous cavities. Another source of false positive results include tumours in the upper respiratory tract or mouth. Among the cytological methods employed, the best results are obtained by aspirates from lung, lymph node and other involved sites.[12]

Fluid after bronchial washing and bronchial brushing can be used for cytodiagnosis.[49,50] Cytological positivity in bronchial brushing and washing specimens is very poor.[12] The material is stained with Papanicolaou technique. The nuclei of the malignant cells exhibit hyperchromatism, large nucleoli with irregularly placed chromatin. Exfoliative cytology is of value particularly when bronchoscopic bite biopsy is not possible or the tumour is at the periphery.[51]

Absolute Lymphocytopenia

Absolute lymphocytopenia has been suggested to be a diagnostic indicator in patients of bronchogenic carcinoma. The pathogenesis of lymphocytopenia is unclear but decrease occurs possibly in response to elevated levels of cortisols which is seen in these cases of bronchogenic carcinoma.[30]

Lung Scan

To know the extent of perfusion in the lungs the perfusion lung scan is performed. There is a significant decrease in the perfusion of the lung when the tumour approaches the hilum and involves the vessels.When the relative perfusion of the affected lung is less than one-third of the total perfusion the tumour is likely to be inoperable.

The spread of malignancy can be studied by Gallium (GA) scan. Though the isotope is taken by carcinoma, it is also concentrated in the inflammatory parenchymal disease. But uptake by pulmonary infiltrations or embolus is unlikely.[2]

Endoscopy

Tumour in the bronchial and segmental bronchi are visualised by bronchoscopy, even when plain X-ray does not cast any shadows. Fiberoptic bronchoscopy has offered many advantages over a rigid bronchoscope. The ease of introduction, offers greater visibility of the bronchial tree and has increased patient tolerance.[2]

Bronchoscopy

Bronchoscopy helps to stage lung cancer and decide operability.

The bronchial brushings are used for cytology and for culture.[92,93] The biopsy specimen can be used for histo-pathological study.

The bronchoscope can be easily manoeuvred. The patient tolerates the procedure well and is safe. It causes minimum discomfort. Its flexibility and small size has increased the range of visibility of bronchi and subsegmental bronchi and the upper lobes can be seen easily. Oxygen can be administered through nasal prongs through one of the nostrils as hypoxaemia quite often occurs during the procedure.[2]

A premedication of 50 to 75 mg meperidine, 50 to 75 mg hydroxyzine and 0.6 mg atropine is generally administered half an hour prior to the procedure. Four per cent lidocaine solution is instilled intra-trachealy and sprayed into the nose and oropharynx before the introduction of the scope. The distal end of the scope is smeared with lidocaine jelly, the scope is introduced intranasally or orally and 2 ml of 2 per cent lidocaine is instilled above the vocal cords. Then the scope is advanced into the trachea, carina and the bronchi and segmental bronchi on either side. The secretions are collected for cytology and culture. A differential cytology is necessary when the sputum has shown positive results for malignant cells in the absence of a radiological shadow. The suspected area can be brushed using the brush attached at the end of a flexible wire, introduced through the channel of bronchoscope. A biopsy is taken when the growth is visible or under fluoroscopic control when it is located in the periphery. Fine needle aspiration cytology technique combined with bronchial brushings or forceps punch biopsy improves diagnosis from 65 per cent to 76.6 per cent in centrally located bronchial carcinoma with little risk of complications.[51] A widening of the main carina indicates metastasis in the subcarinal lymph nodes.[2]

The frequent diagnostic indications for bronchoscopy are cough, haemoptysis, radiologic abnormalities suggestive of tumour, unresolved pneumonia, bronchial obstruction, atelectasis and localised wheezing.[50] The instrument can be introduced into the segmental and subsegmental bronchi. Its small size and manoeuvrability have enabled one to explore the upper lobes and the periphery of the lung which are inaccessible to the rigid bronchoscope. The endobronchial lesions can be visualised and the BALF and biopsy can be obtained for diagnostic purpose. It is also useful in conditions with a stiff neck due to ankylosing spondylitis affecting the cervical spine and other disorders preventing extension of neck and aortic aneurysm and in debilitated individuals. It can be used to perform tracheobronchial toilet in patients who are mechanically ventilated. The selective culture can be obtained in unresolved pneumonia. Fiberoptic bronchoscopy is useful in cases exhibiting positive cytology without any radiological abnormality.[2,50] The histocytological yield of the diagnosis with flexible fiberoptic bronchoscope can be as high as 84 per cent.[12]

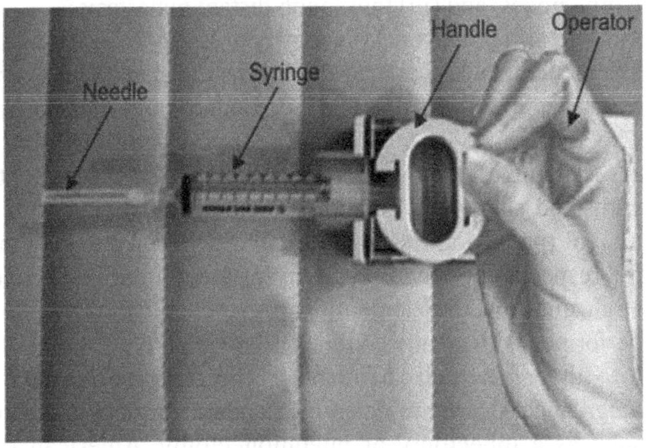

Fig. 6.1: Fine needle aspiration cytology (injection-needle and syringe fitted with a handle to perform FNAC).

However the rigid bronchoscope has its therapeutic value in removal of the foreign body, in patients with massive haemoptysis and in small children.[2]

Laryngoscopy

Vocal cord paralysis due to involvement of the recurrent laryngeal nerve is diagnosed by laryngoscopy.

Mediastinoscopy

It is useful in visualizing the growth if extended into mediastinum. The metallic tube can be introduced through a parasternal approach, for the left upper lobe lesions and through suprasternal approach for the evaluation of the right lung lesions. The histological metastasis in the mediastinal lymph nodes indicates inoperability of the growth. The demonstration of spread of the disease by mediastinoscope curtails the need for thoracotomy. Vagotomy on the right side can be performed with mediastinoscopy if an inoperable carcinoma is associated with hypertrophic osteoarthropathy.[2]

CT Scan

CT scan can detect unsuspected calcification and small nodules that are missed by standard chest radiograms. CT scan thin sections are sensitive in identifying the presence of mediastinal adenopathy. The procedure is preferred to mediastinoscopy. Mediastinal metastasis in malignancy of the lung obviates thoracotomy. The whole body CT scan is essential procedure in staging of bronchial carcinoma. Squamous cell carcinoma of lung can also rarely produce an air bronchogram sign on CT scan of thorax.[52] Also both CT scan and MRI are very useful in distinguishing solid and cystic lesions.[12] MRI is better than CT in the chest wall tumours. Features of CT scan are listed in Table 6.13.

Table 6.13: CT scanning: Few facts

1*	Can demonstrate metastasis as small as 3-6 mm size.
2*	May not distinguish metastatic deposits, tuberculoma and fungal granuloma (in these cases).

Biopsy

The bronchial biopsy obtained through bronchoscope helps in establishment of the diagnosis. Fluoroscopic control is essential in peripheral lesions when transbronchial biopsy is performed. The biopsy forceps is advanced during inspiration and is closed during expiration. It enables the cutting of the bonchial wall demonstrating the suspected growth.

Aspiration Biopsy

The growth can be biopsied using Vim-silverman needle or trephine biopsy when the growth is within 3 cm of the pleural surface. A transthoracic fine needle aspiration biopsy (Thoracoscopy) under fluoroscopic guidance helps in obtaining the tumour tissue and it is preferred. Pleural biopsy using flexible fiberoptic pleuroscope reveals the spread of the growth to the pleura.[2] The biopsy of the palpable cervical and scalene nodes helps in establishing the tumour spread.

Scalene Node Biopsy

No invasive diagnostic procedure should be done prior to a good history. A thorough physical examination, sputum cytology and X-ray review should be done because these baseline studies help to decide which invasive procedure will be most suitable for the patient. Further the invasive procedures should begin with the least traumatic one first. The importance of this simple procedure therefore is that it may save the patient from a major surgical trauma in the form of an exploratory thoracotomy, that has to be performed if the diagnosis remains unconfirmed.[2]

Methodology of Scalene Node Biopsy

Biopsy can be done under local anaesthesia both on an in-patient or out-patient basis. Before attempting the procedure, however the young surgeon must know the regional anatomy to avoid complications like massive haemorrhage, air embolism, chylous fistula, pneumothorax etc.

Scalene lymph nodes are lower deep cervical glands lying lateral to the internal jugular vein, on the scalenus anterior muscle. A three inch incision centered on the lateral border of the sternocleidomastoid is made parallel to and about 3/4 inch above the clavicle. Skin and deep fascia are divided. The omohyoid is pulled upward and the sternocleidomastoid medially. The lymphoid and fatty tissue lying on the scalenus anterior and that in the jugulosubclavian junctional angle is identified and removed for histopathology in case the glands are not found.

In cases where the lesion is in the lower two thirds of the lung fields, the biopsy can be performed bilaterally because the lymphatics from the lower two thirds of the lung drain to the lymph nodes at the carina from where they can drain to either side.

Scalene lymph node biopsy is a good diagnostic procedure in the setting of a centrally placed or upper lobe suspicious lesion which has not been diagnosed. It can also be done to assess the resectability of an intrathoracic neoplasm even if nodes are not palpable because lymph nodes can be discovered on operation in many of these cases. A positive biopsy report may alter the line of action of the thoracic surgeon and radiotherapist.

Elevated hormone levels like human chorionic gonadotropin in 12.14 per cent, luteinizing hormone in 26.6 per cent, follicular stimulating hormone in 4.4 per cent, prolactin in 37.8 per cent, thyroid stimulating hormones in 3.2 per cent and cortisol in 30 per cent of cases has been observed in patients of bronchogenic carcinoma.[53] Blood DNA levels in cancer patients are low and in 16 per cent of cases, the RNA levels are higher.[54] FDA approved indication of FDG PET/CT scan in lung cancer in non-small cell in initial staging and in non-small cell for diagnosis, staging and restaging being used. Even, the characterization of solitary pulmonary module to differentiate from malignancy from inflammation has also been used.

In non-small cell cancers, showing sensitivity of 75-91% in nodal metastases, with higher specificity for bone, adrenal and distant metastases.

Response to chemotherapy and recurrence can also be evaluated.[55]

Staging of Lung Cancer

Earlier bronchogenic carcinoma used to be placed into three general categories as (i) those with a peripheral lesion without evidence of spread to the regional lymph nodes or distant metastasis, (ii) those with spread beyond the lung to the regional lymph nodes, and (iii) those with distant metastasis.

The introduction of a battery of investigations and treatment regimens has made it necessary to classify lung cancer by its histologic cell types and the extent or stage of the disease. The location of the tumour (anatomic staging) and the assessment of the cardiovascular status of the patient to withstand single and combined methods of treatment of the tumour (physiologic staging) are to be evaluated to determine the respectability and operability of the tumour respectively. High quality CT examinations have enabled staging to be performed with greater confidence.

But for small cell carcinoma, it is necessary to find out if the lung cancer can be resected by standard surgical procedures such as a lobectomy or pneumonectomy. American joint committee for cancer staging and end results reporting recommended TNM (Tumour-nodal involvement-metastasis) system of staging of cancer, and it has been replaced by a new international staging system. It provides a basis for categorising the location and extent of malignant lesion according to stages of development and various letters stand for the following: The letter T denotes the extent of the primary tumour and the number in the same line as the letter refers to an increasing size of the tumour and its extension into the adjacent structure; the letter N with appropriate numbers describes the absence (N_0) or presence (N_1 to peribronchial and or ipsilateral hilar lymph nodes, N_2 to ipsilateral mediastinal and supraclavicular lymph nodes) of regional lymph nodes involvement and the letter M with appropriate numbers refers to the absence (M_0) or the presence (M_1) of distant metastases. This classification system with clinical relevance is employed to the treatment planning and to the estimation of prognosis. Although overall survival rate is not altered, yet 1985 TNM staging allows greater prognostic accuracy.[55]

Primary Tumour (T)

TO	No evidence of primary tumour.
TX	Occult cancer remain bronchial washing cytologies but not seen on X-ray or bronchoscopy.
TIS	Carcinoma in situ.
T_1	Tumour less than ≤ 3 cm
T_2	Tumour >3cm with atelectasis, obstructive pneumonitis, extending to hila.
T_3	Tumour of any size with direct extension to chest walls, diaphragm, mediastinum, pleura, pericardium, heart, vessels, trachea oesophagus, vertebrae.
T_4	Tumor of any size with invasion of mediastinum or other organs as stated in T_3 or with presence of malignant pleural effusion.

Regional Lymph Nodes (N)

N_0	No demonstrable metastasis to regional lymph nodes.
N_1	Metastasis to peribronchial or ipsilateral hilar area.
N_2	Metastasis to ipsilateral mediastinal or subcarinal lymph nodes.
N_3	Metastasis to contralateral mediastinal, hilar, scalene, supraclavicular or ipsilateral scalene node.

Distant Metastasis (M)

M_0	No known distant metastasis.
M_1	Distant metastasis present with site specified *e.g.* brain.

Stage grouping using new ISS

Occult carcinoma	*TX*	*NO*	*MO*
Stage 0	TIS	Ca in situ	
I	T_1	N_0	M_0

Contd.

Contd.

	T_2	N_0	M_0
II	T_1	N_1	M_0
	T_2	N_1	M_0
IIIa	T_3	N_0	M_0
	T_3	N_1	M_0
	T_3	N_2	M_0
IIIb	Any T	N_3	M_0
	T_4	Any N	M_0
IV	Any T	Any N	M_1

Primary tumour is referred to a TX (occult carcinoma proven by the presence of malignant cells in bronchopulmonary secretions but not visualised either by radiography or bronchoscopy), T_0 (No evidence of primary tumour), TIS (carcinoma in situ), T_1 (tumour 3 cm or less in diameter without evidence of invasion), T_2 (tumour more than 3 cm or of any size with evidence of invasion into the visceral pleura, or of obstruction), T_3 (tumour of any size with extension into the chest wall, diaphragm, or mediastinal pleura or pericardium or tumour in the main bronchus within 2 cm of the carina), or T_4 (tumour of any size with invasion into the mediastinum or involving heart, great vessels, trachea, oesophagus, vertebral body or carina or presence of malignant pleural effusion).

The stage grouping of TNM subsets is as follows: occult carcinoma (TX, N_0, M_0). stage 0 (TIS), stage I (T_1 N_0 M_0, T_2, N_0 M_0, stage II (T_1 N_1 M_0, T_2 N_1 M_0) stage IIIa (T_3 N_0 M_0, T_3 N_1 M_0), $T_{1\text{-}3}$ N_2 M_0), stage III b (any TN_3 M_0,T_4 any N M_0) and stage IV (any T and N M_1). Stage grouping is significant for all histologic cell types except small cell carcinoma wherein there is no significant relation between stage and survival rates. In that cell type it is described as a limited-extensive system. It is called a limited disease when the disease is confined to one hemithorax excluding cytology-positive pleural effusion, but including ipsilateral mediastinal, scalene or supraclavicular lymph nodes.[52] In recent years, the definition includes bilateral supraclavicular lymph nodes. All forms of disease not defined above are called extensive disease. Various signs of spread of bronchial carcinoma are shown in Tables 6.14 to 6.17.

Prognosis

Bronchogenic carcinoma are considered extremely virulent tumours, since the different histologic types have a tendency to metastasize as well as to spread locally. Many a times the diagnosis is made late when the dissemination has already taken place. The life expectancy in such instances is measured in months. The age and performance status of the patient, the histologic type of tumour, the extent of spread and the presence of symptoms, weight loss and spread to nervous system influence the survival. Thus a patient with a small tumour in the lung, not invading the mediastinum or metastasizing distally,

Table 6.14: Signs of spread of bronchial carcinoma

1. Hilar and mediastinal lymph nodes enlargement through lymphatic spread.
2. Pleural effusion
   a. Due to malignant pleural involvement
   b. Due to associated lung infection
   c. Large effusion or effusion on the opposite side strongly favour malignant spread.
3. Mediastinal involvement: Suggested by mediastinal widening and elevation of a hemidiaphragm due to phrenic nerve involvement by tumour. CT helps in assessing mediastinal invasion as an accurate and more sensitive method.
4. Chest wall invasion: Rib destruction adjacent to primary pulmonary shadow is diagnostic of bronchial carcinoma. CT can demonstrate soft tissue invasion even before bone is not eroded.
5. Rib metastasis: Bone destruction may be seen in lung carcinoma. Sclerotic secondary deposits from lung carcinoma are rare.
6. Pulmonary metastasis: Metastasis to other parts of the lung from primary lung carcinoma are occasionally seen.
7. Lymphangitis carcinomatosa: This occurs due to blockage of pulmonary lymphatics by carcinomatous tissue. The signs are identical to those seen in interstitial pulmonary oedema (septal lines, loss of vessels and peribronchial thickening). But if heart size is normal, with hilar adenopathy and lobar consolidation, diagnosis of lymphangitis carcinomatosis is more favourable. This is further helped by clinical history of gradually increasing breathlessness over few weeks, compared to sudden dyspnoea in pulmonary odema.

Table 6.15: Pulmonary metstasis

1. Seen as rounded multiple shadows of different sizes in both the lungs.
2. Occasionally may have irregular borders.
3. Clearly visible when measuring more than a centimeter.

Table 6.16: Pleural metastasis

1. Usually give rise to pleural effusion.
2. The individual pleural metastasis are quite rare.

Table 6.17: Rib metastasis

1. Commonly seen in tumours metastasizing to bone, *e.g.*, breast, bronchus, thyroid, kidney, prostate.
2. All produce lytic metastatic deposits except breast and prostate.
3. Sclerotic metastasis in an elderly suggest primary prostatic cancer.
4. Sclerotic or mixed lytic and sclerotic metastasis in a female points toward a primary breast cancer.

has a 70 per cent five years survival. However, once mediastinal pleura, chest wall or ipsilateral lymph nodes are affected, five year survival rate falls to18 per cent. Early diagnosis and specific cell typing is important for both the treatment and prognosis.

Surgery is the treatment of choice in patients with non-small cell carcinoma. Radiation helps in few surgical treatment offers good results especially in squamous cell carcinoma, compared to small cell carcinoma where chemotherapy is useful. However less than 25 per cent of bronchogenic carcinoma appear resectable at the time of diagnosis. It is worth noting even among those undergoing resection, the five years survival rate is only about 25 per cent. The five years survival rate for all patients is less than 9 per cent whereas five years survival rate for squamous cell carcinoma and adenocarcinoma is 10 per cent, it is only 3 per cent with undifferentiated lesions. The mean survival in oat cell carcinoma, despite radiotherapy and chemotherapy, is about one year.

Squamous cell carcinoma has a long symptomless phase. The symptoms of bronchial obstruction appear early and metastasis occurs late. Small cell carcinoma has a poor prognosis as it grows rapidly and metastasizes early. Local forms of treatment such as surgery and/or radiotherapy infrequently produce long-term survival. The addition of combination chemotherapy has significantly changed the clinical course of small cell carcinoma,[2] improving median survival at least four to five-fold.[56]

Treatment of Lung Cancer[57]

Lung cancer continues to occur in epidemic proportions in the United States. According to American Cancer Society estimates for 1991, it is the second most common cancer among men and women combined. Furthermore, because it is seldom diagnosed early, when prospects for cure are high, lung cancer is the most common cause of death both in men and women.[58]

The cause of this epidemic is not mysterious. About 95 per cent of lung cancers in men and 80 to 85 per cent of lung cancers in women result from cigarette smoking. The dose-dependent relationship and relative risk of death from lung cancer, has increased upto 25-fold for men who smoke 25 to 40 cigarettes per day compared with never smokers. Both cigarette consumption per capita and the percentage of current smokers and women have declined over the past two decades.[59] Even if all cigarette smokers discontinue their habit today, the major health care burden from long cancer would persist for many years.

The 5 years survival of Americans afflicted with lung cancer improved only slightly, from 12 per cent to 13 per cent, from 1974 through 1987.[60]

The incidence is also increasing fast in developing countries including India.[61] Symptoms of early stage disease are non-specific and are ignored by the patients as being due to smoking or other non-malignant diseases, particularly chronic bronchitis and pulmonary tuberculosis. By the time manifestations are severe enough to force the patient to seek medical advice, the disease is usually advanced. Complete surgical resection is possible in less than 30 per cent of cases and the overall probability of surviving lung cancer for 5 years is less than 15 per cent. The median survival of untreated patients is only a few weeks. Three primary modes of therapy are available, viz. surgery, radiotherapy and chemotherapy, depending upon the cell type.

From the management point of view, lung cancer can be divided into small cell lung cancer (SCLC), consisting of the three major WHO histological types, viz., squamous or epidermoid cell type, adenocarcinoma and large cell carcinoma. Small cell carcinoma has a different cell of origin and biological behaviour, has early dissemination, produces ectopic hormones and peptides, and has a better response to radiotherapy and chemotherapy as compared to NSCLC.

Small Cell Lung Cancer

Small cell lung cancer (SCLC) is characterized by its relatively rapid growth rate and propensity for distant metastasis. About two thirds of patients have distant metastatic disease at the time of diagnosis, compared with less than half in NSCLC. In the absence of treatment, median survival in SCLC is only a few months. Demise can be equally rapid in patients with NSCLC, but a minority of patients experience a relatively idolent course, and in fact there are rare five-year survivors who never receive any treatment. Because of its tendency to metastasize, SCLC can rarely be treated surgically, while upto one third of NSCLC patients are surgically resectable at diagnosis. However, tumour regression with chemotherapy or irradiation occurs much more frequently in SCLC than in NSCLC.[62-64] As patients with lung cancer present very late in the course of their disease, surgery cannot be offered to these patients, even in the western countries, in more than 80 per cent of cases compared to 95 per cent of the Indian patients[21] Only 3 per cent of patients have a resectable tumour. Management of SCLC is described below heading Small-Cell Lung Cancer.[26]

Non-Small Cell Lung Cancer

In NSCLC, therapy is greatly influenced by the extent of tumor dissemination at diagnosis. One third of patients or fewer present with localized cancer confined within the pleural reflection (stage I and II, according to the new international staging system.[125] Approximately one third have locally or regionally advanced disease (stages IIIa and IIIb) which has directly extended through the pleural reflection or metastasized to the mediastinal lymph nodes. The final one third to one half have clinically detectable distant metastasis (stage IV). The 5 years survival rate (which generally indicates cure of the original neoplasm) in the first group is approximately 40 per cent; virtually all patients who live 5 years will have undergone surgical resection. For the second group, 5-year survival is at most 6 per cent to 8 per cent; most survivors will have received chest radiation and some will have had surgery. For the final group, 5-year survival is less than 1 per cent.[64] Thus, the great majority of patients who are cured of NSCLC receive surgical treatment.

NSCLC histology is 5-8 times more common than SCLC.[7] Treatment of NSCLC is essentially surgery, but most of the patients present late in the course of their disease. In operable stage I and II disease, a 5-year survival has also been observed in 70 per cent and 35-38 per cent of cases respectively according to the cell type.

Five years survival rate approaching 30 per cent can be achieved in patients in whom complete resection of primary tumor and mediastinal metastasis is possible. Unfortunately, such patients represented only 9 per cent of NSCLC cases in one institutional study. Some patients present with occult lung cancer, in which cytologic analysis of the sputum is positive without an obvious tumour appearing on a chest roentgenogram or apparent on bronchoscopic examination. These tumors, which are usually of the squamous cell type, can be identified by meticulous fiberoptic bronchoscopic examination, sometimes aided by fluorescent techniques using hematoporphyrins. Most of such patients treated surgically prove to have localized stage I cancer that will not recur in the majority of cases. However, they are at risk for developing a second lung cancer at rates as high as 5 per cent per year. Therefore, the surgical procedure of choice in occult lung cancer or in poor-risk patients with peripheral, roentgenographically apparent stage I NSCLC has become the minimum operation (often a segmental or wedge resection) needed to resect tumor completely while preserving the maximum amount of functional lung tissue. This approach reduces post-operative morbidity and mortality while making later lung resection, should another cancer mandate, more feasible. Only a quarter of the cases will be suitable for surgical intervention at the time of presentation, since majority of patients in India appear for treatment when the disease is far advanced.

The extent of the lung resection depends on the site of the growth. Lobectomy will suffice for the lesions confined to one lobe. Pneumonec tomy is required for the growths involving the main bronchus. Growth involving the orifice of the lobar bronchus requires removal of the involved lobe and a cylinder of the main bronchus (sleeve resection). In all these methods, paratracheal, subcarinal and para-aortic lymph nodes are removed. The survival rate following lobectomy is higher than that of pneumonectomy and it has a lower post-operative mortality.

Absolute contraindications for surgery include distant metastasis, involvement of trachea, carina and within 2 cms of origin of the main stem bronchus, evidence of spread into mediastinum (oesophagus, superior vena cava, recurrent laryngeal nerve, phrenic nerve and pericardium), and brachial plexus, extensive invasion of the chest wall, malignant pleural effusion, positive mediastinoscopy with tumour in contralateral lymph nodes, undifferentiated small cell carcinoma, coexistent cardiorespiratory diseases (chronic bronchitis, ischaemic heart disease) and poor respiratory reserve. Advanced age over 70 years, local chest wall invasion, Pancoast tumour, mediastinoscopy with microscopic evidence of tumour in ipsilateral lymph nodes and pleural effusion from relative contra-indications for surgery.

Adjuvant therapies like pre- and post-operative radiotherapy have not shown any benefit as regards the median survival. Similar observations have also been made with the use of adjuvant immunotherapy like intrapleural BCG, BCG cell wall skeleton and levamisol.

Chest irradiation, sometimes given in high doses with curative intent, is probably the most commonly administered initial therapy for patients with stage III NSCLC. It is also used for patients with earlier-stage neoplasms who cannot undergo thoracotomy for medical reasons.[57]

Higher rates of tumour regression and better control of disease in the thorax has been observed with higher doses, but there is no difference in survival, which was 5 per cent at 5 years, irrespective of dose.

Radiotherapy is given as palliative measure: (i) for relief of symptoms of superior vena caval obstruction; (ii) major airways obstruction; (iii) for relief of excruciating intense pain from bone secondaries; (iv) for control of intractable cough and haemoptysis; and (v) for treatment of Pancoast tumour. Often irradiation makes the patient sick with weakness, nausea, anorexia and dysphagia. Radiation pneumonia may reduce the respiratory reserve.

Large pleural effusion, extensive invasion of the mediastinum, or chest wall, large sized tumour and presence of distant metastasis form contraindications for radiation.[2]

Laser Therapy

Patients with malignant airway obstruction in squamous cell carcinoma may manifest shortness of breath, haemoptysis and cough. Airway palliation and debulking of the lesion in technically inoperable patients can be undertaken by external beam irradiation, laser treatment or endobronchial brachy-therapy. External beam irradiation is useful in those with bulky extraluminal disease and obstructing peripheral disease involving multiple airways. Neodymium YAG (yttrium-aluminium-garnet) laser is utilised to debulk intraluminal tumour situated in the lobar bronchus or larger airways. Brachytherapy can be used as an adjunct to the above two methods of treatment[50] where a nylon after loading catheter is placed through a flexible bronchoscope for low dose rate iridium 192 given in a dose of 3000 cGry to 5 mm radii over 20 hours in the bronchus.[2]

However, the exact dose and the overall advantage is not yet certain. Recent potential advances in radiotherapy are the intratumour implant of iodine 125, iridium 192; laser therapy for central obstructive growths; photodynamic therapy with haematoporphyrin derivatives; the technique of LET irradiation; and the use of hypoxic cell radiosensitizers, neutrons and hypothermia. Response rates to chemotherapy of upto 35 per cent or more have been achieved. Whether such regimens favourably influence survival in patients with widespread NSCLC is still not established.[57] Either of two cisplatin-based combination chemotherapy programmes produces modest but statistically significant survival benefits compared with a policy of supportive care alone.

A positive controlled trial that evaluated this strategy was reported in 1990.[65] Because only uncontrolled studies of preoperative chemotherapy have been performed, its survival benefits are uncertain. In NSCLC, only two controlled randomized studies, conducted by the Lung Cancer Group in patients whose tumours had been marginally or completely resected, compared combination chemotherapy with no further treatment and with immunotherapy, respectively. In addition. all marginally resected patients received post-operative irradiation. In both trials, cisplatin-based chemotherapy significantly improved recurrence-free survival, although survival benefits were of only marginal statistical significance.

Doubts have been expressed about its usefulness[66] and justification, particularly when its toxicities are taken into account. Studies on human lung cancer being conducted in some centres for the establishment of cell lines, heterotransplant of tumour material (xenografts in nude mice), and direct coloning of tumour cells using a soft agar assay, might help to improve selection of drugs for clinical use in the future.

With chemotherapy the results are not very impressive but treated patients have had better survival than untreated patients.[67]

Small Cell Lung Cancer

For therapeutic purposes, most physicians divide SCLC patients into two categories: those with limited disease and those with extensive disease. Chest irradiation is a stage-specific adjunctive therapy often administered in limited disease.

The role of radiotherapy as the primary mode of therapy has been doubted recently[68] although SCLC is the most radiosensitive. Chemotherapy is the primary mode of treatment for this type of lung cancer. Prophylactic cranial irradiation for those who achieve complete remission after 2-3 months of chemotherapy has received attention recently.[69]

Chemotherapy leads to substantial prolongation of survival in SCLC. In the prechemotherapy era, median survival of approximately 3 months in limited-stage and 1.5 months in extensive-stage patients was commonly observed. Because of the nearly universal presence of occult distant metastasis, surgery and radiotherapy had little effect on median survival in patients with limited disease, although less than 1 per cent who had surgery and 3 per cent who had radiotherapy were 5-year survivors.[62] Prognosis is very poor if the lesion is extensive. Ten per cent of limited-stage patients and 5 per cent of all patients have survived free of cancer for 10 years or longer.[70] Only one third of patients who are 2-year cancer-free survivors suffer relapse of their SCLC, although these individuals are still at high risk of dying of other causes, principally smoking-related illnesses such as cardiopulmonary disease and new primary malignancies, especially NSCLC.[70]

SCLC is said to be a limited stage disease when the tumour is situated in one hemithorax with metastasis to one or both supraclavicular glands. Extensive stage disease includes all other forms of the disease.[55] A number of agents are known to be active against SCLC, like vincristine, vindesine, VP-16, VM-26, cyclophosphamide, iphosphamide, nitrogen mustard, hexamethylamelamine, cisplatin JM-8, doxorubicin, CCNU and methotrexate. Gemcitabine, vinorelbine, paclitaxel and docelaxel in combination with cisplatin gives higher level of response, longer median survival and better side effect profile.[71] Chest radiography, apart from bone scintigraphy and liver ultrasonography, is useful guide both in pre and post treatment of SCLC.[72]

Current trials in patients aged 70 years or less provide a median survival of 14-16 months and 2 years' disease-free survival in 10-20 per cent of cases with limited stage disease; for extensive stage disease the values are 8-11 months and 1-2 per cent respectively. The other prognostic factors besides stage and age of the patient are performance status, sex and serum LDH levels.[55] Several studies have suggested means to improve the results of chemotherapy. They are (i) use of alternating non cross-resistant chemotherapy, (ii) administration of drugs according to the cell cycle kinetics; (iii) incorporation of new drugs like VM 26 and JM 8 having high activity, (iv) intensive high dose chemotherapy with or without bone marrow transplantation, (v) simultaneous use of synergistic compounds, (vi) use of drugs according to the cell culture and sensitivity, (vii) use of anticoagulants (warfarin). However, these methods are investigational at present and therefore, cannot be recommended for routine use.

Use of simple two-drug regimen of etoposide and cisplatin has become common and, in randomized clinical trials, give better survival when used in conjunction with other combination drug programmes. Lower, less myelosuppressive doses of these drugs proved both equally effective and much less toxic than higher doses,[73] adoption of shorter durations of drug treatment is useful. There is no survival benefit from chemotherapy given for more than 4 to 6 months. Even single-agent etoposide or its analogue teniposide, sometimes given orally, produces response rates as high as 80 per cent without obvious compromise in survival.[74] Such simple, modestly toxic treatment has not been shown to yield therapeutic results equivalent to combination chemotherapy, but is clearly an acceptable option for patients at increased risk of drug toxicities.

Tumour regression occurs with chest irradiation alone in 90 per cent of patients with newly diagnosed SCLC. Whether adding chest radiotherapy to chemotherapy provides survival benefit beyond that produced by chemotherapy alone in limited disease, however, has been controversial.[55] Improvement has been observed when radiotherapy was given either concurrently with chemotherapy or in a split-course, alternating fashion that did not delay administration of drug treatment.[75] However, the toxicities of combined treatment, particularly increased pulmonary, oesophageal, and myelosuppressive side effects, have somewhat compromised its advantages.[64] Recent uncontrolled data suggest that etoposide and cisplatin can be given concurrently with chest radiotherapy, not only with more acceptable toxicity but also with considerably improved survival. Promising results have been reported both in a cooperative group setting with conventional daily radiation fractionation[76] and in single-institution trials with twice-daily radiation treatments.[77]

Surgery in SCLC has a limited role since more than 95 per cent of cases will be inoperable. In the small number of cases where it has been tried (T_1/T_2, N_0 M_0 disease) an improved survival has been seen when chemotherapy followed surgery.[78]

Most patients with lung cancer either present with or develop advanced disease and treatment with surgery or radiotherapy will not cure. Non-small cell tumours (80 per cent of the total) respond poorly to chemotherapy—about a third regress for a few months—and a recent consensus conference recommended that chemotherapy for these tumours should be given outside clinical trials.[79] For haemoptysis and bone pain, palliation can usually be obtained by single treatment or short courses of radiotherapy. A Canadian randomised trial compared two regimens of chemotherapy containing cisplatin (CAP and VP) with a conservative policy of *best supportive* for patients with advanced non-small cell lung cancer. All patients were given palliative radiotherapy as required. Patients receiving best supportive care survived for a mean of 24 weeks. Do these benefits justify the toxicity and financial cost of chemotherapy?[80] Chemotherapy has not been extensively used in India. Untreated patients with lung cancer have a median survival of 5 weeks whereas with treatment it is 16 weeks.[12]

The benefits of cancer treatment are longer survival, relief of symptoms, or both. Unrealistic hopes of benefit may lead easily to substantial resources being committed to anti-cancer treatments for patients who are terminally ill. Some purchasing authorities may feel that adjuvant chemotherapy for potentially curable patients is a better buy. They may also be influenced by variations in the cost of potentialy curative treatments.

All treatments of debatable value need economic as well as thorough clinical assessment, and oncologists and their colleagues in the laboratory need to develop better ways of predicting which patients will benefit from them.[80]

Table 6.18: Commonly used combination chemotherapy of SCLC[81]

Regimens	*Dose & schedules*
I. Cyclophosphamide	1 g/M^2 iv day 1, q 4 wks
CCNU	70 mg/m^2 po day 1, q 4 wks
Vincristine	1.3 mg/m^2 iv (maximum 2 mg) day 1, q 4 wks except weekly for first 4 wks
VP 16	70 mg/m^2 po daily on day 1, q 4 wks
2. Cyclophosphamide	1.5 g/m^2 iv
Adriamycin	40 mg/m^2 iv
Vincristine	2 mg/m^2 iv every 3 wks
3. VP16	50 mg/m^2 iv daily x 5 q 3 wks
Adriamycin	45 mg/m^2 iv x 1 q 3 wks
Cyclophosphamide	1 g/m^2 iv q 3 wks

Table 6.19: Selected chemotherapeutic schedule used for treatment of NSCLC[82]

a. Cisplatin 120 mg/m^2 days 1 and 29 and then every 6 weeks Vindesine 3 mg/m^2 or Vinblastin 6 mg/m^2 -iv weekly × 5 and then every other week.
b. Cisplatin as above
+
Vindesine as above + Mitomycin-C8 mg/m^2 on days 1, 29—
c. Methotrexate 40 mg/m^2 + Adriamycin 40 mg/m^2+cyclophosphamide 400 mg/m^2, all iv + CCNU 30 mg/m^2 oral; repeated every 3 weeks.

Considerable progress has been made in the chemotherapy for small cell lung carcinoma. However, this should be cheap, easily available and less toxic, more so when recent reports show late complications of treatment of SCLC, like acute myeloid leukaemia besides the usual toxic reactions.[83] Patients in their terminal illness should be spared of the agony of chemotherapy and should receive symptomatic treatment like local radiotherapy, pain killers, care of infections and nutrition, besides psychological support. Unfortunately, NSCLC has no definite therapy as most of them present very late. Let us concentrate on prevention of such a dreadful disease like lung cancer through an aggressive anti smoking campaign.

Clearly, societal efforts to discourage smoking are effective and deserve continued and enhanced emphasis. Total discouragement of tobacco for the benefit of community health should be adopted as a health policy in the management programme. Secondary prevention, that is, preventing a second lung cancer in patients who have developed and been cured of a first cancer, would also be of value because of the high rate of additional primary lung cancers in surgically treated stage I NSCLC and the small number of 2-year disease free survivors of SCLC. Platinum based doublets in the best accepted regimen for advanced NSCLC with PSO-1 and results in response rate of 25-30% with median survival of 8-11 months. Gene expression might become of primary importance for customized chemotherapy. Target therapies can be used as second line or third line therapy.The successful prevention of second primary cancers with the epithelial differenting agent isotreinoin in patients with treated carcinomas of the upper serodigestive tract[84] should serve as a model for similar efforts in lung cancer patients.[57]

Cytotoxic drugs have increasingly been developed and marketed by multinational drug companies and concern has recently been expressed about the relationship between clinicians, regulatory authorities, and these commercial organisations in the medical journals.[85] A cost-benefit analysis could be built into the original design, though care must be taken to avoid biased analysis.[86] The present means of developing oncological (and many other) drugs is becoming increasingly unacceptable and outdated. Regulation of this market, together with more stringent use of clinical science, can only improve this situation for drug companies, clinicians and patients.[85] Lung cancer is the most common malignancy in the west and is going to become one of the common cancers in the developing countries. Unfortunately most of the patients come in advanced stage when definite therapy like resectional surgery cannot be offered except stage I, where 5-year survival is not 100 per cent. Radiation therapy is a good palliative adjunct to systemic therapy-chemotherapy-that appears more logical theoretically.

Median survival for untreated cases is only 5 weeks; that increases with treatment to 20-25 weeks, in 20 per cent of cases of squamous cell carcinoma and 23 per cent cases of small cell cancer. The picture is brighter in small cell cancer in limited stage disease where median survival of 14-18 months with 10-20 per cent of total patients apparently cured of their disease has been documented. Nevertheless, inextensive stage small cell lung cancer, 3-5 weeks survival is possible with supportive care alone; but with chemotherapy, median survival of 9-12 months with 20 per cent complete response rates has been reported.

With the better understanding of biology of lung cancer and with discovery of activation and mutations of oncogenes such as *ras,* the prognostic markers have been set in. The discovery of loss of suppressor genes like p53 on chromosome 17 and other genes on chromosome 3p has led to new theories of pathogenesis and new potential intervention strategies. The knowledge of peptides, and other growth factors and those of changes of cell surface antigen expression has led to new modalities of treatment like target therapy using monoclonal antibodies. 13-cis-retinoic acid is being studied for its potential in prophylactic therapy. Life shall change for ever with gene therapy. Tumour cells as well as bone marrow is being targeted via retrovirus and liposome mode of delivery to treat cancer through enhancing immune function, tumour ablation, chemoprotection or stem cell-marking.[87]

K ras point mutations and N-CAM expression as measured by Mab l23C3 immunostaining, if present, mark poor survival even after radical resection. Further, high NSE (neurone specific enolase) and LDH (lactic dehydrogenase) levels corelate with increased response of more than 60 per cent to chemotherapy. Increased use of colony stimulation factors like G CSF and GM CSF and serotonin antagonists like ondansatron have reduced the toxicities like myelosuppression and emesis. In future, treatment modalities such as angiogenesis inhibitors, tumour cell euzyne inhibitors, gene therapy, cell culture lines, drug sensitivity to malignant cells, and immunotherapy like INF-alpha and calcium channel blocking agent[87-95] are being developed.

Features to Revise

1. Small cell lung cancers tend to be central with extensive metastatic mediastinal lymphadenopathy and early widespread metastases with a strong link to cigarette smoking.
2. Rate of growth is different, small cell cancers double in size within 30 days, squamous cell is about 90 days and adeno carcinomas take upto 160 days.
3. Sputum cytology of a central lesion gives almost 80% positive response, if 3-4 samples are taken and is lesser with peripheral adeno carcinomas.
4. Bronchoscopic yield is high in central than peripheral lesions while percutaneous needle biopsy may be positive in 85% peripheral lesions.
5. Tumour size, nodal involvement and distant metastases are crucial for lung staging to decide treatment modality and operability.
6. Thoracic CT scan has 88% accuracy and 90% negative predictive value. PEP with 18 FD has greater identifying advantage for distant metastases.
7. Stage 1 and 2 with limited tumour size and gland involvement are considered operable, stage 3 as border line and stage 3B and 4 are considered inoperable.
8. 5-year survival for stage 1 is 40-67% and stage 2 is 25-50% post-operative radiotherapy has adverse effect on survival; some suggest post-operative chemotherapy. Supportive therapy and palliative care has to be considered.
9. Pancoast tumours are not operable.
10. Aggressive radiation in stage 3 inoperable shows 5 to 10 years survival, may offer cure rate of 25%.
11. Small cell cancers stage 1 and 2 need surgery followed by chemotherapy, which may produce 5-10% long term survival.
12. Different schools of thought regarding euthanasia advocate their own views regarding cancer patients.
13. Till now, apart from better screening and early diagnosis and prevention take the lead in lung cancer. Therefore, global initiative on tobacco-ban needs universal support.
14. Phase III trials for small cell lung cancer with BEC2 having GD3 ganglioside found on the tumour incorporated into mouse antibody engineered to resemble human proteins at EORTC 1998.

Bronchioloalveolar Carcinoma[96]

First described by L. Malassez in 1876, bronchioloalveolar carcinoma (BAC) accounts for less than 3 per cent of all primary lung cancers but has attracted disproportionate interest because of its intriguing clinical behaviour and unusual pathological appearance. Indeed, pathologists have been so exercised by this tumour that some have given it 36 different names while others claim that it does not exist at all.[97] In 1960, Leibow coined the current terminology of BAC.

The term bronchioloalveolar carcinoma is confined to those originating in bronchioles or alveoli; it excludes metastasizing adenocarcinomas from the bronchus or distant sites. The tumour may arise from ciliated, mucinous, or clara cells in the bronchiolar epithelium or from type II pneumocytes in the alveolus. The cells all grow as a single layer along the walls of the airspaces, and the unusual environment of the alveolus—with a plentiful supply of food, oxygen, water and space—probably encourages many different cells to grow in the same way.

Smoking and gender appear to be unimportant, while pre-existing lung damage—either local scarring or diffuse pulmonary fibrosis—is definitely associated. Patients at presentation are generally in their 6th or 7th decade, although it can affect younger individuals. Patients may be asymptomatic while peripheral tumour is detected on routine chest X-ray. Other symptoms include chest pain, dyspnoea, weight loss, and productive cough. Haemoptysis can rarely occur. Tumour usually arises in damaged lung or in an area of scar.[98] The strange case report of a man who developed the carcinoma after habitually going to bed with his mouth full of olive oil led to suggestions of a link with the inhalation of oil, although such a history is rare. The pathological similarity between bronchioloalveolar carcinoma and the viral disease of sheep jaagsiekte suggests an infectious cause, but epidemiological evidence does not support this hypothesis.[96] However, immunosuppression precipitates recurrence of BAC in a transplanted lung.[99]

Clinically bronchioloalveolar carcinoma has two distinct forms. More common is an unremarkable focal peripheral lung tumour that may be diagnosed by needle biopsy: metastasis is unusual, and five-year survival after surgery is 70 per cent. The diffuse second form is more distinctive, readily identifiable as typical rosettes in one area of the lung and sometimes presents radiographically as consolidation affecting one or more separate lobes or segments. About 10 per cent of these patients have bronchorrhoea, and spread is assumed to be airborne, although a multifocal origin cannot be ruled out. Increased nuclear expression of p53, p21 and cyclin D_1 has been found in BAC.[100] Currently accepted diagnostic criteria for (BAC) are:[101]

a. Absence of adenocarcinoma elsewhere.
b. Peripheral location.
c. Absence of central malignant bronchogenic focus.
d. Tumour growth along alveolar walls with papillary projections into the alveolar spaces (called Lepidic pattern).
e. Preserved architecture of interstitial lung tissue.

Radiologically, BAC may appear as a single nodule or segmental or lobar consolidation. Lobar consolidation appears as 'angiogram sign' on CT in the form of visible specified vessels after intravenous contrast administration.

Cavitation is uncommon in BAC but a radiologic cavity may be produced by abnormal air collection in and around the tumour, called 'pseudocavity sign' or 'open bronchus sign'.[102] This sign appears because of presence of internal air bronchograms, a finding that is not seen in other types of lung cancers. Other pathological explanations for this abnormal air collection are paracicatricial emphysema, fibrosis with honeycombing and localized bronchiectasis.

MRI appearance of mucinous BAC is specific one, showing the presence of a pulmonary consolidation with a signal intensity comparable with that of static fluid on heavy T_2-weighted MR images and is called 'MR white lung sign'.[103]

Regional and distant metastasis occur less commonly than in other lung cancers.[46] Intrathoracic and extrathoracic spread occurs. Local infiltration on the airways causes mucus production and dermoplasia. Lymphogenous and hematogenous dissemination may be in 50% of cases. Death may therefore be from respiratory failure as more and more of the lung becomes occupied by the tumour. Because this type of bronchioloalveolar carcinoma is widespread surgery is ineffective but eventually appear in upto 45 per cent cases. Neither radiotherapy nor chemotherapy helps. Nevertheless, the tumour may grow slowly, and some patients live for three years after the diagnosis. Both forms of the carcinoma (as well as the metastatic adenocarcinoma) may progress to widespread pulmonary nodules, and at this stage it is uncertain whether spread occurs by blood or airways. Chemotherapy may provide palliation of symptoms and modestly prolong survival.

Recently attempts have been made to classify bronchioloalveolar carcinoma cytologically into mucinous (secretory), non-mucinous (non-secretory), and undifferentiated groups.[104] The mucinous variety tends to associate with multifocal disease, having poor prognosis and the non-mucinous with peripheral nodules, while distant metastasis are more common in the undifferentiated group; but these correlations are imprecise. Since bronchioloalveolar carcinoma represents many tumours with similar histological appearance, clinicopathological correlations will remain difficult until the cell of origin can be identified more reliably. About 5% of large tumours cavitate. Solitary lesion following resection has good prognosis.

Primary Synovial Sarcoma of Lung[105-108]

Synovial sarcoma is a rare cancer occurring near arm, neck or leg. And pulmonary involvement is very rare, i.e. less tham 0.5% of all primary lung cancers. It originates from multipotent mesenchymal cells and has four basic histological variants, namely biphasic, monophasic spindle cell or fibrous, monophasic epithelial and poorly differentiated subtypes; monophasic being the most common.

Patient presents with chest pain, X-ray chest shows lung mass, usually with pleural effusion on affected side. CT guided core biopsy and immuno histochemistry, latter shows tumor cell expressed epithelial membrane antigen, bc12, Vimentin and smooth muscle action and immunonegativity for S-100 and cytokeratin.

Immunohistochemistry in primary synovial sarcoma of lung is usually positive for cytokeratin, EMA, bcl-2, Vimentin, EMA, and negative for S-100 and cytokeratin/desmin.

In majority of cases, balanced translocation exists between chromosomes X and 18,t (X;18) (p 11.2; q 11.2).

No standard treatment is available; surgical excision with adjuvant radiation has been tried. Even chemotherapy with ifosfamide and toxorubicin has been used with success rate of 24%.

Overall 5 years survival in 50% has been observed. Bad prognosis in male gender, older age (>20 years), extensive tumor necrosis and high grade, large number of mitotic figures (>10/HPF) and SYT-SSX1 variant, SYT-SSX2 variant has better prognosis.

Pulmonary Metastasis

Almost all carcinomatous conditions in different parts of the body manifest pulmonary metastasis. The frequency of secondary deposits is estimated to be 20-54 per cent of all patients dying from cancer. Lung is more often affected by metastatic growth than it is a primary neoplasm. Carcinoma as well as sarcoma from anywhere in the body may spread to lung. The common sites of primary growths are uterus, ovary, gastrointestinal tract, breast, prostate, kidney, thyroid, bones and testes. Gestational and teratomatous choriocarcinoma and melanoma may manifest secondaries in the lung. Growth of contiguous tumours into the lungs occur most commonly from oesophageal carcinomas and mediastinal lymphosis.[2] Most metastasis are interparenchymal. Only about 3% of all rejected solitary pulmonary nodules represent solitary metastasis.

Choriocarcinoma usually presents as metastasis after delivery with an incidence of 1 in 1,60,000 live births.[109] After evacuation of vesicular mole or other abnormalities such metastasis may be seen in 4 per cent of cases.[110] Lung is the most common site. The patients present with chest pain, cough, haemoptysis and dyspnoea. It may radiographically show alveolar-snowstorm pattern, rounded opacity, pleural effusion and embolic infarcts in lung.[111] Often pulmonary metastasis are radiologically appreciated, much before the symptoms of primary growth appear. As trophoblastic tumours are supplied by many friable vessels, metastatic lesions are often haemorrhagic, resulting in haemothorax.

There may be no primary lesion in reproductive organs despite widespread metastasis. Severe respiratory distress consequent to extensive intrathoracic bleeding has been reported.[112]

Synovial cell sarcomas are malignant tumours arising in synovial tissues.[113] These neoplasms represent only a small proportion, i.e., only 3.2 per cent. Synovial sarcoma occurs mostly in young patients, between 20-40 years of age and there is a slight male preponderance although female predominance has also been reported. The tumour arises from the lower extremities in 72 per cent of cases. Metastasis occurs most frequently to the lungs (74 per cent to 81 per cent) and may also involve the regional lymph nodes (12 per cent to 23 per cent) and bones (19 per cent to 20 per cent). Treatment of synovial sarcoma is wide local surgical resection followed by irradiation. A 5-year survival of 40 per cent in patients treated in this manner is noted with the recurrence rate of 63 per cent in patients in whom a local resection is not done.

The metastasis is noted in middle-aged and elderly individuals. The malignancy spreads to the lung either by vascular or lymphatic system. Bronchogenic carcinoma spreads locally. Many a times the lung deposits do not exhibit any symptoms. They may clinically manifest progressively increasing dyspnoea and cause great disability. Such manifestations are frequent in lymphangitis carcinomatosis.[28] The metastatic deposits may be multiple and widespread and may occur as a terminal event in the course of the disease.

Radiologically they manifest as well-defined solitary or multiple rounded masses with smooth margins. In a small percentage of cases, they may cavitate. There is no hilar enlargement. Metastatic lesions have spherical and sharp margin on chest X-ray, calcification may occur in metastatic sarcomas and chondrosarcomas, while other pulmonary metastasis have translacent, ground glass appearance. Kerly A and B lines are seen with linear or nodular densities in cases of cancer of breast, kidney, testes colon and rectum and sarcoma of bone and skin. Alveolar snowstorm pattern is seen in secondaries of carcinoma of female genitalia. Multiple miliary nodules are seen in haematogenous spread from cancer of thyroid, breast, prostate and sarcoma. Cannon ball deposits are seen in carcinomas of kidney and testis.[114]

The rate of growth of the tumour deposits is variable. The thyroid secondaries may remain unchanged for a long time and exhibit low grade growth. The activity of secondary deposits is decreased in sarcoma and teratoma. Patients with a solitary secondary havc better prognosis as surgical removal is possible and a long time survival is often noted. They may not have further recurrences. A solitary metastatic tumour may sometimes turn out to be the primary lung cancer.[2]

The treatment of multiple pulmonary metastasis requires either radiotherapy or chemotherapy together with hormones. The entire chest irradiation proves valuable as a palliative measure to reduce dyspnoea and cough. The carcinoma of the breast and prostate are influenced by hormones (androgens and oestrogens). Choriocarcinoma responds well to methotrexate.[2]

Chest Skiagrams in Primary Liver Carcinoma: A Radiological Experience

Hepatic carcinoma is one the most common cancers in the world. Primary carcinoma of the liver, a relatively rare disease in the United States, has a distinct geographic variation in incidence.[115] It is quite common in several countries in the Far East like China, Korea, Japan, Philippines, Singapore, Burma, Indonesia, Nepal and South India.[116] The incidence of primary carcinoma of the liver is high in some countries but little has been described regarding chest skiagram changes in patients with primary liver carcinoma.

Diaphragmatic changes varying from 31.8 per cent, 81.3 per cent, 90 per cent have been described. Only recently[117] Brut and Colon observed localised bulge of right hemidiaphragm in two patients and described it as *humping* of the diaphragm which Sanders reported in seven out of 60 patients. This *humping* was seen in five patients (11.1 per cent) while 36 of them revealed raised right hemidiaphragm. Bulge of right dome as humping has been documented.

The most frequent changes observed in skiagrams of chest are: changes at the right base followed by obliteration of right cardiophrenic angle. The metastatic deposits and pleural effusion however are less common.[116] The pleural effusion is not so common in hepatic malignancy, specially in the primary.

Abnormal opacities at the right base in their chest skiagrams which can be the result of linear atelectasis. This atelectasis results from the obstruction of small subsegmental bronchus producing thin horizontal or plaque like lines referred to as plaque like lobular atelectasis.[117] Raised diaphragmatic hump, obliteration of right costophrenic angle and a reactionary serous effusion may be seen in amoebic hepatic involvement. There might be vasodilation of the peripheral pulmonary arteries possibly associated with the vasodilation known to occur in cirrhosis liver in association with an increased blood flow and/ or arteriovenous communications. An alternative explanation accounted for the increased cardiac output of chronic liver disease where the extra blood is delivered which may cause preferential flow through small pulmonary arterial branches. Well marked peripheral pulmonary arteries and veins both appeared compressed by the elevation of diaphragm and that these lower lobe vessels run more parallel to the diaphragm. Pulmonary deposits as small round multiple shadows without clear margins may be present on both sides. The incidence of pleural effusion of 5-10% and it might be due to secondary deposits and/or hypoproteinemia as a result of massive liver involvement.

Benign Tumours

Lung adenoma is the most common benign tumour. Rarely other tumours like hamartoma, chondroma, lipoma, fibroma, leiomyoma and neurinoma are encountered. Generally these tumours are well localised without exhibiting any spreading tendency because of their slow rate of growth. However bronchial adenomas are considered potentially malignant.[2]

Bronchial Adenoma

It forms 1-5 per cent of the primary tumours of the lung.[28] In adults, 2 per cent incidence is reported.[118] It is observed under 40 years of age, during 3rd to 4th decades of life and women are affected as commonly as men.[2] 90 per cent of patients are less than 50 years of age.[12]

The tumour is situated centrally near the hilum, arising either in the main or lobar bronchus from the duct epithelium of bronchial mucous glands. It may arise from segmental bronchus also. It is recorded more frequently in the right lower lobe.

The tumour looks like a polypoid firm mass and is either pedunculated or sessile. It may obstruct the bronchial passage or grow out as dumb-bell tumour through the bronchial cartilage. The overlying muscosa is smooth and its erosion leads to haemorrhage. The tumour is slow growing, and 10 per cent may metastasize to the regional lymph nodes or distant sites.[2] Even upto 40 per cent metastasis to regional lymph nodes may occur.[28]

It has three histologically distinct varieties, carcinoid, cylindroma and mucoepidermoid tumours. The carcinoid-tumour is more frequent and forms 85-95 per cent of adenoma.

The carcinoid tumour arises from the neural cells of bronchial mucosa and neurosecretory cells (argentaffin) of mucous glands. They consist of a collection of small round cells with deeply stained nuclei and scanty stroma. They resemble carcinoid of intestine. The cylindromatous adenoma is derived from bronchial glands and resembles the salivary glandular pattern histologically with trabeculae and columns and cords of epithelial cells. The cells are large and pleomorphic. The tumour possesses a great malignant potentiality and may infiltrate locally or metastasize to distant organ, having three times greater likelihood of metastasis than does the carcinoid pattern.[28] Mucoepidermoid tumour consists of mixture of squamous cells and glandular elements and is relatively benign.[2]

The clinical features are due to obstruction caused by the growth into the lumen of the bronchus and the infection beyond the obstruction so produced. Initially there may be cough due to the growth as a foreign body, as a dry irritant cough with occasional mucoid expectoration. Haemoptysis which is seen in 50 per cent of cases is a frequent mode of presentation. It occurs from erosion, ulceration and necrosis. It is recurrent. Respiratory passages get impaired drainage, followed by secondary infection. Recurrent episodes of infections may manifest fever, cough and purulent sputum. When the growth is obstructing the bronchus partially, a localised wheeze may be audible and it becomes prominent on expiration. The breath sounds are diminished. Later the signs of collapse supervene. The infection may add the features of consolidation or bronchiectasis. This bronchiectasis, emphysema and actelactasis are all byproducts of intraluminal growth of these lesions. The features of carcinoid syndrome are present only in 2 per cent of cases and may appear when there is a metastatic spread to the liver with secretions of serotonin and kallikreins. There may be attacks of flushing, tremor, fever, wheezing, cyanosis and diarrhoea.[2] Overall, bronchial carcinoids don't have secretory activity.

Chest X-ray shows a collapse or an irregular or round opacity. Laminograms help in demonstrating a rounded density from a tumour encroaching on the air column within the major bronchus. Bronchoscopy confirms the diagnosis as the growth projects into the bronchus. Biopsy of the tissue will be diagnostic. Exfoliative cytology is of no value as growth is covered by an intact bronchial epithelium.

Surgical resection of the lobe is the choice treatment. Often the tumour shows its spread in the lobe or exhibits bronchiectatic changes distal to the growth. A sleeve reaction with bronchoplasty is done in some cases, while an endoscopic removal is done in some cases to save the healthy lung tissue. Though such removal of the pedunculated tumour is possible, the resultant bleeding may be difficult to control and may lead to further aspiration of clots. However, its deeper extension is difficult to remove with such a procedure.[2] Survival is 75 per cent at 15 years. 5 years survival rate is 95 per cent after surgery but decreases to 70 per cent if regional lymph nodes are involved, which happens in 0-10 per cent cases.[119] 68 Ga-DOTATATE has also been tried in lung carcinoid.[120]

Endobronchial Leiomyomas[121]

- Rarest benign tumour.
- Arise in lower respiratory tract.
- Female preponderance.
- Bronchos copy and endobronchial biopsy-diagnostic.
- Conservative line of treatment.

Hamartoma

Albrecht in 1904 first introduced the term hamartoma in order to describe tumour like malformations of liver characterised by haphazard arrangements of its cells. The first reported case of discrete cartilagenous tumour of the lung made by Lebert in 1845 was termed chondroma.[122]

Bayer in 1929 suggested the use of hamartoma to describe chondromas of lung. Goldsworthy proposed the term 'hamartoma chondromatosum pulmonis' and Jaeger in 1953 shortened it as Hamarto chondroma.[123] Currently the terminologies used are hamartoma and chondromatous hamartoma.

Hamartomas are tumour like malformations consisting of an abnormal amount, arrangement and differentiation of normal tissues of the lung. There can be island containing cartilage, fat, fibrous tissue, smooth muscle, nerve, cells and epithelial clefts, with foci of calcification. Generally cartilage predominates.[2] Embryological origin of this tumour is not conclusively proved. According to Antonio and Marcel, *pulmonary hamartomas represent a histologic spectrum of benign mesenchymal neoplasms which originate in the peribronchial connective tissue and incorporate respiratory epithelium as they expand. Thus the present concept is that pulmonary hamartomas are benign mesenchymal neoplasms and not developmental malformations*[124] as it is a disordered growth of bronchial bud.

The incidence of hamartoma in general population according to Young and co-workers is 0.255 while McDonald and Colleagues found the same percentage among 10,000 autopsies performed in Mayo clinic.[123] The incidence of this lesion among all solitary pulmonary nodules on an average is about 6-8 per cent. Most of the pulmonary hamartomas are situated peripherally. Endobronchial hamartomas can occur in 10 per cent of cases.[4] Males are affected two or three times more often than females. It may be found at any age but most commonly between 40-60 years[125] and the lesion continues to grow, suggesting that these benign growths are true neoplasms of the lung rather than true hamartomas. There is no particular lobe predilection for the neoplasm.

Usually the neoplasm is asymptomatic except when it occurs endobronchially. Then the symptoms are cough, haemoptysis, fever and chest pain. Obstruction of bronchus may lead to segmental or lobar emphysema, pneumonitis, atelectasis and bronchiectasis. Hamartoma is a less common cause of solitary pulmonary nodule, after granuloma and carcinoma.[126]

Skiagram chest shows the hamartoma, as a well circumscribed nodule which may be lobulated. There may be areas of translucency or calcification. If *popcorn* calcification is detected by a CT scan it is quite characteristic of hamartoma.[127] Hamartoma enlarges by 1 mm per year but it can rarely grow rapidly.[125] Bronchoscopy except in endobronchial lesion is of no value. Diagnostic yield of 50 to 86% can be obtained both by CT scan and percutaneous needle biopsy. Diagnosis is confirmed by thoracotomy followed by excision of lesion and demonstration of classical histopathological characteristics.

Electron microscopy of the mesenchymal cells show two types of cells. Astellate or irregular cell with features of smooth muscle and a fibrocyte like spindle or stellate cell with a long cytoplasmic process.[124] The significance of these findings is not clear.

Hamartoma is mostly benign. Malignant transformation has remained a controversial issue. Its association with bronchial carcinoma has been put forth as pulmonary hamartoma syndrome. 1.5-8% of all pulmonary hamartomas are endobronchial. Rarely cystic structure or multiple lesions may be seen. Malignant change can occur only very rarely.[128] It scan be enucleated from the parenchyma, from which it is well delineated or removed with the wedge resection of lung. Prognosis is very good.

Fibroma

Pulmonary fibroma is a rare, benign tumour, and may arise from bronchus presenting as a slow-growing endobronchial tumour.[129] It may arise from peripheral parenchyma. It may lie in parenchyma, presenting as an asymptomatic coin lesion,[130] often it is situated posteriorly, near the fissures.

Routine investigations are not much contributory. Plain chest X-ray may reveal a coin-shadow with or without atelectasis. Fibroptic bronchoscopy shows smooth spherical growth. Bronchoscopic biopsy reveals spindle shaped cells, possibly of mesenchymal origin. Often, there is clubbing. If it attains a size of 15-20 cms, it may produce breathlessness.[2] Except hamartomas and carcinoid tumours, benign lung tumours are rare. Pulmonary fibroma (fibrous polyp) can be parenchymal, endobronchial or pleural and rarely mediastinal. It is more common in men, usually asymptomatic, detected on routine chest X-ray.

Endobronchial tumour may produce obstructive atelectasis or pneumonia and rarely haemoptysis. These are spindle shaped fibroblasts like cells embedded in variable amount of collagen, on microscopy. Bronchoscopy is useful in removing the tumour; even Nd: YAG laser can be used to treat. Rarely bronchotomy, sleeve dissection or lobectomy may be required.

Pleural fibromas arise from visceral: parietal pleura in 70:30 percentage ratio, appearing as sharp discrete solitary mass as the lung periphery.[130]

Treatment

Exploratory thoracotomy can be performed. Surgery is usually the treatment of choice but incomplete excision results in recurrence. Fibromas are not sensitive to radiation and mucoid change is common but rarely malignant degeneration may occur, and if calcification occurs, these tumours may become encapsulated.[129]

Lipoma

It is a rare lobulated soft tumour composed of adipose tissue. It exhibits a male sex predominance. It occurs in various places like parenchyma of the lung, pleura, tracheobronchial tree and mediastinum. In the bronchi it arises from submucosal areolar tissue and may expand like a dumb-bell. It can grow to a very big size compared to subcutaneous lipoma which is usually 1-4 cm[131] and manifests dyspnoea or recurrent infection due to obstruction. Pulmonary and pleural lesions do not produce symptoms. Radiologic examination shows it to be a lobulated opacity with clear cut margins. On bronchoscopy it appears as a small glistening tumour. Recurrence after resection is virtually nil.

Reaffirming the Treatment of Lung Cancer

Treatment of lung cancer is essentially palliative—90 per cent of patients die. Prevention is thus vitally important and must always be aimed at reducing the members who smoke. Signs are not all good, smoking among adults has declined, but more among men than women. Dr. Anne Charlton reported on a survey of 15000 school-children aged 9-19 in Cumbria and Tyne and Wear.[132] She found that mostly experimentation with cigarettes starts at between 9 and 11, regular smoking usually starts at about 12 to 13 and children are more likely to smoke if their parents do so. Guidelines for health education on smoking have been developed and Dr. Charlton assessed the impact of a new education programme on smoking.[133] The picture from India, too, is gloomy, since bronchogenic carcinoma in young which form 10 per cent of all cases of bronchogenic carcinoma is being frequently reported and smoking has been the cause in 64 per cent of these who had smoking index of more than 300.[134]

Waled *et al.* have concluded from a recent meta-analysis that people exposed to passive smoking have a small but definite increased risk of developing lung cancer.[135] In addition, the children of smokers have a lower weight at birth, show poorer growth, and are more prone to respiratory problems.[136] Vigorous efforts should be made to persuade especially the elderly smokers to quit.[137] All those concerned including healthy professionals, health organizations, policy makers, health authorities, government and public should play more active role[21] so that the incidence of lung cancer in the world and especially in developing countries like India can be reduced in future, because the ultimate prognosis of the disease is very poor.[12]

The Solitary Pulmonary Nodule[138] (SPN)

The discovery of a solitary pulmonary nodule on a chest radiograph raises important practical problems of management because of the ever-present possibility of malignancy. Early diagnosis is important, particularly in patients with small asymptomatic lesions since the chance of long-term survival in those with malignant disease is greatest in this group.

The prevalence of solitary pulmonary nodules is around 1-2/1000 chest radiography. A solitary pulmonary nodule is a shadow within the lung parenchyma with well circumscribed, although not necessarily smooth borders. It may affect the pleura, mediastinum, or diaphragm and may contain calcium, and cavitation may be present within it.

On a routine postero-anterior chest X-ray examination of asymptomatic individuals, a single, small, circular shadow may be noticed in the lung parenchyma. It is referred to as a coin shadow or coin lésion. John Steele used the term solitary pulmonary nodule (SPN) for such a lesion.[139] Characteristics of SPN[2] include:

1. Solitary.
2. Circumscribed margins.
3. Round, ovoid or slightly lobulated.
4. Completely surrounded by a normal aerated lung.
5. Smooth, spiculated or notched perimeter.
6. Minimal diameter twice the cross-sectional diameter of vessel in its viscinity (1.5 cm).
7. Homogeneous density without cavitation, or presence of large central calcified core.
8. Not associated with infilterations, volume loss, regional lymphadenopathy or significant satellite lesions.

The possible causes[2] of such a shadow are as follows:

1. Bronchogenic carcinoma.
2. Granulomas, tuberculosis, histoplasmosis, Wegener's granulomatosis.
3. Benign tumours—adenoma, hamartoma.
4. Metastatic tumour from a carcinoma in breast, thyroid, kidney, bone.[140]
5. Cyst—hydatid or bronchogenic cyst.
6. Lung abscess before evacuation into a bronchus.
7. Slowly resolving pneumonia, lipoid pneumonia, round pneumonia, paraffinoma.
8. Pulmonary infarct.
9. A.V. fistula.
10. Lymphoma.
11. Rheumatoid nodule, amyloid nodule.
12. Mucoid impaction.
13. Haematoma after trauma.
14. Benign pleural effusion.
15. Infected fluid filled bulla.
16. Chest wall tumours, skin tumour, the nipple.

A patient with chest pain should be considered a case of bronchogenic cyst as differential diagnosis to ischemic heart disease in atypical angina pectoris.[141]

Round pneumonia is common in children, however, a short history of fever with a chest X-ray with SPN and responding to antibiotic therapy with rapid radiological clearance in two weeks in an adult has also been reported, thus saving from cumbersome battalion of investigations.[141,142]

Primary bronchial carcinoma accounts for one third to a half of all solitary pulmonary nodules in patients over the age of 50 years, but it should be noted that this risk falls in patients under the age of 40 years. Malignant nodules have been reported in upto 65% of cases. A great variety of benign tumours have been described and these together with localized infections and granulomas form the majority of non-malignant causes of solitary pulmonary nodules. The high prevalence of fungal infections in North America accounts for the finding of granulomatous lesions in over half the patients studied in large Veterans Administration survey. Tables 6.20 and 6.21 outline some common causes of solitary pulmonary nodules.

Table 6.20: Common causes of a solit ary pulmonary nodule (SPN)

1.	Bronchial carcinoma.
2.	Benign tumour of the lung, hamartoma being the most common.
3.	Infective granuloma, tuberculoma, fungal granuloma.
4.	Metastasis.
5.	Lung abscess.

SPN in a renal transplant recipient may pose diagnosing difficulty because of immunosuppression which interferes with inflammatory responses, leading to blunting of clinical, pathological and radiological presentation.

Direct pathogen detection requires invasive procedure, serological tests are, therefore, often useful in ordinary settings. Within 30 days polymicrobial drug resistant infections are higher, in one to six months, developing of opportunistic infections is higher and after 6 months community acquired viral pneumonias are more.[143]

Management

Obviously it is important to confirm that an opacity lies within the chest and that it is not caused by an overlying object such as nipple, hair plait, button, fibroma, lipoma and so on. Benign pleural thickening with unfolding of a lung segment may also mimic a tumour.

Before embarking on expensive and invasive investigations, the doctor should confirm that the lesion is within the lung. The skin should be examined for any soft tissue mass, and if necessary its relation to the lesion in the radiograph should be investigated by taking repeat films and using a surface marker. A benign pleural plaque may be confused with a solitary pulmonary nodule but may be distinguished by tomography or fluoroscopy: a pleural mass does not move relative to the chest wall with respiration. A full physical examination should be performed on patients with a solitary pulmonary nodule because the nodule may be a metastasis from the breast, kidney, testes, or ovary.

Many attempts have been made to establish radiological criteria for evaluating the solitary pulmonary nodule. Benign nodules are apt to be smaller than malignant lesions. An irregular, lobulated, or spiculated contour is suggestive of malignacy, whereas a smooth contour suggests that the nodule is benign, with few exceptions. The two most useful radiological criteria for excluding malignancy are no growth over two years and the presence of calcium. No growth almost completely rules out malignancy, and hence a comparison with old radiographs may be rewarding. The diagnostic value of calcium depends on the radiological distribution pattern; a dense central nidus or a laminated or diffuse pattern are reliable signs of healed granulomas, but malignancy may still develop in relation to the granulomas. Pepper pot calcification is associated with hamartomas. Calcification may sometimes be seen within a malignant lesion, and so a lesion cannot be diagnosed as benign simply because of calcification. Computed tomography has been proposed as a reliable way of diagnosing benign disease, but early successful studies[144] have not been confirmed.

When a nodule has remained unchanged for more than a year it is unlikely to be due to a malignant tumour and a conservative approach to management may be indicated.[138] An extensive clinical examination is important. A history of previous malignancy should not prevent full investigation since resection of a solitary pulmonary metastasis may carry a good prognosis. Apart from routine haematology, specific precipitin titres (for example for aspergillus or histoplasmosis) or tuberculin testing may be indicated. The measurement of plasma carcino-embryonic antigen has not fulfilled its earlier promise in diagnosing primary lung cancer since false-positive results are obtained. In majority of cases, further investigations are required in order to make a specific diagnosis and to assess the need for thoracotomy. These investigations fall into two groups: radiological and histological.

Imaging Techniques

Plain Chest Radiograph

The posteroanterior film is taken with the patient well positioned and in inspiration. The frequency of bronchial carcinoma has enabled several exhaustive studies of different types of radiological appearance on a plain film. Bronchial carcinomas may vary enormously in shape and radiographic density as well as in size and position.

Over the years, numerous radiographic features have been claimed to be diagnostic; notching in peripheral masses and spiculation or *corona maligna are said to be highly suggestive of malignancy. Such appearances may be indicative but they are not pathognomonic. Cavitation in a thick-walled tumour and atelectasis are features that have been associated with a squamous cell carcinoma. A peripheral nodule is most likely to be due to an adenocarcinoma and that lymphadenopathy is more often associated with small cell undifferentiated carcinomas. However, these features cannot be regarded as sufficiently specific to make a diagnosis.*

The presence of calcification within the solitary nodule is perhaps the most useful indicator of a benign lesion. Several different patterns of calcification are described, such as lamination, punctate, central nidus, or popcorn; these are not always discriminatory features. Calcification can occur in malignant tumours that engulf previously calcified lung tissue such as a Ghon's focus, and some metastasis (for example from an osteosarcoma) may calcify. A tendency, particularly among radiologists, to overdiagnose calcification within nodules has been reported.

Penetrated Film

In addition to the standard views, the so-called *penetrated chest X-ray* can be informative. This is a film taken in the same

Table 6.21: Some causes of solitary pulmonary nodule (SPN)

Common		**Primary bronchial carcinoma**
Pulmonary Manifestations of Extrathoracic Neoplasms (PMEN)	*Metastasis* from	Breast Sarcoma Aminoma Hypernephroma Others
	Infection	Tuberculosis (tuberculoma) Localised pneumonia Abscess
	Hamartoma	
	Bronchial adenoma	
Uncommon	Other benign tumours	Haemoductoma Chondroma Fibroma Haemangioma Leiomyoma Myxoma Neurofibroma Papilloma Thymoma
	Other malignant tumours	Alveolar cell carcinoma/lymphoma
	Arteriovenous malformation	
	Chest wall lesions	Mesothelioma Lipoma Fibroma Others
	Cysts	Bronchiectatic Bronchogenic Hydatid
	Endometriosis	
	Foreign body	
	Infection	Aspergillosis Coccidioidomycosis Histoplasmosis Nocardiosis Cryptococcosis Others
	Intrapulmonary lymph node	
	Pulmonary infarct	
	Pulmonary sequestration	
	Post-traumatic haematoma	
	Rheumatoid nodule/systemic lupus erythematosus	
	Wegener's granuloma	

way as a standard posteroanterior film but exposed at a much higher kilovoltage (and also using an antiscatter device). The radiograph produced is usually darker and it utilizes the properties of X-ray absorption at higher energies to pass through the denser structures of the chest, revealing the anatomy of the tracheobronchial tree within the mediastinum. Such a film may show widening of the carina, bronchial occlusions, or intrabronchial masses within the mediastinum. Abnormal shadows otherwise concealed behind the cardiac silhouette may also become obvious. The penetrated film may reveal either central necrosis and cavitation or calcification within a dense intrapulmonary nodule. Alternatively, it can be particularly useful in demonstrating an air bronchogram, i.e., air contained,[13] within the bronchi in a segment of abnormal lung. The presence of an air bronchogram is conclusive evidence that the lesion is a form of consolidation and that it definitely lies within the lung.

Other Plain Film Views

These can sometimes provide useful information such as the posteroanterior chest film taken in expiration, which effectively alters the mediastinal shape, the filling of the pulmonary vasculature, and the relationship of the lung parenchyma to the adjacent chest wall structure. (This effect can also be obtained with an anteroposterior view). Rarely an intrabronchial mass can lead to a ball-valve effect with air trapping beyond an intermittent obstruction that occurs particularly in expiration.

Decubitus films can be useful in confirming the presence of a liquid pleural reaction; a so-called horizontal beam film can be taken with the patient lying on the affected side, when free fluid drains from the top of the diaphragm along the chest wall where even small quantities may become obvious.

Fluoroscopy

Fluoroscopy is useful in locating abnormal shadows in the anteroposterior plane and detecting the relationship of the suspected lesion to the thoracic cage and the intrathoracic mediastinal structures. Thus for example, pulsation may occasionally be seen, or alterations may be noted into the size or shape of the lesion with changes in the respiratory phase. Such findings suggest a vascular rather than a solid lesion.

Tomography

Tomography cannot produce detail that is not intrinsically present in the lesion; it apparently increases detail by its ability to blur out all planes except the plane of interest. Therefore, the lesions at the apex of the lung that are usually obscured by upper ribs on the standard chest film may be well seen by apical tomography and the anatomy of the carina and bronchi within the mediastinum may be better appreciated when the neighbouring structures have been blurred out of focus. Furthermore, the presence of either flecks of calcium or small cavities can also be revealed by tomography.

Tomography may also be useful in the evaluating equivocally enlarged hilum. In practice, tomography of uncertain hilar shadows usually reveals a rather prominent but otherwise unremarkable pulmonary artery. If the hilar shadow is not definitely abnormal on either frontal or lateral views it is usually also normal on tomography. This technique allows to confirm a lesion that may be only poorly or partially defined on the plain chest films. Whole-lung tomography may be used to exclude multiple lesions, particularly when resection of an apparently solitary pulmonary nodule is being considered.

CT

Since its introduction and successive improvements, CT is now recognized to have certain clear advantages over standard radiographic techniques. Third and fourth generation CT scanners allow increased spatial resolution (together with improved contrast resolution relative to conventional radiography) so that lesions of 3 mm or more can be demonstrated.

Measurement of the tissue attenuation of the solitary nodule can indicate the likelihood of malignancy. The increased sensitivity over conventional radiographic techniques facilitates the identification of a second or multiple nodular lesions in metastatic disease. Metastasis are more commonly found in the lung periphery and, like small pleural effusion, small peripheral metastasis are more radially seen using CT. The procedure is useful in the discrimination of abnormal from normal mediastinal structures, and also usefully distinguishes vascular masses such as aneurysms from solid tumours. It differentiates pleural disease from intrapulmonary disease and effectively supports the need for diagnostic artificial pneumoperitonium or pneumothorax induction; CT can reveal a mass that is otherwise lost within distal consolidation in conventional radiography. Sometimes CT scanning of the patient in both prone and supine positions increases the diagnostic yield by allowing differential aeration of lung tissue. When a bronchial neoplasm has been diagnosed, CT scanning alone cannot be used to assess operability; nevertheless, CT examination of other parts of the body such as the liver may demonstrate metastasis. Uses of CT in SPN are listed in Table 6.22.

Table 6.22: Role of CT in solitary pulmonary nodule

1. CT diagnoses to the nature of the nodule. CT is better able to detect calcification in a nodule than conventional films.
2. To demonstrate the spread of disease in those cases where the nodule is likely to be a primary carcinoma but its precise role is still uncertain.
3. To localise accurately the nodule prior to bronchoscopic or percutaneous needle biopsy in cases where localisation is difficult from conventional films.

Ultrasound

Since only air-free structures can be visualized, ultrasound has a limited use in the assessment of chest pathology. However, pleural masses and effusions are readily seen; as little as 20 ml of free pleural fluid may be detected. Ultrasound guidance may improve the accuracy of needle aspiration or biopsy. Occasionally, ultrasound may be useful in characterizing radiographically demonstrated masses such as cysts, abscesses, or solid tumours when these abut the chest wall.

Radioisotope Studies

Radioisotopes allow the assessment of function rather than anatomy. As such, these techniques are useful in the search for bone, liver and cerebral metastasis. The development and introduction of emission computer-assisted tomography has increased the accuracy of such a preoperative assessment.

Tumour-seeking agents such as gallium may sometimes be useful, particularly in the evaluation of lymphoma. However, the technique is expensive and time-consuming and interpretation may be difficult since this isotope is also taken up in abscesses and pulmonary in flammation, especially sarcoid.

Usually malignant thyroid tissue appears cold on scanning with $I,^{135}$ but this technique can be useful in demonstrating metastasis after the normal thyroid has been ablated. The uptake in metastasis is relative to the differentiation of the thyroid tumour cells.

Lung perfusion scans are most useful in the diagnosis of pulmonary emboli when combined with ventilation studies. Nevertheless, they may also be used in the preoperative assessment of patients with bronchial tumours; a lung cancer may markedly decrease pulmonary vascularity and this may be particularly so when the tumour abuts or lies at the hilum. Isotope angiography is less invasive than conventional arteriographic studies but may lack sufficient anatomical precision. Nevertheless, this technique may be useful to differentiate mediastinal structures from the aorta and major vessels; it allows confirmation of a suspected aortic aneurysm and readily demonstrates superior vena caval obstruction.

Nuclear magnetic resonance (NMR), like ultrasound, is non-invasive and involves non-ionizing radiation. While its clinical application is still in its infancy, NMR allows the production of two-dimensional cross-sectional images derived from the differing proton density of different tissues. As such, its theoretical value in the detection of cancer is obvious since changes occur early at the molecular level and become evident long before the neoplasm shows itself by virtue of the more gross anatomical distortion revealed by conventional radiography. At present the study of intrapulmonary masses surrounded by air-filled lung tissue is less encouraging.

Angiographic Techniques

With the advent of CT, angiography is less used now-a-days. Nevertheless, when there is an abnormal intrathoracic·mass lesion either within or juxtaposed to the mediastinum, aortography is useful in excluding an aneurysm and thus may help in avoiding an unwise biopsy. Furthermore, when an intrapulmonary mass lesion is in fact due to a sequestrated lung segment (it is usually in the left base posteriorly) aortography can demonstrate the feeding arteries that arise from the descending thoracic aorta.

Pulmonary angiography is useful in the very rare cases where a pulmonary artery aneurysms is considered a likely diagnosis.

Various vascular techniques such as subclavian, thyroid and internal mammary arteriography have been used on occasion to demonstrate masses of thymic, thyroid, or parathyroid origin. Rarely, other techniques such as azygos and thymic venography may be of value in specific cases.

Digital vascular imaging is a recent development whereby computerization allows improved acquisition, processing, and display of radiologically obtained data. There is considerable potential for the use of digital image subtraction at different energies in chest radiography in particular, since the detection rate of low contrast intrapulmonary nodules is increased by the suppression of overlying rib detail.

Methods of Making a Histological Diagnosis

Sputum Examination

The presence of pus cells or bacteria may suggest that lesion is inflammatory and following appropriate treatment, serial X-rays should show clearing of the lesion. Malignant cells should always be sought in at least three early morning sputum specimens.

Bronchoscopy

When the suspicion of malignancy remains high, bronchoscopy is usually considered to be the next step. Unless the lesion is clearly inoperable on clinical or radiographic grounds, bronchoscopy is also indicated to assess operability even if sputum cytology reveals malignant cells.

Fiberoptic transbronchial lung biopsy under local anaesthesia has become increasingly popular. The size of each biopsy is smaller but the range of vision, particularly of the upper lobes, is superior. With fluoroscopic guidance, the yield is further improved. The incidence of side effects is low. Pneumothoracis occurs in 1-5 per cent of cases but these rarely require intercostal drainage.

Mediastinoscopy/Thoracoscopy

The insertion of mediastinoscope through a small incision in the suprasternal notch is useful for the examination and biopsy of mediastinal glands. Mediastinal lymph nodes are involved in approximately half of all patients with primary lung cancer.

The creation of a pneumothorax allows the introduction of a thoracoscope into the pleural space. This may be particularly useful in the investigation of pleural effusions and tumours.

Percutaneous Needle Biopsy

This technique is now widely used. It involves the insertion (under local anaesthesia) of a fine 23-gauge aspiration needle or alternatively of a small 20-gauge screw-tipped needle and cannula. While the patient holds his breath the needle is inserted through the chest wall, avoiding the intercostal bundle. Using fluoroscopic control, the needle tip is positioned within the lesion, saline aspiration can be repeated several times; this method gives a better diagnostic yield than the transbronchial approach, with positive results in 80-90 per cent of cases. However, the diagnostic accuracy of cell type may be less.

It is suggested that two negative results of aspiration cytology, when conducted by experienced personnel, make the likelihood of neoplasia extremely remote. The risk of both haemorrhage and pneumothorax is increased if the nodule contains a cavity. Spread of infection and seeding of tumour cells along the needle track are insignificant risks. Both transbronchial and percutaneous lung biopsy are contraindicated if it is through a pneumothorax and might prove fatal in the presence of a bleeding diathesis. Peripheral lesions over 2 cm in diameter are the most suitable for this technique.

The marriage of radiology and cytology has produced a major advance in the diagnosis of a solitary pulmonary nodule. The direct aspiration of intrathoracic lesions enables the diagnosis of primary carcinoma of the lung to be made with a high degree of accuracy. The positive recognition of the benign nature of a lesion may be made by the cytologist and, furthermore, culture of percutaneous aspiration samples may reveal the nature of an infecting organism.[145]

A doctor has three possible options in managing a solitary pulmonary nodule: to do nothing, to undertake invasive investigations, or to perform a thoracotomy. As an operation offers the only chance of curing local malignant disease the initial approach is determined by the probability of malignancy and the possibility of surgery. Primary bronchial malignancy is rare in non-smokers and patients under 35, but the possibility of a solitary secondary tumour from a breast or testicular primary tumour or a lymphoma must not be ignored. Geographical and ethnic factors may point towards granulomatous or hydatid disease.

Controversy exists whether biopsy should be performed before a surgical operation. A negative result seldom excludes malignancy, and a positive results in a fit patient leads to a thoracotomy. Therefore if a lesion seems to be operable and the patient could tolerate a thoracotomy, perform a computed tomography of the abdomen and thorax. If no distant or mediastinal metastasis are found then thoracotomy is recommended for a *cure* or definitive diagnosis. The patient should be made aware of the diagnostic aspect of the operation and apprised of the possibility of some of the lung being resected despite benign disease. Thus in the patient with operable disease, the lesion must be assumed to be malignant unless it can be proved to be benign or the chances of malignancy are so low that a short period of careful observation can be justified.

In the patient for whom an operation is contraindicated for poor lung functions, age, coexistent cardiovascular disease, or by the results of computed tomography, further management is influenced by symptoms and the probability of malignant disease. In an older patient with no symptoms, it is always better to watch and wait. In younger patient or a patient with symptoms, further management will be influenced by whether malignancy is positively diagnosed. Bronchoscopy is safe and well tolerated but depends on the chance of reaching a bronchus that will lead into the lesion. Biopsy or needle aspiration through the bronchoscope with fluoroscopy improves the chances of a positive diagnosis. A diagnosis may be made by transbronchial lung biopsy in a quarter of cases in which the nodules are smaller than 2 cm and in about two thirds of cases in which they are larger. CT scan is informative and CT guided fine needle aspiration biopsy is diagnostic particularly for malignant lesions.[145] Percutaneous needle biopsy is simpler but is contraindicated in case the patient has a bleeding diathesis, severely compromised lung functions, pulmonary hypertension, or suspicion of an hydatid cyst, arteriovenous malformation, or a sequestrated lung segment. In malignant lesions the diagnostic yield from needle biopsy increases with increasing size, reaching 80-90 per cent for single sample from tumours larger than 3 cm and further potentiated to 95 per cent for two or three samples. Transoesophageal ultrasound guided biopsy of lesions in mediastinum is a minimal invasive method for staging of lung cancer.[146,147]

PET scan is highly informative regarding origin of malignant lesion, its dissemination and evaluation of management modalities.[148]

An attempt has been made to evaluate the effect of these three management strategies (an operation, biopsy, or observation) on life expectancy by using decision analysis.[149] The results vary with the management strategies that produced the longest life expectancies for smokers at specific ages and with tumours of different diameters. The most interesting finding is that the differences between the strategies was surprisingly small. Therefore, the patient's own preference may thus be given considerable weight in reaching the final decision on what to do.

Bronchogenic Carcinoma and Pulmonary Tuberculosis

The co-existence of pulmonary tuberculosis and bronchogenic carcinoma has been known since 1810, when Bayle included *Cavitation Cancereuse* as one of the six types in his classification of tuberculosis. Penard gave the first clear pathologic description of these entities in a single patient in 1846. Recognition of carcinoma co-existing with pulmonary tuberculosis is of practical importance, because there is a better chance to cure pulmonary tuberculosis, than to treat malignancy.

In 1919 Broders summarised all the available data and found that two diseases were associated in 16.3 per cent of cases. Barron incriminated old tuberculosis scars and cavities as precancerous lesions, and Fried supported this opinion and blamed the proliferation of bronchial epithelium of tuberculous cavities as the exciting cause of carcinoma. He pointed out that secondary to tuberculosis could be bronchial irritation, parenchymal scarring by healed focus, local bronchiectasis aiding the localisation of tar from cigarette smoke and the carcinogenic activity of cholesterol frequently seen in healed foci. There is an undeniable implication that tuberculosis among other scar producing diseases may excite the formation of some pulmonary carcinomas.

Many reports of association between pulmonary tuberculosis and lung cancer described benign and malignant tumours arising at the site of long standing tuberculous bronchial scars produced by perforations from tuberculous lymph nodes. Such scars are usually covered by metaplastic squamous epithelium.

In an important investigation Gekzer (1956) found that the originating scar tissue was tuberculous in 79.5 per cent and 78 per cent of peripheral cancers in upper lobes. Bergel and Themel (1958) have confirmed that so called scar cancer develops mostly from healed tuberculosis lesions (33 out of 37 cases).[150] comparison percentage of different studies has been shown in Table 6.23.

Table 6.23: Association of tuberculosis with cancer of lung

Author	*Year*	*Percentage of patients with lung cancer having tuberculosis as well*
Anastastu	1959	8.4
Bariety	1963	9.6
Criniquette	1961	7.1
Criniquette	1962	8.86
Khiefets	1962	31.00
Mody	1963	14.9

The interval between diagnosis of tuberculosis and earliest roentgenographic evidence of cancer may vary from 3 years to 14 years. The age of patients at the time of diagnosis of carcinoma varies from 42 years to 72 years, mostly in males.

There are many difficulties associated with diagnosis of lung cancer in patients with tuberculosis. The tuberculous process dominates the picture for a number of years so that development of malignant growth is overlooked and symptoms are erroneously attributed to original disease.

Symptom-wise, persistent dull and poorly lacalised chest pain in the absence of pleural complication; localized persistent unilateral wheeze not heard previously; paroxysmal dysponea out of proportion to lung involvement; and profuse haemoptysis occurring in a patient with limited tuberculosis is particularly suspected to be caused by complicating carcinoma. Changes in character of expectoration, marked weight loss and anaemia, are also pointers.

Radiologically, appearance of new lesion in patient with negative sputum is suggestive of malignancy. Secondly, the earliest shadow might readily be mistaken for spread of disease, but shadow due to carcinoma is more homogenous rather than mottled. It shows rapid increase in size. There is unilateral enlargement of hilar gland. There can be segmental atelectasis to start with, later on lobe or entire lung may become opaque. Emphysema may be present. Diaphragmatic paralysis, retraction of ribs and at times erosion of ribs may be seen. Diagnosis of bronchogenic carcinoma superimposed on healed tuberculosis requires high degree of awareness of this possibility. Malignancy should be suspected in an elderly patient who has a change in old lesion after many years. Latest molecular techniques have been tried to establish link between tuberculosis and lung cancer.[151]

Aetiology

i. Possible bronchial irritation by calcified lymph nodes.
ii. Parenchymal scarring by healed focus.
iii. Localised bronchiectasis as a sequelae of tuberculosis aiding in localisation of tar from cigarette smoke.
iv. Carcinogenic activity of cholesterol found at the site of tuberculous scar.
v. Chemotherapy.

vi. Radiation due to repeated X-ray and fluoroscopic examination specially during chemotherapy as done previously.
vii. Immunological relationship.

Role of Isoniazid

Isoniazid, which has revolutionized the treatment of pulmonary tuberculosis, was introduced in Britain in 1952 and came into general use in 1953. It is a cheap, highly effective drug of low toxicity. It has a very important role in the control of tuberculosis in many parts of the world. However, there is now substantial evidence that in high dosage it can produce tumours of lung in mice of different strains.[152] Further it has been shown that certain metabolites of isoniazid also produce same type of tumours in mice but differ in their carcinogenic activity. Hydrazine—a hydrolysis product of isoniazid is more carcinogenic than the parent substance, however hydrolysis of isoniazid to hydrazine is a very minor pathway in man. Adenomatous hyperplasia of bronchus in patients who had been treated with isoniazid is reported. A rapid progression of the carcinoma of lung in a patient given a very high dose of isoniazid is also described.[153]

There is another possible explanation with immunological background. It may be that persistent viable tubercle bacilii provide a continuing immunological stimulus which later prevents the initiation of malignant disease. In the early days of chemotherapy more patients might have been left with viable bacilli following treatment (and thus with a potentially better immunological defence mechanism) than in later period when chemotherapy is more likely to be bactericidal.

Management of Symptoms in Advanced Cancer[154]

Success in controlling symptoms lies in time honoured medical care allied with detailed attention to therapeutics. Invasive diagnostic procedures, for example, taking blood or other time-consuming actions should be kept to a minimum.

Advanced cancer is an acute disease, the clinical picture may change rapidly, so patients must be reassessed regularly to plan for treatment and drugs adjustment. First rate nursing care is essential. Drugs must be constantly reviewed to avoid iatrogenic problems contributing to the patients' misery. Most of the patients' symptoms can be controlled most of the time by the proper use of a few well-known drugs.

Pain

Pain is the most dreaded symptom of advanced cancer and its frequency and severity increases as the disease progresses. Pain is almost always associated with a solid tumour or multiple myeloma, being uncommon in the lymphomas and leukaemias.

No patient who has cancer should die in unrelieved pain. Pain that is difficult to control occurs in about 5-10 per cent of patients. Pain due to extensive bone metastasis or pain in young patients may present problems.

Opioids

The best results are obtained by giving the drugs orally, tailoring every dose individually by titrating it against the pain, and giving the drug regularly (usually every four hours). Dosing round the clock that is, giving scheduled doses even when there is no pain, is a key concept.

A second key concept in using opioids is the use of *rescue* analgesics for breakthrough pain. The drug used as a rescue can be as simple as paracetamol 500-1000 mg or perhaps 10-25 per cent of the current dose of opioid given by mouth every four hours. Depending on the circumstances, rescue analgesics can also be given sublingually, rectally, or by injection. The dose of the rescue analgesic is adjusted according to the severity of pain breakthrough.

These simple ideas are followed and explained clearly to the patient. Opioids are most effective against pain of visceral origin and relatively ineffective against pain due to bone metastasis or nerve destruction. Opioids must always be accompanied by a regular laxative to prevent the otherwise inevitable constipation.

Morphine

Morphine is the drug of choice for chronic severe pain in advanced cancer. It is flexible and has been in use for a long time. Morphine is used like insulin in diabetes mellitus, except that instead of being titrated against the blood concentration of glucose, the dose is titrated against the pain reported by the patient. Morphine in aqueous solution is given every four hours in five to six doses/24 hours.

Most patients need one of the smaller dosage to control pain. If 30 mg every four hours is ineffective it is wise to review the diagnosis and treatment to ensure that nothing has been over looked; for example, non-steroidal anti-inflammatory drugs for painful bone metastasis.

Morphine has the advantage that it can also be given sublingually, rectally, and by continuous subcutaneous or intravenous infusion. Intermittent subcutaneous injection should be used only for moderate or severe breakthrough pain in patients who have reached the terminal stage and cannot swallow. Bolus intravenous injections should not be used for routine pain control, as they provide poor control of pain with maximum side effects. Every effort must be made to control pain using oral medications. Continuous subcutaneous infusion of morphine and other opioids is a useful approach in those who have poor control of pain and are unable to swallow, or suffer from severe nausea or vomiting.

Heroin and hydromorphine are useful alternative drugs for parenteral use, as they are highly potent; that is, they have a greater analgesic effect for each mg administered. They can therefore be given in small volumes, which are less distressing for intermittent subcutaneous or intravenous injection and more convenient for continuous infusion. Heroin, however, has no advantage over morphine in terms of its analgesic efficacy or side effects.

Side Effects of Morphine

Provided that the oral route and tailored individual doses are followed, the use of morphine as described above is safe. Overdosed patients become confused and restless. Though patients may become physically dependent on opioids, that is, develop a withdrawal syndrome if the drug is abruptly withdrawn—addiction (drug seeking behaviour) is rare provided that adequate dose of opioids are given. Opioids can in fact be withdrawn in steps similar to the method used for withdrawing corticosteroids. Withdrawal symptoms after accidental withdrawal from oral opioid are surprisingly mild. Naloxone should be used only for specific indications, as it can produce a massive withdrawal syndrome with severe pain breakthrough.

The three common side effects of opioids are constipation, nausea or vomiting, and drowsiness. Constipation is inevitable and must always be anticipated when regular administration of opioids begins. Both nausea or vomiting and drowsiness tend to be mild and transient. They often clear, even with the continued use of morphine, after a few days. An antiemetic for example prochlorperazine 5.0 mg orally every four hours— is often prescribed routinely for a week after morphine is started. Drowsiness is troublesome in only a few patients. Excessive sedation may require a reduction in the dosage of morphine; some doctors add a stimulant—for example, amphetamine. Metoclopramide (given regularly every eight hours) is a good choice.

Non-steroidal Anti-inflammatory Drugs

Aspirin and related drugs are used in two main ways in treating pain in cancer. Firstly, they seem to have a specific effect on pain caused by bone metastasis by interfering with the production of prostaglandin. This is doubly important, as this type of pain responds poorly to opioids. For those patients who have diffuse bone metastasis and in whom chemotherapy, hormonal treatments, and radiation treatment are ineffective, non-steroidal anti-inflammatory drugs are the treatment of choice. Non-steroidal anti-inflammatory drugs vary in effectiveness, but gratifying responses do occur within 48-72 hours. Secondly, non-steroidal anti-inflammatory drugs have a general non-specific analgesic effect. The combination of one of these drugs and an opioid will provide better pain relief than either drug used alone. In patients who have cancer and who are thrombocytopenic, they are best avoided because of the risk of haemorrhage. It is worth maximising the dosage of individual agents and changing drug if side effects are problem or if a poor response is obtained.

Psychotropic, Anti-epileptic and Psychostimulant Drugs

In pain from cancer, an opioid sparing action has been claimed for both groups of drugs. There is now evidence that tricyclic anti-depressants do have a co-analgesic opioid sparing effect. Curiously, this action does not affect mood. Phenothiazines are sedative, antiemetic, and possibly co-analgesic. They are also useful for helping to control anxiety and agitation in the terminal stages. Burning pain is said to respond to anti-depressants, whereas stabbing pain may respond to phenytoin or carbamazepine. Psychostimulants like methylphenidate are useful in those complaining of chronic weakness or if there is excessive sedation induced by opioids.

Corticosteroids

Corticosteroids seem to help pain that is caused by the destruction of nerves—for example, damage to the brachial or lumbosacral plexus. Their mechanism of action is unknown. Relief of pain is difficult to separate from their psychostimulating, anti-anorexic, and strength improving action, which are all beneficial in advanced cancer. Nevertheless, the side effects of corticosteroids are well-known.

Anorexia

Anorexia is a common but poorly understood complaint. Many find it as distressing as pain. In some patients who have cancer it is related to previous chemotherapy or radiation treatment and if so usually improves once this treatment has been completed. Abnormalities in the sensation of taste are common in patients who have cancer and contribute to the problem.

A multi-vitamin tablet should be given daily to those who are unable to eat normally. Megavitamin treatment is best avoided, it is ineffective and can be dangerous. There is no evidence that zinc supplements help. Patients who have cancer show a diurnal variation in appetite, their appetite is often best in the morning, and if so appropriate adjustments in the diet should be made. Changes in food preparation or additives help those with abnormalities in taste—for example, reducing salt in cooking food that tastes too salty.

Corticosteroids

They are very effective in anorexia, and most patients will respond to them. The disadvantage of their use is steroid effects, which are common, though usually minor. Oral thrush should be routinely looked for and dosage adjusted for the optimal effect at the lower dose.

Alcohol

This is readily available and is a familiar effective appetite stimulant.

Metoclopramide

10 mg orally every six hours seems specifically to help those who have symptoms of gastroparesis—that is, early satiety—but may help others too. Those who respond will be less anorexic and gain weight.

Cyproheptadine

Cyproheptadine may be tried if corticosteroids are ineffective, but its record is unimpressive.

Nausea and Vomiting

Nausea and vomiting are common (in 60 per cent) in advanced cancer mostly in elderly women. Among those given opioids vomiting is also more common in women and is more likely to create difficulties in treatment. It is important to exclude common remediable causes such as faecal impaction. Sometimes it may be appropriate to investigate and then attempt to control uremia or hypercalcaemia or their underlying cause.

Some patients whose vomiting is induced by opioids, respond well to metoclopramide, possibly because of its action in helping gastric motility. If vomiting is severe or persistent and unresponsive to single antiemetic, a combination of drugs with different sites of action—for example, metoclopramide plus prochlorperazine—should be tried. Cyclizine or an anticholinergic such as hyoscine can also be added. This approach is often effective, and there are theoretical reasons to support it.

Cough and Dyspnoea

Dyspnoea is common (incidence 40 per cent) even in patients who have cancer without obvious cardiorespiratory disease. In those who have considerable or recurrent pleural effusions and dyspnoea, thoracentesis followed by teracycline pleurodesis can be performed if the likely survival time of the patient is weeks or months. Morphine in small doses (sustained release morphine 10 mg twice daily) is effective. Dyspnoea due to lymphangitis carcinomatosis is difficult to treat but may respond to a combination of morphine, bronchodilators and systemic corticosteroids.

Cough is usually treated with codeine when it is an isolated symptom. The opioids are cough suppressants but are best used only if the cough is causing distress, for example, disturbing sleep. There is probably little difference between the opioids in terms of their effectiveness as cough suppressants.

Steam inhalations help those whose cough is due to difficulty in expectorating sputum. Cough *mixtures* are best avoided. In resistant cases, prednisolone 10 mg orally is worth trying every eight hours.

Constipation

Constipation is common in the elderly, in patients who are bedridden or receiving inadequate diets, and in those taking a variety of drugs (opioids, anticholinergics, sedatives). Regular bowel motions should continue even if there is little dietary intake. They should be instructed also to take as required a stimulant (senna) or osmotic (milk of magnesia) laxative.

Itch

Severe itch is very distressing and in advanced cancer is usually due to cholestasis. Good nursing care and topical treatment of the skin is vital, whatever the cause. Calamine lotion and menthol creams reduce itch by cooling the skin. Antihistamine and phenothiazines are only partly effective, largely because of their antipruritic effect that is mediated through sedation. Hydroxyzine orally 25-50 mg every six hours is a useful agent.

Cholestyramine 4 mg every six hours is effective for itch caused by incomplete biliary obstruction, but gastrointestinal upset may occur, and it interferes with the absorption of some drugs and the fat soluble vitamins. Dosage should therefore be reduced once a therapeutic response occurs. The itch of lymphomas responds to effective treatment of the lymphoma or, failing that, to non-steroidal anti-inflammatory drugs. Antihistamine ointments are valuable in severe cases. Lignocaine gel applied topically may be tried in desperate cases.

Depression

Sadness and anxiety are common among patients who have advanced cancer. Severe depression is uncommon, and suicide is rare. About 40 per cent of patients show some evidence of depressive illness. Non-somatic symptoms (particularly feelings of guilt and worthlessness) are helpful in diagnosing depression. Sympathetic support must be offered. Involvement of the family can be therapeutic. Morale is helped by relief of other symptoms and good patient-doctor relationship. Unspoken fears—for example, about dying—should be gently inquired about.

If an anti-depressant is required, it is best to start with a low dose—for example, imipramine 12.5 mg at night—as side effect can be a problem. This is particularly true in patients already taking opioids.

Terminal Phase

The final hours or days of life are indicated by fluctuating consciousness and increasing detachment from the surroundings. Agitation is not uncommon, and in those who are unconscious, pain should be assumed to be the cause, and they should be treated by analgesic suppository or injections. A distended bladder or impacted rectum should be treated appropriately. If no cause can be found, sedation with a phenothiazine can be used to avoid distressing relatives.

Few patients die dramatically, but it is wise to have morphine 10 mg and chlorpromazine 25 mg to hand in a syringe to be given quickly by a nurse (or competent relative if the patient is at home) should thereby any dramatic distress or terminal event for example, massive haemoptysis. Hyoscine 0.4 mg is a useful addition to help the *death rattle.* Most patients prefer to die at home and their wishes should be respected whenever possible.

Terminal Decisions

In the recent years, people have become increasingly concerned that the dying process is too often needlessly protracted by medical technology and is consequently marked by incapacitation, intolerable pain and indignity.[155] In one public opinion poll, 68 per cent of respondents believed that *people dying of an incurable painful disease should be allowed to end their lives before the disease runs its course.* A number of comparable surveys indicate similar public sentiment.

A change has been observed in the death-place as well. Earlier, the vast majority of deaths occurred at home. Now most people die in hospitals or long-term care facilities. Approximately 75 per cent of all deaths in 1987 occurred in hospitals and long-term care institutions, up from 50 per cent in 1949, 61 per cent in 1958 and 70 per cent in 1977. This transition from the privacy of the home to medical institutions has increased public awareness and concern about medical decisions near the end of life. *Since deaths which occur in institutions are more subject to scrutiny and official review, decisions for death made there are more likely to enter public consciousness*).[156]

The availability of sophisticated life support technologies now enables medicine to intervene and forestall death for most patients. Do-not-resuscitate order are now common place. In 1988, 3775 to 6575 persons were dependent on mechanical ventilation and 1404500 persons were receiving artificial nutritional support.[157] This growing capability to forestall death has contributed to the increased attention to medical decisions near the end of life.[156]

Opinions on withdrawing and withholding life-prolonging treatment from patient who are terminally ill or permanently unconscious and reports concerning do-not-resuscitate orders,[158] euthanasia and withdrawal of life-prolonging treatment from permanently unconscious patients,[159] are published. The issue of decisions near the end of life for incompetent patients is addressed in a separate report.[160] The decisions near the end of life examined in this report are those decisions regarding actions on intentional omission by physicians that will foreseeably result in the deaths of patients. In particular, these decisions concern the withholding or withdrawing of life-sustaining treatment, the provision of a palliative treatment, that may have fatal side effects, euthanasia and assisted suicide.

Life sustaining treatment may include, but is not limited to, mechanical ventilation, renal dialysis, chemotherapy, antibiotics and artificial nutrition and hydration. At one time, the term passive euthanasia was commonly used to describe withholding or withdrawing life-sustaining treatment. However, many experts now refrain from using the term passive euthanasia.

The provision of a palliative treatment that may have fatal side effects is also described as double effect euthanasia. The intent of the treatment is to relieve pain and suffering, not to end the patient's life, but the patient's death is a foreseeable potential effect of the treatment. An example is gradually increasing the morphine dosage for a patient to relieve severe cancer pain realizing that large doses of morphine may depress respiration and cause death.

Euthanasia is commonly defined as the act of bringing about the death of a hopelessly ill and suffering person in a relatively quick and painless way for reasons of mercy.

Voluntary euthanasia is euthanasia that is provided to a competent person on his or her informed request. Non-voluntary euthanasia is the provision of euthanasia to an incompetent person according to a surrogate's decision. Involuntary euthanasia is euthanasia performed without a competent person's consent.

Euthanasia and assisted suicide differ in the degree of physician participation. Assisted suicide occurs when a physician facilitates a patient's death by providing the necessary means and/or information to enable the patient to perform the life-ending act (e.g., the physician provides sleeping pills and information about the patient may commit suicide).

Competence can also refer to a legal standard regarding a person's soundness of mind. Decision-making capacity signifies the ability to make a particular decision and is not considered a legal standard.

Physicians are healers of disease and injury, preservers of life, and relievers of suffering. Ethical judgements become complicated, however, when these duties conflict. The instances in which physicians might act to hasten death or refrain from prolonging life involve conflicts between the duty to relieve suffering and the duty to preserve life, are: (i) the principle of patient autonomy and the corresponding obligation of physicians to respect patients' choices; (ii) whether what is offered by the physician is sound medical treatment; and (iii) the potential consequences of a policy that permits physicians to act in a way that will foreseeably result in patient's deaths. We demonstrate respect for human dignity when we acknowledge *the freedom (of individuals) to make choices in accordance with their own values.*

Generally, a treatment that is likely to cause the death of a patient violates the principle of non-maleficence, and a failure to save a patient's life is contrary to beneficence. Policies governing decisions near the end of life must also be evaluated in terms of their practical consequences. The withdrawing or withholding of life-sustaining treatment is not inherently contrary to the principles of beneficence and non-maleficence. The physician is obligated only to offer sound medical treatment and to refrain from providing treatments that are detrimental, on balance to the patient's well being. When a physician withholds or withdraws a treatment on the request of a patient, he or she has fulfilled the obligation to offer sound treatment to the patient. The obligation to offer treatment does not include an obligation to impose treatment on an unwilling patient. In addition, the physician is not providing a harmful treatment. Withdrawing or withholding is not a treatment, but the forgoing of a treatment.[43]

Others may argue that if a physician has a strong moral objection withdrawing or withholding life-sustaining treatment, the physician may transfer the patient to another physician who is willing to comply with the patient's wishes.

The distinction between *ordinary* vs *extraordinary* treatments has been used to differentiate ethically obligatory vs ethically optional treatments. In other words, ordinary treatments must be provided, while extraordinary treatment may be withheld or withdrawn. Criteria proposed to distinguish ordinary from extraordinary treatment include customariness, naturalness, complexity, expense, invasiveness, and balance of likely benefits vs. burdens of the particular treatment. The ethical significance of all these criteria essentially are subsumed by the last criterion—the balance of likely benefits vs. the burdens of the treatment. Artificial nutrition and hydration have frequently been cited as an objectively ordinary treatment and can be very burdensome to patients. There is also no ethical distinction between withdrawing and withholding life-sustaining treatment.

However, as most bioethicists now recognize, such a distinction lacks ethical significance.[159,160] The physician must ensure that the patient has the capacity to make medical decisions before carrying put the patient's decision to forgo (or receive) life-sustaining treatment.

Palliative care has assumed significance in end of life care, especially when curative care is not useful/feasible in an elderly patient. Psychological and socio-spiritual support offers real help to patient as well as family members, especially when applied appropriately and skillfully.[161, 162]

Pain is *one of the most pervasive causes of anxiety among patients, families and the public.* The level of analgesia necessary to relieve the patient's pain, however, may also have the effect of shortening the patient's life. The principle of respect for patient's autonomy and self-determination requires that patients decide about such treatment. The patient has a right to decide either to risk the side effects or to forgo the treatment. It does not follow from this reasoning that a patient also has a right to choose euthanasia as a medical treatment for their suffering.

Euthanasia

Euthanasia is the medical administration of a lethal agent in order to relieve a patient's intolerable and untreatable suffering. Whether or not a physician may use the skills or knowledge of medicine to cause an *easy* death for a patient who requests such assistance, has been debated as early as the time of Hippocrates. Recently, euthanasia has been gaining support from the public and some in the medical profession. In the Netherlands, while physician-performed euthanasia remains illegal, physicians have not been prosecuted since 1984 when they follow certain criteria.[163] These criteria include that (i) euthanasia is explicitly and repeatedly requested by the patient and there is no doubt that the patient wants to die; (ii) the mental and physical suffering is severe with no prospect for relief; (iii) the patient's decision is well informed, free and enduring; (iv) all options for alternate care have been exhausted or refused by the patient; and (v) the physician consults another physician.[164] The first nationwide study of the practice of euthanasia in the Netherlands estimated the incidence of euthanasia to be 1900 persons per year.[163]

In the United States there has been growing public support for legalized euthanasia. The Hemlock Society, an organization dedicated to legalizing voluntary euthanasia and assisted suicide, has doubled its membership in the past 5 years to approximately 33000. Recently, an initiative in Washington State that would have legalized euthanasia for terminally ill patients was put to a vote. Although the initiative was unsuccessful, 44 per cent of the voters supported the initiative. The question remains whether it is ethical for a physician to agree to perform euthanasia.

Can euthanasia ever constitute sound medical treatment? Any treatment designed to cause death is generally considered detrimental to the patient's well being, and therefore unsound. However, proponents of euthanasia argue that euthanasia is a sound treatment of last resort for the relief of intolerable pain and suffering. From the perspective of competent patients who request euthanasia in the face of such suffering, death may be preferable, on balance, to continued life.

On the other hand, most pain and suffering can be alleviated. The technology of pain management has advanced to the point where most pain is now controllable. The success of the nospice movement illustrates the extent to which aggressive pain control and close attention to patient comfort and dignity can ease the transition to death.[165]

There may be cases, however, where a patient's pain and suffering is not reduced to a tolerable level and the patient requests a physician to help him or her die.[166] If a patient's pain and suffering are unrelievable and intolerable, using medical expertise to aid an easy death on the request of the patient might seem to be the humane and beneficent treatment for the patient. However, there are serious risks associated with a policy allowing physician-performed euthanasia. There is a long-standing prohibition against physicians killing their patients, based on a commitment that medicine is a profession dedicated to healing, and that its tools should not be used to cause patients' deaths. Weakening this prohibition against euthanasia, even in the most compelling situations, has troubling implications.[167] Though the magnitude of such risks are impossible to predict accurately, the medical profession and society as a whole must not consider these risks lightly.

If euthanasia by physicians were to be condoned, the fact that physicians could offer death as a medical treatment might undermine public trust in medicine and dedication to preserving the life and health of patients. Some patients may fear the prospect of involuntary or non-voluntary euthanasia if their lives are no longer deemed valuable as judged by physicians, their family, or society. Other patients who trust their physicians' judgements may not feel to resist the suggestion that euthanasia may be appropriate for them.[168]

Another risk is that physician and other health care providers may be more reluctant to invest their energy and time serving patients whom they believe would benefit more from a quick and easy death. Caring for dying patients is taxing on physicians who must face issues of their own mortality in the process, and who often perceive such care as a remainder of their failure to cure these patients. In addition, the increasing pressure to reduce health care costs may serve as another motivation to favour euthanasia over longer-term comfort care.

Allowing physicians to perform euthanasia for a limited group of patients who may truly benefit from it will present difficult line-drawing problems for medicine and society. In specific cases it may be hard to distinguish which cases fit the criteria established for euthanasia. Determining whether a patient will benefit from euthanasia requires an intimate understanding of the patient's concerns, values and pressures that may be prompting the euthanasia request. More broadly, the line-drawing necessary in the establishment of criteria for euthanasia is also problematic. If competent patients can receive euthanasia, can family members request euthanasia for an incompetent patient?

Since it is unclear at this time where these lines should be drawn, the proposition of allowing euthanasia is particularly troublesome. Furthermore, in the United States there is currently little data regarding the number of euthanasia requests, the concerns behind the requests, the types and degree of intolerable and unrelievable suffering, or the number of requests that have been granted by health care providers.

In June 1990, Dr. Jack Kevorkian assisted the death of a person with the use of a *suicide machine* which he invented, has been criticized by many.[158] A physician who described his role in assisting his patient's suicide,[169] the care and compassion evidenced by the physician and the reasoned decision making process of the patient marked this account as truly compelling.

There is an ethically relevant distinction between euthanasia and assisted suicide that makes assisted suicide an ethically more attractive option. Physician-assisted suicide affords a patient a more autonomous way of ending his or her life than does euthanasia. However, the ethical objections to physician-assisted suicide are similar to those of euthanasia since both are essentially interventions intended to cause death. While in highly sympathetic cases physician-assisted suicide may seem to constitute beneficent care, but due to the potential for grave harm the medical profession cannot condone physician-assisted suicide at this time.

Issue of End-of-Life-Care

Areas of conflict exist in DNR (Do not resuscitate) order. A consent or decision by family members and attending doctor can help in training DNR orders. But a valid guideline is needed urgently in India to avoid lot of troubles often seen in hospital ICUS. We talk of dignity in death but where are the fool-proof guidelines of end-of-life-care? At present, advanced directives are not recognized by the legal system in India. Doctors can discuss with patient's relatives about the futility of further expensive treatment which prolongs death rather than prolonging life in a particular grim situation. Since chronic diseases are on the rise, available medical services do demand for saving life, and for adding more years as life expectancy is increasing. Technical working committee must work with MCI to formulate recommendations with concurrent supervision or even involvement of our Supreme Court to bring forth guidelines on end-of-life-care issue. Let government comes forward to take faster and proactive decision in this regard before it culminates into serious problem.

The weakness of system and helplessness of the caregiver should see some light and clear guidelines so as to bring to zero the fear of legal harassment to physicians to passively allow terminat patient to leave against medical advice (LAMA) or discharge against risk bonds (DARB).

REFERENCES

1. Alder I., Primary malignant growths of lungs and bronchi, London, Lungman Greens 1912; 3.
2. Shankar P.S., Neoplastic disease: In Chest Medicine; Oxford and IBH Publ. Co. (P) Ltd. 1994, 4th ed.
3. Kar M., Early diagnosis of lung cancer; In; M. Panja; ed.; Med update;API 2001;11:53-58.
4. Parikh P.M., Abhyankar D., Lung cancer and chemo prevention; In: Panja, M., ed.; Med. Update; API 2001;11:90-95.
5. Arora V.K., Seetaraman M.L., Ramkumar S., *et al.* Bronchogenic Carcinoma—Clinico pathological pattern in South Indian population, Lung India 1990; 7: 133-36.

6. Jindal S.K., Malik S.K., Malik A.X., Kartar Singh, Gujral J.S. and Sodhi J.S., Bronchogenic carcinoma—A review of 150 cases. Ind J. Chest Dis. and All Sci. 1979; 21(2): 59-64.
7. Dhabhar B.N., Malhotra M. and Advani S.H. Incidence of lung cancer, JAPI 1991; 40: 493.
8. Jain N.K., Madan A., Sharma T.N., *et al.* Bronchogenic carcinoma, A study of 109 cases, JAPI 1989; 37: 379-82.
9. Behera D. and Kashyap S., Pattern of malignancy in a North Indian hospital, J. Ind. Med Assoc. 1988; 86: 28-29.
10. Bhatia R.S., Pattern of respiratory diseases from a private clinician Ludhiana; Lung India 1995;13: 125-26.
11. Becher J.R., Worldwide variation in the sex incidence of bronchial carcinoma. Paper presented in the Annual Conference of British Thoracic and Tuberculosis J. Chest Dis 1971; 13: 34-35.
12. Behera D., Balamugesh T., Lung cancer in India; Ind J. chest Dis All Sci 2004; 46: 269-81.
13. Bhatia R.S. Rising trend in respiratory disorders; In; Das S., ed.; Med update; API 2003; 13: 260-67.
14. Jain S.R.; An overview of lung cancer; INI Med update API; EDJ S R Joshi; 2014; 24:781-86.
15. Clark A. Ronald, Lung cancer—Past, present and future; B.B. Takur (ed.); P. G. Med., API 2002;16: 365-67.
16. National Research Council, Emson mental tobacco smoke, Measuring exposure and assessing health effects, Washington D.C., Natl. Acad. Press 1986.
17. Jindal S.K. and Malik S.K., Smoking index—A measure to quantify cumulative smoking exposure, Lung India 1988; 6: 195-96.
18. Jindal S.K., *et al.*, Lung Cancer in North India in relation to age, sex and smoking habits, Eur J Resp Dis 1987; 70: 23-28.
19. Pakhale S.S., *et al.,* Chemical analysis of smoke in Indian cigarettes, bidis and other indigenous forms of smoking levels of steam volatile phenol, hydrogen cyanide and benzo (a) pyrene, Ind J Chest Dis and All Sci 1990; 32: 75-81.
20. Bhatia R.S., Vijayan V.K., Tobacco and health: What can the medical profession do? Lung India 1994; 12(4):178-85.
21. Bhatia R.S., Smokeless tobacco; Cardiovascular and pulmonary effects: A short review; IJCP 1995; 6(5): 82-85.
22. Chatterjee T., *et al.*, A study on habits of tobacco use among medical and non-medical students of Kolkata; Lung India 2011; 28:5-10.
23. Turakhia D.P., To breathe air that is free of tobacco smoke—A forgotten light, JAPI 1990; 38: 190-91.
24. Colditz G.A. Stamfer M.J. and Willett W.C., Diet and lung cancer, Arch Internal Med 1987; 147: 157-60.
25. Gupta M.P., *et al.,* Effect of cigarette smoke inhalation on benzo (a) pyrene induced lung carcinogenesis in vitamin A deficiency in the rat, Cancer Letters 1990; 55: 83-88.
26. Fadlo R.K., Lippman S.M., Lung cancer—Chemo preservation; Semi Surg. Oncol. 2000; 18: 100-05.
27. Aronchick J.M., Semi Roentgen 1990; 25:5-11.
28. Rawat J., *et al.,* Clinic pathological profile of lung cancer in Uttarakhand; Lung India 2009; 26: 74-76.
29. Crippi M.A., Semi Roentgen 1990; 25:12-24.
30. Rao S., Absolute lymphocytopenia as a diagnostic aid in bronchogenic carcinoma, JAPI 1994; 42 (3): 199-200.
31. Pietra G.G. The pathology of carcinoma of the lung; Semin Roentgenol 1990; 1:.25-33.
32. Woodring J.H., Pitfalls in radiological diagnosis of lung cancer AJR 1990; 54: 1165-75.
33. Woodring J.H., Sterring C.B., Adenocarcinoma of the lung; A tumour with changing pleomorphic character, AJR 1983; 140: 657-64.
34. Sundram P., Joshi J.M., Adenocarcinoma of the lung; pleomorphic rodiographic appearances; JAPI 1996; 44 (4): 291.
35. Jussawala D.J., Yeole B.B. and Natekar M.V., An assessment of cancer mortality in Greater Bombay. Indian J. Med. Res 1982; 75: 68-82.
36. Jayant K. and Yeole B.B., Cancers of the upper alimentary and respiratory tracts in Bombay, India, A study of incidence over two decades, Br. J. Cancer 1987; 56: 847-52.
37. Behra D., *et al.,* Galactorrhoea with gynaecomastia in a male with lung cancer, Ind J Chest Dis and All Sci 1987; 29: 112-14.
38. Peter Coy, Elwood J. Mark and Andrew J Coldman, Clinical indicators of profuse unresected lung, Cancer 1981; 80: 453-458.
39. Crofton J. and Douglas A., Respiratory Disease, 2nd ed., Blackwell, Oxford, 1971; 526.
40. Telerman A., Gerard B., Venden Heule B. and Bleiberg H., Gastrointenstinal metastases from extra-abdominal tumours, Endoscopy 1985; 17: 99-101.
41. Kapoor A.S., Clinical manifestation of neoplasia of the heart. In Kapoor, A.S. Ed: Cancer and the heart. New York, Springer-Verlag 1986; 21-25.
42. Lopez J.M., Delgado J.L., Tovar E. and Gonzalez A.G., Massive pericardial effusion produced by extracardiac malignant neoplasms Arch Intem Med 1983; 143: 1815-16.
43. Sharma S., Balaney B. and Mandke J.Y., Cardiac temponade as a presentation of muco epidermoid bronchogenic carcinoma, JAPI 1989; 37: 183-85.
44. Coombs R.C., Metabolic manifestations of cancer J. Appl. Med. 1982; 361-68.
45. Calman K.C., Cancer cachexia, J. Appl. Med. 1982, 369-373.
46. Roy T., Mukherjee A., Choudhuri M., *et al.,* Metastatic and non-metastatic complications in a case of bronchial carcinoma, JAPI 1991; 39: 414-16.
47. Ammanagi A.S., *et al.*, Sputum cytology in suspected cases of carcinoma of lung; Lung India 2012; 29:19-23.
48. Choi Y.D., *et al.*, Effectiveness of sputum cytology using thin prep method for evaluation of lung cancer; Diagn Cytopathol 2008;36:167-71.
49. Bhatia R.S., BAL: Indications and present status; Lung India 1994; 12: 27-29.
50. Bhatia R.S., Sibia S.S., Therapeutic uses of FOB; Lung India 1994; 12:138-39.
51. Gupta P.K., *et al.,* FNAC through bronchoscopy in a central lung lesion a comparison with brushing and punch biopsy, Lung India 1993; 11: 17-21.
52. Sengupta A., *et al.,* Squamous cell lung cancer producing bilateral air bronchograms on CT scan thorax; JAPI 2013; 61: 839-41.
53. Behera D., *et al.,* Circulating hormones in lung cancer, Ind J Med Res 1984; 79: 636-40.

54. Behera D., *et al.,* Circulating blood RNA in lung cancer, JAPI 1986, 34: 579-80.
55. Tilve G.H., *et al.,* Utility of PET in medicine, IN; MS Rao: ed; Med update; API 2010; 20 : 645-49.
56. Bhatia R.S., *et al.,* Lung Cancer. Indian scenario; Med Pulse 1998;5: 36-39.
57. Albert Y., Lin M.D., MPH, Daniel C. and Ihde M.D.,Recent developments in the treatment of lung cancer, JAMA 1992,267: 1661-64.
58. Boring C.C., Squires T.S. and Tong T., Cancer statistics, 1991, CA 1991; 41: 19-36.
59. Garfinkel L. and Silverberg E., Lung cancer and smoking trends in the United States over the past 25 years, C.A. 1991; 41: 137-45.
60. Ries L.A.G., Hankey B.F., Miller B.A., Hartman A.M. and Edwards B.K., Cancer Statistics Review 1973-88 Bethessda, Md: National Cancer Institute, NIH publication 1991; 2789.
61. Jindal S.K., Malik S.K, Dhand R., Gujral J.S., Malik A.K. and Datta B.N., Bronchogenic carcinoma in Northern India, Thorax 1982; 37; 343-47.
62. Neal J.W., *et al.,* Current management of small cell lung cancer, Clin Chest Med 2011;32:853-63.
63. Isobe T., *et al.,* Current management of advanced NSCLC: Target therapy, Semin Oncol 2005;32:315-28.
64. Soon Y.Y., *et al.,* Duration of chemotherapy for advanced NSCLC—A systemic review and metaanalysis of randomized trials, J Clin Oncol 2009;27:3277-83.
65. Dillman R.O., Seagren S.L., Propert, K.J., *et al.,* A randomized trial of induction chemotherapy plus high-dose radiation versus radiation alone in stage III non-small cell lung cancer. N. Engl. J. Med. 1990; 323: 940-45.
66. Anonymous. Aggressive treatment of inoperable lung cancer—How much benefit for the patient? (Editorial), Lancet 1986; i:722.
67. Klastersky J., Paesmans M., Response to chemotherapy quality of life benefits and survival in advanced NSCLC: Review of literature results; Lung cancer 2000; 34: S95-S101.
68. Southami R.L., Geddes D.M., Spiro S.G., *et al.,* Radiotherapy in small cell cancer of the lung treated with combination chemotherapy: A controlled trial. Br. Med. J. 1984; 288: 1643-46.
69. Pedersen A.G., Kristjansen P.E.G. and Hansen H.H., Prophylactic cranial irradiation and small cell lung cancer, Cancer Treat Rep. 1988; 15: 85-103.
70. Hohnson B.E., Grayson J., Makuch R.W., *et al.,* Ten years survival of patients with small-cell lung cancer treated with combination chemotherapy with or without irradiation J. Clin. Oncol 1990; 8: 396-401.
71. Bhattacharya G.S., Sarkar D., Medical management of NSCLC; IN; SB Gupta; ed; Med update; API 2005; 15: 805-12.
72. Rubens R.D., Towlson K.E., Ramirez A.J., *et al.,* Appropriate chemotherapy for palliating advanced cancer, BMJ 1992; 304: 35-40.
73. Ihde D.C., Mulshine J.L., Kramer B.S., *et al.,* Randomized trial of high vs standard dose etopside (VPI6) and cisplatin in extensive stage small cell lung cancer. Proc. Am. Soc. Clin. Oncol. 1991; 10: 240.
74. Bork E., Hansen M., Dombernowsky P., Hansen S.W., Pedersen A.G., Hansen H.H., Teniposide (VM-26), an overlooked highly active agent in small cell lung cancer, results of phase II trial in untreated patients, J. Clin. Oncol. 1986; 4: 524-27.
75. Perry M.C., Eaton W.L., Propert K.J., *et al.,* Chemotherapy with or without radiation therapy in limited small cell carcinoma of the lung. N. Engl. J. Med. 1987; 316: 912-18.
76. McCracken J.D., Janaki L.M., Crowley U., *et al.,* Concurrent chemotherapy/radiotherapy for limited small cell lung carcinoma: A Southwest Oncology Group Study. J. Clin. Oncol. 1990; 8: 892-98.
77. Ihde D.C., Grayson J., Woods E., *et al., Twice daily chest irradiation as an adjuvant to etoposide cisplatin therapy of limited stage small cell cancer.* In: Salmon S.E., Ed. Adjuvant Therapy of Cancer VI Philadelphia, Pa: WB Saunders Co. 1990; 162-65.
78. Osterling K., Hansen H.H., Roth M., Hansen M. and Dombernowsky P., Treatment policy of surgery in small cell carcinoma of the lung. A retrospective analysis of a group of 874 consecutive patients, Thorax 1985; 40: 272-77.
79. Timothy A.R., Ashq D., Corris P., *et al.,* Workshop on consensus guidelines for management of lung cancer. Clin. Oncol 1990; 2: 97-101.
80. Rees G.J.G., Cancer treatment, deciding what we can afford, BMJ 1991; 302: 799-800.
81. Hansen H.H., Chemotherapy of small cell carcinoma, a review. QJ Med. 1987; 63: 275-82.
82. Kris M.G, Gralla RJ., Wertheim M.S., *et al.,* Trial of combination of mitomycin, vindesine and cisplatin in patients with advanced non small cell lung cancer. Cancer Treat Rep. 1986; 70: 1091-96.
83. Pedersen-Bjergaard J., Osterling K., Hansen H.H., *et al.,* Acute non-lymphocytic leukaemia, preleukaemia and solid tumours following intensive chemotherapy of small cell carcinoma of the lung. Blood 1985; 66: 1393-97.
84. Hong W.K., Lippman S.M., Itri L.M., *et al.,* Prevention of second primary tumours with siotretinoin in squamous cell carcinoma of the head and neck. N. Engl. J. Med. 1990; 323: 795-801.
85. Mead G.M. and Williams C.J., Developing new drugs for cancer, BMJ 1991; 303: 1005-06.
86. Hillman A.L., Eisenberg J.M., Pauly M.V., Bloom B.S., Glick H., Kinosian B., *et al.,* Avoiding bias in the conduct and reporting of cost effectiveness research sponsored by pharmaceutical companies, N. Engl. J. Med. 1991; 324: 1362-65.
87. Mishra S., Human gene therapy—A brief overview of the genetic revolution; JAPI 2013;61:41-47.
88. Sozzi G., *et al.,* Detection of micro satellite alterations in plasma DNA of non small cell lung cancer patients; a prospect for early diagnosis; Clin Cancer Research 1999; s(10): 2689-92.
89. Minamato T., *et al.,* K-ras mutation; early detection in molecular diagnosis and risk assessment of colorectal, pancreas and lung cancer—A review; Cancer Detection and Prevention 2000; 24(1): 1-12.

90. Staber P., *et al.*, CYFRA-21-1 in the early diagnosis of recurrent disease in non small cell lung carcinoma; Anti Cancer Research 1999; 19/4A: 2665-68.
91. Lippman S.M., *et al.*, Cancer chemoprevention: Progress and promise; J. Natl. Cancer Inst 1998; 90: 1514-28.
92. Sikara K., Cancer screening; Med. International 1999; 21: 35-38.
93. Lam S., Shibuya H., Early diagnosis of lung cancer; Clinics in Chest Med 1999; 20(1): 53-61.
94. Ferreira C.G., *et al.*, Noval approaches to the treatment of NSCLC; Crit Rev, Oncol; Haematol 2002; 41: 57-77.
95. Landis S.H., *et al.*, Cancer statistics, 1998; CA Cancer J. Clin. 1998; 48: 6-29.
96. Bhattacharya A.K., Bronchoalveolar cell carcinoma; Lung India 2009; 22: 60-62.
97. Carter D. and Eggleston J.C., Atlas of tumour pathology, Second series, fascicle 17, Washington D.C., Armed forces Institute of Pathology 1980; 127-47.
98. Guleria J.S., Pulmonary tumours; In: G.S. Sainani, *et al.*, ed., API Textbook of Medicine 1999; 6th ed.; 270-75.
99. Robert I. Graver, *et al.*, BAC recurs in transplanted lung; New Eng. J. Med 1999; 340: 1071-74.
100. McDonald J.W., Pilgram T.K., Nuclear expression of p53, p21 and cyclin D1 is increased in BAC; histopathology 1999; 34: 439-46.
101. M. Hodges, Gregory P., Kalemkerian BAC masquerading as pneumonia; Primary Care and Cancer 2000; 20: 7.
102. Weisbrod G.L., *et al.*, Cystic change (pseudocavitation) associated with BAC: A report of 4 patients; J. Thorac Imaging 1995; 10(2): 106-11.
103. Gaeta N., *et al.*, MR white sign: Incidence and significance in pulmonary consolidations; J. Comput. Assist. Tomoyra 2001; 25(6): 890-96.
104. Travis W.D., *et al.*, The new IASLC/ATS/ERS international multidisciplinary lung adenocarcinoma classification; J. Thorac Oncol 2011; 6:244-85.
105. Rong R: *et al.*, Metastatic poorly differentiated monophasic synovial sarcoma of lung with unknown primary–A molecular genetic analysis: Int J Chin. Exp Pathol; 2010; 3:217-21
106. Raizada N; *et al.*, A rapidly developing lung mass diagnosed as desnoplastic small sound cell tumor; Lung India; 2011;28:287-90.
107. Roy P; *et al.*, A primary synovial sarcoma of lung; N Amer J Med Sir; 2012;4:241-43.
108. Devleena; *et al.*, primary synovial sarcoma of lung; Lung India; 2014;31:277-79.
109. Kistner R.W., Gynaecology Principles and Practice, 4th Edition. Year Book Medical Publishers Inc., Chicago, London 1982; 491-525.
110. Berkowitz Goldstein, Pathogenesis of gestational trophoblastic neoplasm. Pathobio Ann 1981; 11: 39-41.
111. Sung H.C., Wu P.C., Hu M.H., Roentegenologic manifestation of pulmonary metastases in choriocarcinoma and invasive mole, Am J Obst, Gynaecol 1982, 141: 89-97.
112. Shah S.Y., Potdar P.V. and Kamat S.R., Metastatic choriocarcinoma with repiratory distress and haemoperitonium JAPI 1988; 36: 454-55.
113. Aggarwal P., Sharma S.K. and Verma K., Synovial cell sarcoma with pulmonary metastasis, JAPI 1988; 36: 617-18.
114. Bhatia R.S., Pulmonary manifestations of extrathoracic neoplasms; IN; Manoria PC; ED; Medicine Update; API, Bombay 1996; 6: 229-33.
115. Blake Cady, Natural history of Primary and Secondary tumours of the liver, Seminar in Oncology 1983; 10: 127-135.
116. Tandon B.N. and Nundy S., Hepatocellular carcinoma and other tumours of the liver in Hepatobiliary Diseases Text Book of Topical Gastroentrology, 1st Edition, Delhi, Oxford University Press 1988; 1: 218-27.
117. Nigam P., Chaturvedi A.K., Sharma S.P., *et al.*, Appearance of chest skiagrams in primary liver carcinoma, Lung India 1990; 7: 137-41.
118. Donahue J.K., Weichert R.F. and Ochsner J.L., Bronchial adenoma, Ann, Surg 1986; 167: 873-80.
119. Mathur R.S., Pandit A., Ahuja H.S., *et al.* Collapse of left lung secondary to bronchial carcinoid tumour, JAPI 1988; 36: 233-35.
120. Bhoil A., *et al.*, Is 68 Ga-DOTATATE the answer in lung carcinoid? Case report and review of literature, Lung India 2012; 29:378-80.
121. Swarnakar R, Sihna S; End bronchial leionayoma-a rare and innocent tumour of the bronchial tree; Lung India; 2013; 30: 57-60
122. Newland O. Jr., Young W.G. Jr. and Sealy W.C., Hamartoma of the lung. J. Thoracic. Cardio Vase. Sug 1967; 53: 735-42.
123. Kutras P., Urschel H.C. Jr. and Paulson D.L., Hamartoma of the lung, J. Thorac. Cardivasc. Surg 1971; 61: 768-76.
124. Perez-Atayde A.R. and Seller, Pulmonary hamartoma—An ultra-structural study, Cancer 1984; 53:485-92.
125. Murry and Nadel, Hamartoma In. Text Book of Respiratory Medicine, Vol. 2., W.B., Saunders Company 1988; 1262-63.
126. Joshi J.M., *et al.* Pulmonary hamartoma; JAPI 1995; 43(10): 712-13.
127. Alfred P., Fishman Hamartoma In: Pulmonary disease and disorder. Second edition, Vol. 3, Mc Graw Hill Book Company 1989; 2020.
128. Ravindran P., *et al.*, Hamartoma of the lung, Lung India 1990; 8: 207-209.
129. Shah A.A., *et al.*, Pulmonary fibromas—A rare tumour, JAPI 1995; 43(1):61-62.
130. Das S.K., *et al.*, A case of haemoptysis due to endobronchial fibroma; Lung India 2008; 25:25-27.
131. Robbins S.L. and Cotran R.S., Clinical aspects of neoplasia, In; Pathologic basis of disease, W.B.Saunders Co., Japan, Ind. ed., 1981; 206, 208.
132. Charlton A., Children's advertisements—Awareness related to their views on smoking, Health Education Journal 1986; 45: 75-78.
133. Charlton A., Evaluation of a family-linked smoking programme in primary schools. Health Education Journal 1986; 45: 140-144.
134. Rao S., Rau P.V.R. and Sahoo R.C., Bronchogenic carcinoma in the young, Lung India 1992; 10: 101-102.
135. Wald N.J., Nanchahal K., Thompson S.G and Cuckle H.S., Does breathing other people's tobacco smoke cause lung cancer, Br. Med. J. 1986; 293: 1217-22.

136. Williams C.J., Preventing lung cancer, BMJ 1987; 295: 1433-34.
137. Higgins Millicent W., *et al.,* Smoking and lung functions in elderly men and women, JAMA 1993; 269: 2741-48.
138. Dunlop B., The solitary pulmonary nodule, J.Appl. Med 1982; 8: 969-977.
139. Sahu G.N., *et al.,* Aetiological diagnosis of SPN—A five-year study; Lung India 2002; 20: 80-82.
140. Bhatia R.S., Pulmonary manifestations of extrathoracic neoplasms; Curl Med Journ 1996; 2(4):25-28.
141. Michels G., *et al.*, Bronchogenic cyst mimicking H.D., Lung India 2012; 29:376-77.
142. Rose A.R., *et al.,* Round pneumonias in adults; JAPI 2002; 50: 285-86.
143. Soman R; *et al.,* A puzzling pulmonary nodule in a renal transplant recipient; JAPI; 2014; 62:38-42
144. Zerhouni E.A., Stitik F.P., Siegelman S.S., *et al.* Computed tomography of the solitary pulmonary nodule. A national cooperative study, Radiology 1986;160: 319-27.
145. Rupak Singla, Ramesh Chakhani, Anand Jaiswal, *et al.* Pulmonary tuberculosis minicking metastatic nodule, Ind. J. Tuber. 1991; 38: 33-36.
146. Puri R., Vilman P., Transoesophageal ultrasound guided biopsy of lesions in mediastinum—A minimal invasive method for primary diagnosis of unknown mediastinal lesions and staging of lung cancer; JAPI 2009; 57:467-71.
147. Rawat J., *et al.,* Clinicopathological profile of lung cancer in Uttrakhand, Lung India 2009; 26:74-76.
148. Tilve G.H., *et al.,* Utility of PET in medicine; In: M.S. Rao; ed., Med Update, API 2010; 20:645-49.
149. Cummings S.R., Lillington G.A. and Richard R.J., Managing solutary pulmonary nodules, Am. Rev. Respir. Dis. 1986; 134: 453-60.
150. Burgel E. and Themel K.G., Zur Pathologic Und klinic des Lungennarbeaukazinmous, Oncologia 1958; 11: 254.
151. Sekhon J.S., Dhimas A., TB and lung cancer; IN; R.S. Bhatia; ed; Tuberculosis; Peepee Pub. N. Delhi 2007; 9: 55-56.
152. Peacock A. and Peacock P.R., The results of prolonged use of isoniazid to mice, rats and hamsters, British Journal of Cancer 1966; 20: 307.
153. Berenci G., Entz A. and Vajkscy A., Quoted by leading articles Ruft Isonikotins aurehydrazid Tumoren Hervor? Deutsche Medizinche-Wochenschrift 1960; 85: 1955.
154. Walsh T.D. and West T.S., Controlling symptoms in advanced cancer, BMJ 1988; 296: 477-81.
155. Decisions near the end of life, Council on ethical and judicial affairs, Amer. Med. Assn. JAMA 1992,267: 2229-2233.
156. Capron A.M., Legal and ethical problems in decisions for death, Law Med. Health Care 1986; 14: 141-44.
157. Office of Technology Assessment Task Force. Life sustained Technologies and the Elderly, Philadelphia. Pa. Science Information Resources Center, 1988.
158. Council on Ethical and Judicial Affairs. Guidelines for the appropriate use of do-not-resuscitate orders, report D, In: Proceeding of the House of Delegates of the AMA, December 1990; Chicago III, 180-85.
159. Council on Ethical and Judicial Affairs and the Council on Scientific Affairs. Persistent vegetative state and the decision to withdraw or withhold life support, Joint report, In: Proceedings of the House of Delegates of the AMA, June 1989; Chicago III, 314-18.
160. Council on Ethical and Judicial Affairs, Decisions to forego life-sustaining treatment for incompetent patients, report D. In: Proceedings of the House of Delegates of the AMA, June1991; Chicago III, 261-69.
161. Mathur A., Geriatric care giver training; J Ind Acad Geriatr 2007; 3: 03-04.
162. Kar M; Roy R; Recent changes in lung cancer; IN; SB Gupta; ed: PG Med, API; 2014; 28:487-93.
163. De Wachter M.A.M., Active euthanasia in the Netherlands, JAMA 1989; 262: 3316-19.
164. Van der Mass P., Van Delden J., Pinjnenborg L. and Looman C., Euthanasia and other medical decisions concerning the end of life, Lancet 1991; 338: 669-74.
165. Gelman D. and Springen K., The doctor's suicide van, Newsweek, June 18, 1990; 46-49.
166. Jindal S.K., Issues in the care of the dying; Ind J. Med Ethics 2005; 2: 79-80.
167. Sprung C.L., Changing attitudes and practices in foregoing life-sustaining treatment, JAMA 1990; 263: 2211-15.
168. Wolf Susan M., Physician-assisted suicide; Clin. Geriatr Med 2005; 21:179-92.
169. Quill T.E., Death and dignity, a case of individualized decision making. N. Engl. J. Med 1991; 324: 691-94.

PULMONARY PLASMA CELL GRANULOMA

Pseudotumor

Plasma cell granuloma is a benign lymphoproliferative disorder of mature plasma cell infiltration[1] that usually occurs below the age of 30 years in 2/3rd of the cases, while 1/3rd presenting below 10 years of age. Both the sexes are equally affected and in children below 15 years of age it is said to be the most common primary tumor like lesion of the lung.[2] The aetiology still remains unclear and is thought to be a post-inflammatory process.[3] It most commonly presents as a solitary well defined rounded mass or a coin lesion which may grow insidiously, to occupy whole of the lung. Occasionally areas of cavitation or calcification may develop. However, pleural effusion has not been reported so far. Other presentation includes pneumonic consolidation/atelectasis, mediastinal pseudomass which may then involve the adjacent lung.[4] Treatment is by surgery.[5]

Plasma cell granuloma is one of the pulmonary pseudomasses which pose a diagnostic challenge radiologically.[1] The common causes of pulmonary pseudotumor include, interlobar pleural effusion, pulmonary sequestration, pulmonary artery aneurysm, pulmonary hemangioma, pulmonary venous varix, aneurysm of the thoracic aorta/bronchiocephalic artery and pulmonary lymphoproliferative disorders like pseudolymphoma and plasma cell granuloma.

REFERENCES

1. Kapoor A. and Setia V., Pulmonary pseudotumor J. Med. and Surg 1991; 30: 10-11.
2. Glickstein M., Kornstein M.J. and Petro G.G., Non-lymphomatous lymphoid disorders of lung, Amer. J. Med 1986; 147: 227-237.
3. Bahadori M. and Leibow P., Plasma Cell granuloma of the lung cancer 1973; 31: 191-208.
4. Hutchins G.M. and Eggleston J.C., Unusual presentation of pulmonary inflammatory pseudotumor (plasma cell granuloma) as oesophageal obstruction, Amer. J. Gastroent 1979; 71: 501-04.
5. Mandelbaum I., Brachean R. and Hull M., Surgical treatment and course of pulmonary pseudotumors, J. Thorac. Card. Vas. Surg 1981; 82: 77-82.

OTHER TUMORS

Midline Granuloma[1-3]

An uncommon disease characterised by localised inflammation and destruction of the tissues of upper respiratory tract and face.

Aetiology is not known. Initially thought to have granulomatous immunogenic or neoplastic origin. Recently, it is considered to be part of spectrum called angiocentric immunoproliferative lesions.

Pathology[4,5]

Acute or chronic inflammation with necrosis and superadded bacterial infection may be the histological findings. Primary vasculitis is rarely seen. A non-caseating granuloma with or without giant cells form the pathological hallmark.

Clinical Presentation[6,7]

It occurs in 5-6th decades, but no age is exempted. More commonly, it is seen in females with recurrent sinusitis and allergic rhinitis. Nasal and buccal mucosa including gums are affected. Regional lymph nodes are enlarged only when secondary infection occurs. X-ray shows parasinusitis with areas of destruction of bone in advanced cases.

Treatment

1. Antibiotics for superimposed infection.
2. Steroids have no value.
3. Few reports of response to cytotoxic agents.
4. Surgery may cause rapid progression of the disease.
5. Radiotherapy is useful.[8,9]

Dose of 50000 rad (50000m Gy) is useful and remissions of 20 years have been reported. Recurrence is common with low dose radiation. Reconstructive and plastic surgery can be done after one year following irradiation.

REFERENCES

1. English G.M. (ed), Oncolaryngology (Rev. ed), N. York, Harper and Row, 1989.
2. Frick W.E. and Busse W.W., Respiratory infection, Their role in airway responsiveness and pathogenesis of asthma, Clin. Chest. Med 1988; 9: 539.
3. Gwaltney J.M., Sinusitis, In: Principles and practice of infectious diseases, 3rd ed, Manden G.L., *et al.* (ed), N. York, Churchill Livingstone 1990; 510-14.
4. Hilovinen P., *et al.* Pharyngitis in adults, the presence and coexistence of viruses and bacterial organisms. Ann. Intern. Med 1989; 110: 612.
5. Lucent F.E. and Hyams V.J., Inflammatory and neoplastic disorders of the nasal mucosa, Clin. Dermatol 1987; 5: 35.
6. Naclerio R.M., The pathopysiology of rhinitis, Impact of therapeutic intervention, J. Allergy Clin. Immunol 1988; 82: 927.
7. Togias A., *et al.* Studies on allergic and non-allergic nasal inflammation. J. Allergy Clin. Immunol 1988; 81: 782.
8. Fauci A.S., *et al.* Radiation therapy of midline granuloma, Ann. Intern. Med 1976; 84: 140.
9. Fichner R.E., Lamppin D.W., Midline malignant reticulosis, Arch Otolaryngol 1972; 95: 467.

PRIMARY PULMONARY NON-HODGKIN'S LYMPHOMA

Primary Pulmonary Non-Hodgkin's Lymphoma (PPNHL) is an uncommon neoplasm constituting only 0.3 per cent-0.4 per cent of primary tumour in lung.[1] The true incidence of primary pulmonary non-Hodgkin's lymphoma is difficult to determine, largely because of variable criteria used in establishing pathological diagnosis. Small lymphocytic forms of non-Hodgkin's lymphoma are characterised by pleuro-parenchymal involvement. The reported frequency of pleural effusion associated with non-Hodgkin's lymphoma is 6 to 19 per cent,[2] frequency of pleural effusion as presenting manifestation is variable and cytological evidence of lymphoma in pleural fluid is exceptional. The prognosis of non-Hodgkin's lymphoma is very variable, if confined to lung.[1,3]

Clinically patient gives history of reduced appetite, weight loss, shortness of breath, fever, fatigue and one-sided chest pain without sweating. There may be previous history of treatment, for pulmonary tuberculosis with pleural effusion. ESR is increased. Radiological examination of the chest reveals an opacity without cavitation or calcification, with or without pleural effusion. In the right lateral view, wedge-shaped opacity with apex towards the hilum may be seen. C.T. scan chest shows consolidation with pulmonary mass and pleural effusion without hilar or mediastinal lymphadenopathy.

Fiberoptic bronchoscopy shows erythematous appearance at the upper lobe orifice, cytological examination of bronchial brushings and washings may not reveal any malignant-tumour cells. Serum protein estimation shows decreased albumin and increased globulin, serum protein electrophoresis shows M peak in the gamma-region-IgM gammopathy.

Pleural fluid analysis shows highly cellular monomorphous small lymphocyte like cells, dispersed singley, mixed with a few plasma cells, without reactive mesothelial or inflammatory cells.

Pleural biopsy reveals focus of dense aggregate of monomorphous small lymphoid cells. Fine needle aspiration cytology performed under fluoroscopic guidance and cytology reveals *low grade B cell type lymphoplasmacytoid lymphoma.* Estimation of lymphocyte associated antigen in serum and pleural fluid may be mildly positive, indicating that the mass in lung can be a lymphoma.

As a therapeutic measure, stage by stage thoracentesis can be done. Combination chemotherapy with inj. vincristin (2 mgm) I.V. on day one and eight, Chlorambucil 5 mgm twice daily for seven days; Procarbazine 50 mgm × three times daily for seven days; Allopurinol 100 mg × 2 times daily for seven days; Corticosteroids 20 mgm × 3 times daily for seven days can be started. Continuous treatment must be kept depending upon restrictive pattern of interstitial lung disease.

Lung is an unusual primary site for lymphomas.[4] Non-Hodgkin's lymphoma (NHL) in lung are rare and are vexing lesions.[4] Only 3.6 per cent tumours originating from lower respiratory tract,[5] and 3.6 per cent originating in lungs, pleura or trachea[6] have been described. Between 55 per cent and 72 per cent of pulmonary lymphomas are of small cell type and are asymtomatic and the lesions are found in routine chest skiagram, and if symtoms are present, they are related to chest.[7]

The diagnosis of non-Hodgkin's lymphoma may be established by Fine Needle Aspiration Cytology (FNAC) of lung but it is usually open lung biopsy or lobectomy that provides highest diagnostic yield and allows exact histological typing of lesion.[8]

Pleural effusion in non-Hodgkin's lymphoma is infrequent,[3,7,9] the reported frequency being 6-19 per cent.[2,10] The frequency of a pleural effusion as a presenting manifestation in non-Hodgkin's lymphoma is variable.[2] Pleural fluid cytology showing lymphoma cells is exceptional.[8] In the pleural fluid cytology, presence of highly cellular monomorphous small lymphocyte like cells, is an exceptional feature.[8]

Aspiration biopsy cytology—a well established diagnostic technique for solid neoplasm has controversial value in lymphoma[11] and is of value, if lymphoma is of high grade type.[9]

Tumours cells derived from B lymphocytes sometimes produce typical IgM serum protein spikes,[12] as a supporting evidence for the diagnosis of lymphoma, most frequently of plasmacytoid lymphocytic type.[1,7] Patients with macroglobulinaemia of Waldenstron, may initially have lymphocytic plasmacytoid lymphoma, limited to lung[5,7] with pleural effusion that can occur, though it is uncommon.[5,7]

The detection in the serum and pleural fluid of Lymphoma Associated Antigen (LAA) is a supporting evidence for the diagnosis of lymphoma.[13,14]

The presence of pleural effusion in initial chest skiagram is a significant predictor of poor prognostic sign in lymphoma, especially if malignant cells are present in the pleural fluid, and probably shortens survival.[10] The presence of IgM in serum may indicate a lower median survival, than those patients without evidence of paraproteinemia.[15] Response to therapy also appears to indicate a better prognosis.[10,16]

REFERENCES

1. Frazer Pare Generau. Lymphoreticular neoplasm and leukaemia in neoplastic disease of lungs. In Diagnosis of Diseases of the Chest, 3rd Ed, 1989; Vol. III, Philadelphia, W.B. Saunders Company, 1535-52.
2. Kapoor R., Karol A., Das O.K. and Saha M.M., Ultrasonic visualization of pleural masses in non-Hodgkin's lymphoma, Ind. J. Chest. Dis. All Sci. 1990; 32: 150-58.
3. Weick J.K., Kielu J.M., Harrison E.G., Carr D.T. and Scanlon P.W., Pleural effusion in lymphoma, Cancer 1973; 31: 848-53.
4. Koss M.N., Nochholazer L., Nichols P.W., Wehunt W.O. and Lazarus A.A., Primary non-Hodgkin's lymphoma and pseudo lymphoma of lung—A study of 161 patients, Human Pathology 1983;14: 1024-38.
5. Costa J. and Martin S.E., Pulmonary lymphoreticular disorders. In Major problems in pathology. Ed. Jaffe Elain, Vol.16, Philadelphia, WB Saunders Company, 1985; 282-97.
6. Carr J. and Holoyoke P.Y., Miscellaneous malignant tumours in neoplasms of lungs. Textbook of Respiratory medicine. Ed. Murray J.F. and Nadel J.A., Philadelphia, WB Saunders Company, 1988; 1251-60.
7. Koss M.N., Lymphoproliferative disorders of lung, In surgical pathology of Lung Neoplasms. Ed. Marchevsky A.M., New York Marcel Dekker. The Lung Biology in Health and Disease1990; Vol. 44: 433-86.
8. Scully R.E., Mark, E.J., Mc Neely W.F. and Mc Neely B.U., Case records of the Massachusetts General Hospital Case 26,1 1991; New Eng J. Med. 1991; 324: 1876-84.
9. Strauchen J.A. and Kleinerman J.I., Lungs in malignant haematologic disease. In Pulmonary Diseases and Disorders. Ed. Fishman A.P., 2nd Ed, Vol.3 McGraw Hill Book Co. 1988; 2045-68.
10. Manoharan A., Pitney W.R., Schonell M.E. and Bader L.V., Intrathoracic manifestations in Non-Hodgkin's lymphoma, Thorax 1979; 34: 29-32.
11. Singh M.K., Verma K. and Kapila K., Value of aspiration cytology in diagnosis and subtyping of malignant lymphomas. Ind. J. Med. Res. 1988; 87: 32-36.

12. Colby T.V. and Carrington C.B., Pulmonary lymphomas—Current concepts, Hum. Path 1983; 14: 884-87.
13. Udaychander M., Meenakshi A, Ansamma J. and Muthiah R., Lymphoma associated antigen (LAA), Isolation characterization and clinical evaluation, Br. J. Cancer 1983; 48: 717-25.
14. Udaychander M., Meenakshi A, Ansamma J., Muthiah R. and Sankthivel, Development of a radioimmunoassay Diganostic and Therap 1984; 5: 201-05.
15. Kennedy J.L., Nathwani B.N., Burke J.S., Hill L.R. and Rappaport H., Pulmonary lymphomas and other pulmonary lymphoid lesions—A clinicopathologic and immunologic study of 64 patients, Cancer1985; 56: 539-52.
16. Vijaylakshmi Thanasekaran, Deivanayagam C.N. and Venugopalan K., *et al.*, Primary pulmonary Non-Hodgkin's lymphoma—A case report, Lung India 1992; 10:140-44.

BRONCHIAL EPITHELIAL-MYOEPITHELIAL CARCINOMA[1,2]

This is an extremely rare tumour first described by Donath in 1972, representing only 0.5% of all salivary tumors. Tracheobronchial submucosal glands are pulmonary analogue of minor salivary glands of oral mucosa from which salivary type of tumours arise. Few reports are available in literature about this tumour arising from bronchial mucosa and having low grade and low metastatic potential, showing local or regional aggressiveness.

There is no history of chest pain, dyspnoea, haemoptysis, loss of weight or loss of appetite. On examination, there is no palor, cyanosis or clubbing. Few coarse crepitations are present over the area of tumour.

Routine investigations are non-contributory. Bronchoscopic biopsy clinches the diagnosis. Histopathology shows lobulated tumour having biphasic proliferation of inner small cells lining duct-like spaces with outer large cells with clear abundant cytoplasm. Outer cells are S-l00 protein and smooth muscle action positive, confirming their myoepithelial nature and inner cells are cytokeratin positive, as is evident by immunohistochemsitry.

REFERENCES

1. Nistal M., Garcia-Vera M., *et al.*, Epithelial-myoepithelial tumour of the bronchus; Amer. J. Surg. Pathol 1994; 18: 421-25.
2. Shanks J.H., Haslecton P.S., *et al.*, Bronchial epithelial-myoepithelial carcinoma; Histopathology 1998; 33: 90-91.

TRACHEAL TUMOURS[1,2]

These are quite rare, comprising only 1.2% of all lung tumours. 85% of these are carcinoid tumours, 10% are adenoid cystic carcinomas and 5% are mucoepidermoid tumours. Mixed tumours are rare.

Patients often present with cough, wheeze, dyspnoea and hemoptysis. Often symptomatlogy mimics chronic bronchitis or bronchial asthma and even temporarily respond to bronchodilator and anti-inflammatory therapy, thus, further delaying the real diagnosis.

Adenoid cystic carcinoma is also termed as 'cylindroma' because of classical tubular structures formed by epithelial cells of mucus glands surrounding rounded spaces filled with eosinophilic or basophilic material which is mucopolysaccharide or mucoprotein. It is a slow growing endophytic tumour, having intact overlying respiratory epithelium. Affecting both the sexes, it commonly occurs in 6th or 7th decades of life. Metastasis occurs in lungs and bones. Recurrence is common after resection, possibly because of perineural and intraneural infiltration. Surgical resection and radiation if used early yields remission for many years. Endotracheal radioactive iridium insertion gives dramatic palliative results in case of recurrence of tumour.

REFERENCES

1. Cleveland R.H., Nice Jr. C.M., Ziskind L., Primary adenoid cystic carcinoma of the trachea; Radiology 1997; 122: 597-600.
2. Baydur A., Gottlieb L.C., Adenoid cystic carcinoma of the trachea masquerading as asthma; JAMAs 1995; 234:829-31.

PRIMARY ADENOID CYSTIC CARCINOMA

Frequency of primary adenoid cystic carcinoma among lung cancer patients is 0.3%. Tobacco and biomass fuel smoke are potential risk factors.[1,2]

REFERENCES

1. Cortes-Telles A., Mendoza-Posada D., Primary adenoid cystic carcinoma of tracheobronchial tree; Lung India 2012;29: 325-28.
2. Jaso J., Malhotra R., Adenoid cystic carcinoma; Arch Pathol Lab Med 2011;135:511-15.

Disorders of Airflow Obstruction

7

CHRONIC OBSTRUCTIVE PULMONARY DISEASE

INTRODUCTION

COPD has silently grown in magnitude and impact. In fact, it has become the 4th leading cause of death worldwide. That is why WHO in collaboration with the US National Heart, Lung and Blood Institute has initiated a global response for COPD called GOLD. Effectively acting against the recognised factors such as tobacco, occupational dusts and chemicals and pollution from biomass fuels in poorly vented dwellings would be the real response to the challenge of GOLD.[1,2] GOLD criterion of using FEV_1/FVC value below 70% as an indicator of airway obstruction cannot be applied as a general rule of thumb to general population, with false positive results in older adults and false negative results in young adults.[2] Chronic obstructive pulmonary disease (COPD) is a disorder characterised by abnormal tests of expiratory flow that do not change markedly over periods of several months' observation. In fact combination of chronic bronchitis and emphysema is equated with COPD, but disorders like emphysema, peripheral airways disease and chronic bronchitis are included in COPD. Five distinct clinical phenotypes of airways disease have been defined. The definition does not include variable airways obstruction from bronchial asthma and other specific causes of air flow obstruction such as localised disease of the upper airways, bronchiectasis and cystic fibrosis. National burden of COPD in 1996 was estimated at over 12 million, having smoking association in a ratio of 2.65. This study also demonstrated relationship of environmental tobacco smoke (ETS) passive smoking exposure with COPD in non-smoker population. In 2006, prevalence of COPD has been estimated to be 4.1%, although objective spirometry (which in gold standard in any COPD prevalence study) as required to support the available epidemiological data which, right now, is very thin.[3]

Airways obstruction is better called air flow limitation (CAL). The name chronic obstructive pulmonary disease itself suggests a slowly progressive indolent airway problem with airflow limitation. It may result from occupational exposures as well. The chronic irritation out of smoke may lead to airway inflammation, hypersecretion of mucous and ciliary dysfunction. Cardinal symptoms of CAL are shown in Table 7.1.

Table 7.1: Cardinal symptoms of CAL
1. Cough
2. Sputum production
3. Dyspnoea

Chronic bronchitis and emphysema are two important members of the group of disease described under the title *chronic obstructive pulmonary disease.* Their classification into *pink and puffing* and *blue and bloated* originally suggested by Dornhorst is now widely accepted. Recent postmortem studies have, however, shown no clear cut difference in the degree of mucous gland hyperplasia or emphysema in the sections from lungs of the cases belonging to the two types during life. The two conditions co-exist in the majority of cases though one or the other of the pathological processes may dominate.

There is a constant and yet diffuse obstruction of airways. The condition makes a slow progress over years. It forms the most important cause of chronic corpulmonale. The term COPD (synonyms, chronic obstructive lung disease, COLD; chronic obstructive airways disease, COAD; chronic airflow obstruction, CAO) includes those patho-physiologic processes contributing to the syndrome—chronic bronchitis, emphysema and small airways disease.

In COPD, *the abnormalities that result from chronic bronchitis cannot be separated from those which result from emphysema and those which result from a combination of both.* COPD also include a small group of patients who do not have airways obstruction as determined by the FEV_1, but have clinical, or radiologic features of chronic bronchitis or emphysema respectively.[4]

Usually employed pulmonary function tests to determine airways obstruction, the FEV_1 (forced expiratory volume in 1 second) and PEFR (peak expiratory flow rate) actually measure airflow limitation produced by both loss of elastic recoil of the lung from destructive changes in the parenchyma of the lung (emphysema) and/or pathologic narrowing of central conducting airways (chronic bronchitis). Hence the chronic airflow obstruction (CAO) means an impaired pulmonary function from obstruction within the airways and from impaired elastic recoil.[5]

Classification

COPD is broadly defined as *a disorder characterized by abnormal tests of expiratory flow which do not change markedly over long periods of observation.*[5] COPD includes chronic bronchitis, emphysema and small airway disease.

Chronic Bronchitis

There is chronic or recurrent excess mucous secretion into the bronchial tree sufficient to cause cough and sputum on most days for at least three months of the year and for at least three consecutive years in the absence of any specific cardio-respiratory disease.[6] It results in expiratory airflow obstruction. Its significance varies depending upon whether it is being described by the clinician, the pathologist, the radiologist or the pulmonary function analyst. Pathologically there is an increased thickness of the layer of mucus glands in the bronchi. The radiological criteria for the diagnosis of the condition are less clear and is not diagnosed radiologically.

Chronic bronchitis may be simple with mucoid expectoration, mucopurulent with persistent or intermittent mucopurulent expectoration due to infection or obstruction with persistent widespread narrowing of intrapulmonary airways leading to an increased resistance to the expiratory flow of air.

Aetiology

It is often seen in adult males belonging to the lower socio-economic class. It is prevalent among tobacco smokers and city dwellers irrespective of social status. The bronchial irritation either from environmental atmosphere pollution (rich in sulphur dioxide) due to smoke and fog or personal atmospheric pollution from tobacco smoking acts as the initiating factor for hypersecretion of mucus in the bronchial tree and increased airway resistance. Female gender with COPD has more morbidity and less mortality as compared to male gender, perhaps showing higher tolerance to disease (Celli, *et al.*, Amer J. Resp Crit Care Med 2011; 183: 317-22).

The incidence of the disease is closely related to the duration of smoking. It increases with increase in the amount smoked. It was previously considered that smoking was merely an aggravating factor. Recent studies, however, point to an important role for it in the causation also; lung function estimations support this concept.

Cigarette smoking is prevalent mainly in adult males mostly belonging to the lower socio-economic class. There is a linear increase in incidence of chronic bronchitis with increased smoking. Daily cigarette consumption and the number of years smoked have a direct bearing on the COPD morbidity and mortality.[7] The risk of death from chronic bronchitis and emphysema in patients smoking 30 cigarettes daily is 20 times that of non-smokers.

Tobacco smoke impairs ciliary activity and the bacterial action of macrophages, thus exposing the alveoli to the direct effects of inhalants and the bronchial tree to infection. There occurs hyperplasia of the bronchial mucous glands and squamous metaplasia of the epithelium of the airways. The oxidant radicals generated due to cigarette smoking may increase airways reactivity. Smoking increases the activity of alveolar macrophages which in turn produce a large amount of superoxide.[8] Superoxide may have a direct or indirect effect leading to lung injury and diminished activity of antiprotease respectively.

$Alpha_1$-protease inhibitor (A_1-P_1) is responsible for inhibition of proteolytic activity in the serum. It is susceptible to oxidative inactivation by compounds present in tobacco smoke, ozone, industrial gases and oxidants released by macrophages. There occurs an imbalance of elastase and/or antielastase which could help in development of emphysema.[9,10]

The influence of atmospheric pollution compared to cigarette smoking is said to be less marked. Carbonaceous particles, sulphur dioxide, hydrocarbons, nitrogen dioxide, ozone, aldehyde and other chemicals present in industrial dusts and automobile exhausts leading to urban air pollution appear to play an additive role in smokers for hypersecretion of mucus in the bronchial tree and increased airway resistance and may be partly responsible for progression of disability in patients with COPD.[7] Only recently effect of automotive exhaust resulting into chronic bronchitis and emphysema has been reported,[11] while others have not confirmed the effects. Exposure to smoke by burning cow dung and hay sticks in kitchen leads to development of airways obstruction in many women.[12] 1/5th of population in Bangladesh after the age of 40 suffer from COPD. Mostly rural, exposure to biomass burning and tobacco are significant risk factors.

Infection from bacteria, mycoplasma and viruses are known to cause acute exacerbations of already established obstructive lung disease and lead to the progression of disability. Atopy or multiple infections in childhood have also been incriminated as the factors making the host tissues particularly vulnerable.

There may be some constitutional differences between individual smokers to the stimulus of irritation from smoke. The cigarette smoke impairs ciliary activity and the bactericidal actions of macrophages, thus exposing the alveoli to the direct effects of inhalants and the bronchial tree to infections. Nearly 15% of COPD patients develop pulmonary hypertension.

The environmental pollution and viral infections possibly lower the resistance of the bronchial tree. Seasonal rise in the degree of pollution and the corresponding rise in morbidity and mortality have been noted. Occupations involving exposure to dust, fumes and other environmental pollutants have been shown to be associated with increased prevalence. In actual practice, however, barring coal mining and a few other dusty occupations air pollution has caused a rising trend in airflow respiratory disorders[13] but it is a much less important factor than cigarette smoking.

Periodic infection from H. influenzae and Strep. pneumoniae may lead to acute exacerbations. Complicated cases of COPD have higher levels of ILI-Beta and CRP while severe cases have higher levels of CRP and TNF-alpha.[14]

In India, a tertiary care centre patients show clinical profile of chronic airflow limitation as asthma (35%), COPD and obliterative bronchiolitis (15%), bronchiectasis (5%) and occupational airway disease (1%).

85% of tobacco inhalers are bidies smokers. 15% of COPD cases develop pulmonary hypertension.

Table 7.2: Risk factors for COPD

1. Cigarette smoking
2. Environmental and genetic factors
   a. Air pollution, auto exhaust
   b. Occupational
   c. Talcosis
   d. Alpha$_1$ antitrypsin deficiency
3. Demographic factors
   a. Age—lower respiratory tract infection infancy
   b. Family history of COPD
   c. Male sex

Pathology

Normal bronchial secretions amount to 100 ml in 24 hours. It has important functions of humidification of inspired air and removal of particulate material from the respired air in conjunction with the ciliary mechanism. In chronic bronchitis there is increased secretion of mucus in the bronchial tree.

The bronchial epithelium responds to bronchial irritation due to atmospheric pollution (rich in sulphur dioxide) and tobacco smoking. The immediate effect of smoking a cigarette is a sudden increase in airways resistance, but in many years, it acts as an important direct irritant—an inciting factor in the mucus hypersecretion. The bronchial epithelium is not under control of the vagus nerve and responds reflexly to the inciting factors of surface epithelium. The goblet cells are stimulated by irritants directly. The mucous glands situated in the submucosa of large cartilagenous airways show hyperplasia and hypertrophy. The glands increase in their size and even protrude between the cartilaginous plates.[15] Number of acini and mucous glands are increased. The mucus is rich in uraminidase resistant acid mucopolysaccharide.

Ratio of the thickness of the submucous glands to that of the bronchial wall (from the basement membrane of epithelium to cartilage)[16]—Reid Index—is increased. The ratio is virtually the same in all individuals *from a child of four years to the adult stage* and it constitutes one-fourth of the thickness (less than 0.4). In chronic bronchitis the gland thickness may exceed two-thirds of the total thickness (increased to 0.7 to 0.8). The lumen of the proximal airways due to increased thickness of the glands and their hypersecretion is decreased.[5]

Mucus secretion also increases in small non-cartilagenous airways by an increase in the number of goblet cells. The lining epithelium is covered with this secreting layer. It is not uniform in all the regions. The goblet cell secretion is mainly responsible for blockage of peripheral airways. There is no gross cellular infiltration indicating that the condition is not due to infection. The infection occurs later, causing damage to the bronchioles and alveoli.[3]

Airways get obstructed by the increased secretion. This provides good nidus for infection. The ciliary mechanism loses its working efficiency, and lowers the resistance. It allows the entry and growth of microorganisms.

The infection is followed by infiltration of the walls with inflammatory cells, oedema, abscess and ulceration. On healing it is replaced by squamous epithelium. The infection may extend downwards. It leads to narrowing and distortion of bronchioles and repeated infections lead ultimately to the destruction and scarring. The infection may extend to the alveoli causing damage to the alveolar walls. It may lead to fibrosis without disturbing its architecture.[3] These patients become respiratory cripples from severe airways obstruction and they may not exhibit any structural emphysema. Others (20 to 25%) may develop mild to moderately severe emphysema, due to the destructive mechanism from recurrent micro-abscesses at the junction of bronchioles and alveoli. It contains a mixture of centriacinar and panacinar emphysema. The distribution is irregular. The major site of airflow obstruction is small airways. The secretions, infection and bronchospasm cause great disability in these sites unlike the disease that is confined to the larger airways. The onset of emphysema leads to a progressive reduction in effective alveolar surface.

There is a relation between mucous gland enlargement (volume density of mucous glands) and sputum production, but no significant relation between the FEV_1 and either the volume of sputum production or any of the indices of mucous gland enlargement.[17]

Emphysema

It is defined morphologically as a condition of the lung characterised by abnormal permanent enlargement of the airspaces distal to the terminal bronchioles (acinus: respiratory bronchiole, alveolar ducts, alveolar sacs and alveoli) accompanied by the destruction of their walls and without obvious fibrosis.[18] Pathological features of emphysema are listed in Table 7.3.

Table 7.3: Pathological features of emphysema

1. Loss of alveolar capillary bed
2. Abnormal, permanent enlargement of air spaces distal to terminal bronchioles.

Due to destruction of alveolar septa, total surface area for gas exchange is reduced alongside loss of alveolar capillary bed. Hence there is reduced diffusion capacity, although lung volume is increased. Elastic recoil property of the lung is also reduced.

Emphysema forms a respiratory airspace enlargement without fibrosis. Differential diagnosis include Down's syndrome or congenital lobar hyperinflation where acinus enlargement pattern is without any destruction. Nevertheless, airspace enlargement with fibrosis can occur in fibrotic states such as interstitial fibrosis, tuberculosis, sarcoidosis etc.

Airspace enlargement may develop due to hypoplasia of alveoli, atrophy of the alveolar walls, overinflation or and destruction of the alveolar wall.[19]

Because of alveolar septal destruction, total gas exchange surface is reduced, alongwith loss of alveolar capillary bed. Thus, despite increased lung volume, diffusion capacity is reduced. Elastic recoil property of lung is also reduced. Emphysema is an important subcategory of respiratory airspace enlargement without fibrosis. However, airspace enlargement with fibrosis can be seen in interstitial fibrosis, tuberculosis, sarcoidosis etc.

With advancing age there is thinning of the alveolar walls resulting in the enlargement of alveoli and bronchioles. Though there is reduction in the surface area of the alveoli, it does not cause any disability. The total lung capacity remains the same, without any airways obstruction. These atrophic conditions are seen classically in the aged lung (senile emphysema).

The overdistension, a relatively benign condition, is characteristically seen in compensatory emphysema. The air passages and air spaces undergo inflation following removal of a lung or a lobe. It is also seen in the collapse of the lung. There is neither parenchymal destruction, nor any airways obstruction. It does not cause severe functional disturbances. Such an over-distension of air space is also seen following foreign bodies inhalation but it is associated with airways obstruction. In emphysema the lesions develop in the following manner, enlargement of some alveoli in the acinus; loss of alveoli on the respiratory bronchioles; fusion of enlarged alveoli into tiny cysts, formation of pyramidal cysts from fusion of respiratory bronchioles with its alveolar ducts and sacs; and, collapse of respiratory bronchioles. The fusion of cysts progresses in a centripetal direction.[5]

Emphysema is further classified into three subtypes, according to the part of the acinus involved: (i) Centriacinar (proximal acinar, centrilobular) affecting the center of the secondary lobules; (ii) Panacinar (paraseptal or distal acinar) affecting the entire acinus; (iii) Periacinar (Paraseptal or distal acinar) affecting the periphery of the acini and the part related to lobar septa.

More than one morphological variety of emphysema may be present at one time in lung with emphysema. Centriacinar and panacinar subtypes are most important varieties[20] and are generally found (mixed morphological pattern) together in patients with bronchitis and emphysema, thus suggesting the likelihood of a common pathogenesis.

Centriacinar Emphysema

This primarily affects the proximal part of the acinus. There is destruction of the walls of respiratory bronchioles of the first or second order as well as of peribronchiolar alveoli and of the alveolar ducts and they are converted into abnormal air spaces. Generally they are surrounded by some normal lung parenchyma. These changes vary from acinus to acinus and lobule to lobule. Cut surface of the lung exhibits multiple punched out holes and are separated by a relatively normal lung. Upper zones are commonly affected and it may even be noted uniformly throughout the lung. Centrilobular emphysema is the most common form of centriacinar emphysema, seen commonly in smokers,[21] which occurs mostly in men and is associated with chronic bronchitis. The bronchioles supplying the air spaces generally exhibit inflammation (bronchiolitis). There is peribronchiolar infiltration with polymorphs or lymphocytes or they may even be obliterated.[5] Such airways cause air-trapping from expiratory collapse of the bronchial wall. The inhalation of coal dust also cause dilation of respiratory bronchioles with accumulation of dust-laden macrophages in and around respiratory bronchioles (focal emphysema).

Panacinar Emphysema

This destructive emphysema affects all components of the acinus in a uniform manner. The wall of alveolar ducts and alveoli are also destroyed. There is total disorganisation of acinar architecture that results in large airspaces of acinar architecture of irregular size and shape which compress the respiratory bronchioles during expiration. The condition does not exhibit presence of any normal alveoli. Though the changes occur in an unselective manner, these changes begin at the lung basis. The condition may occur with centrilobular emphysema, in smoker's lungs.[5] There is bronchiolar obliteration without any evidence of inflammation, 60 to 70 per cent of the affected individuals are male. Panacinar emphysema is commonly associated with $alpha_1$ antiprotease (antitrypsin) deficiency[20] young. Patients may or may not be smokers.[21] Such patients are homozygous for the deficiency state (Pi type 22). Heterozygous patients (Pi type MZ) though do have diminished level of $alpha_1$ antiprotease, may not have increased tendency for emphysema when compared to normal persons (Pi type MM).[22]

Paraseptal or Distal Acinar Emphysema

The distal part of the acinus, alveolar ducts and sacs are predominantly involved. Since the distal acinus abuts on pleura, vessels and airways, emphysema is more severe in those areas. There is no airways obstruction. The condition manifests spontaneous pneumothorax or bullous disease of the lung.[5]

The lace-like architecture of the normal lung is destroyed resulting in a loss of gas exchanging surface. The loss of elastic recoil results in poor emptying. During expiration there is collapse of bronchioles due to loss of elasticity of the supporting lung and loss of tethering effect of alveolar attachment. It acts like a flap valve and does not allow air to get out. The intra-alveolar pressure thus rises during expiration which further leads to disruption and destruction of alveolar walls.

The basic defect in emphysema is elastic fragmentation of alveolar architecture. Expiration is normally a passive process and it is dependent on elastic recoil of the lungs from their inspiratory inflating. In emphysema, the morphological changes result in premature narrowing or collapse of airways or both during expiration. Thus, expiration remains no longer a passive event. There is airflow obstruction due to extramural bronchial compression and collapse caused by overdistended alveoli in which air has been trapped during expiration. Lung volumes change due to loss of elasticity and expiratory obstruction. T.L.C. and R.V. are increased. There is decrease in the surface area of the capillary bed.[5]

Variants of Emphysema

Macleod's Swyer-James's syndrome—A unilateral emphysema may be an incidental X-ray finding. The airways are normal both in number and structure but the alveoli are reduced. This occurs before the age of 8 years when alveoli are normally increasing in number. This is not a true emphysema as overdistension and alveolar septal destruction is not present. Repeated infections press for surgical excision.

Scar Emphysema

Overdistension and alveolar septal destruction in the lung regions surrounding scar tissue is called scar emphysema. If present along the borders of acinus, it is called paraseptal emphysema that may predispose to spontaneous pneumothorax.

Congenital Lobar Emphysema

A rare form where infants develop a check valve mechanism in lobar bronchus which leads to immediate overdistension, which is life threatening.

Bronchiolitis Obliterans

A widespread inflammatory and fibrotic destruction of small airways, which was thought to be due to parainfluenza viral infections in children, has recently been described in adults with rheumatoid arthritis. Response to bronchodilators is poor and fatal respiratory failure occurs within 2 years. Huge airways obstruction may develop, complicate without the evidence of this syndrome in the recipient of bone marrow transplants.

Small Airways Disease

Many pathologic changes are noted in the peripheral conducting airways (non-alveolated airways of less than 2 mm internal diameter and the respiratory bronchioles) of the lungs in patients with COPD and the term *small airways disease* has been applied to describe them.[23] Inflammation, fibrosis, smooth muscle hypertrophy, pigment depositing in the airways walls, goblet cell metaplasia and desquamation of the epithelium of the terminal bronchioles and inflammatory changes in the respiratory bronchioles lead to a marked increase in airflow resistance causing airflow obstruction. Small airways disease appears to play a more important role than chronic bronchitis in causing airflow obstruction.

The development of small airways disease has been associated with exposure to cigarette smoking which is also associated with the development of emphysema and chronic bronchitis. If smoking is stopped in the early stages of the disease, the inflammation is reversible. The abnormality in small airways contributes to mild spirometric and other functional abnormalities in young smokers. The progression of the disease leads to squamous cell metaplasia and fibrosis of the bronchial walls. It results ultimately in airflow limitation in advanced COPD.[15]

There is obstruction and marked slowing of forced expiration (FEV_1) which can happen from: (i) loss of elastic recoil of the lung allowing marked narrowing of airways during expiration, and (ii) from narrowing in the bronchitis in the form of inflammation, mucous gland hypertrophy and accumulation of mucus. There is premature airways closure to cause marked airtrapping (increased RV) and loss of elastic recoil of lung (increased TLC, increased RV/TLC). Around the scar tissue which has resulted from inflammation, infection and infiltration (granuloma, silicosis), emphysematous changes develop irregularly. However, the condition is rarely symptomatic.

Patient with chronic bronchitis may be disabled from airways obstruction and die of cor pulmonale without any evidence of emphysema at autopsy, although a quarter of the cases develop emphysema. Nevertheless, there may be severe emphysema clinically without any accompanying chronic bronchitis as in primary emphysema. On the other hand, primary emphysema may coexist in some chronic bronchitis, where the latter is not responsible for the structural emphysema.

Pathogenesis

It is believed from the days of Laennec that emphysema occurs due to mechanical overdistension of the lung tissue. Also frequently it may arise from inflammation and infection and can even be enzyme-induced emphysema. Centriacinar emphysema arises following an early bronchiolitis. There occurs inflammation of the bronchioles and a significant number of neutrophils in the alveoli arising from respiratory bronchioles can be seen. This condition is seen in males predominantly over 40 years of age. Air pollution and tobacco smoking are the provocative factors.[24] Tobacco smoke attracts a large number of alveolar macrophages to collect around small terminal bronchioles. They release neutrophil chemotactic factors which attract polymorphonuclear leucocytes to that site. Polymorphs then release a proteolytic enzyme, human neutrophil elastase which initiates the tissue destruction. This can lyse all the macromolecules forming the lung interstitium: elastin, collagen, proteoglycans, fibronectin and laminin. This enzyme activity of human neutrophil elastase is prevented during health by alpha$_1$ protease inhibitor molecule close to its binding site for elastase. The oxidants present in cigarette smoke oxidise the methionine, thereby rendering elastase inactive.

Thus emphysema may be caused by an imbalance of proteases and antiproteases in the lung. However, distinct biochemical abnormality without much inflammation is shown only in patients with homozygous alpha$_1$ antiprotease deficiency. Apart from cigarette smoke, there are some unknown risk factors or some structural abnormalities in the lung accounting for the effects of smoking.[5]

Possible mechanisms of airway obstruction: The resistance of the peripheral bronchi and bronchioles is much less compared to larger airways is normal individuals. The resistance in the peripheral airways is greatly increased in obstructive pulmonary disease. This appears to occur from three different mechanisms such as: (i) loss of lung elastic recoil, (ii) destruction of alveolar support, and (iii) inflammation in the airways, and they develop in the background of heavy tobacco smoking.[25]

There is a loss of elastic recoil of the lungs in emphysema and destruction of supporting alveolar attachments, leading to airways narrowing. The chronic inflammatory process in the airways causes thickening of the wall and narrowing of the lumen of the distal airways, rather than the changes in the lung parenchyma.[14]

The inflammatory process causes vascular congestion and damage to the mucus-secreting epithelium of the airways. There is shedding of the epithelial cells and excess secretion of mucus. There occurs exudation of plasma and cells from the vascular spaces migrate into the interstitial spaces at the site of damage. There is release of potent mediators from plasma-derived proteins such as the complement, kinin, and coagulation from fibrinolytic systems and from mast cells which control the exudation. Polymorphonuclear leucocytes and mononuclear cells migrate into the damaged site, followed by organisation of the exudate. Metaplasic replacement of shed epithelium occurs by either squamous or goblet cells. The smooth muscle and sub epithelial connective tissue show hyperplasia leading to contraction of the tissue and fixed narrowing of the airway lumen.

Thus, COPD requires cessation of smoking, removal of irritants and adequate medical therapy. Air contaminate with tobacco smoke causes low grade continuous inflammation which may be overwhelming in those with deficiency of serum antiproteolytic enzymes.

Factors affecting the course of disease (COPD) are listed in Table 7.4.

Table 7.4: Factors affecting the course of the disease (COPD)

1. Cessation of smoking
2. Removal of irritants
3. Adequate medical therapy for acute exacerbation

Pulmonary Hypertension in COPD

The process of progressive elevation of pulmonary arterial pressure starts early but manifests in severe COPD.

Pulmonary vascular bed is reduced due to an extensive destruction of the parenchyma of the lung. The arterioles and capillaries undergo destruction in the process. The airways obstruction results in the elevation of the mean intra-alveolar pressure especially during expiration. It causes compression of the pulmonary arterioles thereby increasing the pulmonary vascular resistance. BODE index used in assessing COPD shows a positive corelation with number of exacerbations and development of pulmonary hypertension.

Three factors namely hypoxaemia, hypercapnia and acidaemia noted in the course of chronic bronchitis have a great functional effect. The hypoxaemia noted episodically during acute infective exacerbations causes pulmonary hypertension by its vasoconstrictor effect at the level of small arteries and arterioles. Progressive rise in pulmonary arterial pressure is commonly accompanying COPD. Several mechanisms interplay such as loss of vascular bed, hypoxemia induced erythrocytosis and hyperviscosity and many other contributing factors. Later with exacerbations, it becomes widespread. Persistence of hypoxia when hypoxia has persisted for a long time has distinctly effected the walls of the vessels. The muscular pulmonary arteries undergo thickening of their walls, without intimal fibrosis. The arterioles closely related to the airspaces undergo marked thickening with an appearance of smooth muscle in their walls and thickening of elastic laminae. As the disease progresses and involves widespread regions, the structural changes appear more and more.

High $PaCO_2$ tension and acidosis also contribute in the production of pulmonary hypertension. Polycythaemia is seen in a small group of chronic bronchitis as a compensatory mechanism to increase the oxygen carrying capacity of the blood. It also contributes to accentuation of hypertension by increasing the viscosity of the blood. It may lead to enhanced tendency for thrombosis. Novel therapies include tyrosine kinase inhibitors and autologous endothelial progenitor cells in the treatment of pulmonary artery hypertension.[26]

Chronic bronchitis alone or in combination with emphysema is able to produce cor pulmonale. As chronic bronchitis is associated with severe blood gas abnormalities, the heart failure develops early. The hypoxia leads to the occurrence of pulmonary hypertension. Hypoxia also reduces proficiency of myocardium. The right ventricular hypertrophy (cor pulmonale) and its ultimate failure occurs because of the increased work-load against rising pressure.

Cor pulmonale occurs in diseases affecting the parenchyma of the lung (chronic bronchitis bronchiectasis, asthma, emphysema and fibrosis) or its vasculature (massive or recurrent small thromboembolism) or from the abnormalities of thoracic cage (Kyphoscoliosis). The cardiac output is normal or slightly reduced when the heart is affected in bronchitis.

Clinical Features

The initial features of COPD are commonly cough and expectoration to be followed by appearance of wheeze and dyspnoea. The condition generally referred as *smoker's cough* and lasts for many years without causing much disability. It starts worsening during winter with cough and sputum, steadily increasing in its severity in succeeding winters. There is no history of haemoptysis. There is sometimes tightness in the chest. The patient begins to cough out large quantities of sputum in the morning and also during the night while lying down. The quantity of sputum increases during exacerbations and infections, becoming mucopurulent or purulent in character. Streaky hemoptysis is also known. COPD exacerbation can occur by presence or worsening of left ventricular diastolic dysfunction and may have reversible myocardial ischemia. Breathlessness increases, as the disease advances, and is relatively constant unlike the day-to-day variability noted in bronchial asthma.

Chronic airways obstruction can be categorised as chronic bronchitis and emphysema.[20] Bronchitis shows marked involvement of airways with less marked anatomical abnormality unlike emphysema. There is hypoventilation and retention of carbon dioxide. The emphysematous patient associated with destruction of the lung, is able to hyperventilate to keep $PaCO_2$ down either to normal or below normal level until late in the course of the disease. During the course of the disease the patient though may progress to either direction, many exist as an intermediate group between these two polar forms of the disease.[15] However, five distinct clinical phenotypes of airways disease have been defined by cluster analysis to form basis of a modified taxonomy for disorders of airways obstruction (Eurp. Resp. J; 2009; April 8).

The essential anatomical and functional abnormality seen in chronic bronchitis is the chronic airflow limitation leading to poor alveolar ventilation. There is history of smoking and air pollution. The condition manifests with cough and expectoration showing exacerbations during winter because of recurrent infection. Recurrence of such episodes lead to cor pulmonale later. Often these patients are obese, plethoric and do not appear obviously short of breath. As they get used to high level $PaCO_2$, they are not distressed. These patients are able to walk and continue to work. They are prone to greater risk of chest infection that precipitates hypoxia and cardiac failure. They complain of headache and become disoriented and progressively drowsy that may lead to coma. The hypoventilation and mismatched ventilation and perfusion leads to arterial hypoxaemia (PaO_2 45 to 50 mm Hg or even less) with CO_2 retention (50 to 60 mm Hg or even high) while breathing room air. This gives rise to blue and bloated appearance of an advanced chronic bronchitis patient. The patient becomes cyanotic. Central cyanosis occurs which can be best appreciated on the out-stretched tongue seen in good light. It indicates an arterial oxygen desaturation with atleast 1.5 gm of reduced haemoglobin in 100 ml of arterial blood.[20]

Emphysema patient is able to keep $PaCO_2$ level down by fighting for breath and often show visible dyspnoea. The condition starts with middle age and there is exertional dyspnoea. It progresses slowly and is often present even when at rest. If the patient is a smoker, there may be a history of cough and sputum.[5] On examination, the breath sounds are weak, there is no wheeze neither any added sounds in the chest.

By virtue of increased respiratory efforts, these emphysema patients washout PCO_2 in the blood. They may have erythrocytosis. But despite hypoxemia, they donot show cyanosis. There is tachypnoea, with prominent accessory muscles. Pink and puffing implies to such patients. The condition is rarely seen in women. There is hardly any cyanosis or oedema. They hold the chest in a state of inspiration and encourage breathing with the use of accessory muscles to keep the chest blown to make it as large as possible to breathe the tidal volume. There is a downward and lateral pull from the diaphragm. With an effort, the patient is able to keep the chest against the elastic recoil.[15] When the muscle exhaustion sets in and the patient becomes highly short of breath and finds it difficult to carry on with his routine.

The clinical chest examination reveals generalised restriction of the movements. Due to airflow obstruction, the accessory muscles of respiration are active. The sternomastoid, scalenus anterior and trapezius muscles contract to move the whole chest upwards and forwards during inspiration. The typical barrel shape or square chest with increased anteroposterior diameter may be seen in the later stages as evidence of emphysema. A barrel shaped chest may also result from airways obstruction with overinflation. Overinflated chest may not be seen in all the patients with chronic bronchitis. There is reduction of the cricosternal distance, bilateral inspiratory indrawing of supraclavicular fossae and intercostal spaces over the lower portion of the chest, and widening of the subcostal angle.[14] Overinflation may not be seen in bronchitis.

Patient becomes tachypnoic in emphysema. The chest is resonant on percussion with encroachment of a resonant note over hepatic and cardiac dullness. The breath sounds are generally distant and the expiratory phase is prolonged. Sometimes the breath sounds are inaudible; poor breath sounds reflect poor regional ventilation. Rhonchi may be heard over wide areas in the basal region and they are made audible on forced expiration. Basal crepitations are audible due to cardiac failure or from infections. On deep and rapid breathing with an open mouth, the breath sounds are heard distantly. Normally it is possible to empty the lung in four to five seconds, but a patient with airflow obstruction shows a prolonged expiratory time on auscultation, corresponding to the decrease in FEV_1 compared to normal emptying of lungs in 4-5 seconds.

The jugular veins stand filled during expiration due to a rise in the intrathoracic pressure to expel the air. The veins become engorged during inspiration, as heart failure develops. Transcutaneous jugular vein flow velocity measurement may be applicable to bedside prediction of pulmonary hypertension in COPD patients. The supraclavicular fossa and suprasternal fossa are hollowed out during inspiration from the fall in the intrathoracic pressure. The costal margin is drawn inwards (costal paradox) during inspiration due to inward traction from the low, flat everted diaphragm (Hoover's sign).[5]

Because of hyperinflation, the apical impulse is typically difficult to locate. Right ventricular heave is inconstant. There may be tachycardia. A collapsing pulse is noted when $PaCO_2$ level is high and the hands turn warm. The cardiac dullness is obliterated. The heart sounds are distant and are better audible in the epigastric region. The pulmonary component of the second sound is accentuated with the onset of pulmonary hypertension. The augmented atrial contraction leads to gallop rhythm and is heard in the lower end of the sternum during cardiac failure. The features of tricuspid incompetency may appear.

The liver may be palpable by descent of diaphragm or may be enlarged and tender as an evidence of heart failure. Finger clubbing is not a feature. Oedema, disproportionate to the degree of elevated venous pressure, is present. Fundoscopy may reveal engorged veins and papilloedema due to CO_2 retention and raised C.S.F. pressure. In terminal stage, muscles get fatigued of exacerbated workload, CO_2 starts getting retained in the system, with concomitant development of co-pulmonale and right ventricular failure. Response to treatment fails and patient needs ventilation support to tide over the crisis.

Clinical symptoms of acute respiratory failure appear as a result of the precipitating event and others due to hypoxaemia and hypercapnia. Muscle twitching and tremors in outstretched hands are due to respiratory failure. Other features of CO_2 retention include high volume pulse, sweating, progressive drowsiness with subsequent occurrence of coma with abdominal distension and paralytic ileus. These signs and symptoms occur from chronic airway narrowing with forced expiratory volume in first one second in patients with even mild airway disease and should lead to suspicion of alveolar hypoventilation.[15]

Evaluation of COPD mainly include the following:

1. Pulmonary function tests.
2. Blood gas analysis.
3. Haemodynamic profile.

Spirometry is useful in COPD in making diagnosis, assessing severity, response to drug treatment and lung age, detecting upper airway obstruction and also in making preoperative pulmonary evaluation. In cases of asthma/COPD overlapping, certain biomarkers such as sputum cytology and cytokine analysis, measuring fraction of exhaled nitric oxide, and proteomics and gene expression microassays and additionally CRP, plasma fibrinogen, interleukin-6 and other cytokines and copeptins are useful.

Pulmonary Functional Abnormality

Normally expiration is a passive event and expiratory airflow is limited by the mechanical properties of the lung and airways over the lower 75 per cent of the vital capacity. Maximal expiratory flow is directly proportional to the elastic recoil of the lungs from their inspiratory inflation and inversely proportional to the airways resistance. Pulmonary elastic tissue is fragmented causing disruption of alveolar architecture in emphysema, which causes airway narrowing or collapse or both during expiration. Expiration remains no longer a passive event. The airways have lost support from radial traction by the elastic parenchyma.

The condition is associated with increased airway resistance or decreased elastic recoil or both, flow rates at all lung volumes during maximal forced expiration are generally below than normal. The degree of airflow limitation is assessed either from the spirogram plot of forced expiratory volume against time.

The main functional disturbance in chronic bronchitis is airflow limitation which is generalised due to obstruction from the secretions in the lumen of the bronchi and its narrowing by the hypertrophy of mucous glands. A short course of corticosteroids will be beneficial in chronic bronchitis to note the existence of reversibility of airways obstruction. As the disease progresses, airways obstruction becomes fixed due to gross distortion of bronchial passages, infection and fibrosis. Emphysema if present, adds further to the airways obstruction. The natural retractibility of the lung is, thus, decreased due to loss of elasticity.

FVC (forced vital capacity), FEV_1 and MEFR (maximum mid-expiratory flow rate, forced expiratory flow measurement over the mid-50 per cent of vital capacity) and peak flow are useful to detect the airflow limitation. There is reduction in FEV_1 in less than 80% and FEV_1/FVC ratio is less than 70 per cent indicating airways obstruction. It declines further with the progress of the disease. The patient takes a longer time to expel the vital capacity forcibly from the chest. The airflow limitation is considered severe if FEV_1 is less than 50 per cent of the predicted value where the patient experiences exertional dyspnoea. The patient will have dyspnoea at rest when FEV_1 less than 1 litre, and the FEV_1/FVC ratio is markedly low (around 30 per cent). MVV and MEFR are also diminished due to obstruction to airflow. Peak expiratory flow rate (PEFR) is low. Repeat daily measurement of PEFR shows little variability.[5]

The bedside airflow obstruction is measured by forced expiratory time (the time taken to perform a complete forced expiration after a maximal inspiration). Such a forced vital capacity is measured by placing the diaphragm of the stethoscope over the cervical trachea. Normally airflow is complete in 3 seconds or less. It takes a longer time in airflow obstruction.

Lungs are over-inflated in emphysema. The total lung capacity (TLC) and RV (residual volume) are increased due to air-trapping and alveolar distension. RV/TLC ratio is also increased in emphysema. Alveolar fragmentation leads to decrease in surface area of the capillary bed in emphysema which is evident by a reduction of diffusing capacity for carbon monoxide.

Therefore, inspiratory flow rates remain normal. The bronchi are anatomically of normal caliber in emphysema. In chronic bronchitis, inflammatory changes in the bronchial wall result in a narrowing of the bronchial lumen. Excessive production of viscous mucus results in expiratory obstruction as in emphysema but also inspiratory obstruction. Lung volumes remain essentially preserved, so also the diffusing capacity for carbon monoxide.[5]

Gold staging of severity of COPD is as follows:

Stage	Severity	Manifestative chronic cough sputum production	FEV_1/FVC	FEV_1% predicted
0	At risk	— ±	< 70%	> 80%
I	Mild			
II	Moderate	+	< 70%	< 80%
III	Severe	++	< 70%	< 50%
IV	Very severe	+++	< 70%	< 30%

Gas Exchange

In chronic bronchitis there is diffuse bronchial narrowing and mucus plugging are responsible for marked abnormalities in gas exchange. It causes alveolar hypoxaemia and hypercapnia that result in pulmonary hypertension. Any acute exacerbation causing deterioration of gas exchange results in an acute increase in pulmonary hypertension. It leads to right ventricular hypertrophy, right ventricular failure and oedema. Such patients are referred to as *blue bloaters.*

Because of the anatomic abnormalities the regional changes in ventilation are matched by regional changes in perfusion in emphysema, the pulmonary gas exchange is preserved. These patients maintain normal or near normal arterial oxygenation by hyperventilation, despite moderate to severe dyspnoea. Often they are called *pink puffers.* A pink puffers will have a large dead space whereas blue bloater will have a large blood flow to the alveoli receiving little ventilation (physiologic shunt).[5] In them, mild-to-moderate hypoxaemia exists. There is an increased alveolar air to arterial blood oxygen difference (A-aO_2), signifying poor distribution of ventilation with respect to perfusion.

Despite hypercapnoea, the respiratory drive is not augmented in chronic bronchitis as respiratory centre is lazy. Hypoxemia is only the stimulus working in such patients. Over correction of hypoxemia with uncontrolled oxygen therapy may cause further depression and even respiratory arrest in these patients. Similarly use of respiratory depressants/sedatives can lead to respiratory failure and carbonacosis. Since respiratory centre is alert and alive in emphysema, the phenomenon is unlikely in these patients.

Estimation of arterial blood gases confirms respiratory failure in COPD. Hyperaemia and hypercapnia are present both in acute and chronic respiratory failure. In acute respiratory failure there is acidosis, exhibiting low pH while in chronic respiratory failure, pH is near normal as bicarbonate is retained to compensate for high $PaCO_2$. An elevated $PaCO_2$ results in a fall in pH and respiratory acidosis. If there is persistence of hypercarbia, kidneys compensate by excretion of hydrogen ions and reabsorption of bicarbonate, leading to rise in plasma bicarbonate. When respiratory failure develops suddenly, the rise in $PaCO_2$ is associated with only a slight rise in bicarbonate, which is not sufficient to prevent a fall in pH, while a gradually developing respiratory failure gives time for renal compensatory changes.[15] Hence there is an increase in bicarbonate and usually a near normal pH.[19]

Investigations

Radiology

Chest X-ray is normal in early stages of chronic bronchitis. The changes are seen in about 15 per cent of cases following the onset of emphysema. Chest X-ray may remain normal even with advanced disease.

In panacinar emphysema and in advanced disease, an increased translucency is observed. The diaphragm is low and flat with maximum curvature of the right dome, less than 1.5 cm, and is invariably below the anterior end of the seventh rib or lower. The intercostal spaces are wide and so is the retrosternal translucent area (normal 2.5 cm). The cardiac silhouette is long and narrow with normal or prominent hilar vessels. Sometimes the pulmonary trunk is prominent. The peripheral vascular markings are small and thin in the lung fields. These alterations are not uniform and different zones are affected to a variable extent. In widespread emphysema, the vessel changes are seen in more than four zones. There may be complete local loss of vessels in a well-demarcated hyperlucent zone as in bulla or in an ill-defined bullous area. There is an arterial deficiency pattern in the upper zones in centriacinar emphysema and in the lower zone in panacinar emphysema.[5]

The features of emphysema get obscured with the onset of heart failure. The cardiac shadow appears enlarged with dilation of pulmonary trunk. A chink of air below the apex or inferior cardiac surface could be present, the apex of heart may also appear slightly lucent. Features commonly associated with cor pulmonale have been listed in the Table 7.5.

The presence of pulmonary artery hypertension, the width of right descending (interlobar) pulmonary artery in an upright chest radiograph in the postero-anterior projection exceeds 16 mm.[26] The width of 20 mm or more helps in separating patients with pulmonary hypertension from those without hypertension.[27]

The normal clouding of the lungs, noted during expiration, does not appear on screening, because of air-trapping from airways obstruction. There is marked reduction in the excursion of the diaphragm.

Bronchography reveals marked distortion, dilatation and irregularity of the bronchial tree. The bronchial lumen is narrowed with peripheral poor filling. The ducts of mucous glands often are filled with radio-opaque material. Bronchiography is not advised in cases with marked airways obstruction, specially in chronic bronchitis.

Computed tomography (CT) is more sensitive than chest radiography and can be obtained during breath-holding at end-inspiration. It demonstrates the presence of areas of abnormally low attenuation in emphysema. The pixels in the display with low-density values are highlighted by white dots.[15] In emphysema the total lung size increases due to overinflation. The destruction and dilation of terminal airspaces result in a decrease in lung density.[28]

Sputum Examination

Presence of pus in the sputum is considered as the outward sign of bacterial infection. It may be purulent, mucopurulent or mucoid. Treatment with antibiotics causes disappearance of purulence while the mucoid sputum does not require any treatment with antibiotics.

The bacterial species usually found are H. influenzae and S. pneumoniae. Other organisms known to produce acute exacerbations are S. viridans, Staph. aureus, Klebsiella, and B. catarrhalis. The sputum is sent for culture and sensitivity to various antibiotics.[29]

Electrocardiogram

ECG offers a good diagnostic screening test in addition to other clinical investigations in COPD patients. Changes of non-ischemic etiology such as COPD include p-pulmonale, rightward displacement of QRS and T-wave axes, low voltage QRS in limb leads and S_1 S_2 S_3 pattern with large S-waves in V_5, V_6.

With cardiac involvement in cases of COPD, electrocardiogram shows clockwise rotation of the heart, right axis deviation. R/S pattern in chest leads, peaked 'p' waves, qR pattern in AVR and V_1, ratio of R/S less than 1 in V_5, prominent S wave in L_1 and incomplete right bundle branch block.[30]

Haematologic Changes

An increase in red cells may occur due to secondary erythromytosis polycythemia. Noctural hypoxaemia may lead

Table 7.5: Chronic cor pulmonale: Import ant radiological signs

1. In PA view:	(a)	Bulge in the region of main pulmonary artery, along the left border of heart, below the pulmonary artery.
	(b)	Widening of heart shadow in the region of conus.
	(c)	Prominence of hila due to posteroanterior enlargement.
	(d)	Pulmonary emphysema usually present.
	(e)	Transverse cardiac diameter is not increased.
2. In the right anterior oblique position:	(a)	Anterior bulge of conus.
	(b)	Increased oval density of pulmonary trunk at its bifurcation.
	(c)	Encroachment by heart upon retrosternal space.
	(d)	Lack of significant displacement of oesophagus in the region of left atrium.
3. In the left anterior oblique position:	(a)	Encroachment on the retrosternal space by enlarged left ventricle.
	(b)	Interventricular groove displaced posteriorly and upwards.
	(c)	Increased circular density at the bifurcation of the pulmonary trunk.

to elevated haemoglobin concentration. The acute exacerbation due to infection may be reflected in leucocytosis and ESR may not be high in the presence of polycythemia.[5]

Serum Mg^{2+} levels are significantly lowered in acute exacerbation of COPD.

Complications

Complications of COPD occur as a consequence of structural and functional changes in the disease. These include:

a. Cor pulmonale.
b. Respiratory muscle dysfunction.
c. Acute exacerbation
   - Infective
   - Non-infective
   - Pneumothorax
   - Pulmonary embolism
   - Neuromuscular dysfunction (secondary to nutritional deficiency, hypothyroidism)
d. Respiratory failure with carbonarcosis

Pulmonary hypertension and cor pulmonale are the main complications. Pulmonary vascular bed is grossly reduced due to an extensive destruction of lung parenchyma. The arterioles and capillaries undergo destruction in the process. The airways obstruction results in elevation of the mean intra-alveolar pressure, especially during expiration. It causes compression of the pulmonary arterioles, hence the pulmonary vascular resistance is increased.

However, with the development of pulmonary artery hypertension and cor pulmonale, cardiomegaly with widening of cardiac shadow can be seen. Enlarged pulmonary trunk and increased bronchovascular markings can also be observed.

Triad of hypoxaemia, hypercapnia and acidaemia noted in the course of chronic bronchitis has a great functional effect. The hypoxaemia noted episodically during acute infective exacerbations causes pulmonary hypertension by its vaso-constrictor effect at the level of small arteries and arterioles. It is a very potent factor in the elevation of pulmonary artery pressure. Longstanding hypoxia has a direct effect on the walls of the vessels, causing thickening of the muscular pulmonary arteries. Widespread structural changes are noted with the progress of the disease. Raised arterial carbon dioxide tension and acidosis also contribute in the production of pulmonary hypertension. Thus chronic bronchitis or emphysema alone or in combination is able to produce cor pulmonale. Non-invasive tests including M-mode echocardiography have been extensively used to detect the presence of pulmonary hypertension. Higher prevalence of osteoporosis and osteopenia in advanced COPD patients has been observed.[31]

Cardiovascular Functions in COPD

COPD leads to severe haemodynamic consequences such as pulmonary artery hypertension. It occurs due to hypoxic pulmonary vasoconstriction mediated by contraction of smooth muscle in the walls of small pulmonary arterioles. Reduced pulmonary vascular surface area from structural derangement of the pulmonary parenchyma hypoxaemia—a potent pulmonary vasoconstrictor—further adds to pulmonary hypertension. Resting pulmonary arterial pressure in patients with COPD is inversely related to the level of arterial oxygen tension. Both acidosis (from elevated arterial CO_2 tension) as well as hypoxia acts synergistically to cause a significant increase in pulmonary artery pressure and pulmonary vascular resistance.

Raised pulmonary artery pressure and pulmonary vascular resistance induce an increased afterload that leads to right ventricular dilation and hypertrophy and ultimately to right-sided congestive cardiac failure. The right ventricular distension causes distortion of the geometry of the interventricular septum and impaired left ventricular ejection fraction.[15] Myocardial efficiency is also decreased because of hypoxia.

Breathing During Sleep in Patients with COPD

Sleep-onset insomnia with frequent or early morning awakenings or both is common in patients with COPD. There is worsening of hypoxaemia during sleep in patients with chronic airflow obstruction. It is particularly noted during REM sleep and hypoxaemia is more severe during periods of intense eye movements.[32] There can be mild hypercapnia.

In a sleeping COPD patient with hypoxaemia and hypercapnia alveolar hypoventilation occurs from a lowered ventilatory drive, decreased respiratory muscle tone and activity, increased work of breathing, reduced FRC, blunted hypercapnic ventilatory response and probably ventilation to perfusion mismatching. These factors contribute to sleep hypoxaemia.[33] This may be exacerbated in patients with concomitant sleep apnoea or nocturnal hypoventilation.

Significant cardiac and haemodynamic changes occur due to hypoxaemia. Pulmonary hypertension noted in COPD is due to nocturnal desaturation to some extent. A fall in SaO_2 (arterial oxygen saturation) by 1 per cent is likely to cause an elevation of pulmonary arterial pressure by 1 mm.[34] Effect of recurrent nocturnal oxygen desaturation, and to some extent, hypercapnia, together play a major role in the progression of the disease and development of pulmonary hypertension.[35] There is increased frequency of occurrence of premature ventricular contractions during sleep. These patients have an uncomfortable sleep and show arousals during episodes of desaturation.[36]

Respiratory Muscle Dysfunction in COPD

The increased resistance to airflow in COPD increases the work and energy needed for breathings. Hyperinflation imposes limitations on respiratory muscle function and there occurs mechanical disadvantage. Diaphragm, which plays a central role in normal breathing, is displaced downwards, therefore its operating length is shortened. Lung volume is increased and the inspiratory muscles are passively shortened by their own elasticity rather than by active contraction. Hence they are forced to function on the unfavourable portion of their length-tension curves.

About 2 per cent of their total oxygen is required for respiratory muscle function in a normal person while patients with COPD may require upto 60 per cent as the work of breathing is markedly increased. Accessory muscles of inspiration notably sternomastoid and scalene muscles swing into active operation to overcome the mechanical disadvantage, even at rest. The patient finds it harder to breathe, having rapid, and shallow breathing. There are asynchronous, alternating and paradoxical movements of the rib-cage and abdomen due to an increased respiratory load. The situation, if not relieved, leads to muscle fatigue and muscle failure.

Respiratory tract acute infection by viruses, mycoplasma and bacteria results in tracheobronchitis and pneumonia and is responsible for exhibiting either chronic or recurrent purulent sputum production. Bronchopulmonary infection possibly plays a role in the development of COPD as well as in its frequent exacerbations. During an acute exacerbation, there is change in the colour or consistency of sputum or increase in cough and amount of sputum. Increasing dyspnoea may be present in many; however, fever, chills or signs of systemic toxicity or leucocytosis may not be present.

Sputum cultures often yield Streptococcus pneumoniae and Haemophilus influenzae during the episodes of purulent sputum production. Electrolyte disturbance, hypothyroidism, nutritional deficiency and neuromuscular dysfunction do contribute to acute exacerbations in COPD.

Acute exacerbations can be linked to viral infections during winter. Inhalation of irritants such as cold air, smoke, ozone, sulphur dioxide, nitrogen dioxide, pollens and moulds can result in acute inflammation.

Respiratory Failure in COPD

Respiratory failure in COPD develops either due to increased workload for breathing which is abnormally exacerbated or due to neuromuscular efficiency being further jeopardized.

Hypoventilation developing out of imbalance can lead to type II respiratory failure, possibly due to respiratory depression occurring from overzealous oxygen therapy or use of sedatives in COPD patient. Even aminoglycoside induced neuromuscular weakness can lead to CO_2 retension.

However, in many instances, ventilation perfusion mismatch that leads to primary type I respiratory failure may go to type II. Retained secretions, infection pneumothorax, pulmonary embolism etc. commonly act as precipitating factors for ventilation perfusion mismatch. Degree of distress or disability largely depends on the dimension of precipitating event and the functional status of the patient.

Pneumothorax

Pneumothorax is less common, but the resultant lung collapse can cause further elevation of already increased pulmonary arterial pressure by direct vascular compression and hypoxic reflex constriction of vessels on the affected side. Blood flow of the unaffected side is diverted and may result in elevation of pulmonary arterial pressure. The increased intrathoracic pressure from tension pneumothorax impedes venous return, decreasing preload to the right heart which in turn exhibits a decreased ability to pump blood through the pulmonary vascular bed.[3]

Pulmonary Embolism

Inactivity in patients with cor pulmonale make them prone to an increased risk of development of pulmonary embolism that may result in profound dyspnoea which is unresponsive to bronchodilators. Every patient of pulmonary hypertension or right ventricular dysfunction in COPD must be looked for pulmonary embolism.

Acute exacerbations in COPD may also occur secondary to electrolyte disturbance, neuromuscular dysfunction, hypothyroidism and nutrients' deficiency.

Carbon Dioxide Narcosis

Narcotic analgesics, sedatives and hypnotics are respiratory depressants. They lead to decreased central respiratory drive and subsequent hypoventilation. Uncontrolled administration of oxygen to a patient with COPD, retaining CO_2 results in severe hypoxaemia and carbon dioxide narcosis. Hypoventilation leads to hypercapnia and acidosis. A metabolic alkalosis compensating for chronic hypoventilation-induced respiratory acidosis may also be seen in patients with severe COPD. It gets worsened with administration of diuretics which cause chloride deficit. It contributes to a depression of ventilatory drive and increased retention of CO_2.[5] Comorbidities in COPD are listed in Table 7.6.

Table 7.6: Comorbidities in COPD
• Cardiovascular disease
• Skeletal muscle dysfunction
• Insulin resistance
• Osteoporosis (in almost 70%)
• Depression
• Anemia

Prevention

There is no reservation in saying that chronic obstructive pulmonary disease is essentially preventable. Cessation of cigarette smoking and control of atmospheric pollution works. Cigarette smoking causes, maintains and aggravates COPD. On discontinuation of smoking, beneficial effects like decrease in airway irritation, decreased production of sputum and decrease in coughing can be obtained. Continued smoking deteriorates the respiratory functions and ultimately meet a fatal end. As health and disease go hand in hand and doctors are meant for both,[37] doctors can play a significant role in guiding their patients. The patients can well be persuaded to stop smoking. Honb'le Supreme Court orders may prove an excellent surrogate step to control tobacco use in the society.[38]

Patients can be benefited by shifting from polluted environment or changing the employment. As infections cause an exacerbation of the disease, and are usually responsible for irreversible progression of the disease, protection of the chronic bronchitis against influenza with flu vaccine annually, may reduce the chance of an acute exacerbation.

An intermediate deficiency of alpha[1] antiprotease (heterozygous) should be detected at an early age as these persons can be protected from development of the disease.[39] Like others they should be advised to avoid smoking and dusty occupations and promptly given antibiotics for any infections. Genetic counselling has its place in these patients.[5,15] Preventive measures have been listed in Table 7.7.

Table 7.7: Preventive measures for chronic airflow limitation (CAL)

1. Prevention of precipitating and risk factors
2. Prevention of progression of CAL
3. Prevention of acute exacerbations
4. Prevention of complications particularly cor pulmonale

Management[5]

Tobacco smoke has been the chief culprit in COPD. Therefore, deterioration of patients with COPD as well as deterioration in their lung functions can be prevented by cessation of smoking by control of atmospheric pollution and by treatment of symptoms with drugs like bronchodilators, antibiotics and oxygen. Again treatment mainly stresses on stoppage of smoking in total. Spirometric early detection of asymptomatic smokers for COPD ultimately reduces the burden of disease.[40] Goals of therapy and treatment strategies are listed in Table 7.8.

Table 7.8: Goals and modalities of therapeutic strategy

Goals
a. Treat acute deteriorations or exacerbations.
b. Treat reversible components of the condition.
c. Prevent progression of chronic airflow limitation.
Modalities
1. Pharmacologic therapy
2. Pulmonary rehabilitation
3. Domiciliary management—home oxygen therapy
4. Care of comorbidities of complications

Bronchodilators

Beta-adrenergic bronchodilators, anticholinergic bronchodilators and corticosteroids can be administered in the form of aerosol to relieve airways obstruction. The fine particles of medication (1 to 5 millimicrons) get deposited by gravitational sedimentation in all parts of the lungs following administration by pressurised meterdose inhaler (MDI). Aerosols can be produced by jet nebulisers or ultrasonic nebulisers to give most efficient delivery of inhaled drugs to the lungs.

The aerosol is released from a sealed canister at some distance from the open mouth. A steady inhalation has to be synchronized with actuation. A slow, deep inspiration should be followed by holding breath for an optimal period of 10 seconds to allow sedimentation. This enables nearly 10 per cent of the drug to reach the lungs. Those who find difficulty in activating MDI at the appropriate time, especially during an acute exacerbations of COPD, or patients who are usually dyspnoeic and tachypnoeic, a spacer (reservoir) device is used where patients fix MDI into the spacer before inhaling from it. This is useful for children and elderly patients.

Beta-adrenergic bronchodilators (salbutamol, terbutaline, orciprenaline, fenoterol) have bronchodilator effects by acting directly on the small muscle beta-adrenoceptors present in high density in small airways. The dose given by inhaler is smaller than that taken orally. Each puff of aerosol supplies the following concentrations of medication: Salbutamol 0.1mg, terbutaline 0.25 mg, orciprenaline 0.75 mg, fenoterol 0.2 mg, termiterol 0.2 mg and salmeterol 0.1 mg. They induce a significant bronchodilation. Long acting drugs have also come up, having action from 12 to 24 hours. To achieve success of inhalation therapy, fluticasone proprionate, as an anti-inflammatory, has been successfully used in combination with salmetrol.[41]

Salbutamol (2 to 4 mg) and terbutaline (5 mg) can be administered orally. The beta-2-agonists cause bronchodilation by relaxing the bronchial smooth muscle, increasing mucociliary transport and by inhibiting release of inflammatory bronchoconstrictor mediators. Tremors, nervousness and tachycardia occur as side effects. Such side effects are much less noticeable when they are administered by inhalation, as drug goes directly into the lungs and that, too, only 10% of the total drug administered.

Ipratropium: Acetylcholine stimulates muscarine receptors present in the smooth muscle of bronchial passages are stimulated resulting in bronchoconstriction and mucus secretion. The synthetic congener of atropine, ipratropium bromide, 18 mcg per puff, increases the airflow by cholinergic blockage. Prolonged bronchodilation is obtained by anticholinergic and beta-2 adrenergic in combination in COPD patients.[42]

$Beta_2$ receptors and anticholinergic receptors can cross-talk and may show some autonomy, synergy or could antagonise at times; i.e. is why B_2 agonists does not work at times and anticholenergics may offer better result than B_2 agonists in some situations.

Theophylline: In COPD by slow-release oral theophylline, continuous bronchodilation is provided by a sustained level of 10-20 mcg/ml in the serum throughout the 24 hours. Though absorption of theophylline is better on an empty stomach, it is often erratic due to poor solubility. Theophylline improves airways conductance. Generally the treatment is initiated at low doses orally (400 mg a day) and it is gradually increased if tolerated. It can be combined with an inhaled beta-2 agonist, or an inhaled ipratropium bromide or steroids.

Bronchodilation by inhaled $beta_2$ agonists is potentiated by ipratropium bromide,[43] theophylline[44,45] and all the three together.[46,47] Adding steroid in a high topical dose may yield further bronchodilation in chronic bronchitis.[48] The combination of theophylline (oral) and $beta_2$ agonists (inhalation) in chronic bronchitis with emphysema may improve marginally respiratory muscles function.[49] As oral theophylline passes into lung lining fluid and can halve the bacterial activity of alveolar macrophages,[50] it may not be prudent to use theophylline to improve respiratory muscle function in acute exacerbations as acute exacerbations of respiratory failure often arise from infection in these patients.[51]

As mentioned earlier, corticosteroids are beneficial in a very small group of patients with COPD as these are potent anti-inflammatory compounds. It must show a 20 per cent increase in FEY_1 to be considered beneficial.[52] In such patients the dose of prednisolone is tapered to a maintenance level to obtain the benefit of therapy. Inhaled fluticasone propionate may have important role in the long-term management of COPD. During acute exacerbation of bronchitis with worsening of symptoms, a short course of intravenous or oral corticosteroids may be indicated. Antibiotics may be required to prevent secondary or super added bacterial infections. Inhaled corticosteroids offer no added advantage in COPD patients; rather predispose to local ADRS such as oral candidiasis.

Association between hypomagnesium and COPD[53] and an improvement in respiratory parameters after magnesium therapy[54] have been documented.

Antibiotics

Exacerbations of COPD are a major cause of morbidity in these patients and about 5 lakh of such patients are hospitalised in USA every year. About 50% of these exacerbations are caused by bacterial infections, 3% by viral infections and remaining are caused by atypical infections and allergic exposure. Infective exacerbations of chronic bronchitis associated with H.influenzae, Moraxella catarrhalis and Strep. pneumoniae, and the presence of pus in the sputum indicates the need for antibiotic therapy. Bactericidal agents are capable of bringing down the viable count of bacteria, as they inhibit the growth of bacteria and make the sputum mucoid.

In the early stages of the disease, a short course of antibiotics is effective in controlling the infection while in advanced stages of the disease, the infections become frequent and persistent due to impaired defence of the host. Thus administration of antibiotics for a longer period is required. Stagnant secretions and blockage of small airways make it quite difficult to eradicate the infection completely. Ampicillin, tetracycline, co-trimoxazole or pefloxacin are effective in controlling the infection.

Unanimity has not been reached on the value of short-term use of antibiotics in acute exacerbations and the prophylactic use of antibiotics to prevent exacerbations.[55,56] Antibiotics are quite commonly used in treating infection in COPD patients. In (Expert Opin. Pharmaco Therap 2009:10: 1173-82), acute exacerbations of chronic bronchitis show better outcome with quinolones than macrolides. Erythromycin is advocated when mycoplasma infection is suspected.

Other drugs used are as follows:

(a) Influenza and polyvalent pneumococcal vaccinations are cost effective in preventing COPD exacerbation.
(b) Bronchovoxom–A mixture of bacterial products that activates macrophage function, may reduce severity of acute exacerbation.
(c) Mucolytics have also been tried to ease mucus expectoration.
(d) Antioxidants also reduce frequency and severity of acute exacerbation in COPD.
(e) Management of cor pulmonale includes:
    - Oxygen therapy (Maximum 30% O_2).
    - Diuretics.
    - Digoxin and ACE inhibitors.
    - Venesection if haematocrit is very high.

Prognosis is 30% mortality within one year and 40% survival rate of 5 years. Urgent management of infection holds the key as it helps to avoid acute exacerbations to cut down deterioration of respiratory reserve and preventing disability in COPD patients by preventing complications such as respiratory failure and cor pulmonale.

Other Drugs Used in COPD

- Bronchovoxom.
- Mucolytics.
- Antioxidants.
- Influenza and polyvalent pneumococcal vaccine.
- Inhaled corticosteroids.

- PDE 4 inhibitors (Anti-inflammatory).
- Immunomodulators.
- Antiproteases.
- PPAR agonists.
- Statins.
- NRF-2 activators.
- Stem cell therapy.
- Anti-ageing therapy.

Oxygen Therapy

Inadequate gas exchange may lead to acute respiratory failure (type I respiratory failure) and/or inadequate ventilation (type II respiratory failure, hypercarbic respiratory failure, ventilatory failure). COPD forms a very important cause of type II respiratory failure, wherein the PaO_2 is reduced and $PaCO_2$ is elevated. Patients with COPD develop chronic respiratory failure due to smouldering disease in the lungs.[56] Acute respiratory failure often gets superimposed on chronic respiratory failure.

An arterial oxygen tension ranging from 80 to 95 mm Hg while breathing ambient air is able to maintain adequate tissue oxygenation. Hypoxaemia is considered to be present when PaO_2 is less than 80 mm Hg. The brain, heart, pulmonary vasculature, liver and kidney are extremely sensitive to lack of oxygen. Hypoxaemia is potentially lethal. Unlike hypoxaemia, the body can tolerate an elevation of CO_2 for hours or days. This is what is happening to patients with COPD. Hypoxaemia occurs in COPD due to mismatched ventilation and perfusion (normally ventilated lung may be poorly perfused or area of lung with good perfusion may be poorly ventilated). There is inefficient gas exchange. In situations of acute respiratory failure in COPD, there is also hypoventilation.

Management has two aspects: relief of hypoxaemia by means of oxygen and at times, ventilatory intervention and reversal of the precipitating process responsible for the respiratory failure. Oxygen therapy is indicated in all disorders accompanied by a low PaO_2. Controlled oxygen therapy is advocated in acute respiratory failure following acute exacerbations of COPD. Oxygen has to be administered in a concentration greater than that found in the ambient air to achieve satisfactory levels of PaO_2, to avoid pulmonary oxygen toxicity noted after prolonged inhalation of high concentrations of oxygen and attenuation of the hypoxic drive to ventilation. Oxygen therapy helps to relieve hypoxaemia by increasing alveolar oxygen tension to reduce the work of breathing and to decrease the work of the myocardium.[57]

CO_2 retention and hypoxaemia is a feature of severe disease. The arterial oxygen tension falls linearly and the level of CO_2 rises in an hyperbolic way. During acute exacerbations of COPD following infection, or an uncontrolled administration of oxygen or use of sedatives, the chemoreceptor drive for ventilation is eliminated and there is reduced alveolar ventilation. Generally, administration of oxygen through ventimask is begun in a concentration of 24 per cent which is only 3 per cent higher than that of fresh air. It improves oxygenation without losing the respiratory stimulant effect. A minimal dose of oxygen raises the arterial oxygen tension as the gas exchange occurs on the steep part of the oxygen dissociation curve.

A known fixed concentration of oxygen can be delivered to the patient with venturi mask regardless of the oxygen flow rate to the mask and the minute ventilation of the patient. It fits lightly over the nose and the mouth and gives a blast of fresh air over the face, and has a soothing effect. Oxygen flowing at a high velocity (4-8 litres/min in the form of a jet through a narrow orifice in the base of the mask) creates negative pressure, entraining atmospheric air through the perforations in the face-piece, and there is no re-breathing. Additional humidification, is not required as room air is already mixing with it.[14]

A variety of masks are available to deliver low fixed concentrations of oxygen at 24 per cent, 28 per cent, 35 per cent and 40 per cent. However, the mask is somewhat uncomfortable to the patient and it has to be removed while eating, drinking and coughing.[57]

A low concentration of oxygen has to be administered continuously through nasal catheter or nasal cannula or double nasal prong. If it is given at 1, 2 or 3 litres per minute, a concentration of 24 per cent, 28 per cent or 35 per cent can reasonably be achieved as described earlier. However, FiO_2 delivered to the lungs varies with patient's breathing pattern. FiO_2 in these situations is $20 + 4 \times O_2$ flow (litres/min).[3] Availability of this non-invasive mechanical ventilation serves most of the patients, saving them from mechanical ventilation and intubation if refractory acute respiratory failure gets superimposed.[58,59]

Oxygen delivery should not be stopped abruptly until the patient has made recovery. At the same time, intermittent administration of oxygen in patients with CO_2 retention is dangerous, as it results in an immediate fall in arterial oxygen concentration. Unlike a large store of CO_2 in the body fluids, the body cannot store oxygen. Sudden discontinuation results in washing out of meagre body stores of oxygen leading to fall in alveolar oxygen tension. CO_2 is eliminated slowly and its level in the alveoli continues to remain high. It dilutes alveolar gas, causing a decline in oxygen tension. Hence continuous or oxygen therapy is suggested. Oxygen has to be administered preferably by a 24 per cent venturi mask or through nasal prongs or catheter at the rate of 2 litres per minute, and it usually brings the PaO_2 into an acceptable range. Oxygen should not be given intermittently to these patients retaining carbon dioxide as it will cause further fall in PaO_2 while breathing air. Its level will be lower than that found during oxygen administration. There is need to make repeated measurements of arterial blood gases in patients with acute respiratory failure on initiation of oxygen therapy. Blood gas analysis is found to be compatible with clinical status in 3/4th of cases and influences the treatment in

Table 7.9: Hyperbaric oxygen therapy

(A) Beneficial effects	(B) Complications	(C) Toxic effects on respiratory system
1. Correction of hypoxia	1. Pain in ears	1. Irritating cough
2. Inhibition of bacterial growth by affecting their metabolism	2. Rupture of tympanic membrane	2. Dyspnoea
3. Enhancing fibroblastic activity	3. Haemorrhage in the ear	3. Substernal pain
4. Promoting gas exchange in the appropriate direction	4. Surgical emphysema of mediastinum	4. Breathing discomfort
	5. Pneumothorax	5. Bronchopneumonia (prolonged exposure)
	6. Rupture of pulmonary cavities	
	7. Arterial air embolism	

1/3rd of cases. The goal is to maintain an arterial oxygen tension of at least 60 mm and arterial pH has to be watched.[5,15]

A small increment in arterial oxygen tension results in a significant rise in the saturation of haemoglobin. Under normal situations, no additional benefit is secured by raising PaO_2 level to greater than 60 to 80 mm Hg. An increase of 1 per cent of inspired oxygen concentration elevates oxygen tension by 7 mm Hg. It is necessary to maintain normal haemoglobin level in the presence of respiratory failure as proper oxygen transport to the tissues is to be maintained. Benefits, complications and toxic effects of hyperbaric oxygen therapy are shown in Table 7.9.

With the controlled oxygen therapy, most of the patients with hypercapnia and hypoxaemia secondary to chronic obstructive pulmonary disease during episodes of acute respiratory failure can be managed. In a review on respiratory disorders, non-invasive ventilation offers better long-term survival, especially in those cases of COPD with documented cause of respiratory failure.

Mechanical ventilation should be avoided in acute respiratory failure secondary to COPD as weaning from the ventilator is very difficult in these patients. However, it is indicated when cough becomes inefficient, or when the pH falls below 7.25 or when mental status shows a deterioration or when dyspnoea occurs or coma supervenes.[5] Major targets to be achieved by therapy in CAL are listed in Table 7.10.

Table 7.10: Major goals in the management of the p atients with chronic airflow limitation

1. To reduce the work of breathing.
2. To maximise the ability to perform daily activities.
3. To prevent acute exacerbations as far as possible.

Pulmonary Rehabilitation (PR)

American Thoracic Society in 1981 recommended that rehabilitation really means providing good comprehensive care for patients with pulmonary impairment. PR has significantly contributed in caring of patients with chronic lung disease. It increases functional ability and improves quality of life despite having irreversible abnormalities of lung architecture.

PR varies from patient to patient, and disease to disease, e.g., a COPD patient requires gradual exercise training programme, an environmental issue-based education has to be imparted to a patient of asthma to avoid exercise-induced spasm (trigger) and a modified training with varied intensity has to be given to a patient with interstitial lung disease to avoid exercise-induced hypoxemia. Prior to PR, an assessment criteria are applied to have base line exercise capacity along with muscle strength, health and nutritional status, emotional status and cognitive function. Main stress is laid on the following:

1. Exercise training, its intensity, specificity and strength-training.
2. Respiratory muscle training.
3. Maintenance of training effect (Training reversibility).
4. Education.
5. Use of oxygen during training.
6. Psychosocial support.

Exercise training for 20-45 minutes gradually for 4-5 days a week, utilising upto 6% of the basal capacity over a period of 3-4 months forms an important part of PR and results are favourable in providing benefits in the form of improved exercise ability, general well-being, decrease in dyspnoea and improved general health status.

COPD—a leading cause of disability, morbidity and mortality—being a chronic, progressive disorder, requires treatment of reversible airflow obstruction, management of complications and relief of symptoms. Despite therapy, many patients with advanced disease exhibit severe impairment because of destructive changes. It has been found that there are almost 6 lakh patients of COPD in UK, most of whom report to the doctor after the age of 40 years.[60] Women patients of COPD have fastly reached almost equal to men.[61] Minimal exertion causes exertional dyspnoea due to an increased metabolic demand. They get adapted to dyspnoea by becoming inactive in the home. They require pulmonary rehabilitation. A multidisciplinary programme to create an improved sense of well-being, decreased hospitalization requirement and an improved tolerance for exercise is needed. However, it does not reverse the structural damage associated with COPD. Pulmonary rehabilitation includes physical therapy, respiratory therapy, psychologic support, vocational counselling and education.

Other measures which form important constituents of physiotherapy programme are as follows:

Energy Conservation

COPD patients have limited reserve and they have to be taught to utilise it in such a way as to conserve energy. Energy expenditure has to be reduced and energy conservation techniques are to be incorporated into the daily activities and work.

Chest Physical Therapy

COPD patients have decreased vital capacity and flow rates. The mucociliary and cough mechanisms are not effective to clear the secretions from the lower respiratory tract. The secretions get accumulated and worsen airflow obstruction. Chest physical therapy provides mechanical and gravitational assistance to an ineffective cough mechanism through cough stimulation, postural drainage, chest percussion and chest vibration.[62]

COPD patients with pulmonary hypersecretion will be benefited from chest physiotherapy. Clearance of bronchial secretion improves pulmonary ventilation and facilitates better action by antimicrobial agents. The patient should lie on a firm mattress with 15° head down tilt in both lateral decubitus positions, supine and prone positions, spending 10 minutes in each position, and cough up the secretions. Postural drainage preceded by administration of aerosolised bronchodilators and followed by controlled coughing is useful.[5]

Postural drainage clears large amounts of secretions by gravitational force, and enables breathing to occur more freely. While the patient adopts different positions, the chest may be percussed with a rapid vibration tap or tapped with cupped hand.

Breathing Retraining Exercise

To lessen the work of breathing and to decrease respiratory discomfort with improved breathing techniques, breathing retraining is advocated. As the chest is hyperinflated in COPD and diaphragm is low and flat and there is loss of its elasticity, diaphragm becomes a weak inspiratory muscle. The accessory muscles of inspiration swing into action when diaphragm is fatigued. There is asynchronous thoracoabdominal movement with paradoxical inward motion of abdominal wall during inspiration. The increased work and cost of breathing is manifested by increased rate of respiration, increased sensation of air hunger, greater anxiety, fatigue and air-trapping.[5]

Muscle relaxing exercises do benefit. Breathing requires retraining in advanced stages to decrease the rate of respiration, to improve alveolar ventilation and to restore the diaphragmatic function. The patients are instructed to breathe through their nose and breathe out twice as long as they breathe in. The lips should be kept firmly together except in the centre. While exhaling air, it should be blown out slowly in a firm steady stream through the centre of lips.[63]

The strength and coordination of breathing muscles can be improved with breathing exercises. Deep breathing helps in opening the poorly ventilated areas. The diaphragm and abdominal muscles should play an active part. After deep inspiration, the patient has to exhale slowly to prevent collapse of the airways.[63] During exhalation, the patient has to press the hands placed in the lower thoracic cage inwards and upwards firmly so as to contract the abdomen and to push the diaphragm upwards to expel the trapped air.

Exercise Conditioning

Exercise performance in emphysema can be improved by pulmonary rehabilitation programme. Exercise training helps in improving oxygenation of tissue. It helps to build endurance and strength, and reduce dyspnoea.[64] Exercise training methods using treadmill or bicycle ergometer or 12 minutes' walking are useful to patients. Benefits of walking are known to medical fraternity since ages.[65] Walking improves mobility and arm exercises maintain strength and endurance of upper extremities. Walking a distance covered in a 12 minutes time period is a simple, efficient and inexpensive method. It can be carried out without additional equipment and supervision.[66]

In blue-bloater chronic obstructive pulmonary disease (COPD) patients, the pathology primarily involves the airways. There is minimal damage to lung parenchyma till late.[67] The large respiratory reserve, remains unutilised as the airways obstruction, leads to reduced autonomic drive with consequent hypoventilation and inefficient pattern of breathing.[68] The disease progressively increases to cor pulmonale and death. Progress of the disease can be altered and theoretically there is scope for functional improvement by training the patient to breathe deep and slowly voluntarily, overcoming the reduced autonomic drive.[67] Based on this assumption, a variety of measures have been tried so far.[69-73] All have beneficial effects. However, the methods and apparatuses used in these studies are impractical for day-to-day use and uninteresting and unconvincing to the patients. A simple and handy electronic device has also been tried.[74] There may or may not be an increase in VC. Reduction in air trapping is suggested by the decrease in the mean RV, with corresponding increase in ERV, while the TLC remains unchanged.[75]

There is change in FEV_1/FVC ratio. There is uniform improvement in the objective parameters as well as subjective parameters.[71] The results are achieved in a short duration of six weeks[71] with a simple and handy electronic device. The respiratory progress as monitored by the lighting panels of the spirocare, that motivates and encourages the patient to achieve the set goal. The achievement results in a sense of accomplishment and hence the patient does better in next attempt. By avoiding the use of force during expiration, the patient learns to postpone dynamic compression and corrects his inefficient pattern of breathing. This results in improved emptying of the lungs and avoids air trapping. The unchanged FEV_1/FVC ratio indicates that there is no change in the obstruction of the airways when force is applied during expiration.[74] Incentive-breathing exercises are a more practical and effective method for respiratory training in patients of COPD. Cheaper devices can be developed based on the same principles of functioning for the domiciliary use, especially for the people of developing countries.

Respiratory Muscle Training

There is shortening of muscle fibres of diaphragm in COPD and it results in reduction in tension-generating capability of the diaphragm. Maximal inspiratory pressure is also decreased. The inspiratory muscle strength and endurance can be improved by inspiratory muscle training wherein the patient is encouraged to inspire against progressively increasing resistance loads.[73]

Respiratory Therapy

Administration of aerosols and use of supplemental oxygen by severely hypoxic patients with COPD can help in the reversal of many of the adverse effects of chronic hypoxia.

Home Oxygen

The United Kingdom MRC Multicenter trial and the United States Nocturnal Oxygen Therapy trial have clearly demonstrated decreased cardiovascular complications and increased survival of patients with COPD exhibiting severe resting hypoxaemia following oxygen supplementation.[76,77]

Continuous oxygen therapy is considered for patients with severe resting hypoxaemia. Those exhibiting an arterial PO_2 of less than 55 mmHg three weeks or more while in a stable clinical state, or having pulmonary hypertension, cor pulmonale or secondary polycythemia or impaired neuropsychiatric function, with a PaO_2 between 55 and 59 mm Hg in a stable state are considered candidates for home oxygen therapy. Such patients do not have the ability to adapt to even a moderate degree of hypoxaemia.[78] Exacerbations of bronchitis or heart failure have to be ruled out. They should exhibit the above findings on two separate occasions, preferably three weeks apart, under optimal medical therapy and after discontinuing smoking and while breathing room air.[79]

COPD is a progressive disease that leads to marked limitation of exercise tolerance in some individuals and virtually they become respiratory cripples with profound hypoxaemia at rest and during exercise. Long-term oxygen therapy benefits such chronically hypoxaemic individuals and enables them to carry out their daily living activities. Supplemental oxygen reduces haematocrit, improves neuropsychiatric function, and reduces pulmonary artery pressure, thereby improving the overall survival and quality of life. Oxygen has to be delivered by nasal cannula at 1 to 2 liters per minute with additional 1 litre per minute flow during conditions of exercise and while sleeping to prevent hypoxaemic episodes as discussed earlier. Such a therapy has shown to improve the end-organ function (mental, cardiac and renal functions). Survival is better with either 12 or 15 hours oxygen and best with more continuous (20 hours) oxygen in selected patients with advanced COPD. Patients with normal oxygen tension at rest may show frequent and sometimes more severe desaturation during activities of daily routine, thereby making the prescription of oxygen difficult as supplemental oxygen has not shown that much of benefits but recent guidelines of Royal College of Physicians have clearly mentioned its benefits if there is significant desaturation of SPO_2 less than 90%. The administration of oxygen must begin quite earlier at night as hypoxaemia worsens during sleep.

Both stationary (compressed gas high pressure cylinders or tanks and oxygen concentrators) and portable (transfilling gaseous or liquid system) oxygen systems are available for use in the home for patients receiving long-term oxygen therapy. Bedridden patients or those who are confined to home, do not require a portable system, and a stationary source with a 13 metres extension tube is adequate.

A portable system is necessary for ambulatory patients including those who are able to work for several hours each day, away from home. This is very expensive and is useful to those who stay away from home for a longer period. Though portable liquid oxygen weighs about the same as the compressed gas system, it holds nearly twice as much oxygen. Therefore it is easier to carry with shoulder strap or wheels.[14]

Single prong nasa cannula, oxygen coserver cannula having a reservoir system enabling storage of oxygen during exhalation and delivery of a small bolus or enriched oxygen during inhalation, electronic demand oxygen delivery system supplying a short bolus of enriched oxygen early in inspiration on triggering of the inspiratory sensor by negative nasal pressure to avoid oxygen waste indeed-space gas and during expiration, and the use of transtracheal oxygen administration through a small polyethylene transtracheal catheter are being advocated to improve efficiency of oxygen delivery, to reduce cost of oxygen delivery and to improve cosmetic appearance, for ambulatory patients requiring long-term oxygen therapy.[80] Rehabilitation programmes for lungs in COPD patients have to be applied for life long, sticking to exercise training.[81] Lung volume reduction surgery has also been found to show improvement in FEV_1, health status and exercise performance, perhaps more than obtained by rehabilitation alone but surgery can be applied to a few selected patients only.[82,83] Trans-bronchial decompression of emphysematous bullae has been successfully applied.[83]

Psychologic support: Patients with COPD are psychologically deranged since the disease has impaired their full ability. Because they are unable to conduct the normal activities of daily living, they feel dependent and depressed. They need encouragement and support, both at family as well as community level.[5]

Vocational counselling: The vocational retraining improves the ability to perform daily activities both at home and work.

Education: Education of patient and the family helps to allay anxiety about the disease and improves patient's compliance. Cessation of smoking, therefore, is to form important part of health education.[85] Black tea is useful in COPD for the role of polyphenols.[86] Complications of COPD are given below in Table 7.11.

Table 7.11: Complications of COPD

1. Cor pulmonale.
2. Respiratory muscle dysfunction.
3. Acute exacerbation
   a. Infective.
   b. Non-infective.
   c. Pneumothorax/pleural problem.
   d. Pulmonary embolism.
   e. Neuromuscular dysfunction due to:
      1. Dyselectrolytemia.
      2. Nutritional deficiency.
      3. Hypothyroidism.
4. Respiratory failure with carbanosis.

Surgical Management

Surgical management includes:

a. Bullectomy that allows decompression of adjacent lung tissue by removal of large bullae.
b. Lung transplantation is considered in irreversible, progressively disabling end-stage pulmonary disease exhibiting respiratory failure unresponsive to conventional medical treatment and a poor quality of life. Obstructive lung diseases like end-stage emphysema, especially $alpha_1$, anti-proteases deficiency, form one of the indications for lung transplantation. Double-lung transplantation is advised in patients aged less than 50 years with end-stage emphysema. The lung implanted in COPD is smaller than the larger diseased lung.[87,88] Following transplantation, the overinflated chest cavity decreases in size as air-trapping no longer exists. Single lung transplantation offers 80% survival for one year and 42% survival for 5 years in COPD patients.
c. Lung volume reduction surgery helps in increasing elastic recoil, correction of ventilation-perfusion mismatch, improvement in functions of respiratory muscles and improvement in right ventricular functions.[89] At present, this is not recommended for emphysema. Newer pharmacotherapies are emerging.[90]

Bronchoscopic lung volume reduction using multiple valve implants to cause distal collapse and volume reduction in severe emphysema has been tried. Long-term results and complications of such implants would show the right path.

End of life care becomes essentially important. Ethical issues crop up but humanistic guidelines to deal such situations when patient thrives pathetically with respiratory distress, recurrent infections, immobility, depression and other comorbidities.

POINTS TO REMEMBER

I. *Symptoms of COPD*—History of tobacco smoke, other dusts or smoke, cough, sputum production, exertional dyspnoea.
Cough—Chronic, intermittent, seldom nocturnal.
Sputum production—Chronic with repeated episodes of acute bronchitis.
Dyspnoea—Persistent, progressive, worsens with exercise and during respiratory infections.
COPD is redefined as a disease state characterised by (a) airflow limitation, and (b) not fully reversible.

II. *COPD Severity and Survive—Classification*

Stage 0	—	Normal spirometry with chronic cough and sputum production.
Stage I	—	$FEV_1/FVC < 70\%$.
	—	$FEV_1 > 80\%$ predicted with or without symptoms.
Stage II	—	$FEV_1 < FVC < 70\%$.
	—	$30\% < FEV_1 < 80\%$ predicted.
Stage III	—	$FEV_1 / FVC < 70\%$ $FEV_1 < 30\%$ predicted respiratory failure or signs of right heart failure.

Survival Rate

Age	*FEV_1*	*3 years*
<60	>50%	90%
>60	40-50%	75-80%

III. *Differential Diagnosis of COPD*

COPD—Onset in midlife, slowly progressing symptoms, chronic smokers, exertional dyspnoea; irreversible air flow limitation, airway hyperresponsiveness absent, inflammatory cells involved are neutrophils.

Asthma—Onset early in life (childhood), history of anergy or eczema or family history of asthma is present. Variable symptoms from day-to-day; reversible airflow limitation, inflammatory cells are eosinophils and airway hyperresponsinevess is present.

CHF—Fine basal crackles, no airflow limitation, X-ray chest shows dilated heart, pulmonary odema, PFTs indicate volume restriction.

Bronchiectasis—Purulent copious sputum-coarse crackles, clubbing often present. Chest X-ray reveals bronchial dilation and bronchial wall thickening.

Tuberculosis — All ages affected, infiltrate or nodular lesions in X-ray chest. Microbiological confirmation.

Obliterative Bronchiolitis—Younger age onset in non-smokers, history of rheumatoid arthritis or fume exposure, hypodense areas in CT on expiration.

Diffuse Panbronchiolitis—Male non-smokers with history of chronic sinusitis. HRCT and chest X-ray reveals diffuse small centrilobular nodular opacities and hyperinflation.

IV. *Comorbidities in Elderly COPD Patients*

a. Atherosclerosis: Smoke, sedentary life style, systemic inflammation.
b. Aortic aneurysm: Smoke, steroids, Beta agonists (slowing expansion of aneurysm with Beta blockers); Loss of elasticity of vessels.
c. Cardiac dysfunction: Rt. ventricle dysfunction; cor pulmonale multifocal tachyarrhythmias.
   Cachexia: Ducts circulating cytokines, catabolic hormonal activity, lack of exercise, drug induced steroids, hypoxia related slowed down digestion, depression.
   Cataract: Old age, steroids, hypoxemia.
   Cancer (lung): Smoke, chronic inflammation.
d. Depression: Old age.
   Dementia: Hypoxemia, hypercapnea, cognitive impairment of memory.
   Diabetes: Old age, steroids.
e. Hypertension: Old age: steriods.
f. Osteoporosis: Inactivity, old age, catabolic status, steroids, malnutrition.
   Obstructive sleep apnoea: Old age.
g. Pulmonary embolism and thrombophlebitis: COPD is associated with thrombophilic status.

V. *Differences and Similarities Between Asthma and COPD*

Asthma	**COPD**
↓	↓
Sensitizing agent	Noxious agent
↓	↓
CD4 T cells Eosinophils	CD8 T cells Macrophages, Neutrophils
↓	↓
Completely reversible airflow limitation	Completely irreversible airflow limitation
↓	↓
Steroid response	No steroid response

VI. *Management of COPD*

More than 7 lakh people die per annum, 6 lakh males and 1 lakh females due to diseases related to tobacco. India is likely to bring a bill in Parliament to make India Tobacco free zone as there is law in Germany, France and England. A campaign has been started in Delhi University campus, and in Delhi after 31st of May to pay a fine of Rs 100 and then 200 on second time and then 500 or more on third time if found smoking at public place.

1. So, avoidance of risk factors including influenzae vaccination may have a place in preventing COPD.
2. Short acting bronchodilators.

Differences Between Asthma and COPD

	Asthma	*COPD*
Anatomic site	Airways	Airways and lung parenchyma
Age of onset	Early childhood, onset at any age	Mid-late adult life
Smoking history	Non-, ex- or current smoker	Usually smoker or ex-smoker
Nature of inflammation	Eosinophilic, CD4 driven, LTD4, IL-4, IL-5, Eotaxin, RANTES	Neutrophilic, CD8 driven, LTB 4, TNF-alpha, IL-8
Decline in lung function	Normal or slightly accelerated	Accelerated
Reversibility of airflow obstruction	Mostly reversible	Irreversible
Exacerbations	Occur at all levels of severity	Increases with increasing severity
What is not reversible	Airway remodeling	Remodelling, loss of alveolar attachments
Objective of treatment	Reducing inflammation	Relieving symptoms
Inhaled corticosteroids	+++	+ (In patients $FEV_1 < 50\%$)
Oral corticosteroids	++ (severe asthma)	Contraindicated
β_2-agonists, theophylline, anticholinergics	+++	+++

3. Rehabilitation including exercise training, education and nutrition.
4. Inhaled glucocorticoids if repeated exacerbations (antibiotics for repeated airway infection). Acute infective exacerbations lead to marked deterioration of respirative reserve. Therefore, urgent treatment of infection holds the key, to prevent pulmonary damage which leads to respiratory failure and cor pulmonale.
5. Treatment of complications.
6. Noninvasive positive pressure ventilation in acute exacerbation.
7. Long-term O_2 therapy (if respiratory failure).
8. Surgical modalities.[91]

Complex comorbidities, metabolic syndrome and even obesity with COPD have been interlinked.[92,93,94] Use of antipneumoccocal vaccine has shown clinical efficacy in patients with COPD.[95]

REFERENCES

1. Culver BH; Interpretation of spirometry – We can do better than the GOLD standard; Resp Care 2006; 51: 719-21.
2. Agarwal AN; How appropriate is the GOLD standard for diagnosis of airway obstruction, Lung India 2008; 25: 139-41.
3. Dipika A, Udwadia ZF; Burden of undiagnosed airflow obstruction in India; JAPI 2007; 55:742.
4. William Mac Nee, Rubin M Tuder; New paradigms in the pathogfenesis of COPD; Proct Amer Thorac Soc 2009; 6: 527-31.
5. Shankar P.S., Chest Medicine; Oxford and IBH Publ. Co. (P)Ltd., N.Delhi, 1994, 4th ed.
6. Terminology, definitions and classification of chronic pulmonary emphysema and related conditions. A report on the conclusion of the CIBA Guest symposium. Thorax 1959; 14: 286-99.
7. Lambert P.M. and Reid O.D., Smoking, air pollution and bronchitis in Britain, Lancet 1970; 1: 853.
8. Richter A.M, Abbound R.T., Johal S.S., Erz. T.A., Acute effects of smoking on superoxide production by pulmonary alveolar macrophages, Lung 1986; 1964:233-42.
9. Khan H, *et al.*, Alpha-1 antitrypsin deficiency in emphysema; JAPI 2002;50: 579-82.
10. Tabin M.J., Hutchinson D.C.S., An overview of pulmonary features of alpha-1-antitrypsin deficiency: Arch Inter Med 1982; 142: 1342.
11. Shankar P.S., COPD-etiopathogenesis: Interplay of environmental and genetic factors; Lung India 2006;23:15-19.
12. Bhatia RS, *et al.*, Effect of smoking and kitchen environments; Med. Pulse 1997;4:65-66.
13. Bhatia RS; Rising trends in pulmonary disorders–Reasons and remedies; In; Selected topics in Chest Med; Arora Publ 2005; 4: 23-24.
14. Amer MS, *et al.*, Proinflammatory cytokines in Egyptian elderly with COPD; Lung India 2010; 27: 225-29.
15. Gothi D., *et al.*, Clinical profile of diseases causing chronic airflow limitation in a tertiary care centre in India; JAPI 2007;55;551-55.
16. Reid L., Measurement of the bronchial mucous gland layer. A diagnostic yardstick in chronic bronchitis,Thorax1960; 15: 132-41.
17. Jamel K., Cooney T., Fleetham J.A. and Thurlbeck W.M., Chronic bronchitis: Correlation of morphologic findings to sputum production and flow rates, Am. Rev. Respir. Dis 1984;129:719-22.
18. National Heart, Lung and Blood Institute, Division of Lung Diseases, Workship Report. The definition of emphysema. Amer. Rev. Respir. Dis 1985;132: 182-85.
19. Reid, Lynne Pathology of Emphysema, London, Blackwell, 1967.
20. Niewoehner D.E., New messages from morphometric studies of chronic obstructive pulmonary disease. Sem. Respir. Med 1986; 8: 140-46.
21. Bhatia R.S., Sibia S.S., Sibia H.K., Bedi P.S., COPD and kitchen education; paper selected for award session of ICS; 1995.
22. Taylor DR, Pavord D; Biomarkers in assessment and management of airways disease; PG Med J 2008; 628-34.
23. Hogg J.C., Macklem P.T. and Thurlbeck W.M., Site and nature of airway obstructive lung disease, N. Engl. J. Med 1968:278: 1355-66.
24. Hunninghake G.W., Cristal R.G., Cigarette smoking and lung destruction: Accumulation of neutrophils in the lungs of cigarette smokers, Amer. Rev. Respir. Dis 1983; 128: 833-38.
25. Hogg J.C., Mechanisms of airways obstruction in COPD, Pulm. Perspectives 1990; 7:1-3.
26. Natarajan R; Recent trends in pulmonary arterial hypertension; Lung India 2011; 28: 39-48.
27. Chetty K.G., Brown S.E. and Light R.W., Identification of pulmonary hypertension in chronic obstructive pulmonary disease from routine chest radiographs, Am. Rev. Respir. Dis 1982;126:328-34.
28. Bergin C., Muller N., David M., *et al.,* The diagnosis of emphysema. A computed tomographic-pathologic correlation, Amer. Rev. Respir. Dis 1986; 133:541-46.
29. Haas H., Morris J.P., Samson S., *et al.*, Bacterial flora of the respiratory tract in chronic bronchitis. Compression of transtracheal fiber bronchoscope and oropharyngeal sampling methods, Am. Rev. Respir. Dis 1977;116: 41-47.
30. Agarwal RL; *et al.*, Diagnostic values of ECG in COPD; Lung India 2008; 25: 78-81.
31. Bhattacharya P., *et al.*, Prevalence of osteoporosis and osteopenia in advanced COPD patients; Lung India 2011; 28; 184-86.
32. Douglas N.J. and Flenley D.C., Breathing during sleep in patients with obstructive lung diseases, Amer. Rev. Respir. Dis 1990, 141: 1055-70.
33. Martin R.J., The sleep-related worsening of lower airways obstruction: Understanding and intervention, Med. Clin. North Amer 1990; 74: 701-14.
34. Boysen P.G., Block A.J., Wynne J. W., Hunt L.A. and Flick M.E., Nocturnal pulmonary hypertension in patients with chronic obstructive pulmonary disease, Chest 1979; 76: 536-42.
35. Kinsman R.A., Varoush R.A., Fernandez E., *et al.,* Symptoms and experience in chronic bronchitis and emphysema, Chest 1983; 83: 755-71.
36. Tirlapur V.G., Mir M.A., Nocturnal hypoxaemia and associated electrocardiographic changes in patients with chronic obstructive airways disease, N. Engl. J. Med 1982; 306: 125-130.

37. Bhatia R.S., Smoking: A challenge for doctors, Curr. Med. Pract 1992;36: 85-86.
38. Singh V; Tobacco use among medical students and surrogate control of tobacco in India; Lung India (Ed) 2011; 28: 01.
39. Tabin MJ, Hutchison DCS; An overview of pulmonary features of alpha-1 antitrypsin deficiency; Arch Inter Med 1982; 142: 1342.
40. Barthwal MS, Singh S; Early detection of COPD in asymptomatic smokers using spirometry; JAPI 2014: 62: 38-42.
41. Calverley PM, *et al.*, Salmetrol and fluticasone propionate and survival in COPD; N Eng. J Med 2007: 358: 775-89.
42. Guleria R., Behera D. and Jindal S.K., Comparison of bronchodilatation produced by an anticholinergic (ipratropium bromide), a beta-2, adrenergic (Fenoterol) and their combination in patients with chronic obstructive airway disease, J. Assn. Phys. India 1991; 39: 680-82.
43. Brown I.G., Chan C.S., Kelly C.A., *et al.*, Assessment of the clinical usefulness of nebulised ipratropium in patients with chronic airflow limitation, Thorax 1984;39: 272-76.
44. Svedmyr K. and Svedmyr N., Does theophylline potentiate inhaled beta-2 agonists? Allergy 1982;37: 101-10.
45. Taylor D.R., Buick B., Kinney C., *et al.*, The efficiency of orally administered theophylline, inhaled salbutamol and a combination of the two as chronic therapy in the management of chronic bronchitis with reversible airflow obstruction, Amer. Rev. Resp. Dis 1985;131: 747-51.
46. Cartwright A.C., Controlled release—A regulatory dilemma, Manufacturing Chemist 1987, March, 33.
47. Kethy H.W., Theophylline toxicity, In, Jenne J.W., Murphy S. Ed, Drug therapy for asthma, lung biology in health and disease; New York; Marcel-Kekker 1987; 31: 925-51.
48. Flenley D.C. and Whyte K.F., Topics in chronic bronchitis and emphysema, IN: Flenley D.C., Petty T.L.; Ed; Recent advances in respiratory medicine; Churchill Livingstone, Edinburg 1986; IV: 193-216.
49. Mahler DR; Effect of inhaled beta-2 agonists on clinical outcome in COPD; J Allergy Clin Immunolo 2002; 110(S6); 298-303.
50. O'Neill S.J., Sitar D.S., Klass D.J., *et al.*, The pulmonary disposition of theophylline and its influence on human alveolar macrophage bactericidal function, Amer. Rev. Resp. Dis 1986;134: 1225.
51. Warren P.M.A., Miliar J.S., Flenley D.C., *et al.*, Respiratory failure revisited, acute exacerbations of chronic bronchitis between 1961-68 and 1970-76, Lancet 1980; 1i: 467-71.
52. Chhabra SK, Ailawadhi M; Effect of prednisolone on lung functions and bronchodilator responses in stable COPD; Lung India 2006; 23: 8-14.
53. Rolla G., *et al.*, Hypomagnesemia in COPD; Effect of therapy; Mag. Trace. Exam 1990; 9: 132-36.
54. Molloy D.W., *et al.*, Hypomagnesemia and respiratory muscle power; Amer. Rev. Resp. Dis 1984;129: 497-98.
55. Rodrigues Poision R; COPD exacerbations: Management, Thorax 2006; 61:535-44.
56. Decremes M; *et al.*, Targeting COPD exacerbations; J Resp Med 2008; 102 (S II): 453-515.
57. O' Neill B., *et al.*, Short burst oxygen therapy in COPD; Resp Med 2006:100:1129-38.
58. Leger P., *et al.*, Acute respiratory failure in COPD patients treated with non-invasive intermittent mechanical ventilation with nasal mask; Amer. Rev. Resp. Dis 1998;137:A63.
59. Hira H.S., *et al.*, Efficacy of non-invasive nasal mechanical ventilation in acute respiratory failure: Monitored by breathing pattern; JAPI 2000; 48: 1164-69.
60. Calverly P.M.A., Bellamy D., The challenge of providing better care for patients with COPD; the poor relation of airways obstruction; Thorax 2000; 55: 28-82.
61. Soriano J.B. *et al.*, Recent trends in physician diagnosed COPD in women and men in UK; Thorax 2000; 55: 769-79.
62. Rochester D.F. and Goldberg S.K., Techniques of repiratory physical therapy, Am. Rev. Respir. Dis 1980; 110: Part I: 133.
63. Mueller R.E., Petty T.E. and Filley G.F., Ventilation and arterial blood gas changes induced by pursed lip breathing, Jour. Appl. Physiol 1970; 28: 384.
64. Bhatia R.S., Cardiopulmonary disease testing; Indications and contraindication; How to improve upon? IJCP 1996; 6(9): 36-40.
65. Bhatia R.S., Batta S. and Wander G.S., Let us walk for the nation, Curr. Med. Pract 1991; 35: 190.
66. McGavin C. R., Gupta S.P. and Mc Hardy G.J., Twelve-minute walking test for assessing disability in chronic bronchitis, Brit. Med. Jour 1976; 1: 822.
67. Cotes J.E., Lung function, assessment and application in medicine, 4th ed., Oxford, Blackwell Scientific Publication, 1979; 417: 490-91.
68. Parot S., Breathing pattern and hypercapnoea in patients with obstructive pulmonary disease, Am. Rev. Respir. Dis 1980; 121: 985-91.
69. Kant S., Singh G.V., Breathing exercises as adjuvant in the management of COPD–An overview; Lung India 2006; 23:165-69.
70. Sinclair D.J.M. and Ingram C.C., Controlled trial of supervised exercise training in chronic bronchitis, Br. Med. J 1980; 280: 519-21.
71. Belman M. L. and Mittman C., Ventilatory muscle training improves exercise capacity in chronic obstructive pulmonary disease patients, Am. Rev. Respir. Dis 1980; 121: 273-80.
72. Thomas R.L., Stoker G.L. and Ross J.C., The efficiency of pursed lips breathing in patients with chronic obstructive pulmonary disease, Am. Rev. Respir. Dis 1966; 93: 100-06.
73. Kulpati D.D.S. and Kamath R.K., The influence of physical conditioning by yogasanas and breathing exercise in patients of chronic obstructive pulmonary disease, Lung India 1982; 1: 35-38.
74. Tiwary R.S., Lakhere S.C., Kain T.C. and Sinha K.C., Effect of incentive breathing on lung fuctions in COPD; J. Assn. Phys. India 1989;1: 689-91.
75. Pardy R.L., Rivington R.N., Despas P.J. and Macklem P.T., The effects of inspiratory muscle training on exercise performance in chronic airway limitation, Amer. Rev. Respir. Dis 1981; 123: 426.
76. The Medical Research Council Working Party, Long term domiciliary oxygen therapy in chronic hypoxia cor pulmonale complicating chronic bronchitis and emphysema, Lancet 1981;1: 681-86.
77. Carison J.L., *et al.*, Cycle ergometer and inspiratory muscle training in COPD; Amer. J, Resp. Crit, Care Med 1999; 160: 500-07.

78. Garrod R., *et al.*, Randomised controlled trial of domiciliary NIPP ventilation and physical training in severe COPD; Amer. J. Resp. Crit. Care Med 2000; 162: 1335-41.
79. Revill S.M., *et al.*, Randomised controlled trial of ambulatory oxygen and an ambulatory ventilator on endurance exercise in COPD; Resp. Med 2000; 94:778-83.
80. Shigeoka J.W., Oxygen concentrators, home oxygen prescriptions and the role in the respiratory care practitioners, Respir. Care 1991; 36: 178-83.
81. Kant S, Singh GV; Breathing exercises as adjuvant in the management of COPD–An overview; Lung India 2006; 23: 165-69.
82. Geddes D., *et al.*, Effect of lung volume reduction surgery in patients with severe emphysema; N. Eng. J. Med 2000; 343: 239-45.
83. Drazen JM; Surgery for emphysema–not for everyone; N Eng J Med 2001; 345-1126-27.
84. Bhattacharya P., *et al.*, Transbronchial decompression of emphysematous bullae–A new therapeutic approach; Eur Respir J 2007; 29: 1003-06.
85. Bhatia R.S., Vijayan V.K., Tobacco and health; What can the medical profession do? Lung India 1994; 12(4): 178-85.
86. Tabak C., *et al.*, COPD and the role of catechins, flavonols and flavones—The Morgan study; Amer J. Resp. Crit Care Med 2001; 164: 61-64.
87. Misra S., Human gene therapy–A brief overview of the genetic revolution; JAPI 2013;61:41-47.
88. Arcasry SM, Kotloff RM; Lung transplantation; N Eng J Med 1999; 340: 1081-91.
89. Fein A.K., Lung volume reduction surgery: Answering the crucial question: Chest 1998;113:2775-2825.
90. Barnes PJ; Emerging pharmacotherapies for COPD; Chest 2008; 134: 1278-86.
91. Drazen JM; Surgery for emphysema–not for everyone; N Eng J Med 2001; 345: 1126-27.
92. Marquis K., *et al.*, Metabolic syndrome in patients with COPD; J cardiopulm. Rehabil 2005; 25: 226-32.
93. Fabbri LM; *et al.*, Complex chronic comorbidities of COPD. Eurp. Resp. J 2008; 2 : 351-74.
94. Sood A; Obesity, adipokines and lung disease; J App. Physiology 2010; 108: 744-53.
95. Alfagent I., *et al.*, Clinical efficacy of anti-pneumococcal vaccine in patients with COPD; Thorax 2006; 61: 189-95.

UNILATERAL HYPERRADIANT LUNG

Unilateral hyperradiancy of the lung was described in a child in 1953 and in adults in 1954. It is a condition of air flow trapping with poor ventilation and perfusion occurring in a small unilateral transradiant lung or lobe.[1] This is an acquired condition possibly due to end result of a severely occurring patchy obliterative bronchiolitis in childhood. Often there is a past history of viral or mycoplasmal infection, causing patchy obstruction. There occurs a ball-valve effect which is responsible for air trapping, interfering with the alveolar ventilation. Lungs get damaged due to infection hindering in the physiological development of pulmonary artery which in turn hinders postnatal development of lung. Panacinar emphysema usually accompanies hypoplastic lung. Patients do not have any symptoms unless complicated by chronic bronchitis. There is diminished lung expansion on the affected side, so are the breath sounds. Clinically there is no cyanosis.[1]

The lung may be small but with a marked increase in its transradiancy. The hilar shadow is small and pulmonary vascular markings are significantly reduced. There is a mediastinal shift to the opposite side during expiratory phase and upward movement of the diaphragm is restricted. As normal side deflates on expiration, air gets trapped on the affected side which can be demonstrated on chest screening. Classical terminal bronchiectatic pattern with poor peripheral filling is demonstrated by bronchogram. Proximal filling may be normal while peripherally it may manifest as spidery bronchioles and irregular dilatations. The blood flow is reduced on the affected side because of hypoplastic pulmonary artery with diminished vascular pattern. Both ventilation (because of severe non-valvular obstruction of small airways) as well as oxygen uptake are diminished.

Differential diagnosis of unilateral hyperlucency of the lung without vascular abnormality includes congenital absence of pectoralis major, muscle wasting, post mastectomy etc. Such changes can be seen in parenchymal abnormalities like compensatory emphysema, foreign body inhalation, causing ball-valve obstruction of main bronchus with air trapping, during an attack of asthma and in emphysematous bulla. In congenital absence of pulmonary artery neither the transradiancy is prominent nor is there any trapping of air. Unilateral translucency of the lung may also occur in case where there is vascular occlusion due to extrinsic compression of proximal pulmonary artery by fibrosing mediastinitis or by an embolus. Even mediastinal irradiation has been reported to cause unilateral hyperlucent lung disease.[2] Presence of infection and bronchospasm demands antibiotics and bronchodilators respectively. Surgical lung resection is indicated in cases of haemoptysis, recurrent chest infections and progressive dyspnoea.[1]

REFERENCES

1. Shankar P.S., ed., Chest Medicine, 4th ed, Oxford and IBH Pub. Co. P. Ltd., N. Delhi, 1994.
2. Wencel M.L., Sitorin R.G., Amer. Rev. Resp. Dis 1988;137: 955-57.

BRONCHIAL ASTHMA

Introduction

Bronchial asthma is an important cause of pulmonary disability seen in this part of the tropics affecting both sexes and age is no bar to this. In India, asthma imposes a substantial burden, prevalence being 2.38% (ICMR).[1] The term bronchial asthma, breathlessness or shortness of breath, refers to one of the episodic manifestations of obstructive pulmonary disease with episodes of wheeze and dyspnoea. The old physiological definition has been redefined by American Thoracic Society as a clinical syndrome where tracheobronchial tree has hyperresponsiveness to variety of stimuli manifesting physiologically by generalised airways obstruction, responding either to some primary treatment or spontaneously over a short period of time and clinically by paroxysmal attacks of cough, wheeze, dyspnoea, heavy chest etc.[2]

Tobacco smoke has adverse association with asthma. Drugs requirement is increased. Airway remodelling, fixed airway obstruction and an exaggerated lung function decline develops as a result of tobacco smoking.[3] Incidence of bronchial asthma to the tune of 25.2% has been reported from a private clinic in Punjab.[4] Asthma which was considered to be of allergic origin only, has recently been understood to be heterogeneous disorder in which episodes of airways hyper-responsiveness and obstruction occur predominantly due to inflammation.[5]

Aetiology, Pathophysiology and Clinical Varieties

Bronchial asthma is a chronic persistent inflammatory disease of the airways. It is a complex disorder involving heterogenous group of patients where airways hyper-responsivenss occurs due to airways inflammation, leading to airways obstruction, in response to varied variety of exogenous and endogenous stimuli, which are infact responsible for precipitation of an episode. This leads to narrowing of airways which is reversible. The neuro-immunoclinical mechanisms cause contraction of airways smooth muscles and inflammation, leading to mucosal cellular infiltration, mucosal odema, and accumulation of mucus because of excessive bronchial secretions and their impaired clearance, epithelial damage and basement membrane thickening.[6] It is now established that although mast cells play an important role in the immediate response to allergen, and in the late response of bronchial hyper-responsiveness, macrophages and eosinophils have important role[7] to play. Pathological changes in the airways in bronchial asthma are shown in Table 7.12.

Table 7.12: Pathological changes in the airways in bronchial asthma

1. Patchy to complete denudation of epithelial lining.
2. Mucosal and submucosal filtration with leucocytes, predominantly eosinophils, platelets and monocytes.
3. Degranulated mast cells.
4. Epithelial basement membrane thickening.
5. Bronchial smooth muscle hypertrophy.
6. Mucus glands hyperplasia.
7. Airway occlusion with mucus, serum proteins and cellular debris.
8. Some degree of peribronchial fibrosis.

The heterogenicity[2] of the patients can be explained on the basis of:

1. Precipitating factors—extrinsic, intrinsic or both as shown in Table 7.13.
2. Site of airways affected—obstruction of large, small or both the airways.
3. Reversible or not—If reversible, complete or incomplete.
4. Frequency of attack—daily, monthly, yearly etc.

Table 7.13: Possible precipitating factors

1. Air pollutants.
2. Allergens as shown in Table 7.14.
3. Emotional stress.
4. Exercise, sleep, oesophageal reflux, menstruation.
5. Environmental factors (Tobacco and diesel fumes, household chemicals and smoke, air, fog, wind, gases, like SO_2 etc).
6. Chemical sensitizing agents as shown in Table 7.15.
7. Dust and fumes.
8. Food preservatives like tartrazine, monosodium glutamate, metabisulphite.
9. Bronchopulmonary aspergillosis.
10. Recurrent sinus infection, viral infection etc.
11. Occupational/Industrial exposure as shown in Table 7.16.

5. Degree and depth of episode—mild, moderate or severe and frequent or infrequent.
6. Time of onset—periodical, seasonal, diurnal variation, postural etc.
7. Symptomatology—cough is overwhelming or breath-lessness and vice versa.
8. Treatment response—immediate, delayed or late.

Global rise in bronchial asthma in the last decades in the age group of under four and in persons near 40 years of age has been observed. Hospitalisation and fatality among young adults has also risen, owing to lack of knowledge about the disease and its care and certain behavioural problems. Half of the younger asthmatics have remission after the age of 16 years and half of these still flare up again in middle age. In others, long standing damage with or without permanent scarring has been produced by bronchial asthma.[8] Copy number variation of different immune response, inflammatory and airway modeling genes can also contribute to the susceptibility for bronchial asthma.[9] Polymorphisms in the interlukin-4 (IL-4) gene have also been described, associated with greater output of IL-4. Number of cytokines such as MIP-1 alpha, MCP-1 and TGF-beta that recruit inflammatory cells and stimulate extracellular matrix production are produced by myofibroblasts.[10] Matrix tissue is also regulated by metalloproteinases, collagenase and growth factors from eosinophils.

Strenuous exercise at low temperature entailing breathing large volumes of cold air is the suggested explanation of bronchial hyperresponsiveness, asthma like syndrome and persistent asthma in cross country skiers.

Table 7.14: Overall predominant allergens

D+Antigens	*% age*	*I+Antigens*	*% age*
Cotton dust Gynandropsis Helminthosporium House dust mite House dust Wheat dust	15% to 30%	Gundropsis House dust Xanthium Cotton dust House dust mite	15% to 20%
Lawsonia Cassia Cynodon Argemone	12% to 15%	Argemone Helminthosporium Cassia Brassica Cynodon	12% to 15%

Table 7.15: Respiratory tract irritants

1. Mucosal irritation	Nose, Throat, e.g., Acids, SO_2, NH_3, Cl, Isocyanates, Aldehydes
2. Irritation of lower airways	Petroleum products, NO_2, Phosgene, MIC, Cl
3. Lungs	Pesticides, NO_2, Cl, SO_3, MIC
Mechanism of action through O_2 deficit	CO, N, NO_2, CO_2, Aniline, Cyanide

Table 7.16: Hazardous industrial substances

1. Organic	Polymer, Synthetic Fiber, Cotton, Sugarcane, PVC
2. Inorganic	Asbestos, Coal, Synthetic fiber, Cement stone, Gold, Berillium
3. Chemicals	a. **Inorganic:** CO_2, CO_2, Pb, Hgce, NH_3, CCl_4 b. **Aromatic:** Acids, Methane, Benzene, Drugs, Aldehydes, Aniline, Xylene, Toluene c. **Pesticides:** BHC, DDT, MIC, Malathion, Carbamates d. **Fertilizers:** Nitrate, Urea, Phosphate, Biologic
4. Pollutants	**Air:** SO_2, CO, O_3, NO_2, SO_3, POM, S.P.M. **Water:** Oxygen demand, Chemicals, Bacteria **Soils:** Chemicals, Parasites, Pesticides, Salinity, Fluoride

Exacerbating factors include:

A. Acid reflux, which is present in asthmatics with enhanced gastric secretions and relaxed gastroesophageal sphincter due to bronchodilator therapy. This reflux causes bronchoconstriction as a result of cholinergic reflex (the reflux reflex) leading to hyper-responsiveness of airways through unknown mechanism. Even a close link between fall in oesophageal **pH** and increased bronchoconstriction exists in asthma. However, asymptomatic gastroesophageal reflux is unlikely to be the cause of poorly controlled asthma.[11]

B. Chronic sinusitis, possibly causing a postnasal drip and inflammation of respiratory tract and is generally associated with poorly controlled asthma. Cure of rhinitis would prevent only some cases of new-onset-asthma.[12]

C. Occupational asthma is underdiagnosed, a long list of the sensitizing agents, has been listed in Table 7.16. A rising trend of bronchial asthma is attributed to rise in air pollution.[13]

D. Foods like nuts, strawberries and shellfish are commonly implicated. Even increased dietary salt is contributory to severity of asthma. Food additives possibly act through stimulation of nerves and monosodium glutamate is implicated in 'Chinese restaurant asthma'. Tartrazine probably acts as a histamine releaser.

E. In few patients, infections like C. pneumoniae may initiate asthmatic symptoms.

Psychogenic influence in asthma is poorly understood but bronchoconstriction may be induced by suggestion. Treatment modalities in such cases has been shown in Table 7.17.

Systemic diseases like thyrotoxicosis may upset control of asthma possibly through an altered steroid metabolism, and treatment of thyrotoxicosis reduces severity of asthma.[14]

Asthma may be a prominent feature of systemic diseases like eosinophilia with pulmonary infiltration, Churg-Strauss syndrome and carcinoid syndrome. Prevalence and severity of asthma increased in persons with abnormal α_1 antitrypsin deficiency phenotype.[15]

The effect of overweight on asthma has been examined in several epidemiological studies. Obesity impairs ventilatory

Table 7.17: Treatment of emotional component s in asthma

The relationship between asthma and emotionality has for long been the topic of discussion and debates. Till date, views regarding this link still remain controversial. Hence, treatment of this emotional component is also empirical and varies with the numerous variables outlined. The treatment strategies include:

1. Stress not associated with bronchoconstriction	Psychotherapy may not be beneficial
2. Association between stress and exacerbation of asthma	Psychotherapy beneficial
3. Negativity resulting from asthmatic symptoms	Psychotherapy not beneficial
4. Patients with high levels of panic-fear	Psychotherapy
5. Patients with symptoms of anxiety	Educate patients regarding side effects of anti-asthmatic drugs and reduce dose if possible

Ref: Current Medical Science 1993; 8(6): 2.

functions, reduces muscle strength of respiratory muscles, decreases thoracic cage compliance and impedes diaphragmatic excursion. This may result in dyspnoea, which is not asthma. Asthma in obesity is related to genetics, increased pro-inflammatory adipokines, reduced anti-inflammatory adiponectins and other obesity related biochemical changes.

Increased levels of adipokines such as eotaxin, visfatin, complement, plasminogen activator inhibitor and TNF alpha have been implicated. Role of lepin in augmenting ozone or allergen induced airway inflammation has been suggested.

Asthma is more difficult to control in obese than lean asthma patients. Weight reduction through diet, drugs or surgery improved airways functions in asthma patients.

Table 7.18 and Figure 7.1 show symptoms and triggers that precipitate bronchial asthma.

Table 7.18: Bronchial asthma

Symptom	*Feature characteristic*
• Cough	• Episodic
• Wheeze	• Variable
• Breathlessness	• Nocturnal (Triggers' induced)
• Tight chest	

Trigger Factors

Allergic	*Non-allergic*
• House dust mite	• Exercise
• Pollen	• Food
• Fungal spore	• Blisters
• Pet	• Drugs
	• Viral infection
	• Air pollution
	• Tobacco smoke
	• Psychological factors
	• Climatic changes
	• GERD
	• Occupational factors

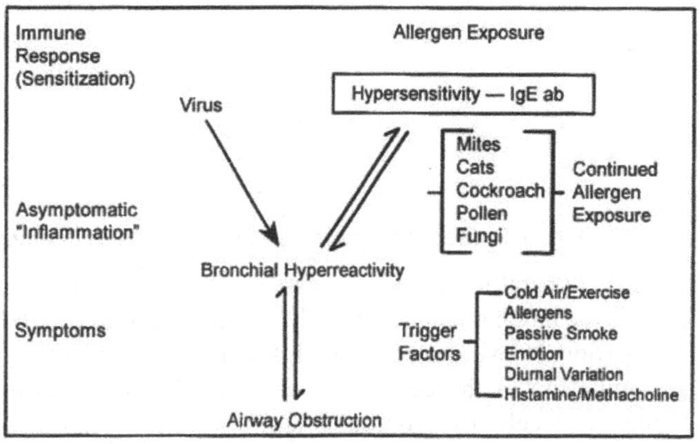

Fig. 7.1

Clinical Differentiation of Asthma

Extrinsic Atopic Asthma

This is commonly seen in young adults and children, may occur in adults with declining atopic status. There are known external allergens to which body shows production of large amount of reaginic antibodies through its inborn ability. There is a positive family history of eczematous dermatitis, allergy, asthma etc. Mostly the allergens are inhalants, some time eatables may behave the same way, especially in children. There is often seasonal variation and many a times, remissions are observed at puberty. Even hyposensitisation works equally good. Chlamydia pneumoniae infection, as demonstrated by their antibody titre, may have a casual association with asthma and asthmatic bronchitis.

In atopic individuals, the exposure to antigen stimulates peripheral lymphoid tissues to synthesise reaginic antibodies. These reagins are called immunoglobulins-IgE. Normally the mean IgE level in adults is 200 ng/ml (1 ng=1/1,000,000 mg). The level of IgE in individuals of extrinsic asthma is five to seven times the normal. The increased IgE levels along with positive skin grades suggest their atopic significance.[16] This is shown in Figure 7.2. The reagins possess two Fab and Fc pieces. They get fixed by a Fc piece to the mast cells situated just beneath the bronchial epithelium and blood vessels and to the circulating basophil leucocytes. The mast cells is filled with metachromatically staining cytoplasmic granules, which appear

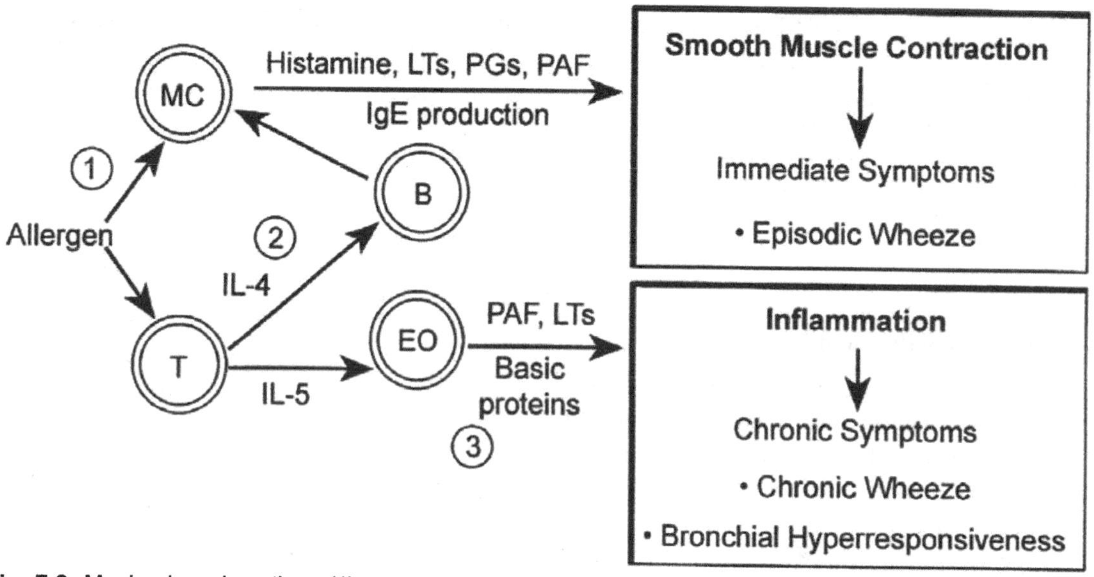

Fig. 7.2: Mechanisms in asthma (1) as seen in atopics (2) as seen in non-atopics (3) late phase reaction

as whorls or parallel lines. Further exposure to the same antigen leads to the union of antigen with the antigen receptors on the Fab portion of two molecules of IgE antibody. It results in degranulation of the cells by exocytosis. The contractile elements of cells (microtubules and microfilaments) also participate in this process and get aggregated. Entry of calcium into the mast cells induces the contraction of microfilaments, thereby releasing mediators of anaphylaxis[2] (Fig. 7.3).

Allergen extracts provocation can cause a rapid onset of bronchoconstriction reaching a maximum of 15 to 30 minutes after challenge and recovering over the following one to two hours. Bronchoconstriction which begins four to six hours after challenge and lasts for 12 hours as a late responses occur as a result of cellular and biochemical mechanisms and are

Antigen-IgE Reaction on Sensitised Mast Cell

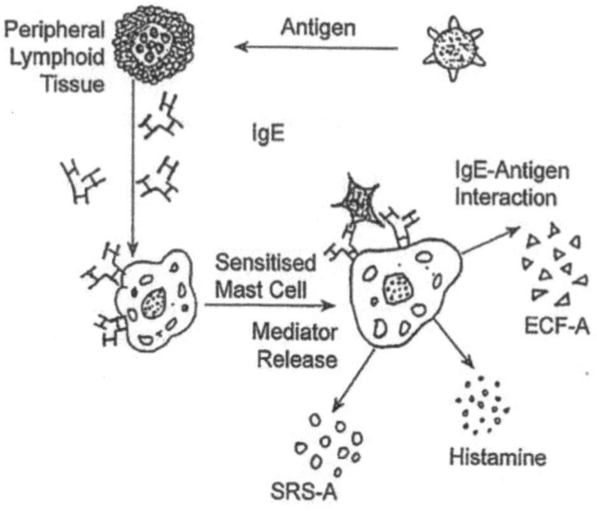

Fig. 7.3

accompanied by an increased bronchial responsiveness. The condition may be seasonal or perennial. Variations depending upon the time of exposure to the offending allergen are known.[2] Inflammatory cells and chemical mediators involved in bronchial asthma are listed in Table 7.19.

Table 7.19: Bronchial asthma: Cellular and chemical mediators

Inflammat(ory) cells	*Chemical mediators*
Mast cells	Leukotrienes
Macrophages	Platelet activating factor
Eosinophils	Cytokines (interleukins)
Neutrophils	Neuropeptides
T. lymphocytes	
Platelets	

The mediators play an important role in the pathogenesis of asthma. Histamine is a preformed granule, associated with powerful bronchospastic mediator. It is found in mast cells and basophils. Its actions are mediated via membrane associated H_1 receptors. There is bronchial smooth muscle contraction, increased vascular permeability, increased airways mucous production and production of prostaglandins. The cross linkage of cell bound IgE is responsible for activating a series of enzymes which mobilize arachidonic acid from membrane phospholipids. Oxidative metabolism of arachidonic acid via either the cyclo-oxygenase pathway produces prostaglandins (PGE_2, PGF_2, alpha PGD_2 and PGI_2) and thromboxenes (Tx), or lipoxygenase pathway produces hydroxy-fatty acids and leukotrienes (LTC_4, LTD_4 and LTE_4). Classical and alternative pathways have been shown in Figures 7.4 and 7.5.

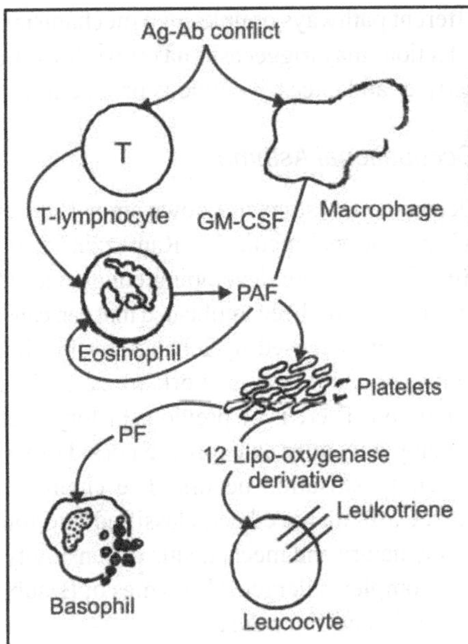

Bronchial Asthma

Inflammatory Cells	Chemical Mediators
Mast Cells	Leukotrienes
Macrophages	Platelet Activating Factor
Eosinophils	Cytokines (Interleukins)
Neutrophils	Neuropeptides
T. Lymphocytes	
Platelets	

Fig. 7.4: Interplay of cells and cytokines in asthma

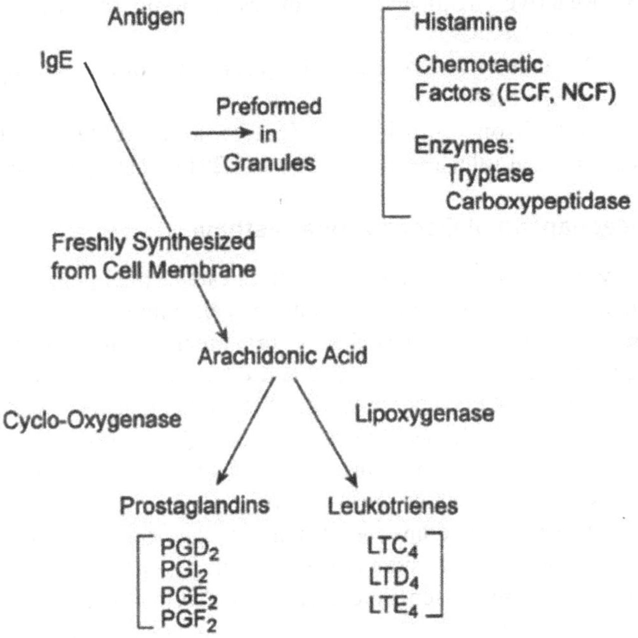

Fig. 7.5: The classical and alternative pathways in asthma

PGE_2 and PGI_2 cause relaxation of airways smooth muscle, whereas PGF_2 alpha and TX_{A2} cause contraction of smooth muscle, PGE_2 and PGI_2 cause vasodilation, and vasoconstriction is caused by TX_{A2}. PGD_2 increase vascular permeability and stimulates neutrophil chemokinesis. Leucotrienes (earlier referred to as a slow reactive substance of anaphylaxis SRS_{-A}) LTC_4, LTD_4 and LTE_4 are potent contractors of airways smooth muscles. They cause vasoconstriction, increase vascular permeability and stimulate mucus production. Platelet activating factor acether (originally called platelet activating factor, PAF) released from lipid membranes causes bronchoconstriction, increased vascular permeability and vasoconstriction. It causes aggregation and activation of inflammatory cells. In addition there is release of a variety of chemotactic mediators like eosinophil chemotactic factor-A (ECF-A) and neutrophil chemotactic factor (NCF) in the lung. Bradykinin, a peptide split product of plasma kininogen by the effect of enzyme kallikrein causes vasodilation and increased vascular permeability. Serotonin is released by neuro-epithelial bodies situated in the bronchial and alveolar walls and also by the aggregation of platelets. They cause bronchial smooth muscle contraction, increased vascular permeability and increased bronchial secretion.

Histamine, prostaglandins and leukotrienes derived from activated mast cells account for the early response with allergen inhalation. Mediators released from activated mast cell triggered by an IgE-dependent mechanism is inhibited by beta 2-adrenoceptor stimulants, sodium cromoglycate and nedocromil sodium.

In a late reaction, there is an increased bronchial responsiveness which can be inhibited by sodium cromoglycate and corticosteroids. There is airflow limitation in smaller airways which is characterised by mucosal oedema, hypersecretion of mucus and exudation of plasma proteins. The contraction of airways smooth muscles play a minor role.

Mast cells have been found to be increased in immediate response to allergen but the late response does not seem to be mast cell dependent.[7-17] Macrophages are activated by IgE dependent mechanisms, and are involved in late phase in- flammatory reaction, releasing mediators.[19] Eosinophils are increased only in last asthmatic reaction, releasing variety of mediators. T cells perpetuate the inflammatory response and platelets are also implicated, releasing variety of mediators. Neutrophils are involved in certain occupational asthmas.[7] Influx of eosinophils and polymorphs into bronchial epithelium and leukotrienes and PAF-acether lead to mucosal oedema and exudation of plasma proteins. In fact, asthma could be regarded as a chronic eosinophilic bronchitis where several inflammatory cells contribute to bronchial hyper-responsiveness and chronic asthma.[18]

Nonatopic Extrinsic Asthma

Mostly seen in adults with a positive family history of allergy, urticaria and atopic dermatitis or asthma. A variety of allergens exposure may stimulate sufficient number of antibodies which in combination with inhaled allergens form immune complexes, which in turn fix and activate the complement and bring about type III reaction which are precipitin mediated. Skin test is positive and gives a late reaction, 6 hours after the challenge and is often associated with fever and leucocytic reaction. Response to bronchodilators is less satisfactory.

Intrinsic Asthma

It occurs in middle aged patients, with a prior history of upper respiratory tract infection. The episodes are quite continuously occurring and there is hardly any family history of allergy or bronchial asthma. No particular external allergen is pointed out to which these symptoms can be attributed. Common allergens don't show any immediate type of hypersensitivity on skin testing. Blood IgE levels may not be elevated since the attack is not mediated through IgE, although same chemical mediators may be responsible for the attack. No organ specific auto-antibodies can be demonstrated in patient's serum.

Blood test shows eosinophilia. Even sputum and nasal secretions may have eosinophils. The response to corticosteroids is good.

Clinical Types

The clinical types of asthma are essentially based on specific or non-specific the stimulators of bronchoconstriction. The airways exhibit hyper-irritability for a variety of stimuli. Any alteration in the balance of sympathetic control of bronchomotor tone causes an increase in the airways resistance, leading to airways obstruction. The airways obstruction occurs through mechanisms based on immunological reactions with the presence of reaginic and non-reaginic antibodies or pharmacological reactions from release of pharmacologically active chemicals eliciting smooth muscle contraction or neurological mechanisms from stimulation of parasympathetic efferent pathways or unknown mechanisms.[2] Respiratory viral infections may trigger asthma probably by increasing cholinergic activity and excessive mucus production.

Occupational Asthma

Occupational asthma is known since 18th century when "Father of occupational medicine" Ramazzini recognised that workers shifting grains are developing cough and wheeze.[19] More than 200 agents have been implicated that can cause occupation related asthma. It is caused by inhalation of airborne dusts, vapours, fumes encountered in work place and asthma develops in adulthood. There is no previous history of atopy and symptoms develop only after an exposure period of weeks to years during which sensitisation occurs. The chemical substances which induce asthma have been classified into four categories[2] based on the nature and mechanisms of sensitivity as follows:

1. Complete allergens: Enzymes of B. subtilis, animal dander, grain and flour dusts.
2. Non-reactive chemicals forming haptenes: Antibiotic dust, halide salts of platinum, nickel.
3. Reactive chemicals: Isocyanates, phthalic anhydrides, ethenolamines.
4. Wood dust: Western red cedar (Prevalence of this type of asthma is 5%).[20]

Definition, aetiological factors and incidence of occupational asthma are listed in Tables 7.20 to 7.23 respectively.

Mechanism of Occupational Asthma

Several mechanisms have been implicated, including non-immunological as well as immunological. Immune mediated occupational asthma is due to IgE mechanism. Role of glycoproteins, polysaccharides and other proteins has been demonstrated. Even possible role of IgG is being investigated. Non-immunologic mechanisms include:

1. Stimulation of irritant receptors by toxic or irritant substances such as plicatic acid.
2. Actuation of serum complement by classical or alternate pathway, e.g., western red cedar; and
3. Direct pharmacologic effect such as by toluene di-isocyanate.

Goldsmith often use nitric acid in making certain jewellery. Toxic gases, are often released during the process. Nitrogen dioxide is most toxic of all. It cause eye irritation, dry cough, chest tightness. Deterioration of lung functions occurs. Deep lung irritation can be fatal due to pulmonary odema.

Acute respiratory illness may present with dyspnoea, and dry cough. Auscultation would yield bilateral crepitation and rhonchi. Removal from source, hospitalization, oxygen administration, nebulized bronchodilators, corticosteroids and antibiotics for prevention of secondary infection are important for favourable outcome.

Table 7.20: Definition of occupational asthma[21]

Occupational asthma has been defined as a disorder of variable airflow obstruction and airway hyper-responsiveness to the causes and conditions that are attributable to a particular occupational situation and that excludes those that are due to non-work place exposure. It can be caused by both allergic and non-allergic causes.

Table 7.21: Causes of occupational asthma[22]

Class	*Agent*	*Representative occupation or industry*
A. Natural organic		
1. Animal proteins	Laboratory animals	Drug, research, breeders
Bovine proteins	Dairy workers	
Egg white/yolks	Egg processing workers	
Prawns	Prawn workers	
2. Enzymes	Subtilisin	Detergent
	Trypsin	Drug
	Pancreatin	Drug
	Papain	Food processor
3. Insects and ascardies	Grain mites	Granary workers
	Silkworm	Sericulture
	Fowl mites	Poultry workers
	Cockroaches	Laboratory workers
4. Plant proteins	Cereal grains	Granary workers, millers
	Wheat flour	Bakers, millers
	Buck wheat	Food processors
5. Legumes	Coffee beans	Food processors
	Soyabeans	Farmers
	Castor beans	Fertiliser handlers
6. Seeds	Cottonseed	Cottonseed oil producers
	Linseed	Linseed oil producers
	Flax seed	Flax seed workers
7. Vegetable gums	Karaya	Hair dressers
	Tragacanth	Printing, hair dressers
8. Wood dusts	Western red ceder	Carpenters
	African maple	Wood workers
9. Organic dyes	Azo- and anthraquinone	Cloth dyeing
	Methyl blue, black	
	G-R dyeing	
10. Miscellaneous	Tobacco leaf	Tobacco farmers and processors
	Garlic	Food workers
	Latex	Nurses, surgical glove manufacturers
	Colophony	Electronics mechanics
B. Pharmaceuticals	Penicillin	Pharmaceutical
	Spiramycin	Pharmaceutical
	Tetracycline	Pharmaceutical
	Piperazine	Pharmaceutical
C. Organic chemicals		
1. Anhydrides	Phthalic anhydride	Plastics, drugs
	Trimellitic anhydride	Epoxy resins, plastics
	Hexahydraphthalic anhydride	Plastics
2. Diisocyanate	Toluene diisocyanate	Isocyanate manufacturing
	Hexamethylene diisocyanate	Paint, plastics
3. Miscellaneous	Ethylenediamine	Beauty, plastics
	Chloramine-T	Pharmaceutical
	Triethylene tetramine	Epoxy resins
D. Inorganic chemicals		
1. Metal salts	Platinum salts	Platinum refining
	Nickel salts	Metal plating
	Chromium salts	Cement, tanning

Table 7.22: Incidence of occupational asthma in high-risk occupations[23]

Occupational group	*Rate/Million/Year*
Welders/solders/electronic assemblers	159
Laboratory technicians and assistants	204
Metal making and processing	409
Bakers	409
Chemical processors	405
Coach spray painters	639
Other painters	104

Bronchiolitis obliterans may occur 2-6 weeks later. Regular follow up is important.[24,25]

a. Physiologic Testing

Pre and post-shift spirometry, PEFR, methacholine testing and specific inhalation challenge testing are methods that have been utilized to evaluate occupational asthma. Intrashift decrement in FEV of atleast 10 per cent are considered significant, especially if these can be correlated with symptoms at work. Methacholine inhalation test is a sensitive screening test for occupational asthma. A negative methacholine test at work essentially excludes occupational asthma.

b. Immunologic Studies

In vivo and in vitro, immunologic methods can readily detect specific IgE to HMW proteinaceous antigens. Various tests that can be employed for the detection of antibodies include radioallergosorbent assay (RAST), radioimmunoassay and enzyme linked immunosorbent assay. Specific IgG antibodies to occupational antigens have also been studied, but the significance or usefulness of these measurements is uncertain.

Management

Medical management is similar to management of any asthmatic. Obviously, a team work required to properly assess and place the worker at the proper place or work. Unlike western countries, medicolegal implications in terms of compensation, have not received much attention in India.[27]

Prognosis

Respiratory symptoms and airway hyper-responsiveness continue for several years after avoidance of exposure in many cases of occupationally induced asthma. The symptoms and non-specific bronchial hyper-responsiveness do not recover completely even after avoidance of exposure to a casual agent. So limitation of everyday activity is expected in about half to three fourth of the cases.

Table 7.23: Occupational asthma among health care workers [21]

Substance	*Occupation*	*Department*
(A) HMW substances		
Animal proteins	Lab. workers	Research lab.
Ipsaghulla	Nurses	Geriatrics
Pancreatic extracts	Nurses	Paediatrics
Bromelian	Lab. technician	Blood bank
Bovine serum	Lab. technician	Pathology
Albumin		
Latex	Nurses	Surgery
Allergens	Technician	Respiratory medicine starch
Corn starch	Obstetrician	Obstetrics
(B) LMW substances		
Formaldehyde	Nurses	Renal dialysis unit
Glutaraldehyde	Nurses	Radiology
	Radiographer	Endoscopy
Hexa chlorophene	Nurses	Paediatrics
Chloramine	Lab. technician	Pathology
Methyl-methacrylate	Nurses in OT	Orthopaedics
Methyl blue	Nurses	Cardiology
	ECG technician	
Enflurance	Anaesthetist	Anaesthesia

Ref: IJCP; 1995; 5(9): 70-72.

Prevention

Cessation of exposure is the preferred treatment. Pharmacotherapy is indicated only for the acute attack of occupational asthma. Cromolyn sodium can be considered as a preventive measure for allergen induced occupational asthma. In general, pharmacotherapy is not considered a suitable alternative for reduction of exposure to causative agents. Ultimately early detection and removal from further exposure may be the most useful method of avoiding the development of symptoms of chronic occupational asthma. Diagnosing and managing occupational diseases demands a serious attention at the clinical level as well as creating an opportunity to integrate occupational pulmonary medicine at the educational level in medical schools.[28]

Drug-Induced Bronchospasm

Drugs responsible for inducing bronchospasm are listed below:

1. Aspirin.
2. NSAIDs.
3. Beta blockers.
4. ACE inhibitors.
5. Neuromuscular blocking agents.
6. Laxatives.
7. Antibiotics.
8. Inhalation agents.
9. Food additives.

Bronchospasm is the most common manifestation of drug induced lung disease.[29] Both type I and III immune mechanisms may be involved. Sometimes, bronchospasm may be due to direct stimulation of the parasympathetic bronchomotor tone and at other times, the airways narrowing may be due to interference with arachidonic acid metabolism.

In vast majority, the cause of drug induced spasm remains idiopathic pharmacologic reaction. Suggested mechanisms, however, include:

1. Non-IgE related release of mast cell mediators.
2. Immunoglobulin and IgE requiring mechanisms.
3. Induction of irritating effect via cellular mechanisms ophthalmic agents like pilocarpine, carbachol, methacholine can precipitate bronchospasm. Tartazine–yellow food dye can trigger bronchospasm and even has cross reactivity to aspirin.

Sulfites/metabisulfites, mostly in dry fruits, potatoes, beer and wine and in nebulizing solutions and lidocaine injection can cause bronchospasm.

Aspirin-Induced Asthma

Aspirin-induced asthma generally manifests itself in the third and fourth decades and involves women more frequently than men. There is no history of atopy or asthma. There can be a history of taking aspirin many a times without any reaction. In about ten per cent of adult patients with asthma, aspirin causes airways narrowing which varies in its severity from asymptomatic bronchospasm to fatal status asthmaticus. Urticaria and rhinitis are commonly seen with other symptoms of aspirin intolerance such as watery rhinorrhea and nasal polyps. The aspirin-induced asthma, AIA syndrome, has no clear pathogenesis but it appears to be related to cyclo-oxygenase inhibition, which transforms arachidonic acid into prostaglandin peroxidase, prostaglandins, prostacyclin and thromboxane A.[30,31] This theory draws its support both from animal as well as human studies. Only analgesics with anticyclo-oxygenase activity induce bronchospasm. There is a positive, but weak correlation between the potency of analgesics to inhibit cyclo-oxygenase in vitro and their potency to induce bronchospasm in vivo. It has been suggested that platelets generate chemical mediators following inhibition of cyclo-oxygenase. Salicylates do not affect cyclo-oxygenase activity and prostanoid formation. Sodium salicylate, salicylamide, guainacolic ester of acetylsalicylic acid, dextropropoxyphene and choline magnesium salicylate are well tolerated by patients with asthma.[32] A small number of aspirin sensitive asthmatics may react to drugs that do not inhibit cyclo-oxygenase enzyme.

Ninety-five per cent of reactions occur after ingestion of 5 grams or less of aspirin. There is almost complete cross reaction between aspirin and non-steroidal anti-inflammatory agents. Treatment of aspirin/induced asthma lies in prevention, i.e., avoidance of aspirin and non-steroidal anti-inflammatory drugs. Ibuprofen is reported to cause bronchial asthma.[33] Asthma and angioedema with nimesulide[34] and near fatal asthma with diclofenac sodium tablet on oral ingestion have been reported.[35] Desensitization is a useful therapeutic strategy but caution must be observed as severe bronchospasm may develop with even small doses of aspirin. Aspirin desensitization often protects against reactions to other non-steroidal drugs. Curiously aspirin relieves bronchospasm in some asthmatics.

Indomethacin—an effective anti-inflammatory agent—has been reported to produce fatal airways narrowing in patients with bronchial asthma. Although it is universally known that oral and rectal administration of indocin can cause asthma, Sheehan, *et al.*, have described a 79-year-old patient who developed severe bronchospasm after topical administration of indomethacin eye drops.[36] Hydrocortisone has paradoxically been reported to cause bronchospasm rarely in aspirin-sensitive individuals.

Recent reports of precipitation of allergy, rhino conjunctivitis and asthma with acetaminophen have appeared too (Am J Resp Crit Care Med 2011; 183: 165-70 and 171-78).

Beta-Blockers

Life-threatening bronchospasm with beta-blockers can occur in patients with underlying airways hyperactivity. Individuals from atopic family background, but with no prior history of asthma, may occasionally succumb to bronchospastic episodes. Although the mechanism of beta-blocker induced bronchospasm is not thoroughly understood, it occurs only with L-isomer of propranolol and not with the D-isomer. Beta-blockers induce bronchoconstriction either by enhancing cholinergic tone or by enhancing the release of mediators from the mast cells. Anti-cholinergic agents and pre-treatment with disodium cromglycate blocks propranolol-induced bronchospasm. Inhaled anti-cholinergic drugs form treatment of choice for beta-blocker-induced bronchospasm.

An extremely non-selective B_1-B_2 adrenergic antagonist, Timolol is about six times more potent than propranolol in causing bronchospasm. About twenty per cent of the patients who use Timolol either orally or as eye drops develop bronchospasm.[37] Elderly patients, particularly those with asthma and airways obstruction are more susceptible. Since a respiratory arrest may occur with the first dose of Timolol, it is strongly recommended that ophthalmic beta-blockers should not be given to patients with bronchial asthma, chronic obstructive lung disease and latent bronchial hyperactivity. If the use of the drug is unavoidable, then it should be given under strict medical supervision with means of controlling bronchospasm at hand.[3] Atenolol is considered to be a less potent bronchoconstrictor. Various drugs causing vasoconstriction have been listed in Table 7.24.

ACE Inhibitors

Cough is a well-recognized side effect of angiotensin converting enzyme (ACE) inhibitors. Although the incidence of cough varies, it commonly affects women. The mechanism of this cough remains clouded, but, the underlying bronchial hyperactivity appears to be a predisposing factor. An increase in bradykinin concentration in upper airways has been mooted. ACE inhibitors may uncover an asthmatic tendency in patients with pre-existing bronchial hyperactivity by permitting asthma developing de novo. Enalapril precipitating an attack of asthmaticus bronchitis has been reported.[38]

Inhalation Agents

Following the use of metered dose inhalers, bronchospasm may be related either to the non-specific irritant effect of the inhaled particles, or to inert propellants and dispersant or to sulfate sensitivity. Isoproterenol, metaproterenol, albuterol, beclomethasone dipropionate, ipratropium bromide and aerosolized pentamidine have caused bronchospasm in susceptible individuals.[39]

Neuromuscular Blocking Agents

D-tubocurarine, alcuronium, atracurium, vecuronium and pancuronium have been incriminated causing histamine related bronchospasm.

Laxative Related Asthma

A number of laxatives contain extracts from seeds of the psyllium plant, a member of the plantago weed family. Psyllium has been identified as causing occupational asthma in pharmaceutical industries manufacturing such laxatives. Also asthma may occur in individuals and nurses exposed at home and in nursing homes preparing psyllium. Sensitization to psyllium is an IgE mediated reaction which is initiated by inhalation of psyllium powder. However, the ability of this laxative to induce respiratory symptoms when ingested by

Table 7.24: Drugs causing bronchoconstriction

1. Analgesics and anti-inflammatory		
Opiates	Morphine	
NSAID	Aspirin	Flurbiprofen, ibuprofen
	Indomethacin	Mefenamic acid, diclofenac sodium
	Naproxen	Nimesulide
2. Autonomic system modulators		
Beta blockers	Propranolol	Oxyprenolol
	Timolole	Metprolol
Anticholin esterase	Echothopate	
3. Antibiotics		
Penicillins		Tetracyclines
Cephalosporins		
4. Others		
ACE inhibitors		Rifampicin
Cromoglycates		Tartrazine
Griseofulvin		Clozapine
Pancreatic extracts		Sulfates
Iron dextran		Aminophylline
Iodinated contrasts		

sensitized subjects indicates that individuals exposed to psyllium by respiratory route, e.g., nurses and pharmaceutical workers should avoid laxatives containing psyllium.[40]

Antibiotic and Other Drugs

Antibiotics (Penicillin, cephalosporin etc.), Anti-tuberculosis drugs (Rifampicin), Antifungal (Griseofulvin), Choline esterase inhibitors (Neostigmine), Parasympathomimetic drugs (Carbachol), Analgesics (Pentazocine) are known to cause bronchospasm. Different varieties of bronchial asthma are listed in Table 7.25.

Table 7.25: Variants of bronchial asthma
1. Nocturnal asthma
2. Exercise induced asthma
3. Drug induced asthma
4. Occupational asthma
5. Local asthma
a. Tokyo Yokohama
b. New Orleans
c. Bombay (Mumbai)

Certain ophthalmic agents such as timolol and betaxolol (beta blockers), and parasympathetic drugs like pilocarpine, carbachol, methacoline can also precipitate bronchospatua in susceptible subjects. Yellow food dyes can trigger bronchospasm in asthma patients.

Sulfiting agents through liberation of sulfur dioxide can induce acute asthma in susceptible patients. These agents are found in processed potatoes, beer, wine and dry fruits and also in nebulizing solutions and lidocaine injectable preparations.

Exercise-Induced Asthma (EIA)

Exercise can initiate or exacerbate bronchospasm. This may be an occult manifestation of hyperactive airways. During exercise, there is hyperventilation, decrease in airways temperature and respiratory tract water loss. There is mouth breathing because of increased oxygen demand that is aggravated. Possibly, the rewarming of respiratory tract during cessation of exercise may be responsible for bronchoconstriction.[41] Odema from hyperaemic of microcirculation may partially contribute to bronchial obstruction. Rebound hyperaemia from hyperplastic capillary bed, that occurs, may contribute to airways odema and the bronchial obstruction. In addition, there can be thermally-sensitive neuroreceptors, hyperplastic capillary bed and generalised allergy; that plays a crucial role.[42] These patients get exacerbation of dyspnoea on exposure to cold as well. Dyspnoea, wheeze and chest tightness 3 to 5 minutes after exercise is experienced. The mechanism of cooling of airways mucosa and loss of airways heat may release mast cell mediators, stimulate oropharyngeal irritant receptors and induce local intrathoracic stimulation causing bronchospasm.[2] Beta$_2$ agonists if inhaled, 1/2-1 hour prior to exercise, can prevent EIA in 3/4th of cases.

Nocturnal Asthma

Nocturnal asthma is common and quite troublesome. Although the syndrome has been recognized for centuries, its pathogenesis remains unclear.

In 1698, John Floyer, himself an asthmatic, remarked, *I have observed that fit always to happen after sleep in the night, when the nerves are filled with windy spirits.* Recently, Janson and colleagues have shown that asthma patients do not sleep and they have more periods of wakefulness than non-asthmatics.[43]

These sleep disturbances could be related to nocturnal cough and bronchoconstriction. Many asthma patients remain totally asymptomatic during the day but develop wheezing during the night or early morning. Several hypotheses have been put forward, including the influence of sleep in supine posture, circadian variation in circulating adrenaline, histamine, cortisol levels, gastroesophageal reflux (GER) and the effect of drugs,[44] as shown in Table 7.26.

Table 7.26: Factors related to nocturnal asthma
1. Night bronchoconstriction experienced by normal individuals
2. Sleep
3. Posture
4. Alteration of circadian rhythm
5. Autonomic nerve activity
6. Gastroesophageal reflux
7. Secretion and airways inflammation
8. Drugs: Anticholinergics, theophylline, calcium-channel blockers.

Nocturnal bronchoconstriction is a normal phenomenon. The extent of decrease in expiratory flow rate, however, is minimal and inconsequential in normal individuals. In asthma patients, on the other hand, the bronchoconstriction reflects the severity of hyperreactivity. If the airways are markedly hyperresponsive, the episodes of nocturnal bronchoconstiction tend to be severe. Change of environment reduces hyperresponsiveness and lessens bronchoconstriction. Bronchial reactivity increases in normal individuals and in patients with asthma at night. Nocturnal bronchospasm can be attributed to an exaggeration of abnormal circadian rhythm in airways caliber in patients with labile airways. The biological clock during the peak rhythm has not been identified. Although overnight changes in peak flow rate reflect changes in corticosteriod levels, neither stabilization of 11-hydroxycorticosteroid level by hydrocortisone infusion, nor high dose steroid therapy, nor adrenalectomy prevent morning dip in peak flow rate.[40] The circadian rhythm of corticosteriod secretion does not appear to be the main cause of nocturnal and early morning asthma. If patients are kept awake at night, the nocturnal dip in peak flow rate is significantly reduced. Nevertheless, in a truly awake patient bronchospasm does not completely disappear, indicating that other factors also play some role. The circadian rhythm in peak flow is often in phase with the timing of sleep, but sleep does not cause nocturnal asthma.[45] EEG studies have shown that in asthmatic children bronchospasm does not occur during phase IV of rapid eye movement (REM) sleep. It is conceivable that certain phases of sleep could, nevertheless, cause nocturnal asthma.

Bronchial smooth muscle is supplied by the parasympathetic and non-adrenergic non-cholinergic (NANC) nervous systems. An increased parasympathetic tone may contribute to nocturnal bronchoconstriction. The effect of sympathetic and nonadrenergic noncholinergic nerves and diurnal variation of airways oedema and inflammatory mediators in nocturnal asthma may be of relevance for future research. Alteration in the vagal tone may be caused by cold, snoring or GER. The increased vagal tone may be blocked by cholinergic blockers like atropine or ipratropium bromide.

It is well known that GER causes aspiration and a constellation of respiratory disorders including recurrent pneumonia, atelectasis, asthma and fibrosis. Acid infusion into the esophagus can produce bronchoconstriction. A high incidence of GER has been observed in patients with nocturnal asthma. In such patients the use of H_2-receptor blocker has been shown to improve asthma symptoms. It appear that GER in most of the asthmatics do not immediately precipitate asthma, although it does seem to influence vagal bronchomotor tone as has been demonstrated by the low morning peak expiratory flow rate. Anticholinergic drugs, calcium-channel blocking agents and theophylline may exacerbate GER. During sleep, mucocilliary clearance is impaired. The resulting accumulation of mucus is associated with mucosal oedema and may contribute to airways narrowing.

Steps to Control Nocturnal Asthma

1. Optimum control of daytime asthma, using $beta_2$-agonists, inhalation of steroids and cromolyn sodium.
2. Long-acting $beta_2$ agonists: 1 to 2 tablets orally before going to bed.
3. Single dose, prednisone, 20 to 30 mg orally at bed time (in extreme cases).

It is important to give these drugs regularly throughout the day in order to stabilize the airways even in apparently asymptomatic subjects. When a properly administered $beta_2$ agonist drug regimen does not produce effective relief of bronchospasm, aerosolized corticosteroids should be prescribed to suppress the airways inflammation that appears to underline the severe bronchial hyperactivity in asthma. Oral theophyllines and oral $beta_2$ agonist can markedly reduce symptoms of nocturnal asthma. However theophylline tends to disturb sleep, releases oesophagal sphincter (aggravating the GER) and causes psychological impairment in children. Controlled release $beta_2$ agonists are as effective as theophylline, and without the serious side effects of theophylline. Weiner and colleagues suggest that a single oral dose of prednisone is effective in controlling nocturnal asthma.[46]

Respiratory Infections and Asthma

The upper respiratory tract infections particularly of rhino virus, respiratory syncytial virus, parainfluenza and influenza virus often cause exacerbation of asthma. There is change in airways reactivity and increased airways resistance. Airways lumen is narrowed by inflammatory exudate. There is epithelial destruction leading to increased sensitivity of airways irritant receptors and their stimulation.

Aspergillus Sensitivity and Asthma

Exacerbation of asthma may be related to inhalation of aspergillus spores especially in an atopic patient with a long history of asthma. There is an interplay of immune mechanism with underlying asthma. The vicid mucus may facilitate growth of inhaled fungus to which the patient becomes sensitised.[2]

Reflux triggered brochospasm may occur because of retrograde flow of gastric contents into oesophagus because of lack of competent gastroesophagal junctions, especially in patients with reactive airways, when they sleep in supine position.[2]

Rubber Glove Asthma

Apart from rhinitis and anaphylaxis, asthma can be provoked by vapours given off by rubber gloves.[47] Even washing powder perfume provoking asthma has been observed.

Bhopal Gas Effect

An asthma like syndrome has been reported as Reactive Airways Dysfunction Syndrome.[48]

Mediators of Asthma

The release of mediators is a non-cytolytic process requiring energy and calcium ions. It is influenced by cyclic nucleotides.

An increase in the level of CAMP (cyclic adenosine 3' 5' monophosphate) inhibits secretion; whereas its diminished level results in an enhanced secretion of mediators. An increased level of CGMP (cyclic guanosine 3' 5' monophosphate) increases the secretion of mediators. A diminution in the content of CGMP is associated with diminution in the secretion of mediators (Fig. 7.6).

Biosynthesis of Cyclic AMP

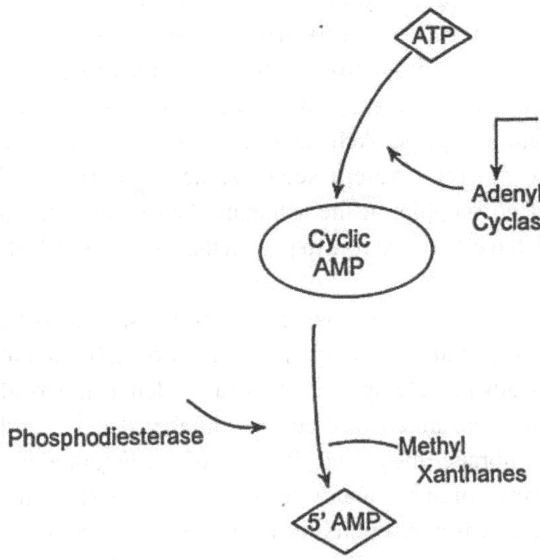

Fig. 7.6

The enzyme-adenylate cyclase (AC) and guanylate cyclase (GC) catalyse the biosynthesis of CAMP and CGMP from ATP (adenosine triphosphate) and GTP (guanosine triphosphate) respectively. Cyclic nucleotide phosphodiesterase (PD) causes selective degradation of CAMP. Thus the levels of CAMP and CGMP regulate the function of the cells in a bi-directional manner with an opposing effect on generation and release of mediators of asthma. These substances appear following an autonomic stimulation. An autonomic imbalance associated with decreased beta adrenergic responsiveness, alters the relative concentration of cyclic nucleotide (CAMP, CGMP), in turn release of substances of hypersensitivity.

The synthesis of CAMP is augmented by stimulation of adenylate cyclase by endogenous hormones (beta catecholamine, prostaglandins and histamine). The level of CAMP is decreased by the action of alpha catecholamines. The level of CGMP is increased on stimulation of guanylate cyclase enzyme coverting GTP to CGMP by cholinergic agents (acetyl choline).[2] These have been discussed in detail in the following text under sub-heading 'Mechanism'.

Pathophysiology[2]

The pathophysiological changes occur essentially in the bronchial lumen and its walls. The medium and small bronchi are filled with thick viscid yellow plugs of mucus.[49,50] They are rich with a large number of eosinophils and clusters of disquamated bronchial epithelial cells. The bronchi and bronchioli are markedly thickened. The number and size of bronchial glands and goblet cells are increased. Bronchial epithelium is lost in many places, with marked thickening of basement membrane. The wall and peribronchial tissues show marked infiltration with eosinophils, lymphocytes and mononuclear cells and smooth muscle hypertrophy.

Airways obstruction is essentially brought about by the mucosal oedema, sticky mucus in the bronchial lumen. There is hyperplasia of goblet cells and an inability of smooth muscle relaxation. There is vascular congestion of mucosa and submucosa. The marked hypertrophy of smooth muscles also contributes to the spasm. There is an increased airways resistance as well.

The airways obstruction causes an increased resistance to airflow during both phases of respiration resulting in air trapping and hyperinflation of lungs. The uneven ventilation does not match to blood flow. Lot of ventilation is washed. There occurs hypoxemia. Patients hyperventilates, arterial CO_2 ($PaCO_2$) is reduced initially. Functional residual capacity increases, necessitating an increase in transpulmonary pressure to produce an adequate tidal volume. The work of breathing is loaded further, creating the demand of oxygen. The minute ventilation is thus increased to compensate for the increase in wasted ventilation and CO_2 production. This adds workload on respiratory muscles further, causing their fatigue. Persistent airways obstruction results in retention of CO_2 and respiratory acidosis and anaerobic metabolism causes metabolic lactic acidosis.

Mechanism[2]

The human airways are controlled by myogenic, neurogenic and chemical mechanisms. The activity originates in the smooth muscles. Small airways inflammation and obstruction is an important site involved in asthma and COPD and needs to be exposed further to evolve better pharmacotherapy.[48] Neurogenic control occurs through the vagus nerves innervating the muscles. Chemical control is blood-borne and is via a locally-derived substance.

Bronchial hyper-responsiveness: The mechanism of bronchial asthma have shown that bronchial hyper-responsiveness is the essential pathophysiologic abnormality. The responses are two-fold as (a) bronchoconstriction and (b) airways inflammation. Triggers are provoking agents. They may be specific such as antigens that act through an immunologic mechanism or non-specific physical or chemical agents such as exercise, cold air, emotion, environmental pollutants, aspirin, non-steroidal anti-inflammatory drugs, sulphur dioxide, beta blockers and metabisulphite. Viral respiratory tract infections, chemical sensitizing agents and allergens act as inducers of asthma effectively enhancing the responsiveness to other stimuli.

Airway inflammation: Marked inflammation is present in the airways with infiltration of inflammatory cells especially eosinophils, epithelial cell sloughing into lumen and plugging of the airway lumen by viscous mucus. There is smooth muscle hyperplasia. Biopsy study of airways in mild asthmatics has revealed airways shedding of ciliary epithelium, collagen deposition beneath basement membrane, partial mast cell degranulation and eosinophil cell infiltration of lamina propria.

Immune mechanism: Allergenic substance when inhaled into the lower respiratory tract may produce in a small group of population immunoglobulin E (IgE) antibodies. Any subsequent exposure to such substance produces a series of immunologic and biochemical reactions leading to occurrence of asthma. Protein substances such as pollens, grains, weeds, moulds, house dust, mite, animal dander and non-protein substances like platinum salts, toluene diisocyanate and trimellitic anhydride elicit immunologic response via IgE dependent interaction. Mast cells are present in the lining of the bronchioles and bronchi beneath basement membrane and adjacent to the capillaries. Mast cells probably are also involved in the immediate response to other non-IgE mediated stimuli. However mast cells are not involved in infection and intrinsic asthma.

Inflammatory cells: Previously asthma was seen merely as allergen induced mast cell degranulation resulting in the release of mediators such as histamine and slow reacting substance of anaphylaxis (SRS-A) and chemotactic factors for neutrophils (NCF) and eosinophils (ECF). Currently asthma is considered as a chronic inflammatory disease involving multiple interacting cells. Each cell covers the other and sends messages. A wide variety of inflammatory mediators are released by the cells that activate several trigger cells in the airway, resulting in bronchoconstriction, microvascular leakage and oedema, mucus hypersecretion and stimulation of neural reflexes. Inflammation and inflammatory mediators appear to underly bronchial hyper-responsiveness. Neural mechanisms may contribute to or modify these inflammatory events. The inflammatory stimuli to the airways activate cells normally found in the lungs referred to as primary effector cells. They are mast cells, basophils, alveolar macrophages, epithelial, and endothelial cells of the airways. On activation they release mediators that are chemotactic for cells in the circulation. They are referred to as secondary effector cells and include eosinophils, neutrophils, T-lymphocytes and platelets. These cells and their mediators modulate airways reactivity. Macrophages present in the airway lumen get activated by IgE dependent mechanisms. They release a large amount of mediators such as thromboxene, prostaglandins, and platelet activating factors (PAF). Macrophages are likely to initiate late response and bronchial hyperresponsiveness. The asthmatic airways are characteristically infiltrated by eosinophils. There is marked increase in eosinophil count and bronchial hyperresponsiveness. Eosinophils release a variety of mediators such as leukotriene C_4PAF, oxygen radicals and basic proteins (major basic protein and eosinophil cationic protein). The latter being toxic to airway epithelium causes its damage. Though there is neutrophil infiltration, their role is not determined. Lymphocytes may have a regulatory influence on the inflammatory response. Activated CD_4^+T lymphocytes have the capacity to orchestrate a selective accumulation and activation of eosinophils in the asthmatic bronchial mucosa and also they have a critical role to play in the regulation of IgE synthesis.

Airway obstruction: Following factors are shown to be operative in the production of airways obstruction in bronchial asthma: Smooth muscle spasm, mucosal oedema, mucosal cellular infiltration, mucus secretion, epithelial damage and basement membrane thickening. Release of mediators along with the infiltrate of inflammatory cells especially eosinophils and to some extent neutrophils in the airway wall provide a potent stimulus for the pathologic alterations in asthma.

Inflammatory mediators: A wide variety of inflammatory mediators have been implicated in asthma and they bring about inflammatory changes and cause hyperresponsiveness of the airways. Histamine, in a preformed granule, is a powerful bronchospastic mediator, and is found in mast cells and basophils. Its actions are mediated via membrane associated H_1 receptors. There is bronchial smooth muscle contraction, increased vascular permeability, increased airways mucus production and production of prostaglandins. The cross linkage of cell bound IgE activates a series of enzymes which mobilize archidonic acid from membrane phospholipids. Oxidative metabolism of arachidonic acid via either the cyclo-oxygenase pathway produces prostaglandins (PGE_2, PGF_2, PGD_2 and PGU and thromboxenes (Tx), or lipo-oxygenease pathway produces hydroxyfatty acids and sulphidopeptide leukotrienes (LTC_4, LTD_4 and LTE_4). PGE_2 and PGI_2 cause relaxation of airways smooth muscle whereas PGF_2 alpha Tx_{A2} cause contraction of smooth muscle-PGE_2, and PGI_2 cause vasodilation and vasoconstriction is caused by Tx_{A2}. PGD_2 increases vascular permeability and stimulates neutrophil chemokinesis. Leucotrienes (earlier referred as slow reactive substance of anaphylaxis SRS-A) LTC_4, LTD_4 and LTE_2 are potent contractors of airway smooth muscle. They cause vasoconstriction, increased vascular peremeability and stimulate mucus production. Platelet activating factor acether (originally platelet activating factor, PAF) released from lipid membranes causes bronchoconstriction, increased vascular permeability and vasoconstriction. It causes aggregation and activation of inflammatory cells. In addition there is release of a variety of chemotactic mediators like eosinophil chemotactic factor-A (ECF-A) and neutrophil chemotactic factor (NFC) in the lung. Bradykinin, a peptide split product of plasma kininogen by the effect of the enzyme kallikrein causes vasodilation and increased vascular permeability. Serotonin is released by neuro-epithelial bodies situated in the bronchial and alveolar walls and also by aggregation of platelets. They cause bronchial smooth muscle contraction, increased vascular permeability and increased bronchial secretion. Histamine, prostaglandins and leukotrienes derived from activated mast cells account for the early response with allergen inhalation. Mediators released from activated mast cells triggered by an IgE dependent mechanism is inhibited by $beta_2$ adrenocpetor stimulant, sodium cromoglycate and nedocromil sodium. In late reaction, there is an increased bronchial reponsiveness that can be inhibited by sodium cromoglycate and corticosteroids. There is airflow limitation in smaller airways. It is characterized by mucosal oedema, hypersecretion of mucus and exudation of plasma proteins. The contraction of airway smooth muscles play a minor role. The late reponse does not appear to be a mast cell dependent event. Macrophages, monocytes, eosinophils, T-lymphocytes and platelets are capable of expressing receptors for IgE on their cell surface and are able to respond to IgE dependent stimulation with mediator release following a suitable stimulus. There is an influx of polymorphonuclear leucocytes and eosinophils into the bronchial epithelium and lumen. Leukotrienes and PAF-acether lead to mucosal oedema and exudation of plasma proteins.

In non-atopic persons, the non-reaginic mechanisms showing type II hypersensitivity reaction, that is precipitin mediated and manifestations of asthma occurs in 5-6 hours after exposure to allergen. The inflammatory mediators increase permeability of the epithelium by disrupting the tight junctions between epithelial cells. There is microvascular leakage in airways at postcapillary venules. Consequently, epithelial shedding, exudation of plasma and oedema of airways occurs. Plasma provides inflammatory mediators that react with mucous to produce mucus plugging and cause obstruction of peripheral airways. The epithelial damage is responsible for airways hyperresponsiveness. They remove protection to airways smooth muscles, cause loss of relaxing factors, release mediators chemotactic to inflammatory cells and nerve endings as well as irritant receptors are exposed to physical agents and inflammatory mediators, leading to activation of neural reflexes.

A strong mediator of inflammation is platelet activating factor (PAF, PAF-acether), which is a complex phospholipid, that causes inflammation, leading to bronchial hyperresponsiveness. PAF is not released from mast cells; and is produced by platelets, vascular endothelial cells and variety of leucocytes like macrophages, monocytes, neutrophils and eosinophils. PAF is a molecular link connecting various inflammatory cells and eosinophils are strongly attracted and activated by it. PAF releases eosinophil chemotactic factor of anaphylaxis-A (ECF-A) and leukotriene B^4 (LTB^4). PAF induces bronchoconstriction, bronchial oedema, bronchial epithelial dysfunction and mucus hypersecretion.

Neural mechanisms: An abnormality in autonomic neural control in the form of an imbalance between excitatory and inhibitory pathways results in contraction of airways. Respiratory tract smooth muscle is under control of both parasympathetic (cholinergic) and hormonal (adrenergic) nerves. Resting tone in a normal airways is vagally mediated. Its stimulation results in bronchoconstriction. Certain neuropeptides also act as neurotransmitters for bronchial hyperresponsiveness. Muscarine, cholinergic, alpha-adrenergic and non-cholinergic pathways are excitatory, causing hyperresponsiveness and contraction of airways smooth muscles. Beta-adrenergic and non-adrenergic pathways are inhibitory to airways, causing its relaxation. An increased response to the former and decreased response to the latter bring about airway constriction, however, these changes appear to be secondary and not primary. There may be some interaction between neural and inflammatory mechanisms. Many inflammatory mediators bring about release of neuro-transmitters. Cholinergic mechanism forms the dominant neural bronchoconstrictor pathway in human airways. Many stimuli that produce bronchospasm also stimulate afferent receptors and may lead to reflex cholinergic bronchoconstriction and facilitate release of acetylcholine from motor nerve endings in the airway. Since anticholinergic drugs are not very effective in asthma, cholinergic mechanism does not appear to play an important role. Adrenergic mechanism involves sympathetic nerves. They do not directly control airway smooth muscle and the circulating catecholamines particularly epinephrine may play an important role in regulation of bronchoconstrictor tone. Inflammatory mediators also enhance alpha adrenergic receptor function and cause bronchoconstriction. However the effect is insignificant.

Vasoactive intestinal peptide (VIP) is a powerful relaxant of airways and if it is degraded rapidly by enzymes released from inflammatory cells, it causes exaggerated broncho-constrictor response. Other neuropeptides such as substance P, neurokinin A and calcitonin gene related peptide could be released by a local axon reflex following damage to airway epithelium exposing the afferent nerves to the effect of inflammatory mediators. It results in bronchoconstriction, microvascular leakage and mucus secretion.[2] Various mediators involved in bronchial asthma are listed in Table 7.27.

Table 7.27: Bronchial asthma: Mediators
A. *Causing bronchoconstriction*
Prostanoids PGD_2, PGF_2 alfa
Leukotrienes LTC_4, LTD_4
Adenosine
Bradykinin
Thromboxane A_2
Substance P
Plate activating factor (PAF)
Calcitonin gene related peptide
B. *Causing inflammation*
Leukotrienes LTB_4
Bradykinin
Adenosine
High molecular weight neutrophilic
Chemotactic factor of anaphylaxis
Lymphocytic chemotactic factor
Eosinophilic chemotactic factor
C. *Causing enhanced mucus secretion*
Leukotrienes
PAF
D. *Causing increase in capillary permeability*
PAF
Prostanoids (prostacycline)

Clinical Features

There are recurrent attacks of dyspnoea, cough and wheeze. The attacks of breathlessness persist for a time varying from a short duration to a long duration of hours or days as in status asthmaticus. Initially the attacks may come at longer intervals or in different seasons, as noted during summer in those sensitive to pollen and fungal spores.

As the disease progresses, the period of freedom from dyspnoea decreases and becomes perennial. There is a nocturnal wheeze. Cough often accompanies it. The latter is marked because of accompanying infection and is associated with mucopurulent or purulent expectoration.

Precipitation of the attacks may occur by inhalation of allergens like pollens of grass, weed, or trees or fungi (seasonal prevalence), house dust (nocturnal or on coming in contact with animals like dogs, cats, horses or birds). There may be a contact of feathers, fur, leather, flour or face powder of orris root. Rarely it can be precipitated on ingestion of food (egg, wheat, fish, milk, potato), especially in children. Those attacks are associated with gastrointestinal manifestations or urticaria. The infection in the nose or in the upper respiratory tract or anxiety or psychological stress or an incompatible situation in the family or place of work may precipitate an attack of asthma.

Severe attacks may last for several hours or days. The patients during such episodes get exhausted greatly. They may be cyanosed and become dehydrated from hyperventilation. This is described under acute severe bronchial asthma.

Clinical examination during attack reveals evidence of over-inflation of the lungs. There is diminished expansion of the chest. The accessory muscles of respiration come into action to enhance the force of expiration. There is an increased resonance over the chest with decreased vocal fremitus and vocal resonance. Stethoscopic examination reveals rhonchi over wide areas of the chest which are expiratory in character.

In severe attacks there is an increased work of breathing with flaring of nostrils, poorly moving low diaphragm, wide intercostal spaces, retraction of sternomastoid and intercostal regions during inspiration and unequal intensity of breath sounds. Expiratory wheeze is high pitched with tachypnoea, tachycardia, hypoxemia and often dehydration. There may be pulsus paradoxus from high intrapulmonary pressure. Cyanosis, systemic hypertension and arrhythmia may occur. In between the attacks, the lungs reveal no abnormality but the forced expiration reveals appearance of wheeze. Overinflation may be present in long standing cases. Fischl index—a scoring system,[51] using seven criteria, each being equal to one point—it is used to predict severity of disease. There is a need for hospitalisation if an index of four points or more is positive. The seven points parameters are as follows: (1) Pulse rate of 120 beats per minute; (2) Respiratory rate more than 30 breaths/minute, (3) Pulsus paradoxus more than 18 mmHg; (4) Peak expiratory flow rate less than 130 liters/minute; (5) Moderate to severe dyspnoea (resting); (6) Wheeze; and (7) Accessory muscles of respiration in action. Signs and differential diagnosis of bronchial asthma have been listed in Table 7.28.

Table 7.28: Bronchial asthma: Signs and dif ferential diagnosis (DD)	
Signs:	Barrel chest
	Harrison's sulcus
	Hypoventilation
	Rhonchi
DD:	Bronchitis
	Carcinoma lung
	CCF
	Emphysema (Obstruction)
	Pulmonary embolism
	Tuberculosis

Investigations:

Table 7.29 shows common investigations done in a bronchial asthma patient.

There is reversible airways obstruction, air trapping and hyperinflation in bronchial asthma which causes pulmonary function abnormalities. Peak expiratory flow (PEF) which can

Table 7.29: Common investigations in asthma

- Spirometry
- Peak flow meter testing
- Bronchoprovocation test (To measure hyper responsiveness of airway)
- Exhaled nitric oxide test (To measure airway inflammation)
- Sputum test (After inhaling hypertonic saline) for cytology, eosinophils and cytokines (measure of airways inflammation)
- Chest X-ray
- Eosinophil count
- Total IgE
- Prick test
- Specific IgE allergen test (ELISA)

easily be measured with a peak flow meter, is quite valuable in assessing a patient of asthma as well as evaluation of response to the therapy. How to use peak flow meter has been shown stepwise in the following Figures from 7.7 to 7.10.

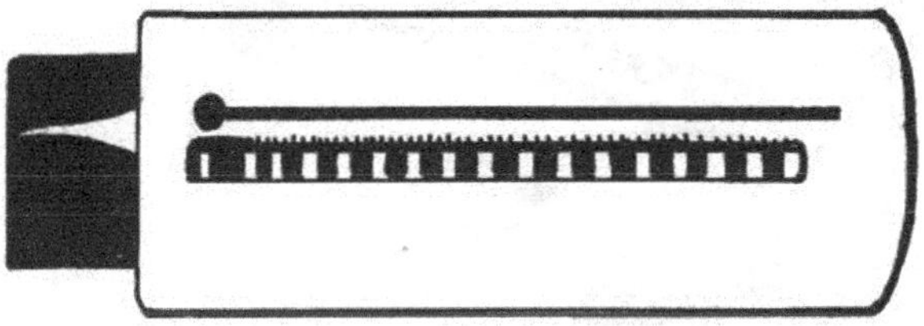

Fig. 7.7: How to use peak flow meter

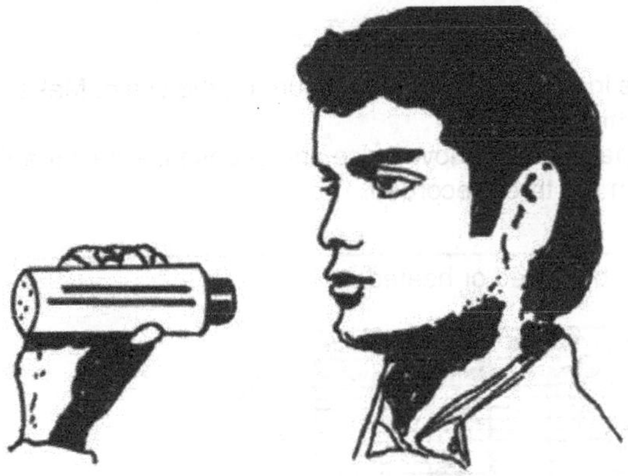

1. Make sure that the indicator on the Peak Flow Meter is at the end of the scale (zero position) nearest to the mouthpiece.

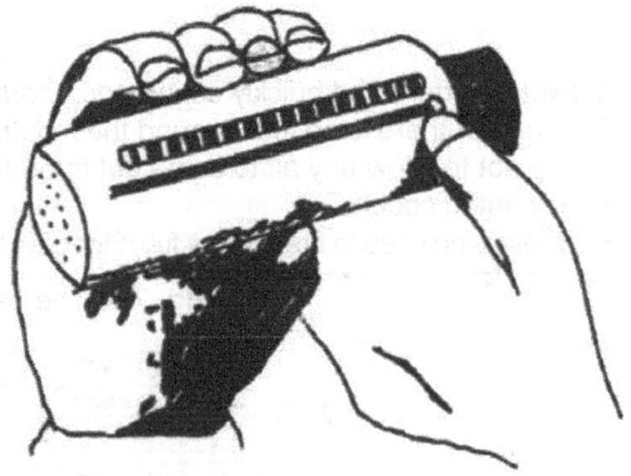

2. Hold the Peak Flow Meter with the scale pointing away from the mouth.

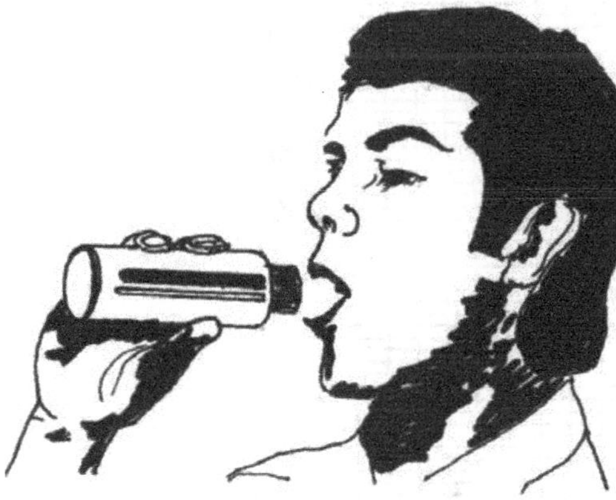

3. Breathe in as deeply as possible. It does not matter if it is through mouth or through nose. Most people find it easier to breathe in through the mouth.

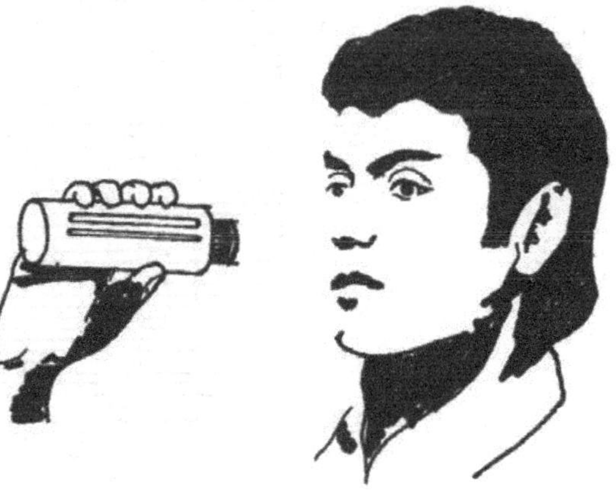

4. Hold breath for a moment and do not allow any air to escape. Now immediately place the end of the mouthpiece into the mouth and make an air-tight seal with lips around the mouthpiece.

Fig. Contd.

Fig. Contd.

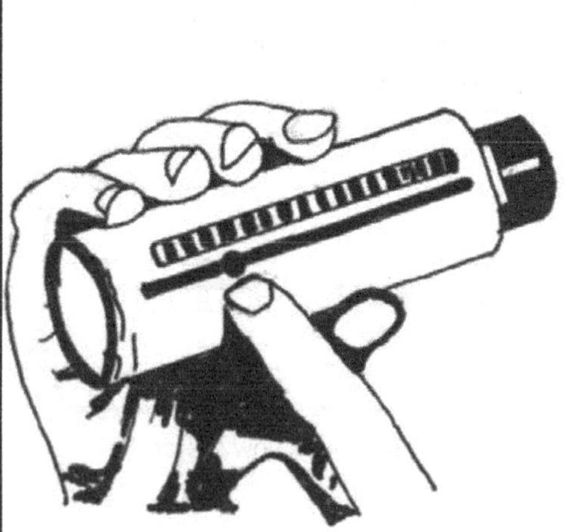

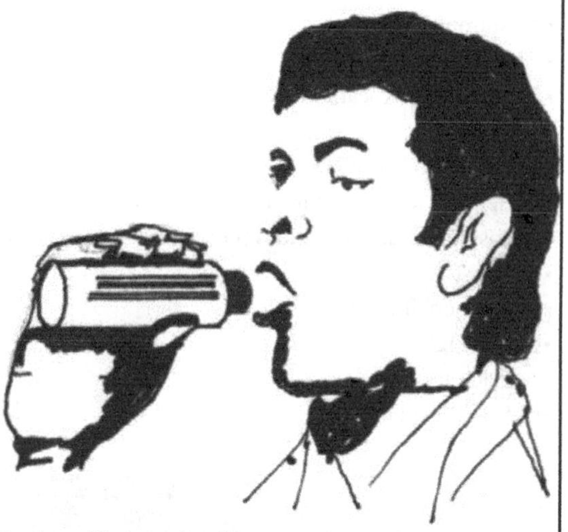

5. Blowout as hard and quickly as in *one short sharp* blast. Ensure that there is no leak around the mouthpiece.
   - Try not to allow any air to come out through the nose.
   - Try not to cough.
   - There is no need to breathe out fully Stop after the initial blow.
6. The indicator will stop at a figure on the scale. Make a note of this reading.
7. Repeat all the above twice and choose the best reading from the three recorded.

Fig. 7.8: The peak flow meter must not be boiled or heated

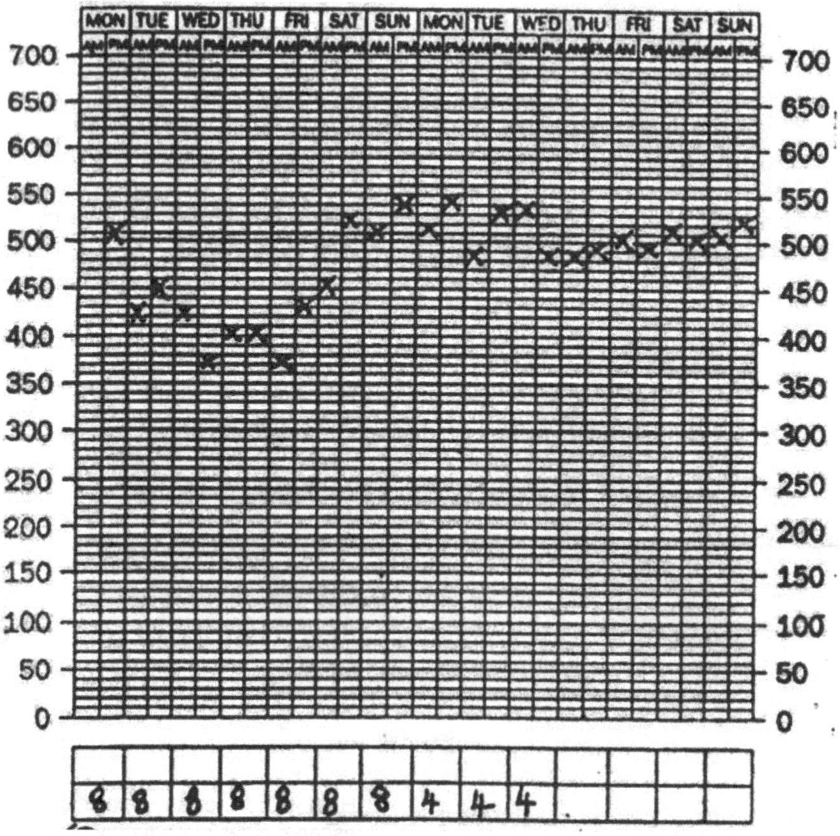

(Prednisolone tablets 5 mg)

Fig. 7.9: Peak flowchart showing an acute asthma attack, which resolves with a short course of oral steroids

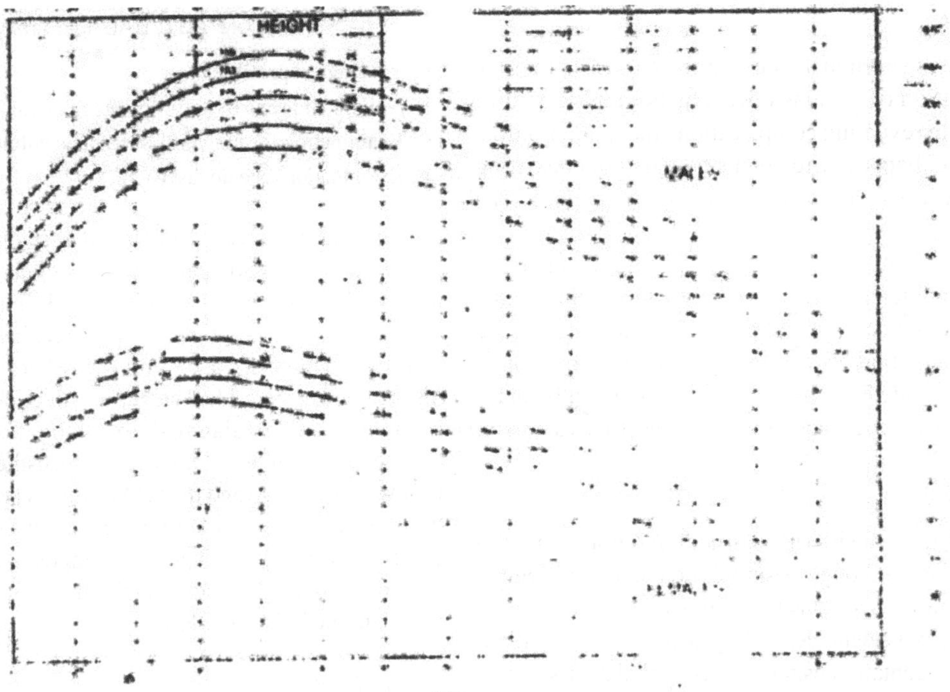

Fig. 7.10: Normal peak flow values

PEAK FLOW METER: CLEANSING AND CARE

It is important that the peak flow meter should be kept clean to ensure proper functioning. The white mouthpiece should be cleaned regularly in warm water to remove accumulated foreign matter (mucus, dust etc.). The body of the peak flow meter should be wiped with a clean cloth to keep it dust-free. However, do not disturb or adjust the delicate inner parts of the instrument.

A peak flow of less than 100 liters/minute is observed in an acute attack of asthma, which correlates with a forced expiratory volume in one second (FEV_1) of less than 0.7 litres.[49] So one measurement of FEV_1 and FVC gives an indication of severity of the airways obstruction. There exists hypoxemia because of imbalance in ventilation and perfusion. The situation worsens in the presence of intrapulmonary shunts, consolidation, atelectasis and pneumothorax. The CO_2 retention occurs when FEV_1 is 750 ml and is associated with acidosis because of fall in arterial PH. A rise in $PaCO_2$ by 10 mm of Hg is associated with a fall in arterial pH by p.08 units. Coexisting metabolic acidosis is to be suspected when reduction in PH is out of proportion to the alteration in $PaCO_2$. Peak flow rates and symptoms amongst patients with bronchial asthma have also been studied.[52]

Pulmonary Functions[2]

The measurement of FEV_1 and PVC gives an indication of the severity of airways obstruction. There is a fall in FEV_1/FVC ratio and it is less than 70 per cent during an attack. Based on FEV_1, the severity of asthma has been classified into three categories: Mild 50 per cent or more predicted FEV_1, moderate 25 to 50 per cent predicted FEV_1 and severe less than 25 per cent predicted FEV_1. There is a rough correlation between FEV_1 and PaO_2. A fall FEV_1 below one litre is likely to be associated with PaO_2 less than 60 mm Hg 1.

The daily estimation of PEFR helps in evaluating the response to the treatment. The ratio of FEV_1/FVC must show an improvement of atleast 15 per cent after bronchodilator aerosol. Exercise or a challenge with allergen can provoke pulmonary functional abnormality. There is a fall in FEV_1 on exercise. There is a marked ventilation-perfusion imbalance during acute attack of asthma resulting into hypoxemia. A linear relationship between the severity of hypoxemia and the airways obstruction exists. Patient may be hyperventilated in the initial stages of attack. CO_2 is eliminated by normally ventilated alveoli due to its linear relationship of CO_2 content to $PaCO_2$. There occurs a fall in $PaCO_2$. If airways obstruction persists there is a fall in total ventilation. It is associated with a rise in $PaCO_2$ and fall in PaO_2. Fall in pH may result in severe acidosis.

Anion gap metabolic acidosis may result from accumulation of lactate in severe asthma. A non anion gap metabolic acidosis may also be seen in asthma patients who hyperventilate secondary to renal loss of bicarbonate in compensation for prolonged hypocapnia. However there may be a slight fall in plasma ionized calcium. Hypoxia may result from the areas poorly ventilated relative to their perfusion resulting into bronchoconstriction. As mentioned earlier, intrapulmonary shunts, atelectasis, pneumothorax or pneumonic consolidation may further worsen the situation. RV and FRC are increased due to overinflation from premature airways closure and increase in airways resistance.

X-ray and ECG

Chest X-ray may be normal in uncomplicated cases or it may reveal overinflation of the lungs. Roentgenographic studies may be helpful in revealing complications like pneumonitis, pneumothorax, collapse due to mucus plugging or coexisting changing shadows of aspergillosis or pulmonary tuberculosis.

Electrocardiogram (ECG) may reveal supraventricular tachycardia, p-pulmonale, right axis deviation, right bundle branch block and right axis deviation. These abnormalities are reversible. One may find T wave changes, ventricular ectopic, sinus tachycardia and ST-changes due to drugs like salbutamol or ephedrine taken as repeat dose prior to the electrocardiogram.

Laboratory Tests

There may be leucocytosis with eosinophilia more than 500 cells/cumm at least, although eosinophilic count may remain normal in some cases. ESR may be slightly more. Sputum may be mucoid or mucopurulent, depending on associated bacterial infection. Sputum contains eosinophils, epithelial debris, creola bodies in some cases due to detachment of epithelial cells of lower respiratory tract and sometimes Curshmann's spirals and Charcot-Leyden crystals due to breakdown of eosinophils.

Bronchoscopy

Bronchoscopy reveals congested bronchial mucosa and tenaceous secretions plugging many a times in the lumen. The bronchial mucosa is highly inflamed with or without membrane in bronchial mucosa. In few cases, there may not be any abnormality.

The bronchoalveolar lavage (BAL) can be obtained and subjected to cytological examination. The common cellular yield obtained is shown in the Table 7.30. Asthmatics having high eosinophilic count in BAL do not respond to conventional bronchodilators but show good symptomatic response to corticosteroids. At the same time BAL eosinophils count is reported to be proportional to severity of asthma. Other part of BAL fluid can be sent for culture and sensitivity for pyogenic, fungus and acid fast bacilli, as shown in the Table 7.31.

Table 7.30: BAL fluid–common cytological yield

1. Neutrophils
2. Lymphocytes
3. Monocytes
4. Eosinophils
5. Epithelial cells
6. Alveolar macrophages
7. Goblet cells

Table 7.31: BAL fluid analysis

1. Cytological profile
2. Culture and sensitivity for pyogenic organisms
3. Examination for fungus by smear and culture
4. Examination for acid fast bacilli

There is an increased number of eosinophils in BAL fluid at base line in asthmatic patients[53] especially in allergic asthma. Increased number of neutrophils in BAL fluid in asthma patients before and after an antigenic challenge, is because of its being an inflammatory disease[54] and partly because of chronicity of disease and superadded bacterial infection.[55] The procedure involves clinical diagnosis of asthma,[56] written consent, bronchoscopy of both lungs under anaesthesia, i.e., inspection followed by lavage and thus BAL fluid is procured. It is filtered through two layers of surgical gauze to remove mucus, total cell count is done with haemocytometer and differential count by microscopic glass cover technique. Only few BAL studies are available in Indian literature.[56]

Bronchial Biopsy

It shows activated mast cells, eosinophils and lymphocytes; epithelial shedding and fragility and thickened basement membrane. The (inflammatory) changes are seen in all types of allergic, non-allergic and occupational asthmas and help to distinguish asthma from other inflammatory diseases of the airways.[57]

Skin Tests

These tests are helpful in recognising atopic subjects but the positivity of the tests need to be correlated with the history of the patient.

Prick test is performed by placing a drop of allergen fluid in the forearm, followed by pricking by fine needle to introduce the contents into the superficial epidermis. An urticarial wheal within ten minutes is a positive reaction which disappears in 1-2 hours. The reaction can be read easily with a glass slide and can be suppressed with corticosteroids. Antihistaminics and bronchodilators are helpful. Similar reaction can be obtained through bronchial challenge but there is always danger of provocation of an acute attack of asthma.[2]

Similarly food allergy causing bronchospasm can be ruled out by a trial diet based on provocation and elimination diet tests, especially in children.

Serum IgE Levels

These are found to be similarly raised both in extrinsic and intrinsic varieties of asthma and are inversely related to lung function. So there is a steeper FEV_1 decline with an increased level of IgE.[58]

Differential Diagnosis

Tropical Eosinophilia

Dyspnoea may not be that severe and blood test shows eosinophilic count of more than 2000 cells/cumm. There is hardly any precipitating factor and the response to bronchodilators is not satisfactory.

Cardiac Asthma

Generally it is seen in adults with a history of noctural episode of dyspnoea. Hypertension or other cardiac abnormality like congestive cardiac failure may be associated. Auscultation reveals creptitations at the bases of the lungs.

Chronic Bronchitis

History of attacks of cough and dyspnoea, especially in the morning is positive. Blood test may show mild eosinophilia, while no eosinophils are found in the sputum. It may partially respond to corticosteroid therapy.

Extrinsic Allergic Alveolitis

Differentiating features are shown as follows:

Sr.No.	*Bronchial asthma*	*Extrinsic allergic alveolitis*
1.	Pulmonary involvement only	Pulmonary as well as severe systemic upsets present
2.	Chest-examination reveals Ronchi+++	Crepts +++
3.	Lung functions tests (LFTs) show reversible airways obstruction	LFTs reveal restrictive pattern
4.	Eosinophils ±	No eosinophilia

Allergic Bronchopulmonary Aspergillosis

This can be differentiated from bronchial asthma by skin test for A. fumigatus (immediate reaction), total IgE levels more than 1000 ng/ml, increased antibodies to A. fumigatus and eosinophils may not essentially increase. 6-8 weeks corticoids and 12-16 months 200 mg/day itraconazole is recommended.

Complications of bronchial asthma may include pneumonia, pneumothorax, aspergillosis and fractures. Chronic cases may develop cor pulmonale. Even growth in the children may be retarded due to the disease.

Prognosis

Bronchial asthma follows a variable course. Children show improvement with age as airway becomes larger and as they achieve an ability to tackle the psychological precipitating factors. In atopic individuals the causal allergen has to be detected, better to be avoided and hyposensitisation has to be carried out against it. The treatment remains palliative in other patients. Mortality has tremendously decreased by use of steroids in the management of acute asthma and it is to be used as a long term maintenance therapy.

Management

Management of asthma includes role of preventive medicine as well. Proper guidance regarding disease and drugs would cut down deaths due to asthma which is on the rise.[59,60] Total abstinence of smoking is useful.[59] Avoidance of cold environments is also helpful since inhalation of mild cool air may be an important risk factor for asthma exacerbation.[60] Symptoms and peak-flow rates have been studied in pre and post menstrual states in females. Education and guidance regarding disease do help.[61] Tables 7.32 and 7.33 depict aims of management and determinants of successful management of bronchial asthma.

Table 7.32: Management aims in asthma

The management of asthma essentially aims at:
- Reversing of disturbed lung function to as close to normal as possible, with drug dosages short of producing serious side effects. In difficult cases one may have to be satisfied by just keeping the patient functional so that the daily chores of life is not seriously disturbed.
- Encouraging the child patient to participate in activities indulged in by other school mates.

Table 7.33: Determinants of successful management of asthma

I. Understanding of pathophysiology of asthma
II. Education of patient with special attention to objective measurement of peak expiratory flow rate (PEFR); and correct aerosol inhalation techniques
III. Attempts to identify the cause(s)
IV. Preventive measures
V. Treatment modalities according to severity of the disease.

In atopic asthmatics, damp dusting has to be carried out, preventing exposure to the dust and the contact with domestic pets needs to be avoided. The offending food is to be eliminated from the diet. The patients exhibiting aspirin and NSAIDs sensitivity should avoid their use; instead acetaminophen and propoxyphane can be used as analgesics in case it is essential.

Allergy to pollens or house dust (Figs. 7.11 and 7.12) is to be treated by hyposensitisation, to stimulate the production of antibodies belonging to the IgG class. These will compete with IgE as blocking antibodies and bind the allergen to eliminate it without causing any symptoms of allergy. The amount of

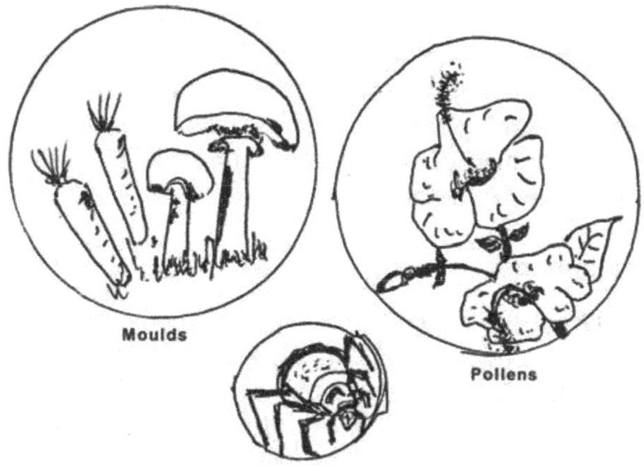

Fig. 7.11: House dust mite

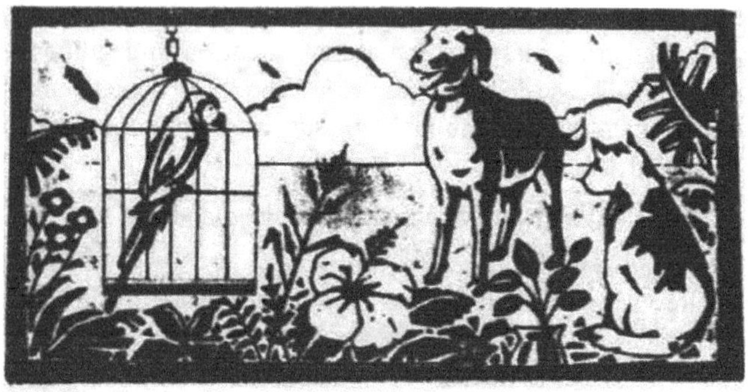

Flora and fauna

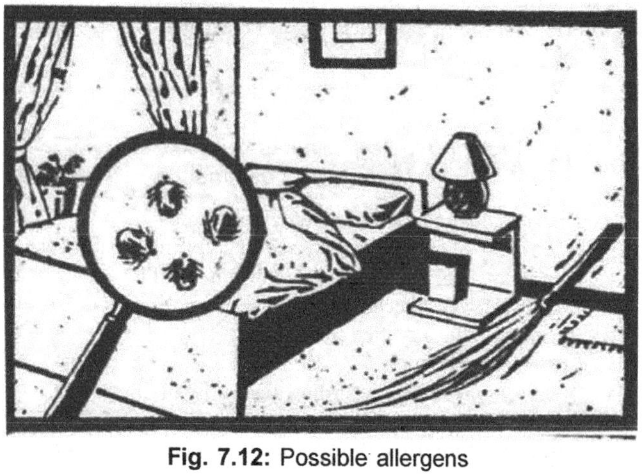

Fig. 7.12: Possible allergens

histamine liberated with IgG is 500 times less than that of IgE.[2] The hyposensitisation is carried out pre-seasonally and can be repeated in the next season. It is done with the use of aqueous solution containing pollen extract and is injected subcutaneously in gradually increasing doses over weeks.

Antibiotics are to be used only in case there is coexisting infection. The psychological make-up of the individual has to be assessed and any such problem which is likely to trigger asthma, has to be tackled. Regular breathing exercises enabling the active use of diaphragm and abdominal muscles during expiration are advised (Fig. 7.13).

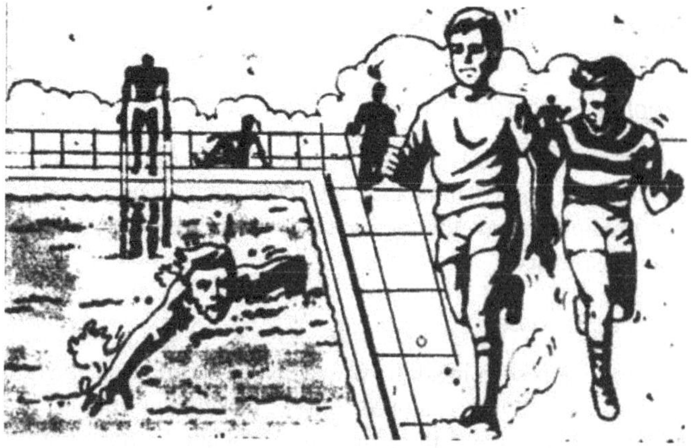

Fig. 7.13: Regular exercise help in preventing bronchial asthma

The management during the acute attack directed to keep the airways patent, to maintain proper ventilation and to reduce the bronchospasm and mucosal oedema to prevent air trapping.[3] Indicators of response of therapy in bronchial asthma are listed in Table 7.34.

Table 7.34: Indicators of response of therapy in bronchial asthma

1. Cough
2. Sputum
3. Dyspnoea (resting)
4. Dyspnoea (exertional)
5. Sleep

Supportive Therapy

Adequate oxygenation and hydration is to be maintained. Humidified oxygen at a flow of 2-6 liters/minute and 2 liters of 5% glucose or glucose saline over 24 hours normally provides oxygenation and corrects hypovolemia and also provides intravenous line to administer bronchodilators and other drugs. 75-100 ml of 7.5% sodium bicarbonate helps in correcting metabolic acidosis.

Bronchodilator Drugs

The inhibition of mediator release (increase in CAMP and decrease in CGMP) occurs with beta adrenergic stimulants (Isoproterenol, Isoprenalin) and their modified beta$_2$ adrenergic stimulants stimulating enzyme adenyl cyclase (salbutamol, isoetherine, terbutaline metaproterenol, orciprenalin, prostaglandin E_2) or with drugs inhibiting the breakdown of CAMP by phosphorelation (methyl xanthines, aminophylline). Atropine release of mediators (CGMP) by vagal blockage. Corticosteroids stabilize adenyl cyclase and potentiate the action of catecholamine. The release of mediators is enhanced (increase of CGMP and fall of CAMP) by alpha adrenergic receptor stimulants, beta blockers (propranolol), vagal stimulants and calcium.[2]

The sympathomimetic drugs relieve bronchospasm by acting on the adrenergic receptor sites and result in vasoconstriction and relaxation of the bronchial smooth muscles.

Various drugs used have been listed in Table 7.35.

Table 7.35: Beta agonists—Available compounds

1.	Indirect sympathomimetic agent—ephedrine (not used)
2.	Non-selective sympathomimetic agents (alpha and beta effects)—adrenaline
3.	Non-selective beta agonist—isoprenaline
4.	Partially selective beta agonists—orciprenaline, fenoterol
5.	Selective beta-2 agonists—salbutamol, terbutaline, rimiterol
6.	Long acting salbutamol, salmeterol, bambuterol, formeterol

Old conventional therapy includes ephedrine hydrochloride 30 to 60 mg given orally thrice a day. This is no longer in use these days.

Adrenaline 1 in 1000 dilution (0.1 per cent) 0.5 ml is administered subcutaneously in severe cases. It has rapid action and can be repeated every 10 minutes upto a dose of 2 ml. In acute severe bronchospasm, adrenaline may be continuously given in a dose of 1 minim a minute till relief is obtained (Hurst method). It may be necessary to alter the site of injection to avoid delay in absorption from local vasoconstriction. Though adrenaline relieves airway obstruction, it has not much effect on hypoxemia. An undue increase in cardiac rate warrants discontinuation of its administration.[62] Adrenaline which was chemically understood in 1902[63] has its value in angio-oedema and infantile asthma even to date.[64]

The aerosol as shown in the Figure 7.14 is a suspension of fine liquid (mist) or solid (dust) particles in air and it gets dispersed over a wide surface.[2] Since the dose is small, the systemic absorption is quite minimum and the side effects are not of much significance. The drugs exhibit their action immediately. The inhaler therapy is effective and ideal as shown in Table 7.36, provided aerosol has been inhaled properly into the lungs. Unfamiliarity of the wide range available and lack of knowledge to doctors regarding proper using technique of inhalers may be one of the reasons of reluctance of usage of inhalers.[65] It is used to administer drugs such as beta-adrenergic bronchodilators, anticholinergic bronchodilators, sodium cromoglycate and corticosteroids for prevention or reversal of airways disease.

The particles having a size of 1 to 5 millimicrons are in a respirable range and they get deposited by gravitational sedimentation in all parts of the lung including large airways, small airways and alveoli. Drug can be administered by using pressurised metered dosc inhalers or dry powder inhalers. Aerosols can be produced by jet nebulisers or ultrasonic nebulisers.Using a compressor pump or an intermittent positive pressure breathing device, the medication can also be nebulised. The metered dose inhalers (MDI) are commonly used for inhaler therapy.[2] The correct use of MDI is shown in Table 7.37.

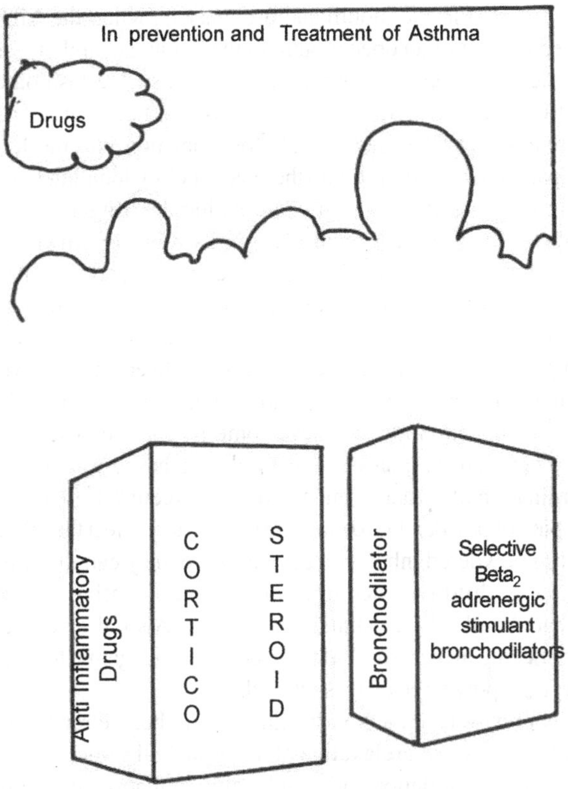

Fig. 7.14: Aerosols locally available

Table 7.36: Aerosol method of administration

1.	Does not require co-ordination at the time of administration.
2.	Delivers particles that are all within the 1-5 millimicrons size range.
3.	Is quick and easy to use.
4.	Delivers a high fraction of the dose into the airways.
5.	Is easy to carry along.
6.	Is environmentally acceptable.

Table 7.37: Instructions to patients on correct use of metered dose inhaler

1.	Start to breathe in at the time of actuation.
2.	Breathe in slowly and deeply (to the top of the lungs).
3.	Hold breath for few seconds before breathing out.

The aerosol release in front of the mouth from the MDI followed by a steady inhalation has to be synchronised with actuation. It should be swallowed by holding of breath for an optimal period of 10 seconds to allow sedimentations. This enables nearly 10 per cent of the drug to reach the lungs.

An Extension Device

Spacers have improved both the drug delivery as well as patient compliance. Aerosols generated by an MDI come out from the nozzle at high velocity and large particles of 10 to 20 m diameter get deposited in the mouth and oropharynx, when the MDI is placed in front of an open mouth. In the holding chambers, such particles are deposited within the device in such a fashion that only a stable aerosol of small particles of less than 5 m diameter are released to become available for inhalation into the lungs. The patient fires the MDI into the spacer before inhaling from it. This avoids the necessity of coordinating the triggering of the MDI with the commencement of a long slow breath, which many patients find difficult.[2] The spacer device thus has a major advantage that breathing and release of drug need not be synchronised and drug delivery to lungs is ensured.[66] Comparison of different modes during delivery are shown in Figures 7.15 and 7.16. Recent addition of micromised dry lung powder inhalation devices have come up for use. The patient compliance and response is improved with these preparations as coordination of actuation/inhalation is not required.[67] However, damping of powder due to moisture may greatly affect the efficacy of drug powdered inhalation devices. Also, they cannot be used in young children, incompetent or uncooperative patients, intubated and severe asthmatic patients.[68] Also, the powdered drug sticking in the throat has to be removed with gargle following everytime powdered drug is inhaled.

Isoprenaline sulphate can stimulate all beta adrenoceptors powerfully causing relaxation of the bronchial smooth muscle, myocardial stimulation and peripheral vasodilation. Its frequent administration in large doses in an exercise to achieve its effectiveness is likely to have cardiovascular side effects like tachycardia, hypertension and arrhythmia and may lead to death.

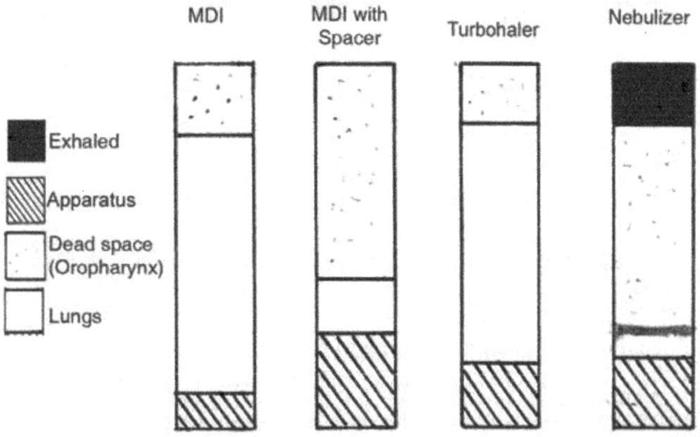

Fig. 7.15: Aerosols and proportional deposition

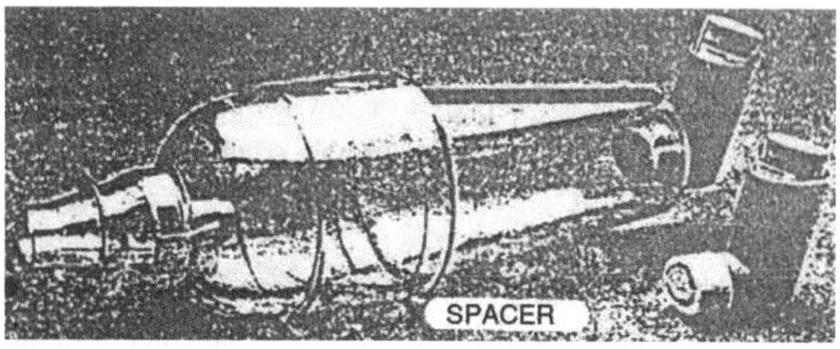

Fig. 7.16

Beta-adrenergic bronchodilators (salbutamol, terbutaline, orciprenaline, fenoterol) have bronchodilator effects by acting directly on the smooth muscle beta-adrenoreceptors. Various actions of beta 2 agonists in lungs are listed in Table 7.38. The dose given by an inhaler is smaller than that taken orally. When two puffs of salbutamol (200 ug) are taken, only 10 per cent (20 ug) of the medication reaches the lungs and is active. It has a rapid topical effect. Each puff of aerosol supplies the following concentration of the drug: Isoprenaline 0.1 mg; isoetherine 0.1 mg; salbutamol 0.1 mg orciprenaline (metaproterenol) 0.75 mg; terbutaline 0.25 mg; fenoterol hydrobromide 0.2 mg, rimiterol 0.2 mg and salmeterol 0.1 mg. A significant bronchodilation is noted 30 minutes after its administration which lasts upto six hours. $Beta_2$ adrenoceptor stimulants may produce minimal side effects and are dose related as well as affected by route of administration as shown in the Table 7.39 and Figure 7.17. There can be nervousness, skeletal muscle tremors, headache, tachycardia and flushing. Terbutaline may exhibit cardiovascular side effects like tachycardia and increased pulmonary artery pressure in doses recommended for clinical trial.[2]

Orciprenaline (20 mg), salbutamol (2 to 4 mg) and terbutaline (5 mg) can be administered orally. Salbutamol administered in doses of 100 of 300 mcg intravenously in acutely ill patients with severe asthma has shown to produce good bronchodilator

Table 7.38: Beta agonist's action in lungs

a. Relaxation of bronchial smooth muscle—Beta agonists cause relaxation of bronchial smooth muscles irrespective of the bronchoconstrictor stimulus, hence the name "functional antagonists".
b. Inhibition of vagal tone-beta agonists modulate cholinergic neurotransmission in autonomic ganglia and thus inhibit vagal tone to the airways.
c. Inhibition of mediator release from mast cells and possibly other mediator releasing cells—Pretreatment with beta agonists inhibits the release of histamine and other mediators after antigen challenge.
d. Mucociliary clearance—Ciliary beat frequency and mucus production is increased with beta agonists.

Table 7.39: Side effects of salbutamol therapy commonly seen and route of administration

	Route of administration		
	Oral (4 mg) T.I.D.	*Inhalation (200 ug) T.I.D.*	*Intravenous (500 mcg) T.I.D.*
1. Headache	10%	10%	10%
2. Tremors	15%	—	10%
3. Palpitation	10%	—	10%
4. Tightness in chest	—	—	10%
5. Agitated behaviour	—	—	10%
6. Ventricular premature beats	—	—	5%

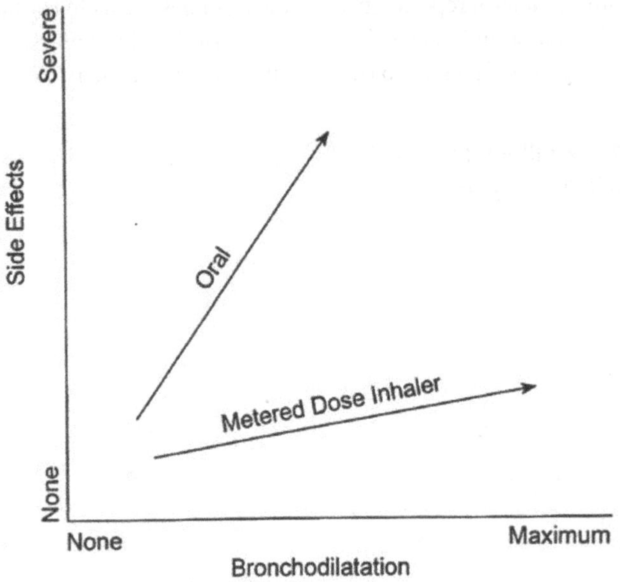

Fig. 7.17: Side effect and route of administration

response. Intravenous infusion of rimiterol hydrobromide appears to benefit patients refractory to routine bronchodilators. Terbutaline can be administered in doses of 0.25 mg subcutaneously in severe attacks of asthma.[2] Tremors and tachycardia, the major side effects, are much less noticeable when beta 2 agonists are administered by inhalation. Tremors present a common situation found in clinical practice. Classification of tremors as well as factors affecting physiological tremors have been listed in the Tables 7.40 and 7.41.

Table 7.40: Classification of common tremors

1. Tremors at rest
Parkinson's disease
2. Postural tremors
Physiological tremor
Exaggerated physiological tremor
Essential tremor
Tremor with basal ganglia disease
Parkinson's disease
Dystonia
Wilson's disease
Cerebellar postural tremor
Tremor with peripheral neuropathy
Hereditary peripheral neuropathy
Acquired neuropathy
Post traumatic tremor
Dicholoric tremor
3. Kinetic tremors
Cerebellar kinetic (intention) tremor
4. Task-specific tremors
Primary writing tremor
Focal tremor
Orthostatic tremor
5. Hysterical tremors

Table 7.41: Physiological tremors

1. Emotion
Anxiety, stress, fear
2. Exercise, fatigue
3. Hypoglycemia
4. Thyrotoxicosis
5. Pheochromocytoma
6. Hypothermia
7. Withdrawal from alcohol
8. Drugs
a. Beta-adrenergic (isoproterenol, amretamine)
b. Dopaminergic
c. Anticonvulsant (Valproate)
d. Lithium
e. Neuroleptic
f. Tricyclic
g. Methylxanthine (caffeine, theophylline)

It has been found that inhaled terbutaline affects the platelet activity indirectly by suppressing release of platelet activating factor from periobronchial mast cell that reduces airways inflammation, reverse the bronchospasm and help in preventing development of chronic airflow obstruction (CAO).

With the introduction of isoprenaline as a selective beta stimulant and the pressurized metered dose aerosol in the mid and late 1960s respectively and an epidemic of asthma deaths were linked to the over prescribing and indiscriminate use of isoprenaline although even to this day the debate continues as to whether there was a true or casual association,[69] the risk of asthma death was attributed to including induction of cardiac arrhythmia, overdependence on symptomatic treatment in a situation of deteriorating asthma, and toxic effects of the chlorinated fluorocarbons. Concern is once again being expressed over the environmental consequences of carbofluorocarbons (CFCs), and there has been an upsurge in the use of powder devices, already well established in the market as dry powder inhalers, together with the newer systems, having multidose presentations. New oral $beta_2$ agonists are also available and although these are by no means as effective as the inhaled formulations for relieving acute airways obstruction, they have found use as preventive agents particularly for nocturnal asthma. The encapsulation of salbutamol in an osmotic, slow-release tablet[70] and that of bambuterol, produce bronchodilation sustained for upto 24 hours.[71] Arformoterol–along acting beta-2 agonist, has a rapid onset and long duration of action, has been used for non severe asthma.[72]

The most significant advance in $beta_2$ agonist therapy for asthma has been the discovery of the long acting inhaled drugs. Salmeterol and formeterol, when administered by inhalation, both drugs are reported to produce prolonged bronchodilation and therefore might be considered for once or at the most twice daily use.[73] In the case of formeterol, the prolonged duration of action relates to its high affinity for $beta_2$ receptors and its slow absorption and degradation. Salmeterol consists of salbutamol attached to a long hydrophobic chain containing an oxygen bridge and a benzene group at the distal end. The side effect with salmeterol reported from clinical studies are tachycardia, mild tremor and insignificant fall in diastolic blood pressure. Chemistry and pharmacology of salmeterol are shown in Figures 7.18A and B.

Chemically, salmeterol is 4-hydroxy-x [[[6-(4-phenylbutoxy) hexyl] amino]-methyl]-1, 3 benzene dimethanol, 1-hydroxy-2-naphthoate

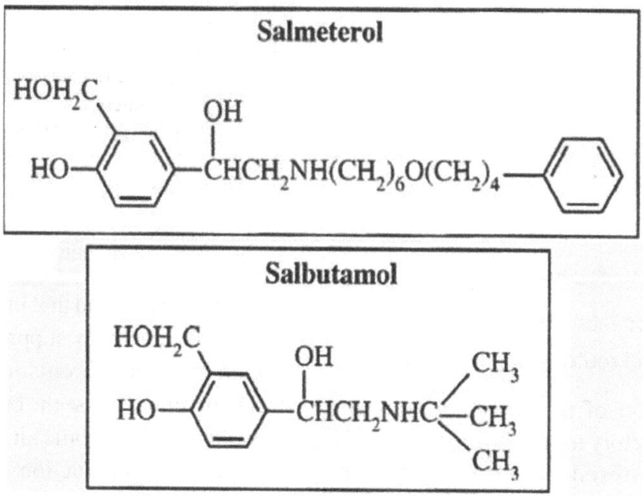

Structural formulae of salmeterol and salbutamol

Fig. 7.18A: Chemistry of salmeterol

Salmeterol is a selective B_2—adrenoceptor agonist which binds firmly to B_2-adrenoceptor protein and produces bronchodilation via a mechanism common to salbutamol and other B_2-agonists. Briefly B_2-agonists stimulate production of cyclicAMP by activation of the enzyme adenyl cyclase. CyclicAMP then triggers a sequence of intracellular events, ultimately producing bronchodilation.

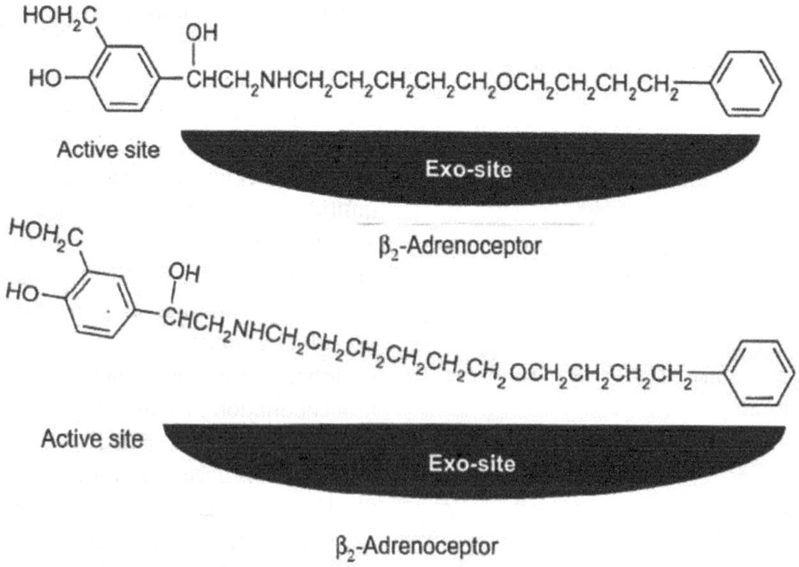

Fig. 7.18B: Pharmacology: Mechanism of action

Diagrammatic representation of the exo-site hypothesis for the mode of action of salmeterol showing the phenylethanolamine head structure at the active site of the B_2—adrenoceptor and the long non-polar tail attached to the exo-site.

HOW TO USE THE INHALER CORRECTL Y (Figs. 7.19 to 7.23)

Important

Use the inhaler only as directed by doctor. If the recommended dose does not provide relief of symptoms or symptoms become worse, consult the doctor.

Warning

The metal canister of your inhaler is pressurised. Do not puncture or burn it even when empty.

Keep away from eyes.

Keep away from children.

Storage

Store the inhaler in cool place, but do not freeze.

Two different modes of inhaling drug

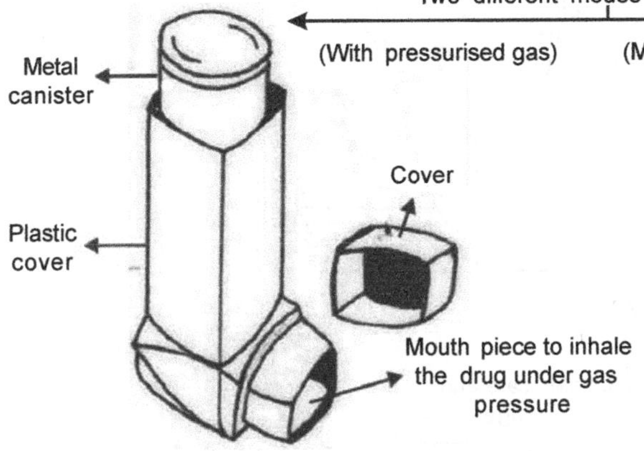

Fig. 7.19A: Inhaler

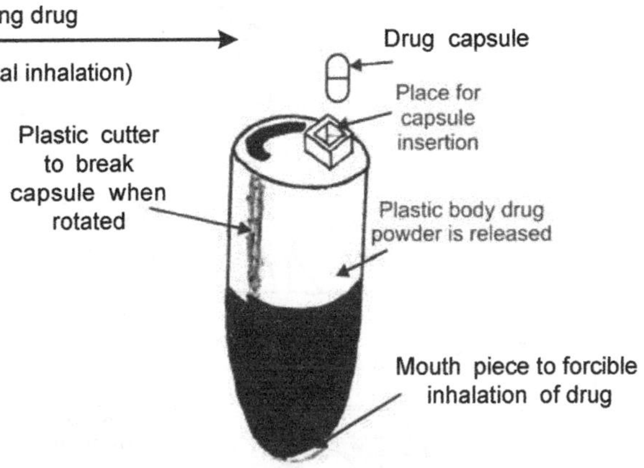

Fig. 7.19B: Rotahaler

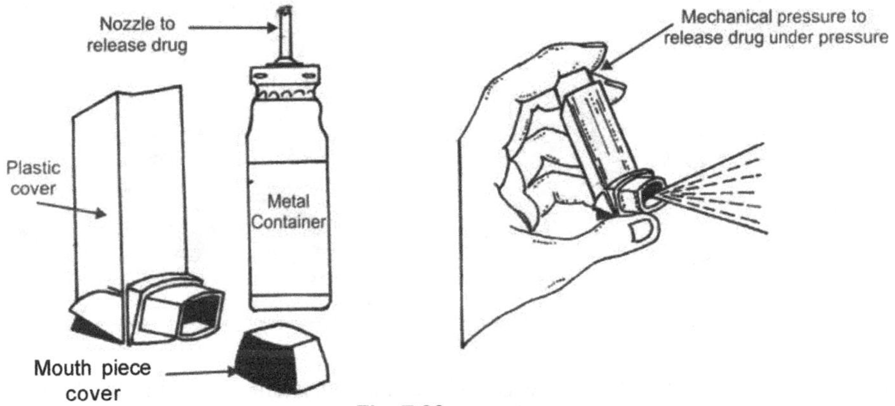

Fig. 7.20

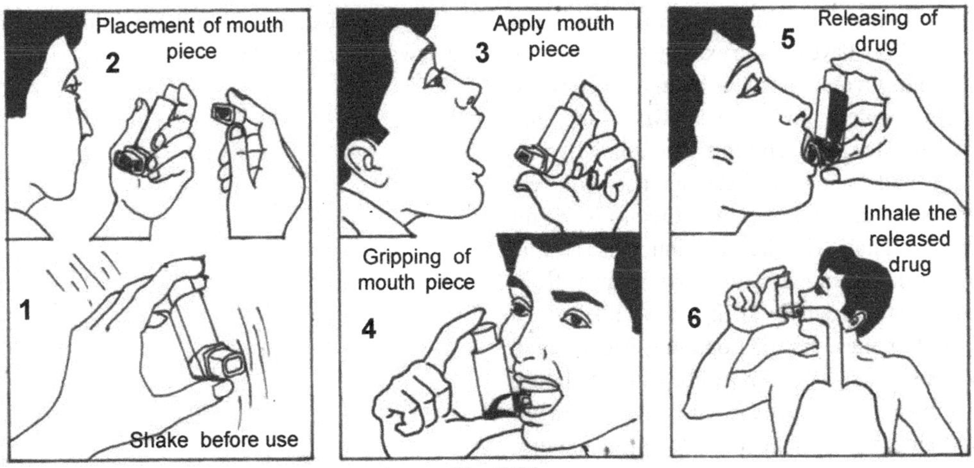

Fig. 7.21

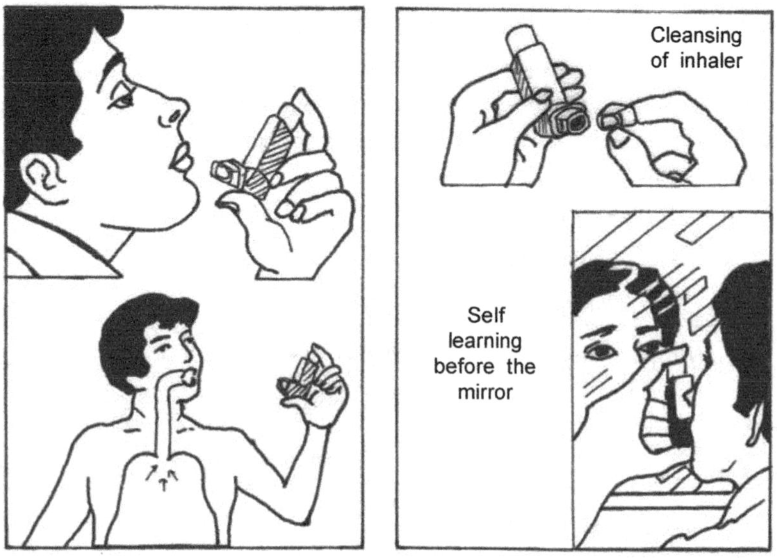

Fig. 7.22

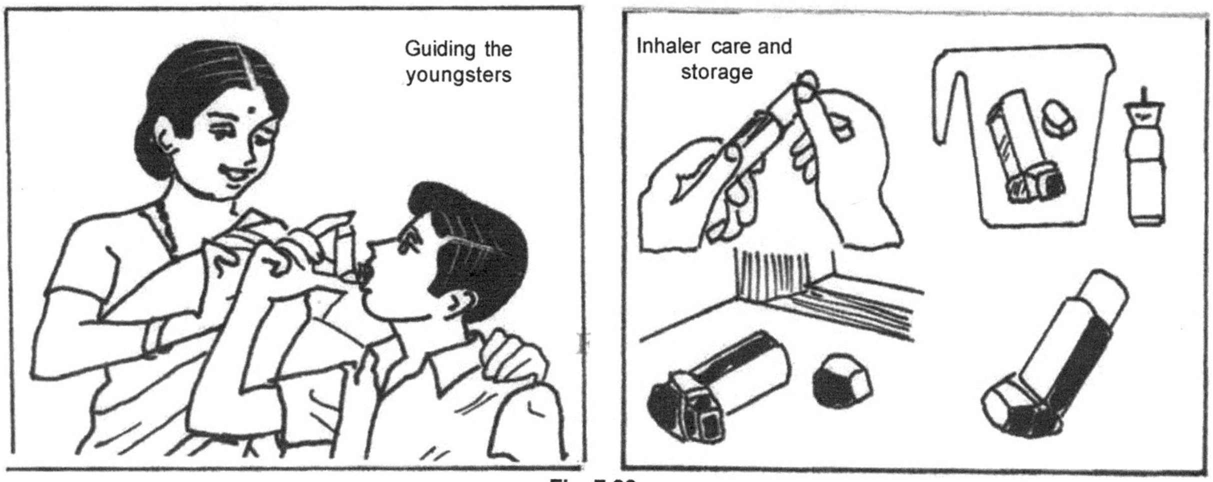

Fig. 7.23

Both salmeterol and formeterol protect the airways of asthmatics against the constrictor effects of histamine or methacholine for upto 14 hrs and in this capacity are serving as functional antagonists. They have proven extremely efficacious in the treatment of asthma symptoms when administered twice daily.[74,75] When given regularly for four to six weeks and then stopped abruptly, they lead to rebound bronchial hyper-responsiveness.[76] It is widely held that $beta_2$ agonists will treat only the symptoms of asthma and not the underlying inflammatory response. Thus, with their continued use as sole therapy in the face of deteriorating asthma, withdrawal from their protective effect (for example at night) would lead to catastrophic attacks. For these reasons opinion leaders have expressed the view that first-line therapy for asthma should include disease-modifying drugs such as inhaled corticosteroids, sodium cromoglycate, or nedocromil sodium. Nevertheless, $beta_2$ agonists now have a firm place in the armamentarium of asthma treatment. In combination with steroids, salmeterol and formeterol have successfully been used.

Salmeterol xinafoate (formerly salmeterol hydroxynahoate) is a new long acting inhaled $beta_2$ agonist (Fig. 7.24). Salmeterol

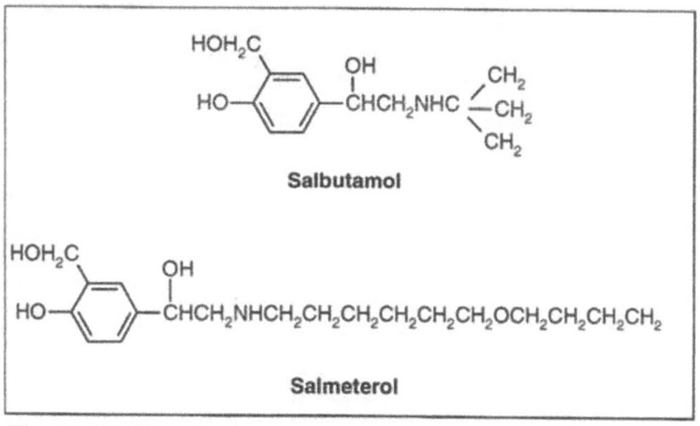

Fig. 7.24: Chemical structure of salbutamol and salmeterol

provides 12 hours bronchodilation from single dose.[72] It is suitable for adult patients requiring to use their inhaled bronchodilator atleast once daily or who have night-time exacerbations of asthma. Features, comparison of adverse effects and compliance of both these drugs have been shown in Tables 7.42 to 7.45.

Table 7.42: Comparison of adverse symptoms

Adverse symptom	*Salbutamol*	*Salmeterol*
Tremor	10-6%	3-4%
Cough	3-4%	
Headache	3-4%	2-4%

Table 7.43: Comparison of the pharmacological predictive adverse events seen with salmeterol 150 mcg bd and salbutamol 200 mcg over one year period

	Number of patients (%) experiencing a particular adverse event	
	Salmeterol 50 mcg bd	*Salbutamol 200 mcg qds (3 months) 200 mcg bd (9 months)*
Tremor	3.6%	2.1%
Palpitations	3.9%	1.8%
Tachycardia	0.6%	0.9%
Headache	12.3%	12.9%

Table 7.44: Status of compliance of the patients in two groups

Status	*Salbutamol*	*Salmeterol*
Compliant	70-75%	90%
Non-compliant	25-30%	10%

Table 7.45: Features of salmeterol

1. It has longer duration of action.
2. No need to reduce dose in the elderly or in patients with renal impairment.
3. Hypokalemia may occur in severe asthma.
4. Observe caution in-thyrotoxicosis while using salmeterol.

Hypothesis for mechanism of action (Fig. 7.25) includes its binding to the exosite, the salmeterol molecule is able to engage and re-engage itself with the beta$_2$ receptor. Evidence for engagement and re-engaging comes from its in vitro binding studies.

The time to onset of action of salmeterol has been studied by assessing both time to peak bronchodilation and time to 15% increase in FEV_1.

Salmeterol is found to be equipotent with isoprenaline and more potent than salbutamol against histamine, leukotrienes (C.D.E.) and prostaglandin D_2 release from human neutrophils and attenuate the influx of neutrophils in guinea pig lung following challenge. In addition, in vitro work has also demonstrated attenuation of eosinophil infiltration in the lungs

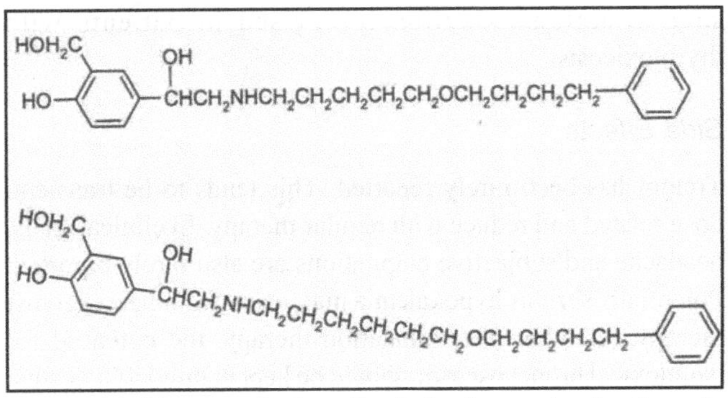

Fig. 7.25: The exo-site hypothesis for the mode of action of salmeterol

of guinea pigs following allergen and PAF (platelet activating factor) challenge.

Study of the effects of salmeterol on the alveolar macrophage reveals that salmeterol caused a significant inhibition of thromboxane B_2 release of 37% which was not reversed by propranolol. Salmeterol might inhibit some of the inflammatory features of the late phase response.

Salmeterol acts locally in the lungs after inhalation, therefore, plasma levels are not predictive of therapeutic effect. Only small amounts are detectable in the plasma.

The recommended dose for mild to moderate asthmatics is 50 mcg bd. No further benefit in lung function was gained by increasing the dose of salmeterol from 50 mcg bd to 100 mcg bd. It has shown to improve objective sleep quality also.

The most common adverse events associated with salmeterol are the extrapulmonary reactions. Although hypokalemia is a recognised effect of beta$_2$ agonists, this has not been seen as a clinically significant problem with salmeterol 50 mcg bd.

No treatment related ECG abnormalities are seen in patients with mild to moderate or moderate to severe asthma. In the comparative study with a theophylline, both drugs are well tolerated and the incidence and nature of adverse events is similar in the two groups. However, patients receiving theophylline experience a slightly higher incidence of nausea, vomiting, headache and palpitations.

Salmeterol is administered by inhalation as a pressurised inhaler or as a dry powder inhaler. In adults: The daily regimen is:inhaler: One blister (50 mcg) twice daily. Metered dose inhaler: Two inhalations (2 × 25 mcg) twice daily. There is no need to reduce the dose in the elderly or in patients with impaired renal function.

In children, there is insufficient data to recommend the use of salmeterol in children at present.

Hypokalemia may occur, particularly in severe asthma. It may be potentiated by xanthine derivatives, steroids, diuretics and hypoxia. Serum potassium levels should be monitored in such situations. Caution is advised in patients with thyrotoxicosis.

Side Effects

Tremor has been rarely reported. This tends to be transient, dose related and reduce with regular therapy. In clinical trials, headache and subjective palpitations are also rarely reported. Potentially serious hypokalemia may result from beta$_2$ agonist therapy. As with other inhalation therapy, the potential for paradoxical bronchospasm, should be kept in mind. If it occurs, the preparation should be discontinued immediately. Experience of the use of salmeterol during pregnancy or lactation is limited.

Many muscarine receptors are present in the muscues of trachea and bronchi, often stimulated by acetylcholine resulting into bronchoconstriction and mucus secretion. Anticholinergic drugs like atropin, ipratropium bromide etc. induce bronchodilation. However effect of ipratropium is less effective then beta$_2$ agonists in asthma, compared to equally effective in certain chronic bronchitic patients. Dry mouth and cough are commonly encountered side effects.[2]

Disodium Cromoglycate

Cromolyn sodium is a kellin compound containing the active principle of Ammi Visnaga. It acts on tissue mast cell and stabilises its cells membrane. It prevents the degranulation and influx of calcium required for activation of microfilaments as shown in Figure 7.26. It prevents the release of histamine and other tissue mediators involved in the pathogenesis of asthmatic attacks. It blocks the immediate and late asthmatic reactions.[2]

As sodium cromoglycate does not prevent the union of antigen and the cell bound antibody (IgE), it should be present prior to occurrence of such a union to demonstrate its effectiveness. Then only can it prevent the release of mediators from such union. It has been shown to be equally effective in extrinsic and intrinsic asthma.[2] As it does not relieve the asthmatic attack once it has developed, hence it is considered to be a useful prophylactic drug.[77]

Metered dose inhalers are available for its administration. The inhalation of the powder may induce transient bronchoconstriction in a few patients. It is prevented by addition of 0.1 mg of isoprenaline sulphate. Its action begins to occur in 10 minutes after its administration and it lasts for four hours. It is eliminated in the urine without any change. Cromoglycate can cause dryness and irritation of throat and trachea in some patients; otherwise it has no toxic side effects. Long term use of chromoglycate does not alter its efficacy.

Ketotifen: Like disodium cromoglycate, it also prevents mediator release. It is an H$_1$ antihistaminic (structurely similar

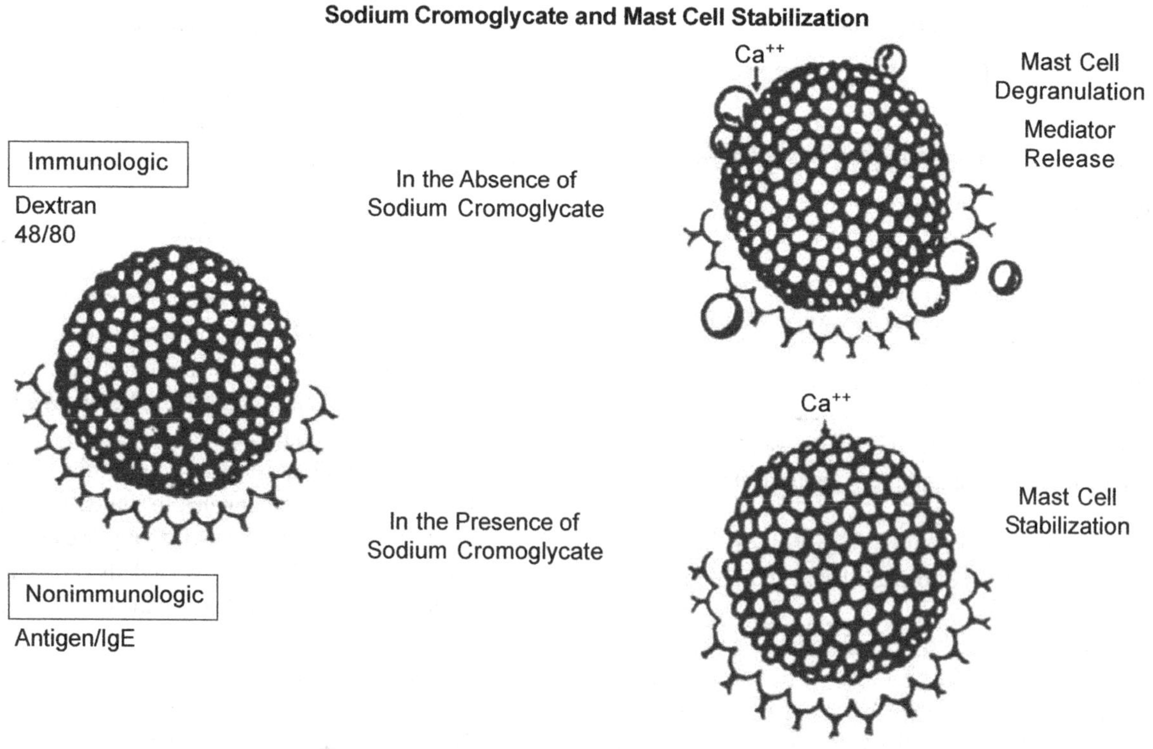

Fig. 7.26: The protective effect of sodium cromoglycate on the mast cell from the immunologic and non-immunologic triggers

to cyproheptadine) and inhibits phosphodiesterase.[78] It has a prophylactic role in extrinsic bronchial asthma.

Nedocromil sodium (Fig. 7.27): It is a salt of a pyranoquinoline dicarboxylic acid rigid molecule that appears to be suitable for direct delivery to the bronchial mucosa by pressurized metered dose aerosol. It is administered in a dose of 2 to 4 mg, two or four times a day. It is excreted rapidly from the body mostly, unchanged. Occasionally it produces an unpleasant taste. It is not recommended for children below 12 years of age.

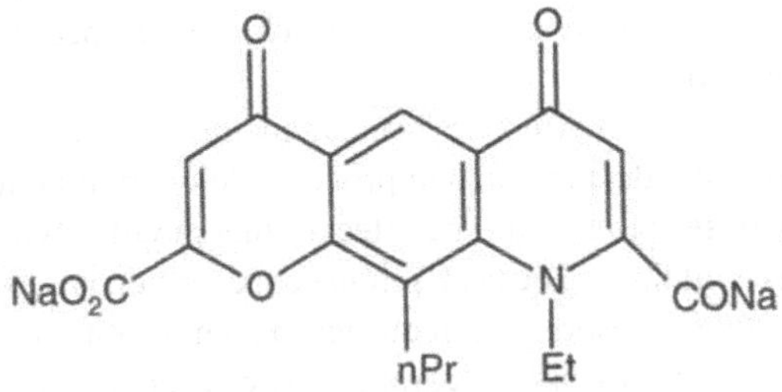

Fig. 7.27: Nedocromil sodium

Nedocromil sodium has an anti-inflammatory activity in patients with reversible obstructive airways disease. It inhibits immediate and late bronchoconstriction provoked by inhaled allergen or by exercise, when administered 10 to 15 minutes prior to provocation. This effect appears to be related partly to its selective capacity to inhibit mediator release from activated mast cells in the bronchial mucosa and partly to its inhibitory effect on neural reflexes in airways. Nedocromil sodium may be useful to replace or reduce the dosage of inhaled steroids. It appears to have more potent anti-inflammatory effect than sodium cromoglycate[79] in relieving airways obstruction triggered by non-immunologic stimuli and useful as a prophylactic drug in adult asthma. (a) Nedocromil sodium has a proven anti-asthma effect, (b) It is a partial replacement to rest of bronchodilator therapy, (c) It cannot replace inhaled corticosteroid, (d) It does not have an oral steroid sparing effect, especially in patients of chronic steroid dependent asthma, (e) It is a potential drug, but no clear cut advantage over disodium chromoglycate has been demonstrated, (f) It is not comparatively cost effective. But it can be substituted in case chromoglycate sodium doesn't suit.[80]

The *antihistaminics* are not effective but prescribed in routine from practitioners to specialists in this part of the tropics. Morphine is contraindicated as it is a respiratory depressant. Tranquillisers are only of use in highly emotional or restless patients during an attack.

Children become acidotic from respiratory distress, hypoxemia and lactic acid accumulation. It makes them non-responsive to bronchodilators and the bronchospasm tends to be prolonged. It is corrected by administration of soda bicarbonate in a dose of 2 mEq/kg intravenously over five minutes to be followed by a similar dosage over the rest of the hour. In rare occasions when the condition does not improve even after steroids, exhibiting hypoxemia, acidosis and hypercapnia, patient requires endotracheal intubation and mechanical ventilation till the normal ventilatory pattern is re-established.

The inhalation form of therapy is very well accepted, even then oral forms of beta$_2$ agonists are in use till date. They are continuously used (1) they may possibly tolerate-precipitate and expose to sensitizing agents. (2) Long acting B_2 actrenergic drugs are not a substitute as they suppress the symptoms such as morning dyspnoea.[81] (3) Their use without the additional anti-inflammatory drugs like corticosteroid may accelerate decline in ventilatory functions.[82]

Theophylline[2]

Theophylline (1, 3 dimethlyl xanthine) and its derivatives probably cause bronchial smooth muscle relaxation by inhibition of degradation of phosphodiesterase, an enzyme that catalyses the breakdown of cyclic AMP (CAMP). However the degree of such inhibition is miminal at therapeutic concentrations. Other mechanisms have been proposed to explain its action: translocation of intracellular calcium ions, prostaglandin antagonism, stimulation of endogenous catecholamine release, beta agonist activity, inhibition of cyclic guanosine monophosphate metabolism, increased binding of cyclic AMP with AMP binding protein, and adenosine receptor antagonism. Though these effects appear to be less prominent within the therapeutic range, each may contribute in causing bronchodilation. This is shown in Figure 7.28. Bronchodilator effect of theophylline is possibly due to adenosine receptor antagonism.[2] Various effects of theopylline have been shown in Table 7.46.

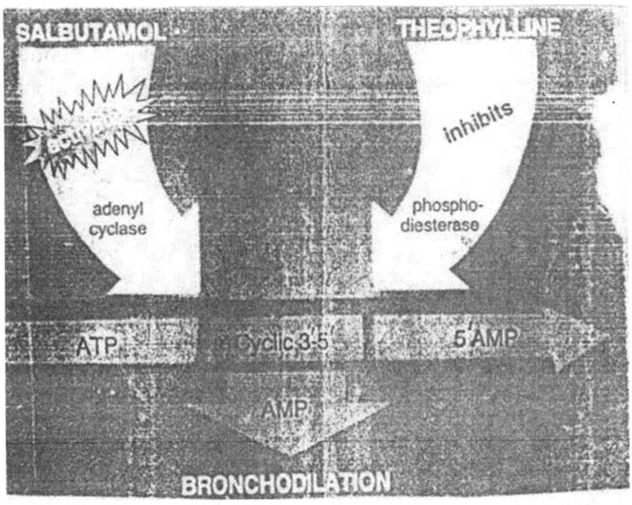

Fig. 7.28: Bronchodilation

Table 7.46: Possible theophylline actions in asthma

1.	Stabilizes inflammatory cells
2.	Stabilizes barrier function
3.	Reduces plasma leakage in the airways
4.	Prevents bronchoconstriction

Theophyllines may be given orally in the form of tablets and solutions, intravenously, intramuscularly or rectally, but they are not effective when inhaled. The clinical effects of various methylxanthine preparations are dependent on the amount of anhydrous theophylline (84 per cent in the salts containing ethylenediamine and 64 per cent in choline theophylline) and the rate of absorption from the gastrointestinal tract.

The sustained release preparations are given every 12 hours. Though absorption of theophylline is better on an empty stomach, it is often erratic due to poor solubility. It can be taken after milk, food or antacid, in those complaining of gastrointestinal upsets like nausea, vomiting and epigastric discomfort. Choline theophyllinate (oxytriphylline) has greater acquous solubility and is absorbed better. Dyphylline is stable in acidic medium and is less irritant to the gastric mucosa.

Theophylline enemas and suppositories can be used to avoid the unpleasant side effects of oral therapy. The absorption rate is unpredictable with suppositories (500 mg). Aminophylline given as a retention enema (200 to 300 mg) gets absorbed quickly and reaches the pulmonary circulation. It relieves moderate attacks of asthma.

Nearly 40 per cent of theophylline on absorption is bound to plasma protein and the remaining free drug gets distributed throughout the body fluids. Nearly 90 per cent of theophylline undergoes biotransformation through the oxidative pathway by the action of cytochrome oxidase in the liver and gets metabolised into its relatively inactive metabolites. Nearly 10 per cent is eliminated unchanged in the urine. The clearance of theophylline varies from person-to-person. It is dose dependent and is decreased at extremes of age (infants and elderly patients) and in conditions like congestive heart failure, acute pulmonary oedema, cor pulmonale in the presence of chronic airflow obstruction, decompensated cirrhosis of the liver, acute hepatitis, febrile viral respiratory tract infections and simultaneous intake of ciprofloxacin, erythromycin or oral contraceptives. This drug-interaction necessitates decrease in dosage of theophylline to prevent toxic reactions.

Theophylline clearance (Table 7.47) is increased during childhood and adolescence, with cigarette smoking, coexisting disorders such as cystic fibrosis, and hyperthyroidism and intake of phenytoin, phenobarbital, carbamazepine and rifampicin. Therefore large doses are required to achieve therapeutic serum concentrations.

The drug is an effective bronchodilator. Its specific effect on airways conductance and improved pulmonary function and toxicity dose are related. The effect of theophylline with beta-agonists is additive. The peak serum concentration is dependent on dose, rate of absorption, frequency of administration, hepatic biotransformation and clearance. The drug has a narrow therapeutic range. The dose is altered according to the relief of symptoms and occurrence of side effects, in different persons.

In acute bronchial asthma, aminophylline (85 per cent theophylline and 15 per cent ethylene diamine) is administered intravenously, it is given in a loading dose of 5.6 mg/kg over a period of 30 minutes in patient not receiving theophylline, to be followed by a maintenance dose of 0.5 (non-smoker) to 0.9 (smoker) mg/kg/hour depending on the smoking status. Patients who are already taking oral preparations of theophylline may receive intravenous aminophylline at a dose equivalent to their previous maintenance dose. A loading dose of 250 mg aminophylline dissolved in 50 ml of 25 per cent glucose is to be administered intravenously over a period of 30 minutes. This will help in achieving a serum level of 10 ug/ml rapidly in those who are not on theophylline therapy. In the present era where patients have been given corticosteroids and other bronchodilators, the bronchodilator effect of aminophylline becomes questionable where fullest bronchodilation has already been achieved through $beta_2$ agonists and corticosteroids.

Table 7.47: Factors influencing plasma theophylline clearance

	Increased clearance	*Decreased clearance*
1. Age	1-15 years	Less than one year
2. Diet	Low carbohydrates, high protein	High carbohydrates, low protein
3. Diseases	Cystic fibrosis	Cirrhosis liver Congestive heart failure Pneumonia Viral infection
4. Drugs	Phenobarbitone Phenytoin Rifampicin Carbamazepine	Erythromycin Cimetidine Propranolol Oral contraceptives
5. Smoking	Yes	

Each mg/kg of theophylline administered will increase the serum concentration on an average by 2 ug/mg. The loading dose has to be followed by a continuous drip wherein 250 mg 10 aminophylline is administered at six hours interval, producing satisfactory serum level of 10 to 20 ug/ml in most patients. This is given as 250 mg/10 ml aminophylline in 5% glucose 500 ml to be given to patients already receiving theophylline preparation, to avoid side effects.

The sustained release theophyllines which reduce asthmatic response to allergen challenge, are useful in noctural attacks of bronchospasm and are administered twice a day. They avoid swings in serum levels and provide more stable serum concentrations with longer dosing intervals. The greatest benefit may be derived from sustained release theophylline administered on an evening dosing schedule. It has shown a significant reduction of night time or early morning wheezing and awakenings, greater patient compliance and increased peak expiratory flow rate capacity.

The adverse effects of theophylline are dose related (Fig. 7.29). These are in the form of anorexia, nausea, vomiting, abdominal discomfort, diarrhoea, tachycardia, systremma, central nervous system stimulation (irritability, nervousness, insomnia and tremors). These may occur in therapeutic concentrations of theophylline. Gastrointestinal side effects occur from excess plasma concentration and not from local irritation. There can be life threatening adverse manifestations in the form of seizures, supraventricular tachycardia and cardiac arrhythmias.[2] These are noted when theophylline concentration is more than 20 ug/ml. Minor toxic symptoms do not proceed life threatening seizures or arrhythmias. Aminophylline suppositories may cause granular proctitis. Theophylline causes sleep disturbance, poor concentration and impaired learnmg in children.

Corticosteroids

Steroids are useful both in extrinsic as well as intrinsic type of acute attack of bronchial asthma. Treatment is directed as

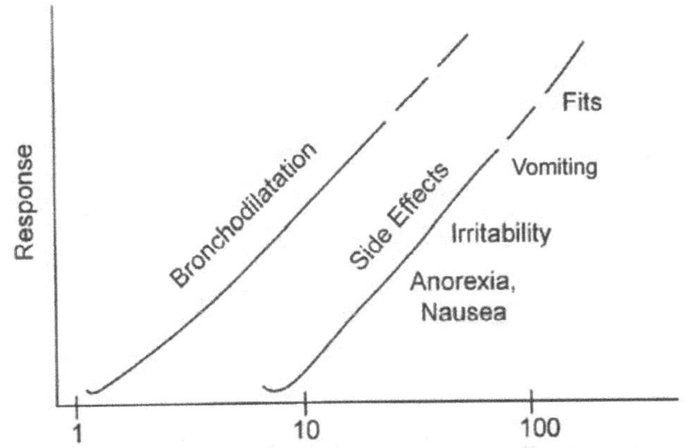

Fig. 7.29: Relationship of theophylline serum levels, efficacy and side effects

outlined in GINA guidelines.[83] These are life saving in life threatening situations like status asthmaticus, with respiratory failure and physical exhaustion. They are useful in all intractable cases, not responding to bronchodilator therapy. Corticosteroid preparations stabilise adenyl cyclase in the bronchial smooth muscle, thus potentiating the action of catecholamines. Hyperaemia and mucosal oedema are reduced. Betamethasone and dexamethasone have longer duration of action and have greater suppressive action on hypothalamus-pituitary-adrenal (HPA) axis. Their biological half life is 36 hours while plasma half life is 300 minutes. Short acting (hydrocortisone) and intermediate acting (prednisolone, prednisone and methyl prednisolone) have no such prolonged suppressive effect on HPA axis. The short acting steroids have a biological half life of 8 to 12 hours and plasma half life of 50 minutes. The intermediate steroid has a biological half life of 30 hours and plasma half life of 200 minutes. Prednisolone is cheap and does not have a prolonged suppressive effect on HPA axis and is often preferred. Prednisone is biologically inactive and gets converted into prednisolone in the liver to exhibit its activity. Generally there is no difficulty in such conversion except in chronic active hepatitis. During a severe attack of bronchial asthma and in situations where asthma is getting progressively worse, corticosteroids need to be administered to secure prompt relief. High dose oral or I/V steroids are recommended in acute severe asthma. Nevertheless, these are routinely used in mild cases of asthma which is unfair.[2]

Acute asthma attack becomes refractory only because of the airways obstruction which is initially partly due to smooth muscle spasm but later on mucosal oedema and mucus plugging play a dominant role. The refractory asthma need a course of corticosteroid along with bronchodilator. Early introduction of anti-infammatory drug in the treatment, especially the inhaled steroids,[84] not only effectively control symptoms but also they bring back proper pulmonary functions through anti-inflammatory effect as well as by increasing the beta adrenergic responsiveness. Their possible mechanism of action is as under: (1) On leucocytes: (a) They alter migration capacity and cytotoxicity. (b) Cause destruction of specific cell types. (2) On mediators of inflammation: (a) They decrease action of histamines, kinin and arachidonic acid. (b) They stabilise lysosome. (3) On adrenergic system: (a) They increase adenylcyclase activity. (b) They increase beta receptors. (c) They decrease phosphodiesterase and CAMP activity. 125 mg of hydrocortisone hemisuccinate 6 hourly intravenously for 48-72 hours generally tide over acute phase, although response may vary from person to person. The side effects of steroids therapy are not related to duration of therapy. The beneficial effect of steroids may take 4-6 hours to exhibit their peak effect.

Hence, other forms of therapy need be continued along with. The parenteral therapy is replaced by oral and tapered off as soon as the clinical improvement is observed. Those who had never used steroids are tapered off the drug within a week's time, others may take longer period, to avoid drug withdrawal syndrome.

Aerosols: Inhalation of corticosteroids forms the cornerstone of treatment in bronchial asthma. This anti-inflammatory drug has to be dispensed as maintenance therapy. The inhalation of aerosols of betamethasone dipropionate and betamethasone valerate in a dose of 100 mcg (two puffs) from a press pressurised inhaler four times a day has shown to be useful in the maintenance treatment of asthmatics in whom long-term corticosteroid therapy is contemplated. In addition to them, tramcinolone acetonide, flunisolide and budesonide aerosols have also shown marked topical effect in bronchial asthma. They do not suppress HPA axis and are not associated with side effects of steroids.[2] Fluticasone propionate is a noval inhaled steroid with improved efficacy and safety profile. Dry powder inhalation, which is convenient to use, has shown almost similar beneficial results with budesonide in a mild to moderate reversible airway obstruction. The acceptability of dry powdered inhalation preparation by patients is expected to increase in future and would prevent the damage to the ozone layer caused by metered dose inhalor propellants. Mechanism of action and effect of corticosteroids on airway inflammation are shown in Figures 7.30 and 7.31.

The topical steroids are effective at every stage of inflammatory and immunological reactivity. They decrease cellular chemotaxis and histamine release. Oropharyngeal candidiasis is a frequent side effect. It is usually self-limiting.

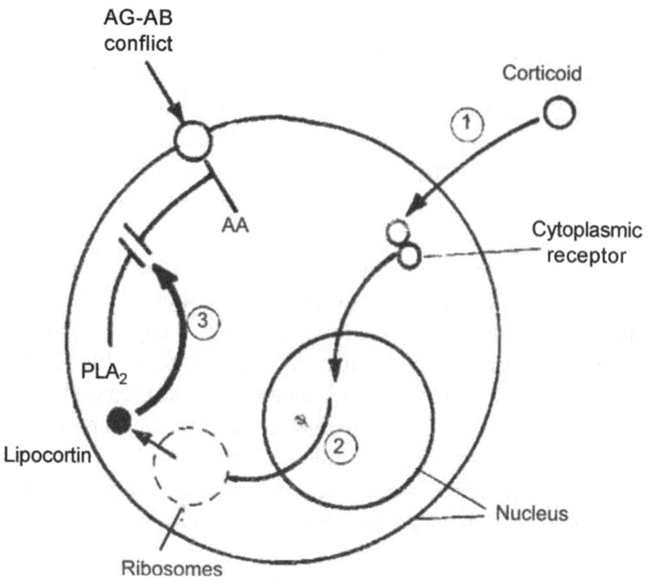

Fig. 7.30: Mechanism of action of corticosteroids

That is why mouth washing after every inhalation is advised. There can also be dysphonia from bilateral adductor vocal cord paresis with deformity and bowing of the cords and weakness (reversible steroid myopathy). There are reports like bone and skin thinning, easy bruising and cataract formation. Use of large volume spacer, mouth rinsing after dry powder inhalers, using low dose steroid inhalers and when appropriate using steroid sparing medications like cromolyn and nedocromil sodium, help in reducing the systemic effects of inhaled steroids.[85]

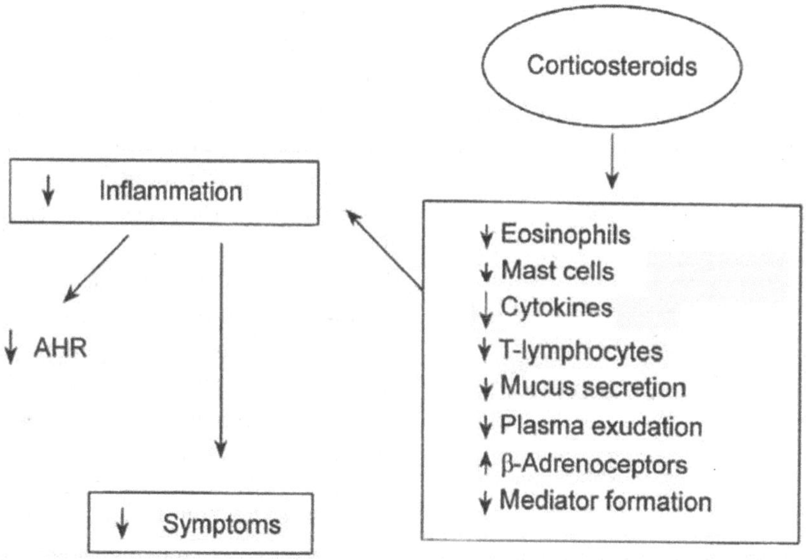

Fig. 7.31: Effect of corticosteroids on airway inflammation airway hyperresponsiveness (AHR) and symptoms
Ref: Annu Rev. Med. 1993 44: 229-42

As described earlier, nearly 80 to 90 per cent of inhaled steroid is deposited in the oropharynx and only 10 per cent enters the lungs like other aerosol inhalations. Less than 3 per cent reaches distal airways and alveoli. It fails to control exacerbations of asthma. It fails to stabilise brittle, highly variable asthma or morning dipping and acute severe asthma. Therefore guidance and education to the patient, regarding when to go for hospitalization is equally important and must be imparted by the attending physician.

In children the administration of corticosteroid on a long term basis is not advisable though it may be given only for a short interval during a severe episode. If it is given in young age it retards the growth and the suppression is dose related.[86] Nevertheless, 400 micro gm/day inhaled budesonide does not stunt growth in children with asthma.[87] In spite of increased availability of drugs prescriptions for asthma in children, they continue to miss classes because of untreated or undertreated wheezing.[88]

Patients showing hypercapnia $PaCO_2$ of more than 60 mm Hg, exhaustion and clinical deterioration despite rigorous medical support (treatment), require ventilatory support along with other forms of treatment. Patient is sedated, soft cuff endotracheal-intubation is done and ventilation is done by volume-cycled ventilator with a low inspiratory pressure and a total volume of 12 mg/kg body weight at a respiratory rate of 10/ minute. Spontaneous ventilation has to be paralysed by pancuronium bromide—a neuromuscular blocking agent. Weaning from ventilator is done on improvement in arterial blood gases with a fraction of inspired oxygen of 0.5 or less and when the patient is awake, alert and able to double his resting minute ventilation. Fiberoptic bronchoscopy may help in removing the excessive mucus plugging and bronchial lavage with solutions containing N-acetyl-L-cysteine that may sometimes become necessary in such patients.[2] To sum up, acute severe asthma can be made completely reversible with prolonged aggressive treatment. Recent evidence suggests that frequent or regularly scheduled therapy with specific inhaled $beta_2$ agonists is associated with diminished control of asthma and increased risk of near death or death. At the same time, $beta_2$ agonist bronchodilators are available without prescription in United States and many patients use them several times without concomitant use of anti-inflammatory agents.[89] The 72-page report by International Consensus on diagnosis and management of asthma (Table 7.48) from international asthma management project, a working group of 18 physicians and scientists convened by the National Heart, Lung and Blood Institute, Bethesda, MD recommends regular use of anti-inflammatory agents preferably inhaled corticosteroids (Fig. 7.32) as first line therapy for anything more than occasional mild asthma and $beta_2$ agonist bronchodilators are endorsed only for pretreatment of exercise induced asthma or for symptomatic relief of acute exacerbations.[89]

Table 7.48: International consensus report on diagnosis and management of asthma 1992 [89]

'Regular use of anti-inflammatory drugs, preferably inhaled corticosteroid, as first line therapy for anything more than occasionally mild asthma. $Beta_2$ agonist bronchodilators, commonly used in United States as regularly scheduled first line therapy, are endorsed only for the pretreatment of exercise-induced asthma and for the symptomatic relief of acute exacerbation, or "asthma attacks", when anti-inflammatory therapy is insufficient.'

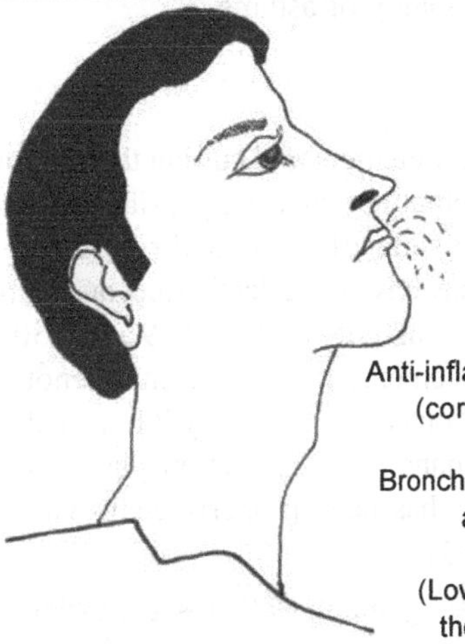

Fig. 7.32: Management of bronchial asthma

Antibiotics

They do not form part of anti-asthma treatment. Even purulent sputum merely reflects presence of eosinophils. If there is coexisting bacterial infection, antibiotics need be used. However, these are being routinely prescribed in this part of the tropics.

H_1 Receptor Antagonists

Keeping in view the mast cell-dependent release of mediators like histamine in the pathogenesis of exercise induced bronchoconstriction, H_1 receptor antagonists prevent release of inflammatory mediators from IgE sensitised mast cells and basophills. Their modest dose related bronchiolator effect, however does not form first line treatment for acute or chronic asthma.

Anti Leukotrienes

These drugs are used in patients with moderate asthma. Their established role is yet to be asserted. These are used in adult patients but for monteleukast which can be used in children above 6 years of age. Hepatic drug effect is still under observation. These drugs are struggling to find a place in the management of asthma. Experimentally, these drugs significantly inhibit, in a dose dependent manner, the bradykinin-induced contraction of tracheal smooth muscle in guinea pig and allude to an interaction between bradykinin and leukotriene medimators.[90] Nevertheless, these are useful in asthma with

IgE raised levels, especially in decreasing the dose of $beta_2$ agonist and even corticosteroids.[91]

Nonpharmacological Management

Acupuncture

Acupuncture gives modest improvement in objective parameters, but the mechanism by which it works needs to be further investigated to have better understanding of this technique in the pathophysiology of asthma.[92]

Yoga

Reduction in panic of anxiety element and cutting the viscious circle of aggravating bronchial obstruction, possibly appears in relieving the acute episode of asthma through yogic exercises.[93] 'Pranayama' may have beneficial effect on asthma by reducing bronchial hyperreactivity (Tables 7.49 and 7.50).

Obesity and asthma has emerged as a different phenotype of asthma, where improved outcomes are likely if both asthma and obesity are properly managed.[94] An action plan to deal with various trigger factors has been properly dealt with, as shown in (Tables 7.51 to 7.53).

Table 7.49: Asthma management: Patient's education

1. Patient requires a good understanding of the disease and its management.
2. In view of level of literacy, patients are required to be educated about the disease according to their ability to understand.

Table 7.50: What patient needs to know

1. That the disease is chronic, requiring prolonged treatment.
2. Treatment to be continued even when symptoms have abated.
3. PEFR measurement to be done to assess asthma.
4. Appropriate measures to be taken when asthma control deteriorates.
5. About 'triggers' that precipitate asthma attack.
6. Advantages of inhaled route over oral use of medicine.
7. About drugs—protectors, relievers and preventors.

Table 7.51: At the first sign of breathlessness what to do: Guidelines to the patient

1. Do not panic.
2. Take the medicine you have been advised to use correctly.
3. Take slow deep breaths.
4. Use pursed lip-breathing.
5. Check your breath with a peak flow meter if advised by your doctor.
6. Inform your relative or friend.
7. If you have difficulty in speaking, call a doctor immediately.

Table 7.52: Patient's self-assessment: Recognising signs when asthma worsens

- More frequent and more troublesome wheezing or shortness of breath.
- Being woken at night by shortness of breath and coughing.
- Increased shortness of breath on walking.
- Less complete relief of symptoms after use of your medicines (or a more frequent need for it).
- A reduction in your peak expiratory flow rate (PEFR) and an increasing difference between the morning and evening readings.

Table 7.53: Useful tips for a patient of bronchial asthma to lead a normal life

- Use the medicines recommended by your doctor regularly. Avoid self-medication.
- Do breathing exercise and other general exercises to keep fit.
- Take light meals at night and try to sleep early.
- Drink plenty of water.
- Try avoiding dust, cigarette smoke and smoky surroundings.
- Avoid cold water baths.
- Avoid cold, deep fried or sour food.
- Avoid keeping pets such as dogs, cats, etc.
- Avoid smoking and alcohol.

$Beta_2$ agonists are found to increase airway reactivity and detrimental in asthma control if regularly used and may add to morbidity and mortality due to overuse in acute asthma.[95] Hence use of inhaled steroids has been emphasised.

Theophylline is extensively used but has a narrow therapeutic range and need to be avoided in epilepsy, peptic ulcer, hepatic and heart ailments. Dose has to be halved in febrile cases. Low dose has been found to be suitable for maintenance.[96] The concept of 'hormesis' explains that how the low dose can be effective, further explaining that a drug can give biopositive results with low dose while can become bio-negative in the higher doses.

Steroids inhalation therapy is the first line therapy in asthma, supplimented by $beta_2$ agonists if needed. They are essential in nocturnal asthma to control the inflammatory process to avoid day time fatigue. Optimal asthma education has to be an integral part of asthma management to reduce asthma related morbidity and increase knowledge regarding inhalation technique.[97] These patients already have poor lung functions. Levoalbuterol has an additional advantage in reducing the dose of corticosteroids in nocturnal symptoms or exercise induced spasm. Systemic corticosteroids for a short duration are useful in acute exacerbation of asthma. Oral and intravenous administration of corticosteroids have similar efficacy in the treatment of adult acute attack of bronchial asthma.[98] Leukotrienes receptor antagonist are especially helpful in aspirin sensitive asthmatics. A monoclonal antibody against IgE are effective in reducing exacerbations.

Acupuncture, hypnosis and ionization has minimal or no beneficial effects. Stepwise slowing of breathing (pranayamic breathing), supported by study of airway models has been found to be a good adjuvent.[99] Longitudinal slitting of hypertrophied circular bronchial muscles with controlled radiofrequency via bronchoscope is bronchial thermoplasty, being worth a look for patients above 18 years where typical inhalational bronchodilator and anti-inflammatory medication is not working.[100] Important points have been listed in Table 7.54. and 7.55 regarding management.

Table 7.54: Management of acute bronchial asthma

Initial Assessment

History, examination, use of accessory muscles, heart rate, respiratory rate, PEF or FEV_1, oxygen saturation, ABG analysis etc.

Initial Treatment

- O_2 therapy to achieve O_2 saturation ≥90% (95% in children).
- Rapid acting β_2 agonist continuously for one hour.
- Systemic corticosteroids if poor response.
- Sedation—Contraindicated.

Reassess after one hour:

- Physical examination.
- PEF.
- O_2 saturation.

Criteria for

Moderate	Severe
Accessory muscles	Chest retraction at rest
PEF 60-80% predicted	PEF < 60% predicted

Treatment

- O_2 therapy.
- B_2 agonists and anticholinergic inhalation, every hourly.
- Oral glucocorticoids.
- Intravenous magnesium.

Reassess after one hour:

Good response PEF < 70%

O_2 saturation > 90%

- Can be discharged with follow up treatment.

Incomplete Response

PEF < 60%

O_2 saturation not improving

- Aggressively treat; monitor PEF, O_2 saturation, pulse

Poor Response

Drowsiness

Confused patient

PEF < 30%

PCO_2 > 45 mm Hg

PO_2 < 60 mm Hg

- Intensive care; consider intravenous glucocorticoids, B_2 agonists and theophylline.
- Possible intubation and mechanical ventilation if exhaustive fatigue, and CO_2 > 60 mm Hg despite rigorous medical management.

Oral intubation is preferred. Sedation an relaxation before intubation with midazolam, ketamine and vecuronium. High pressures used to achieve normal alveolar ventilation may result in high mortality due to barotrauma, which can be reduced by permissive hypercapnia. On improvement when patient is awake and alert and is able to double his resting minute ventilation as well as ABG with a traction of inspired O_2 of 0.5 shows improvement^{+}, patient is weaned off.

Table 7.55: Other modalities/measures

- Bronchoscopy may be required.
- No role of anti-histaminics or mucolytics.
- Nitric oxide is of value and is recommended but not as a routine therapy.$^{+}$
- Magnesium therapy and heliox therapy have also been successfully utilized.$^{++}$
- Non conventional measures like use of anaesthetics, hypothermia and extracorporeal life support and bronchoscopic therapeutic lavage have also been tried.$^{+}$
- NIPPV has no advantage.

Bronchial asthma, which affects 5% of industrialised nations, the poor compliance due to social factors is one of the important causes of treatment failure. In developing countries the undereducation. Compliance can be improved through education and use of spacer devices to decrease oropharyngeal side effects. Assessment of severity, reasons for non-responsiveness and indications for hospitalisation are shown in Tables 7.56 to 7.58.

Table 7.56: Causes of non-responsiveness to drug therapy in bronchial asthma

Conditions associated with bronchial asthma or which may complicate asthma or which mimic asthma and hamper response to treatment

1. Gastro-oesophageal reflux.
2. Frequent exposure to allergens: Dust mites, fungi including aspergillus, occupational allergens.
3. Non-specific irritants like chemicals.
4. Food allergens: Nuts, shells, fruits, metabisulphite used as preservative, tartrazine used as colouring agent, monosodium glutamate.
5. Chronic sinusitis and ear, nose and throat infections.
6. Thyrotoxicosis and adrenal insufficiency.
7. Asthmatic pulmonary eosinophilia and Churg-Strauss syndrome.
8. Airway obstruction: Foreign body, granulomas, metastatic malignant tumours, variable airway obstruction like in vocal cord palsy.
9. Left ventricular failure.
10. Hypersensitivity pneumonitis.
11. Bronchiectasis.
12. Acute pulmonary embolism.
13. Sarcoidosis.
14. Hyperventilation due to any cause, when associated with asthma, e.g., high grade fever, metabolic acidosis.

Contd.

Contd.

Drug related
1. Poor compliance with therapy.
2. Steroid resistance.
3. Use of beta blockers, aspirin, indomethacin, ibuprofen, naproxen.
Psychological factors
Special types of bronchial asthma which are difficult to control.
1. Brittle asthma
2. Premenstrual asthma
3. Fixed asthma
Ref: Prabhudesai P.P., JAPI 1994, 42: 56-59.

Table 7.57: Bronchial asthma: Assessment of severity

The severity of asthma—the disease–can on the other hand be assessed on the basis of the following:

- Duration of disease.
- Frequency of acute exacerbations.
- Response to non-steroidal treatment.
- Need for steroids to relieve an attack, or steroid dependence.
- Number of hospitalisations and/or emergency treatment received despite routine care, more than 2 visits per year indicates severe disease.
- Diurnal variations in PEFR—greater the variation, the more severe is the disease.

The more severe disease as a rule requires more aggressive therapy.

Table 7.58: Indications for hospit alisation

The indices to recognise acute severe asthma, and life threatening features, as well as indications for hospitalisation.

Recognition of acute severe asthma	*Life threatening features*
Too breathless to talk	PEFR < 30% of best
Too breathless to feed	Cyanosis
Respiratory rate >50 breath/min	Fatigue/exhaustion
Heart rate >140 beats/min	Agitation/reduced level of consciousness
PEFR < 50% of best	Blood gases are helpful in deciding initial management

Varieties of Difficult Asthma

Unstable Asthma

It is commonly seen in young women. Since it is difficult to manage, it may be called *Brittle* asthma. It shows sudden and unpredictable fall in lung function tests, which may be normal in between the attacks. It may not respond to bronchodilators and may require ventilation in some cases. Possibility of neurogenic origin cannot be ruled out. Beta$_2$ agonist subcutaneously may be effective. Salmeterol inhalation may be of use. Even dramatic improvement with intramuscular injections of progesterone[101] or lutenising hormone releasing hormone analogue have been reported[102] in these cases.

Steroid Dependent Asthma

These asthmatics are controlled only with oral steroids. Being less than 1 per cent of all asthma patients, steroids in these patients can be weaned off under medical supervision. Others may require steroids sparing treatments like methotrexate. Severe refractory steroid resistant asthma is likely to be targeted towards cytokines and bronchial thermoplasty.[103]

Steroid Resistant Asthma

Those who don't respond to even higher doses of steroids despite a considerable bronchodilation, are included in this group. These patients, who were responding to oral steroids in the past, become steroid resistant, possibly through a cellular defect in the response of monocyte to steroids. Long acting beta$_2$ agonists may be of help, in treating such patients. Interleukin: 25 induced hyper cytokine production have been linked with exacerbations of asthma in steroid resistant cases.[104]

Some patients who are not responding to corticosteroid inhalation therapy may actually need coadministration of antibiotics as there is co-existing neutrophilic airway inflammation due to H. influenzae and other bacteria which lead to development of a phenotype of steroid neutrophilic resistant asthma (Thorax; 2012:67:588-99). Asymptomatic GER is not a likely cause of poorly controlled asthma. Proton-pump inhibitors should not be routinely prescribed for asthma symptoms.[105]

Fixed Asthma

In these patients airways obstruction becomes less reversible with time, possibly through structural changes in the airways due to chronic inflammation. These cases can't be differentiated from COPD with chronic bronchitis. Bronchial thermoplasty may be the answer in severe persistent asthma.[106]

Bronchial Asthma in Childhood

Asthma is the most common chronic disease of childhood and it affects about 10 per cent of school children. Factors influencing asthma among school children in rural areas have been documented.[110] About 80 per cent of children with asthma have the first symptoms before the age of 5 years and at least 1/2 will stop having attacks when they become adults. The symptoms of bronchial asthma in childhood are caused by narrowing of the bronchi and bronchioles by mucosal swelling and contraction of muscles in their walls, with viscid secretion obstructing the lumen (Figs. 7.33 and 7.34). The muscle contraction is reversible by bronchodilators which belong to two main groups: adrenoceptor stimulants such as salbutamol

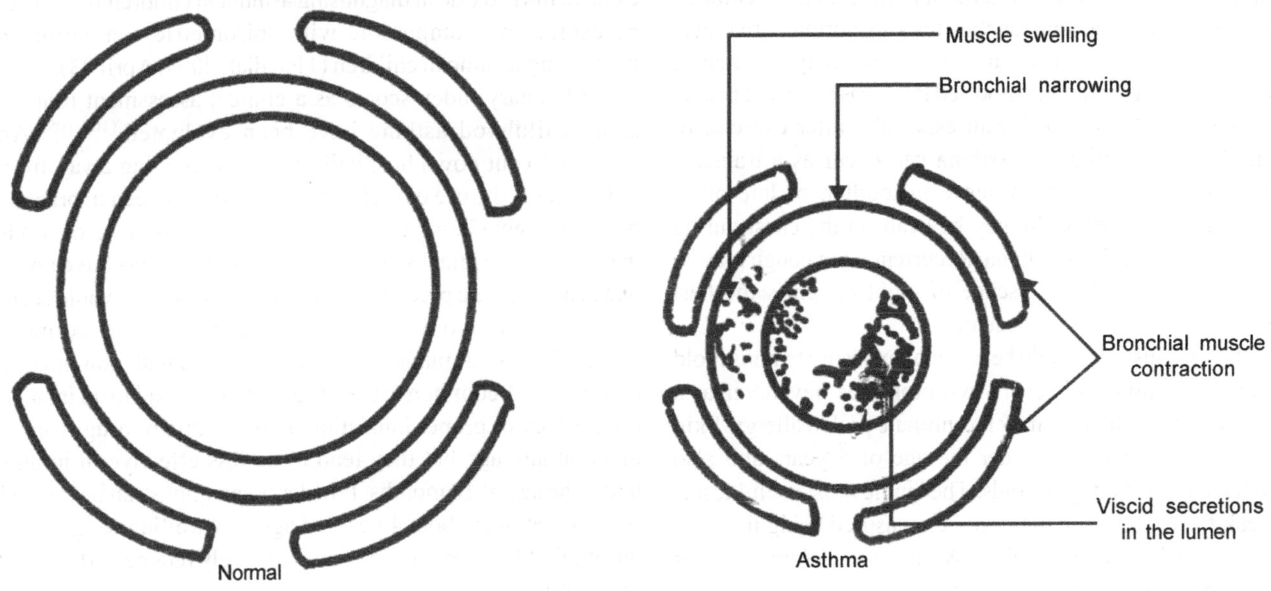

Fig. 7.33: Bronchial inflammation and bronchoconstriction

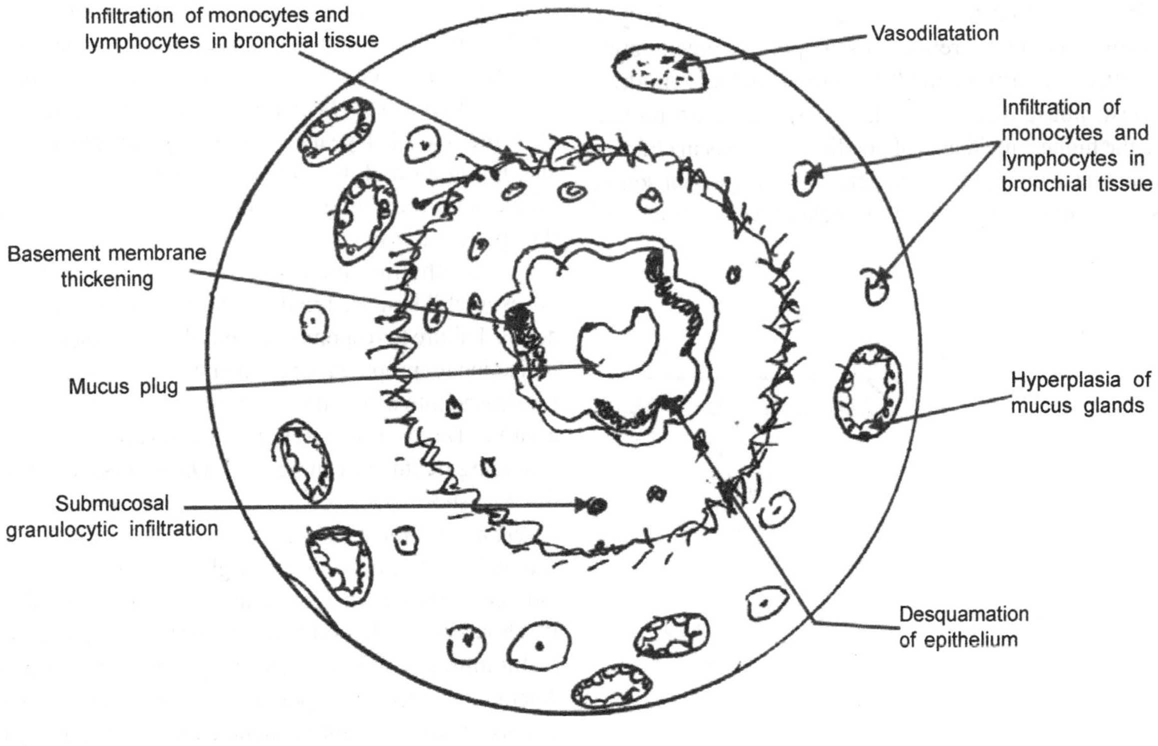

Fig. 7.34: Pathological changes in asthma

or xanthine derivatives such as aminophylline. In most children with bronchial asthma, lung function tests are normal. Treatment needs to be reviewed regularly as the severity fluctuates. Bronchial asthma should be suspected if there is recurrent cough, wheezing, or shortness of breath especially after exercise or during the night. Childhood asthma can occur as a transient infant wheeze, non atopic wheeze in toddler, or late onset childhood asthma. Rhonchi may be heard in the chest during and in between attacks of asthma. Recurrent night cough may be the only feature and the absence of night cough is the best evidence that treatment is adequate.

A detailed history should be taken of exposure to household pets or other animals. Severe symptoms or hay fever at a particular time of the year may incriminate pollen allergy. Skin tests tend to be negative under the age of 5 years and also when the child is taking steroids. The single most useful test is the peak flow reading, which can be measured using the low-range (30-370 L/m) mini-alright peak flow meter. Normal ranges are related to the height of the child. In children over the age of 5 years, especially in those in whom the diagnosis is not clear, fall in peak expiratory flow rate of 15 per cent or more after exercise to a similar rise with a bronchodilator confirms the diagnosis. A chest radiograph is taken at the initial assessment to exclude a foreign body in the lung or oesphagus, but further films are usually not helpful. Sweat test excludes cystic fibrosis. The importance of psychological factors inducing attacks of asthma is difficult to determine. Virus infections especially of upper respiratory tract, are the most important precipitating cause of attacks of asthma in 80-85% of school age children. House dust, house dust mite (Fig. 7.35) and grass pollens produce the highest incidence of postline skin tests in children with bronchial asthma. Felted carpets are an important source of house dust mite. Measurement of higher levels of tractional exhaled nitric oxide in diagnosing asthma in children is found to be useful and comparable with spirometric evaluation in diagnosing asthma in children (J Paediat; 2009: April 23).

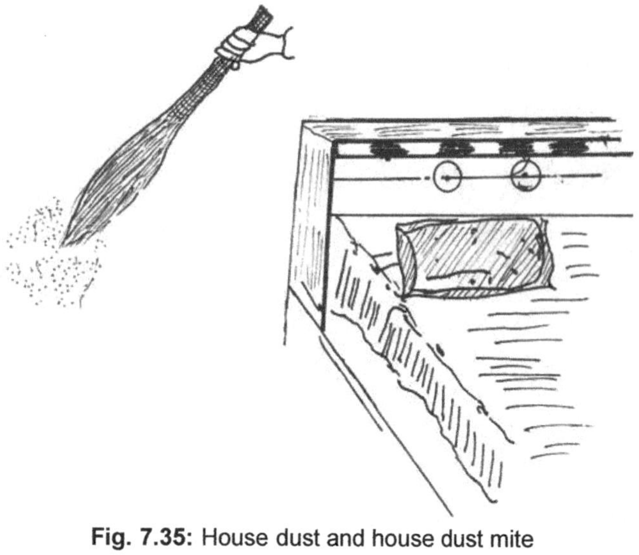

Fig. 7.35: House dust and house dust mite

Pulmonary index scores as a clinical assessment tool for acute childhood asthma have been evaluated.[108,109] An exercise to cut down hospitalisation, a step going away from guidelines is the use of oral corticosteroids has been in practice but at the same being questioned.[110] The importance of foods in precipitating attacks are controversial. If parents have noted that symptoms are precipitated by particular food, it would seem reasonable to avoid that food. Anemic children are more susceptible to asthmatic attacks as compared with non-anemic children.[111] A common cause of failure to respond to an inhaled drug is lack of proper inhalation. Bronchodilator drugs can be given at any age but they tend to be less effective in infants under the age of 18 months. Powder preparations can be inhaled by children over about 4 years of age. Controlling weight gain during first few years of life can effectively reduce or delay the incident of asthma.[112]

The metered dose can be released into a plastic disposable cap or plastic container and younger children can inhale a drug through a valve but this technique may not be effective. Children who have frequent attacks (more than once in six weeks) need a prophylactic drug continuously for at least a year. The choice is between sodium cromoglycate and long acting theophylline preparations. Sodium cromoglycate has been used for over 15 years and the rare side effects like candida of the mouth or a cough during inhalation of the powder which can be eliminated by reducing dose of bronchodilator have been noted. Children usually have to be over the age of 4 years, before they can grasp the idea of sucking in air and powdered cromoglycate through the spin inhaler into their lungs. A whistle device can be attached to the spin inhaler to check correct technique.

In theophylline, prescribing the exact dose is difficult. The doses in children are relatively high compared with those for adults. Failure to respond to cromoglycate or theophylline is an indication for prophylactic inhaled steroids (Fig. 7.36). The dose is released into a container and is inhaled by the child through a valve. Delay in appreciating the severity of the attack or providing treatment can be fatal. Drowsiness, cyanosis of the lips and shortness of breath during speaking are the signs of severe attack. Tachycardia is often a side effect of drugs. Child should be encouraged to sit upright in position that makes him most comfortable. This is usually done with his elbows forward. If 2 hours have elapsed since the previous dose of nebulized salbutamol, a further dose may be given with oxygen. Alternatively, nebulized ipratropium bromide can be given. These drugs can have an additive therapeutic effect and may be given alternatively or together. If patient is deteriorating the following are given (Fig. 7.37).

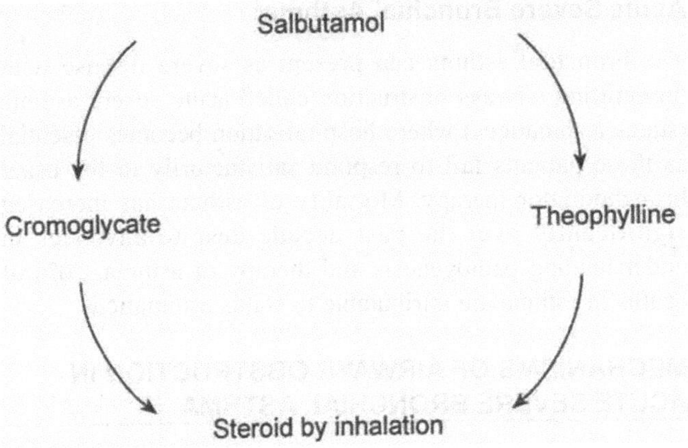

Fig. 7.36

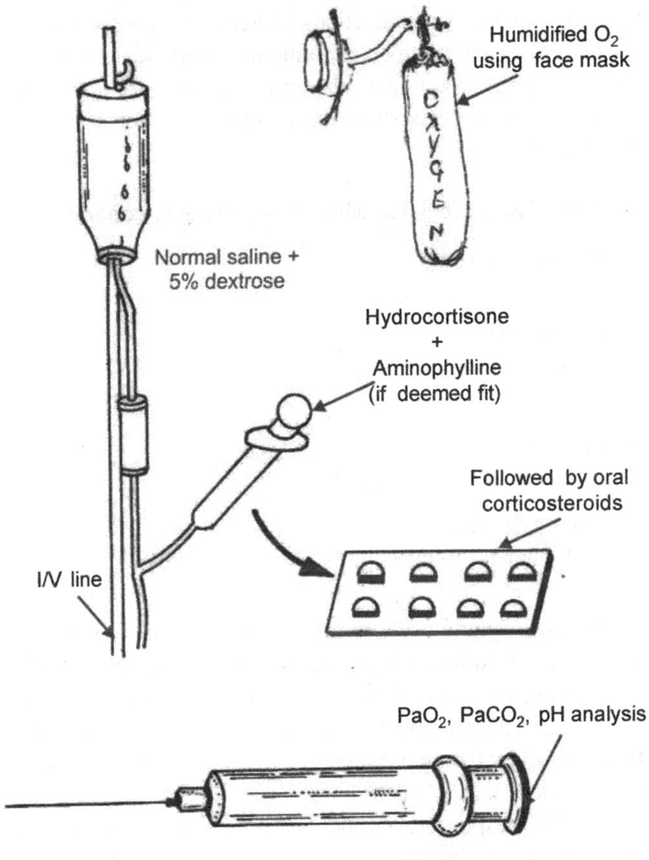

Fig. 7.37: Active management of bronchial asthma

1. Intravenous fluids are started with sodium chloride 0.18 per cent and glucose 5 per cent. In addition for the maintenance of volume, extra fluid may be needed as the child may be dehydrated.
2. Hydrocortisone is given in a dose of 100 mg intravenously every 3 hours for 3 doses and then every 6 hours for a total of 24 hours. The dose is not related to the body weight.
3. If an aminophylline preparation has not been given previously, then a single intravenous dose of 3 to 5 mg/kg body weight can be given. It must be given slowly, followed by an infusion of aminophylline at a lower dose of 1 mg/kg/hr for further 8 hours. When hydrocortisone has been given, use of aminophylline does not offer any further bronchodilation.
4. Prednisolone 2 mg/kg/24 hours by mouth should replace the intravenous hydrocortisone as soon as the child can swallow. This is gradually reduced and stopped within a week.
5. Humidified oxygen at a concentration of 100 per cent is given by face mask or other method acceptable to the child.
6. If the child is drowsy or becoming exhausted, he should be admitted to the intensive care unit, where arterial blood needs to be taken for urgent estimation of PaO_2, $PaCO_2$, pH, and plasma sodium and potassium concentration. The most suitable site for obtaining arterial blood is radial artery and the femoral artery should be avoided. Deterioration may occur rapidly and the same observer should attend all the patients at least half hourly. The investigations need to be repeated every two hours or whenever the child's condition becomes poor.

Artificial ventilation is indicated if the $PaCO_2$ is rising or is above 9KPa (67 mm Hg). Steroids do not have a maximal effect before 6 to 8 hours. Indications for admission to intensive care units (ICU), preferably intensive care pulmonary units, are given in Table 7.59. If the attack is severe and does not respond quickly to treatment, a chest radiograph should be taken to exclude pneumothorax or pneumonia.

Table 7.59: Indications for admission to ICU
• Need for immediate intubation
• Possible need for mechanical ventilation
• Rising, near normal, or elevated arterial carbondioxide tension
• Change in mental status: Confusion or drowsiness
• Severe fatigue, exhaustion, feeble respiration
• Metabolic acidosis
• Profound hypoxaemia
• Failure to respond to initial treatment

There is no reason why an asthmatic mother should not take theophylline, and $beta_2$ and corticosteroids in an inhalation form. Those who are taking oral steroids should be given hydrocortisone 100 mg 6-8 hourly during delivery, discontinuing 24 hours after delivery. Sodium chromoglycate inhalation can safely be used in pregnancy as a prophylactic agent, as it doesn't cross placenta under recommended inhalation dose. All mothers on regimens of $beta_2$ agonist inhalation, theophylline and oral or inhaled corticosteroids can safely breast feed their babies.

Other Measures

a. *Cromakalim:* A potassium channel activater has been used in a noctural asthma.
b. Immunosuppressive therapy has been used in intrinsic asthma, where further treatment with steroids is not advisable in certain cases. Chlorambusil 90 mg or azathioprine 150 mg is added, side by side gradually tappering off the steroids.
c. *Prostaglandins:* They have bronchodilator activity in bronchial asthma. However, they are irritant when inhaled.

New Modalities in Future

Seratrodast is a thromboxane A_2 receptor blocker, an oral medication for the management of asthma, recommended by GNA and Japanese guidelines.[113] Selective (type IV) phosphodiesterase inhibitors have inhibitory effects on inflammatory cells. LTD antagonists and 5-lipoxygenase have inhibitory effect on allergens. FK 506, an immunosuppressant and drugs to act against Th_2 lymphocytes are promising possibilities for future in the management of asthma. Role of immune agents such as IL-4, IL-5 and IL-13 in bronchial asthma are being investigated.[114] Anti-IgE improves markers of bronchial asthma when added to oral or inhaled steroids in moderate to severe asthma and also help in decreasing the dose of corticosteroids, in addition to reducing the number of exacerbations.[115] Humanized monoclonal antibodies (MAbs), which are more specific and less toxic and have fewer adverse effects are being used in the treatment of bronchial asthma, in addition to treatment of cancer, infections, graft rejections, autoimmune disorders and various cardiopulmonary disorders.[116] Even cold water bath has been suggested to prevent asthma attack and reduce the need of medication in asthmatics aging 4 to 20. A small subset of patients may respond to desensitization by the allergens.[117] Nitric oxide has been found to be useful in asthma; long acting preparations may be of interest in future.[118] Even role of naloxan in the management of asthma has been put forth.[119,120] Role of fish oil is being explored.[121] Methotrexate and cyclosporin in refractory asthma have been studied. Possibly they inhibit both neutrophil chemotaxis and wheel and flare response and may suppress the generation of inflammatory mediators such as lipoxygenase products.[122] Newer modalities being studied in bronchial asthma are shown in Table 7.60.

Table 7.60: Newer modalities being studied in bronchial asthma
i. Target inhibition of IL-4, IL-5, IL-13 is being investigated.
ii. Anti TNF α antibody is associated with higher incidence of cancer and reactivation of TB.
iii. Anti-IgE humanized monoclonal antibody has been approved in severe allergic asthma.
iv. PDE4 inhibitors have severe nausea, vomiting, headache.
v. Kinase inhibitors to improve corticoid action in steroid insensitivity in asthma are being studied.

Acute Severe Bronchial Asthma[2]

The bronchial asthma can present as severe disease with unremitting airways obstruction called acute severe asthma (status asthmaticus) where hospitalisation becomes essential as these patients fail to respond satisfactorily to the usual bronchodilator therapy. Mortality of asthma has increased significantly over the past decade despite advances in understanding pathogenesis and therapy of asthma. 20% of deaths in asthma are attributable to status asthmaticus.

MECHANISMS OF AIRWAYS OBSTRUCTION IN ACUTE SEVERE BRONCHIAL ASTHMA

Hypersensitivity of airways leading to acute attacks with severe airways obstruction is precipitated with hyperirritable airways by viral respiratory tract infections, exercise, allergens, emotional stress, cold air, environmental pollutants, pharmacologic agents such as aspirin or non-steroidal anti-inflammatory drugs, and chemical sensitizing agents. Aggravating conditions are given in Table 7.61.

Table 7.61: Bronchial asthma: Aggravating conditions
• Psychiatric disorder
• Hyper gastroesophageal reflux
• Cardiac disease
• Apnoea
• Obesity
• Pregnancy
• Sinusitis with nasal polyps
• Aspirin allergy
• ACE inhibitor therapy

The neuro-immunochemical mechanisms cause contraction of bronchial smooth muscle, oedema, mucosal cellular infiltration, excessive bronchial secretion and its impaired clearance, epithelial damage and basement membrane thickening. Because of persisting airways obstruction and an increase in mucosal oedema and mucus plugging, the attack becomes more severe. The response to bronchodilators changes as they can only reverse the bronchospasm, and cannot clear the mucus plugging and mucosal oedema. The latter needs corticosteroids administration.

CLINICAL FEATURES OF ACUTE SEVERE BRONCHIAL ASTHMA

The patient presents with increasing breathlessness and wheeze as an emergency. He has difficulty to talk or walk. Clinical examination shows tachypnoea with a respiratory rate more than 30 breath/minute, tachycardia with heart rate persisting more than 110 beats/minute. There may be cyanosis, systemic hypertension and arrhythmias. There is an inspiratory fall in systolic blood pressure (pulsus paradoxus) of more than 10 mm Hg. Chest is overinflated with wheeze. Expiratory phase of respiration is prolonged. Sometimes the chest may be silent from markedly decreased airflow, but the patient is in a grave situation, in that situation a silent chest on auscultation, poor respiratory efforts, cyanosis, bradycardia, exhaustion, confusion, agitated behaviour or unconsciousness are life threatening features requiring emergency management.

Investigations

Airway obstruction, air trapping and hyperinflation are responsible for pulmonary abnormalities. Peak expiratory flow (PEF) is measured with peak flow meter, even in severely dyspnoic patient. There may be peak flow of less than 100 litres/minute in an acute attack of asthma, that correlates with forced expiratory volume in one second (FEV_1) of less 0.7 liters. There is carbon dioxide retention, hypoxaemia and fall in arterial pH, and the fall of 0.08 units in arterial pH is associated with a rise in $PaCO_2$ by 10 mm Hg. And if the fall in pH is out of proportion to the alteration in $PaCO_2$, a co-existing metabolic acidosis is to be suspected.

Overinflated lungs can be seen on chest X-ray. Pneumonic patch, pneumothorax or collapse due to mucus plugging may also be present. Reversible electrographic changes may be seen such as p-pulmonale, supraventricular tachycardia, right ventricular hypertrophy with right axis deviation and right bundle branch block. Better tools for assessment and monitoring of asthma are needed.[123]

Management

Acute severe bronchial asthma requires specific as well as supportive treatment. Aims of the treatment are to quickly relieve airflow limitation and hypoxemic, urgently restoring lung functions and simultaneous health education of the patient to prevent future relapses of acute emergency. Patient is referred to hospital when there is lack of response to intensive therapy, persistence of confusion, increasing hypoxemia or suspected respiratory arrest. Signs of impending respiratory arrest are listed in Table 7.62.

Table 7.62: Signs of impending respiratory arrest in acute severe bronchial asthma

1. Altered consciousness
2. Tachycardia or bradycardia and pulsus paradoxus
3. Exhaustion and difficulty in speech
4. Cyanosis
5. Silent chest, tachypnoea, low arterial pH and high $PaCO_2$

Adequate oxygenation has been suggested to be first step in tackling acute (severe) asthma. Humidified oxygen at the rate of 4-6 liters/minute is to be delivered by nasal route. Proper hydration is essential,[124] keeping a precaution of overhydrations correcting the hypovolaemia by two liters of glucose saline or 5 per cent glucose intravenously over 24 hours. Metabolic acidosis can be corrected with 75-100 ml of 7.5 per cent sodium bicarbonate. Antibiotics need to be administered if infection is suspected.[125] Chest physiotherapy is not beneficial.

Specific therapy includes $beta_2$ agonist like 0.1 per cent adrenaline salbutamol or terbutaline 0.25 mg subcutaneously and to be repeated every 20-30 minutes in case there is no improvement.[126] A combination of beta adrenergic agonist by a compressed air-driven nebulizer and intravenous aminophylline dissolved in 50 ml of 25 per cent of glucose can be administered over a period of 25 minutes, as a loading dose.

Corticosteroids form the cornerstone of asthma therapy through their anti-inflammatory effect on airways as they enhance beta adrenergic receptor responsiveness as well as decrease the release of lipid mediators in the areas of inflammation. A higher dose may be necessary in patients who are already taking high dose of steroids. High dose (amount given at a single time) is not related to the side effects of corticosteroids; rather these are related to the duration of therapy. Nevertheless, higher dose may act as double edged sword, precipitating acute hypokalemia in susceptible patients (vomiting, diarrhoea) through its mineralocorticoid effect,[127] slowing initial response (improvement), deteriorating on 3rd day with peripheral weakness, abdominal distension and difficultly in breathing.[128] Acute severe asthma needs I/V fluids with correction of hypokalaemia caused by use of Beta-2 agonists/steroid treatment. Clinical improvement demands tapering off the dosage gradually over a period of 7-10 days. Others may require a longer period to tapper off to avoid precipitation or acute exacerbation of asthma.

Clinical deterioration, excessive fatigue and hypercapnoea (CO_2 more than 60 mm Hg), despite rigorous medical management, may require ventilatory support[129] along with rest of the treatment. Severity of asthma has been listed in Table 7.63.

Table 7.63: Severity of bronchial asthma

Moderate	PEF < 70% of predicted
Severe	PEF < 50% of predicted value
Very severe	PEF < 150-200 l/min

Patient is sedated and intubated. Spontaneous ventilation is paralyzed by neuromuscular blocking agent. On improvement, when the patient is awake, alert and is able to double his resting minute ventilation and the arterial blood gas with a fraction of inspired oxygen of 0.5 or less shows improvement;[130] patient is weaned from the ventilator. Mortality of status asthmaticus in unintubated patients is 1-3% and increases upto 3% in those who need mechanical ventilation. Sometimes, bronchoscopy may be required to clear the excessive plugging mucus that is interfering with proper ventilation. Mucolytics have no role, antihistaminics are not effective and sedation is strictly avoided.

As such it cannot be recommended as therapy in acute asthma, although nitric oxide has been found to be of value in acute asthma.[131] The effect is short lived; preparations with sustained effect are expected to be in use in future. Magnesium therapy has shown good results in controlled trials in life threatening asthmatic attacks. Although inhalational and intravenous magnesium is being used in the management of asthma, actual prevalence of hypomagnesemia in bronchial asthma is not known.[132] Heliox therapy has also been suggested to have some role.[133] Bronchial thermoplasty has been tried in patients with severe asthma, not responding to typical asthma treatment. For how long its benefit will last, still remains debatable. But current results show 32% reduction in asthma symptoms, 84% reduction in emergency room visits, 73% reduction in hospitalisation and 66% reduction in loss of days from school/work place. Treatment involves a controlled application of radiotherapy to hear and slice the smooth muscle mass in distal airways. The resulted acute epithelial destruction is replaced by connective tissue as airways smooth muscle has no capacity to regenerate.

Procedure is contraindicated in patients having pacemaker, internal defibrillator or any other implanted electronic device. Also it is better avoided during acute exacerbation of symptoms and also in patients with coagulation disorders.[134,135]

Salient Points: Management of Acute Severe Asthma[136,137]

- 100% oxygen
- Salbutamol nebulisation
  0.5 mg/20 minutes × 3
  0.15 mg/kg/20 minutes × 3 (children)
- Prednisolone
  60 mg orally
  1 mg/kg (children)
- Ipratropium
  0.5 mg/every 30 minutes × 3
  0.25 mg/every 30 minutes × 3 (children)

Additionally

- Epinephrine 0.3 mg subcutaneous/every 20 minutes × 3
  0.01 mg/kg subcutaneous/every 20 minutes × 3 (children)
- Magnesium sulfate 2 gm I/V
  40 mg/kg I/V (children)
- Aminophylline 6 mg/kg/I/V, followed by 0.9 mg/kg/hour
  0.7 mg/kg I/V, followed by 0.5 mg/kg/hour (children)

REFERENCES

1. Vora C Agani; Bronchial asthma; JAPI 2014: 62: 5-6.
2. Shankar P.S., Airflow obstruction; In: Chest Medicine; Oxford and IBH Publishing Co. (P) Ltd., 4th ed., 1994.
3. Jindal SK; Effects of smoking on asthma; JAPI (S) 2014; 62: 32-37.
4. Bhatia R.S., Respiratory disease pattern at a private clinic in Ludhiana, Punjab; Lung India 1995,13:125-26.
5. Paul M. O'Bryne, Fredrick E Margreave, John Kirby, Airway inflammation and hyperresponsiveness; Amer. Rev. Respir. Dis 1987; 135: 535-37.
6. Shanker P.S., Mechanism of bronchial asthma; In: Update in Internal Medicine; Assn Phys, India, Bombay 1990; 1: 87-92.
7. Peter J. Barnes New concepts in the pathogenesis of bronchial hyperresponsiveness and asthma; J Allergy Clin Immunol 1989; 83: 1013-26.
8. Sarnaik R.M., New developments in bronchial asthma; the pathways from science to clinical; IN; B. B. Thakur, ed.; PG Med 2002; 16: 91-104.
9. Kumar A, Ghosh B; Genetics of asthma—A molecular biologist's perspective; Clin Mol Allergy 2009;7: 7-15.
10. Hisada T., *et al.*, Cysteinyl-leukotriences partly mediate eotaxin-induced bronchial hyperresponsiveness and eosinophilia in IL-5 transgenic mice; Amer. J. Resp. Crit. Care Med 1999; 160: 571-75.
11. Kumar S, Gupta D; Asthma and GER: End of the balance game; Lung India 2009; 26: 100-101.
12. Mehta P; Allergic rhinitis and bronchial asthma; JAPI (S) 2014; 62: 23-26.
13. Bhatia R.S., Rising trend in respiratory disorders and their prevention; IN; Das S. ed. Med Update: API 2003; 13: 260-67.
14. Setipane CA; *et al.*, Asthma and hyperthyroidism; J Allergy Clin Immunol 1972; 49: 348-55.
15. Khan H., *et al.*, Alpha-1 antitrypsin deficiency in emphysema; JAPI 2002; 50: 579-87.
16. Jaju M., Vijayalakshmi Y., Reddy P. S., Jain S. N., Murthy K.J.R., Intradermal skin testing, Total IgE levels and atopic status in asthmatics, Lung India 1991;10: 61-64.
17. Rishi J.P., Govil A., Agarwal A., Arya A., Goyal M., *et al.*, Bronchoalveolar lavage cells in bronchial asthma; Lung India 1991;9: 49-51.
18. Hargreave F.E., Dilorich O'Byrne P.M., *et al.*, The origin of airway hyperresponsiveness; J Allerg Clin Immunol 1986;78: 825-32.
19. Ramazzini B., In de Morbis Artificum Diatriba; Translated by Wright WC; 1940; Uni. of Chicago Press.
20. Frew A.J., *et al.*, Mechanisms of red cedar asthma; J Allergy Clin. Immunol 1993; 92: 466.
21. Gaude G.S., Diagnosis of occupational asthma, IJCP 1995; 5(a), 69-76.

22. Hayes J.P. and Litzgerald M.X., Occupational asthma among hospital care personnel, a cause for concern, Thorax 1994; 49: 198-200.
23. Malo J., Ghezzo H., Larcheveque J., *et al.*, Is the clinical history a satisfactory means of diagnosing occupational asthma? Amer. Rev. Resp. Dis 1991; 43:528-32.
24. Singh Neelima., *et al.*, Nitrous fumes induced acute lung injury in a goldsmith; JAPI 2013; 61: 290.
25. Sahu S; *et al.*, Assessment of lung function status of goldsmiths working in an unorganized sector of India; Lung India 2013; 30: 33-37.
26. Berustein D.I., Berustein I.L., In: Allergy; Principles and Practice; ED; Middleton E., *et al.*, 1994; 4th ed; Mosby.
27. Om Parkash, Clinical approach to occupational asthma; Ind. J. Clin. Pharmcol and Therap 1997; 18: 11-13.
28. Mishra NP; Diagnostic approach to bronchial asthma; IN; S. Venkataraman; Ed; Med update API 2004; 14: 227-30.
29. Meeker D.P., Wiedemann M.D., Drug induced bronchospasm, Clin Chest Med 1990; 11: 163-74.
30. Szczeklik A., The cyclo oxygenase theory of aspirin induced asthma, Eur Resp Journ 1990; 3:588-93.
31. Szezeklik A., Mechanism of aspirin induced asthma; Allergy 1997; 52:613-19.
32. Szczeklik A., Nizankowska E. and Dworski R., Choline magnesium trisalicylate in patiens with aspirin induced asthma, Eur Resp Journ 1990; 3: 535-39.
33. Mathur S.L., Ibuprofen in bronchial asthma, J Assn Phys India 1988; 36:523.
34. Magalvadhekar S.S., *et al.*, Bronchial asthma and angioedema with nimesulide; JAPI 2000; 48:548.
35. Gupta D., *et al.*, Near fatal asthma following ingestion of diclofenac sodium tablet; JAPI 2000; 48: 258-59.
36. Sheehan G. J., Kutzner M. D. and Chin W. D., Acute asthma attack due to ophthalamic indomethacin, Ann Intern Med 1989, 114:337-38.
37. Bhatia RS, Surya Kant; IN; Bronchial Asthma; Peepee Pub. N. Delhi 2008.
38. Bhatia R.S., Enalapril precipitating an attack of asthmaticus bronchitis; JAPI 1994; 42:506.
39. Shim C.S. and Silliams M. H., Jr., Cough and wheezing from beclomethasone dipropionate aerosol are absent after triamcinolone acetonide, Ann Intern Med 1987, 106: 700-03.
40. MC Connochie K., Edward J.H., Fified K., Ispaghula sensitization in workers manufacturing a bulk laxative, Clin Experi Allergy 1990, 20: 199-02.
41. Dhar HL, Joshi SV; Recent advances in exercise induced bronchospasm; IN; S. Venkataraman; ed; Med Update; API 2004; 14: 235-37.
42. Sahoo RC; Current Concepts in the pathogenesis of bronchial asthma; IN; S. Das; ed; Med Update API 2003; 13: 207-209.
43. Janson C., Gislason T., Bowman G., Hetta J. and Roos B.E., Sleep disturbances in patients with asthma, Resp Med 1990, 84: 37-42.
44. Gupta KB, Tandon S; Nocturnal asthma; Lung India 2000; 18: 16-20.
45. Morrison J.F.J., Teale C., Pearson S.B., Marshall P., Dwyer N.M., Jones S. and Dean H.G., Adrenaline and nocturnal asthma, Brit Med J 1990;301:473-76.
46. Weiner D.E., Moore E.G., Pak J. and Martin R.J., A single evening dose of prednisone alters the nocturnal asthma response; Amer Rev Resp Dis 1990; 141 (Suppl 4: Part 2) A 23.
47. Rubinfield A.R., Wagner P.D. and Turnbull J., Rubber glove asthma, BMJ 1988; 296:531-32.
48. Vijayan Y.K., Bronchial asthma; problems and challenges; Lung India 1996; 14: 57-59.
49. Jill R Johnson, Qutoyba Hamid; Appraising the small airways in asthma; Curr Opin Pulm Med 2012;18:23-28.
50. Williamson P.A., *et al.* Assessment of small airways disease using alveolar nitric oxide and impulse oscillometry in asthma and COPD; Lung 2011;189:121-29.
51. Fischl M.A., Pitchemik A., Gardner L.B., An index predicting relapse and need for hospitalization in patient with acute bronchial asthma, N Eng J Med 1981; 305: 783-89.
52. Nowack R.M., Pensler M.J., Sorkar D.D., *et al.*, Comparison of peak expiratory flow and FEV_1 admission criteria for acute bronchial asthma, Ann Emerg Med. 1982;11: 64-69.
53. Tandon N., Saha G.K., Modak A., Maitra S.B., Kundu S.C. and Batabayal S.K., Mites in house dust as a cause of bronchial asthma, J Assn Phys India 1988; 36: 141-44.
54. Lall B., Gupta K.B., Sharma R. and Sethi K.G., Cytologic profile in bronchoalveolar lavage of bronchial asthma patients, Ind J Tuber 1991; 38:95-98.
55. Surya Kant, Bharadwaz P; BAL; J Intern Med, India 2003; 6i 99-104.
56. Wardlaw A.J., Dunnette S., Gleich G.J., Collins J.V., Kay A.B., Eosinophils and mast cells in bronchioalveolar lavage in subjects with mild asthma, Amer Rev Resp Dis 1988; 137: 62.
57. Rishi J.P., *et al.*, BAL in bronchial asthma; Lung India 1991; 9: 49-51.
58. Sandeep T., *et al.*, Evaluation of serum IgE levels in bronchial asthma; Lung India 2010; 27:138-40.
59. Bhatia R.S., Smoking—A challenge for doctors; Currt Med Pract 1992, 36: 85-86.
60. Saxena T, *et al.*, Mild Cool air–A risk factor for asthma exacerbations–Results of a retrospective study; JAPI 2011; 59: 624-28.
61. Kaur S, Behera D; Pre and post menstrual peak flow rates and symptoms amongst patients with bronchial asthma; JAPI 2010; 58: 331.
62. Bhatia R.S., Bronchial asthma, Current management, Currt. Med Prac 1991; 35: 227-28.
63. Stempal D.A., Reding G.J., Management of acute asthma; Paed. Clin. North Amer 1992; 39: 1311-25.
64. Takamine D.J., Adrenaline—the active principle of the suprarenal gland; Scot Med J 1902;10: 131-38.
65. Kristjansson S., Wennergren G. and Sten G., Effects of inhaled recemic adrenaline in acute asthma in early childhood, Clin Exp Allergy 1990; 20 (Suppl, 1): 95.
66. Schecker M.H., *et al.*, A device for overcoming discordination with MDI; J. Allergy Clin. Immunol 1993; 92: 783-89.
67. Jayakrishnan B., Aerosol systems in asthma; selection and practice; JAPI 1996; 44(3): 186-88.
68. S.V. Shah and Bhatia R.S., Aerosol bronchodilators: Practical considerations, Lung India 1996; 14(3): 133-35.
69. Jackson R.T., Beaglehole R., Rea H.H. and Sutherland I.C., Mortality from asthma; A new epidemic in New Zealand, Brit Med J 1982; 285: 771-74.

70. Maesen F.P.V., Smeets J.J., Comparison of a controlled-release tablet of salbutamol given twice daily with a standard tablet given four times daily in the management of chronic obstructive lung disease; Eur J Clin Pharm 1986; 31:431-36.
71. Persson G. and Pahlm O., Efficacy and safety of bambuterol once daily in comparison with terbutaline TID, Clin Exp Allergy 1990; 20 (Suppl 19): 35-37.
72. Das SK; *et al.,* A comparative study of efficacy and safety of arformoterol and salbutamol nebulization as rescue therapy in acute non-severe asthma; Ind J Pharm 2011; 43: 463-65.
73. Deinte F.L., *et al.,* Effect of single dose of salmeterol on the increase in airway eosinophils induced by allergen challenge in asthmatic patients; Thorax 1999; 54: 622-24.
74. Roberts J.A., *et al.,* The long acting beta$_2$ agonist salmeterol xinafoate; Effects on airway inflammation in asthma; Eur. Resp. J 1999; 14: 275-78.
75. Pearlman D.S., *et al.,* Inhaled salmeterol and puticasone; A study comparing monotherapy and combination therapy in asthma; Ann. Allergy Asthma Immunol 1999; 82: 257-65.
76. Wallin A., *et al.,* The effects of regular inhaled formeterol, budesonide and placebo on mucosal inflammation and clinical indices of mild asthma; Amer. J. Resp. Crit. Care Med 1998; 158: 79-86.
77. Vathenon A.S., Knox A.J. and Higgins B., Rebound increase in bronchial responsiveness after treatment with inhaled terbutaline; Lancet 1988; i: 554-58.
78. Fanta CH; Drug therapy, Asthma; N Eng J Med 2009; 360: 1003-14.
79. Martin U. and Romer D., The pharmacological properties of a new orally active antianaphylactic compound, Ketotifen—A benzocycloheptathiophene, Drug Res 1978; 28:770-81.
80. Thomson N.C., Nedocromil sodium, An overview, Resp Med 1989; 83: 269-76.
81. Jain S.K., Nedocromil—Expert's viewpoint, Ind J Clin Pract 1991; 2:59.
82. Crompton G.K., Beta$_2$ agonists in asthma, Lancet 1991; 337: 43-44.
83. Mehta S; *et al.,* Chronic stable asthma: JAPI 2014; 62 (S): 12-14.
84. Van Schayck C.P. Graafsam S.J., Visch M.B., Dompeling E., Vanweel C. and Van Herwaarden C.L.A. Increased bronchial hyperresponsiveness after inhaling salbutamol during one year is not caused by subsensitization to salbutamol; J Allergy Clin Immunol 1990; 86: 793-800.
85. Vijayan V.K., *et al.,* Characterisation of airway inflammation in stable bronchial asthma; Lung India 1995;13:132-35.
86. Singh V, Singh A; Role of inhaled steroids in bronchial asthma/ COPD; IN; S. Venkataraman; ed; Med Update, API 2004; 14: 231-34.
87. Wolthers O.E. and Pedeson S., Growth of asthmatic children during treatment with budesonide—A double blind trial, Brit Med J 1991; 303: 163-65.
88. Bhattacharya P; Short term adherence to inhalation therapy in asthma treated at a tertiary clinic, Lung India 2007; 24: 79-80.
89. Hill R.A., Williams J., Britton J.R., Tattersfield A.E., Can morbidity associated with untreated asthma in primary school children be reduced? A controlled intervention study, Brit Med J 1991; 303: 1169-74.
90. Noor A., *et al.,* Effect of montelukast on bradykinin induced contraction of isolated tracheal smooth muscle of guinea pig; Ind J Pharm 2011; 43: 445-49.
91. Tan R.A., Role of antileukotriences in asthma management; Curr. Opin. Pulm. Med 1998; 4 (1): 25-30.
92. Bhatia R.S., Singhal M., Bronchial asthma; Current trend; Med. Update 1999; 6:817-18.
93. Joshi J.M., Acupuncture in bronchial asthma, J Assn Phys India 1992; 40: 327-31.
94. Baruwa P., Sarmah K.R; Obesity and asthma; Lung India, 2013; 30:38-46.
95. Spitze W.O., Suissa S., Ernst P.J., *et al.,* Use of beta agonists and risk of death and near death from asthma, NEJM 1992; 326: 501-06.
96. Bhatia RS; Low dose theophylline in asthma; JAPI 2003; 51: 53-54.
97. Barthwal MS., *et al.,* Impact of optimal asthma education programme on asthma morbidity, inhalation technique and asthma knowledge; JAPI 2009; 57: 574-79.
98. Demla G., *et al.,* Oral versus I/V steroids in acute exacerbation of asthma–randomized controlled study; JAPI 2011; 59: 621-23.
99. Chhabra S.K., An epidemiological investigation into nocturnal asthma; J. Asthma 1995; 32: 147-50.
100. Cox G., *et al.,* AIR$_2$ Trial–execution of a sham-controlled double blind study of a novel device for the treatment of severe asthma; Amer J Respir Crit Care Med 2009; 179: A 2787.
101. Bhatia RS, Bharadwaj BL; Pulmonary changes during perimenstrual period; IN; SB Gupta; Ed; Med Update, API 2005; 15: 565-68.
102. Perrin B., Bousquet J., Michel F.B., *et al.,* Severe premenstrual asthma, Lancet 1988, ii: 843.
103. Luhadia SK; Steroid resistant asthma; JAPI (S) 2014; 62: 38-40.
104. Bryan CP, *et al.,* Interleukin: 25 induces type 2 cytokine production in a steroid resistant interleukin-17 RB myeloid population that exacerbates asthmatic pathology; Nature Med 2012; 18: 751-58.
105. Mastronarde JG; *et al.,* Efficacy of esopmerazole for treatment of poorly controlled asthma; M Eng J. Med 2009; 36: 1487-99.
106. Cayetano KS; *et al.,* Bronchial thermoplasty–A new treatment paradigm for severe persistent asthma; Clin Rev Allergy Immunol 2012; 43: 184-93.
107. Ganesh KS; *et al.,* Prevalence and factors associated with asthma among school children in rural Pondicherry, India; Curr Pediatr Res 2012; 16: 159-63.

108. Hsu P; Pulmonary index score as a clinical assessment tool for acute childhood asthma; Anu Allergy Asthma Immunol 2010; 105: 425-29.
109. Gowin S; *et al.*, Prospective evaluation of two clinical scores for acute asthma in children 18 months to 7 years of age; Acad Emerg Med 2010; 17: 598-603.
110. Self TH; *et al.*, Preventing emergency department visits and hospitalisations for asthma by use of oral corticosteroids at home; Are we adhering to national guidelines?Asthma 2010; 47: 1123-27.
111. Ramakrishnan K, Borade A; Anemia as a risk factor for childhood asthma; Lung India 2010; 27: 51-53.
112. Gupta PR; Asthma in the obese: Yet another reason to lose weight; Lung India 2008; 25: 01-03.
113. Dewan B; Thromboxane A_2 receptor blocker seratrodast—A novel controller medication for the management of asthma; INC; M. Panja; ED; PG Med; API 2013; 27:232-44.
114. Shankar PS; New strategies in the management of asthma; JAPI (S) 2014; 62: 41-45.
115. Abramson MJ; *et al.*, Injection allergen immunotherapy for asthma; Cochrane Database Syst Rev 2010; 8: CD 001186.
116. Jasleen Kaur; *et al.*, Monoclonal antibodies: Pharmacological relevance; IJP 2010; 42: S_2-S_{11}.
117. Srivasthava DN; Singh BP; Current immunological approaches for management of allergic rhinitis and bronchial asthma: Inflamm Research 2009; 58: 523-26.
118. Das U.N., Clinical significance of L-Orginine: Nitric oxide system, JAPI 1995; 43(2): 122-26.
119. Bhatia R.S., Aerosol bronchodilators—Practical considerations; Med Update 1998; 6:431-33.
120. Bhatia R.S., Naloxan in bronchial asthma; can we use it? Curr Med Pract 1991; 35: 327.
121. Gupta KB, Verma M; Nutrition and asthma; Lung India 2007; 24: 105-14.
122. Bhatia RS; Corticosteroid-dependent asthma and immunosuppressive agents: Beneficial role if any? Lung India 2005; 22: 99-100.
123. Vora A; Therapeutic options for uncontrolled asthma; IN; A. Muruganathan; ED; Med. Update; API 2013; 23: 464-72.
124. Tillie-Leblond I, *et al.*, Inflammatory events in severe acute asthma; Allergy 2005; 60 (1): 23-29.
125. Bedi RS; Managing acute severe asthma–nebulizer or MDI; Lung India 2005; 22: 04.
126. Bhatia R.S., Status asthmaticus, Management, Curr Med Pract 1991; 35: 274.
127. Narsimhan R, Gayathri AR; Acute severe asthma; IN; SB Gupta; ed; Med Update; API 2005; 15: 501-05.
128. Bedi RS; Managing acute severe asthma: Nebulizer or MDI; Lung India 2005; 22: 04.
129. Drazen Jeffrey M; Asthma treatment; 2004; IN; SB Gupta; (ed); Med Update, API 2005; 15: 506-10.
130. Narsimhan R, Gayathri AR; Acute severe asthma; IN; SB Gupta; ed; Med Update; API 2005; 15: 501-05.
131. Bhatia RS; Magnesium in cardiopulmonary disorders; Ind J Clin Pract 1994; 47-48 (Special Issue).
132. Das SK; *et al.*, Serum magnesium and stable asthma: Is there a link? Lung India 2010; 27: 205-08.
133. Rodrigo GJ, *et al.*, Use of helium oxygen mixture in the treatment of acute asthma—A systemic review; Chest 2003; 123(3): 891-96.
134. Cox G, *et al.*, AIR_2 Trial; Amer J Respir Crit Care Med 2009; 179: (A_2) 787.
135. Cox G., *et al.*, Asthma Control during the year after bronchial thermoplasty; N Eng J Med 2007; 356: 1327-37.
136. Charles B Cairns; Acute Asthma management; IN; Clinical Asthma; Mosby 2008; 22: 199-204.
137. Gopinathan UP; Management of acute severe asthma; IN; MS Rao; ed; Med Update 2010; 20: 784-85.

Diseases and Disorders of Pleura, Mediastinum and Diaphragm

8

PLEURAL DISEASE

The lungs are encased in and covered with serous membranes called visceral pleura and the chest cavity is lined by a similar membrane called parietal pleura. The visceral pleura envelops the surface of the lung including the interlobar fissures and sends prolongation into the parenchyma of the lung. The parietal pleura lines the inner surface of the chest wall, cervical tissues, mediastinum and diaphragm, and there is connective tissue layer with collagen and elastic fibres, beneath it. These membranes with a single layer of nucleated, flat mesothelial cells enclose a potential space—pleural cavity that normally contains 10 ml of transudate of low protein and cell concentration. The pleural spaces is like an interstitial space which becomes real when fluid or air separates the two layers of the pleura.[1]

The visceral pleura receives its major blood supply from the branches of pulmonary arteries. The pleura around the hilum is supplied by the bronchial arteries. The parietal pleura is supplied by the intercostal arteries and the branches of internal mammary artery. The venous drainage is through pulmonary veins from the visceral pleura and the drainage from the parietal pleura is to the systemic veins.

The lymphatic drainage from the visceral pleura is to the hilum. 90 per cent absorption is by lymphatics, rest by connection across the mesothelium into the lungs or chest wall. The intercostal, parasternal and paravertebral lymphatics drain the costal pleura and the drainage from diaphragmatic and mediastinal pleura is to the posterior mediastinal lymph nodes. Sensory nerve fibres are absent over visceral pleura. The costal pleura receives the fibres from the spinal nerves. The pleuritic pain probably originates in the endothoracic fascia rich in intrapleural nerves. The central part of the diaphragm is supplied by phrenic nerve and its peripheral part by the intercostal nerves. The pleural fluid is being constantly formed and reabsorbed mainly through the subpleural capillaries and pleural lymphatics. The intracellular junctions offer a gap for diffusion of solutes and molecules.[1] The accumulation of fluid in the pleural space depends according to Frank-Starling relationship among capillary permeability,[2] the opposing hydrostatic and oncotic (colloid osmotic) pressures acting on the visceral and parietal pleura. Normally the oncotic pressure on either side of the visceral and parietal pleura is equal. The plasma oncotic pressure (34 cm H_2O) exerted by albumin and other protein molecules in the intravascular compartment help in absorption of the pleural fluid at both the parietal and visceral pleura. The pleural fluid oncotic pressure (8 cm H_2O), the negative intrapleural pressure (-5 cm H_2O at mid-chest, more negative at the top of the lung than its base) and the capillary hydrostatic pressure are responsible for the formation of the pleural fluid. These pressures are equal both at the visceral and parietal pleura except the capillary hydrostatic pressure. It is greater at the parietal (30 cm H_2O) than at the visceral pleura (11 cm H_2O) as the parietal pleura is supplied by systemic vessels. This pressure difference is responsible for the formation of the fluid at the parietal pleura. Thus the pressure contributing to the formation of fluid at the parietal pleura is 9 cm H_2O (43-34) and the pressure favouring absorption of pleural fluid at visceral pleura is 10 cm H_2O (34-24). Very little fluid is present in the pleural space normally as the capacity to produce liquid (hydrostatic and oncotic pressure) and its drainage (lymphatic system) is well balanced in the pleural cavity.[1]

Normally the fluid secreted at the parietal surface gets absorbed by the visceral surface. Lymphatics of lower mediastinal pleura absorb proteins and red blood cells.[3] Electron microscopic study has shown that microvilli are present on the surface of the mesothelial cells.[4] They are in greater number on the visceral pleura compared to the parietal pleura. It gives support to the view that the parietal surfaces secrete and the visceral surfaces absorb the fluid. The number of microvilli increase in the pleural effusion. Respiratory movements help in reabsorption of the fluid.

The fluid can accumulate in the pleural space—pleural effusion—in situations like congestive heart failure (increased capillary hydrostatic pressure due to excessive back pressure from visceral surface), cirrhosis of the liver, nephrotic syndrome, severe hypoproteinaemia (decreased colloid osmotic pressure due to significant decrease in serum proteins), pneumonia, inflammation, infarction, immunologically related diseases and malignancy (increased capillary permeability due to pulmonary inflammation and lymphatic obstruction,[2] collapse (increased intrapleural negative pressure) and mediastinal involvement of carcinoma (decreased lymphatic drainage). Exudative pleural effusion can also occur in ALP poisoning.

Pleural Effusions in ICU Patients

a. Most of them are small.
b. 2/3rd are non-infectious.
c. Most of them resolve following treatment of primary pathology.

Pleurisy (Pleuritic Pain)

Pleural inflammation begins as an acute fibrinous (dry) pleurisy. It is secondary to the underlying diseases of the lung such as tuberculosis, pneumonia, infarction or bronchogenic carcinoma. It may complicate lung abscess, and bronchiectasis as a result of injury over the chest or as an acute benign pleurisy from Coxsackie B virus infection (Pleurodynia). Hyperaemia of the pleural surfaces is followed by deposition of fibrin over the surfaces, resulting in the loss of their normal shining appearance. They become dull, shaggy and rough.[1]

There is a sudden onset of pleuritic chest pain overlying the lesion in the chest, aggravating on deep breathing and coughing. The pain is often severe, sharp and unilateral and the patient tries to restrict the movement of the chest by lying on the affected side or by elapsing the area with his hand. In diaphragmatic pleurisy, the pain is referred to the shoulder or abdomen depending on the affection of central or peripheral parts of the diaphragm respectively. It is associated with dry cough, rapid, shallow breathing and moderate fever.

Chest examination reveals restricted movement of the affected side and friction fremitus may be felt with localised tenderness. Auscultation reveals existence of pleural rub having a superficial, rubbing sound of scratchy character over a localised area, both during inspiratory and expiratory phase, and not altered on coughing. It increases in intensity on pressing the chest piece of the stethoscope. The breath sounds are decreased in that area.[1] As the pleural fluid accumulates in the space.[2] Friction rub disappears after its transitory appearance.

The disease may follow different course, depending on the underlying cause. It may clear completely or thc fibrinous exudate may organise to result in adhesions or progress to serofibrinous stage with accumulation of fluid. Local application of heat or by use of hot water bottle or kaoline poultice gives the relief of pain. The movements are restricted by strapping. Analgesics are useful to relieve pain and cough is suppressed by linctus codeine. The underlying disease needs specific therapy.[1]

Pleural Effusion

Pleural effusion is a collection of fluid in the pleural space. It develops generally due to an underlying lung disease or systemic disease. The accumulation of fluid as a result of increased transudation is referred to as hydrothorax. Transudation denotes systemic disease while exudation fluid collection in the pleura usually implies disorder.[2] Pleural effusion usually occurs in cases of idiopathic and familial pulmonary arterial hypertension (Chest; 2009: April 24). When it results as an exudation from the pleural surface it is referred to as pleurisy with effusion. An exudate is present when the total fluid serum protein ratio exceeds 0.5 or the pleural fluid LDH levels exceed 60 per cent of the serum level.[2] Often it is the progressive stage of dry pleurisy. Sterile effusion in tropical myositis probably due to allergic inflammation has also been reported.[5]

A battery of tests are available but 100 per cent sensitivity and specificity are lacking.[6] Causes and types of pleural effusion have been shown in Tables 8.1 to 8.3.

Table 8.1: Causes of pleural effusion[7]

1. Increase in hydrostatic pressure in systemic capillaries.
2. Decrease in colloid pressure of blood.
3. Increase in pleural capillary permeability secondary to inflammation or neoplastic involvement of the pleura.
4. Obstruction of lymphatics.

Table 8.2: Transudative pleural effusion[7]

A. Cardiothoracic
   1. Cardiovascular diseases
      a. Congestive heart failure
      b. Fluid overload
      c. Constrictive pericarditis
      d. Superior vena cava obstruction
   2. Thoracic
      a. Pulmonary atelectasis
      b. Mediastinal fibrosis
      c. Pulmonary oedema
B. Liver diseases
   a. Cirrhosis
   b. Chronic hepatitis
C. Renal diseases
   a. Nephrotic syndrome
   b. Acute glomerulonephritis
   c. Urinary tract obstruction, i.e., hydronephrosis
   d. Peritoneal dialysis
D. Miscellaneous
   a. Myxoedema
   b. Postpartum state
   c. Meig's syndrome
   d. Sarcoidosis
   e. Iatrogenic

Table 8.3: Exudative pleural effusion
A. Infections
a. Bacterial: empyema; parapneumonic
b. Tuberculosis
c. Viral
d. Fungal
e. Parasitic
f. Mycoplasma
g. Rickettsial
B. Neoplastic
a. Direct pleural involvement
i. Metastasis
ii. Direct invasion from surrounding structures
iii. Primary pleural neoplasm
b. Indirect causes
i. Lymphoma
ii. Meig's syndrome
C. Thromboembolism
a. Pulmonary embolism
b. Pulmonary infarction
D. Immuno-mediated
a. Rheumatoid arthritis
b. Systemic lupus erythematosis
c. Wegener's granulomatosis
d. Sarcoidosis
e. Post cardiac injury syndrome
f. Sjögren's syndrome
g. Progressive systemic sclerosis
E. Intra-abdominal diseases
a. Pancreatitis
b. Subphrenic abscess
c. Intrahepatic abscess
d. Post abdominal surgery
F. Drug induced
a. Nitrofurantoin
b. Methysergide
c. Dantrolene
d. Bromocriptine
e. Practolol
f. Methotrexate
G. Inhalation of organic dust
a. Asbestos
H. Miscellaneous*
a. Oesophageal perforation
b. Post-endoscopic sclerotherapy
c. Uraemia
d. Radiation
e. Familial Mediterranean fever
f. Radiation pleuritis
g. ALP poisoning

*May be exudative or transudative

Collection of pus, blood or chyle is referred to as emphyema, haemothorax or chylothorax respectively and the term pleural effusion is not applied to these conditions. Pleural effusion in different disorders is shown in Table 8.4.

Accumulation of fluid occurs in the lower part of the pleural cavity and causes compression of the lung. Large effusions displace the mediastinum to the contralateral side. Clinically, it presents with breathlessness and pleural chest pain, depending on the size of the collected fluid and functional status of the underlying lung. Other manifestations depend on the cause of effusion.

The clinical signs of pleural effusion depend on the size of the effusion and the degree of lung compression. The physical signs are elicited only when the fluid is 300 ml to 500 ml, in the form of diminished expansion with fullness of intercostal spaces, decreased vocal fremitus, stony dull percussion note with its level being high in the axilla and decreased or absent breath sounds and decreased vocal resonance, sometimes E to A change from the lung just superior to the fluid level.[2] Contralateral mediastinal shift is not noted even though the fluid is large in situations of carcinoma of the main bronchus with collapse of the lung, a fixed mediastinum from malignant lymph nodes and malignant mesothelioma.[1] Features of pleural effusion are listed in Table 8.5.

Pleural fluid may be localised in the pleural cavity or in the interlobar fissure or rarely it may be confined to the mediastinal or intrapulmonary pleural spaces. These pleural fluid collection may give rise to pulsus paradoxus.[8]

Types: Pleural effusions may be transudate or exudate.

Transudates

Fluid may accumulate in the pleural space from the passive transudation of fluid and the pleura itself is not affected by disease (Hydrothorax). It is noted in congestive heart failure (increased pulmonary capillary pressure), nephrotic syndrome and cirrhosis of the liver with ascites (hypoproteinaemia and sodium retention). It may be a manifestation of a systemic disease. Transudation of fluid is also noted in myxoedema, Meig's syndrome (benign ovarian tumour, ascites and pleural effusion) and in peritoneal dialysis.[1]

The fluid may be unilateral or bilateral. It can be unilaterally right sided in congestive heart failure and in cirrhosis of the liver. In congestive heart failure the effusion resolves after administration of diuretics generally and it does not require aspiration.[1] The transudate fluid is quite huge in congestive cardiac failure followed by parapneumonic, malignant and pulmonary embolism associated effusions, in descending order.[2] There is no fever.

Exudate

These are secondary to the involvement of the pleura as in pulmonary tuberculosis, pneumonia (increased capillary permeability), pulmonary infarction, malignancy (bronchogenic

Table 8.4: Pleural effusion in different disorders[1]

Conditions	*Typical findings*
Congestive heart failure	Transudate: protein may increase with diuresis or chronicity; right side more frequent but often bilateral: may localize in fissure (pseudotumor).
Pneumonia	Exudate: bacterial infections: in 1/3rd of patients (more with pneumococcus and gram-negatives) cells mainly mononuclear; may be eosinophilic (>10%) in either; designated an empyema when organisms present or gross purulence.
Malignancy	Exudate: lymphocytic, often hemorrhagic, with malignant cells in fluid or on pleural biopsy; often large and symptomatic; frequency; lung>breast>lymphoma>others.
Pulmonary embolism	Exudate (75%) or transudate (25%): may be hemorrhagic; occurs in 1/3 to1/2 of patients.
Tuberculosis	Exudate: lymphocyte-predominant, high-protein; eosinophilia (>10%) rare, unilateral; small to moderate in majority; usually not associated parenchymal abnormality on chest radiograph; tubercle bacilli demonstrable in 10% on smear, 25% on culture, 50-75% on pleural biopsy; presentation either acute (>1 week), fever, chest pain or subacute; can be asymptomatic.
Cirrhosis	Transudate: usually right-sided: can be massive and symptomatic, even without marked ascites.
Rheumatoid arthritis	Exudate: leukocyte count variable: glucose often very low (<15 mg/dl.); LDH may be very high; may contain high cholesterol level and/or crystals; effusion occurs in 5% of patients, more commonly in men; may persist for months and require repeated drainage.
Systemic lupus erythematosus	Exudate: leukocyte count variable; glucose near serum level; fluid complement levels (C_3, C_4 components) typically low; LE cells may be present; effusion occurs in 1/3 to 1/2 of patients; often bilateral, usually small and of short duration.
Drug-induced effusion	Exudate: in drug-induced lupus, characteristics are similar to those in naturally occurring lupus; uncommon otherwise; often eosinophilic.
Dresser's syndrome	Exudate: in setting of pleuro pericarditis following myocardial infarction, trauma, or surgery involving pericardium.
Benign asbestos-related effusion	Exudate: cells variable, often serosanguineous; may be eosinophilic (>10%); sometimes bilateral can recur; usually small to moderate in size; asymptomatic in 2/3; related to amount of exposure; shorter lag time than with other asbestos-related conditions.
Pancreatitis	Exudate with high amylase (of pancreatic origin); usually small-to-moderate size; typically left-sided but may be bilateral.
Intra-abdominal abscess	Exudate: leukocyte count (polymorphonuclears) often very high; glucose >60 mgdL; sterile.
Oesophageal perforation	Rapidly increasing exudate, often with air fluid level; epithelial cells; sometimes with food particles; high amylase (of salivary origin); may be either side or bilateral; usually acute presentation with severe pain, toxicity, prostration.

Table 8.5: Features of pleural effusion

1. Chest wall movements restricted
2. Vocal fremitus reduced
3. Percussion note dull
4. Breath sounds decreased
5. Chest X-ray is helpful

carcinoma, metastatic carcinoma), congenital neuroblastoma,[9] neonatal and adult neuroblastoma,[10,11] ganglioneuroblastoma in adults[12,13] and connective tissue diseases (rheumatoid arthritis and systemic lupus erythematosus). Fluid can accumulate in the pleural space in viral diseases, fungal and parasitic diseases.[14] Pleural effusion may occur in uremic pleurisy, post-myocardial infarction syndrome, sarcoidosis, asbestosis, late stages of atelectasis, lymphatic abnormality, chylothorax and hypersensitivity response to drug (nitrofurantoin). The diseases below the diaphragm such as subphrenic abscess, hepatic amoebiasis and pancreatitis may lead to the appearance of fluid in the pleural cavity. Pleural effusion may occur following a chest injury.

Bilateral pleural effusion can occur in collagen diseases, miliary tuberculosis, lymphoma, lymphangitis, carcinomatosis and congestive heart failure.[1]

Radiology[15]

Pleural effusion is the most significant abnormality encountered in day-to-day practice. The healthy normal pleura are almost too fine and thin to be radiologically visible, although interlobar fissures are accurately demonstrated when viewed end-on. In approximately 90 per cent of the instances, the plain chest radiograph is the only imaging study needed. A vaiety of other imaging technique can be used to evaluate the pleura and pleural space. Computed Tomography (CT), Ultra Sonography (US) and Magnetic Resonance Imaging are other imaging techniques. CT and US are only complementary to the standard radiographs.

Before the appearance of radiological shadow at least 300 ml of fluid must be present in the pleural space. It is collected initially in the posterior recess and presents as a uniform density on the upright X-ray. There is only blunting of the costophrenic angle when the amount is small. As the amount increases the shadow covers the diaphragm in addition to the costophrenic angle and extends laterally towards the axilla with concavity of the shadow (miniscus) towards the hilum. However, chest X-ray in lateral decubitus with affected area dependent is helpful to indicate mobility and localisation of the fluid. Small effusion (even 100 ml) which are not evident on routine upright films as in subpulmonic effusion (fluid situated between the base of the lung and the diaphragm) can be appreciated.

Shadows from underlying lung disease or from coexisting interlobar effusion may also be seen. The lateral film localises the interlobar effusion. Massive effusion will appear as a complete opacity on the affected side of the thorax with shift of the mediastinum to the contralateral side. The encysted fluid in the pleural space including the interlobar fissure may present as a circular shadow (pseudo tumour).[1] The radiological detection of pleural fluid, therefore, depends on the size of effusion, patient's position, radiological technique and film used.

Invasive Tests in Patients with Undiagnosed Exudative Pleural Effusion

Needle Biopsy of Pleura

It is a bedside technique. In thoracentesis along with pleural biopsy, the diagnostic yield is high, particularly in tuberculosis and malignancy. Specimens of parietal pleura is taken either with Abram's or Cope's needle.

Indications

Undiagnosed lymphocytic exudate, e.g., malignancy (57%) TB (75%) fungal disease of pleura, sarcoidosis, rheumatoid pleurisy and parasitic diseases.

Contraindications

(1) Bleeding diathesis (2) Patients on anticoagulant therapy (3) Uncooperative patient.

Complications

Pneumothorax/local pain/vasovagal reaction/local haematoma/ bleeding/subcutaneous emphysema.

Visceral pleural biopsy, using modified Prabhudesai, *et al.*, technique[16] along with parietal pleural biopsy helps in establishing differential diagnosis in most of the cases of idiopathic pleural effusion.[17]

Pleural fluid cytology is > sensitive than pleural biopsy for the diagnosis of malignancy.

Pleural fluid cytology and pleural biopsy can give definite diagnosis. Pleural fluid ADA $\geq$ 70 u/L is almost diagnostic of tuberculosis and may not require pleural biopsy.[18]

Pleuroscopy or Thoracoscopy

Thoracoscopy should be choice investigation in undiagnosed pleural effusion as it gives good yield with minimal complications. Induce pneumothorax on the side of pleural effusion and then introduce rigid fiberoptic bronchoscope under local anaesthesia with minimal damage.[19] Diagnostic pleuroscopy with biopsy improves diagnostic yield as shown in Table 8.6.

Table 8.6: Diagnostic pleuroscopy or thoracoscopy

Indications	:	TB or malignant pleurisy
Advantages	:	1. 10-20 biopsies can be obtained
		2. Direct visualisation of the pleural surface

Open biopsy of the pleura: Open biopsy is the gold standard against which if closed pleural biopsy and thoracoscopy are compared. A diagnostic yield of 30-90 per cent is reported in selected groups. *Indication:* Undiagnosed pleural effusion. *Advantage:* This can be combined with open lung biopsy.

Fiberoptic bronchoscopy: When there is suspicion of malignancy and pleural fluid is non-diagnostic, then endobronchial lesions can be diagnosed with fiberoptic bronchoscopy. CT thorax should be performed before fiberoptic bronchoscopy. Pulmonary function testing shows a restrictive defect (reduced total lung capacity and vital capacity with normal ratio of forced expiratory volume in one second to forced vital capacity). The severity is related to the degree of lung compression caused by effusion.

Pleural Fluid Analysis

As described earlier, the pleural fluid may be exudate or transudate. It may be haemorrhagic or chylous in appearance. The exudate is straw yellow or amber coloured, thick and clots on standing. Differentiating details are shown in Table 8.7.

Cytologic Studies[20-22]

Neutrophils predominate in acute inflammatory diseases affecting the pleura including pneumonia, pulmonary infarction, tuberculosis and lupus pleuritis, and mononuclear cells predominate in trasudate effusions and in chronic exudative effusions such as those associated with carcinoma, tuberculosis and rheumatoid arthritis. Later the mononuclear cells make their appearances and become predominant cells type. It is noted in tuberculosis, carcinoma, lymphoma, rheumatoid pleurisy and uraemic pleurisy. A Wright's stain of centrifuged pleural fluid is helpful in distinguishing neutrophils from mononuclear cells. The predominant presence of small lymphocytes (50% of cells)

Table 8.7: Pleural fluid[2]

	Transudate	*Exudate*
Typical appearance	Clear	Clear, cloudy or bloody*
Specific gravity	< 1016	> 1016
Protein absolute value	< 3.0 g/dL	>3.0* g/dL
Pleural fluid/serum ratio	< 0.5	>0.5
Lactic dehydrogenase		
Absolute value	200 IU/L	>200 IU/L*
Pleural fluid/serum ratio	0.6	> 0.6 (7)
Glucose	60 mg/dL (usually same as in blood)	Variable; often < than 60 mg/dl
Leukocytes	1000 cells/cmm	> 1000 cells/cmm
Polymorphonuclear	50%	Usually 50% in acute inflammation
Erythrocytes	5000 cells/cmm	Variable
Pleural biopsy mediated	No	Parapneumonic/other acute inflammation chronic/ subacute or undiagnosed effusion

*pH of transudate is greater than 7.4

in an undiagnosed pleural fluid has been suggested as an indication for pleural biopsy to search for malignancy or tuberculosis.

Eosinophils are not seen in tuberculosis. They are noted in hydropneumothorax or haemothorax, pulmonary infarction, parasitic and fungal lung disease. Pleural fluid eosinophilia (more than 10% of total leukocytes) commonly occurs in patients with effusion due to asbestosis. It occurs in less than 5 per cent of exudative malignant or tuberculous effusions. Giardiasis as a possible aetiology of bilateral eosinophilic pleural effusion has been documented. Present more than 1 per cent of mesothelial cells in pleural fluid indicates a non-tuberculous cause, and presence of lupus erythematosus cells in pleural fluid is considered to be diagnostic of systemic lupus erythematosus. Polymorphonuclear cells predominate in pleural fluid of Wegener's granulomatosis. Cytogenetic analysis of pleural fluid and DNA analysis using flow cytometry will aid in the diagnosis of malignant pleural diseases. The presence of red blood cells varying from 5000 to 10000 cell/cmm makes the fluid haemorrhagic. It can be due to pulmonary infarction, malignancy or trauma pulmonary infarction in unlikely when the RBC count exceeds 100,000 cell/cmm. The traumatic haemorrhagic fluid clots unlike other situations where it is defibrinogenated.[1]

Biochemical Markers

A low pleural fluid glucose less than 60 mg/dl or a pleural fluid to serum glucose ratio of less than 0.5 is encountered in exudative pleural effusion secondary to rheumatoid pleurisy, empyema rupture of oesophagus, lupus pleuritis and in some cases of bronchogenic carcinoma and tuberculosis. Glucose concentration of pleural fluid to serum ratio is decreased in tuberculosis, malignancy, rheumatoid disease, parapneumonic effusion and anaerobic empyema. Pleural fluid acidosis (pH less than 7.30) has been found in systemic acidosis, empyema, malignancy, rheumatoid arthritis and tuberculosis. Adenosine deaminase or adenosine aminohydrolase catalyzes conversion of adenosine to inosine which is required in lymphocyte differentiation; its activity is high in diseases where cellular immunity is stimulated such as typhoid fever, infectious mononucleosis, brucellosis Mediterranean spotted fever, tuberculosis, malignancies, lupus erythematosus, and rheumatoid arthritis. Determination of pleural adenosine deaminase activity (ADAP), pleural lysozyme (LP) and the pleural lysozyme/serumlysozyme ratio (LP/LS) help in the differential diagnosis between tuberculous and non-tuberculous pleural effusions and indirectly between tuberculosis and malignancies. Tuberculous pleural effusion will exceptionally show an ADAP less than 33U and LP/LS ratio less than 1.2 and the malignant effusions will rarely show an ADAP greater than 33U and LP/LS ratio greater than 1.2 except in some adenocarcinomas. Protease inhibitors are found in the human body which constitute 10 per cent of about total plasma proteins. Release of proteases from micro organisms are inhibited by the protease inhibitors. Alpha-l antitrypsin levels are elevated in tuberculous effusion but not in malignant effusion or in pyothorax. Increase in the activity of ADA and elevated levels of antitrypsin help in diagnosis of tuberculous pleural effusions. Diagnostic sensitivity is varying from 60-90% and specificity from 50-75%. Coinfection with HIV further reduces the value of ADA.

Extracellular phospholipase A_2 has been detected and characterized in pleural effusions of tuberculous patients. Activity of isoenzyme of lactate dehydrogenase is high and LDH_5 occupied about 50 per cent of total activity in tuberculous effusion patients, whereas in negative cases levels are low and consist mainly of LDH_2.

Among the tumour associated proteins and the concentration of carcinoembenic antigen (CEA) and cancer antigens 125, 15-3 and 19-9 are elevated in pleural effusions assoicated with cancer whereas particularly neurone-specific enolase is elevated in small cell lung cancer. Tumour associated trypsin inhibitor (TAT) which reflects an acute phase reaction is elevated in pleural fluid of patients with malignant gynecologic tumours, hepatocellular, gastric, pancreatic and lung cancers, renal insufficiency and biliary obstruction. Higher levels of cholesterol and phosphate levels aid in differentiating tuberculous effusions from transudative effusions. The pleural fluid amylase is elevated in acute pancreatitis, rupture of oesophagus and carcinoma of the lung. Ratio of pleural to serum amylase tends to be higher in pancreatitis-associated effusions whereas pleural fluid is rich in salivary isoamylase in bronchogenic carcinoma. The higher concentrations of two eosinophil cationic protein (ECP) and eosinophil protein (EPX) are found in eosinophilic than in non-eosinophilic pleural effusions. Pleural fluid salic acid content is higher in malignant neoplasms than that found in other diseases. The concentration of lysoxyme in the pleural fluid and in plasma is similar but in certain pleural diseases (tuberculosis, empyema) a very high concentration may be found in the pleural fluid.

Immunological Markers[23]

Most inflammatory pleural effusions contain a high proportion of T cells and the ratio between T and B lymphocytes is greater than in peripheral blood.[10] Similar changes are also seen in neoplastic effusion. In transudates, the percentage of T & B cells are almost the same as in the pleural fluid and peripheral blood. Immune alterations in pleural fluid occur during the course of many diseases. There is an increase in the percentage of T_3 and T_4 lymphocytes and an elevated T_3/T_4 ratio in the pleural fluid compared with the values in the peripheral blood of tuberculous and malignant effusions. There is an increased response of T cells with PPD in tuberculous pleural effusion. IFNy levels are found to be elevated in tuberculous pleural effusion, while in other effusions (malignant, idiopathic, parapneumonic and transudates) it is almost undetectable. B cell percentage in blood of patients with effusion has increased as compared to controls. High PF/serum ratios of IgG, IgA and IgM effusions are found in malignancy. Interleukin 5 (IL-5) levels are elevated in the pleural fluid and in the serum samples of a patient with pulmonary infiltration with eosinophilia (PIE) syndrome. Interleukin 6 (IL-6) levels are singnificantly higher in tuberculous effusion. Circulating immuno complexes (CTC) are detected in exudative pleural effusion.

Pathogenesis[7]

Transudative Pleural Effusions

This occurs as a result of three basic mechanisms: systemic venous hypertension, pulmonary venous hypertension and reduced plasma oncotic pressure. Rarely, transudation can occur as a result of direct leakage of fluid from the interstitial space of the lungs. Because the pleural membranes are not affected, the pleural fluid red cells, white cells, proteins and glucose levels are not affected much.

Congestive Heart Failure

About 60-70 per cent of patients with symptomatic congestive heart failure, pleural effusion is present. In this condition, elevation of systemic as well as pulmonary venous pressures increase the formation of fluid by the parietal pleura and decrease absorption by the visceral pleura. High systemic venous pressure impends lymphatic drainage also. In the presence of pulmonary oedema, pleural effusion may arise due to shift of fluid from the interstitial space to the pleural cavity. Pleural effusion is common when both systemic and pulmonary venous pressures are elevated. In cor pulmonale and isolated mitral stenosis which produce elevated systemic venous pressure and pulmonary venous pressure respectively, pleural effusion is uncommon.

Cirrhosis

Pleural effusion occurs in about 5 per cent cases of cirrhosis with ascites and is very rare in the absence of ascites. It occurs primarily because of direct passage of ascitic fluid across the diaphragm either through defects in the diaphragm or through transdiapragmatic lymphatic channels, because, low plasma oncotic pressure due to hypoproteinemia may contribute to formation of pleural effusion. Rarely it may be massive, causing acute dyspnoea, requiring pleurodesis with instillation of talc.[24]

Renal Diseases

Pleural effusion can occur in patients with nephrotic syndrome, acute glomerulonephritis, urinary tract obstruction and also in patients who are on peritoneal dialysis. In nephrotic syndrome, about 20 per cent of the patients develop effusion. It is mainly due to reduction in plasma oncotic pressure due to hypoproteinemia though increased hydrostatic pressure from salt and water overload may be contributory. In nephrotic syndrome due to renal vein thrombosis, pulmonary embolism is responsible for pleural effusion in about 20 per cent of the cases. In children, about 50 per cent cases of acute glomerulonephritis have pleural effusion (urinothorax). Pleural effusions are very common in patients undergoing peritoneal dialysis. The mechanism is similar to that for effusion in cirrhosis with ascitis. It results from fluid overload and increased systemic venous pressure. Urinary tract obstruction is a rare cause of effusion. However, when urine extravasates into the retroperitoneal space, it may lead to pleural effusion.

Pulmonary Embolism

In about 25 per cent cases of pulmonary embolism, transudative pleural effusion occurs. It is due to elevation in systemic venous pressure as a result of right ventricular failure secondary to multiple pulmonary emboli.

Iatrogenic Effusion

Misplacement of central venous line into the pleural cavity or mediastinum and subsequent infusion of fluids can lead to effusion.

Superior Vena Cava Obstruction

SVC obstruction due to any cause leads to elevation in systemic venous pressure, thereby producing effusion.

Exudative Pleural Effusion

This occurs as a result of increased pleural capillary permeability, reduced reabsorption of fluid by visceral pleura, reduced absorption of proteins, cells and fluid by the pleural lymphatics and abnormally subatmospheric pleural pressure due to local or generalized reduction in lung compliance.

Tuberculosis

It occurs as a hypersensitive reaction to tubercular protein following primary tuberculosis or as a result of an extension of caseous primary focus or rupture of caseous lymph node or from the infection of the pleura from miliary tuberculous cavity may result in effusion. The condition may develop within a year of primary infection or within few weeks following steroids. Haematogenous spread may cause bilateral pleural effusion. Pleural tuberculosis with large hemorrhagic effusion or pleural masses and without visible parenchymal lung disease is not uncommon in developing countries.[25] The onset may be acute with constitutional symptoms of fever, loss of apetite, weakness or loss of weight. In addition, pain of pleuritic nature, dry cough, and gradually increasing dyspnoea may be present. It leads to increased pleural capillary permeability and decreased clearance of proteins through lymphatics resulting in accumulation of pleural fluid which usually contain relatively few tubercle bacilli. The occasional occurrence of a negative tuberculin test may be due to compartmentalization of sensitized lymphocytes in the pleural fluid or with very high levels of suppressor T cells in the blood. Occasionally, tubercular empyema occurs due to rupture of a caseous lesion or lung cavity.

The pleural fluid is straw coloured exudate with a high protein content and contains a large number of white cells predominantly lymphocytes. The centrifuged specimen in one fifth of the cases may show tubercle bacilli on staining with Ziehl Neelsen stain. The pleural biopsy with Abrams or Copes needle is useful as it gives histologic confirmation of caseating granuloma in pleural tissue. When the pleura is thickened, Vim Silverman needle may be used for biopsy. ESR is elevated and tuberculin test is positive.[1] Estimation of pleural adenosine deaminase[26] in pleural fluid is suggested to be a safe, simple, non-invasive adjuvant test in distinguishing tubercular from non-tubercular pleural effusion.

The condition needs active treatment with anti-tuberculosis drugs even in the absence of pulmonary lesions as there is always a chance of late appearance of pulmonary tuberculosis. It prevents subsequent development of pulmonary lesions in such instances. To relieve the effects of pressure on the lung and to prevent the occurrence of pleural thickening, aspiration of the fluid has to be done using a syringe connected with a bi-way needle. The paracentesis thoracis is done in the mid-auxillary line at the site of maximum dullness.

During the process of aspiration the patient may complain of discomfort in the chest and cough, when the fluid is removed in large amounts quickly. Such instances may lead to the occurrence of pulmonary oedema and circulatory collapse. It should therefore be performed slowly under complete asepsis with all precautionary measures to prevent entry of air or infection. Air embolism may occur when the pleura is thickened and inelastic.

Corticosteroids are useful to facilitate rapid absorption and reduce the incidence of pleural thickening allowing an early expansion of the lung. Daily 20 to 30 mg of prednisolone is given in divided doses for two to three weeks and is tapered later. In addition 4 to 8 mg of dexamethasone may be injected into the pleural cavity after aspiration. It hastens recovery and prevents adhesions.

Resolution is generally complete and in some cases as a hallmark of old pleurisy, there may be an organisation of the exudate with obliteration of costophrenic angle, irregular or raised diaphragm, thickening of pleura, contraction of hemithorax and calcification. Pleural adhesions are commonly seen in tuberculosis.[1]

Pneumonia

Country specific guidelines are of immense importance. Recently guidelines have been laid down for diagnosing and management of community acquired and hospital acquired pneumonia in adults in India.

Factors Responsible for Non-resolving Pneumonia

1. COPD
2. Diabetes mellitus
3. Tobacco smoking
4. Immunosuppression

Common Causes of Non-resolving Pneumonia

1. Tuberculosis	36%
2. Malignancy	27%
3. Bronchiectasis	9%
4. Pneumocystis pneumonia	7%
5. BOOP	6%
6. Antibiotic resistant pneumonia	14-15%

An exudative turbid fluid accumulates in the pleural cavity with a large number of neurophils in pneumonia. The fluid has high protein content, normal glucose and a pH greater than 7.3. The fluid has high contents of lactate and needs antibiotics to prevent the occurrence of empyema and localisation. Those with a small collection of fluid get absorbed with effective therapy and may not require aspiration. About 50 per cent of all bacterial pneumonias are associated with parapneumonic pleural effusions which are exudative and usually contain no bacteria. It is because of inflammation of the pleura over an area of parenchymal infection resulting in the leakage of fluid, proteins and cells. In few patients, bacteria invade the pleural space resulting in formation of empyema. Viral infections are common causes of exudative pleural effusions. This is due to increased permeability of pleural capillaries. About 20 per cent of patients with mycoplasma pneumonia have pleural effusion. Pleural effusions are occasionally seen in patients with fungal infection like aspergillosis, cryptococcosis, coccidioidomycosis and others. Most cases of pulmonary actinomycosis and about 25 per cent cases of nocardiosis have pleural effusion. About 35 per cent of patients with amoebic liver abscess develop pleural effusion. This is most often as a result of subphrenic inflammation.

Rupture of abscess into the pleural cavity results in typical *anchovy sauce* like effusion. Inflammatory exudate can also occur in malignancy of the lung. The pneumonic lesion distal to the obstruction of neoplasm can result in a pleural effusion that is neither haemorrhagic nor does it recur.[1]

Infarction

The fluid is generally small in volume, exudative and blood stained. It contains a large number of eosinophils. It is due to increased capillary permeability secondary to release of inflammatory mediators from the platelet rich thrombi. Ischaemia of visceral pleura consequent to pulmonary artery occlusion plays a minor role in the development of effusion in this setting because the capillaries are supplied by the bronchial circulation. The diagnosis of pulmonary infarction is probable when pleuritic pain is accompanied with a basal pulmonary infiltrate, raised diaphragm and a small pleural effusion. Management includes administration of anticoagulants.

Connective Tissue Disease

Involvement of respiratory system in rheumatoid arthritis frequently accompanies pleural effusion. It is more frequent in males with active articular disease. The effusion is unilateral and may be recurrent. Pleural effusion exists often without parenchymatous lung disease. The fluid is turbid with a high leucocyte count. It has a very low glucose content (less than 30 mg/dl). LDH level is high. A low glucose content may be due to an enhanced glycolysis by the pleural membrane and to an impaired glucose transport into the pleural space by the mediators released from the inflammed pleural rheumatoid reaction.[27]

The effusion in systemic lupus erythematosus is frequently bilateral and may even accompany pericarditis. The effusion is recurrent and manifests pleuritic chest pain. It also occurs in drug-induced SLE. Common drugs are isoniazid, procainamide, hydralazine and phenytoin. Other collagen vascular disorders which can produce pleural effusion are Wegener's granulomatosis, Sjögren's syndrome and familial Mediterranean fever. The effusion is small or moderate in amount. The straw coloured fluid contains many mononuclear cells and LE cells may be demonstrated. Immune complexes are present in pleural fluid in SLE and rheumatoid arthritis. The concentration of immune complexes is similar in the blood and pleural fluid in SLE, and is higher in pleural fluid than blood[1] in rheumatoid arthritis. Resolution occurs on administration of corticosteroids or spontaneously.

Malignant Pleural Effusions

There is a rapid recurrence of accumulation of pleural fluid in malignancy, requiring repeated aspirations. The fluid in majority of cases is blood stained and the accumulation is associated with unpleasant pain. Demonstration of the presence of malignant cells in the pleural fluid and biopsy establish the diagnosis.

The pleural effusion may be presenting feature of bronchogenic carcinoma of any histologic type situated in the periphery of the lung or it may appear later with other manifestations of the disease. Radiation therapy can lead to effusion due to impaired mediastinal lymphatic drainage while some chemotherapeutic agents like methotrexate and cyclophosphamide can also cause effusion.

Malignancy related effusions occur in lung cancer (35 per cent of such effusions), breast cancer (25 per cent) and lymphoma (10 per cent), generally due to local effect of the tumour causing lymphatic obstruction and systemic effect like pulmonary embolism secondary to hypercoagulability.[2] Nearly 50% of patients with disseminated lung cancer develop pleural effusion during the course of illness. Presence of malignant cells in the pleural fluid signifies inoperability.[28] Diagnostic difficulty arises in pleural based mass when the lesion may be in pleura or lung parenchyma. Chest X-ray can classify parenchymal and extraparenchymal lesions. CT guidelines help in separating pleural or extraparenchymal lesions through their obtuse angles with chest wall from the parenchymal lesions which form usually an acute angle with chest wall. But pleural lymphomas and neurogenic neoplasms are mistaken for pleural fluid. Ultrasound guided biopsy of solid mass (fine needle aspiration) for cytology is safe, complication free and high yield diagnostic facility for evaluation of such lesions. Infact CT guided biopsy for all thoracic lesions that are visible on CT scan regardless of their size or position is recommended. Chemical pleurodesis with tetracyclines is the choice procedure in such cases as both systemic chemotherapy and radiotherapy are ineffective.[2]

The mechanism responsible for the occurrence of pleural effusion in pulmonary malignancy are: pleural spread of malignancy from peripherally located malignant tumours and obstruction to lymphatic drainage by tumour at the hilar region. The fluid can also accumulate from pneumonia or atelectasis occurring as a result of obstruction from the neoplasm arising in the bronchial tree and impaired bronchial drainage. Other causes are obstruction of the superior vena cava by tumour, direct damage to the subpleural capillaries by the tumours, pulmonary infarction and hypoproteinaemia.[29] Ig indices, as shown in the Table 8.8, are increased in malignancy, due to increased capillary permeability associated with malignant deposits and active synthesis as well as secretions of local immunoglobulins by these deposits.[30] Chemotherapy or radiation therapy may also be followed by pleural effusion.

Table 8.8: Ig indices

Ig index	*Malignant disorder*	*Non malignant disorder (mainly tuberculosis)*
IgG index	More than 0.6 (100%)	More than 0.6 (16%)
IgA index	More than 0.6 (100%)	More than 0.6 (24%)
IgM index	More than 0.5 (100%)	More than 0.5 (Nil)

Haemorrhagic fluid may be obtained from a traumatic thoracentesis. However it clots within several minutes. The fluid initially withdrawn is bloody, and it clears as more fluid is aspirated. The haemorrhagic fluid caused by pleural disease does not clot as it is defebrinated.[1] The malignant effusion may be associated with the shift of the mediastinum to the same side from bronchial obstruction and collapse of the lung.

Malignant pleural effusion can occur in metastatic *pleural malignancy from breast, ovary, uterus, and stomach or lymphoma, or in primary pleural mesotheliomas.* Mesothelioma is closely related to asbestos exposure especially erionite, and is associated with marked wasting, cough, increasing dyspnoea and chest pain. Incidence of malignant pleural mesothelioma is IIA/million in males and 2.8/million in females. Even those living near asbestos mines are said to have higher risk of developing malignant pleural mesothelioma. Cytological variants include epithelial, fibrosarcomatous, mixed 11.4 polygonal (polyhedral) type. A cancerous proliferation affecting large extent of pleural cavity often presents with refractory, massive haemorrhagic pleural effusion, that includes differential diagnosis of pleural effusion, that includes differential diagnostics of pleural alerio carcinoma, benign asbestos pleurisy, benign pleural fibrous mesothelioma.[31] Demonstration of the presence of malignant cells in the pleural fluid and biopsy establishes the diagnosis. Differential diagnosis includes adenocarcinoma involving pleura, benign asbestos pleurisy, benign fibrous mesothelioma and other pleural lesions. Utilising flexible fiberoptic bronchoscope as pleuroscope, the whole of the pleural cavity can be explored and biopsies of any suspicious lesions under direct vision. Malignant pleural mesothelioma is said to be incurable; surgery, radiotherapy and chemotherapy have been tried. Vinorelbine has been tried with success as chemotherapy in malignant pleural mesothelioma.[32]

The treatment of malignant pleural effusion is essentially for the relief of symptoms. Rapidly accumulating effusion needs immediate treatment for relief of respiratory distress. Repeated pleural aspirations may be required. However if the fluid accumulates rapidly, a chest tube may be inserted into the pleural space, to drain the fluid. If the reaccumulation of the fluid is less than 100 ml/24 hours, the chest tube may be removed in 48 hours. To prevent accumulation of fluid in the pleural space, pleurodesis may be undertaken to induce adhesion of parietal and visceral pleural surfaces. After drainage of pleural effusion, an irritant substance is instilled into the pleural space to produce pleural irrigation, fibrosis and adhesion. A variety of chemicals such as nitrogen mustard, cyclophosphamide, quinacrine hydrochloride, doxorubicin, cisplatin, bleomycin sulphate, iodised talc, radioactive colloid gold and yettrium have been used to encourage pleural adhesions with variable success. Talc usually requires a single administration with highest success rate. Even micro organisms like Corynebacterium parvum or B.C.G. cell wall skeleton have been used to induce pleurodesis.[33] Now tetracycline is commonly preferred for pleurodesis. After thoroughly draining the pleural space, tetracycline mixed with 50 ml of 5 per cent normal saline is injected through the tube into the pleural space and the tube is clamped for 24 hours. After injection, the patient is encouraged to change his posture every five minutes in such a way as to allow chemical spread to all surfaces of the pleura. After 24 hours the chest tube is removed. It facilitates pleurodesis.[1]

Gastrointestinal and Intra-abdominal Disorders

Pleural effusion develops in about 15 per cent of cases of acute pancreatitis. It is due to transdiaphragmatic passage of exudative fluid from the abdominal cavity to the pleural cavity. As this fluid is rich in enzymes, pleural inflammation occurs which results in further accumulation of pleural fluid. Sometimes, there is formation of a pancreatopleural fistula which results in massive pleural effusion. Oesophageal perforation is a rare cause of pleural effusion. Subphrenic abscess can lead to pleural effusion due to inflammed diaphragm and increased permeability of diaphragmatic pleural capillaries. Similarly intrahepatic abscesses are associated with pleural effusion in about 20 per cent of patients. Small effusions are common after abdominal surgeries.

Miscellaneous Causes

Uraemia can produce pleural effusion in about 30 per cent of cases. In Meig's syndrome, pleural effusion occurs as a result of passage of ascitic fluid across the diaphragm. Ascitis occurs due to generalized secretion of exudative fluid, from the tumour. Rarely, it may produce transudative effusion. In sarcoidosis, pleural involvement is uncommon. It occurs as a result of granulomatous involvement of the pleura. Drug induced pleural disease may be in the form of pleuritis, pleural effusion with or without pleural thickening.[34] Lupus-pleuritis and effusion that occurs due to drugs like procainamide, hydralazine, chlorpromazine, phenytoin, quinidine, isoniazid and methyl dopa. It improves on discontinuation of the offending drug.

Eosinophilic pleural effusion can occur with dantrolene without any pulmonary infiltrations, with valoric acid with parenchymal infiltrates and with nitrofurantoin. Nitrofurantoin given for a longer period may result in interstitial pneumonitis and fibrosis and without pleural effusion. Bromocriptine, isotretinoin and propythiouracil also produce eosinophilic pleural effusions.

Chemotherapy of malignant conditions by bleomycin, cyclophosphamide, methotrexate, mitomycin and procarbazine may result in pleuro pulmonary manifestations either as a hypersensitivity reaction or due to direct cytotoxicity, resulting into pleural effusion with or without pleural thickening.

Cardiovascular drugs such as amiodarone, minioxidil and practolol may result in pleural effusion with or without interstitial lung disease and pleural thickening.

Ergoline drugs such as bromocriptine and methysergide may cause pleural effusions with fibrosis.

Pleural effusion may be produced by variety of agents such as sodium morrhuate and absolute alcohol, metronidazole, acyclovir, sclerotherapeutic agents, recombinant interleukin-2 and rarely with the use of D-penicillamine, itraconazole, simvastin, L-tryptophan, granulocyte colony-stimulating factor and clozapine. Withdrawn of offending agent and administration of corticosteroids in refractory cases forms the essential management.

Chylothorax

This rare condition with accumulation of chyle in the pleural cavity may result from the rupture of the thoracic duct (carries lymph from the entire body except the right side above the diaphragm) or of a large lymphatic channel following closed chest injuries, intrathoracic operations, bronchogenic carcinoma or lymphoma affecting the thoracic duct, filariasis and thrombosis of subclavian vein. It can occur without damage to the thoracic duct as in lymphangiectasis associated with incompetent valves leading to a chylous reflux or from a development deficiency causing a downstream obstruction to the lymphatic drainage called yellow nail syndrome. The condition referred to as yellow nails, has lymphoedema and pulmonary complications such as pleural effusion, bronchiectasis, bronchopneumonia and malignancy. The nails are thick, yellowish-brown, slow growing and exhibit an increased transverse curvature. The effusion is yellow pleural exudate. Lymphangioleiomyomatosis occurring in young women may be associated with chylothorax. Bilateral chylothorax secondary to tuberculosis has also been documented.[35]

In traumatic causes, there is sudden development of chylous effusion leading to sudden onset of dyspnoea, emaciation, signs of malnutrition and thirst. It is frequently right sided as the thoracic duct is in contact with pleura on the right side upto T5 vertebra.

In chylothorax, the pleural fluid is milky white in appearance due to a high fat and triglyceride content. The protein level is elevated. The cells are mainly lymphocytes. The fluid is sterile. On standing there is formation of creamy top layer, and the milky colour clears on addition of ether to the fluid. The fluid is rich in chylomicrons and they can be seen accumulating on the top as whitish layer in a centrifuged specimen of the fluid drawn following a meal. The fat globules stain positively with Sudan III dye. The total lipid content is more than 400 mg/dl. The level of triglycerides is generally greater than twice that present in the serum (more than 110 mg/dl). The cholestrol concentration is low.[2] The pleural fluid becomes red on consuming Sudan III dye.[1]

Chylous effusion has to be distinguished from chyliform effusion (pseudochylothorax), in which the effusion is long standing and it is due to tuberculous pleurisy, rheumatoid pleurisy or carcinoma. Often pleura is thickened and may even be calcified.[36] The concentration of cholesterol is high and it is due to degeneration of cells, mainly lymphocytes. This increased lipid content mainly cholesterol gives a milky or oplascent appearance to the pleural fluid. The fluid may show typical rhomboid cholesterol crystals. The triglyceride content is low (less than 50 mg/dl). There are no chylomicrons and the Sudan III stain of the pleural fluid is negative.[1]

Chylous effusion can be controlled by repeated thoracentesis or thorocostomy tube drainage as there is a chance of spontaneous closure of traumatic lymph fistula. Spontaneous recovery has been reported in 50 per cent of cases in children under one year of age. Surgery may be necessary in post traumatic chylothorax if chyle drainage doesn't stop even after 10 days.[2] A fat free, high carbohydrate and high protein diet is advised. Radiation therapy is advised for lymphoma affecting hilar and mediastinal lymph nodes but usually therapy fails in cases of chylothorax due to malignancy. Ligation of thoracic duct, first described by Lampson in 1948, can easily be done through right thoractomy. Thoractomy is successful in 80 per cent of cases.[37-39] Failures are common in non-traumatic chylothorax.[40] Frequent accumulation of the effusion and rapid loss of weight may necessitate pleurodesis by injection of sclerosing agents like nitrogen mustard or iodised talc into the pleural space, or ligation of the thoracic duct. A pleuroperitoneal shunting device in the absence of infection or renal failure may help in keeping the pleural space free of fluid.

Pulmonary Lymphangioleiomyomatosis[1]

It is a rare disease seen in females in the child bearing age and shows a rapid progression during pregnancy. It may co-exist with tuberous sclerosis. It consists of a triad of ILD, pleural effusion and pneumothorax. Recurrent pneumothorax can be seen in 50% of cases. Clinically, there may be progressive dyspnoea with chylous effusion. Haemoptysis may occur in few; but clubbing is absent. Chest X-ray shows diffuse parenchymal infiltration, coarse reticulonodular shadows and pleural effusion. HRCT demonstrates diffuse, small thin walled cysts and ground glass appearance. Pathologically, entire pulmonary interstitium is involved by smooth muscle cells called LAM cells. Collagen deposits are present between the muscle cells; however fibrosis is absent. LAM cells may penetrate vessel wall causing secondary microscopic haemorrhages. Peribronchiolar proliferation may narrow bronchioles.[41] Initial restrictive pattern becomes obstructive on PFTs, as the disease advances. Lung biopsy is diagnostic. Patients can be stabilised by progesterone therapy or oophrectomy. Prognosis is variable. Respiratory failure and death are the ultimate of this slowly progressive disorder.

Hemothorax

This is a gross bloody pleural effusion with hematocrit at least 25 per cent of that in the peripheral blood.[1] Its usual cause is penetrating or non-penetrating chest trauma, but it may also be iatrogenic (following central line placement, thoracentesis, or pleural biopsy, especially in patients with coagulopathy) or may occur in association with spontaneous pneumothorax, where it may be called hemopneumothorax. Rupture of an aneurysm is unlikely to be a cause in childhood.[42] Therapy consists of thoracostomy tube drainage, both to remove the blood and to monitor the rate of bleeding. Passive or persistent blood loss indicates need for thoracotomy.

Re-expansion Pulmonary Edema[43-47]

Introduction: This life threatening complication can occur during treatment of pleural effusion, lung collapse, pneumothorax and even after lobectomy. Exact mechanism is not clear, but enhanced capillary permeability due to depleted surfactant or hypoxic capillary damage have been implicated. Unlike animal model, where negative pressure is applied to pleural space, re-expansion pulmonary edema in human beings can occur even without negative pressure that occurs during treatment of pleural effusion.

Pathogenesis

Enhanced pulmonary vascular permeability and not the difference in hydrostatic pressure, is responsible for increased leakage to result in edema. Oxygen free radicals and reperfusion add to lung injury, since re-expansion pulmonary edema can be prevented by oxygen inhalation as FiO_2 0.4 when lungs are setting re-expanded.

Clinical Features

Apart from asymptomatic cases, sudden onset of respiratory failure with circulatory shock are also seen. Cough or tight chest following chest tube placement or thoracentesis, with pinkish, frothy, copious sputum should arouse suspicion of re-expansion pulmonary edema. Tachypnoea, tachycardia, dyspnoea, nausea and vomiting, followed by hypotension, hyperthermia and even cyanosis are seen. Chest X-ray may reveal pulmonary edema. Mortality is as high as 20%. But timely treatment is rewarding with total recovery.

Treatment

Thoracentesis or tube thoracotomy are the modes of management, keeping in mind the duration of pleural effusion or pneumothorax. Negative pressure should be avoided and under water-seal drainage remains the choice. Independent risk factors, however, remain the younger age extent of lung collapse.

Supportive therapy includes oxygen, morphine and intravenous fluids. Unlike cardiac unilateral pulmonary edema, diuresis better be avoided in re-expansion pulmonary edema. Non-invasive positive pressure oxygen can be used. Severe situation may require mechanical ventilation.

REFERENCES

1. Shankar P.S. Chest Medicine; Oxford and IBH Publ. Co. (P) Ltd., 1994; 4th ed.
2. Harrison's principles of internal medicine, Wilson J.D., et al. ed, 12th ed, McGraw Hill, New York, 1991.
3. Emerson P.A., The pleura and its effusions. In: Fifth Symposium on Advanced Medicine. Williams, R. (ed) Pittman Medical, London 1986, 23.
4. Wang N.S., Mesothelial cells in situ. In: Pleura in health and disease. Chretein, J., Bignon J. and Hirsch A., Marcel Dekkar, New York 1986, 23.
5. Kulpati D.D.S., et al. Tropical myositis with pleuropericardial effusion. JAPI 1990, 38: 184-85.
6. Bhatia R.S. et al. Diagnostic value of ELISA and ADA in TB: JAPI 1998;46: 574.
7. Wali J.P., Aetiopathogenesis of pleural effusion In: Shankar, P.S: ed, Medicine Update, API Bombay 1995, 5: 440-445.
8. Kulkarni S.G., Pulsus paradoxus with tense pleural effusion, JAPI 1990, 38: 818.
9. Minola E. and Gambacorta M., Hemothorax in congenital neuroblastoma, Tumor 1987, 73: 81-83.
10. Ekloof and Fritis M., Thoracic neuroblastoma of the neonate, Acta Rad (Diagn) 1985, 26: 441-46.

11. Radhakrishanan S., *et al.* Recurrent pleural effusion due to thoracic neuroblastoma, Ind. J. Chest. Dis. All Sci 1979;21: 48-51.
12. Reed J.C., *et al.* Neural tumours of the thorax. Review; J, Radiol 1978; 126: 9-17.
13. Aggarwal P., *et al.* Adult thoracic ganglio neuroblastoma with massive pleural effuison, JAPI 1993; 41: 306-07.
14. Thippanna G. and Vidyasagar G., Pulmonary hydatid cyst presenting as a massive effusion, Lung India 1987, 5: 74-76.
15. Thanasekharan V., Imaging and tests in massive pleural effusion, In: Shankar P.S., ed; Medicine Update, API Bombay 1995; 5: 460-64.
16. Prabhudesai P.P. *et al.;* Percutaneous visceral pleural biopsy with penetrated cup biopsy forcep; Thorax 1992; 47: 753-54.
17. Jain N.K. *et al.;* Comparative study of visceral and parietal pleural biopsy in the etiological diagnosis of pleural diseases; JAPI 2000;48: 776-80.
18. Pandit S.; *et al.,* Role of pleural biopsy in etiological diagnosis of pleural effusion Lung India 2010; 27: 202-04.
19. Parsad BNBM; Medical thoracoscopy in the management of pleural diseases; Pulm and Crit Care Bull 1996(6):55-56.
20. Ghelani D.R. *et al.* Diagnostic significance of immumoglobulin and ADA in pleural effusion; JAPI 1999; 47: 787-90.
21. Good J.J., *et al.* Diagnostic value of pleural fluid, Chest 1980;78: 55-59.
22. Singh U; *et al.,* Eosinophilic pleural effusion and giardiasis–A causal or a casual relationship? Lung India 2013; 30: 69-71.
23. Bousquet J., Michel F.V., Gauci L. and Clot, J., The immunological basis of pleural reactions In: Disease of pleura. Chretein J., Bignon, J. and Hirsch A., (eds). New York: Masson 1983, 233.
24. Milanez J.R.C.; *et al.,* Intrapleural talc for prevention of recurrence in benign or undiagnosed pleural effusion; Chest 1994; 106: 1771-75.
25. Patel A; Choudhary S; Pleural TB presented as multiple pleural masses–An atypical presentation; Lung India 2013; 30: 54-56.
26. Nagaraja M.V., *et al.,* ADA in pleural effusions, JAPI 1992; 40: 157-59.
27. Sahn S.A., Malignant pleural effusion, Semin Resp Dis 1987, 9: 43-53.
28. Reshad K., *et al.,* Treatment of malignant pleural effuison, Chest 1985;88: 393.
29. Sahn SA, Clin. Chest. Med 1985; 6: 113.
30. Gupta S., Brali A.J., Prakash K., Immunological study in pleural effusion, JAPI 1993,41: 641-43.
31. Mitschell Margolis; MPF; In; Pulmonary diseases & disorders. Alfred P Fishman(ed); 2nd ed; Tata Mcflraw-Hill 1998; 284-89.
32. Steele; Phase II Study in patients with MPF: J Chin. Oncol 2000;18:3912-17.
33. Dhillon D.P. and Spiro S.G., Malignant pleural effusions; 1. Appl. Med 1984; 10: 13-17.
34. Morlock S.Y., Shan S.A. Drugs and the pleura; Chest 1999; 116: 212-21.
35. Kant Surya, *et al.,* Development of bilateral chylothorax in a younger female secondary to tuberculosis; Lung India 2011; 28: 56-59.
36. Saccon E.S. and Light R.W., Chylothorax and pleurochylothorax Clin. Chest. Med 1985; 6:163.
37. Ribonson C.L.N., The management of chylothorax, Ann Thorac, Surg 1985; 39: 90.
38. Watson E.H. and Foster L.F., Spontaneous chylothorax in infancy, prognosis and management, Amer. J. Dis. Child 1946; 72:89.
39. Strausser J.L. and Flye M.W., Management of non-traumatic chytothorax, Ann.Thoraci. Surg 1981; 31:520.
40. Ferguson M.K., Little A.G., *et al.* Current concepts in the management of postoperative chylothorax . Ann. Thoraci. Surg 1985;40:520.
41. NHLBI workshop summary: Report on lymphangio-leiomyomatosis; Amer. J. Resp. Crit. Care Med 1999;159: 679-83.
42. Nelson W.E. (ed), Textbook of Paediatrics, Philadelphia, WB Saunders, Co 1987.
43. Murat A; *et al.,* Re-expansion pulmonary edema; Acta Radiol 2004; 45: 431-33.
44. Beng ST, Mahadevan M; An uncommon life threatening complication after chest tube drainage of pneumothorax; Amer J Emerg Med 2004; 22: 615-19.
45. Volpicelli G; *et al.,* A case of unilateral re-expansion pulmonary edema successfully treated with non-invasive continuous positive airway pressure; Eurp J Emerg Med 2004; 11: 291-94.
46. Bhatia RS; Khan G; Aetiopathogenesis of spontaneous pneumothorax; IN; Pulmonary Medicine; Peepee Publ 2007; 6: 38-59.
47. Singh SP; *et al.,* Cardiogenic unilateral pulmonary edema; JAPI 2007; 55: 672.

PNEUMOTHORAX

The collection of air in the pleural space is called pneumothorax. Air (gas) can enter the pleural space either from the lung parenchyma and airways (intrernal) or from outside (external) artificially, traumatically or spontaneously.[1]

Aetiology and Pathogenesis

It may occur suddenly as in spontaneous pneumothorax or it may develop following injuries over the chest or rib fractures (traumatic pneumothorax) where the sharp bony spicules lacerate the underlying lung. The air may reach the pleural space by alveolar overdistention and rupture, direct laceration of the lung by fractured rib or foreign object, or by entry of air directly through the chest. Treatment is by tube thoracostomy. If there is a large air leak and the lung fails to re-expand with suction, injury to the trachea or main bronchus should be suspected. Hydropneumothorax after closed-chest injury may be a sign of oesophageal rupture, a diagnosis further suggested if the fluid contains high levels of amylase. Common causes of pneumothorax are shown in Table 8.9.

Table 8.9: Common causes of pneumothorax

1. Emphysema, bronchial asthma
2. Trauma
3. Certain forms of pulmonary fibrosis, cystic fibrosis
4. Tuberculosis, suppurative pneumonia, lung abscess, bronchiectasis
5. Bronchogenic carcinoma, metastasis, rarely

Iatrogenic Pneumothorax[2]

Probably more common than all forms of spontaneous pneumothorax combined, this develops as a result of direct puncture or laceration of visceral pleura (during attempts at central line placement, percutaneous lung aspiration, thoracentesis, or closed pleural biopsy), transbronchial lung disruption (bronchoscopic forceps biopsy or brushing), or direct alveolar overdistention (anesthesia, cardiopulmonary resuscitation, or mechanical ventilation). Iatrogenic pneumothorax is a recognised complication[3] of subclavian cannulation, intercostal nerve block, chest aspiration lung biopsy[4] supraclavicular brachial plexus block,[5] and fine needle aspiration cytology in diagnosing breast lumps.[6] The diagnosis should be suspected in a patient who develops respiratory distress or hemodynamic deterioration following day of the above procedure. It is also commonly detected for the first time on a postprocedure or routine chest radiograph. Treatment differs from that for spontaneous pneumothorax; in that prevention of recurrence in not a concern. Pneumothorax developing in a patient on mechanical ventilation should always be treated with chest tube drainage if the patient cannot be removed from the ventilator. Other patients may be observed without treatment if the pneumothorax is small and asymptomatic, or the air may be aspirated using a small catheter as described for primary spontaneous pneumothorax. Tube thoracostomy may be required if the latter is unsuccessful.

Catamenial Pneumothorax

This is rare condition in which spontaneous pneumothorax (usually right sided) occurs in women over 25 to 30 years of age in association with menstruation. Whether it is the result of minute diaphragmatic endometrial implants or of passage of air from the peritoneal cavity via a small diaphragmatic dent is controversial. The diagnosis should be considered if spontaneous pneumothorax develops within 48 hours of the onset of a menstrual period. Ovulation-suppressing drugs are the preferred treatment as the condition characterstically recurs and otherwise requires surgical exploration. Pleurodesis may be the treatment of choice, especially if the woman wants to conceive.

Primary (Simple) Spontaneous Pneumothorax

This is a disorder most commonly affecting tall, and slender men between 20 and 40 years of age; the male to female ratio being 6:1 and is believed to occur within subpleural pulmonary bullae. Although the pathophysiology is uncertain, the blebs occur, may be as a consequence of the increased traction placed on the uppermost parts of the lung, during maximal inflation. From 30 to 50 per cent of affected individuals experience a recurrence (75% ipsilateral, 25% contralateral), and after one recurrence subsequent episodes are much more likely. Chest pain and dyspnoea are the usual symptoms. It is not a totally benign disease.[7] Management is designed both to re-expand the affected lung and to decrease the likelihood of a recurrence on that side. Features of spontaneous pneumothorax are shown in Table 8.10.

Table 8.10: Spontaneous pneumothorax

Features	Amphoric or cavernous breathing Apex beat and tracheal displacement Hypo or hyperventilation Thoracic tympany or vocal fremitus
Chest X-ray is diagnostic	HRCT has additional diagnostic value
Differential diagnosis	Chest trauma Asthma, bronchitis, emphysema Pleurodynia Tuberculosis Pulmonary abscess Pulmonary infarction

Only recently shouting induced primary spontaneous pneumothorax has been reported.[9]

Pneumothorax is common in men of the age group 20 to 40 years. It can be recurrent, but rarely bilateral in silicotic alveolar proteinosis.[8] Spontaneous pneumothorax presents a common clinical condition secondary to underlying pulmonary lesions such as congenital weakness of the pleura, rupture of subpleural tuberculous focus or cavity or emphysematous bulla or congenital cysts in the lungs.

Secondary (Complicated) Spontaneous Pneumothorax

Unlike primary spontaneous pneumothorax, a generally benign condition which occurs in otherwise healthy young individuals, development of pneumothorax in a patient with underlying pulmonary disease is more serious and frequently life-threatening. Virtually all patients have dyspnoea, chest pain, and cyanosis and hypotension occurs in perhaps in 10 per cent. Chronic obstructive pulmonary disease is the most common associated condition, although secondary pneumothorax is also a recognized feature of asthma, cystic fibrosis, idiopathic pulmonary fibrosis, tuberculosis, sarcoidosis, lung abscess, pneumocystis carinii pneumonia, and several other pulmonary diseases. It is also common in the adult respiratory distress syndrome. In each instance the primary event is believed to be overdistention and rupture of an alveolous with dissection of air into the pleural space. The rupture may be directly across the visceral pleura, or air may dissect into an adjacent bronchovascular sheath, with subsequent centripetal air dissection to the root of the lung, and thence into the mediastinum and pleural space. This diagnosis should be considered whenever a patient with chronic lung disease develops sudden clinical deterioration. There is a history of tobacco addiction and emphysematous disease. Mechanism is probably the pleural endometriosis and small perforations of the diaphragm. Tube thoracostomy should be performed promptly in all cases. Failure of complete lung re-expansion and persistent bronchopleural air leak (bronchopleural fistula) are more common than with primary spontaneous pneumothorax. Sclerosis of the pleural surfaces using tetracycline or another agent should immediately be done after the first episode, because of the seriousness of the condition. Surgery is indicated for a massive air leak with failure of lung expansion or as smaller leak persisting even after one week. Complication like emphysema or hemothorax may need drainage. Pleurectomy can also be done. 90-95 per cent success rate is reported.

Lung cancer and pneumothorax rarely occur simultaneoulsy, in patients who are generally above 40 years of age.[10] Spontaenous pneumothorax may be presenting feature of an advanced lung cancer, incidence being 0.03 to 0.05 per cent,[11,12] even as high as 0.16 per cent from a short study have been reported.[13] Cause of spontaneous pneumothorax in lung cancer may be due to (1) Rupture of dilated alveoli distal to tumor into the pleural space (2) Rupture into pleural space of those alveoli which have become distended in compensation to atelactesis due to obstruction casued by the tumor (3) Bronchopleural fistula secondary to rapid invasion of the pleura (4) Associated diseases like chronic bronchitis, emphysema, asthma etc.; disturbed pulmonary architecture due to cancer may rupture these emphysematous bullae. Incidence of 0.45 per cent has been reported.[14] Both a giant cell and a primary bronchogenic carcinoma with ipsilateral spontaneous pneumothorax have been reported.[13,15] Cases with primary lung cancer[16] and with bronchoalveolar carcinoma,[17,18] have been reported as well. In an interesting series,[14] pneumothorax has been the first manifestation of lung cancer in 78.3 per cent of cases, which conclude that spontaneous pneumothorax in association with lung cancer is not a rare complication but a serious one, occurring at an advanced stage of the disease and if the patients happen to be above 40 years of age, with recurrent pneumothorax, neoplasm should be suspected.

The association of *spontaneous pneumothorax* to primary lung neoplasm is very uncommon, and is extremely rare in the presence of metastatic tumours of the lung.[19] Thornton and Bigelow were the first to report the occurrence of spontaneous pneumothorax secondary to metastatic sarcoma.[20]

The incidence of pneumothorax in reported series of malignant neoplasms averages 1.4 per cent.[19] Simultaneous occurrence of lung cancer with spontaneous pneumothorax *seems extremely low,* occurring in approximately one of every 2000 patients with lung cancer.[21] Spontaneous pneumothorax to be a rare feature of primary pulmonary malignant neoplasm.[22] Although spontsneous pneumothorax can occur with any type of pulmonary metastasis, there is distinct preponderance for sarcoma metastasis to be associated with this condition.[23] Osteogenic sarcoma followed by Wilms tumour are the most common malignant metastatic neoplasms associated with pneumothorax.[24] Sherman and Brant reported the first case of cancer metastasis causing spontaneous pneumothorax.[23] The occurrence of bilateral pneumothorax complicating secondary deposits is very rare. Only 25 such cases have been reported in the literature.[1] O'Leary and team reported bilateral pneumothoraces from synovial cell sarcoma.[25] Rarely, the spontaneous pneumothorax may precede the development of roentgenographically demonstrable pulmonary metastasis.[22] The exact mechanism of the pneumothorax is not clear.[26] Accepted explanation is that in most of the cases it is not due to necrosis of the tumour nodule with the production of the bronchopleural fistula.[27] Even drug like, adriamycin has been reported to be associated with pneumothorax.[28,29]

Pneumothorax can occur as a complication of bronchial asthma or rupture of staphylococcal pneumatocoele. It can be a manifestation of honeycomb lung or cystic fibrosis. The condition is rarely seen in bronchogenic carcinoma, silicosis, coal workers' pneumoconiosis, fibrosing alveolitis and sarcoidosis.[30] Pneumothorax may be precipitated during corticosteroid therapy, positive pressure breathing, use of positive and expiratory pressure (PEEP)[31] or menstruation. Spontaneous pneumothorax as a complication to desquamative interstitial pneumonia and hydatid pulmonary diseases has been reported.[32,33] In some instances, especially in young patients with a previous record of good health and no underlying lung lesion demonstrable, the air enters through a subpleural bleb situated in the upper regions of the lung which may give way under mechanical stress producing pneumothorax.

Normally a negative pressure of -2 to -7 cm of water exists intrapleurally and the visceral and parietal pleura remain in close contact. With the entry of air, it is converted into a real cavity and the two layers of the pleura are separated.[30] In the west, AIDS related pneumothorax is a common entity where pneumocystis carinii pneumonia often gets complicated by a virulent form of necrotizing subpleural necrosis, resulting in diffuse air leaks.[34]

Depending on intrapulmonary disturbances, three types of pneumothorax are recognised, i.e., closed, open and valvular.[30] In closed (simple) type the opening is sealed by deposition of fibrin. Generally the pleural pressure is negative and the lung re-expands without any sequelae. In an open pneumothorax, the communication between the lung and the pleural space remains patent and is relatively large allowing free movement of air in and out of pleural cavity during respiration thus leading to wastage of ventilation. It prevents re-expansion of the lung. The opening may be in the pleura or in the lung. Occasionally a communication may develop between a bronchus and the pleural space to result in a bronchopleural fistula. The intrapleural pressure remains atmospheric. In the valvular type, the flap of opening acts as a check valve at either the internal or external site, allowing entry of air into the pleural cavity during inspiration. Its escape is prevented during expiration. It results in a progressive increase in the size of pneumothorax to a great extent and the intrapleural pressure becomes positive. There is a complete lung collapse with shift of the mediastinum to the opposite side compressing the opposite lung and the great vessels leading to marked cardiorespiratory embarrassment (tension pneumothorax).[30]

Clinical Features[35]

The clinical features and functional abnormalities directly correspond to the size of the pneumothorax, amount of collapse of the lung and on the pre-existing lung diseases. In valvular pneumothorax there is rapidly progressing dyspnoea. It may be associated with severe pain and sensation of tightness over the affected side of the chest. There may not be any history of extra strain as the condition can occur while the patient is sitting quietly. In closed pneumothorax, acute symptoms subside within few hours. But with tension pneumothorax, the individual becomes increasingly short of breath, restless, anxious and cyanotic. The respiratory distress is marked when it complicates bronchial asthma, chronic bronchitis and emphysema. Shock and circulatory failure may occur.

Physiological Abnormality[30]

Pneumothorax alters the intrathoracic pressure. It reduces the gas exchanging parts of the lung following its collapse. Lung volume is reduced with restrictive ventilatory insufficiency and reduced diffusing capacity. Cyanosis disappears later due to reduction in the perfusion of the collapsed lung. The arterial oxygen tension is also reduced markedly in those with the underlying lung disease.

Physical Signs[30]

Clinical examination reveals cyanosis, rapid shallow breathing and tachycardia. Movement of the chest are restricted in the affected side, with fullness of intercostal spaces. Contralateral mediastinal shift is seen in gross penumothorax. Percussion reveals a hyper resonant note which encroaches on the liver or cardiac dullness depending on the side affected. It may even be tympanic in character. The vocal fremitus and vocal resonance are reduced. The breath sounds are markedly diminished or absent, and without any added sounds. In persistent opening, an amphoric breath sound with metallic tinkle may be heard. Coin sounds are audible clearly on performing coin test. The signs of a small pneumothorax are not obvious.

A shallow left sided pneumothorax with at least 300 to 500 ml of air in the pleural cavity may produce crunching or clicking sounds near the apex of the cardia (systolic clicks), often referred to as noisy pneumothorax. Even the patient may complain of a clicking sound, audible without a stethoscope, gets accentuated as the patient leans towards the left side and exhales.

When there is fluid in the pleural cavity (hydro-pneumothorax), dullness on percussion with a horizontal upper limit is noted in the lower part and it shifts on change of posture of the patient. A succession splash is elicited on shaking the patient. Hydropneumothorax may be iatrogenic while aspirating the pleural fluid, following the tear of pleural adhesions and laceration of its vessels.

When pneumothorax is secondary to tuberculosis, history of fever, cough, sputum and haemoptysis, positive evidence of tuberculosis in the lung, fluid in the pleural cavity, and apical adhesions may be evident. In emphysema, pneumothorax is generally a shallow one. The lung fails to collapse completely as it has lost its elasticity. The onset may not be striking. An increasing shortness of breath without much cough must lead to its suspicion. The breath sounds are weak generally even in emphysema and the mediastinal displacement may not be striking. Another differential diagnosis is, bronchial asthma, where the history of attacks of dyspnoea, wheeze and rhonchi may be contributory.

Investigations

The chest X-ray reveals hyperlucency at the periphery of the lung without any lung markings. The margin of the collapsed lung can be clearly defined. Increased vascular markings and congestion due to increased blood supply may be seen in opposite lung. There may be herniation of the pleura to the opposite side as a translucent shadow.[30] Lateral neck X-ray to screen spontaneous pneumo-mediastinum in patients with dysphagia is very useful.[36]

Chest X-ray in an erect patient, a pneumothrax is usually apical and is comparatively easy to detect as an apicolateral transradiancy devoid of vessels, bounded on its inner side by the visceral pleural line.[37] When the patient is supine, pneumothorax may truly be undetectable in the radiograph or it may be manifested by one or more subtle signs—namely, relative transradiancy of the lower chest and upper abdominal quadrant;[38] deepening of the lateral costophrenic sulcus;[39] the appearance of the anterior costophrenic sulcus as an oblique interface extending downwards and outwards across the diaphragm;[40] sharp delineation of the diaphragm[38] and cardiac border, particularly the apex, with apical pericardial fat pads sometimes appearing as lobulated discrete opacities;[41] and a vertical line on the right, just inside and parallel to the chest wall, caused by retraction of the middle lobe from the chest wall.

The lower border of this air is formed by the reflection of the parietal pleura off the diaphragm and on to the chest wall anteriorly.[8] It appears as a line rather than an interface because of gas lying below in the stomach and colon. The dome of the diaphragm can be seen to lie much higher, a finding which has been referred to as the *double diaphragm* sign.[41] A horizontal ray decubitus radiograph with the patient lying on the unaffected side should confirm the diagnosis.[37] On screening, the mediastinum moves towards side of pneumothorax on inspiration and it moves to the healthy side on expiration. The size of the pneumothorax is graded in terms of the percentage of the hemithorax it occupies. In hydropneumothorax, a uniform opacity with a fluid level is noted with a translucency above the horizontal opacity.[30] HRCT improves diagnostic yield in secondary spontaneous pneumothoraces which were earlier labelled as primary. HRCT can also detect eosinophilic granuloma and lymphangio leiomyomatosis.[42] HRCT also improves diagnostic yield of pulmonary tuberculosis where chest X-ray is reported normal.[43]

Complications

Pneumothorax gets rarely infected. In open pneumothorax, infection secondary to tuberculosis or staphylococcal infection may develop empyema and bronchopleural fistula. The secretions occlude the bronchus causing lung collapse.

Hydropneumothorax mostly gets absorbed and may require to be aspirated, if there is a delay. When bleeding occurs as a complication, early aspiration is required and may even require thoracotomy. The lung collapse may persist rarely. Pneumothorax persisting for more than three months becomes chronic. Respiratory failure may be precipitated by pneumothorax in patients with poor respiratory function. Recurrent pneumothorax within one year is common, especially on the same side.

Prognosis

The prognosis is good in young adults without any underlying lung disease, while mortality is higher in the elderly with airway obstruction. With lowered morbidity and proven safety, VATS can be used in elderly and paediatric population.[44] The tension pneumothorax may be rapidly fatal for want of treatment.[32] Death may be due to acute respiratory failure. The occurrence of haemothorax is hazardous.

Management

The treatment lies in obtaining rapid re-expansion of the collapsed lung. The methodological strategies depend on the size and type of pneumothorax, extent of the lung collapse, existence of the underlying or systemic diseases and the age of the patient. The mechanical removal of offending material, or the unilateral lung lavage when the contralateral lung is isolated and ventilated by double lumen endotracheal tube. Appropriate treatment depends not just on the size of a pneumothorax on chest X-ray, but more importantly on the clinical status of the patient.[45] Bed rest, sedatives and morphine is given if there is no chronic obstructive lung disease (COPD).[30] Oxygen administration is necessary. In tension pneumothorax, in a high concentration if there is no disease of airways. Controlled oxygen therapy is required in those with airways obstruction. Conservative line of treatment is adopted in shallow or small pneumothorax causing no respiratory embarrassment, especially in healthy young adult. Air gets spontaneously reabsorbed. In those situations with closure of the opening, the absorption of air occurs gradually within three to four weeks. Repeated chest X-ray may be required to observe re-expansion of lung. Manual exertion has to be avoided for several weeks although complete bed rest is not essential. In those, secondary to tuberculosis anti-tuberculosis drugs have to be given simultaneously.[30] Active management is required in case there is associated lung disease with reduced respiratory reserves or there is lung collapse more than 20% per cent of its normal volume.

In closed pneumothorax the expansion of the collapsed lungs is 1.5 per cent of its radiological lung volume per day and with a moderate or massive collapse of the lung it takes a longer time to re-expand. In such cases, active measures have to be taken using intercostal intubation to remove the air, to facilitate lung expansion.[46] Emergency treatment is instituted in cases of tension pneumothorax, to remove air and facilitate early lung expansion so as to relieve acute pain, dyspnoea and cyanosis. Needle aspiration of tension, pneumothorax can be a life saving temporizing maneuver.[47,48]

A wide bore needle has to be introduced into the pleural cavity above the rib to prevent injury to the intercostal vessels as an emergency to equalise the pressure with that of atmosphere. As there is a chance of injury to the expanding lung from the tip of the needle, an intercostal catheter is introduced and is connected to a water seal which promotes pleural adhesions from the reaction at the site of intubation and prevents the collapse of the lung. Recently simplified procedure of using disposable sterile jelcos has been suggested.[49] Chest X-ray is not as effective as CT. Therefore, for secondary pneumothoraces, intercostal tube drainage offers better option for those with a distance of more than 2 cms, above which the volume of pneumothrorax will be more than 50%.[42] A passage is created through trocar and cannula or with an artery forceps in the fifth or the sixth interspace anteriorly under local anaesthesia and a self-retaining Malecot catheter or a soft rubber catheter is inserted into the pleural space and is fixed to the skin with a stitch on one end and connected to the longer arm of the glass tubing of an under-water seal drainage bottle on the other end. It acts as a one-way valve, allowing escape of air from the pleural cavity while preventing entry of air through the system. If pneumothorax is localised, intubation has to be carried out in that area.[30,32]

The thoracostomy tube drainage is the most common treatment used[49] and results in re-expansion of the collapsed lung, in three to four days and the tube is kept in the pleural cavity for 48 hours after the last air bubble has come out. It encourages development of adhesions between the layers of the pleura. A sedative is given before withdrawal of the tube. If the bubbles still continue to come out without stopping as in open pneumothorax, suction with a negative pressure of -2 to-10 cm Hg may be tried by connecting the open end of the water seal to a suction pump, which is necessary in secondary pneumothorax that may be noted in patients on ventilators.

While both air and fluid are being drained, an increased resistance is encountered that can be minimised by adding a dry trap bottle between the patient and underwater seal bottle. The trap bottle further facilitates the measurement of fluid collected. Sometimes the air bubbles stop coming out from a kinked tube or from obstruction in the drainage tube by a clot of blood, or in the bronchus from a mucus plug. Expectoration of secretions should be encouraged by stimulating cough or with physiotherapy or removed by bronchoscopic aspiration, to facilitate the re-expansion of the collapsed lung. If the drainage tube is blocked with the exudate, it has to be replaced by another tube in an intercostal space lower than the previous one. During the respiratory movement and coughing, the movement of the miniscus of water column indicates patent communication.

Repeated check X-rays are necessary to recognize the expansion of the lung. Though intubation may cause pain, but it is quite safe and effective. There is likelihood of blockage if there is coexistent fluid in the pleural cavity and the fluid has to be aspirated.[30] Pyopneumothorax if develops as a complication, has to be drained and antibiotics are to be given. Sometimes rib resection may be required to achieve adequate drainage of pus. In chronic pneumothorax and recurrent pneumothorax, re-expansion of the lung becomes difficult, even after intercostal intubation for several days, possibly due to pulmonary collapse from retained secretions or a persistent air leak or a bronchopleural fistula. The retained secretions have to be aspirated through a bronchoscope. The persistent air leak or a bronchopleural fistula requires thoracotomy and closure of the opening and fistula.[30] 10 to 30 per cent of cases of pneumothorax are likely to have a recurrence within a year either on the same or the other side. VATS is indicated for spontaneous pneumothorax with giant bulla which can itself be manifestation of lung carcinoma or a focus for recurrent infection.[50] Pleurectomy is effective but has more morbidity and needs to reserved for extreme cases. Either of the methods has 90-95 per cent effectiveness.[47] Combined VATS bullectomy with surgical pleurodesis reduces recurrence rate in primary spontaneous pneumothorax in the range of 1.7-5.7%.[51] Lesser shoulder dysfunction and pain medication requirements are observed with VATS as compared to post lateral thoracotomy during postoperative period.[52]

In those without any lesions, pleurodesis is done by inducing chemical pleuritis. Due to the inflammatory reaction, the visceral and parietal pleura get adherent, thus leading to pleural symphysis, particularly useful in patients with emphysema. Iodised talc, camphor in oil, silver nitrate, patient's own blood, olive oil, hypertonic saline, glucose, turpentine or kaoline can be introduced to induce pleural irritation. The procedure is painful and causes thick adhesions. The introduction of 1 per cent camphor in oil is painless and preferable. Five to 10 mg of 1 per cent iodised talc can be introduced through thoracoscope. Quinacrine hydrochloride, 600 to 800 mg dissolved in 60 ml sterile water can be introduced into pleural space in two to three fractional dose. Recurrence of pneumothorax even after intubation and chemical pleurodesis requires pleurectomy. The parietal pleura is stripped from the chest wall and the upper mediastinum following thoracotomy and it leaves behind a raw surface to which visceral pleura adheres.[30]

In AIDS related spontaneous pneumothorax, aggressive stepped care with large bore tube drainage, chemical pleurodesis and an early video assisted talc powder age is recommended.[53]

Re-expansion Pulmonary Edema[54-57]

It is a rare but life threatening complication of treatment of diseases like pleural effusion, lung collapse, pneumothorax and even after lobectomy. It results from increased fluid leakage due to increase pulmonary vascular permeability and not due to difference in hydrostatic pressure. Cases without any symptom as well as with respiratory failure and circulatory shock are documented. Copious, pinkish cough with nausea/vomiting, dyspnoea, tachycardia, hypotension, fever and cyanosis following thoracentesis or chest tube placement pointers towards re-expansion pulmonary edema which is evident on plain X-ray. Timely management is rewarding. Mortality occurs in 20% of cases.

Thoracentesis or tube thoracotomy are the management modalities. Negative pressure should be avoided. I/V fluids, morphine and oxygen form supportive therapy. Diuresis has to be avoided. NIPPV is useful; mechanical ventilation may rarely be required in severe situations.

Empyema Thoracis

Empyema thoracis is a suppurative condition associated with collection of pus in the natural anatomical space[49] called pleural space. It is generally unilateral. It may occupy whole (total) or part (encysted) of the space.

Aetiology[33]

Empyema has a variable aetiology and results commonly from infections in the surrounding structure, mostly from lungs. The use of antimicrobial agents for common infections has greatly reduced empyema, still it is seen due to irregular or improper treatment. Empyema occurs as complication of pneumonia in the form of a synpneumonic process in infections associated with streptococcus or staphylococcus or as a metapneumonic process following infection from streptococcus pneumoniae. Pulmonary tuberculosis, lung abscess and bronchiectasis can lead to the development of empyema as a complication. The bronchogenic carcinoma associated with obstruction and collapse may lead to distal suppuration. Rarely hydatid cyst or actinomycosis may also result in empyema.

The subphrenic abscess and amoebic liver abscess can burst through the diaphragm and infect the pleura. The infection from the exterior can be introduced following penetrating chest injuries, or as an extension of infection of the chest wall like osteomyelitis of the rib or as an iatral phenomenon while performing paracentasis of the pleural cavity without proper aseptic precautions. Rarely it can appear as a complication of pneumonectomy or perforation of oesophagus or pyaemia. The coexistent pneumothorax or haemothorax is readily susceptible for bacterial infection. Gram negative, fungal and enterococcal aetiology has recently been observed.

Pathology

Streptococcus pneumoniae, streptococci and staphylococci are the common pyogenic organisms. In infants staphylococcus aureus forms the common cause. The coliforms, anaerobic streptococci or E. histolytica can enter pleura through the diaphragm. The chest wall infection is commonly caused by staphylococci.[30] Mixed infection is found in empyema secondary to lung abscess and bronchiectasis.

Anaerobic streptococci, spirochaetes and fusiform bacilli in the pleural cavity lead to formation of foetid pus in empyema. Pleural infection either by direct or by lymphatic spread, leads to exudation into the pleural cavity. It contains a large number of bacteria and polymorphs. The pneumococcal infection leads to the formation of a thick greenish-yellow exudate. The amount of protein is high and adhesions occur between the pleural surfaces following deposition of fibrin. In streptococcal infection, the serofibrinous fluid becomes purulent later. The fluid initially lies in the posterior recess of the pleural cavity, and then increases in its amount.

Large infective exudative effusion is rich with leucocytes.[58-60] The fibrinous adhesion succeeds in limiting the involvement to just one or more loculated compartments. The capability of lung to expand and obliterate potential space plays an important role in confining the infection and preventing fibrous *peel* prunation over visceral pleura that can permanently restrain lung in a partially collapsed configuration (Trapped lung). The expanded lung enhances pleural ability to resolve infection. However, infection is potentiated by an air leak (bronchopleural fistula) and by pneumonectomy in posterosection empyema.[1]

Empyema may compress the underlying lung leading to the displacement of the mediastinum. Under tension it can open through the lung into a bronchus leading to a bronchopleural fistula or furrow through the chest wall into the subcutaneous tissue as a swelling (empyema necessitatis) and can burst open discharging the contents through a sinus. Division of acute and chronic empyema is arbitrary.

The acute empyema gradually becomes chronic if left untreated or following delayed institutions of therapy or inadequate therapy. During organization, pleural ring is formed. It persists if there is a bronchopleural fistula or underlying disease or foreign body or infection from tuberculosis or actinomycosis.[30] Tuberculous empyema is an important etiology in country like India and differs from non-tuberculous empyema in age profile, clinical presentation and management and may have poorer outcome.[58]

Pathogenesis

Initial inflammatory phase has increased permeability of pleuro-pulmonary capillaries and influx of polymorphs and plasma clotting factors. In fibrin purulent phase, fibrin is deposited. Loculation may occur, a limiting membrane is formed in this transition phase. The exudate is slowly organised with deposition of fibrin. It encases the cellular debris on the pleural surface. The pleura is not thickened but a great amount of fibrin material is deposited in the space as a tough, rigid peel, restricting the movement of the lung. It is avascular.

Clinical Features

The symptoms overlap the features of preceding infection. Therefore, clinical features are variable. In pneumonic process, the fever may stay or recur after some improvement. The fever is high and remittent and is associated with rigors, weakness and loss of appetite. Pleuritic chest pain may be felt initially and with accumulation of fluid there is increasing discomfort and breathlessness. Cough is not an early symptom. When empyema ruptures through a bronchus, there is sudden expectoration of profuse amount of pus. There may be haemptysis. Those who have a faulty treatment or no treatment, suffer from chronic ill-health accompanied by fever, cough, and pus from time to time. Persistence of pus for more than three months leads to a chronic stage while toxaemia persists.[30] Loss of weight sets in.

Pus from the pleural cavity under tension usually empties into bronchus resulting in broncho-pleural fistula. Rarely, instead, it can burrow through chest wall and present as empyema necessitans. It usually points anteriorly close to the sternum near fifth costochondral junction, where the chest wall is thinnest due to deficiency of external intercostal membrane anteriorly or very rarely in mycotic and tuberculosis, empyemas can track down caudally behind the diaphragm to point posteriorly. It is obvious that pus of spontaneous pyopneumothorax can easily discharge into bronchus and therefore seldom necessary for it to manifest as *empyema of necessity*.[61] Because of the reinforcement of latissimus dorsi aponeurosis and thickening of lumbar fascia and skin posteriorly, there is no pointing of the abscess.[62]

Patient looks pale. Clubbing can be seen after some time. The examination of the chest reveals signs of pleural effusion with diminished movements, dullness, decreased VF, VR and absence of breath sounds. Bronchial breathing, if there is compression collapse of underlying lung with patent bronchus, is common in children.[30] The mediastinal shift is variable. With a fixed chest by adhesions or associated collapse, there may not be any contralateral shift or it may be drawn towards the affected side. The occurrence of pyopneumothorax is common in children from staphylococcal and clostridium[60-66] infections. The chest may become flattened on the affected side especially in a chronic stage. When it is interlobar, infrapulmonary or mediastinal empyema, the physical signs reveal no abnormality over the chest. In empyema necessitatis, a tense swelling appears commonly in the region of the fifth costochondral junction. An impulse may be seen on coughing and later pus may discharge through a sinus.[30] Even a case of tuberculous pyopneumothorax necessitans has been reported,[67] A massive empyema necessitans in a case of pseudotumour of the chest wall has also been documented.[68] Amyloidosis is a late complication of the disease.[30]

Complications

Complications in empyema occur only when the treatment is delayed or treatment is ineffective, they add significantly to the existing morbidity. Common complications are bronchopleural fistula, trapped lung, empyema necessitans, fibrothorax, amyloidosis, pericarditis, rib osteomyelitis, and infection reaching to mediastinum, meninges and even peritoneum.

Investigations[30,69,70]

Diagnostic aspiration is the choice. The needle is inserted in the region of maximum dullness. The fibrin tends to sediment at the bottom. The fluid shows a large number of polymorphs greater than 15,000 cells and gram stain and culture reveals causative organisms and the sensitivity to antibiotics respectively. Culture may be sterile following treatment with antibiotics or when secondary to tuberculosis. Serofibrinous fluid may be aspirated initially in streptococcal infection and it becomes purulent later. The pH of the pleural fluid is less than 7.2 compared to benign pleural effusions. There is polymorphonuclear leucocytosis and ESR is elevated.

The chest X-ray reveals a dense opacity with obliteration of costophrenic angle and concave shadow towards hilum. Postero-anterior and lateral views are necessary to localise the collection. When the fluid is encapsulated, there is convex opacity towards the hilum. An encysted fluid in the interlobar region shows an elliptical shadow in line with fissures or a shadow continuous with mediastinum in the mediastinal empyema or as a rounded hump over the diaphragm in the infrapulmonary empyema. Pleural calcification may be noted in long-standing cases.

The bronchopleural fistula which is common in tubercular and fungal infections, can be confirmed by injection of 2 ml of 1 per cent methylene blue into the pleural cavity. The blue dye is coughed up in the sputum when there is a fistula. Bronchoscopy and bronchogram may be necessary to delineate the underlying lesion and introduction of contrast medium (dionosil) helps in outlining the lower limit of the empyema cavity. In chronic cases, the ribs are crowded, with shift of mediastinum to the same side and the diaphragm is elevated. Differential diagnosis includes lung abscess, infected congenital cyst, and infected bulla (Pyocyst).

Management

Empyema can be managed by the control of infection, and removal of pus from the pleural cavity, thus obliterating the empyema space to enable the apposition of the visceral and parietal pleura and improvement of general health with supplements of protein, vitamins and minerals and physiotherapy and active breathing exercises to enable the expansion of the collapsed lung. The underlying source of infection has to be detected and treated.

A wide bore needle and appropriate antibiotic has to be given parenterally and injected into the pleural space. Penicillin does not penetrate the pleural surface readily unless high concentration is given. In children repeated aspiration gives good results than in adults. Alternatively an intercostal catheter can be inserted at the most dependent position continuously. Such closed water seal drainage depends on the thickness of pus. The response to therapy is assessed when daily aspiration is performed and there is gradual thinning of the fluid. Antibiotics are selected according to their sensitivity. Specific therapy is needed in conditions secondary to tuberculosis and amoebiasis.

A proper drainage of the pleural cavity can prevent it from becoming chronic. It should be performed under CT scan guidance to avoid inadvertent tube drainage of parenchyma. Thoracocentesis gives 0-12 per cent success rate. When the pus is very thick or when pus is obtained even after two weeks of aspiration or when the patient becomes actually ill from its effects, an open drainage by rib resection is necessary. The tube may get blocked in intercostal tube drainage and may be painful for pressure on the intercostal nerve. A rib resection with open drainage externally is better. It can be done under local anaesthesia if there is bronchopleural fistula or under general anaesthesia if there is no bronchopleural fistula.

Close tube drainage with antibiotic irrigation is more acceptable, especially with thoracoscopy which aids in achieving an optimal tube position as well as lysis of the intracavitary loculations.[71-76] Chest tube insertion may have complications like, bleeding, secondary infections and pneumothorax.

Decortication involving excision of empyema is necessary in chronic empyema with a large collection of thick pus and organisation of fibrin as well as in loculated empyema while drainage is not possible. Success rate of decortication is 80-100 per cent and often shortens patient's hospital stay. Forzen shoulder—a common complication of chronic empyema should be prevented with regular arm exercise. The pulmonary resection becomes necessary, to which thoracoplasty and intrathoracic rotating muscle flaps added to help obliterate the remaining space.[49] In bronchopleural or tubercular aetiology, pneumonectomy may become necessary.[77] Nevertheless, complete resolution has been obtained with appropriate antimicrobial in adequate dose without intervention in bilateral loculated pyopneumothorax with total radiological clearance.[78]

Pleural Plaques and Calcfication[47]

Pleural plaques are idiopathic thickening of parietal pleura, usually white, smooth and generally calcified. These are white bilaterally symmetrical densities measuring 1-5 mm, which don't occur at the apex or on the visceral pleura.

Calcified plaques occurring in the course of healed inflammatory or traumatic lesions are generally larger and unilateral. It has no relation with mesothelioma or other neoplasms. It is a uniform diffuse thickening with calcification of parietal pleura, presenting with chronic pleuritis, may occur in tuberculous or non-tuberculous empyema or from infective pleuritis, or pleuropneumonitis. A chronic calcified pleura wall may also result in active empyema. Such cases virtually require resection, decortication, pleurectomy and thoracoplasty.

MEDIASTINITIS

Inflammation of the mediastinal structure is usually of infectious aetiology and is classified into *acute* and *chronic* categories.

Acute Mediastinitis[2]

Acute mediastinitis is more frequently encountered in the era of endoscopy and median sternotomy, and treatment is more often successful. Perforation of the oesophagus can occur, either *spontaneously* following forceful vomiting with a full stomach (Boerhaave's syndrome), as a result of penetrating trauma or instrumentation, or by an eroding carcinoma. Common causes include post sternotomy for cardiac surgery, eosophaged perforation due to difficult endoscopy, forceful omiting, foreign body or carcinoma oesophagus and direct extension of infection from neck, retropharyngeal, space, lung, pleura or pericardium and osteomyelitis spine. Rare causes include tooth abscess, supraglottitis and laparoscopic chole cystectomy.[79-83]

Rupture of the oesophagus unrelated to foreign bodies, direct external trauma or instrumentation is termed *spontaneous* and constitutes about 15 per cent of the total cases.[84] Spontaneous perforation may occur in association with vomiting, parturition, severe coughing, seizures or weight lifting. The common denominator is a precipitous rise in intra-adominal pressure which is transmitted to the relaxed oesophagus against a closed glottisy.[85] It is a life threatening surgical emergency. The common mode of presentation is severe substernal or epigastric pain following a violent bout of vomiting. About 90 per cent of patients develop a concurrent pneumothorax, pleural effusion or hydropneumothorax.[86] Shock occurs in 25 per cent of cases and mediastinal crunch (Hamman's sign) is heard in 20 per cent.[87] The diagnosis may be missed for many days or even weeks.[88]

The trachea can be disrupted. Infection can also extend directly into the mediastinum from lung, pleura, and from elsewhere both above and below the diaphragm. The onset of acute mediastinitis is sudden and traumatic, with chills, fever, apprehension, and prostration. Tachycardia, tachypnoea and systemic toxicity are prominent findings, and subcutaneous emphysema may be present. Pain is referred to left hypochondrium, left shoulder and is so characteristic as to be diagnostic as 90 per cent of cases have left sided manifestations. Classical sign is seen in 66 per cent cases.[89] Hamman's sign (a crunching sound heard over the anterior chest in synchrony with cardiac systole) is characteristic but not invariably present. Radiographic hallmarks include mediastinal widening, air in the mediastinum and soft tissues, and pneumonia or hydropneumothorax. Contrast studies of oesophagus, methylene blue test and oesophagoscopy contribute to diagnosis.[90] Therapy consists of prompt surgical drainage of both mediastinum and pleural cavities, along with appropriate antibiotics. Initial management may be conservative which includes intravenous fluids, antibiotics, nasogastric suction and/or T-tube drainage combined with gastrostomy or feeding jejunostomy and adequate pleural drainage.[91,92] This has to be followed by an elective surgical repair without which survival is extremely uncommon. A delay in the diagnosis of oesophageal rupture often leads to death because of sepsis, mediastinitis and empyema.[91] Mortality may be as high as 75 per cent when surgery is delayed, but can be reduced to 25 per cent or less if drainage is achieved within 24 hours of the precipitating event. Broad spectrum antibiotics including anaerobic cover can bring down mortality due to infection.[93]

Mediastinitis following cardiac surgery has become an important entity occurring after 1 to 2 per cent of procedures. It tends to be a less fulminating condition than acute mediastinitis in other settings. Most patients have drainage from the sternotomy incision and other localized signs of infection, and the diagnosis is generally made by re-exploration of the wound. Treatment consists of surgical debridgement and adequate drainage with appropriate antibiotic therapy.

Chronic Mediastinitis

Granulomatous mediastinits and mediastinal fibrosis represent the ends of a spectrum of chronic inflammation that causes varying degrees of host reaction and progresses in some cases to a largely acellular fibrosis. Granulomatous mediastinitis, most often due to histoplasmosis or tuberculosis is usually asymptomatic and is detected as a mediastinal mass on chest X-ray. The end stage of mediastinal fibrosis can also be caused by drugs (especially methysergide), as a part of so-called multisystem fibrosing, silicosis, malignancy, syphilis, radiation, and other processes. This condition presents with symptoms, of which those of superior vena caval obstruction predominate. Compression of the oesophagus, tracheobronchial tree, pulmonary vessels, and mediastinal nerves can also occur. Patients with chronic mediastinitis present with the superior vena caval syndrome (giddiness, headache, epistaxis, facial puffiness, cyanosis and distended veins in face, neck and arms) or with mediastinal widening detected on chest radiograph. Computed tomography reveals the extent of involvement but often cannot distinguish between benign and malignant processes and in most cases, flexible (fiberoptic) bronchoscopy, followed by surgical exploration, is required. No therapy is of definite help. Amphotericin and other specific therapies for presumed causes of chronic mediastinitis are generally ineffective.

Pneumomediastinum (Mediastinal Emphysema[2])

Air may appear within the tissue planes of the mediastinum spontaneously, in association with blunt or penetrating trauma, following instrumentation of the airways or oesophagus, or because of disease above the thoracic outlet or below the diaphragm. It occurs with sharply raised intrathoracic pressure, as in strenuous vomiting or coughing, or marked pressure swings from positive to negative, as in acute severe asthma. In the absence of any predisposing disease or trauma, it is called primary spontaneous pneuomediastinum. Alveolar over-distention and a pressure gradient from alveolus to bronchovascular sheath lead to dissection of air via the interstitium to the hila and mediastinum. From there, if it does not rupture into the pleural space to cause a pneumothorax, the air instead may spread into the subcutaneous tissue of the neck, chest and elsewhere. Reterosternal pain, fever and dyspnoea are the usually symptoms, and physical examination may reveal Hamman's sign and subcutaneous emphysema. Chest pain may mimick myocardial infarction or pericarditis with exacerbation on movement and deep breathing and relief on leaning forward in sitting position. Dyspnoea, dysphagia and dysphonia are common. Chest radiographs in the postero anterior and lateral positions confirm the diagnosis. Leucocytosis may occur. Pulsus paradoxus may be felt and cardiac sounds may be indistinct. Rarely cardiovascular collapse has been reported.

Pneumomediastinum may develop under three circumstances:[94] (i) Mediastinal sepsis from gas forming organisms introduced from infected soft tissues nearby, commonly the head and neck; (ii) Traumatic disruption of large gas containing structures (oesophagus, trachea), frequently in association with positive pressure ventilation, or from the retero-peritoneal space; (iii) Damage to alveoli and to bronchioles, allowing gas to leak along the bronchovascular bundle towards the mediastinum. Rupture of the alveoli is usually precipitated by straining with breath held in inspiration and may therefore be seen in labour[95] or in any lung disease, in which acute airway obstruction is combined with severe cough, e.g., bronchial asthma, bronchiolitis, whooping cough, following pulmonary function testing and in mountain climbers. Rupture of the alveolus occurs into the interstitial space surrounding the airways and blood vessels. The pressure within the mediastinum is lower than in peripheral lung parenchyma and thus air dissects along the bronchovascular bundles in a continuous pathway towards the mediastinum and reaches the hilum from where it extends into the mediastinum. It can be said that the air is *milked* by continuous respiratory efforts to the mediastinal structures. It then tracks along the tissue planes into the neck and has access to the subcutaneous tissues elsewhere in the body.[96] Mediastinal emphysema may also be seen in muconium aspiration syndrome[94] and in patients with anorexia nervosa or in those who engage in vigorous retching and emesis.[97]

Luis Bourgeois who was midwife to the Queen of France was the first to observe the occurrence of pneumomediastinum presenting as the stabbing pain in the chest and subcutaneous crepitus during childbirth due to extreme effort.[98] The development of spontaneous pneumomediastinum in adults is usually associated with substernal pain or it may be virtually symptomless in many of the cases.

Spontaneous Pneumomediastinum (SPM)

Spontaneous pneumomediastinum (SPM) is a benign condition where air presence is observed in mediastinum without any obvious cause.[99] It is a rare condition, noted as 1 in 30,000 emergency attendance, first case being reported in 1939 by Hamman.[100] Known risk factors include asthma, drug abuse, tobacco smoking and activities triggering valsalva maneuver. Secondary pneumomediastinum such as chest injury, pulmonary/mediastinal infection or oesophageal rupture following vomiting must be ruled out before diagnosing spontaneous pneumomediastinum.

Pathophysiology of spontaneous pneumomediastinum includes an acute rise in intra-alveolar pressure which results in alveolar rupture, allowing the air to ascend along the mediastinum towards cervical subcutaneous space causing cervicofacial subcutaneous emphysema. Illicit drug use, bronchial asthma, forceful straining, coughing, sneezing, vomiting and during child birth, all activities requiring valsalva maneuver, involving intense exercise and breathing that predisposes to SPM.[101] Other predisposing factors include malnutrition with anorexia nervosa and self implicated oral injury.[102]

Clinical presentation includes an acute central chest pain radiating to the lower mandible, neck, as well as both anteriorly and posteriorly with cutaneous swelling and hoarse voice are the most common symptoms. Dysphagia, cough, odynophagia and dysphonia are less frequent presentations. 40-100% of patients develop cervical subcutaneous emphysema. In 12% of cases, Hamman's sign is recognized by a distinctive crunching/ bubbling sound which is synchronous with heartbeat.[101]

Radiological diagnosis is the mainstay. However, one third of cases may have normal plain chest X-ray. CT scan of chest is considered the gold standard in diagnosing pneumo-mediastinum. Oesophagogram, oesophagoscopy and even bronchoscopy may complement the diagnosis and even help to rule out spontaneous Boerhaave syndrome or post traumatic rupture of oesophagus or tracheobronchial tract. In addition, lateral cervical X-ray is quite useful in pin pointing spontaneous pneumomediastinum.[103]

Conservative management yields good outcome. A case of pneumo-mediastinum occurring after a transbronchial biopsy in a woman with pulmonary fibrosis, which was confirmed with CT scan.[104] Large amounts of air in the mediastinal tissue may produce compression effects. Air tamponade is rare and is found in cases of tension pneumomediastinum interfering with cardiac filling and thus output. *Air block* describes the splinting action of peribronchial air which induces further occlusion of airways.

Associated pneumothorax is an obvious cause for concern. Pulmonary vascular compression by interstitial air collection could cause pulmonary arterial hypertension.[105] Hamman's sign is present in only 50 per cent of the cases.[90] Pressure effect on the subcutaneous nerves is considered responsible for the pain. Various radiological signs that characterise the mediastinal emphysema have been extensively reviewed by Beyers *et al.*[106] Some of these include vertical translucent steaks that outline the soft tissue layers and structures of the mediastinum, pneumopericardium (air extending between the pericardium and the diaphgram gives rise to the continuous diaphragm sign,[106] *ring around the artery* sign (air around the right pulmonary artery in frontal view) and the V sign (the confluence of innominate veins outlines in frontal view). The treatment to pneumomediastinum varies from reassurance and mild analgesia to energetic measures directed towards managing hypoxia and shock.[96] In most of the cases spontaneous absorption of air occurs within a week.[107,108] It has also been shown to improve by breathing 95 per cent oxygen replacing nitrogen by rapid absorption of oxygen and it has been suggested that non-surgical pneumomediastinum would probably respond favourably to hyperbaric oxygen therapy.[109]

Tumors and Cysts of Mediastinum

The most practical means of classifying mass lesions in the mediastinum is according to their location, as shown in Table 8.11. The most common mediastinal mass in the adult are

Table 8.11: Tumors and cysts of the mediastinum[1]

A. Masses occurring in the anterior mediastinum
- Thymoma
- Germ cell tumors: teratoma; seminoma; embryonal cell carcinoma; choriocarcinoma
- Lymphoma
- Mesenchymal tumors: lipoma; fibroma; others
- Thyroid
- Parathyroid

B. Masses occurring in the middle mediastinum
- Lymph nodes: lymphoma; metastatic cancer; granulomatous disease
- Developmental cysts: pericardial; bronchogenic; enteric
- Vascular masses and enlargements
- Diaphragmatic hernias

C. Masses occurring in the posterior mediastinum
 a. Neurogenic tumors
  1. Arising from peripheral nerves: neurofibroma; neurolemmoma; neurosarcoma
  2. Arising from sympathetic ganglia, ganglioneuroma: ganglioneuroblastoma; neuroblastoma; sympathicoblastoma
  3. Arising from paraganglionic tissue: pheochromocytoma; paraganglioma (chemodectoma)
 b. Oesophageal lesions: neoplasms: achalasia; hiatal hernia
 c. Diaphragmatic hernias
 d. Miscellaneous conditions: primary carcinoma or sarcoma; pseudocyst; thoracic duct cyst, extramedullary hematopoic meningocele.

neurogenic tumours, thymomas, and developmental cysts,[110] which together account for approximately 60 per cent of all cases. Lymphomas and germ cell tumors such as teratoma and seminoma account for another 25 per cent and the other 15 per cent is made up of a large number of reported lesions.[2]

At least half of all mediastinal masses are asymptomatic, and of these some 90 per cent prove to be benign. On the other hand, masses that produce symptoms for which the patient consults a physician, at least half are malignant. Symptoms usually caused by invasion or compression include cough, dyspnoea, recurrent respiratory infections, dysphagia, and chest pain. Superior vena caval syndrome, hoarseness due to vocal cord paralysis, Horner's syndrome, phrenic nerve involvement, and spinal cord compression are other presentations, mediastinal tumors are associated with systemic syndromes. These include myasthenia gravis (thymoma), pure red cell aplasia (thymoma), Cushing's syndrome (thymoma; carcinoid), gynecomastia (certain germ cell tumors), hypertension (pheochromocytoma, ganglioneuroma), and hypercalcemia (lymphoma, parathyroid adenoma) along others. Non-invasive diagnosis is non-contributory.[111]

Non-Hodgkin mediastinal lymphoma (mass) needs aggressive approach as has an excellent response to chemotherapy. TB forms important differential as effusion is lymphocytic rich with higher levels of ADA in both conditions.

Diagnostic evaluation depends on tissue diagnosis. Because most lesions should be removed, even if benign, surgical exploration is considered by many to be the right and judicious approach. Chest X-ray, CT, differential diagnosis and relation to expiration of mediastinal masses are listed in Tables 8.12 to 8.16.

Table 8.12: Mediastinal masses: Plain chest films in mediastinal masses

- Lymphadenopathy is the most common cause of a mediastinal mass.
- Neurogenic tumours are by far the most common posterior mediastinal lesions.
- Certain tumours such as dermoid cysts and thymomas are confined to the anterior mediastinum.
- Calcification occurs in many conditions but never in malignant neoplastic lymphadenopathy.
- A mediastinal mass due to hiatus hernia is usually easy to diagnose on plain films.
- Masses in the right cardiophrenic angle anteriorly are virtually never of clinical significance.
- A mass in the superior mediastinum that extends into the neck and displaces the trachea is likely to be goitre.

Table 8.13: Mediastinal mass: Differential diagnosis

a. Accurate detection by X-ray or CT scan
b. CT scan and MRI can accurately position them and may sometime be able to determine its structure.

Superior mediastinal mass:	
	Bronchogenic cyst
	Ectopic thyroid
	Oesophageal enterogenous cyst
	Reterosternal goitre
Inferior mediastinal mass:	
	Abscess
	Hiatus hernia
	Pericardial cyst
Posterior mediastinal mass:	
	Aortic aneurysm
	Neurogenic tumours, neurofibroma, neuroblastoma
	Paravertebral abscess
Anterior mediastinal mass:	
	Aortic aneurysm
	Dermoid cyst
	Germ cell tumour
	Thymic tissue, thymoma, thyroid tissue (ectopic), teratoma
Varied mediastinal position:	
	Hodgkin's disease
	Lymphoma
	Metastatic carcinoma
	Sarcoidosis
	Tuberculosis

Table 8.14: Jacobsen Holdsnedt phenomenon

The phenomenon is positive if mediastinum is displaced away from affected side on expiration, while comparing both chest X-ray films on inspiration and expiration. *Positive:* Unilateral obstructive emphysema which has occurred due to valve-like mechanism created by foreign body or tumour.

Table 8.15: Hering-Breuer reflexes

The desire to inspire when the breath is held in expiration and vice-versa. It has no clinical significance.

Table 8.16: CT of mediastinal masses

1. Abnormalities can be accurately localised.
2. Occasionally the density of the abnormality reveals its nature:
   a. Fat can be recognised as such.
   b. Intravenous contrast enhancement permits ready differentiation of aneurysms.
   c. Calcification is more readily seen at CT.
   d. Cysts containing clear fluid e.g. pericardial cysts and some bronchogenic cysts can be recognised as such.

Mediastinal Lymphangiomas[112]

They account for 0.7-4.5% of all mediastinal tumours and mostly occur in the anterior compartment of superior mediastinum. They are congenital hamartomatous malformation which result from a localised failure of developing lymphatic system to communicate with its venous counterpart. Occasionally, they may arise from multiple sites. They are classified simple, cavernous and cystic. Cystic forms (often called cystic hygroma) arise in cervix of infants and may extend (in 10% of cases) to superior mediastinum.

They are benign lesions, often multiloculated, comprising endothelial lined spaces with supporting connective tissue stroma which contains smooth muscles round cells and lymphoid tissue. They may contain clear or dark brown fluid.

Most of the patients are asymptomatic. Pain occurs due to infection, rapid extension or haemorrhage into the cyst. Pressure symptoms such as dyspnoea or dysphagia may occur. Rupture into the pleural space causing chylothorax and into the pericardium causing tamponade, are other complications.

A well defined homogenous round opacity with defined borders is noted in superior mediastinum on routine chest X-ray. CT shows a smooth spherical lesion, and ultrasound and MRI demonstrate a water filled mass. Differential diagnosis includes mediastinal cysts, haemangiomas. Asymptomatic cases are left as such.

Surgical excision requires both cervical and thoracic approach. Often there is a damage to phrenic or vagus nerve. Sclerosis with tetracycline, irradiation or steroid injections have no benefit. Injection of bleomycin, fat emulsion or intralesional streptococcal lysine have eradicated the lesion.

Liposarcoma of Mediastinum

It arises from soft tissue fat and is potentially malignant. Annual incidence is 2.5 cases per million, 5 years survival is less than 50% lung and liver receive metastasis.

Clinically fever, chest pain, dyspnoea and dry cough are encountered. Chest X-ray/CT thorax show homogenous opacity and a pearl shape lesion from thoracic wall. CT guided biopsy reveal spindle cell sarcoma. Surgical resection and pharmacotherapy is the treatment options for this underdiagnosed tumour.

Teratomas[113]

They are most common forms of germ cell tumours, consisting of disorganized mixture of ectodermal derivatives. The tumour usually contains skin and its appendages, cartilage, bone, neurovascular, intestinal and respiratory epithelium. It commonly occurs in young adults, affecting both sexes. 80% of teratomas are benign; 20% are teratocarcinomas which are rapidly spreading neoplasms with poor prognosis.

Small teratomas are usually asymptomatic. Pressure symptoms such as pain, cough and dyspnoea may occur. Haemoptysis occurs if tumour erodes into the bronchus. Pleural space erosion may result in acute respiratory distress. Recurrent attacks of hypoglycemia are relieved after surgical excision of the tumour.

Chest X-ray reveals a smooth rounded, well circumscribed lesion if cystic in nature, while solid forms are seen as lobulated asymmetric, homogeneous opacities. Presence of teeth in the tumour is often seen. In patients with malignant teratomas, serum levels of alpha-fetoprotein and carcinoembryonic antigen levels are usually raised.

Treatment is surgical. Cure is complete with resection in benign forms. Prognosis is poor in malignant teratomas; combination chemotherapy does not offer much help.

THE DIAPHRAGM

Diaphragmatic Paralysis[2]

Unilateral diaphragmatic paralysis is caused by interruption of the phrenic nerve, occasionally by trauma but most commonly by invading tumor (chiefly bronchogenic carcinoma). Often it may prove to be idiopathic, despite extensive diagnostic evaluation. Unilateral diaphragmatic paralysis is usually asymptomatic, discovered on a routine film or during evaluation of lung cancer, although some patients may complain of dyspnoea. Pulmonary function is only mildly affected. The diagnosis is confirmed when an elevated diaphragm is shown on fluoroscopy to move paradoxically (that is upward) during the "sniff" manoeuver. No treatment is known.

Although less common, bilateral diaphragmatic paralysis is a much more debilitating condition and frequently leads to hypercapnic respiratory failure, and may occur because of cervical spinal cord trauma, cord cardioplegia, dystrophia myotonica, cardiac surgery, motor neuron disease, polyneuropathy, poliomyelitis, or mediastinal malignancy.

Most patients complain of severe dyspnoea that worsens when supine and paradoxical (inward) motion of the abdomen is observed during inspiration when the patient is in the supine position. The vital capacity is severely reduced, more so in the supine position, but the *sniff test* under fluoroscopy may not reveal abnormal motion. Measurement of trans diaphragmatic pressure changes during inspiration using oesophageal and gastric balloons which can help to confirm the diagnosis. Assisted ventilation for all or part of each day is the treatment of choice.[114,115]

Diaphragmatic Hernias

Herniation of the stomach or other viscera into the chest through the oesophageal hiatus is by far the most common of the diaphragmatic hernias. Hernias through the foramen of Bochdalek occur in the posterolateral chest, usually on the left, and are most often seen in infants. They may contain fat, the upper pole of the kidney, or occasionally the spleen. Anterior diaphragmatic hernias through the foramina of Morgagni occur most often in patients with increased intra-abdominal pressure or marked obesity. Nearly always asymptomatic, they may contain omental fat, bowel, stomach or even liver. Radiographically they appear as an anterior rounded density in the region of the right cardiophrenic angle. Diagnosis may be aided by radiographic contrast studies or by computed tomography. Although strangulation of the hernia's contents has been reported, both types of diaphragmatic hernias are nearly always asymptomatic and require no treatment. However, surgical exploration may become necessary to exclude other diagnosis.

Bochdalek Hernia

Closure of the posterolateral portion of the diaphragm by fusion of the pleuro-peritoneal membrane with the septum transversum normally occurs by the eighth week of foetal life. Diaphragmatic hernia is more common than herniation through foramen of Morgagni and paraoesophageal foramen. Bochdalek described the hernia in 1848. Boch and Zimmerman found an incidence of Bochdalek hernia of four to eight per 10,000 live births.[116] 80 to 90 per cent of Bochdalek hernias occur on left side partly because of the fact that the defects in the right hemidiaphragm are protected by the liver and partly due to the earlier closure of the pleuro-peritoneal canal on the right side. These hernias are devoid of hernial sac.[117-119]

Bochdalek hernia (now also called congenital posterolateral diaphragmatic hernia) manifests acutely in neonates or infants and causes high mortality. Symptoms include vomiting and respiratory distress. In older children and adults, this condition is rare and symptoms are insidious and are related to respiratory and gastrointestinal system.[120-123] Rarely, Bochdalek hernia can be discovered on routine check up late in life.[124,125]

Because of higher mortality rates and complications like strangulation or obstruction of intestines,[126,127] diagnosis of these cases is of utmost importance. In case of left-sided Bochdalek hernia, diagnosis is often made by finding gas and fluid levels in herniated intestinal loops located in the thorax but the diagnosis of right sided Bochdalek hernia may be difficult both clinically and radiologically.[128,129]

In infants herniation through Bochdalek foramen is not only the most common form of diaphragmatic hernia but also the most serious. In most cases there is no hernial sac, communication between pleural and peritoneal cavities being wide open. When the defect is small, a sac lined by pleura and containing retroperitoneal fat may be the only abnormality discernible.[130,131] The intra abdominal pressure elevation due to defecation or repeated vomiting may lead to herniation.[132]

Herniation of lung may be defined as protrusion of pulmonary tissue covered by parietal pleura and visceral pleura, through an abnormal aperture in thoracic wall. Herniation may develop in cervical, thoracic and diaphragmatic area. They are classified as congenital and acquired hernia. Acquired hernias commonly occur as a result of trauma when the parietal pleura has been damaged.

Ectopic herniation of a pulmonary cavity appears to be a very rare entity. Three cases have been reported in medical literature, namely, air trapped in bronchogenic cyst presenting as a cervical mass in newborn, cervical bronchial cyst and ectopic herniation of pulmonary cyst.[133-135]

More-Lavallee classified lung hernias according to aetiology as below:[136]

1. Congenital: Due to defect in the thoracic wall.
2. Acquired:
   a. Traumatic: Due to fracture rib penetrating lesion—surgical intervention.
   b. Consecutive: Some time after localised trauma and following healing of wound.
   c. Spontaneous: Due to local impairment of the thoracic wall with increased intrathoracic pressure by protracted cough, weight lifting, etc.
   d. Pathological: Thoracic wall has been weakened by a pathological process, *i.e.,* lung abscess penetrating the chest wall, an abscess of the wall or caries of a rib.

Two-thirds of the post-traumatic hernias, occur due to injury, and most common site is through anterior chest wall, adjacent to the sternum where intercostal musculature is thinnest.

Sometimes weakened area is the result of inflammation adjacent to the thoracic cage. Three factors which control the tendency towards protrusion, are the parietal pleura, the neck muscles and the Sibson's fasciae. A deficiency or weakness in any of these structures creates a predisposition to hernia.

Clinically, lung hernias are diagnosed by:[137]

i. Presence of soft, crepitant protrusion, reducing in size on quiet respiration and again bulging on coughing.
ii. Defect in chest wall which can often be palpated.
iii. Radiological demonstration of protrusion of pulmonary tissue on tangential exposure.

Treatment is mainly surgical repair, although they may rarely disappear spontaneously without surgical intervention.

Gorham's Disease[138-140]

This is a disease of bony cage. It is a rare disorder characterized by vascular channels' proliferation that results in destruction and resorption of osseous matrix, rarely ending with chylothorax and osteolysis of ribs.

REFERENCES

1. Krishna Dass K.V., Textbook of Medicine; J.P. Bros. (P) Ltd; 3rd ed 1996.
2. Wilson J.D., *et al.* (ed) Harrison's principles of internal medicine, 12th ed, Vo1.2, McGraw Hill, New York 1991.
3. Gatelay C A., *et al.* Pneumothorax, acomplication of fine needle aspiration of the breast, BMJ 1991; 303: 627-28.
4. Leahy B.C. and Stretton T.B., Pleural disease, Medicine International 1989; 35:1446-51.
5. Thompson A.M., Newman RJ. and Semple J.C., Brachial plexus anaesthesia for upper limb surgery, are view of eight years' experience. J. Hand Surg. (Br) 1988; 13: 195-98.
6. Dixon J.M., Immediate reporting of fine needle aspiration of breast lesions, BMJ 1991; 302:428-29.
7. Janameja A.A., *et al.,* Analysis of 100 cases of spontaneous pneumothorax; Lung India 1995; 13: 12-16.
8. Arora V.K., *et al.,* 'Silicotic alveolar proteinosis with bilateral spontaneous pneumothorax, JAPI 1992; 40: 760-62.
9. Taneja A., *et al.,* Shouting induced pneunmothorax; Lung India 1994; 12; 204-20.
10. Gupta S., Pneumothorax; In: Bansal B.C., Ed: PG Med; API, Bombay 1997; 11:334-38.
11. L. Hyde C.I. Rare occurnce of simultaneous pneumothorax and lung cancer; J Amer Med Assn 1978; 239: (4):1421-22.
12. Woodring J.H., Unusual radiographic manifestations of lung cancer, Radiol Clin North Amer 1990; 28(3):608-09.
13. Gaude Gajanan, *et al.,* Spontaneous pneumothorax, a rare complication of bronchogenic carcinoma, Lung India 1993; 11:23-26.
14. Steinhauslin C.A., Cuttat J.F., Spontaneous pnemothorax—A complication of lung cancer, Chest 1985; 88:(5)709-13.
15. Mahajan V., *et al.* Pneumothorax—A rare manifestation of lung cancer, Chest 1975; 68:730-32.
16. Citron K.M., Spontaneous pneumothorax complicating bronchogenic carcinoma; Tubercle 1956; 40:384-86.
17. Bouros D. and Anchianopoulo E., Spontaneous pneumothorax—A complication of lung cancer; Chest 1986; 90:926.
18. William H.O., Kindnery P.H., Alveolar cell carcinoma presenting as pneumothorax, Amer. Rev. Resp. Dis 1971;103: 108-12.
19. Raj Kapoor, Gupta N.C. and Saha M.M., Bilateral spontaneous pneumothorax due to metastatic synovial sarcoma. Ind. J. Chest Dis. All Sci 1988; 30: 273-75.
20. Thornton T.F. and Bigelow R.E., Pneumothorax due to metastatic sarcoma (report of 2 cases), Arch Path 1944; 87: 334-36.
21. Wright F.W., Spontaneous pneumothorax and pulmonary malignant disease—A syndrome sometimes associated with cavitating tumours, Clin Radiol 1976; 27:211-12.
22. Dines D.E. Cortese, D.A. Brennan, M.D., Hahn R.G. and Payne W.S., Malignant pulmonary neoplasm predisposing to spontaneous pneumothorax, Mayo Clin Proceed 1973;48: 541-44.
23. Sherman R.S. and Brant E.E., An X-ray study of spontaneous pneumothorax due to cancer metastasis to the lung, Dis. Chest 1954; 26: 328-37.
24. Seremetics M.G. and MacDonald J.C., Spontaneous pneumothorax and carcinoma of the lung—A case report. Milt Med 1970; 135: 898-900.
25. O'Leary C., Elsoussi M. and Cowie J., Spontaneous bilateral pneumothoracis from synovial cell sarcoma. Resp Med 1991; 85(6): 533-34.
26. Gajanan S., Gaude, *et al.,* Bilateral spontaneous pneumothorax secondary to metastatic osteogenic sarcoma; Lung India 1992; 10: 79-80.
27. Janetes G.P. and Ochaner S.F., Bilateral pneumothorax in metastatic osteogenic sarcoma, Am. Rev. Respir. Dis 1963; 88: 78-76.
28. Loh K., Dahl O. and Vigander T., Pneumothorax during combination chemotherapy, Cancer 1981; 47:1743-45.
29. Smevik B. and Klopp O. Risk of spontaneous pneumothorax in patients with osteogenic sarcoma and testicular cancer. Cancer 1982; 49: 1734-37.
30. Shankar P.S., Chest Medicine; 4th ed; Oxford and IBH Publ. Co. N. Delhi. 1994.
31. Crofton and Douglas Resp. Medicine, Seaton A., Seaton D and Gordon Leitch A; ed., 4th ed 1989, Oxford University Press, Delhi.
32. Bhatia R.S., Sibia S.S., Spontaneous pneumothorax. JAPI 2003; (In press).
33. Vidyasagar, *et al.* Spontaneous pneumothorax caused by ruptured pulmonary hydatid cyst, Lung India 1988,6: 79-80.
34. Motorsky M.L., *et al.,* AIDS related spontaneous pneumothorax; Chest 1995; 108:946-51.
35. Light R.W., Pneumothorax; In: Textbook of Resp. Medicine; Murray J.P., Nadel J.A. (ed), Saunders, Philadeplhia 1988.
36. Cho Taejin, Kim Hoon; Unusual presentation of spontaneous pneumomediastinum; Lung India 2010; 27: 239-41.
37. Cummin R.C., *et al.,* Pneumothorax in the supine patient, BMJ 1987; 295:591-92.

38. Rhea J.T., Van Sonnenberg E. and McLoud T.C., Basilar pneumothorax in the supine adult. Radiology 1979; 133: 593-95.
39. Gordon R., The deep sulcus sign. Radiology1980, 136: 25-27.
40. Tocino I.M., Miller M.H. and Fairfax, W.R., Distribution of pneumothorax in the supine and semi recumbent critically ill adult, AJR 1985; 144: 901-05.
41. Ziter F.M.H. and Westcott J.C., Supine subpulmonary pneumothorax; AJR 1981; 137:699-701.
42. Bauman M.H., *et al.* Management of spontaneous pneumothorax; An ACCP Delphi conseusus statement; Chest 2001; 119; 590-602.
43. Collins J., *et al.* CT pattern of bronchiolar disease; What is 'Tree-in-bud'? AJR 1998; 171: 365-70.
44. Yim A.P.C. VATS in Asia; its impact and implications; Aust NZ J Med 1997; 27; 156-59.
45. Henry M., *et al.*, BTS guidelines for the management of spontaneous pneumothorax; Thorax 2003; 58; ii 39-52.
46. Butland R.J.A., Spockett G.P., seaton D.A survey of management of primary spontaneous pneumothorax in UK; Thorax 1987; 42; 226.
47. Noppen M., Manual aspiration vs chest tube drainage in first episode of primary spontaneous pneumothorax; Amer J Resp Crit Care Med 2002; 165; 1240-44.
48. Masood Imrana; *et al.*, Role of simple needle aspiration in the management of spontaneous pneumothorax; JAPI 2007; 55: 628-29.
49. Saraswat D.K., *et al.*, Simplified emergency procedure for treatment of tension pneumothorax; JAPI 1994; 42:336.
50. Ng C.S.H., *et al.*, Giant pulmonary bulla; Canad; Resp J 2001; 8: 369-71.
51. Ng C.S.H., *et al.*, VATS in spontaneous pneumothax; Canad Resp J 2002; 9; 122-27.
52. Li W.W.L., *et al.*, The impact of thoracic surgical access on easly shoulder function; VATS vs posterolateral thoracotomy: Eur J cardiothoracic lung 2003; 23: 390-96.
53. Wait M.A., Dal-Nogare A.R. Treatment of AIDS related spontaneous pneumothorax; MA decade of experience; Chest 1994; 106: 693-96.
54. Murat A; *et al.*, Re-expansion pulmonary edema; Acta Radial 2004; 45: 431-33.
55. Beng ST, Mahadevan M; An uncommon life threatening complication after chest tube drainage of pneumothorax; Amer J Emerg Med 2004; 22: 615-19.
56. Volpi Celli G., *et al.*, A case of unilateral re-expansion pulmonary edema successfully treated with non-invasive continuous positive airway pressure; Eurp J. Emerg Med 2004; 11: 291-94.
57. Bhatia RS, Khan GQ; Aetiopathogenesis of spontaneous pneumothorax and its management; IN; RS Bhatia, GQ Khan; ed; Pulmonary Medicine; Peepee Publ 2007; 6: 38-59.
58. Kundu S; *et al.*, Adult thoracic empyema: A comparative analysis of tuberculous and non-tuberculous etiology in 75 patients; Lung India 2010; 27: 196-201.
59. Le Roux B.T., *et al.*, Suppurate diseases of the lung and pleural space Part I, Empyema, Curr. Probl. Surg 1986, 23: 1.
60. Bhatia R.S.; Respiratory disease pattern in a private clinic in Ludhiana; Lung India 1995; 13: 125-26.
61. Yelvin E.N., Marks I. and Theoddrec and Elckhoffam Empyema necessitans; Ame. Rev. Resp. Dis 1970; 101:159-61.
62. Last R.J. Anatomy-Regional and Applied 7th Ed. English Language Book Society, Edinburgh, Churchill Livingstone 1984; 308.
63. Mertin J., Raff. Judith D., Johnson Deepak Nagar, Fred Z Ferris and Mary L., Macormick Spontaneous clostridium empyema and pyopneumothorax. Rev. Infect. Dis 1984; 6(5):715-19.
64. Arnold S., Bayer Stephen,C., Nelson Jefrey E.Gal P.N., Anthon W., Chow and Lucein R. Guzo, Necrotizing pneumonia and empyema due to Clostridrium infection, Report of a case and review of literature, Am.J.Med 1975; 59: 851.
65. Geunanovikh, *et al.*, Pneumoperitoneum as a complication of tension pyopneumothorax in a child, Cumulated Index Medicus 1986, Subject Index, Vol 127, p, 9505 (Vestn khir) 1985; 135 (a): 97-98.
66. Robert G. Frasen, Peter Pare, J.A., Pare P.O., Richard S., Fraser and George, P. Genereux., Diagnosis of the Diseases of the Chest, 3rd Ed., Vol. II, W,B. Saunders Company, Philadelphia 1986; 876.
67. Natrajan A.S., *et al.*, Tuberculous pyopneumothorax necessitans M case report, Lung India 1990; 8: 146-48.
68. Behera George D'Souza and Malik, S.K., Pseudotumor of the right chest wall MA case of massive empyema necessitans, Ind. J., Tuberc 1988; 35:206-07.
69. Heffner A., A successful approach to empyema; Contemp. Int. Med.; 1991; June 95.
70. Swain J.A., Empyema; an update on diagnosis and management; pulmonary aspects; Amer. Col.Chest Phys 1992; 9:6.
71. Chen LE; *et al.*, Management of late-stage parapneumonic empyema; J Paediatr Surg 2002; 37: 371-74.
72. Frimodt-Moller P.C. and Vejlsted H., Early surgical intervention in non-specific pleural empyema; Thor. Cardiovas Surg 1985; 33: 41.
73. Hakim M., Milsterin B.B., Empyema thoracis and infected pneumonostomy space; case for cyclical irrigation, Ann Thorac. Surg 1986; 41:85.
74. de Campos JR; *et al.*, Thoracoscopy talc-pondrage–a 15-year experience; Chest 2011; 119: 801-06.
75. Ronson RS; Miller JI, Jr; Video-assisted thoracoscopy for pleural disease; Chest Surg Clin North Amer 1998; 8: 919-32.
76. Lemmer J.H., *et al.* Modern management of adult thoracic empyema, J. Thorac Surg 1985; 90: 849.
77. Iseman M.D., Madsen L.A.; Chronic tuberculous empyema with bronchopleural fistula resulting in treatment failure and Progressive drug resistance; Chest 1991; 100: 124.
78. Verma SK; Mahajan V; Complete radiological clearance in bilateral loculated pyopneumothorax managed conservatively; Lung India 2009; 26: 55-56.
79. Furst, *et al.*, A rare complication of tooth abscess M Ludwig's our give and mediastinitis; J. Can Dent Assoc 2001; 67: 324-27.
80. Coales U.F. lolomons N. Supraglottitis complicated by media stinitis; J Laryngolotol 2001; 115:321-23.
81. Furst I., *et al.*, unusual complication of endothracheal intubation; Retropharyngeal space abscess, mediastinitis and empyema; J Otolarygol 2000; 29: 309-11.

82. Rehring T.F., *et al.*, Osteomyelitis and mediastinitis complicating blunt sternal fracture; J Trauma 1999; 47: 594-96.
83. Hejjel, *et al.*, Fatal mediastinitis after routine laparoscopic Cholecys tectomy; Surg Endosco 2000; 14: 296.
84. Bladergroen M.R., Lowe J.E. and Postlethwait R.W., Diagnosis and recommended management of oesophageal perforation and rupture. Ann Thorac Surg 1986; 42: 235-39.
85. Michel L., Post-emetic laceration and rupture of the gastro-oesophageal junction, Acta Chir, Beig 1982; 82: 13-24.
86. Gupta K.L., *et al.* Spontaneous rupture of oesophagus presenting as pyopneumothorax, JAPI 1991; 39: 211-12.
87. Jaworski A., Fisher R. and Lippman M; Boerhaave's syndrome, computed tomographic findings and diagnostic consideration. Arch Intern. Med 1988; 148: 223-24.
88. Singh G.S. and Slovis C.M., Occult Boerhaave's syndrome. J. Img Med 1988; 6:13-16.
89. Naclerio E.A., The V signosis in the diagnosis of spontaneous rupture of the oesophagus (an early roentgen clue). Am J. Surg 1957; 93: 291-98.
90. Palekar S.N., *et al.* Boerhaave's syndrome, JAPI 1991;39: 348-50.
91. Saario I., Kostianien S., Salo J.,Meurala H. and Eerola S., Treatment of spontaneous rupture of the oesophagus, Acta Chir Scand 1983; 149: 771-74.
92. Walker W.S., Cameron E.W.J. and Warbaum P.R., Diagnosis and management of spontaneous transmural rupture of the oesophagus (Boerhaave's syndrome). Br. J. Surg 1985;72: 204-07.
93. Parkash A., *et al.*, Mediastinitis presenting as PUO; JAPI 2003; 51: 405-07.
94. Baruwa P, Sarmah KR; Obesity and asthma; Lung India 2013; 30: 38-46.
95. Jensen H., Labour complicated by spontaneous mediastinal emphysema, Acta Obstet. Gynae Scand 1987; 66(6):567-68.
96. Mausuda J., Tension pneumomediastinum secondary to muconium aspiration syndrome. Crit Care Med 1984; 12(11): 1009-10.
97. Overby K.J. and Litt J.D., Mediastinal emphysema in an adolescent with anorexia nervosa and self-induced emesis. Paediatrics 1988; 81(1): 134-36.
98. Gilhotra R. and Malik S.K., Pneumomediastinum complicating status asthmaticus, Lung India 1986; 4(1): 35-37.
99. Newcomb AE, Clarke CP; Spontaneous pneumomediastinum–a benign curiosity or a significant problem; Chest 2005; 128:3298-302.
100. Hamman L; Spontaneous mediastinal emphysema: Bull Johns Hopkins Hosp 1939; 64: 1-21.
101. Macia I; *et al.*, Spontaneous pneumomediastinum–41 cases; Eurp. J Cardiothorac Surg 2007; 31:1110-14.
102. Van Veden I, *et al.*, Pneumomediastinum–A rare complication of anorexia nervosa in children and adolescents: A case study and review of literature; Eurp J Paediatric 2008; 167: 171-74.
103. Cho Tj, Kim H; Unusual presentation of spontaneous pneumomediastinum; Lung India 2010; 27: 239-41.
104. Naughton M., Irving L. and Mckenzie A., Pneumomediastinum after a transbronchial biopsy, Thorax 1991; 46: 606-07.
105. Cooley J.C. and Gillespie J.B., Mediastinal Emphysema: Pathogenesis and management, Chest 1966; 49: 104-08.
106. Beyers Z.A. and Melanas C.F., Radiological signs of pneumomediastinum, Br. J. Radial 1987; 60: 877-79.
107. Jabourian Z., Spontaneous pneumomediastinum and subcutaneous emphysema, J. Otolaryngol 1988; 17(1): 50-53.
108. Gajanan S., Guade, *et al.* Pneumomediastinum in acute severe asthma; Lung India 1992; 10: 134-37.
109. Gray J.M. and Hanson G.C., Mediastinal emphysema, aetiology, diagnosis and treatment, Thorax 1966; 21: 325-27.
110. Silverman N.A. and Sabiston D.C., Mediastinal masses; Surg. Clin. North Amer 1980; 60:757.
111. Chauhan M.S., *et al.* Mediastinal tumours and cysts M clinicoradiological study, JAPI 1988; 36: 421-23.
112. Venugopal P., *et al.*, Mediastinal lymphangioma M A_2 rare presentation; Lung India 2002; XX: 9-11.
113. Madhu K., *et al.*, Mediastinal tumourinal 2-year-old boy MA case report; Lung India 2001; XIX:28-29.
114. Tarver R.D., *et al.* Imagine the diaphragm and its disorders, J. Thorac. Imag 1989; 4: 1.
115. Celli B.R., Respiratory muscle function, Clin. Chest Med. 1986; 7: 567.
116. Boch H. Barrett. and Zimmereman J.H., *Study of selected congenital anomalies in Pennsylvania.* Pub Health Rep. 1987; 82: 446, quoted by Fraser and Pare Eds. Diagnosis of Diseases of Chest 3rd Ed vol. III. Philadelphia WB, Saunders, p. 1988; 1881.
117. Harrison M.R. and de Lorimer A.A., Congenital diaphragmatic hernia. Surg. Clin. North Am 1981; 61: 1023-1035.
118. Bingham J.W.A., Herniation through congenital diaphragmatic defect. Br. J. Surg 1989; 47: 1-15.
119. Carter R.E.B., Waterson D.J. and Aberdeen E., Hernia and eventration of the diaphragm in childhood. Lancet, 1962; 1: 656-59.
120. Barret N.R. and Wheaton C.E.W., The pathology, diagnosis and treatment of congenital diaphragmatic hernia in infants, Br. J. Surg 1934; 21: 420-33.
121. Behera D., Malik S.K. Jindal S.K., Kataria R.N. and Kataria, S., Congenital diaphragmatic hernia of Bochdalek type in an adult, Ind. J. Chest. Dist and All Sci 1982; 24: 43-46.
122. Motiani P.D., *et al.* Bochdalek hernia on the right side in an adult, Lung India 1991; 91: 63-65.
123. Krishna A., Bhatnagar V. and Mitra D.K., Diaphragmatic hernia in infants and children, Ind.Paedi 1986; 23: 355-59.
124. Kirkland J.A., Congenital posterolateral diaphragmatic hernia in the adult Br. J. Surg 1959; 47: 16-22.
125. Hanies J.O. and Collins R.B., Bochdalek hernia in an adult simulating a pleural effusion, Radiology 1979; 95: 277-78.
126. Gupta R.L., Gulati S.P. and Garg S.K., Strangulated congenital diaphragmatic hernia in an adult female. J. Ind. Med. Assoc 1966; 46: 20.
127. Cohan D. and Reid J.S., Recurrent diaphragmatic hernia, J.Paed Surg 1982; 16: 42-44.
128. Sandra G., Kirchner M.D., O 'Neil J.A. Jr. and Stahlman M., Delayed radiographic hernia. Radiol 1975; 115:155-56.
129. McSweeny W.J., Radiologic evaluation of newborn with respiratory distress, Radial 1972; 7: 65-83.

130. Le Roux B.T., Supraphrenic herniation of perinephric fat. Thorax 1965; 20: 376.
131. Israel Asselainss R., Uzzan D. and Derrida J., Image pseudotumorable par hernia diaphragmatic de graisse supra renal (Trans diaphragmatic herniation of supra renal fat stimulating tumor mass) J. Franc Med. Chir Thorac 1966; 20: 567.
132. Agnihotri M.S. and Jochi A.K., Delayed appearance of Bochdalek hernia. Ind. J. Chest Dis. and All Sci 1987; 29: 160-64.
133. Robert J. Toulinkian, Air filled bronchogenic cyst presenting as a cervical mass in the newborn. J.Paed.Surg 1982; 17:311.
134. Gessenderfer H., Cervical bronchial cyst. J.Pead.Surg 1978; 8: 435-36.
135. Raj B., Chawala R.K., Bihari Janumeja A.K. and Yadav S.P.S. Ectopic herniation of pulmonary cyst. Ind J. Chest Dis. All Sci 1988; 30:136-40.
136. Bidstrup P., Munck-Nordentoft and Peterson B, Hernia of the lung, brief survey and report of two cases. Acta Radiol 1966; 4: 490.
137. Baldev Raj., *et al.* Ectopic herniation of pulmonary cavity, Lung India 1991; 9: 156-58.
138. Jayaprakash B; *et al.*, Gorham's disease; JAPI 2013; 61; 71-73.
139. Jackson JBS; A boneless arm; Boston Med Surg J 1838; 18: 368-69.
140. Chavanis N; *et al.*, Chylothorax complicating Gorham's disease; Anu Thorac Surg 2001; 72: 937-39.

Pulmonary Embolism

9

INTRODUCTION

Pulmonary embolism—a major health problem has been implicated in 1.5-2 lakh deaths in USA. Diagnosis is frequently missed and oftenly it is difficult to confirm. In untreated cases, mortality is almost 30%, although it can be decreased to 2-8% if proper therapy is instituted at an appropriate time. However, the prevalence at autopsy has not changed in the last three decades.

Pulmonary embolism (PE) and venous thrombosis (VT) constitute one of the most common cardiopulmonary illnesses. Death rate is higher in males than in females and in non-whites than in whites.[1] PE implies impaction of a material, usually a thrombus from leg veins into the pulmonary circulation. Besides thrombus, other embolic substances include vegetations from right-sided infective endocarditis, fat amniotic fluid, tumour cells and air. The clinical features of pulmonary thrombo-embolism may be non-specific and vague in many cases, often making the diagnosis difficult. Available information suggests that an antemortem diagnosis has been made in only 10 to 30 per cent of all cases in which old or recent embolism is demonstrated at autopsy. This emphasises the need for high index of suspicion of PE in patients who are predisposed for deep vein thrombosis in legs. Those at risk include patients having complete bed rest following medical ailments, surgery or trauma, diseases of veins of the lower limbs, congestive cardiac failure, pregnancy, postpartum period, obesity, disseminated malignancy, polycythemia and use of contraceptive pills containing mainly oestrogen.

In a recent study in USA, females compared to males, having less frequency of PE have been reported[2] but PE forms the most common medical cause of maternal mortality associated with live births.[3] Antemortem diagnosis has been difficult especially in elderly and those with underlying cardiopulmonary disease, autopsy studies reveal.[4]

In general, higher incidence of pulmonary embolism has been reported in women than in men,[5] probably due to oestrogen use,[6] child bearing[7] and increased frequency of thrombophlebitis.[8,9] Common risk factors in 75% cases of (females) are oral contraceptives and elective abortion.[6] A postmortem study[10] also showed higher frequency of pulmonary embolism in females (11.1%) compared to males (7.4 %). Deep vein thrombosis (DVT) needs to be mentioned here as it is one of the most important causes of PE. Exact assessment of incidence of DVT cannot be accurately made, but by using objective diagnostic techniques, DVT is detectable in 25-35% cases after operation and 20-25% of patients after myocardial infarction or stroke. Pulmonary embolism kills almost 1/10,000 males and 1.5/10,000 females every year in England and Wales.[11]

Aetiopathogenesis[11]

Venous thrombi are initiated by changes in the coagulation mechanisms of the blood, damage to the endothelial lining of blood vessels, and by reduction in blood flow—the three components of Virchow's triad that was first described in 1846. A fourth component should now be added—the fibrinolytic state of the patient.

Certain factors alter the balance of these mechanisms; immobility is the most important (particularly if it lasts for four days or longer), and a previous deep vein thrombosis will have caused intimal scarring and venous pooling, and therefore, may result in the production of procoagulant material or reduced fibrinolytic activity. Operations are associated with many of the factors—the trauma activating the clotting factors and the stasis occurring during the procedure and recovery period. The extent and duration of the operation also influence the degree of risk. The type of procedure influences the probability of local damage to vessels, which is particularly common in operations on the lower limb and in the pelvic region. Some patients are predisposed to deep vein thrombosis because of deficiencies in blood and tissue factors including antithrombin III, protein C, protein S, and plasminogen activator—a substance released from vein walls and blood, and vital for the activation of the fibrinolytic system. Conversely, high concentrations of plasminogen inhibitor have also been detected in patients with iliofemoral thrombosis.

Many patients will have multiple risk factors, and it is important to realise that the overall risk is the product rather than the sum of the individual factors—thus the risk is greatly increased by the coexistence of two or more factors. More than 90% of pulmonary emboli originate from lower extremities. At the same time, condition is uncommon to occur in healthy people.

There is clearly a need in hospital practice for a procedure that is readily available as well as reliable to cope with the increasingly common diagnostic problem of pulmonary embolism. Despite the development of new diagnostic techniques (some of which are only available in specialist centres) at present there is probably no single test that can be used with an acceptable degree of certainty. Although clinical presentation and history remain the two most important pointers to the correct diagnosis, PE and venous thrombosis can exist in the absence of any detectable physical signs.

Classification[2]

Diagnostic approaches to possible PE depend initially upon the circumstances surrounding its occurrence. PE can be divided clinically into three groups.

Acute non-massive PE is by far the most frequent type; it follows less than 50 per cent obstruction to the pulmonary outflow and is not associated with any haemodynamic disturbance. When accompanied by pulmonary infarction, it can be recognized fairly easily, but signs and symptoms are often more varied and generally less obvious—particularly in the presence of pre-existing cardiorespiratory disease. This group is important because one third of patients with life-threatening massive PE have premonitory (minor) embolism and two thirds of those who ultimately die from PE have previous smaller emboli. Larger emboli in this group are sometimes referred to as acute submassive emboli.

Acute massive PE occurs with obstruction of 50 per cent or more of the pulmonary vascular bed. The signs and symptoms produced are explained by acute right ventricular failure, acute reduction in cardiac output, and ventilation-perfusion disturbances. The onset of symptoms is abrupt in 95 per cent of cases and may include sudden death or a period of cardiovascular collapse. A less common category of subacute massive PE has also been described where the pulmonary obstruction is greater than 50 per cent but the time course is in excess of 2 weeks and no episode of collapse or shock is seen.

In chronic PE (Chronic thromboembolic pulmonary hypertension) repeated small (peripheral) emboli occur over a period of months or years. There is failure of lysis and the appearance of symptoms coincides with the onset of pulmonary hypertension with or without right ventricular failure.

Category PE depends not only on the size of the embolus and the duration of the process but also on pre-existing cardio-respiratory disease. A background of chronic pulmonary obstruction or congestive cardiac failure leads to non-specific symptoms and signs.

Because PE originates from peripheral venous thrombosis, less common causes include tumour, fat, and amniotic fluid emboli. Diagnosis also involves the search for the site of thrombosis. Methods used include venography, Doppler ultrasound, plethysmography, thermography, and isotope scanning with ^{125}I-labelled fibrinogen or ^{99}mTc-labelled urokinase. But venography itself may be followed by an increased incidence of venous thrombosis. Clinically detectable venous thrombosis occurs in less than one third of all cases of PE, and moreover, 50 per cent of patients with deep venous thrombosis on isotope scanning have no symptoms. The large majority of patients with PE have predisposing factors, and an awareness of situations likely to aid in the diagnosis of peripheral venous thrombosis and PE.

The exact overall rate of incidence of PE is unknown. Postmortem studies indicate its presence in 6-20 per cent of hospital deaths but such samples are inevitably biased. The incidence of nonfatal PE seen in clinical practice is estimated at 20 to 1000 hospital in-patients and that of fatal PE as five in 1000. What is clear is that the rate of occurrence is high and, despite considerable energy correctly directed towards prophylaxis, it is still increasing.

Acute Non-massive PE

The clinical syndrome most easily recognized is that of pulmonary infarction. Haemoptysis, pleuritic chest pain and a pleural rub occur frequently, as do fever, phlebitis, and tachycardia. Dyspnoea is also present but is less marked than that following massive PE. In patients with pre-existing cardiorespiratory disease, acute cor pulmonale may be precipitated with signs and symptoms more suggestive of massive PE. Unexplained dyspnoea may be the presenting and the only feature. Sometimes, acute non-massive PE is defined as a patient with shock or hypotension if not caused by new onset arrhythmia, hypovolemia or sepsis.

Factors predisposing to venous thrombosis and PE are given below:

Medical	Bed rest, immobility	
	Myocardial infarction (related to severity rather than bed rest and worsened by associated congestive cardiac failure)	
	Congestive cardiac failure	
	Chronic airway obstruction or cor pulmonale	
	Valvular heart disease	
	Severe infection	
	Carcinoma (especially of pancreas, stomach or lung)	
	Blood dyscrasia	Polycythaemia post-splenectomy
	Diabetes mellitus	
	Nephrotic syndrome	
Surgical	Postoperative	Major abdominal, pelvic, urological or orthopaedic procedure
	Trauma	Lower limb fractures Burns
	Peripheral vascular surgery	
Obstetric gynaecological	Pelvic surgery	
	Pregnancy and delivery	Caesarean section and/or suppression of lactation by oestrogens
Medication	Oral contraception (related to oestrogen content)	
	Corticosteroids (radiographic media during venography)	
Others	Increasing age	
	Obesity	
	Varicose veins	
	Previous thrombophlebitis or PE	
	Genetic predisposition to venous thrombosis	

Overall accuracy in clinical detection of acute non-massive PE is accepted as poor. There is a growing evidence that patients with non-massive PE, who show right ventricular hypokinesia on echocardiography have poor prognosis. This group can be called as sub-massive PE.[13]

Acute Massive PE

It is defined as patient with shock or hypotension (systolic blood pressure less than 90 mmHg or a pressure drop of more than 40 mmHg for more than 15 minutes), if not caused by new onset arrhythmia hypovolemia or sepsis. Syncope and collapse with hypotension are more usually seen following massive PE and are due to an acute reduction in cardiac output and cerebral blood flow. One third of these patients develop circulatory arrest. Central chest pain is experienced in about one third of patients presumably from reduced coronary artery perfusion. Alternatively, pericardial pain or discomfort following sudden distension of the right ventricle can occur. Other features commonly encountered are apprehension, sweating and cough. Haemoptysis in this situation occurs in only 10-25 per cent of patients. Unexplained dyspnoea is also a prominent (and again, sometimes the only) feature of acute massive PE. The mechanism is probably related to arterial desaturation. This dyspnoea differs from that associated with pulmonary venous hypertension in that patients prefer to lie flat with no orthopnoea. The physical signs in acute massive PE are mostly due to acute right ventricular failure, low cardiac output and ventilation-perfusion imbalance. Cyanosis, tachycardia, elevated central venous pressure and a gallop rhythm heard best at the left sternal edge are found in 75 per cent of patients. Blood pressure may be preserved in the supine position but hypotension occurs on sitting upright. Closure of the pulmonary valve, which is initially quiet, characteristically becomes loud and widely split after 24-48 hours due to either a reduction in the obstruction presented to the right ventricle or an adaptation by the right ventricle to meet this obstruction. Wide expiratory splitting of the second heart sound may be an important clue to diagnosis in the absence of bundle-branch block or atrial septal defect. Hypoxia is due to ventilation-perfusion abnormalities, although intrapulmonary shunting can also occur. In addition intra-atrial shunting is possible since the high pressure in the right atrium could cause a right-to-left flow through the foramen ovale which remains patient in 25 per cent of normal people. No single symptom or combination of symptoms is diagnostic of acute PE. Pulmonary infarction, which occurs in acute non-massive PE, can be recognised with reasonable confidence in the clinical situation but diagnostic problems are frequent particularly in those with pre-existing disease or in the elderly.

Certain associations of signs and symptoms are recognized. For example, previous thromboembolism occurs in about a quarter of patients (the majority within the preceding 6 months) and is more likely with non-massive rather than massive PE. Similarly, congestive cardiac failure, oestrogen medication, haemoptysis and pleuritic pain are all related to non-massive PE. Syncope and shock are associated with massive PE but the mortality rate is correlated with pre-existing cardiorespiratory disease, particularly the presence of congestive cardiac failure, rather than the size of the embolus.

Chronic PE

This is much less common and because it differs from acute PE in both aetiology and symptomatology, it is best treated separately. The probable cause has already been given, namely repeated small PEs with a failure of lysis giving rise to progressive obliteration of the pulmonary vascular bed. There is usually a history of venous thrombosis and episodes of haemoptysis or pneumonia.

The main symptom is increasing dyspnoea and reduced exercise tolerance. Pathologically this coincides with the onset of pulmonary hypertension with or without right ventricular failure. The chest X-ray is non-specific and pulmonary angiography shows multiple occlusions of the major branches of the pulmonary artery. Perfusion scanning is markedly patchy with normal ventilation and this combination is usually diagnostic.

On chest X-ray, prominent main pulmonary arteries and an attenuated peripheral vascular pattern are seen in primary or idiopathic pulmonary hypertension. This is a disease of uncertain aetiology with a predilection for young women and a possible familial tendency.

Diagnosis and Differential Diagnosis

Acute pulmonary embolism may present as one of three different clinical syndromes:[14]

a. Acute cor pulmonale.
b. Pulmonary infarction.
c. Acute unexplained dyspnoea.

The pathophysiology, signs and symptoms of these three syndromes are quite different. The differential diagnosis and the appropriate diagnostic work up are also different. The detection of deep venous thrombosis qualifies as an excellent clue to the diagnosis of pulmonary thromboembolism, but its absence does not exclude embolism, as clinical evidence of venous thrombosis is found in less than half of patients of PE. Other *occult* presentation in which embolism should be considered includes syncope suggesting neurological disorder, repetitive bouts of otherwise unexplained supraventricular tachyarrhythmias, sudden onset or worsening of congestive heart failure, sudden deterioration of patients with chronic obstructive pulmonary disease and (as an alternative to the diagnosis) hyperventilation of phychic origin.

Acute Cor Pulmonale

Patients in whom massive pulmonary embolism obstructing more than 60-75 per cent of pulmonary circulation occurs, present with the clinical syndrome of acute cor pulmonale. Normal right ventricle can acutely increase its systolic pressure to above 50-60 mm Hg to overcome the increased resistance in the pulmonary circulation. Acute right ventricular dilatation with increasing filling pressure occurs beyond this level. As right ventricle dilates and fails, its stroke volume decreases leading to decreased cardiac output, hypotension and possible cardiac arrest. Sudden dyspnoea is the most reliable symptom and severe persistent dyspnoea is an ominous sign, for it usually indicates extensive embolic occlusion. Anginal pain due to right ventricular ischaemia may occur. On physical examination vital signs reveal tachypnoea, tachycardia and hypotension. Signs of acute right ventricular failure—distended neck veins, right-sided S3 gallop and a parasternal heave—are usually present. The lungs are clear, signs of deep vein thrombosis may be present. Due to acute fall in cardiac output, patient may present with features of cerebral anoxia with obtundation, convulsions and coma. The differential diagnosis may include acute myocardial infarction, hypovolaemia or sepsis. If the arterial occlusion is massive, death usually occurs within few hours in more than 2/3 of the cases. In those who survive resolution occurs. Nevertheless, recurrent pulmonary embolism is a common cause of secondary pulmonary hypertension.

Pulmonary Infarction or Haemorrhage

Pulmonary infarction rarely follows embolism in less than 10% of cases. This is understandable because lung has three avenues for obtaining oxygen—the pulmonary arterial circulation, the bronchial arterial circulation and the airways. Thus occurrence of infarction means a compromise in bronchial arterial flow and/or airways to the involved areas. Left ventricular failure, mitral stenosis and chronic obstructive pulmonary disease predispose for pulmonary infarction. In such patients its incidence may be upto 30% while it is rare in patients with no cardiorespiratory disease. Cough, pleuritic chest pain and haemoptysis, constitute the clinical triad of pulmonary infarction. Pleural rub may appear after 3-4 days. Signs of consolidation and pleural effusion may develop. The differential diagnosis in patients presenting with pulmonary infarction includes viral or bacterial pneumonitis. A history of a viral prodrome or of a shaking chill with fever or purulent sputum points towards pneumonitis. Complications of pulmonary infarction include secondary infection, cavitation, pneumothroax and haemothorax.

Acute Unexplained Dyspnoea

The sudden onset of dyspnoea may be the most common presenting complaint of patients with submassive pulmonary embolism, who do not sustain pulmonary infarction. On physical examination the only abnormalities may be tachypnoea, possible tachycardia and anxiety. The lungs are clear. There are no signs of right heart failure. Signs of DVT may be present. The differential diagnosis includes left ventricular failure, pneumonia and the hyperventilation syndrome.

Deep Vein Thrombosis[11]

The appearance of common clinical signs of deep vein thrombosis should arouse suspicion, particularly if the patient is in a high risk group, but other conditions may present in similar ways. Fever and tachycardia are of little diagnostic importance; less than half of the patients with local tenderness or Homan's sign have deep vein thrombosis; and only half the limbs, in which there are clinical signs below the knee, contain thrombi. Conversely, more than half of all deep vein thrombosis are clinically silent and are detected only by screening.

The diagnosis should therefore always be confirmed before treatment is started. Ultrasound scanning will show only occlusive thrombi, and is unhelpful if the thrombus is confined to the calf. Venography is the standard technique and provides anatomical information, an estimate of the age of the thrombus, and a measure of whether it is fixed to the wall of the vessel or floating tree. Impedance plethysmography is an accurate, non-invasive diagnostic test for thrombosis at or proximal to the popliteal vein, but false positive results may occur in patients who have arterial insufficiency.

Scanning the uptake of fibrinogen labelled with iodine-125 is a sensitive test, especially for early thrombosis confined to the calf, and permits serial analysis on consecutive days. Preparation for the test includes blocking the uptake of iodine by the thyroid; however, that makes the test suitable only for screening.

Diagnostic Studies

Although the history and physical examination are the means suggesting the diagnosis of pulmonary embolism, a diagnosis on clinical grounds alone is often incorrect. Hence clinical suspicion of embolism requires confirmation by laboratory studies. This is shown in Table 9.1.

Arterial Blood Gases (ABG)

Analysis of ABG in pulmonary embolism typically reveals hypoxaemia, hypercapnia and respiratory alkalosis,[15] in addition to the difference between alveolar dead space. However, a normal PCO_2 does not exclude the diagnosis. The test is not relatable in elderly and those with previous cardiopulmonary disease having lower PO_2.[12]

Electrocardiogram (ECG)

The main value of ECG is to help exclude acute myocardial infarction. Sinus tachycardia is the most common ECG finding in pulmonary embolism. There is an evidence of right ventricular strain. With emboli that provoke a substantial rise in pulmonary arterial and right-sided pressures, patterns of S_1, Q_3, T_3 inverted T waves in V_1-V_3, right ventricular strain, right axis deviation, right bundle branch block and atrial arrhythmias may occur. These changes may be transient.[16]

Enzyme and Biochemical Analysis

Originally, an elevated level of lactate dehydrogenase with a normal asparate transaminase present in PE was used to rule out PE from acute myocardial infarction. Currently, it is accepted that these have little diagnostic significance. Similarly fibrin degradation products lack both sensitivity and specificity.

Table 9.1: Pulmonary thromboembolism (pulmonary infarct)

Investigations:	Chest X-ray	Unreliable
	Total cell count and ESR raised	
	Serum LDH and fibrinogen levels are high	
	Arterial PO_2 is low	
	Technetium 99 scan and pulmonary angiography are helpful	
Differential diagnosis:	Myocardial infarction, pericarditis, aortic aneurysm	
	Acute upper abdominal disease	
	Pulmonary oedema, pneumonitis, asthma, pleurisy	
	Tumours	

Chest Radiograph

Chest film in pulmonary embolism is frequently normal. When the chest radiography is abnormal, there are no findings that can be cited as pathognomonic of pulmonary embolism. Larger the perfusion defect, the less frequent will be radiological abnormality. Similarly a perfusion defect larger than the radiological abnormality is of higher significance than a perfusion defect smaller than the corresponding radiological abnormality which has only a low probability of indicating PE. Presence of bloody effusion is suggestive of PE but bloody perfusion constitute only about 10% of and effusions from PE. In massive PE, X-ray chest may be of considerable value although the signs are quite subtle. Oligremia with a contrast hyperaemia and enlarged hilar shadows can be seen mostly on the right because the left hilum is more difficult to assess. However, changes in pulmonary vasculature are infrequent following non-massive PE. Non-specific infiltrates of virtually any configuration may occur and very few if any are wedge shaped. Characteristically, infiltrates caused by infarction are against the pleura. They do not usually appear until 12-36 hours after the embolism has occurred. Small pleural effusion may occur. Elevation of a hemidiaphragm may occur with or without pulmonary infiltration and is indicative of ipsilateral volume loss.[17] Difference in diameter between vessels that should be of equivalent size should raise the suspicion of embolism. There may be abrupt *cut off* of a vessel, i.e., as the vessel is traced distally, it suddenly disappears. An avascular lung in association with clinical features of pulmonary embolism was described by Westermark in Bostom in 1930s. Rat tail configuration of pulmonary artery, where the vessel is relatively normal, proximally and suddenly tapers to a sharp point, indicates presence of organised clot in the vessel. The laboratory tests discussed thus are far often negative in pulmonary thromboembolism and are relatively non-specific. Therefore, it is usually necessary to proceed to two more definite techniques: isotope lung scanning and the pulmonary angiogram.

Isotope Lung Scanning

Lung perfusion scans are usually carried out using macro aggregates of human albumin that have been labelled with radio technetium 99 m. Isotope lung scanning is simple, safe and rapid. It can be repeated to define resolution or recurrence. A properly performed perfusion scan in multiple views virtually, excludes the diagnosis of clinically significant pulmonary embolism. The lung photoscan demonstrates only abnormalities of the distribution of blood flow. It does not provide anatomic information. An abnormal perfusion scan, therefore, must be interpreted together with the plain X-ray chest, as it lacks specificity and conditions like pneumonia, effusion and fibrosis are likely to cause a local reduction in perfusion. Conditions like emphysema, sarcoidosis, tuberculosis, pneumonia and atelectasis can produce perfusion defects. Although there are no false negative results with perfusion scans, their accuracy is considered to be moderate by some while others consider perfusion scan to be more useful for a firm exclusion of PE since there is significant number of false positive results. One approach to enchancing specificity is to perform ventilation scan using Xenon or Xenon 133. Combined with clinical suspicion, the addition of ventilation scan improves diagnostic accuracy in 66-92% cases but the problem with these investigations (vent perfusion) includes abnormal test results even after recovery from earlier embolism, in 3/4th of patients with previous cardiovascular disease or one half of the cases without such disease, persisting after 1-9 years. To assist in deciding whether a ventilation scan may be useful and when pulmonary angiography is required, two factors should be considered: the size of the perfusion defects and the chest roentgenographic infiltration. Ventilation scan will not be useful and pulmonary angiography is required, if a definite diagnosis is required. On the contrary, if defects are segmental or larger in size and one or more are in areas clear by X-rays, a ventilation scan should be done. If radioactive gas enters *(washed in)* and is cleared *(washed out)* from areas of perfusion defect, this *mismatch* of ventilation and perfusion is characteristic of vascular obstruction. However, if ventilation is also abnormal with ventilation perfusion *match* (if) present, no reliable diagnostic conclusion can be reached and pulmonary angiography is required; PIOPED[18] study is as follows:

The prospective investigation of pulmonary embolism diagnosis (PIOPED) recruited 931 patients, of whom 81 per cent completed mandatory angiography within a day of obtaining an abnormal lung scan. Among 755 patients who completed angiography, 33 per cent had pulmonary embolism. The most important finding in PIOPED is that of the 251 patients with positive angiograms only 102 (41 per cent) had high probability lung scans. In PIOPED, the positive predictive value of lung scanning for pulmonary embolism at angiography was as follows: 87 per cent for high, 32 per cent for intermediate, 16 per cent for near normal scans (Table 9.2).

Pulmonary Arteriography

Pulmonary arteriography is the definitive test for the diagnosis of PE.[19] There is probably no false negative results. The technique, though invasive, expensive and sophisticated, remains a definitive investigation for diagnosis of PE with magnified views. This gives anatomic information about the pulmonary vasculature indicating precisely the severity and extent of pulmonary embolism. This is most useful when active

Table 9.2: PIOPED: Comparison of scan category to angiogram findings in pulmonary embolism

Scan category	*Present*	*Absent*	*Uncertain*	*No angio*	*Total N*
High	102	14	1	7	124
Intermediate	105	217	9	33	364
Low	39	199	12	62	312
Near normal/normal	5	50	2	74	131
Total	251	480	24	176	931

therapy like embolectomy and thrombolytic therapy is contemplated and in doubtful diagnosis when embolism is suspected on the basis of other investigations. Radio opaque material is injected through a cardiac catheter advanced into the pulmonary artery. This procedure is done in cardiac catheterization laboratory by technically skilled personnel and it requires reasonable period for preparation and performance. Being invasive test, it entails more risk than procedures described above.

Suggested indications include: (1) A risk from treatment sufficient to require the diagnosis to be firmly established, especially the exclusion of patients under a strong suspicion of PE on history and an abnormal perfusion scan with a normal chest X-ray film, (2) Planned invasive or thrombolytic therapy, and (3) Uncertain diagnosis. The two diagnostic features of pulmonary embolism on angiography are: (a) filling defects, i.e., embolus produces negative shadow as radio opaque material flows around it, and (b) abrupt *cut off* a vessel at the point of embolic impaction.

Interpretative limitation of angiography are: (1) Injection artifacts, (2) Issnability to evaluate small vessels patency, and (3) Interpretative errors.

An approach to reduce the need for pulmonary arteriography, there can be other studies to investigate the veins of the lower extremities using venography or non-invasive approaches such as impedance plethysmography or doppler study. If these studies demonstrate deep venous thrombosis of popliteal vein or above, one is committed to anticoagulant therapy which is also the main therapy for suspected pulmonary embolism. Negative study of lower extremities veins along with a low probability V/Q scan, excludes pulmonary embolism. While this concept has some merit, one must remember that in 20-30% of patients with proven pulmonary embolism, the studies of lower extremity veins are negative.

DNA Studies

Diagnostic elevation of free plasma DNA levels have been studied in proven cases of PE. But other causes of free DNA like renal failure, connective tissue disorder, steroid therapy, trauma or surgery would limit the value of this test.

Other Imaging Modalities

Echocardiography[20]

Echocardiography features that suggest acute pulmonary embolism include dilated hypokinetic right ventricle, presence of tricuspid regurgitation with increased flow velocity compatible with mild to moderate elevation of pulmonary arterial systolic pressure, absence of right ventricular hypertrophy and absence of important left heart pathological conditions.

Signs of pulmonary embolism on echocardiography are as follows:

a. Thrombus visualisation (rarely).
b. Dilated right ventricle.
c. Right ventricular hypokinesia (Sparing apex).
d. Interventricular septal motion abnormality.
e. Regurgitation of tricuspid valve.
f. Dilated pulmonary artery.
g. Decreased inspiratory collapse of inferior vena cava is lacking.

Digital Substraction Pulmonary Angiography (DSA)

DSA performed via a peripheral vein is useful only in screening patients who present with suspected life threatening pulmonary thrombo embolism having massive central embolism.[21]

Computed Tomography (CT)

CT cannot differentiate between occluded pulmonary segments and normal lung tissue. However, this technique may be appropriate for patients with pulmonary hypertension when the risks of angiography are considered prohibitively high. It is also useful for serial non-invasive evaluation after thrombolysis or surgical embolectomy among patients who have undergone baseline pulmonary angiography.[22]

Magnetic Resonance Imaging (MRI)

This technique is useful for detecting pulmonary embolism and initial case reports have been encouraging. The diagnostic niche for MRI may be helpful in differentiating acute from chronic pulmonary embolism.[23]

Radioisotopic Imaging

Indium-111 platelet scintigraphy, and isotope imaging technique utilising Indium-111 labelled monoclonal antifibrin antibodies and Iodine 125 labelled mutant of tissue plasminogen activator (TPA) have been employed for detection of thrombus in DVT with limited value.

Fiberoptic Angioscopy

After jugular venotomy, the angioscope is guided with fluoroscopic assistance into the right heart and main pulmonary artery. Pulmonary artery branches upto segmental arteries can be examined. This technique may be particularly useful in patients with chronic pulmonary hypertension.[24]

Points to Remember[25]

1. Pulmonary embolism is among the most misdiagnosed and mistreated condition encountered in hospital practice.
2. Pulmonary embolism may present as one of three different clinical syndromes: acute cor pulmonale, pulmonary infarction and acute unexplained dyspnoea.
3. Predisposition for deep vein thrombosis in lower limbs if present offers an additional supporting evidence for the diagnosis of acute pulmonary embolism, and presence of DVT may be confirmed by Doppler or impedance plethysmography.
4. ABG, chest X-ray, E.C.G. as diagnostic aids are not useful as the changes may be non-specific.
5. Isotope lung scans are very useful and a normal perfusion lung scan rules out pulmonary embolism.
6. Pulmonary angiography, though a gold standard in the diagnosis of pulmonary embolism, should only be done in selected cases.

Probability of pulmonary embolism has been classified by Secker-Walker[26] as shown in Table 9.3.

Diagnositc approach to pulmonary embolism is shown in Table 9.4.

Table 9.3: Probability of pulmonary embolism

a. *High probability* of pulmonary embolism (62-90%)
   i. One or more large (> 75% of an anatomic pulmonary segment) of two or more moderate size defect in blood flow (25-75% of an anatomic pulmonary segment) in regions of the lung that have normal ventilation or ventilation that is clearly less severely compromised than blood flow.
   ii. Perfusion defect substantially larger than radiographic abnormality with normal surrounding ventilation.
b. *Intermediate probability* for pulmonary embolism (20-33%)
   i. The presence of severe diffuse airway obstruction regardless of the type of perfusion defect.
   ii. Matched perfusion defect and radiographic abnormality.
   iii. A single moderate sized defect in blood flow in a region of the lung that is normal in chest radiography and which is accompanied by normal ventilation.
c. *Low probability* for pulmonary embolism <10%
   i. Normal perfusion images (probability virtually 0%).
   ii. Small defect in blood flow (<25% of anatomic pulmonary segment).
   iii. Focal defect in blood flow with matched abnormalities of ventilation and no corresponding radiographic abnormalities.
   iv. Perfusion defect substantially smaller than the radiographic abnormalities.

Table 9.4: Diagnostic approach to pulmonary embolism

	Clinical suspicion ABG, ECG and chest X-Ray	Normal (But diagnosis suspected)	
Normal Pulmonary embolism excluded	Perfusion lung scan Ventilation scan	Abnormal	Abnormal
	Ventilation perfusion (V.P.) mismatch Pulmonary emboism	V.P. match (Pulmonary embolism strong possibility) Pulmonary angiography	
		Filling defect (Pulmonary embolism present)	Normal (Pulmonary embolism excluded)

To sum up PE, the most important and consistent symptom of acute PE is the sudden onset of dyspnoea unexplained by pneumonia, heart failure, pneumothorax or exacerbation of airway obstruction. The features such as haemoptysis and pleural rub may be absent in upto two thirds of patients. With previous cardiorespiratory disease, the signs and symptoms become non-specific and a relatively minor PE can produce clinical features more suggestive of a large embolus. Hypoxia and a raised respiratory rate are also suggestive but cannot be relied upon if there is pre-existing cardiorespiratory disease or in the elderly. Although the radiological appearance of an infarct shadow may be recognized, the chest X-ray is frequently non-specific or normal. A negative perfusion scan excludes any significant emboli and an abnormal perfusion scan is suggestive of PE but not diagnostic; its specificity can be increased considerably if facilities are available for a concurrent ventilation scan. A deep venous thrombosis when present is also indicative of PE, although its absence does not preclude the diagnosis. Factors predisposing to deep venous thrombosis are usually present in the patient with PE.

No single diagnostic aid can be relied upon in the diagnosis of PE. As with many illnesses, much of the evidence begins with a careful consideration of the presenting history and physical signs. Further help can be obtained from various investigations, but results must be interpreted with consideration of the patient's age and pre-existing health. The final diagnosis may need to be established by pulmonary angiography.

The selection of investigations must be guided by the general condition of the patient, the degree of necessity for establishing a firm diagnosis and the availability of equipment and personnel for further diagnostic procedures.

Management[11]

General supportive measures include assuring adequate oxygenation and haemodynamic support. Very small fluid less than 500 ml, dopamine and inhalation of NO can be administered in those having low cardiac index and normal blood pressure only. Oxygenation helps in reversing hypoxemia that is present in PE.

The three main aims of treatment of deep vein thrombosis are to prevent extension of the thrombus, to reduce the risk of embolism and to avoid the long-term complications of the postphlebitic limb. The treatment will depend on the site and extent of the thrombus, which should be confirmed objectively. In about 80% of cases the thrombus is confined to the calf veins, but it may propagate into the veins of the popliteal fossa, thigh and pelvis. In some cases the thrombus arises in the iliofemoral segment and may extend distally. Table 9.5 gives certain vital points regarding PE.

Table 9.5: Pulmonary embolism: Points to remember

We should rely on the diagnosis of *pulmonary embolism* on clinical grounds, X-ray examination, ECG findings and on doppler echocardiography and start the lytic therapy as early as possible, unless there is an obvious contraindication to such a form of treatment.

If the thrombi are small and confined to the calf, treatment should be conservative and comprise limb exercise in bed, raising the foot of the bed and wearing elastic compression stockings. For more extensive thrombi, the patient should be given heparin intravenously to maintain the activated partial thromboplastin time at 2-3 times the normal value. Heparin acts by (a) Interaction with antithrombin III that accelerates its ability to inactivate thrombin, factor Xa and factor IXa. (b) Catalyses the inactivation of thrombin by heparin cofactor II and (c) Does not directly dissolve thrombus but allows the fibrinolytic system to reduce the thromboembolic burden. Bleeding and heparin induced thrombocytopenia are the major complications of anticoagulation with heparin.[27]

Accurate diagnosis is essential before instituting heparin therapy, but it should not be withheld waiting for definite diagnosis, atleast in patients with intermediate or high probability of PE. Heparin is initially 80 IU kg, then 181 IU /kg/ hour, to be modified according to activated partial thromboplastin time as recommended by ACCP.

Recent studies, however, have suggested that calcium heparin given subcutaneously may be equally effective in preventing propagation of thrombi. Subcutaneous, unmonitored low molecular weight heparin has been advantageous, efficiently superior with superior bioavailability and anticoagulant response is highly correlated with body weight, thus permitting to use a fixed dose.[28,29] And also it can safely be used in pregnancy.[30] Oral anticoagulant drugs should be started at the same time and continued for 8-12 weeks. Warfarin is given in a loading dose of 20-30 mg and then daily, the dose being adjusted to maintain a prothrombin time of 1.7-3.0 times the normal value by using international reference thromboplastin. It must be noted that initial therapy with oral anticoagulants alone may be less effective and even dangerous. Warfarin induced skin necrosis, occurring in first few days of therapy, must be kept in mind.

Thrombolytic treatment with streptokinase or urokinase should be reserved for more extensive thrombosis. It is most effective when the thrombus is reasonably fresh and only partially occlusive, and may salvage deep veins thus reducing the incidence of postphlebitic changes. These agents require careful monitoring, however, and carry a greater risk of haemorrhage than simple anticoagulant drugs. Furthermore, streptokinase may rarely cause an anaphylactic reaction and urokinase (which does not have this drawback) is quite expensive.

Thrombectomy should be reserved for cases of extensive proximal thrombosis in which anticoagulants are contraindicated or the viability of the limb is threatened. The temporary construction of an arteriovenous fistula, or intermittent pneumatic compression, have been used to maintain venous patency with some success.

Interruption of vena caval flow should be reserved for patients who develop emboli while receiving anticoagulant drugs; those in whom anticoagulation is contraindicated; and, possibly, those with life-threatening, large, proximal, non-adherent thrombi. Early techniques required major operations and resulted in a high incidence of extensive distal thrombosis, peripheral oedema, and postphlebitic change. Modern equipment such as the Greenfield and Gunther filters do not have these disadvantages because they permit continued caval flow and may be inserted through the jugular vein with the patient under local anaesthesia. The management of minor pulmonary emboli is aimed at preventing recurrence or extension. Anticoagulant drugs should be prescribed.

Patients with massive established emboli should initially be resuscitated. Pulmonary arteriography should be considered to confirm the diagnosis and assess the extent of the embolus. If resuscitation has been successful and the patient is stable, treatment is by thrombolytic drugs; if not, pulmonary embolectomy offers the only hope of survival.

Pulmonary Embolism in Children

Although we are not accustomed to considering pulmonary embolism (PE) in children, it occurs more frequently than is generally recognized.[31,32] Based on autopsy data, the incidence of PE in patients younger than 18 years is estimated to be one per 1000 hospital admissions, of which 30% are deemed to be clinically significant. Important risk factors include prolonged immobility, central catheters, heart disease, ventriculoatrial shunts, trauma, neoplasm, and arteriovenous malformations. In the adolescent population, risk factors include oral contraceptive use, trauma to a lower extremity without fracture and abortion. In addition, the Guillain-Barré syndrome has been specifically associated with PE, with fatality rates reported to range from 1.3%[33] to 20%[34] in patients from 1 to 79 years of age.

Despite a paucity of data regarding PE prevention in childhood, the adult experience in which anticoagulation therapy has been demonstrated to decrease the incidence of PE is sufficiently compelling to be utilized in the young.[35] Heparin prophylaxis for a short duration in the patient with paralysis can be given provided there is no coexisting increased risk of hemorrhage due to other medical conditions. Furthermore, additional deep venous thrombosis prophylaxis such as gradient elastic stockings should also be considered.

Given the relatively low frequency of PE in childhood, risk factors for developing PE should be weighed against the risk of heparin prophylaxis.[36] This is of particular concern, since most providers of pediatric care are relatively inexperienced in the use of anticoagulant therapy. More research is needed before firm guidelines concerning the use of heparin, its indications, efficacy and safety in this population can be made.

Prophylaxis[11]

Prophylaxis is probably the most important aspect when considering thromboembolic disease; it is directed towards reducing venous stasis and combating the changes in the blood that promote coagulation.

Venous stasis may be reduced by physical methods, many of which are simple. For patients undergoing operations, carcful positioning of the patient is required on the operating table to avoid pressure on the calves, avoiding restriction of venous outflow and early ambulation after the operation.

External compression by elastic stockings is an inexpensive and safe method of increasing venous velocity but it is important that the compression is graduated. Intermittent pneumatic, compression with a single or multi-chamber device and electrical calf muscle stimulation also improves venous flow.

Of the pharmacological methods available, low dose heparin is the most widely used and has been thoroughly evaluated. The heparin is given subcutaneously in a dose of 5000 units at 8 to 12 hourly intervals starting before the operation and continuing until the patient is ambulant. A large multicentre trial shows significant reductions in the incidence of deep vein thrombosis and pulmonary embolism when patients receiving this regimen are compared with a control group receiving no prophylaxis.[37] The only complication is wound haematoma, and this makes the method unacceptable for neurosurgical operations and operations in which a lot of dissection is necessary. Results have also been, disappointing in the high risk group of patients having hip prosthesis inserted.

Dihydroergotamine causes venous vasoconstriction thus increasing blood flow, and trials have shown that this may be useful when combined with heparin given subcutaneously. Side effects are rare but skin gangrene has been reported, and the drug has to be avoided in patients with myocardial infarction, vasospastic disorders, peripheral arterial disease or sustained hypotension.

Dextran is also effective. Its use does, however, require the intravenous infusion of 500 ml of fluid before and on at least alternate days after operation. This may interfere with fluid balance; furthermore, complications associated with bleeding are common.

In summary, a prophylactic regimen for a particular patient should be adopted after balancing the degree of risk against the potential complications of the prophylaxis. All patients at risk should wear graduated compression stockings and heparin should be given subcutaneously to patients who are particularly at high risk.

To assess the state of the art of venous thrombosis and pulmonary embolism for the medical and other health-related professions, the World Health Organisation (WHO) and the International Society and Federation of Cardiology (ISFC) convened a task force in Geneva, Switzerland. A report was subsequently prepared, revised and the final report was approved by the WHO-ISFC Task Force on pulmonary Embolism Steering Committee. More quantitative information is needed on the frequency of venous thrombosis and pulmonary embolism in hospitalized medical patients as well as in out patients at high risk. Population studies should focus on incidence, survival and long-term complications in different parts of the world with respect to gender and race. Further educational efforts are needed to increase awareness about venous thrombosis and pulmonary embolism prophylaxis. Finally, research into effective techniques for the physicians in practice would be useful.

Epidemiology

Unfortunately, estimated rates for VT and PE in population-based studies have been reported in only a few countries. There is an urgent need to develop clear criteria for assessment of VT and PE. Thus, further information should be collected regarding the frequency of VT and PE among different races and in different parts of the world. Risk factor for VT and PE can be either acquired (Table 9.6) or due to primary hypercoagulable states, which can occasionally be identified (Table 9.7). Pathologic studies have demonstrated that patients with thrombotic PEs have embolization most often to the lower lobes, whereas patients with primary thrombosis of lung blood vessels have pathologic findings more often in the upper lobes of the lung.

Table 9.6: Acquired conditions associated with pulmonary embolism[1]

Surgery
Orthopedic
Gynecological cancer
Major abdominal
Coronary artery bypass grafting
Renal transplantation
Splenectomy
Trauma
Immobilized patients
Cancer
Pregnancy/oral contraceptives
Obesity
Advanced age
Lupus anticoagulant/anticardiolipin antibodies

Table 9.7: Primary hypercoagulable states

Antithrombin III deficiency
Protein C deficiency
Protein S deficiency
Excessive plasminogen activator inhibitor

The risk of VT of the legs[38] and of PE continues for about 1 month after discharge.[39] In a Swedish autopsy study,[40] the overall incidence of VT and PE did not change over a 30-year period. During this time, the proportion of the population aged over 65 years had doubled, and this may have possibly masked the beneficial effects of prophylaxis. Population studies of incidence, survival and long-term complications from VT and PE in different parts of the world are needed to define the extent of the problem in the developing world. Isolated calf vein thrombosis and upper extremity thrombosis may be increasing in importance as antecedents to the development of PE, and their significance should be reevaluated for future plans.[2]

Diagnosis

For diagnosis, PE and VT shall be discussed simultaneously. Clinical examination should include an assessment for findings of VT, such as localized or unilateral swelling of an extremity with or without pain, and for symptoms of PE, such as sudden onset of dyspnoea or pleuritic chest pain. Diagnosis of PE should especially be considered in the presence of predisposing conditions (Table 9.6). Chest roentgenograms and electrocardiograms may demonstrate signs that help differentiate PE from other conditions and reinforce clinical suspicion. Arterial blood gas evaluation may be of adjunctive value when a decrease in the PaO_2 is observed.

When patients present with chronic cor pulmonale, chronic PE should be considered as a possible cause. Chronic PE is difficult to diagnose but is an important entity becuase it may be treatable with pulmonary thromboendarterectomy.

Investigations

Blood Tests

Fibrinogen/fibrin degradation products are elevated.

D-dimer Test

Plasma measurement of D-dimer by the enzyme-linked immunosorbent assay technique may be useful to exclude VT because of the high sensitivity of the plasma D-dimer test (about 95%).[41]

Lung Scanning

As discussed earlier pulmonary ventilation-perfusion lung scanning should be the primary screening technique used to diagnose PE in patients with histories suspicious for PE. High probability scans predict accurately the presence of PE in approximately 90% of patients with this condition and may be accepted as the definitive diagnostic procedure if alternative diagnosis are unlikely.[42] Among patients whose scans show an intermediate probability of PE, other tests, such as pulmonary angiography, contrast venography, compression ultrasound with or without color doppler imaging or impedance plethysmography, are needed to help support the diagnosis of VT.

Perfusion lung scanning is also useful for following up the resolution and/or recurrence of PE during therapy.

Echocardiography

Two-dimensional and the doppler echocardiography may have an important impact on the treatment of patients with suspected PE in selected cases. Doppler echocardiography may also be useful in suggesting alternative causes of hemodynamic impairment when acute PE is suspected, including right ventricular infarction, interventricular septal rupture and chronic pulmonary hypertension. Transoesophageal echocardiography may be especially useful in helping to exclude aortic dissection as well as in obtaining better visualization of proximal pulmonary arteries. As described earlier, there is a growing evidence that patients with non-massive pulmonary embolism who show right ventricular hypokinesia on echocardiography have poor prognosis.

Leg Evaluation

The majority of PEs arise from the deep veins of the legs. Non-invasive studies of the proximal lower leg veins therefore, provide an important adjunctive information in the evaluation of patients with PE.[43] Diagnostic modalities include compression ultrasonography,[44] impedance plethysmography[45] and doppler imaging.[46] Establishing the diagnosis of proximal VT of the legs, although it does not confirm that PE has occurred, has the same therapeutic implications and may in certain instances avoid the need for more invasive studies. Noninvasive modalities, such as compression ultrasonography with color doppler imaging, are more sensitive among patients with symptomatic VT than among those with asymptomatic disease, even in high-risk populations with high rates of proximal leg involvement. Leg examination negative for VT requires additional studies to confirm or exclude the diagnosis of PE. PE should be suspected in hypotensive patients (i) when there is evidence of or there are predisposing factors for VT and (ii) when there is clinical evidence of acute cor pulmonale (acute right ventricular failure), such as distended neck veins, an S_3 gallop, a right ventricular heave, tachycardia or tachypnoea, especially (iii) if there is electrocardiographic evidence of acute cor pulmonale manifested by a new S_1, Q_3, T_3 pattern, new incomplete right bundle-branch block or right ventricular ischemia. When feasible, the diagnosis of PE should be confirmed by pulmonary angiography or should be strengthened by ventilation-perfusion lung scanning or echocardiography.

Pulmonary Angiography

A constant intraluminal filling defect seen in more than one projection is the most reliable feature to diagnose PE among patients undergoing pulmonary angiography. Visualization of thrombi in proximal pulmonary arteries and/or in the right heart cavity by echocardiography in patients with high clinical suspicion may permit initiation of thrombolytic therapy without pulmonary angiography.

Pulmonary angiography can be accomplished with a death rate no higher than 2 to 5 per 1000.[47] Careful right heart catheterization should always be performed prior to injection of angiographic dye. When feasible, hemodynamics should be optimized prior to pulmonary angiography, especially in the presence of elevated right ventricular end-diastolic or pulmonary artery pressures. Technical factors that can enhance the safety of pulmonary angiography include (i) soft-tipped, flexible catheters with side holes or balloon floatation catheters (to avoid right ventricular perforation and pericardial tamponade); (ii) the use of selective and subselective angiography; and (iii) the use of low osmolar (or nonionic) contrast agents to minimize hemodynamic instability and to enhance patient comfort.

Pulmonary thromboembolism implies occlusion of pulmonary artery circulation by clot formed in deep veins of legs (less than 5% in other sites as well). Chest CT has virtually replaced pulmonary angiography (the earlier gold standard).

Prevention in high risk patients and adequate prescription of novel pharmacological and interventional therapeutical optimal techniques shall witness rewarding in future.[48]

Fiberoptic pulmonary angioscopy[49] and intravascular pulmonary ultrasound[50] appear useful in evaluating patients with pulmonary hypertension, who are suspected of having chronic PE and may have a role in the evaluation of acute superimposed on chronic PE. Among these patients, pulmonary angiography may not be definitive. Imaging devices such as magnetic resonance imaging and ultrafast computed tomographic scanning, which may be particularly useful in identifying chronic PE, have high sensitivity and specificity in DVT.[51] To summarize, chest X-ray is the first investigation, though it has low specificity and sensitivity. A normal lung scan rules out clinically important pulmonary embolism. A negative pulmonary angiogram rules out clinically important PE.

Treatment

Treatment, modalities include oxygen, intubation, anti-coagulation therapy, vasoactive medicines, thrombolytic therapy, embolectomy and vena cava filter placement.

Initial Anticoagulation

As discussed earlier, heparin anticoagulation is considered a fundamental therapy for most patients with PE using LMWH, unfractionated 1/4 heparin or adjusted dose subcutaneous heparin.[52] Among hemodynamically stable patients, treatment can consist of thrombolytic agents plus anticoagulation or anticoagulation alone. The risk of bleeding while receiving heparin therapy may be increased by baseline thrombocytopenia, old age, underlying diseases (e.g., undiagnosed colon cancer), and concomitant drug therapy. Heparin therapy may also be associated with a benign thrombocytopenia or, rarely, a life-threatening thrombocytopenia that causes paradoxical arterial thrombosis. Heparin should be administered initially as a bolus, followed by continuous-infusion therapy. The target range for the activated partial thromboplastin time should ordinarily be maintained between 1.5 and 2.5 times control.

Bleeding complications can be reduced by appropriate selection of patients[53] and by minimizing the handling of patients during the thrombolytic infusion. For patients with high clinical suspicion for PE and high-probability ventilation-perfusion lung scans or echocardiographic evidence of thrombi in the main pulmonary arteries or in the right heart cavity, a clinician may elect to proceed with thrombolytic therapy even when the diagnosis has not been confirmed by angiography.[54] Thrombolytic therapy should be administered through a peripheral vein rather than through a pulmonary artery catheter because the latter approach is neither safer nor more effective.[55]

Patients with hemodynamic instability, having hypotension due to PE, (i) heparin therapy and or thrombolysis; (ii) pressor agents, such as norepinephrine, and (iii) hemodynamic monitoring, should be considered. If the systemic arterial pressure is not stabilized promptly in spite of the use of thrombolytic agents, pulmonary embolectomy might be utilized in selected patients. Tenecteplase has successfully been used to treat pulmonay thromboembolism.[56]

Long-term anticoagulation is achieved with oral anticoagulation. In special circumstances such as pregnancy, prior oral anticoagulation failure, or with cancer patients undergoing chemotherapy or suspected of having Trouseau's syndrome (thrombosis that is often migratory or recurrent), long term high-dose subcutaneous heparin therapy may be utilized.

When oral anticoagulation is initiated, the level of protein C may decline, creating a thrombogenic potential. By overlapping heparin therapy and oral anticoagulation for 4 or 5 days, this theoretical procoagulant effect of oral anticoagulation can be counteracted. Oral anticoagulation is usually continued for at least 3 to 6 months but may be administered indefinitely, particularly if underlying risk factors, such as cancer or massive obesity, have not been controlled. For patients who cannot tolerate heparin therapy or oral anticoagulation, an inferior vena caval filter should be inserted.

In a few patients, PEs do not lyse but rather progress to chronic thromboembolic pulmonary hypertension, which is amenable to surgical correction (endarterectomy of chronic endothelialized thrombi). Under optimal circumstances, this operation has a mortality rate of 13%[57] although long-term results from this surgery are outstanding.[58] Catheter embolectomy appears to be a promising technique for future.[59] Catheter tip device for fragmentation of massive PE is safe and useful in patients with contraindication of thrombolytic therapy.[60,61]

Evidence-based recommendations of 6th American College of Chest Physician's (ACCP) consensus conference on anti-thrombolic therapy[52] include:

1. IV heparin adjusted with APTT for DVT and PE.
2. Heparin therapy for five days, with overlapping therapy with oral anticoagulants and discontinuation of heparin.
3. LMWH can be used in place of unfractioned heparin.
4. Long-term anticoagulation should be continued for a minimum of 12 weeks.
5. For patients with recurrent VT, treatment can be continued for indefinite period.
6. Use of thrombolytic agents has to be individualised.
7. Primary therapy should aim at life-saving restoration of blood flow in occluded pulmonary artery or to prevent potentially fatal early recurrences. An IVC filter should not be used routinely as an adjuvant to anticoagulation and systemic fibrinolysis in the treatment of acute pulmonary embolism.[62]

Prevention

It is easier and less expensive to prevent PE than to diagnose and to treat it. Virtually all hospitalized adult patients, particularly after major surgery, and all women after delivery should receive prophylactic measures against venous thromboembolism. The method of PE prevention that is utilized should be based on an assessment of the patient's level of risk for PE and on whether a patient is most likely to benefit from non-pharmacologic (Table 9.8), pharmacologic (Table 9.9), or combined (Table 9.10) modalities. Because the risk of PE continued after discharge from the hospital, prophylaxis should be continued at home among those patients at moderate or high risk for venous thromboembolism.

Table 9.8: Non-pharmacologic approaches to pulmonary embolism prophylaxis

Modality	*Mechanism of action*
Graduated compression stockings (GCS)	Prevent venous stasis
Intermittent pneumatic compression (IPC) boots	Prevent venous stasis, increase endogenous fibrinolytic activity
Inferior vena caval interruption	Prevents pulmonary embolism by mechanical blocking effect but does not prevent deep venous thrombosis
Combined non-pharmacologic methods (e.g., GCS plus IPC boots)	Additive or synergistic effect
Combined non-pharmacologic plus pharmacologic approach (e.g. IPC boots plus low dose heparin)	Additive or synergistic effect

Table 9.9: Pharmacologic prophylaxis

Unfractionated low-dose subcutaneous heparin
Low molecular weight heparin
Dextran
Adjusted-dose warfarin (orthopedic surgery)
Very low dose warfarin

Table 9.10: Recommendations for pulmonary embolism prophylaxis among special high-risk group s

High-risk group	*Recommended pulmonary embolism prophylaxis*
Orthopedic surgery in lower extremity	IPC boots plus pharmacologic prophylaxis, followed by some type of prophylaxis after hospital discharge
Gynaecologic cancer surgery	IPC boots and/or intensive pharmacologic prophylaxis
General surgery	Combined non-pharmacologic or combined non-pharmacologic plus pharmacologic modalities
Immobilized medical patients	Non-pharmacologic or pharmacologic prophylaxis

*IPC indicates intermittent pneumatic compression.

The most commonly used non-pharmacologic measures are graduated compression stockings (GCS) and intermittent pneumatic compression (IPC) boots. Overall, there are five non-pharmacologic approaches to PE prophylaxis, including several strategies that combine various preventive modalities.

Graduated Compression Stockings (GCS)

GCS often have 18 mm Hg of compression at the ankle, 14 mm Hg at the calf, 8 mm Hg at the knee, 10 mm Hg at the lower thigh and 8 mm Hg at midthigh. Among low-risk general surgery patients, GCS can reduce the frequency of VT by more than half compared with no prophylaxis. GCS should be considered as first-line prophylaxis against PE among all hospitalised patients except for those with peripheral arterial disease, whose condition may be worsened by vascular compression. Care should be taken to avoid a tourniquet effect at the proximal portion of the stockings.

Intermittent Pneumatic Compression Boots (IPC Boots)

IPC boots provide intermittent inflation of air-filled cuffs that prevent venous stasis in the legs and appear to stimulate the endogenous fibrinolytic system.

Inferior Vena Caval (IVC) Interruption

IVC interruption is usually accomplished with a filter device that mechanically blocks clinically important thrombus that arises in lower-extremity and pelvic veins thus prevents PE while maintaining patency of the IVC. These devices have no effect on the thrombotic process and do not prevent VT of the upper extremities, pelvis or deep leg veins.

The three main indications for interruption of the IVC[63,64] are (i) contraindication to anticoagulant therapy, (ii) failure of anticoagulation, and (iii) in unusual circumstances, prophylaxis among extremely high-risk patients (e.g., hip fracture surgery after recent PE or chronic severe pulmonary hypertension due to prior PE). Selection of the appropriate filter is crucial.

A well-coordinated team (preferably consisting of a vascular surgeon, interventional radiologist, cardiologist and/or vascular medicine specialist), all comprehensively and specifically trained, is the most effective way to secure the best possible results for the patient and offer learning experience for trainees.

Combined Nonpharmacologic Methods

GCS provide continuous stimulation of linear blood flow velocity and prevent dilation of the venous system in the legs. IPC devices compress the veins more forcefully than GCS but for a relatively brief period. In a randomized trial of patients undergoing general surgery, GCS plus IPC boots are found to be more effective than IPC boots alone in preventing VT.[65]

Combined Nonpharmacologic Plus Pharmacologic Approach

Among patients undergoing general surgery, several studies have demonstrated that GCS plus low-dose heparin is more effective than low-dose heparin alone in reducing the frequency of VT.[66,67]

Pharmacologic Prophylaxis

The most comprehensive randomized controlled trial of low-dose heparin prophylaxis (5000 U of subcutaneous heparin 2 hours preoperatively and every 8 hours thereafter for 7 days) as prophylaxis against fatal postoperative PE was organized by Kakkar in the International Multicentre Trial.[68] Although more wound hematomas occurred among heparin-treated patients, the number of deaths due to hemorrhage was not increased among those who received heparin.

Collins and colleagues[69] confirming the International Multicentre Trial results, showed 40% reduction in nonfatal PE and a 64% reduction in fatal PE among heparin-treated patients.

Low-Molecular-Weight Heparins (LMWH)

Low-molecular-weight heparin therapy has three major potential advantages over unfractionated heparin therapy, (i) a lower frequency of bleeding, (ii) effective prophylaxis with administration only once daily, and (iii) greater efficacy.[70] Current evidence does not indicate an increased risk of bleeding when low-molecular-weight heparins are employed in combination with epidural or spinal anesthesia. However, each of the various low-molecular-weight heparins has a distinct pharmacologic profile and should be standardized against the WHO-endorsed low-molecular-weight heparin standard.[1]

Dextran

This glucose polymer impairs platelet function by causing decreased platelet aggregability. Potential adverse effects include anaphylaxis, volume overload, nephrotoxicity, and paradoxical bleeding. Its particular niche appears to be among patients who require pharmacological prophylaxis but who are unable to receive heparin prophylaxis because of bleeding or other adverse reactions to heparin, such as heparin-associated thrombocytopenia.

Adjusted-Dose Warfarin

In patients at high risk, adjusted-dose warfarin prophylaxis may be appropriate.

Very Low-Dose Warfarin

Further trials, however, are needed before its use is recommended.[1]

Approach for Special High Risk Groups

Orthopedic Surgery

Orthopedic patients should be considered for combined non-pharmacologic and pharmacologic prophylaxis while hospitalized, followed by some form of prophylaxis for approximately 1 month after hospital discharge. Alternatively, predischarge ultrasonography could be performed on all patients, and those without deep VT might not require further prophylaxis.[71] Patients undergoing total knee replacement are at as high a risk of developing PE as patients undergoing total hip replacement.[72]

Gynecologic Cancer Surgery

Patients who develop proximal leg-deep VT and PE after gynecologic cancer surgery often have no evidence of calf vein thrombosis. The thrombi appear to arise de novo in the pelvic or proximal deep veins of the leg.[73] Non-pharmacological prophylaxis, if utilized, should consist of IPC boots. If pharmacological prophylaxis selected, intensive fixed low-dose heparin (5000 U subcutaneously three times daily) is suggested.

Immobilized Medical Patients

Among immobilized patients who are not critically ill, fibrinogen leg scanning identifies deep VT in 13%.[74] Therefore, immobilized medical patients should routinely receive non-pharmacologic or pharmacologic prophylaxis.

Cost-effectiveness of PE Prevention

Prophylaxis not only saves lives but also is cost-effective. In an analysis of patients undergoing major orthopedic surgery, all prophylaxis methods saved health care dollars.[75] In a separate analysis of general surgery patients, the most cost-effective approach was GCS.[76]

New Agents to Prevent VT

Specific antithrombin drugs that are being developed, such as hirudin, have promise in the prevention of venous thrombosis.[1]

Prophylaxis against VT and PE continues to be underutilized, despite the availability of effective non-pharmacologic and pharmacologic methods.[77] The intensification of prophylaxis efforts, with particular attention to special high-risk patients during hospitalization and for the first month after hospital discharge has been endorsed. All clinicians should review the thrombophylaxis policy at their institutions and should devise a system in which the risk for every hospitalized patient is assessed pre-operatively. Especially in high-risk patients, the prophylactic period should be one month minimum.

Pulmonary embolism in the elderly is common due to higher tendency for venous stasis, decreased venous tone, reduced fibrinolytic activity in leg veins and immobility. Prophylactic dose of subcutaneous lower molecular weight heparin is useful.[78]

Pulmonary Embolism and Air Travel[79-81]

Pulmonary thromboembolism (PTE) after air travel was reported in 1954; the term economy class syndrome was coined in 1977 following development of PTE in people after travelling by air in the coach class which has restricted leg space, leading to venous stasis, postulated to be chief precipitating factor, in addition to release of vein wall relaxin factor due to immobility that also enhances venous stasis. Additional factors include dehydration causing hemoconcentration, lowed oxygen tension in the aircraft impairing fibrinolysis as well as activating coagulation process, enhanced fluid retension causing legs-swelling and increased levels of erythropoietin and circulating proteins. There is two to eight-fold rise in (activated) hypercoagulation in the hypobaric aircraft environments. Within one hour the aircraft, hematological changes start appearing. Blood vessel lesions due to seat compression do enhance thrombosis. Thus, Virchow's triad of stasis, hypercoagulability and vessel trauma during air travel enhance the risk of venous thrombosis.

Maintaining good hydration, avoiding leg crossing and tight clothing and completing avoiding tobacco and alcohol help in preventing venous thrombosis.

Short walks, changing leg position and moving left as regular intervals are very useful.

Elastic compression stockings are helpful but may increase the risk of inducing superficial venous thrombosis.

REFERENCES

1. Goldhaber Z. and Molpurgo M., Diagnosis, treatment and prevention of pulmonary embolism, Report of WHO/ International Society and Federation of Cardiology Task Force, JAMA india 1991; 12:29-30.
2. Quinn D.A., Thompson B.T., Terrin M.L., *et al.*, A prospective investigation of pulmonary embolism in women and men, JAMA 1992; 268: 1689-96.
3. Centers for Disease Control. CDC Surveillance summaries, MMWR 1991; 40: 1-13.
4. Karwinski B. and Svendsen E., Comparison of clinical and postmortem diagnosis of pulmonary embolism, J. Clin. Pathol 1989; 42:135-39.
5. Palevsky H.I., Pulmonary hypertension and thromboembolic disease in women, Cardiovasc Clin 1986; 140:667-71.
6. Bernstein D., Goupey S. and Schonberg S.K., Pulmonary embolism in adolescents. AJDC 1986; 140:667-71.
7. Coon W. Epidemiology of venous thromboembolism. Ann Surg 1977; 186: 149-64.
8. Coon W.W., Willis P.W. and Keller J.B., Venous thrombosis and other venous diseases in the Tecumseh community study, Circulation 1973; 48 : 839-46.
9. Breckenridge R.T. and Ralnoff O.D., Pulmonary embolism and unexpected death in supposedly normal persons, N. Engl. J. Med 1964; 270:298-99.
10. Karwinski B. and Svendsen E., Comparison of clinical and postmortem diagnosis of pulmonary embolism, J. Clin. Pathol 1989; 42: 135-39.
11. Goldhaber S_2-; Pulmonary embolism; Lancet 2004; 363: 1295-1305. Piazza G; Goldhaber S_2; Acute pulmonary embolism–Part II–Treatment and proplylaxis; Circulation 2006; 114: e 42-e 47.
12. Sutton P.P. and Clarke S.W., Diagnostic criteria for pulmonary embolism, J. App. Med 1981; 7:893-901.
13. Sinha, N. and Kumar S, Pulmonary embolism management: An update; In; Thakur, B.B. ed.; P.G. Medicine; API; Mumbai 2002, 16: 151-74.
14. Poulose K.P. and Sahajanandan V.K., The incidence and diagnosis of pulmonary embolism, J. Ass. Phys. Ind 1973; 21: 45-49.
15. Bell W.R., Simpon T.L. and Demets D.L., The clinical features of submassive and massive pulmonary embolism, Am. Med 1977; 672:355.
16. Stein P.D., Dalen J.E. and Mcintyre K.M., *et al.*, The electrocardiogram in acute pulmonary embolism, Prog Cardiovas Dis 1975; 17:247.
17. Szucs M.M. Jr., Brooks H., Grossmen W., *et al.*, Diagnostic sensitivity of laboratory findings in acute pulmonary embolism Ann. Intern. Med 1971; 74: 161.
18. The PIOPED Investigators, Value of ventilation perfusion scan in acute pulmonary embolism: Results of the prospective investigation of pulmonary embolism diagnosis PIOPED, JAMA 1990; 263-75.
19. Hull R.D., Hirsh J., Carter C.J., *et al.* Pulmonary angiography; ventilation lung scanning and venography for clinically suspected pulmonary embolism with abnormal lung scan. Ann Intern. Med 1983; 98: 891.
20. Come P.C., Echocardiographic recognition of pulmonary arterial disease and determination of its causes, Am. J. Med 1988; 84: 384.
21. Mussett D., Rosse T., Prtitprez P., *et al.*, Acute pulmonary embolism, diagnostic value of digital substraction angiography, Radiology 1988; 166: 455.
22. Bala Krishnan J., Meziane M.A., Siegelman S.S. and Fishman E.K., Pulmonary infarction, CT appearance with pathologic correlation, J. Comput. Asst. Tomogr 1989; 13:941.
23. Szucs R.A., Rehr R.B. and Ratum J.L., Pulmonary artery thrombus detection by MRI, Chest 1989; 95:232.
24. Shure D., Greogorates G. and Moser K.M., Fiberoptic angioscopy; role in the diagnosis of chronic pulmonary arterial obstruction, Ann. Intern. Med 1985; 103: 844.

25. Shantaran V., PE Clinical recognition and diagnosis, In: Chandrasekharan S., ed, Medicine Update; Assn. Phys India, Bombay 1993; 3:84-94.
26. Secker-Walker R.H. and Roger H., In; Respiratory diseases in clinical nuclear medicine, eds. M.M. Masey, M.E. Britton and D.I. Gliday. Chapman and Hale 1983; 41-58.
27. Warkentin, T.E.; Heparin induced thrombocytopenia; a clinicopathologic syndrome. Throm Haemost 1999; 82. 439.
28. Hull R.D., *et al.*, LMWH vs. heparin in the treatment of patients with PE; American-Canadian Thrombosis Study Group; Arch. Inter. Med 2000; 160: 229.
29. Dolovich L.R., *et al.*, A meta analysis comparing LMWH with unfractioned heparin in the treatment of venous.
30. Vidhya M.R., Sathyamurthy I.; Current status of LMWH in clinical practice; JAPI 2000; 48: 276-320.
31. Byard R.W. and Cutz E., Sudden and unexpected death in infancy and childhood due to pulmonary thromboembolism: An autopsy study. Arch Pathol Lab Med 1990; 1114: 142-44.
32. Bernstein D., Coupey S. and Schonberg K., Pulmonary embolism in adolescents, AJDC 1986; 140: 667-71.
33. Gracey D.R.,McMichan J.C., Divertie M.B. and Howard R.T. Jr., Respiratory failure in Guillain-Barre syndrome, Mayo Clin. Proc 1982; 57: 142-46.
34. Raman K., Blake J.A. and Hanris T.M., Pulmonary embolismin Landry-Guillain-Barrne-Strohl syndrome, Chest 1971; 60: 555-57.
35. Prevention of venous thrombosis and pulmonary embolism, NIH Consensus Conference. JAMA 1986; 256: 144-49.
36. Zerdhling R.G., Pulmonary embolism in children: risks and prevention, JAMA 1991;265, 2888.
37. Bergqvist D. and Lindblad B., A 30-year survey of pulmonary embolism verified at autopsy. An analysis of 1274 surgical patients, Br. J. Surg 1985; 72: 105-08.
38. Scurr J.H., Coleridge-Smith P.D. and Hasty J.H., Deep venous thrombosis: A continuing problem, BM 1988; 297: 28.
39. Huber O., Bounameaux H., Borst F. and Ronher A., Postoperative pulmonary embolism after hospital discharge: An underestimated risk. Arch Surg 1992; 127:310-13.
40. Lindad B., Sternby N.H. and Bergqvst D., Incidence of venous thromboembolism verified by necropsy over 30 years, BMJ 1991; 302: 709-11.
41. Bounanmeaux H., Cirafici P., de Moerloose P., *et al.*, Measurement of D-dimer in plasma as diagnostic aid in suspected pulmonary embolism, Lancet 1991; 337(1) 196-200.
42. The PIOPED Investigators. Value of the ventilation/perfusion scan in acute pulmonary embolism: Results of the Prospective Investigation of Pulmonary Embolism Diagnosis (PIOPED), JAM A 1990; 263: 2753-59.
43. Leclere J.R., Illescas F. and Jarzem P., Diagnosis of deep vein thrombosis, In; Leclere J.R., ed. Venous thromboembolic disorders, Philadelphia, Pa: Lea and Febiger 1991; 176-228.
44. Lensing A.W.A., Prandoni P., Brandjes D., *et al.*, Detection of deep-vein thrombosis by real-time B-mode ultrasonography. N.Eng. J.Med 1989; 320: 342-45.
45. Huisman M.V., Buller H.R. ten Cate J.W. and Vreeken J., Serial impedance plethysmography for suspected deep venous thrombosis in outpatients, N. Engl. J. Med 1986; 314: 823-28.
46. Lensing A.W.A., Levi M.M., Buller H.R., *et al.* Diagnosis of deep-vein thrombosis using an objective doppler method Ann Intern Med 1990; 113:9-13.
47. Stein P.D., Athanasoulis C., Alavi A., *et al.*, Complications and validity of pulmonary angiography in acute pulmonary embolism, Circulation 1992; 85: 462-68.
48. Prasad BN BM; Pulmonary thromboembolism–Indian scenario; IN; A. Muruganathan: ed: Med Update; API 2013; 23: 493-502.
49. Shure D., Gregoratos G. and Moser K.M., Fiberoptic angioscopy, role in the diagnosis of chronic pulmonary arterial obstruction. Ann Intern Med 1985; 103: 844-50.
50. Ricou F., Nicod P.H., Moser K.M. and Peterson K.L., Catheter-based intravascular ultrasound imaging of chronic thromboembolic pulmonary disease, Am. J. Cardiol 1991; 67:749-52.
51. Spritzer C.E. *et al.*, Detection of deep vein thrombosis by MRI; Chest 1993; 104: 54-60.
52. Hirsh T., Dalen T.E., Guyatt G., 6th ed (2000) ACCP guidelines for antithrombotic therapy for prevention and treatment of thrombosis; Chest 2000; 119 (1 suppl.): 15-25.
53. Kearon C., *et al.*, A comparison of three months of anticoagulation with extended coagulation for a first episode of idiopathic venous thromboembolism; M. Eng. J. Med 1999; 340: 901.
54. Hyers T.M. *et al.*, Anti-thrombotic therapy for venous thromboembolic disease; Chest 2001; 119 (1 sypp.): 1765.
55. Verstraete M., Miller G.A.H., Bounameaux H., *et al.*, Intravenous and intrapulmonary recombinant tissue-type plasminogen activator in the treatment of acute massive pulmonary embolism, Circulation 1988;77: 353-60.
56. Sharma A., *et al.*, Pulmonary thromboembolism and right heart thromboembolism—An experience with tenecteplase; JAPI 2012; 60:52-3.
57. Daily P.O., Dembitsky W.P., Iversen S., Moser K.M. and Auger W., Risk factors for pulmonary thromboendarterectomy. J. Throrac Cardiovasc Surg 1990; 99: 670-78.
58. Moser K.M., Auger W.R. and Fedullo P.E., Chronic major vessel thromboembolic pulmonary hypertension, Circulation 1990; 81: 1735-43.
59. Timsit J.F., Reyaud P., Meyer G. and Sors H., Pulmonary embolectomy by catheter device in massive pulmonary embolism, Chest 1991; 100: 655-58.
60. Schmitz-Rode T., *et al.*, Massive pulmonary embolism; percutaneous emergency treatment by pigtail rotation catheter; J. Am. Coll. Cardiol 2000; 36: 375.
61. Kucher N; *et al.*, Massive pulmonary embolism; Circulation 2006; 113: 577-82.
62. Culshanjit Singh; *et al.*, When to intervene in pulmonary embolism and how? IN; SR Joshi ed; Med Update API 2014; 24: 1125-32.
63. Streiff M.B.; Vena caval filters; A comprhensive review; Blood 2000; 95: 3669.
64. Lorch H., *et al.*, Current practice of temporary vena caval filter insertion; a multicenter registry; J. Vasc. Interv. Radiol 2000; 11: 83.
65. Scurr J.H., Coleridge-Smith P.D. and Hasty J.H., Regimen for improved effectiveness of intermittent pneumatic compression in deep venous thrombosis prophylaxis, Surgery1987; 102:816-20.

66. Torngren S., Low dose heparin and compression stockings in the prevention of post operative deep venous thrombosis Br. J. Surg 1980; 67: 482-84.
67. Wille-Jorgensen P., Thorup J., Fischer A., Holst-Christensen J. and Flamsholt R., Heparin with and without graded compresssion stockings in the prevention of thromboembolic complications of major abdominal surgery: A randomized trial, Br. J., Surg 1985; 72:579-81.
68. International Multicentre Trial, Prevention of fatal postoperative pulmonary embolism by low doses of heparin, Lancet 1975; 2: 45-51.
69. Collins R., Scrimgeour A., Yusuf S. and Peto R., Reduction in fatal pulmonary embolism and venous thrombosis by perioperative administration of subcutaneous heparin: Overview of results of randomized trials in general, orthopedic and urologic surgery, N. Engl. J. Med 1988; 318: 1162-71.
70. Verstraete M., Pharmacotherapeutic aspects of unfractionated and low molecular weight heparins, Drugs 1990; 40:498-530.
71. Paiement G.D., Wessinger S.R. and Harris W.H., Cost-effectiveness of prophylaxis in total hip replacement, Am. J. Surg 1991; 161: 519-24.
72. Foley M., Maslack M.M., Rothman R.H., *et al.,* Pulmonary embolism after hip or knee replacement: Post operative changes on pulmonary scintigrams in asymptomatic patients, Radiology 1989;172:481-85.
73. Clarke-Pearson D.L., Synan I.S., Colemen R.E., Hinshaw W. and Creasman W.T., The natural history of postoperative venous thromboemboli in gynaecologic oncology. A prospective study of 382 patients. Am. J. Obstet. Gynaecol 1984; 148: 1051-54.
74. Gulati V; Pulmonary thromboembolism–proplylaxis and management issues; IN; RK Singal, DG Jain: ed: Med Update; API 2007; 17: 155-62.
75. Oster G., Tuden R.L. and Colditz G.A., A cost-effectiveness analysis of prophylaxis against deep-vein thrombosis in major orthopedic surgery, JAMA 1987; 257: 203-08.
76. Oster G., Tuden R.L. and Colditz G.A., Prevention of venous thromboembolism after general surgery: Cost-effectiveness analysis of alternative approaches to prophylaxis, Am. J. Med 1981; 82: 889-99.
77. Anderson F.A. Jr., Wheeler H.B., Goldberg R.J., Hosmer D.W., Forcier A. and Patwardhan N.A., Physician's practices in the prevention of venous thromboembolism, Ann Intern Med 1991; 115: 591-55.
78. Chopra H.K. Acute pulmonary thromboembolism: Management update; IJCP (Cardiology) 1994; 55-70.
79. Lapostolle F; *et al.,* Severe pulmonary embolism associated with air travel; N Eng J Med 2001; 345: 779-83.
80. Bendz B; *et al.,* Association between acute hypobaric hypoxia and activation of coagulation in human beings; Lancet 2000; 356: 1657-65.
81. Bhatia V; *et al.,* Air travel and pulmonary embolism–economy class syndrome; JAPI 2009; 57: 412-14.

Diseases of Undetermined Aetiology

10

SARCOIDOSIS

Sarcoidosis is a granulomatous disorder of unknown aetiology, effecting many systems, mostly in young adults, usually presenting as bilateral hilar lymphadenopathy (BHL) with or without pulmonary parenchymal infiltrates, and characterised by enhanced cellular immune processes at the site of involvement. Recognized by Schaumann in 1917 for multi-system nature of the disorder, Lofgren in 1940 described the classical syndrome of hilar lymphadenopathy and erythema nodosum. Gold standard for diagnosis is based on the presence of compatible clinical illness, the histologic demonstration of non-caseating granuloma[1] and absence of other causes of granuloma formation.

Incidence

It is a global problem but more commonly seen in the Scandinavian countries, the U.K., Northern Europe, the U.S.A. and Australia. A steadily increasing number of cases being documented from India, sarcoidosis in the tropics is no longer considered to be very rare. More than two hundred and fifty cases have already been reported from India itself, including about a hundred in 1984-85. However, cases of paediatric sarcoidosis are still rare in India (six cases reported so far),[2-4] as well as in the West.[5,6] Among the Asian countries, China, Japan, Philippines and Malaysia have reported[7,8] only a few cases. It rarely develops before 10 years and after 60 years of age. In India only six cases of paediatric sarcoidosis (1-15 years) have been detected so far.[9-11] It is common in blacks. Sarcoidosis in India has been reported to be occurring most frequently in adult males above 40 years,[10,11] whereas in the West, women below 40 are the most common victims.[12] Type I sarcoidosis is most common presentation, occurring more in North India and is more amenable to steroid therapy.[13] No such characterisation of paediatric sarcoidosis has yet been possible owing to insufficient material for analysis.

Pathology and Pathogenesis[14]

Widespread, non-caseating granulomas are formed in response to some undetermined stimulus. Pathological features include inflammation in the lung as alveolitis, leading to non-caseating granuloma formation that may resolve or progress to fibrosis. Fine miliary pattern affecting the upper lobes is commonly seen. Pleural involvement many occur in 1/3rd of the cases microscopically, but clinical presentations are uncommon. Pulmonary artery hypertrophy may be seen in the late stage. In sarcoidosis, there is possibly an abnormal immunoregulation. It starts as an inflammatory reaction representing an interaction between the alveolar macrophages, T-lymphocytes and mediators such as interleukin-1, interleukin-2 and gamma interferon to result in an alveolitis, to be followed by formation of a granuloma. There are well-demarcated oval collection of large pale epitheloid cells with abundant cytoplasm and centrally placed multinucleated giant cells surrounded by little cellular reaction[1] of lymphocytes, macrophages, monocytes and fibro-blasts. An intact reticulin surrounds the nodules. There is no caseation and the granuloma is classically non-caseating. A minor degree of fibrinoid necrosis, however, may be seen in the centre. Occasionally, inclusion bodies (crystalline, conchoidal or asteroid) may be seen. The lesions may resolve or progress to non-specific residual hyaline fibrotic lesions.[7]

Clinical Features[12,14]

Clinical presentation includes fever, bilateral hilar lymphadenopathy, ankle pain, erythma nodosum, interstitial lung disease, uveitis etc. The diagnosis rests on a triad of consistent radiology, non-caseating granulomatous inflammation and absence of other causes of granuloma formation such as fungus or mycobacteria. The clinical manifestations of the disease depend on the tissue involvement as well as the degree of inflammation and fibrosis. Intrathoracic involvement is noted in 90 per cent of all patients of sarcoidosis.

About one-third of the patients are asymptomatic and the condition is recognised because of an abnormal chest roentgenogram. Extrapulmonary involvements include skin, eyes, abdomen, heart and CNS. Sarcoid myopathy, cardiomyopathy and neuropathy may also occur. Cardiac involvement in sarcoidosis includes pericardium, myocardium, and conducting system and result in either diffuse microscopic focal infiltrates or larger nodules within the myocardium posterior wall is predominantly affected and mitral regurgitation is not uncommon. Global left ventricular dysfunction and malignant ventricular arrhythmias, mimicking dilated cardiomyopathy may be present with disseminated sarcoidosis. Rarely thromocytopenia may occur in upto 2% of cases, which is immune mediated.[15-17] Depending on the involvement of lymph nodes and lung parenchyma, the radiographic appearances are classified into different disease types.

Type 0

Chest X-ray may be normal and only extrapulmonary disease is evident. This is seen in 5-10% of cases.

Type 1

There is bilateral symmetric hilar adenopathy involving tracheobronchial lymph glands, often accompanied by the right paratracheal adenopathy. Parenchymal infiltration is absent. The condition often remains asymptomatic. There may be associated erythema nodosum or uveitis. This is seen in 40-60% of cases.

Type 2

Both pulmonary parenchyma and nodes are involved. The parenchymal abnormalities may be in the form of fine reticular or reticulonodular infiltrates or alveolar or large pulmonary nodes. The infiltrations may sometimes obscure hilar adenopathy. This is seen in 25-35% of cases.

Type 3

This is a more advanced form of the disease. It exhibits pulmonary parenchymal infiltrates without demonstrable adenopathy. There is pulmonary fibrosis. Marked physiologic abnormalities and pulmonary hypertension may develop in late fibrotic stage. Resolution is infrequent. Progressive lesions may produce cystic changes facilitating colonisation with aspergillus, resulting in aspergilloma. There can be pleural thickening overlying cysts. This is seen in 5-15% of cases. Cases with unilateral hilar lymph adenopathy have also been reported from India.[1] Approximately 50% of patients of sarcoidosis present with stage I disease. Unilateral hilar lymphadenopathy is uncommon being reported in 3-5% of proven cases.[18] Transition from type 1 to 3 is usual but reversal from 3 to 2 or 2 to 1 is unusual. Gradually increasing breathlessness and cough are most common respiratory symptoms.

Acute sarcoidosis has features of erythema nodosum, periarthritis and bilateral hilar lymphadenopathy on chest X-ray.[19] Erythema nodosum as a non-specific hypersensitivity reaction may be noted with fever, polyarthralgia and hilar adenopathy during the early stages of the disease as a characteristic of sarcoidosis. The patients may exhibit periodic fever, fatigue and weight loss as non-specific constitutional symptoms. Haemoptysis may occur when cystic changes and aspergilloma have developed in the lung. Rarely bronchial passages may be narrowed from endobronchial granuloma or from external compression by the glands leading to a sudden onset of breathlessness and wheezing. The sarcoid lymph nodes do not erode the bronchus. There is a dissociation between the marked radiologic changes and a few clinical signs.[14]

Incidence of sarcoid pleural effusion ranges from 0.7 to 4%. Effusion is an exudate containing a predominance of lymphocytes and pleural biopsy shows non-caseating granulomas. Higher incidence of pleural effusion (7%) and pleural thickening (3%),[20] which clears in 4-8 weeks though in some cases, progresses to chronic pleural thickening, have also been reported.

Cutaneous involvements are in the form of granulomatous lesions or granular plaques on the skin (erythema nodosum, persistent violaceous skin lesions and maculopapular lesions). In addition there can be cervical lymphadenopathy, unilateral or bilateral painless parotid gland enlargement, lacrimal swelling, hepatosplenomegaly, involvement of the eyes (uveitis, conjuncival nodules, keratocon (junctivitis sicca), Bell's palsy, involvement of metacarpal, metatarsal bones and terminal phalanges with lattice-like, or punched out cyst-like rarefaction, nephrocalcinosis due to prolonged hypercalcemia and hypercalciuria, renal insufficiency, arrhythmias and heart failure[14] and conduction abnormalities in the heart.

In paediatric sarcoidosis, some of the clinical features are essentially the same as seen in adults, with fever, little incapacitation and arthralgia as prominent complaints. On the contrary, chest complaints have been conspicuously absent as are distinctive biochemical abnormalities.[4] Pulmonary functions show a restrictive element alone or in association with airway obstruction[21] a feature similar to that in adults.[10,11] Kendig and Brummer[22] noted that 9 of 11 children had reduced FVC during acute exacerbation of the disease. Biopsy positivity also appear to be similar as in adults.[23] SACE values have been found to be identical in adults and children in the normal population.[24] Features include abdominal pain and massive splenomegaly. Lymphadenopathy and Sicca syndrome, which are decidedly rare in adults, have been reported in children.[25]

Neurosarcoidosis is rare both in the West (4-7%)[12] and in India (11%).[10,11] There is only one report of neurosarcoidosis in Indian children.[3] The facial nerve, unlike in children, is said to be most frequently involved, causing a lower motor neurone type of palsy with or without impairment of taste sensation.[12] Though arthralgia is one of the most common manifestations of sarcoidosis, such severe pain with effusion is very unusual.[4] Nodule at a Mantoux test negative site[26] is at present regarded as a diagnostic aid in the Indian subcontinent. It does not appear that paediatric sarcoidosis is essentially different from that in adults as a disease entity. The peculiarities found are probably normal variations as has also been found in adults in the form of abdominal mass, isolated unilateral hilar lymphadenopathy, superior vena caval obstruction, etc. However, definite comments are not possible in view of the small number of paediatric cases detected to date.[4] MMR surveys may reveal more asymptomatic cases, as have been done in Japan.[5] Diagnosis will, nevertheless, remain a problem due to lack of awareness amongst physicians in India, prevalence of tuberculosis, the considerable expenses involved in proper investigations and the lack of health consciousness among the population.[4]

Differential diagnosis includes berylliosis, tuberculosis, Farmer's lung, fungal infections, rheumatic fever, rheumatoid arthritis and carcinoma lymph node (lymphoma).

Investigations

An impaired cell-mediated (T-lymphocytes) immunity is shown by deficient delayed cutaneous reactivity and lymphopaenia. There is relative tuberculin anergy. There is cutaneous hyporeactivity to recall antigens like mumps virus, candida, trycophytin and dinitrochlorobenzene. The humoral immunocompetence (B cells) is well-preserved. Hypergammaglobulinaemia is present.

Kveim Siltzbach test[14] is utilized for sarcoid granuloma formation. A papule develops in four to six weeks at the site of intradermal injection of 0.1-0.2 ml of heat sterilised suspension of sarcoid tissue obtained from cervical glands or from spleen. Histologically it demonstrates non-caseating granuloma and it is positive in 80 per cent patients with active sarcoidosis. Lack of adequately standardised material has limited its diagnostic value.

BAL is useful in knowing activity of the disease[27] and reveals cells and substances that reflect inflammation and immune activity. Non-caseating granuloma is classically seen in the biopsy of skin lesions, lymph nodes, conjunctival nodules or transbronchial biopsy of the lung. Serum calcium is raised due to overproduction of vitamin D metabolite with resultant increased intestinal calcium absorption. Hypercalciuria is frequent. Pulmonary function tests show a volume restriction (reduced vital capacity and total lung capacity) and an impaired diffusion capacity that may be seen in 20 to 30 per cent of patients with normal chest X-rays. The physiologic defect may not be significant in spite of dense infiltrates seen radiologically.[14] Serum ACE levels have been found to be significantly higher, compared to pulmonary tuberculosis and normal healthy controls.[28]

Radiological Signs in Pulmonary Sarcoidosis[29]

Sarcoid Sign

In pulmonary sarcoidosis, bilateral hilar lymphadenopathy seen on X-ray chest is in fact due to enlargement of peribronchial lymph nodes: this is best appreciated on the right side. The contour of the outer border of enlarged hila is usually lobulated. A radiolucent area is seen between the medial aspect of the enlarged glands at the hilum and the cardiac border. This represents the bronchus intermedius, suggesting that the enlarged lymph nodes are peribronchially located. When widespread pulmonary shadows are associated with bilateral hilar node enlargement, and particularly when these are set out from the hilar regions in such a way as to show transradient lung between the enlarged glands and the mediastinum, then the features are virtually pathognomonic.

Whereas large masses mimick malignancy, fine nodular shadows simulating a miliary pattern (but without lymph node enlargement) is seen only in less than 2% of cases and has recently been documented.[30]

Egg Shell Calcification

What is appropriately described as egg shell calcification was earlier reported by Scadding.[31] Calcification of hilar lymph nodes has beem reported in roughly 5% of patients. Such calcification is usually a late manifestation of sarcoidosis. It is invariably associated with advance pulmonary disease and in some instances, with steroid therapy.[32]

The pulmonary function studies are used for objective assessment of improvement during therapy with steroids.

In contrast to blood, T lymphocytes are increased in number and function in lavage fluid implying an increased cellular immune activity at sites of sarcoid involvement. There is an increased uptake of Gallium 67 and it may be used to localise the inflammatory process in the hilum and mediastinal lymph nodes and pulmonary parenchyma. This happens in tuberculosis, malignancies etc. It is therefore non-specific.

Prognosis[14]

Spontaneous resolution may occur in sarcoidosis with erythema nodosum, fever and bilateral hilar lymphadenopathy.

The prognosis is good in the younger age group and it may resolve in 50 to 75 per cent of patients with type 1 disease and 25 to 75 per cent of patients with type 2 disease. Resolution is infrequent in type 3 disease.

Treatment

There is no specific treatment.[14] The features, in early stage of disease such as bilateral hilar adenopathy, febrile arthralgia and erythema nodosum can be controlled with the use of anti-inflammatory agents (aspirin, ibuprofen or indomethacin).

Pulmonary granulomatous condition progresses to cause functional abnormality and symptoms of increasing breathlessness, needs corticosteroids as a suppressive therapy. The steroids are indicated on the basis of functional abnormalities and not on abnormal radiological shadows in the lung. Corticosteroids are also used in situations of bronchostenosis and in the treatment of uveitis, hypercalcemia, leptomeningitis and conduction detects.[14]

Corticosteroids appear to suppress granuloma formation and to decrease the immune and inflammatory response. Generally prednisolone is given in a dose of 40 mg a day for four weeks; later the dose is reduced and continued as a maintenance dose of 5 to 10 mg daily for another eight months. Corticosteroids show a beneficial effect in those presenting symptoms. The drug can be stopped on relief of symptoms, regression of radiological shadows and functional improvement. Relapses require reinstitution of high doses of steroids.

For symptomatic relief or for progressive disease, steroids if instituted earlier, will help in stabilisation of disease or reversal of granulomatous process.[33,34] Though it is ameliorative in patients with pulmonary involvement, it is unlikely to prevent pulmonary fibrosis in all cases.

Hypercalcemia and hypercalciuria require reduced intake of calcium and vitamin D. The absorption of calcium from the intestine may be reduced by administration of sodium phytate. The cutaneous manifestations of sarcoid can be suppressed by chloroquine phosphate 500 mg daily for two weeks followed by a maintenance dose of 250 mg for six months. It even regresses radiological shadows in the lung and often dyspnoea is reduced.[35,36] The side effects of chloroquine like myopathy and ocular toxicity should be watched. Immunosuppressive agents have been tried with clinical improvement in some.[14] Cyclosporin, methotrexate, cyclophosphamide have been used as steroid sparing drugs.[37,38]

Levamisole has given good results in one study.[39] Successful transplantation of heart, lung and kidney has been described.[38] Possible beneficial effects of radiotherapy have been documented.[37]

As far as treatment in paediatric sarcoidosis is concerned, it is a reassuring feature that none has yet needed prolonged cortiocosteroids for control. Prolonged steroid use in children is frought with many dangers including growth retardation. Paediatric sarcoidosis may be more responsive. Steroids have to be used as a last resort. Topically active steroid aerosols may be suitable substitutes, if pulmonary affection is predominant —there will be no effect, however, on the multisystem involvement. Since adult patients have little chance of spontaneous remission,[10,11] the paediatric cases will also possibly behave identically. For symptomatic relief, non-steroidal anti-inflammatory drugs like ibuprofen, choloroquine (15 mg/kg/day) or N-phthalylanthranilic acid (20 mg/kg/day) may be initially combined with a short, intensive course of steroid to prevent lung damage by the initial intense alveolitis and to check fibrosis.[4] This may later be substituted by steroid aerosol, if situation permits.[39] Role of antimicrobial therapy in sarcoidosis has recently been reviewed and it gives a definite thought for future.[40]

Coordinated diagnostic approach help in clinching the diagnosis of ILD. VATS gives sizable sample of lung tissue. Corticosteroids are useful in sarcoidosis or certain subsets of ILD. Supportive care for associated pulmonary hypertension. Lung transplantation offers survival for some patients.[41]

Salient Features of Pulmonary Sarcoidosis[42]

- Asymptomatic hilar adenopathy or ILD with alveolitis in 27-45% of Indian sarcoid patients.
- Pleural effusion in 5% of cases.
- Endobronchial involvement in 50% of cases and may lead to airway stenosis in 10% of cases.
- Cough, dyspnea, chest pain, wheeze and lung crackles in 20% of cases.
- Stage 0. Normal.
  1. BHL.
  2. Adenopathy with pulmonary infiltrates.
  3. Pulmonary infiltrates only.
  4. Pulmonary fibrosis.
- Contrast enhanced computed tomography (CECT) is a better modality to look for parenchymal involvement and non-necrotic hilar lymph nodes.

REFERENCES

1. Mathur R.S. and Shah J.R., Unusual manifestations of sarcoidosis, JAPI 1987; 35:855-57.
2. Kashyan S, *et al.*, Clinical profile of sarcoidosis in Himachal Pradesh, Northern India; JAPI 1997; 45 (5):374-75.
3. Gupta Samir K. and Chatterjee S; Systemic and neurosarcoidosis in a child, Indian Pediatrics 1983; 20: 380-81.
4. Gupta Samir K. and Mitra K., Pediatric sarcoidosis, JAPI 1988; 36:150-53.
5. Kendig E.L., The clinical picture of sarcoidosis in children, Pediatrics 1974; 54: 289-92.
6. Jones R.E., Chathem W.W., Update on sarcoidosis; Curr. Opin. Rheum 1999; 11:83-87.
7. Hosoda Y., Kosuda T., Yamamoto M., *et al.*, A co-operative study of sarcoidosis in Asia and Africa: Descriptive epidemiology, Ann N.Y., Acad. Sci 1976; 278: 347-54.

8. Bovornkitti S., Sarcoidosis in Asia. Siriraj Hosp Gaz 1982; 34: 45-48.
9. Gupta Samir K., Sarcoidosis in India, Long term follow-up report of a series. J. Assoc. Phys Ind 1982; 30: 304-08.
10. Gupta Sarnir K., Mitra Koushik, Chatterjee S and Chakravarty S.C., Sarcoidosis in India. Br. J. Dis. Chest 1985; 79:275-83.
11. Gupta Samir K. Mitra Koushik, Roy M. and Dutta S.K., Sarcoidosis in India, Ind. J. Chest Dis. All. Sci 1985; 27: 55-63.
12. Scadding J.G. and Mitchell D.N., Sarcoidosis, London, Chapman and Hall 1985 43-71.
13. Panda B.N.;S arcoidosisinIndia:Anevaluation of 60 cases; Lung India 2000; 18:70-73.
14. Shankar P.S., Sarcoidosis: In: Chest Medicine, Oxford and IBH Publ. Co. (P) Ltd. N. Delhi, 1994; 4th ed.
15. Daniel R.P.; Immunology of sarcoidosis; Semin. Resp. Med 1991; 12: 204.
16. Balbi B., *et al.*, Increased number of T lymphocytes with p and Tantigen receptors in a subgroup of individuals with pulmonary sarciodosis; J Chin. Investi 1990; 85; 1353.
17. Agarwal U *et al.*, Thrombopenia as the presenting mainfestation of sarcoidosis; JAPI 2002; 50:68-69.
18. Kent D.C., Recurrent unilateral hilar adenopathy in sarcoidosis. Am Rev. Resp. Dis 1985; 91: 272-79.
19. Watts Scott DGI; Rashes and Vasailitis; IN; ABC of rheumatology; ED: Snaith L Michael; BMJ 1995;310: 1128-32.
20. Wilen S.B., Rabinowitz J.G., Ulreichs and Lyons H.A., Pleural involvement in sarcoidosis, Am. J. Med 1974; 57: 200-08.
21. Pattishall E.N., Storepe G.L. and Denny F.W., Pulmonary functions in children with sarcoidosis, Am. Rev. Respir. Dis 1986; 133: 94-96.
22. Kendig E.L. and Brummer D.L., The prognosis of sarcoidosis in children, Chest 1976; 70:351-53.
23. Gupta Samir K., Mitra Koushik, Chatterjee S., Banerjee D. and Roy M., Multiple biopsies in the diagnosis of sarcoidosis. J.Chest. Dis 1984; 26: 65-73.
24. Gupta Samir K., Mitra Kaushik and Chakraborty M., Serum angiotensin converting enzyme in respiratory diseases, J. Assoc. Phys. Ind 1985; 33: 651-52.
25. Cohen D.L., Sicca syndrome: An unusual manifestation or sarcoidosis in childhood. Am. J. Dis. Child 1983; 137: 289-90.
26. Gupta Samir K., Mitra Koushik, Roy M. and Dutta S.K., Mantoux test site granuloma in sarcoidosis in India. Sarcoidosis; Lung India 1986; 3: 153.
27. Bhatia R.S.; BAL; Indications and present status; Lung India 1994; XII:27-29.
28. Sainani G.S. *et al;* Serum angiotensin converting enzyme activity in sarcoidosis and pulmonary tuberculosis. JAPI 1996; 44(1): 29-30.
29. Shah J.R. and Mathur R.S., Radiological signs in pulmonary sarcoidosis, JAPI 1989; 37: 547.
30. Gupta D. *et al.,* Bilateral miliary mottling without hilar lymphadenopathy: A rare presentation of sarcoidosis; Lung India 1996; 14(2): 87-88.
31. Scadding J.G., Calcification in sarcoidosis. Brompton Hospital Reports 1961; XXX: 144-64.
32. McLoud T.C., Pulman C.E. and Pascual R., Egg shell calcification with systemic sarcoidosis. Chest 1974; 66: 515.
33. Johns C.J., Michele T.M.; The clinical management of sarcoidosis; A 50-year-experience of John Hopkins Hospital; Medicine 1999; 78: 65-111.
34. Barnard J., Newman L.S.; Sarcoidosis: Immunology, rheumatic involvement and therapeutics; Curr. Opin. Rheumat 2001; 13: 84-91.
35. Baltzan M., Mehta S., Kirkham TH. *et al.*, Randomised trial of prolonged chloroquine therapy in advanced pulmonary sarcoidosis; Amer. J. Crit. Care Med 1999; 160: 192-97.
36. Subhash H.S.; Prolonged chloroquine therapy for thoracic sarcoidosis—a case report; Lung India 2002; XX: 30-32.
37. Jindal S.K., Gupta D.; Diagnosis and management of sarcoidosis; In; Bansal B.C., Post Grad Med 1997; 11: 347-52.
38. Bhatia RS, Khan GQ; Lung transplantation; IN; RS Bhatia, GQ Khan; ed; Selected topics in pulmonary medicine, Peepee Publ.: N. Delhi 2007; 86-97.
39. Selroos O., Use of budesonide in the treatment of pulmonary sarcoidosis in: Advances in the use of inhaled corticosteroids symposium. Excerpta Medica Amesterdam 1986; 1-10.
40. Tercely M; *et al.*, Microbial antigen treatment in sarcoidosis–a new paradigm? Med. Hypotheses 2008; 70: 831-34.
41. Kutty K; Diagnosis and management of ILD. IN; A. Muruganathan; Ed; Med. Update; API 2013; 23: 503-04.
42. Pangtey G, Aggarwal G; Sarcoidosis–An update on recent advances; IN; A. Muruganathan; Ed; Med Update, API 2013; 23: 806-16.

IDIOPATHIC PULMONARY FIBROSIS (IPF) [CRYPTOGENIC FIBROSING ALVEOLITIS (CFA)]

Pulmonary fibrosis may result as part of the healing process following different types of lung injury. Fibrosis occurs when the injury from infections, granulomatous and infiltrative conditions have involved destruction of the alveolar architecture. Many a times the condition may appear as fibrosing lesion from the beginning ('lone' cryptogenic fibrosing alveolitis, CFA).[1]

Recurrent bacterial infections including tuberculosis, mineral dust pneumoconiosis (silica and asbestos), extrinsic allergic alveolitis due to inhaled organic dusts, ingestion of toxic substances (paraquat and drugs such as nitrofurantoin, bleomycin, cyclophosphamide, busulphan, methotrexate and amiodarone), or unknown causes without any external stimulating agents like sarcoidosis, cryptogenic fibrosing alveolitis (idiopathic pulmonary fibrosis), collagen-vascular diseases, histiocytosis X, mesodermal dysplasia (tuberous sclerosis) are some of the common causes of diffuse fibrosis of the lungs. They progress through a common pathway leading to fibrosis of ventilatory parts of the lung.[1] IPF is a disease with non-productive cough and progressive dyspnoea with restrictive pattern on pulmonary functions testing.[2]

Fibrosing alveolitis is an inflammatory process of the lung predominently affecting the most peripheral parts of the lung, the alveolar walls.[3] It is characterised by two histological features: an inflammatory cellular thickening of the alveolar walls with a marked tendency to fibrosis (mural) and the presence of a large number of large mononuclear cells presumably of alveolar origin in the alveolar spaces (desquamative). The original description of the disease as a fulminant, diffuse, interstitial fibrosis by Hamman and Rich,[4] has been considered a variant of this disease having an acute course with a rapid fatal end. CFA runs a chronic course.

Aetiology

Clinically IPF occurs as an isolated lung disorder or it can occur as a part of the other systemic connective tissue disorders like rheumatoid arthritis, ankylosing spondyloarthropathy, progressive systemic sclerosis, Sjögren's syndrome, polymyositis, chronic active hepatitis and honeycomb lungs. Sometimes it may be familial being transmitted as an autosomal dominant trait.[5]

The aetiology is undetermined. An immunological disturbance with deposits of immune complexes appears to be responsible for the initiation of fibrosis of alveolar walls in some cases. Non-organ specific auto-antibodies like anti-nuclear factor, rheumatoid factor and non-organ specific complement fixing auto-antibodies in significant number[1] can be demonstrated in many of these cases.

Several cellular and biochemical processes occur in this interstitial lung disorder. Irrespective of aetiology, parenchymal abnormalities follow a similar progression of inflammatory changes in alveolar walls and adjacent air spaces, laying down an excess amount of connective tissue. The process of injury to fibrosis is very rapid.

Macrophages are activated by FC receptors, induction of activation is done by both local or circulating immune complexes. Alveolar wall B lymphocytes produce antibodies to antigens. Cellular injury is caused by fibronectin and chemoattractants released from activated macrophages. They in turn enhance cell adherance and fibroblasts replication. Neutrophils attracted at the site of injury produce potentially damaging substances, such as elastase, oxygen radicals and platelet derived growth factor. Endothelial cells damage occur involving H_2O_2: iron and xanthine oxidase. Xanthine oxidase also has interaction with chemotactic peptides such as C_{5a} and T_NF-alpha. Lung injury is further produced by role of cytokines and deposition of immune complexes consisting of IgG.[6]

Oxidants, proteases, collagenase and growth factor like mediators produced from activated macrophages and neutrophils modulate fibroblasts growth and collagen deposition, resulting into fibrosis.[7]

In other interstitial lung diseases like hypersensitive pneumonitis and sarcoidosis, it is the lymphocytes which are predominantly involved immune effector cells that are recruited in response to lymphocyte activating factor (IL-l) and chemotactic factor released by activated macrophages.

Pathophysiology

As the pathological changes mostly affect the alveolar walls, the term alveolitis has been suggested. The condition is progressive unlike many other types of fibrosis developing as a part of healing. Characteristically, the most peripheral parts of the lungs are severely affected and the pleura is unaffected in CFA.[1]

Pathogenesis

Changes in lung tissue include interstitial inflammation, increase in plasma cells, muscle cells and fibroblasts, collagen synthesis and fibrosis without granuloma formation. Bronchiolitis obliterans may develop.[2,8] The process begins as reversible alveolar injury, alveolar and interstitial oedema within the alveolar walls forming intra-alveolar hyaline membranes. It is followed by infiltration of inflammatory cells including histiocytes, lymphocytes and plasma cells. Very rarely eosinophils and neutrophils may be seen. Then there is an appearance of an increasing number of fibroblasts together with collagen fibres and elastin to result in gross thickening of the alveolar walls. With further advance in the disease, there is loss of pulmonary epithelium lining cells and extensive area of basement membrane gets exposed. Side by side there is accumulation of variable number of macrophages in the alveolar spaces. Though there may be a small number of neutrophils, eosinophils and occasionally lymphocytes, plasma cells are not found.

As the disease progresses, the alveolar architecture is destroyed to result in extensive fibrosis usually mixed with a cellular exudate of lymphocytes and plasma cells. There may be a proliferation of smooth muscle cells, collection of large number of mast cells and a proliferation of blood vessels arising from bronchial circulation[1] with the persistence of disease, the chain of changes include from increased alveolar-capillary perceivability and desquamation of intra alveolar cells (alveolitis) to mural inflamation and interstitial fibrosis. The activated phagocytes—macrophages—are increased and are capable of producing many cytokines that effect other lung cells and is considered to be hallmark of the alveolitis.[1]

The early *inflammatory* stages are variable. In some there is marked accumulation of lymphocytes and occasionally of plasma cells in the interstitium (lymphocytes or plasma cell interstitial pneumonia). Lymphocytes are usually increased. IPF is part of a collagen vascular disease. There can be a massive accumulation of macrophages in the alveolar spaces with relative little fibrosis (Desquamative Interstitial Pneumonia, DIP). In most cases there is a considerable overlap of cell types and extent of fibrosis.[1]

Several products are released from alveolar macrophages including platelet derived growth factor (PDGF) which chemoattracts mesenchymal cells and stimulates fibroblasts to change from resting cells to cells entering G_1.

With continued activity of macrophages, widespread fibrosis occurs involving vasculature. Functional alveolar tissue changes to scar tissue and cystic areas develop from retraction of terminal airways. In the end stage fibrosis, the histologic changes fail to distinguish the initiating factor.

The monoclonal, antibody staining with peroxidase has shown that the widely scattered lymphocytic infiltration is predominantly made up of T cells.[9] Immunoglobulins are secreted within the germinal follicles. The increase in immunoglobulins, especially the IgG subclass IgG_1 and 3, occurs in response to the initiating factor which is likely to be an antigen and hence the increased immunoglobulin response. These immunoglobulins interact with the surface of the alveolar macrophages either as an opsonin or after becoming part of an immune complex. The chronic inflammation and interstitial fibrosis are characteristically seen in lower lobes. There is an injury of parenchymal cells and connective tissue of alveolar wall with progressive fibrosis of the lung structure. Histopathology includes interstitial pneumonia characterized by thickening of alveolar septal wall with collagenous tissue, infiltration of pulmonary interstitium with fibroblasts and inflammatory cells and both hyperplasia and hypertrophy of alveolar type II cells.

There is a marked change in the alveolar epithelial cells destruction of type I alveolar epithelial cells and repopulation of epithelial surface both by type II alveolar and bronchiolar epithelial cells.

Since type II cells are thought to be progenitor cells of terminal air spaces and alteration in the regenerative functions of type II cells may be responsible for fibrosis, these cells being major source of pulmonary surfactant that reduces surface tension forces and tendency of alveolar spaces to collapse. Reduction of surfactant will promote atelectasis resulting in apposition and fibrotic fusion of denuded alveolar basement membranes. Alveolar epithelium will respond to injury (reflecting the capability of type II cells) and in turn predict the clinical outcome in IPF. Level of surfactant protein-A in the lavage thus represents the collective viability of type II cells in the diseased lung and in turn reflects the regenerative capability of pulmonary epithelium.

Type II pneumocytes are considered passive standby in the alveolar immunologic process and host defence mechanisms. Apart from being involved by the effect of surfactant, these cells also interact with local inflammatory process through the production of mediators. Type II alveolar cells also produce cytokines. Intense staining with anti-TGF-beta antibodies and monoclonal antibody reactive to human TNF-alpha-3 has been demonstrated immunohistochemically, where TNF-alpha-3 has pathogenic role in lung fibrosis.

Thus, surface active material when altered contributes to pathogenesis of IPF, both by increasing the elastic recoil due to surface forces and by promoting alveolar collapse.[10,11,12]

The term *lone* cryptogenic fibrosing alveolitis (CFA) is applied where the lungs alone are affected. The lone CFA demonstrates circulating immune complexes or auto-antibodies which are also a manifestation of certain connective tissue disorders.[1]

Pathology

Initial pathology includes parenchymal inflammation, followed by accumulation of collagen in alveolar lumen and interstitium. Diffuse injury to type I cells and hypertrophy and hyperplasia of alveolar type II cells are early histopathological findings. Role of inflammatory cells mediated oxidants to cause initial injury cannot be ruled out at the same time. An irritant initiates a local immune response and activates macrophages to secrete factors that activate neutrophils and growth factors which are chemotactic for fibroblasts. They release proteases and oxidants that cause parenchymal damage, to which eosinophils also contribute.

Mural and desquamative histological patterns are noted. In the mural pattern, there is fibrous thickening of the alveolar walls with some exudation into the alveolar spaces. The exudate consists of a mixed population of cells, lymphocytes, plasma cells and granulocytes. The changes are irregular and alveolar structure is distorted and hyperplasia of the lymph follicles is not striking. In the desquamative pattern, the striking abnormality is in the alveolar spaces. They are filled with a large number of mononuclear cells. The cells are of the same type and are distributed informally presenting a monotonous picture. Many of them resemble type II pneumonocytes. There is minimal thickening of the alveolar walls from infiltration of cells, alveolar pattern is still retained and there is prominent hyperplasia of the lymph follicles.[1]

These two patterns are regarded as stages of the disease rather than separate diseases. Desquamative interstitial pneumonia appears to be a stage of fibrosing alveolitis simulating desquamative pattern. The end result is a diffuse fibrosis of the peripheral gas exchanging parts of the lung beyond the terminal bronchioles, and honeycomb changes from dilated bronchioles. Classical honeycombing in the form of course, reticular pattern with translucencies indicates severe fibrosis.

Clinical Features[1]

CFA is commonly seen in middle aged and the range varies from infancy to the elderly. The sex distribution is equal. The patient gradually reveals increasing dyspnoea. In some pursuing an acute course, the manifestations begin with fever, cough and tightness in the chest. It is seen in the desquamative pattern and in younger patients.

Initially the dyspnoea is exertional. It takes a long time before profound disturbances occur in the pulmonary function. There is tachypnoea. The low arterial oxygen tension accelerates the ventilatory drive. There is a history of fatigue, arthralgia and loss of weight. Cough associated with scanty mucoid expectoration or dry cough may be the presentation.

Central cyanosis may be noted initially on exercise and later it is apparent even at rest. Clubbing may be seen in 80 per cent of the cases without hypertropic osteoarthropathy. It is more frequent in lone CFA than in CFA associated with connective tissue disease. In the late stage of the disease, cor pulmonale with evidence of pulmonary hypertension may develop.[2]

Lung sounds may be normal initially. Later on, the chest expansion is restricted. There may be an impaired percussion note over the bases with bronchovesicular breath sounds. The distinctive dry or *velcro* crackles are audible at the end of inspiration and they persist after a cough characteristically audible over the lobes posteriorly. There is tachypnoea at rest.

Investigations

The chest X-ray shows bilateral, well-defined, basal non-confluent irregular opacities. Appearance is a ground glass in the early stages and becomes nodular giving appearance of linear opacities all over the lung fields. It is predominant in the basal zones and spreads progressively towards the apices and thus there is a gradual loss of lung volume. Nevertheless, X-ray chest may be normal in 10-15% of cases. The mural type presents discrete small, round opacities or multiple ring shadows or reticular shadows leading to a honeycomb appearance in the end stage disease or Swiss cheese appearance ultimately. In the desquamative type the opacity is irregular with patchy shadowing at the bases. The diaphragm is elevated due to the contraction of the lower lobes. The bronchogram shows contraction of the normal peripheral unfilled zone.[1] Cor pulmonale may be seen in advanced cases. CT scan in early cases of CFA shows loss of sensibility of flow which is present in normal lung, i.e., blood flows greater in dependent areas, i.e., in the supine position, the highest flow is present posteriorly. In prone position, the flow is reversed. The early changes by CT scan are not only basal but also peripheral with selective central sparing. A crescent abnormality affecting the lung periphery in lower zones posteriorly can be demonstrated on CT. As the disease progresses, cystic changes of 1 cm diameter start appearing. HRCT findings include lower zone subpleural reticular pattern with areas of haziness or air space opacification, with or without honeycombing. Bronchi are not affected, pleura are also spared and lymphadenopathy is uncommon in IPF.

Small stiff lungs may be seen in CFA. PFT are normal in early stage, with reduced lung volumes. The total lung capacity is small. The FEV_1 and FVC are lowered equally and the ratio remains normal. The tidal volume is low. The minute ventilation is great at rest and on exercise. There is a restrictive ventilatory defect and a reduced diffusing capacity. The defect in diffusion is greater in the mural type than in the desquamative type and it does not double after exercise. The ventilatory defect is more prominent in the desquamative type. The lung compliance is reduced. There is hypoxaemia while breathing room air due to ventilation-perfusion mismatching and the arterial oxygen tension is reduced further on exercise. The alveolar-to-arterial oxygen tension gradient (A-aDO_2) is further widened on exercise. $PaCO_2$ is normal or low from hyperventilation.[1] Carbon monoxide diffusing capacity is usually reduced by 30-50%. Resting hypoxemia is associated with extensive fibrosis, and pulmonary hypertension and has poor prognosis.

There may be presence of non-organspecific auto-antibodies (anti-nuclear and rheumatoid factors) in the sera in about 10% of patients. Cryoimmunoglobulins may be present and levels of serum immunoglobulins and circulating immunecomplex fibres may be raised. Bronchoalveolar lavage[13] demonstrates an increase in the number of neutrophils with or without associated eosinophils, unlike lymphocytic predominance in sarcoidosis. BAL fluid analysis for surfactant A protein by ELISA showed reduced levels. In CFA there is predominance of neutrophils and in extrinsic allergic alveolitis there is an increase in the number of lymphocytes and plasma cells. The level of IgG is elevated as well as IgG releasing cells. ESR is also elevated.

An open biopsy through limited thoracotomy with subperiosteal rib resection is performed in selected cases. Fibrosis is the end stage of either pattern of diseases. The biopsy of the lung can also be performed through the transbronchial route using fiberoptic bronchoscope.

Differential Diagnosis

Differential diagnostic clues[14] include IPF that is seen more commonly in patients around 50 years of age, compared to young cigarette smokers in histiocytosis, young middle aged adults in sarcoidosis and heavy cigarette smokers in respiratory bronchiolitis with interstitial lung disease (ILD). Lymphangio leiomyomatosis is predominantly seen in women. Examination reveals presence of clubbing and dry end-inspiratory and velcro crepts at lung bases in IPF, compared to absence of these in sarcoidosis.

Similar signs of connective tissue involvement such as arthritis, joints' swelling, photosensitivity, pleuritis, dryness of mouth and eyes, Raynaud's phenomenon and extrapulmonary involvement in IPF is absent as compared to sarcoidosis. ANF and RA factor may be positive with low titre in 20% of cases of IPF as compared to sarcoidosis where these are positive with high titre in 80% of cases.

X-ray findings are given in the Table10.1.

Cryptogenic Fibrosing Alveolitis: Complications

1. Respiratory failure.
2. Cor pulmonale with right-sided heart failure.
3. Secondary pulmonary infections.
4. Spontaneous pneumothorax.
5. Haemoptysis.
6. Death.
7. Bronchogenic carcinoma in 12% of cases.

Recurrent bacterial pulmonary infections are common. Some patients may develop pulmonary hypertension. There is an increased propensity to develop malignancy of the lung. The alveolar epithelium in diffuse interstitial fibrosis exhibits hyperplasia and anaplasia. The rigid lung undergoes honeycomb changes and offers an important background for a typical epithelial proliferation. In the region of severe fibrosis, there appears to be an apparent transition from atypical or dysplastic bronchiolar alveolar epithelium to carcinoma.

Prognosis[1]

The disease has a slow progressive course. The untreated cases show great clinical variability with long periods of remissions. Some cases of desquamative variety may show spontaneous recovery. In older patients the progress is slow to have a more chronic indolent disease. The younger patients present acute picture and in some it may be fatal within six months. Overall improvement in the survival with corticosteroids or immunosuppressants is relatively slight. Pulmonary carcinoma may supervene in individuals with pulmonary fibrosis. Patients with cellular pattern may survive for 10-12 years but in those with fibrotic pattern, survival is reduced to 4-5 years.[6]

Treatment

Overall results depend upon the stage of the disease at which the treatment has been introduced, and in some patients the histological type of the disease. Patients with more cellular appearance and less fibrosis responded better. The desquamative type showed a favourable response to the suppressive effects of steroids compared to the mural type of the disease. The patients with lymphocytic infiltrate of the alveolar walls and slight fibrosis responded better.

A favourable response is noted in the younger age patients, with minimal radiographic abnormalities, shorter history of breathlessness, and a more cellular response on histopathology of a biopsy, implying earlier disease. Those with minimal disability and mild impairment of pulmonary function appear to be ideal candidates for steroid therapy. The response is poor in those with chronic disease. Oral colchicine 0.6 mg in one or two doses per day can be considered as a first line potential alternative treatment to alter collagen synthesis and fibrosis.

Prednisolone 1 mg/kg/day is sufficient to suppress the symptoms for 8-10 weeks. It has to be reduced gradually to a small maintenance dose of 5 mg or less in the patients, as it has to be given for the remaining period of their lives. The sudden withdrawal or reduction of the dose sometimes is associated with exacerbation of the disease. Therefore it has to be tapered off gradually. It has to be stopped in those who have not shown response in six to eight weeks who develop the hazards of long-term treatment with corticosteroids. In such instances immunosuppressive therapy is tried with the use of azathioprine, 2 to 3 mg/kg/body weight or chlorambusil 10 mg or cyclophosphamide 90 mg daily. The dose is reduced on clinical

Table 10.1: X-ray finding: Differential diagnosis

IPF	*Sarcoidosis*	*Other connective tissue disorders and asbestosis*	*Hypersensitive pneumonitis HP*
• Ground glass, nodular, reticular reticunodular and honeycombing • Bilateral, asymmetric, peripheral reticular opacities at lung bases with reduced lung volumes. HRCT-patchy, peripheral subpleural, bibasilar, reticular abnormalities. Traction bronchiectasis and honeycombing seen in 90% of cases.	> 30% of lung shows ground glass opacities in desquamative interstitial pneumonitis, RBILD, HP, Idiopathic-BOOP or NSIP.	Similar to IPF except for presence of fibrosis bands and pleural plaques in asbestosis.	• Upper and middle to be affected • Absent honeycombing

improvement. Cyclophosphamide has shown to be effective or less morbid than glucocorticosteroid therapy. The therapy facilitates a substantial reduction in the steroid dose. It can be started as 1 mg/kg/day, along with low dose of steroids, increasing by 50 mg every week or 10 days.[15] It can suppress the immunologically determined process seen in some cases of fibrosing alveolitis and is evident by lowering of the level of anti-nuclear factors significantly. The occurrence of infections, gastrointestinal disturbances and occasionally thrombocytopaenia may complicate immunosuppressive therapy. The risk of immunosuppression can be minimised by frequent surveillance of the peripheral granulocyte count. It should be maintained at levels above 2000/cm. 'Pulse therapy' with large doses of methyl prednisolone can be used as an effective adjunct to therapy with cyclophosphamides. It is administered in a dose of 10 mg/kg intravenously on three consecutive days after which it is repeated at weekly intervals.[1] It should be noted that both corticosteroids and cyclophosphamide may be useful in the treatment of CFA, but they are not necessarily effective in the same patient.[7] At the same time, complications such as haemorrhagic cystitis and carcinoma bladder have to kept in mind while treating with cyclophosphamide.

Cessation of cigarette smoking is a useful adjuvant therapy. Cautious use of diuretics along with digoxin in cases of right-sided heart failure, although oxygen therapy is the treatment of choice. Bronchodilator for cough and wheeze and prompt management of infections should be done. Pneumococcal and influenza vaccine have been tried prophylactically.[2] Single lung transplantation[16] can be considered in younger patients. Similar results have been reported from an Indian study where 5 years survival has been observed.[17] Antifibrotic drugs are being evaluated. Research has to be continued in the areas of regulation of injury, repair and fibrogenesis in the micro environment of lungs.

REFERENCES

1. Shankar P.S., Chest Medicine; Oxford & IBH Publ. Co. (P) Ltd., New Delhi; 4th ed., 1994.
2. Wilson J.D., Braunweld E., Isselbacher K.J. et al., (ed): Harrison's principles of internal medicine, 12th ed; McGraw Hill, New York, 1991.
3. Crystal R.G., *et al.,* Interstitial lung diseases of unknown cause, Disorders characterised by chronic inflammation of the lower respiratory tract N. Engl. J. Med 1984; 310: 154-235.
4. Hamman L., Rich A.R., Fulminating diffuse interstitial fibrosis of the lungs; Trans. Amer. Clin. Chest Assn 1935; 51: 154.
5. Bitterman P.B., *et al.,* Familial idiopathic pulmonary fibrosis, N. Eng. J. Med 1986; 314: 1343.
6. Behera D., *et al.,* Response to steroid therapy in patients of IPF: A retrospective analysis; J. Chest Dis. Allied Sci 1998; 40: 163-69.
7. Catin A.M., *et al.,* Oxidant mediated epithelial cell injury in IPF; J. Clin. Invest 1987; 79: 1665-73.
8. Epler G.R., *et al.,* Bronchiolitis Obliterans with organising pneumonia, N. Eng. J. Med 1985; 312: 152.
9. Hay J.G. and M.Turner Warwick, Cryptogenic fibrosing alveolitis (idiopathic pulmonary fibrosis) In: Recent Advances in Respiratory Medicine, No 4, D.C. Flenley and T.L. Petty (eds) Edinburgh: Churchill Livingstone 1986; 131.
10. Hamm H., *et al.,* Surfactant: A review of its functions and relevance in adult respiratory disorders; Resp. Med 1996; 90: 251-70.
11. King T.E, Jr., Diagnostic advances in IPF; Chest 1991; 100: 238.
12. Schwartz M.I.; IPF; West Med. J 1988; 149:199.
13. Reynolds H.Y., Idiopathic interstitial pulmonary fibrosis, Contribution of BAL analysis, Chest 1986; 89:139.
14. Kulpati D.D.S.; ILD: IPF; Diagnosis and treatment; in M.M. Panja (Ed.) Med. Update, API 2001;11:70-81.
15. Reynolds H.Y., Idiopathic pulmonary fibrosis, in: Current therapy in allergy immunology and rheumatology, L.M. Lichtenstein, A.S. Fauci (ed) Toronto, Decker 1988; 3: 214-20.
16. Toronto lung transplantation Group; Experience with single lung transplantation for pulmonary fibrosis, JAMA 1988; 259: 2258.
17. Jindal S.K., *et al.,* Fibrosing alveolitis; A report of 61 cases seen over the past 5 years, Ind. J. Chest Dis. and All Sci 1979; 21: 174-79.

LYMPHOCYTIC INFILTRATIVE LUNG DISORDERS (LILD)[1,2]

These are lymphocytic interstitial pneumonias characterised by lymphocytic infiltration of interstitium, mixed with histiocytes plasma cells. They belong to IPF and may also be associated with Sjögren's syndrome or dysproteinemia.

Usually there is a history of chronic cough with recurrent haemptysis. Breathlessness is absent. There is no clubbing or cyanosis. Examination may reveal localised crepitations at the area of involvement. Investigations are non-contributory. Diagnosis is confirmed only after bronchoscopy and histopathology, that reveals patchy lymphocytic alveolitis. Surgical management gives the relief.

REFERENCES

1. Raynolds H.Y. Lymphocytic infiltration disorders of lung; In; Fauci, A.S., *et al.,* (Ed.); Harrison's Principles of Internal Medicine; 14th Ed.; New York, Mc Graw-Hill 1998; 2: 1464.
2. Gupta S.K.; LILD: An isolated entity; JAPI 2002; 50: 1320-21.

SYSTEMIC LUPUS ERYTHEMATOSUS

A disease of unknown aetiology, where tissue and cells are damaged by pathogenic auto antibodies and immune complexes.[1] Systemic lupus erythematosus (SLE) can no longer be considered as a rare disease. It is a frequently diagnosed condition,[2-4] possibly due to greater awareness of its protean manifestations and the availability of anti-nuclear antibody (ANA) as a serological marker.

SLE should be considered in any young female with pyrexia of unknown origin, joint pains/swelling, renal disease with or without other system involvement.[5] *In acute toxic SLE,* prompt diagnosis and adequate treatment often controls the disease in these patients. Other presentations include hair loss, recurrent venous thrombosis and abortions and idiopathic thrombocytopaenic purpura.

There are differences from published western series. While, skin and mucous membrane involvement is quite common, discoid lesions appear rarely. Renal disease is as common if not more common than the black females and appears to be severe too. Haematological abnormalities except anaemia are less common. These differences possibly reflect the influence of genetic, environmental, dietary and socio-economic factors.[6] Lot of work has also been done on Indian soil.[7-16]

Presence of Variant

Mannose binding lectin (MBL) alleles, in immunodeficiency states, HIV/AIDS and chemotherapy induced neutropenia, is associated with more frequent and more severe infections. And deficiency of MBL increases susceptibility to infection, with rapidly progressing lung and liver disease.

It is suggested that MBL deficiency alters the natural history of disease such as cystic fibrosis, immunodeficiency disorders and chronic granulomatous disease such as SLE.[17]

SLE is a disease with continuously changing phenomenon. The severity and activity can change quite dramatically and rapidly. Close and continuous watch is absolutely essential. One of the most important causes of death has been renal involvement, accounting for approximately 40% of SLE deaths; the deaths being maximum in the first year of the illness. Haemodialysis and renal transplantation have reduced renal deaths but not necessarily the overall mortality. Curiously the disease appears to be mild in the elderly. Children and adolescents suffer more. The disease affects females almost 90% during their child-bearing period. Lupus and pregnancy have adverse effects on each other. Drug induced lupus may also occur. Pulmonary involvement may occur during the disease.

Assessment is made according to the revised (1982) criteria of the American Rheumatism Association (ARA) for the classification of SLE.[18]

The routine investigations included complete blood counts, erythrocyte sedimentation rate (Westergren), urinalysis, 24 hours urinary protein excretion, blood urea, serum creatinine and creatinine clearance. A standard twelve lead-electrocardiogram and chest X-ray are also obtained. Immunological investigations include estimation of ANA, rheumatoid factor (RF), serum complement components C^3 and C^4 levels and estimation of total haemolytic activity of complement (CH_{50}).

A percutaneous kidney biopsy is performed in patients with clinical evidence of renal involvement. Tissue obtained is examined by light microscopy as well as immunofluorescence microscopy to detect the presence of immunoglobulin (major classes), C^3 and fibrin deposits. Additional immunological investigations include the antibodies to extractable nuclear antigens (ENA) or soluble cellular antigens (SCA),[10,19] antibodies to double-stranded DNA (ds DNA),[10,11,19] antibodies reactive with single stranded DNA (ss DNA)[12] lupus anticoagulant test (LAC), antiphospholipid antibody and anticardiolipin antibody (ACA).[20]

Based upon clinical and serological activity, patients are categorised into 4 groups and treated accordingly.[3]

Group-I Mild SLE

Mild mucocutaneous, musculoarticular and constitutional symptoms with absence of serositis, nervous system or renal involvement.

Group-II Mild SLE

Mild but unresponsive SLE or with polyserositis.

Group-III Moderately Severe SLE

Prominent general symptoms, mucosal ulcers, rash, musculoarticular symptoms, thrombocytopaenia and/or unresponsive serositis. Patients with acute toxic SLE are also included in this group.

Group-IV Severe SLE

Severe multi organ system involvement including renal and nervous systems. The pulmonary manifestations[22] may occur in the form of acute non-eosinophilic infiltrates, pleural effusion and rarely pulmonary haemorrhage.

Diagnostic significance of various radiological investigations, comparative diagnostic value of abnormal findings on plain chest X-ray, pulmonary function testing and on HRCT[21] have been shown in the following Tables 10.2 to 10.5.

Table 10.2

In SLE–Comparison of abnormal findings favouring diagnosis can be obtained in:

a. Less than 20% of cases on chest X-ray
b. Less than 30% of cases on PFTs.
c. More than 55% of cases on HRCT

Table 10.3

PFTS in SLE can be:

a. Obstructive in less than 3% of cases
b. Restrictive in more than 26% of cases

Table 10.4

Diagnostic Significance

a. Chest X-ray and PFTS–do not exclude early abnormalities.
b. HRCT detects pulmonary involvement in many asymptomatic patients.
c. Pleural abnormalities are less common in SLE.
d. Common HRCT features include interstitial thickening, thickened intralobular septa, parenchymal bands and ground glass opacification–all suggestive of ILD.

Table 10.5

HRCT in SLE

(Usually multiple features are present)

a. Interstitial/Interlobular thickening	– Less than 40% of cases s e p t a
b. Parenchymal bands	– More than 36% of cases
c. Ground glass opacification	– More than 26% of cases
d. Pleural effusion	– More than 10% of cases
e. Bronchiectasis	– Almost 8% of cases (each)
f. Parenchymal micronodules	
g. Sub pleural band	– More than 5% of cases (each)
h. Bullae	
i. Air space consolidation	
j. Thickened pleura	– More than 2% of cases

Non-Eosinophilic Infiltrates and Fibrosing Alveolitis

Though there can be lesions varying from acute alveolitis to an end stage fibrosisin SLE, the occurrence of fibrosing alveolitis is rare. There can be patchy and transient parenchymal infiltrates due to the disease associated with fibrinoid necrosis and vasculitis or to bacterial infection. The predominant pulmonary manifestation is dyspnoea and is often associated with aches in the chest. There may be cough with or without mucoid expectoration. There is tachypnoea, cyanosis and fever. The dyspnoea, though persists for longer duration, is not associated with any abnormal auscultatory signs. Radiologically it shows extensive shadows. The diaphragm is raised and moves sluggishly. Small pleural effusions may be noted during an acute stage. HRCT is very useful.[23]

The progressive fibrosis from chronic fibrosing inflammation and progressive lung destruction leads to a gradual elevation of the diaphragm and shrinkage of lungs. There is reduction in the lung volume with a restrictive defect of ventilation. Deposits of immune complexes around pulmonary capillaries are seen. ANA and LE cells are present. There is raised ESR and leucopenia. Immunologic tests for the presence of precipitins against both double and single stranded DNA (nuclear antigens) are positive. The level of complement components C_3 and C_4 is low. The condition responds to corticosteroids.[22]

Pleural Effusion

About one-third of the patients suffering from SLE have pleurisy with or without effusion. Pleural capillary permeability and circulating immune complexes may contribute in its occurrence. The condition may be unilateral or bilateral. They are small and transient. The incidence is variable and is as high as 3/4 of the patients manifesting pleuropulmonary disease. Pleural manifestations are noted after appearance of the signs and symptoms of disease. Enlarged cardiac size or basal alveolar infiltrate may also be seen on chest X-ray.

The fluid is an exudate, being turbid or yellow in colour. The cell content is high with predominant lymphocytes. Pleural sugar level is usually normal. Rarely the fluid may be a transudate as a complication of renal or cardiac failure. The level of haemolytic complements (C_3 and C_4) is low. LE cells and ANA may be observed. The concentration of immune complexes is similar in blood and pleural effusion. Pleural biopsy reveals non-specific dense infiltrates with lymphocytes and plasma cells. Effusion may resolve spontaneously. Steroids are useful in the management of the large effusions.[22] First report from India appears where SLE has lupus pleuritis as first presenting manifestation,[23] which is otherwise 1-3% although pleural involvement is 50-83% on autopsy and pleural effusion is 35-50%.[24]

Pulmonary Haemorrhage

A massive pulmonary haemorrhage is an occasional feature. However, haemoptysis may be small in relation to the extent of the intrapulmonary haemorrhage. Radiologically it reveals large rapidly changing confluent shadows. Peculiarly the transfer factor is elevated. The level of ANA is high.

Pulmonary involvement 3 is seen in 44% of patients (pleural 36% and/or parenchymal 24%). Exudative pleural effusions, unilateral or bilateral, are found in 21 per cent of patients. Isolated, pleuritic chest pain occur in 15%. Involvement of lung parenchyma is in the consolidation (14%), localised or diffuse rales with a normal chest roentgenogram (9%) and interstitial lung disease (1 %) patient with *shrinking lung* syndrome, has been reported. Elevation of right dome of diaphragm, tension pneumothorax, acute pulmonary respiratory distress syndrome, pleural thickening and respiratory infections are other uncommon respiratory complications.[25,26] Mild weakness of respiratory muscles has also been reported in SLE.[27] There is a restrictive ventilatory defect. Linear atelectasis, infections, pulmonary embolism and pulmonary hypertension have also been reported.[26,28] Pulmonary emergencies in SLE include lupus pneumonitis, the occurrence of which is lesser than infectious processes in SLE, secondly pulmonary haemorrhage—a rare and yet serious complication of SLE, having multisystem involvement; thirdly pulmonary embolism in almost 11% of patients with SLE and lastly pulmonary renal syndrome in SLE; the other causes being Wegener's granulomatosis, microscopic polyangitis and Goodpasture syndrome. Treatment involves high dose steroids and cytotoxic drugs. Refractory cases may benefit from plasmapheresis.[29,30]

Treatment modalities can be as follows: Patients in Group-I are given immunomodulator such as chloroquine (250 mg) or hydroxychloroquine (200 mg) daily for 6 months followed by the same dose on alternate days on a long term basis and non-steroidal anti-inflammatory agents. Six monthly visual field charting using red object and fundus examination should be carried out to detect ocular toxicity of chloroquine. Hydroxychloroquine helps in controlling cutaneous and musculoskeletal manifestations of SLE and also reduce the risk of future thrombosis. Group II patients are given the above drugs and low dose oral prednisolone (7.5-20 mg daily). Group III patients receive moderately high doses of oral prednisolone (1mg/kg/body wt daily). In the absence of a response within one week, *pulse therapy* with methylprednisolone, 250 to 1000 mg or equipotent dexamethasone intravenously over 1 hour upto a maximum of three consecutive days, is instituted. Patients unresponsive to all the above measures and group IV patients are treated with cyclophosphamide (0.5-0.7 g/m^2 body surface area) as an intravenous pulse every 3 weeks upto 6 doses, followed by maintenance pulses given every 6-12 weeks in many patients. This therapy is combined with a low daily or alternate day dose of prednisolone in most of the patients.

In the last group, patients receive alternate cytotoxic drugs (oral) cyclophosphamide 2-2.5 mg/kg body weight or methotrexate 7.5-15 mg weekly orally or intravenously, alone or in combination with prednisolone (0.5-1 mg/kg body weight per day).

Delayed diagnosis for a few months is not uncommon SLE. The clinical pattern of SLE in Indian population appears by and large similar to that seen in caucasians.[2] Just a few differences to note are, a significantly lower incidence of Raynaud's phenomenon and photosensitivity. Nutritional deficiency anaemia is prevalent in Indian female population.[2] The incidence of anti S antibody is known to be much higher in the Chinese SLE population compared to the European.[31] High incidence of renal involvement is reported from Northern India.[3] It must be noted that disease activity in SLE refers to reversible manifestations while irreversible damage refers to non-reversible changes present for atleast 6 months which are not related to active inflammation.

Pulmonary Hypertension in Systemic Lupus Erythematosus

Pulmonary hypertension is a recognised entity in connective tissue diseases but its occurrence in systemic lupus erythematosus (SLE) is infrequent.[32,33] Aetiology of pulmonary hypertension in SLE is not clear. Possible factors in the pathogenesis include vasospasm, arteritis, platelet dysfunction and thromboembolism. Occurrence of primary pulmonary hypertension and Raynaud's phenomenon suggests[34] a link between the two. Although incriminated as a possible cause of pulmonary hypertension, vasculitis may not play a major pathogenetic role. Thromboembolic disease is a well recognised cause of pulmonary hypertension. Venous syndromes and pulmonary thromboembolism are not rare in SLE,[35] and support the postulation of thromboembolism in the pathogenesis of pulmonary hypertension. Tables 10.6 and 10.7 depict clinical profile respiratory emergencies in SLE.

Genetic studies are being done to understand demystified and enigmatic syndrome called SLE, with heterogeneity in genetic complexity and clinical diversity.[36]

Table 10.6: Clinical profile of SLE

A. *Non organ specific manifestations*	
Fever	Lymphadenopathy
Cutaneous lesions	Drug reaction (skin)
Alopecia	Photosensitivity
Oral ulcers	Raynaud's phenomenon
	Panniculitis
B. *Systemic involvement*	
1. *Musculoskeletal*	
Arthritis	
Arthralgias	
Myositis	
Avascular necrosis of bone	
Rupture tendon achilles	
2. *Renal*	
Diffuse proliferative glomerulonephritis	
Mesangial lupus nephritis	
Focal proliferative glomerulonephritis	
Membranous lupus nephritis	
3. *Neurologic*	
Seizures	
Neuropsychiatric	
Cerebrovascular	
Choreothetosis	
Myelitis	
Trigeminal neuralgia	
Mononeuritis multiplex	

Contd.

Contd.

4. *Hematological*
   Anaemia
   Only thrombocytopenia
   Lupus anticoagulant DIC
   Pancytopenia
5. *Pleuropulmonary*
   Pleural effusion and pleuritis
   Restrictive lung function but normal X-ray chest
   Restrictive lung function with reticular shadowing on X-ray chest
   Pneumonia
   Progressive pulmonary hypertension
6. *Gastrointestinal*
   Only hepatomegaly
   Only splenomegaly
   Hepatosplenomegaly
   Ascitis
   Hepatitis
   Enteritis
7. *Cardiovascular*
   Myocarditis
   Pericardial effusion
   ECG changes only

Table 10.7: Respiratory emergencies in SLE

(Critical Care Clinics: SLE in intensive care unit 2002; 18: 781-803)

a. Upper airways obstruction due to:
- Laryngeal inflammation
- Epiglottitis
- Paralysis of vocal cord
- Retropharyngeal abscess

Early recognition and urgent intubation may be required. SLE patients are more susceptible to develop post intubation stricture.

b. Lungs are involved as:
- Lupus pneumonias
- Pulmonary embolism
- Pulmonary hypertension
- Pulmonary hemorrhage
- Acute reversible hypoxemia and shrinking lung syndrome.

In the presence of cough, dyspnoea and hemoptysis, and presence of accompanying features of active lupus, lupus pneumonitis is suspected and diagnosed after exclusion of infective etiology of pneumonia. WBC is normal, cultures are usually negative. BAL and even tissue biopsy may be required. Secondary infections are common and mostly patients may need ventilatory support. High dose steroids along with anti-microbials and immunosuppressive agents are used to treat; however, mortality remains as high as 50%.

Alveolar haemorrhage is another serious complication of SLE seen rarely in SLE patients. Cough, dyspnoea and haemoptysis are presenting symptoms. Mild haemorrhage to life threatening haemorrhage can occur. Clinical trial of haemoptysis, falling haematocrit and pulmonary infiltrates pointer towards pulmonary haemorrhage. Active lupus, usually featuring nephritis, is accompanying. Ventilatory support is essential in case respiratory failure occurs. It has to be differentiated from infection and lupus pneumonias as well as Wegener's granulomatosis and Goodpasture's syndrome. Secondary infections often complicate. Treatment includes high dose glucocorticoids along with antimicrobials and even immunosuppressive therapy.

Pulmonary embolism is usually seen in the context of antiphospholipid syndrome. Patients with pulmonary hypertension have dry cough and progressive dyspnoea. Diagnosis is by excluding cardiac and lung parenchymal etiologies. 2D Echo is usually good enough to confirm. Prognosis remains poor. Calcium channel blockers, anticoagulants, prostacyclin and oxygen are used to treat. Bosentan and sildenafil are being tried.

REFERENCES

1. Gupta P.R., Gupta N., Laryngitis: A rare presentation of SLE; Lung India 1996; 14(2): 89-90.
2. Amin S.N., Angadi S.A., Mangat G.K., *et al.* Clinical profile of systemic lupus erythematosus in western India. J. Assoc. Physicians India 1988; 36: 475-75.
3. Malaviya A.N. Singh R.R., Kumar A., *et al.* Systemic lupus erythematosus in northern India: A review of 329 cases, J. Assoc. Physicians India 1988; 36: 476-80.
4. Madhavan R., Porkodi R., Ramkrishnan S., *et al.* Systemic lupus erythematosis—the Madras experience. J. Assoc. Physicains India 1988; 36: 481-84.
5. Sainani G.S., Mehta P.J., Bichile S.K., *et al.* SLE: No more a curosity (editorial). JAPI 1988;36: 469-70.
6. Bevra H.H., SLE: In: Harrison's Principles of internal Medicine; 13th ed; McGraw Hill, Inc 1994; 1643-48.
7. Malaviya A.N., Bhuyan U.N., Kumar R. and Baliga Shakuntala, Connective tissue disorders in India; clinical and immunological profile of systemic lupus erythematosus, J. Assoc. Physicians India 1978; 26: 461-66.
8. Malaviya A.N., Misra R., Banerjee S., *et al.* Systemic lupus erythematosus in North India Asians—A Prospective analysis of clinical and immunological features, Rheumatol Int 1986; 6: 97-101.
9. Narayanan Kausalya, Rajagopalan Premavathy and Malviya A.N., Immunospecificities of anti-nuclear antibody in systemic connective diseases in India, J. Med. Res 1983;77: 87-95.
10. Malaviya A.N., Bhuyan U.N., Kumar R. and Taneja R.L., Diagnostic significance of anti-DNA antibody in clinical auto-immunity, J. Med. Res 1978; 67: 1001-04.
11. Kumar A., Malaviya A.N. and Ali R., Passive hemagglutination assay for detection and quantitation of autoantibodies reactive with thymus RNA in systemic lupus erythematosus, J. Biochem Biopsy 1983; 20:304-05.
12. Bhuyan U.N., Malaviya A.N., Kumar R., Malhotra K.K. and Tandon H.D., Frequency and severity of renal lesions in systemic lupus erythematosus in North India. J. Med. Res 1977; 66:965-73.

13. Malaviya A.N. and Zaidi Zoya., Connective tissue diseases in India-VIII, familial aggregation J. Assoc. Physicians India 1984; 32: 793-97.
14. Bhuyan U.N. and Malaviya A.N., Deficiency of T-cells in blood and tissues and severity of infections in systemic lupus erythematosus, J. Med. Res 1978; 67: 269-78.
15. Malaviya A.N., Khan M.M., Tiwari S.C. and Bhuyan U.N., Systemic connective tissue diseases in India-VII. Deaths in systemic lupus erythematosus, J. Assoc. Physicians India 1984; 32:313-16.
16. Kumar A., Manchanda S.C. and Malaviya A.N., Left ventricular performanceis systemic lupus erythematosus, J. Assoc. Physicians India 1978; 27:583-84.
17. Pradhan V; *et al.*, MBL in autoimmunity and its role in SLE; JAPI 2010; 58: 688-90.
18. Tan E.M., Cohen A.S., Fries J.F., *et al.* The revised criteria for the classification of systemic lupus erythematosus, Arthritis Rheum 1982; 25: 1271-77.
19. Kakamura R.M., Peebles C.L., Rubin R.L., Molden D.P. and Tan E.M., Autoantibodies to nuclear antigens (ANA), Advances in laboratory tests and significance in systemic rheumatic diseases. Chicago, American Society of Clinical Pathologists 1985; 1-103.
20. Handa R., Wali J.P., Antiphospholipid syndrome—The evolving paradigm; In; M.M. Singh; ed.; Medicine Update; API 1999; 9(1): 343-48.
21. Kakatis; *et al.*, Pulmonary manifestations in SLE with special reference to HRCT; JAPI 2007; 55: 839-41.
22. Shankar P.S., Systemic lupus erythematosus, Chest Medicine: Oxford and IBH Publ Co. (P) Ltd. 1994; 4th ed.
23. Kakati S., Doley B., *et al.*, Pulmonary manifestations in SLE with special reference to HRCT; JAPI 2007; 55:839-41.
24. Goswami R.P., *et al.*, A foe incognito–an interesting case of pleurisy; JAPI 2013; 53-56.
25. Schur P.H., The clinical management of systemic lupusery thematosus, New York, London. Grune and Stratton 1983; 1-290.
26. Wilcox P.G., *et al.*, Chest 1988; 93: 352-58.
27. Martens J., *et al.*, Respiratory muscle dysfunction in SLE; Chest 1984; 84: 170.
28. Hellmen D.B., *et al.*, Fatal in fections in SLE: The role of opportunistic organisms; Medicine1987; 66:341.
29. Handa R., *et al.*, Emergencies in lupus; In: Panja M.; Ed.; Med. Update; API 2001; 11: 206-11.
30. Gupta R.C., *et al.*, Current status of plasmapheresis in medical disorders; In; Y.P. Munjal; ed.; P.G. Med. API 1999; 13: 444-51.
31. Bernstein R.M., Bunn C.C., Hughes G.R.Y., *et al.*, Cellular protein and RNA antigens in autoimmune diseases; Mole. Biol. Med 1984; 2: 105-20.
32. Chandrashekhara Rao A.S., Narayana S., Swamy S.V. and Ramesh B., Pulmonary hypertension in SLE. JAPI 1990; 38: 295-96.
33. Asherson R.A. Mackworth-Young C.G., Boey M.L., *et al.* Pulmonary hypertension in systemic lupus erythematosus. Br. Med. J 1983; 287: 1024-26.
34. Walcott G., Burchell H.B., Brown A.L. Primary pulmonary hypertension, Am. J. Med 1970; 49:70-79.
35. Goldman D.D. and Urowitz M.B., Venous syndromes and pulmonary embolism in SLE, Ann. Rheum Dis 1980; 39: 340-43.
36. Handa R; Genetics of lupus-untying the Gordian knot! JAPI 2012; 60:12-13.

PROGRESSIVE SYSTEMIC SCLEROSIS (PSS)

Progressive systemic sclerosis (PSS) is a generalised connective tissue disorder characterised by fibrosis, atrophy and degenerative changes in the skin and many internal organs.[1,2] In PSS only 8 organ systems are involved. They are skin, vascular, GI tract, cardiac, renal, pulmonary, musculoskeletal, and nervous systems.[3,4] Cardiac involvement may be primary or secondary to renal or pulmonary involvement.[5,6] Pulmonary involvement is rarely a presenting feature of PSS, yet 90% may have pulmonary affliction during some stage of disease. The mean onset is in the age group of 40 to 50 years.[7] Women are affected four times more frequently than men.[8] Raynaud's phenomenon occurs in 90% of the patients with skin changes.[9] With the advent of sophisticated testing techniques, more light has been thrown on its pathogenesis.[10,11]

Aetiopathogenesis

PSS is a disease of unknown aetiology but three factors leading to altered collagen systems, microvascular abnormalities, and possible immunologic derangements have been suggested.[12] Although no clear cut evidence of primary defect in the collagen metabolism has been demonstrated, possibly excessive synthesis[13-15] and decreased degradation due to decreased collagenase activity[16] have been documented. Mononuclear infiltration in the connective tissue following narrowing of small arteries play a part,[17-19] assisted by cell mediated reactions,[20] though triggering factors are unknown. Both interstitial fibrosis and vascular involvement co-exist.

The process begins by cell mediated immune response or inflammatory injury to the endothelial cells of capillaries and small pulmonary arteries which facilitate existence of circulating proteins and possibly cellular elements to result in the proliferation of the connective tissue of the alveoli, leading to fibrosing alveolitis of the mural type.[21] The intimal proliferative thickening, medial thinning and periadventitial sclerosis of pulmonary small arteries and arterioles may lead to vascular occlusion, ischaemia of the alveoli and pulmonary hypertension. The thickening and inelasticity of the muscles of the chest wall and induration of the skin hinder the expansion of the chest.[21]

Clinical Features

The clinical presentation of PSS may be exertional dyspnoea. Pleuritic chest pain and non-productive cough may be noted. Crepitations are audible in the basal regions. Clubbing is usually absent. Pneumothorax and pleural effusion are rarely seen. Pneumonia may occur as a spillover due to oesophageal motility abnormality. Radiologically the interstitial fibrosis tends to involve the lower lung fields predominantly. A honeycombed appearance may be noted in late stages of the disease, along with severe interstitial fibrosis.[20]

Onset of PSS is in the age group of 40 to 50 years. No male patients of PSS below 25 years of age are reported according to Medger and Masi.[4] Epidemiology of 86 patients during the period 1947-1968 according to Mayo Clinic, revealed only 1.2% in I decade and 7.2% in II decade, out of 72 cases. Females are more frequently affected than males in a ratio of 4:1. As described earlier, only 8 organ systems get involved in PSS, but lymph nodes may be significantly involved, the possible explanations can be generalised vasculitis. Even impotency has been reported in PSS.[22]

In the Indian literature, only few studies are available on sclerosis.[23-29] In a recent study, dyspnoea in 82.4%, pulmonary fibrosis in 47%, PFT restrictive pattern in 47%, and pulmonary hypertension in 23.5% cases have been reported.[27] Lungs may be involved in almost ¾th of cases but often patients remain asymptomatic. PFT reveals restrictive ventilatory defect and low diffusing capacity may appear even before the clinical or radiological features appear. Uncommon presentations of PSS are shown in Table 10.7

Table 10.7: PSS: Uncommon factors

1. Asymptomatic pleuritis but histologically positive lesions in 85% of cases.
2. Pneumothorax is a rare and uncommon feature but can be presenting feature.
3. Chest X-ray-reticular or reticunodular shadow in the lower zones in 80% of cases.
4. Bilateral lower lobe interstitial fibrosis evolving into bullous emphysema is common.
5. PSS is a multisystem disorder with irreversible accumulation of fibrous tissue.

Investigations

There can be a restictive lung disease in 25 per cent of the cases; still airflow obstruction is demonstrable in 9 to 16 per cent of the patients. The single breath diffusion capacity is reduced and is unassociated with changes in pulmonary functions. There is poor correlation between the severity of functional abnormality and the extent of pulmonary lesions as noted by echocardiographic and radiological methods. Vascular abnormalities in the lungs may occur in the absence of interstitial fibrosis. It is postulated that it could be related to pulmonary vascular disease,[28] showing intimal proliferation and myxomatous changes in small and medium sized arteries.[29,30] Pulmonary artery hypertension is more frequent in patients with a variance of systemic sclerosis—the CREST (calcinosis, Raynaud's phenomenon, oesophageal dysfunction, sclerodactyly and telangiectasis) syndrome.[21] Pulmonary hypertension may be so sudden that it may constitute a medical emergency in certain cases.[31] Raynaud's phenomenon is a classical feature in 90% of patients with skin changes and may precede other features by months or years.[8] Cases without Raynaud's phenomenon have also been reported.[32] Bronchoalveolar lung lavage (BAL) shows an increased proportion of neutrophils, eosinophils and alveolar macrophages indicating the presence of inflammation. Some cases exhibit an abnormal proportion of lymphocytes also. PFTs show restrictive ventilatory defect.

Treatment[21]

Pulmonary disease in systemic sclerosis is often not rapidly progressive. Prognosis of the patients with isolated pulmonary hypertension is bad. Rarely it may become the seat of malignancy of the lung. The manifestations respond variably to treatment. Occassionally corticosteroids show a beneficial response if given early in the course of disease. Vasodilators such as hydralazine, calcium blockers and ACE inhibitors may decrease pulmonary vascular resistance in patients who have pulmonary hypertension. However, definite benefit has not been confirmed. Ketotifen has been tried. D-penicillamine appears to improve the diffusing capacity and decrease skin thickening.

Prognosis in systemic sclerosis worsens with the development of pulmonary artery hypertension, which does not show any red flag sign in early stages in a significant proportion of patients. Non-invasive screening, therefore, can help in early diagnosis and timely appropriate therapeutic interventions before significant end organ damage occurs.[33]

REFERENCES

1. Nuki George, Progressive Systemic Sclerosis, In: John Macleod, ed. Davidson's Principles and Practice of Medicine, 14th ed. Edinburgh, Hongkong: ELBS/Churchill Livingstone 1984; 575-76.
2. Le Roy E.C., Connective tissue diseases characterised by fibrosis, scleroderma in Kelley W. N., et al., ed, Textbook of Rheumatology, WB Saunders Co, Philadelphia 1985; 994-1036.
3. Suresh K., et al., An unusual presentation of PSS, JAPI 1994: 42: 163-64.
4. Medger Jr. and Masi A.T., Epidemiology of systemic sclerosis. Ann. Intern. Med 1971; 74:714-21.
5. Bulkely B.H.S. and Humphries J.O., The heart and collagen vascular disease, In; J. Willis Hurst, et al., ed. The heart, arteries and veins, McGraw Hill Book Co., New York, 6th ed 1986; 1441-45.
6. Sttolerman G.H., Rheumatic fever and other rheumatic diseases of the heart, Eugene Braunwald, ed., A textbook of cardiovascular medicine; WB Saunders, Philadelphia, 4th 1992; 1721-41.
7. Thomas A., Medger Jr. and Alfose T. Masi, Epidemiology of Progressive Systemic Sclerosis. In: Buchanan Kahn M.F., Veikko Laine; Rodnam G.P., Scott J.T., Zvaifler N.J. eds. Clinics in Rheumatic Diseases, Philadelphia: WB Saunders 1979; 5:

15-25.
8. Rodman C.P., PSS, In: Hollander J.L., Mc Carty D.L., ed, Arthritis and allied conditions; Philadephia, Lea and Febiger, 1979.
9. Bruce C., Gilliland, Mart Mannik, *Progressive Systemic Sclerosis,* In: Petersdorf R.G., Adams R.D., Bruanwald E., Issel bacher K.J. Martin J.B. and Wilson J.D. eds. Harrisons Principles of Internal Medicine, 10th ed., NewYork.Tokyo McGraw-Hill International Book Co 1983; 2002-2006.
10. Follance W.P.,The cardiovascular manifestations of systemic sclerosis, Curr Prob In Cardiolo1986; 11: 244-98.
11. Alaxander E.L. *et al.,* Scleroderma heart disease, evidence of cold induced abnormalities of myocardial function and perfusion, Arch Rheum 1981; 24: 58.
12. Symposium on the fibrotic processes, Ann. Rheum Dis 1977; 36: (Suppl) 2.
13. Herbert C.M., *et al.,* Biosynthesis and maturation of skin collagen in scleroderma and effect of D-penicillamine Lancet 1977: 1: 672.
14. LeRoy E.C., Scleroderma, In; Hugher GRV(ed) Current topics in Rheumatology; London; Heinemann; 1976.
15. Buckingham R.B., *et al.,* Increased collagen accumulation in dermal fibroblast cultures from patients with PSS (Scleroderma), J. Lab. Clin. Med 1978; 92: 5.
16. Brady A.H., Collagenase in scleroderma J. Clin. Invest 1975; 56: 1175.
17. Marichar T. and LeRoy P., Patterns of finger capillary abnormalities in connective tissue disease by wide field microscopy. Arthr Rheum 1973; 16:619.
18. Campbell P.M. and LeRoy E.C., Pathogenesis of systemic sclerosis: A vascular hypothesis; Semin Arthr. Rheum 1975; 4: 351.
19. Segovia A.B., *et al., Immunological aspects of scleroderma;* In; Hughes GRV (ed); Current topics in Rheumatology. London, Heinemann, 1976.
20. Robbins S.L. and Cotran R.S., Scleroderma; In; Pathologic basis of disease; WB Saunders Co., Japan 1981; 2nd ed 308-10.
21. Shankar P.S., PSS; In; Chest Medicine; Oxford and IBH Pub Co (P) Ltd., 1994 4th ed.
22. Nowlin N.S., Brick J.E., Weaver D.J., *et al.,* Impotency in scleroderma, Ann Intern. Med 1986; 104: 794-797.
23. Desai M.M. and Shah D.M., Rheumatic and collagen diseases: A review of scientific papers published during 25 years period, 1944-69; JAPI 1970, 18: 409.
24. Gupta H.L., Balkrishna, *et al.,* Clinical profile of PSS in humans, JIMA 1987, 85:332-41.
25. Ashok Kumar, *et al.,* Clinical and laboratory profile of systemic sclerosis in Northern India, JAPI 1990; 38:765-68.
26. Desai Y., *et al.,* Renal involvement in scleroderma, JAPI 1990; 38: 768-70.
27. Chandalia M.S., *et al.,* Cardiac involvement in systemic sclerosis; JAPI 1993; 41:635-37.
28. Rocco V.K. and Huid E.R., Scleroderma and scleroderma like disorders, Semin Arthrit Rheumato 1986; 16:22-69.
29. Salemi R. *et al.,* Pulmonary hypertension in the CREST syndrome; variant of progressive systemic sclerosis; Ann Inter Med 1977; 86: 394-99.
30. Nath A.R. and Mehta P.J., Scleroderma, the heart and myocardial Raynaud's phenomenon (Editorial), JAPI 1993; 41: 63 1-32.
31. Stupi A.M., Steen V.D., Ownes G.R. *etal;* Pulmonary hypertension in CREST syndrome—variant of systemic sclerosis; Arth Rheum 1986; 29: 515.
32. Narasinhachary N.L., Chandramohan M., Rajesekaran V.N., *et al.,* PSS, JAPI 1987; 35:861-63.
33. Uma Kumar; *et al.,* Prevalence and predictors of pulmonary artery hypertension in systemic sclerosis; JAPI 2008; 56: 413-17.

PULMONARY ANGIITIS AND GRANULOMATOSIS

There is a tissue reactions characterised by focal destructive and infiltrative vascular disease along with granulomatosis in the lung. The aetiology is undetermined. It includes Wegener's granulomatosis, allergic angiitis and granulomatosis and lymphomatoid granulomatosis.[1,2]

Wegener's Granulomatosis

Wegener's granulomatosis (WG) is one of the pulmonary renal syndrome where systemic vasculitides is seen in 50% of cases. It is a disseminated systemic disease characterised by necrotising granulomatous angiitis involving the upper respiratory tract, lungs, glomerulonephritis and small vessel vasculitis. This classic triad may not be present in all the cases. A limited form of Wegener's granulomatosis is associated with lesions restricted to the respiratory tract only. A limited form with minor renal disease have also been described. Neurologic involvement may be seen in the form of CNS involvement, cranial nerve involvement and more commonly peripheral neuropathy. This was initially described by Klinger in Berlin in 1931 but was mistakenly believed to be an atypical form of polyarteritis nodosa.[3] Friederick Wegener later described in 1936 his findings on postmortem in three patients dying of a distinct syndrome consisting of necrotising granuloma and generalised arteritis[4] called Wegener's granulomatosis.

In India, the disease is scantily reported.[5] Lack of availability of serum marker and reluctance of physicians to go for[6] open lung biopsy and the very much of these cases either responding to ATT or being reported as resistant tubercular cases[7] (since tuberculosis is the most common suspected chest infection), these cases of Wegener's granulomatosis remain reported.

Aetiopathogenesis

The aetiology is undetermined, but the presence of primary hypersensitivity suggests that an immunologic reaction triggered by a specific antigen and immune complexes play a role in the pathogenesis. Perhaps, it is a microbial infection which in a susceptible host initiates a cascade of immunological events, resulting in pathological changes seen in the disease.[2] The granulomatosis inflammation suggests an infectious, toxins or autoimmune initiating agent.[8] However, all cultures and microscopic examinations for microorganisms must be negative. Tissue necrosis is followed by migration of mononuclear histiocytes, to form granuloma. Vessels are not involved in the development of parenchymal granulomas.

Pathology: Granuloma has central necrosis, surrounded by a cluster lymphocytes, plasma cells and palisading histiocytes. Vascular lesions are necrotizing angiitis affecting pulmonary vessels. Renal lesions can be segmental glomerulonephritis (with little impairment of renal functions) or necrotising glome-rulonephritis with crescent formation (leading to renal failure).

Clinical Features

The disease is noted in the fourth or the fifth decades, often more in men than in women, although younger patients are also affected.[3] There are non-specific features of systemic inflammation, such as fever, malaise, arthralgia and weight loss. Upper airway complaints include rhinorrhoea, pain in the paranasal sinuses, epistaxis, serous discharge from ears and ulceration in the nasal mucosa which often progresses to perforation of the nasal septum and cartilage causing saddle nose deformity.[9,10] Often there is a secondary bacterial infection. The involvement of the lower respiratory tract is manifested by cough and pleuritic pain. Thus the natural course of the disease may be variable, ranging from rapidly fatal massive pulmonary haemorrhage[11] to indolent sinusitis for several years. Diffuse alveolar hemorrhage is life threatening in Wegener's granulomatosis and urgent pulse cyclophosphamide therapy with steroids is life saving.[11] The pulmonary infiltrates often cavitate leading to expectoration and haemoptysis. The condition is not associated with hypertension, eosinophilia or history of allergy. Renal involvement manifests as glomerulonephritis.[1] Apart from lungs and kidneys, other organs may also have focal or diffuse involvement. Cardiac involvement is uncommon; supraventricular tachycardia may be noted clinically.[12] Subcutaneous nodules,[13] pustules, gingival hyperplasia and very rarely gangrene have been documented.[14,15] Scleritis and blindness may be seen in 50% of cases. Parotids, breast, urethra, cervix and vagina may be involved in 1% of cases.

Diagnosis

Lungs are affected in 45% of patients. The diagnosis of WG is suspected when the following clinical features are encountered:[16]

1. Upper respiratory tract involvement such as paranasal sinus pain with purulent or bloody nasal discharge, nasal mucosal ulceration, saddle nose deformity, serous otitis media, etc.
2. Lung disease manifests as asymptomatic infiltrates or with cough, haemoptysis, dyspnoea or chest discomfort.
3. Evidence of renal disease in the form of proteinuria, haematuria or red cell casts. WG rarely presents as an isolated renal disease.
4. Eye involvement in the form of episcleritis, scleritis, proptosis due to reteroorbital mass, etc.

The diagnosis[17] is confirmed by obtaining histopathological evidence of granulomatous vasculitis or alternatively a picture consistent with WG on appropriate tissue, coupled with a characteristic triad of upper respiratory system involvement, lung involvement and glomerulonephritis.

Differential diagnosis include SLE, Churg-Strauss syndrome, Goodpasture's syndrome, tumours of upper airways and lungs, pulmonary tuberculosis, fungal infections of lungs and midline granuloma. WG relapses are often preceded by a significant rise in ANCA.[18]

Investigations

Chest X-ray shows bilateral nodular infiltrates that often cavitate. Lung biopsy reveals necrotising granulomatous vasculitis with infiltration from neutrophils, lymphocytes, plasma cells, histiocytes and giant cells. There is anaemia and leucocytosis. ESR is elevated. Urine shows protein, RBCs and casts.[1]

The radiological changes in both tuberculosis and WG are similar in many respects.[19] Infiltrates and cavities are major signs for both. However, the infiltrates in WG tend to be nodular, cavitating and sometimes transient, while those in tuberculosis are more linear. The cavitatory lesions of tuberculosis are more often apical while those of WG are more basal. It must, however, be emphasised that no radiologic feature is pathognomonic of WG.[18] WG may present as solitary pulmonary nodule on chest X-ray.[20] Large or moderate pleural effusions are virtually never seen in WG. Even WG granulomatosis responds to anti tuberculosis treatment.[21,22] The major features that can help to separate the conditions are, however, clinical. Upper airway, eye, sinus, skin and renal involvement is rare in tuberculosis and the presence of any of these must alert the physician to the diagnosis of WG.

The diagnosis is confirmed with tissue biopsy.[9] Many involved tissues can be sampled but the highest yield is from the lungs.[23] It was previously believed that the pickup rate of granulomata and angiitis from other tissues was very low. However, recent studies show that a diligent search is frequently rewarding.[24] All involved areas which are easily accessible must be sampled and open lung biopsy should be done more frequently. *Invasive* investigations include open lung biopsy and kidney biopsy. ANCA (anti neutrophil cytoplasmic antibodies) when present, provides further supportive evidence for the diagnosis. Renal biopsy alone does not provide diagnostic information as granulomas and arteritis are rarely seen in biopsy specimen.[17]

ANCA test is carried out using the indirect immunofluorescence method described by Vander Woude, *et al.*,[25] Neutrophils from the blood of a healthy person are separated by density gradient and smears are prepared by cytocentrifugation for 30 minutes. The cells are fixed with chilled absolute alcohol and then incubated with test serum for 30 minutes. After thorough washing in PBS, the smears are incubated with fluorescence isothiocyanate conjugated anti-immunoglobulin for 30 minutes. After washing the PBS, the slides are examined for cytoplasmic staining in an immunofluorescence microscope. A known positive and a negative serum sample are tested with each run. ANCA is a very useful tool in the diagnosis in 85-90% of cases in the classic form with kidney involvement in WG[18] and 67-87% in limited form of WG.[26]

There is some evidence to suggest that WG in India may be more aggressive in its clinical behaviour. It has been observed that the disease usually evolves in a phased manner affecting the upper airways (E) and lungs (L) before going on to the kidneys (K). In developed countries, the ELK pattern is the exception at the time of diagnosis,[27] while it seems to be the predominant pattern in India. This could also be explained for delayed diagnosis (Table 10.8).

Table 10.8: Anatomic extent of Wegener's granulomatosis at the time of diagnosis according to the ELK* system (%)

Patients	*50*	*46*	*77*
Country	USA	Germany	France
E alone	28	59	—
L alone	16	13	8
EL	16	13	16
EK	8	4	—
LK	10	4	16
ELK	22	7	59

*E =Upper airways and related structures, L =Lungs, K = Kidneys.

Prognosis

The course is extremely variable and untreated conditions are fatal from renal or respiratory failure. Rapidly progressive renal failure is present in about 10 per cent of cases. Prognosis of granulomatosis with crescents affecting more than 50% of glomeruli is generally bad. Prognosis is better in patients without renal involvement.[28] Mortality is due to renal failure or infections due to immunosuppression.

Management of vasculitis needs urgent attention, since there is high risk of immediate and irreversible damage of renal physiology. Respiratory failure or massive pulmonary hemorrhage prove fatal. Immunosuppression contribute to infection that might lead to fatal outcome, along with renal failure.[29]

The mean survival of untreated Wegener's granulomatosis may be 5 months[30] with 90% dying within 2 years.[9]

Treatment

Plasma exchange and immunosuppressive drugs are the mainstay in the management. Plasma exchange of four litres with albumin for 2 weeks to cut down antibody titre is useful. In case of coagulopathy, fresh frozen plasma can be used in place of albumin. Inflammatory reactions subsides with steroids; however, the beneficial response is not evident when the disease has progressed. Three pulse doses of I/V methyprednisolone on alternate days, followed by oral prednisolone, which is administered in a dose of 1 mg/kg/day in divided doses. There is rapid amelioration of manifestations and resolution of the lesions with immunosuppressive therapy with cyclophosphamide or azathioprine, begun early in the course of the disease. They are able to suppress antibody formation and tissue injury. Cyclophosphamide (2 mg/kg/day) and prednisolone (1 mg/kg/day) orally for a minimum of one year after remission and initial 3 months respectively. Close monitoring of complete blood counts and urine is done to detect side effects of cyclophosphamide. Total leucocyte count, platelets and polymorphs are maintained above 3500/cmm^3, 10, 10^{5}and 15.0/cmm^3 respectively. Fluid intake has to be increased and patients are advised to avoid holding of urine to minimize the likelihood of haemorrhagic cystitis.[6] Azathioprine can be given in young patients for 3-4 months to avoid gonadal toxicity.

In addition, ESR (Westergren), blood urea, serum creatinine, urine examination and X-ray chest are done periodically to monitor the therapeutic response during follow up. For local upper respiratory tract lesions, radiotherapy can be used as adjuvant therapy.

Criteria for Response[9] (as per NIH Group)

Complete remission can be defined as per the following criteria:

a. Complete absence of general symptoms, such as fever, joint pains, weight loss, etc.
b. Complete healing of pulmonary lesions or stable scarring without signs of active inflammation.
c. Stabilization/improvement of renal function without active renal sediment (mild proteinuria, however may persist).
d. No serositis.
e. Normal ESR.

Partial remission can be defined as per the following criteria:

a. No worsening of any organ-system involvement.
b. Progression towards improvement.
c. Reduction in ESR by at least 50%.

Therapy with cyclophosphamide gives very satisfactory results.[4,6,16] Cyclophosphamide pulse therapy may be advantageous in WG. Both low and high incidence of side effects have been reported respectivley.[6] Current regimen of choice is oral daily cyclophosphamide with oral steroids.[15] C-ANCA estimation helps in titrating immunosuppressive therapy.[29] Plasma exchange may be beneficial in renal involvement.[30]

Vasculitides form a group of rare heterogenous disorders, having diverse etiologies and mainfestations. Clinical presentations are protean depending upon size, site and type of vessel affected in different organs.

Early diagnosis and timely institution of treatment prevents complications, sequelae and mortality which may, otherwise, be higher in the absence of appropriate and adequate therapy in early times.

Pulmonary involvement in vasculitis has been shown in the following table.

Pulmonary involvement in vasculitis[2]

*(Pauci-immune ANCA-associated disorders)

a. **WG (Wegener's granulomatosis)
b. **CSS (Churg-Strauss syndrome)
c. **MPA (Microscopic polyangitis)
   i. **Alveolar haemorrhage** characterized by hemoptysis, anemia and bilateral evanescent lung opacities.
   ii. **Nodules** with or without cavities, infarction.
   iii. **Asthma (CSS)**

* All forms may not always be associated with ANCA.
** Lesion is granulomatous.
• Frequent overlap of small and medium blood vessel involvement.

Deoxysperguralin has been tried in relapsing and refractory cases of Wegener's granulomatosis.[31,32]

SALIENT FEATURES

1. Prevalence is 3/10,000.
2. Focal vasculitis is 5-10% cases has been reported.
3. Upper respiratory tract biopsy is non-diagnostic, lower respiratory biopsies after histologic diagnosis.
4. Immunopathogenesis includes aberrant cell-mediated immune response.

REFERENCES

1. Saigal R, Kansal A; Approach to systemic vasculitis; IN; MS Rao; ed; Med Update 2010; 20: 816-21.
2. Falk RJ, Hoffman GS; Controversies in small vessel vasculitis–comparing the rheumatology and nephrology views; Curr Opin Rheumat 2007; 19: 01-09.
3. de Groot K. *et al.,* Standardised neurologic evaluation of 128 patients with WG; Arch, Neurol 2001; 58: 1215-21.
4. Kaushal R., Dash S.C., Kapoor S., *et al.,* Wegener's granulomatosis in the rapidly progressive glomerulonephritis, J. Assn. Phys. India 1987; 35: 382-84.
5. Sakhuja V., Bamberi P., Mathur R,P., *et al.,* Pulmonary involvement in Wegener's granulomatosis. A report of 4 cases, Indian J. Chest Dis. Allied, Sci 1986; 28: 99-104.
6. Singh Y.N., Malviya A.N., Sharma S.K., *et al.,* Wegener's granulomatosis in northern India; J. Ass. Phys, India 1992; 40:594-96.
7. Bambery P., Sakhuja V., Bhusnurmath S.R., *et al.,* Wegener's granulomatosis—Clinical experience with 18 patients, J, Ass. Phys. India 1992; 40:597-600.
8. Deremse R.A., M.C. Donald T.J. and Louis Weiland, Wegener's granulomatosis: Observations on treatment with antimicrobial agents; Mayo Clinic Proc 1985; 27: 32-60.
9. Leavitt R.A., *et al.,* The American College of Rheumatology 1980: Criteria for classification of WG: Arch Rheumoe 1990; 33: 1101-07.
10. D'Cruz D.P., Baguley E. Asherson R.A. and Hughes G.R.V., Ear, nose and throat symptoms in subacute Wegener's granulomatosis, Br. Med. J 1989; 299:419-22.
11. Mahajan V; *et al.,* Diffuse alveolar hemorrhage in Wegener's granulomatosis; Lung India 2011; 28: 52-55.
12. Goodfield M.E.R., *et al.,* Cardiac involvement in WG; Brit Heart J 1995;73: 110-15.
13. Dawod M.S., *et al.,* Cutaneous WG; J Amer Acad Dermat 1994;31:605-12.
14. Handa R., Wali J.P., WG with gangrene of toes; Scand J Rheum 1986; 25:103-04.
15. Handa R., *et al.,* WG—A Clinicopathologic study; JAPI 1997; 45: 536-39.
16. Fauci A.S., *The vasculitic syndromes.* In: Braunwald E., Isselbacher K.H., Petersdorf R.G., Wilson J.D., Martin J.B., Fauci A.S., Eds. Harrison's Principles of Internal Medicine,Vol.2,New York: McGraw-Hill 1987; 1438-45.
17. Wolff S.M., Fauci A.S., Horn R.G., *et al.,* Wegener's granulomatosis, Ann Intern. Med 1974; 81: 513-25.
18. Jennette J.C., Antineutrophil cytoplasmic antibody associated diseases: A pathologist's perspective; Amer. J. Kind. Dis 1991; 18: 164-70.
19. Bambery P., Katariya S., Sakhuja V., *et al.,* Wegener's granulomatosis in north India: Radiological manifestation in eleven patients, Acta Radial (Diag) 1989; 29: 11-13.
20. Christopher D.J., *et al.,* WG: Two cases presenting with solitary pulmonary nodule; Lung India 1996; 13 (3,4): 141-45.
21. Toyoshima M., *et al.,* Wegener's granulomatosis responding to auntituberculosis drugs; Chest 2001; 119:643-44.
22. Inowe K., *et al.,* Anti-tuberculosis drugs for Wegener's granulomatosis; Chest 2001; 120:2112-13.
23. Hoffman G.S., *et al.,* Wegener's granulomatosis; Ananalys is of 158 patients; Ann. Int. Med 1992; 116:4888-98.
24. Bullen C.L., Liesegang T.J., McDonald T.J. and DcRemee R.A., Ocular complications of Wegener's granulomatosis, Ophthalmology 1983; 90: 279-90.
25. Van Der Woude F.J., Daha M.R. and Van E.S.L.A., The current status of neutrophil cytoplasmic antibodies, Clin Exp. Immunol 1989; 78: 143-48.
26. Kallenbery C.G.M., *et al.,* ANCA—A still growing class of auto antibodies in inflammatory disorders; Amer. J. Med 1992; 93: 675-83.
27. Gross W.L., Wegener's granulomatosis, Sarcoidosis 1989; 6: 15-29.
28. Snaith L., Michael E.D.; ABC of Rheumatology; BMJ 1995; 310: 1128-32.

29. Raju Hari K; Tripathi K; ANCA-associated renal diseases; IN; Manutosh Panja; Ed; PG Med: API 2003; 17: 499-511.
30. Mestri S.G., *et al.,* Disappearing lung lesions in WG; Lung India 2000; 18: 95-96.
31. Flossmann O; *et al.,* Deoxyspergualin in relapsing and refractory WG; Ann Rheum Dis 2009; 68: 125-30.
32. Bande U., *et al.,* Wegener granulomatosis–rare case presentation; JAPI 2012;60:60-63.

ALLERGIC ANGIITIS AND GRANULOMATOSIS (CHURG-STRAUSS SYNDROME)

The syndrome presents with asthma, with subsequent evidence of vasculitis which when develops, asthma abates. A multisystem necrotic vasculitic disorder involving small and medium sized vessels (arteries, capillaries and venules) characterised by bronchial asthma, eosinophilia, eosinophil rich tissue inflammation with infrequent renal involvement.[1-3]

There is a history of asthma and evidence of vasculitis, clinically presenting in the form of fever, weight loss, and anemia. Routine tests show eosinophilia and leucocytosis. ESR is raised, indicating avidity of the disease.[4-7] X-ray chest shows diffuse patchy or nodular infiltrates in 30-80% of cases. The lesions do not cavitate unlike Wegener's granulomatosis. Renal involvement is infrequent and glomerulonephritis is not a feature. There is no destruction of the upper respiratory passages. Skin, nervous system, kidneys and lungs are involved. Dermal leukocytoclastic vasculitis manifests as purpura. The involvement of organ systems is similar to that of polyarteritis nodosa, but the lung is (infrequently involved in the latter condition.[3] Cardiac involvement may occur in l/3rd of cases. Asthma and eosinophilia are distinguishing features and can be seen in almost 80% of cases.[4]

Allergic angiitis and granulomatosis respond to cortisone therapy with or without addition of cyclophosphamide or azathioprine.[3] The condition may prove fatal if not treated energetically.

REFERENCES

1. Langham J.C., Elkon K.B.,. Pusey D.C., *et al., Medicine* (Baltimore) 1984; 63: 65.
2. Leibow A.A., Pulmonary angiitis and granulomatosis; Amer Rev Resp Dis 1973; 108:01.
3. Shankar P.S., Chest Medicine; Oxford and IBH Publ. Co. (P) Ltd; New Delhi; 4th ed; 1994.
4. Harrison's principles of internal medicine. ed; Wilson J.D. Braunwald E., Isselbacher K.J., *et al.,* 12th ed; Vol. 2, McGraw Hill, N. York, 1991.
5. Jadol M., de Strihon C.Y.; Cardiorespiratory system and the kidney; In; Oxford Text book of Clinical Nephrology; 2nd ed; Oxford 1998; 2767-74.
6. Chandler D.B., Fulmer J.D., Pulmonary vasculitis; Lung 1985; 163:257.
7. Edwards C.W., Vasculitis and granulomatosis of respiratory tract; Thorax 1982; 37: 81.

LYMPHOMATOID GRANULOMATOSIS

Lymphomatoid granulomatosis is a separate entity different from lymphoma, to which it simulates histologically, and different from WG, to which it simulates both clinically and histologically.[1] It is a rare condition associated with lymphoreticular proliferation and granuloma formation.[2] There is an infiltration of lymphocytoid, plasma-like cells and macrophages, creating a necrotic granulomatosis inflammatory reaction especially near the blood vessels which is both angiocentric and angiodestructive.

The condition affects primarily the lungs but the skin, kidney and central nervous system may also be involved. It is usually seen in the fourth decade of life. The pulmonary pathology occurs in 50% of cases, having clinical presentation in the form of cough, dyspnoea, fever, malaise and weight loss. Though the condition simulates Wegener's granulomatosis, the involvement of the upper respiratory tract and kidney are rare. Unlike other lymphoproliferative disorders, lymphomatoid granulomatosis does not affect spleen, lymph nodes and bone marrow. Radiologically it presents multiple nodular shadows or ill-defined opacities which often wax and wane.[3] Cavitations are less common.

The condition has a tendency to progress as a lymphoproliferative disorder and may evolve to malignant ly-mphoma in as many as 50% cases. Remissions occur following treatment with steroids and cyclophosphamide and is a good sign as the chances of developing into angiocentric lymphoma are minimised. Patients showing marked cellular atypia need aggressive chemotherapy.

REFERENCES

1. Leavitt R.Y., Fanci A.S., Pulmonary vasculitis; Amer Rev Resp Med 1986; 134:149.
2. Fauci A.S., Haynes B.F. and Costa J., Lymphomatoid granulomatosis Perspective and clinical experience over 10 years, New Engl. Jour. Med 1982; 306: 68.
3. Shankar P.S., Chest Medicine, Oxford and IBH Publ. Co. N.Delhi, 4th ed. 1994.

BENIGN LYMPHOCYTIC ANGIITIS AND GRANULOMATOSIS[1]

Benign lymphocytic angiitis and granulomatosis (BLAG) is a rare disease occurring in the fifth decade of life and is confined to lungs. There is diffuse cellular infiltrate consisting of mature lymphocytes, plasma cells and plasmacytoid lymphocytes that obliterates the alveolar architecture, infiltrates vessels, and invades peripheral airways. There are multiple, loose giant cell granulomas. Necrosis is rarely seen. The patients may be asymptomatic or present with fever, dyspnoea, non-productive cough and chest pain. Bilateral nodular or patchy infiltrates are seen on chest X-ray. An open lung biopsy is diagnostic. It responds to a combination of chlorambusil and prednisolone.

Bronchocentric Granulomatosis[1-4]

Bronchocentric granulomatosis is a necrotizing granulomatous inflammatory process within the walls and surrounding tissue of bronchioles. True angiitis is absent. There is destruction of alveolar walls and of the lung tissue distal to the bronchiolar lesion, leading to pulmonary fibrosis and bronchiectasis. There may be a history of asthma in 50% of patients. The condition appears to be a hypersensitivity reaction to aspergillus and mycobacterial infections. Peripheral eosinophilia is present in 50% of cases, few have positive skin test for serum precipitin to aspergillus. Chest X-ray has variable presentation. Unlike other vasculitides, bronchocentric granulomatosis is not angiocentric or angiodestructive, and involves only the bronchi and bronchioles.

Pulmonary Hyalinizing Granuloma

Pulmonary hyalinizing granuloma is a fibrosing lung lesion, characterized by deposition of lamellar collagen in a haphazard whorl-like fashion.[1] This autoimmune abnormality predominantly affects the middle aged men. The clinical features are cough, breathlessness or chest pain. Sometimes it is asymptomatic. Unilateral or bilateral homogeneous and well circumscribed nodules are seen on chest X-ray, simulating metastatic lung lesion. Diagnosis can be made with the help of wedge biopsy. There may be slow progressive enlargement of the lesion. In some cases it may remain stationary. Associated sclerosing mediastinitis may be seen in 15 to 20% of cases.[1] No treatment is available.[2]

Necrotizing Sarcoid Granulomatosis (NSG)

NSG is a rare pulmonary disease having pathological similarities to Wegener's granulomatosis and sarcoidosis. It affects females, more so in the fifth decade of life. Numerous sarcoid-like granulomas with variable degree of coagulative necrosis and hyalinization in association with vasculitis involving both arteries and veins, are seen histologically; it may present as a rare manifestation of sarcoidosis. The condition may be asymptomatic or may have non-specific presentations like fever, cough, malaise and pleuritic pain. Multiple alveolar infiltrates mostly in the lower lobes can be seen on chest X-ray. The cavitation and hilar adenopathy are uncommon. Course is usually benign. Spontaneous or remission on administration of corticosteroids is known.[2,5]

Idiopathic Bronchiolitis Obliterans Organising Pneumonia

Introduction

Idiopathic Bronchiolitis Obliterans Organising Pneumonia (BOOP)—a term used in USA[6] or cryptogenic organising pneumonia (COP) (synonymous),[7,8] is an infiltrative lung disease with a subacute clinical course.

Pathology

Histologic features of BOOP include patchy bronchiolitis obliterans with organising pneumonia, interstitial mononuclear cell infiltrate, alveolar space foam cells and absence of honeycombing or extensive interstitial fibrosis. There is a tendency for the tissue to be atelectatic in the zones of organisation. BOOP has to be differentiated from IPF and acute interstitial pneumonia as shown in Table 10.9.

In constrictive bronchiolitis obliterans (without organization) which is very rarely seen in BOOP, there is chronic bronchiolar inflammation with constrictive bronchiolar narrowing, submucosal fibrous thickening and mucostasis. Histologic features that go against the diagnosis of BOOP, include hyaline membrane, necrosis, acute inflammation, marked fibrinous alveolar exudates, micro abscess formation, vasculitis,

Table 10.9

Acute interstitial pneumonia	*BOOP*	*Idiopathic pulmonary fibrosis{IPF}*
Uniform diffuse involvement of pulmonary parenchyma	Patchy intraluminal organisation with absence of honeycombing	Varied histology with zones of normal lung, honeycombing and zones of active interstitial widening
Interstitial odematous fibroblastic thickening	Prominent interstitial infiltrate	Prominent paraseptal and subpleural reaction
Residual hyaline membranes present	Cellular bronchiolitis present	Foam cells inconspicuous
Alveolar wall collapsed (microatelectasis)	Alveolar foam cells conspicuous	Focal intra-luminal organising
Paucity of foam cells and chronic-inflammation	Odematous, fibroblastic, interstitial thickening inconspicuous	Odematous, interstitial fibroblastic, thickening present
Absence of cellular bronchitis		

honeycombing, prominent eosinophils, granulomas, marked alveolar lining cells and bronchiolar metaplasia.

The syndrome of unknown aetiology is defined as granulation tissue plugs within lumens of small airways, sometimes with complete obstruction of small airways and granulation tissues may be extending into alveolar ducts and alveoli.[6] Additional features include proliferation of connective tissue that forms intraluminal polyps, fibrinous exudates, alveolar accumulation of foamy macrophages, inflammed alveolar walls and rounded balls of myxomatous connective tissue. There is absence of honeycombing or extensive interstitial fibrosis. However, the background architecture of the lung is preserved.[7-9] Such a proliferative bronchiolitis obliterans lesion may be seen in individuals having history of recent toxic fume exposure or recent infection (adenovirus) or chronic thyroiditis or alcoholic liver cirrhosis or in association with connective tissue disorders or a drug reaction (acebutolol, gold, cyclosporin, sulfasalazine, amiodarone or bleomycin) or radiation therapy or as a myelodysplastic syndrome or following a bone marrow or heart-lung trasplantation. It is an inflammatory lung disease; but in majority of cases the aetiology remains undetemined.[1]

Clinical Features

The illness occurs in men and women aged 20 to 70 years and there is relation to smoking. Most of the patients have a duration of illness of 3 months or less.[9] A preceding flu-like illness and a short history of cough, malaise, fatigue, weight loss and dyspnoea are usually present. Cough is usually persistent and non-productive and dyspnoea is mild. Haemoptysis is very rare.[10] Clubbing may be present in very few.

Investigations

Chest examination reveals fine end-inspiratory crackles. There is no leucocytosis and ESR is raised. Chest X-ray shows bilateral, patchy migratory linear or nodular opacities in the presence of normal lung volumes. Rarely a solitary focal pneumonia pattern may be seen.[11,12] CT scan reveals the air space consolidation sometimes shaped like triangles to be distinctly peripheral in middle and lower parts of the lung with subpleural predominance in 50% of cases. Mild to moderate restrictive ventilatory defect with abnormal diffusing capacity may be found on PFT. Bronchoalveolar lavage cytology shows increase in all cell types, most significantly lymphocytes, foamy macrophages and plasma cells. There is reduction in CD 4^+/CD 8^+ ratio. Because of patchy nature of the disease, bronchoscopic biopsies may not be adequate.[13,14] Open lung biopsy which is rarely required, shows intraluminal changes with buds of granulation tissue within air spaces mostly alveoli but also alveolar ducts and respiratory bronchioles and a variable degree of interstitial infiltration of mononuclear cells and accumulation of foamy macrophages in alveolar spaces.

Differential Diagnosis

Differential diagnosis includes: (a) Idiopathic pulmonary fibrosis which pursues a chronic progressive course that is usually not altered by treatment. It shows heterogenous fibrotic lesions in spatial distribution. (b) Chronic eosinophilic pneumonia exhibits significant infiltrations of eosinophils in the peripheral air spaces and/or the pulmonary interstitium. (c) Extrinsic allergic alveolitis shows a granulomatous interstitial pneumonitis. Diagnosis of BOOP should be made only after excluding other disease states with identical histology, e.g., chemical or drug inhalation injury, infections, irradiation, connective tissue disorder, ulcerative colitis, HIV infection and following bone marrow or lung transplantation.[15] Cases have appeared in Indian literature.[16]

Management

Steroids form the mainstay of treatment. The response of idiopathic BOOP to corticosteroids is good and relapses are unlikely if sufficient therapy is given. Prednisolone is administered in a dose 1mg/kg for 1 to 3 months then tapering doses to 40 mg 3 months, then 10 to 20 mg a day for a total period of one year.[1] Cyclophosphamide has been tried. Complications such as leucopenia, haemorrhagic cystitis and carcinoma of bladder should be kept in mind.

REFERENCES

1. Shankar P.S., Chest Medicine; Oxford and IBH Publ. Co. (P) Ltd; N. Delhi 1994; 4th ed.
2. Sawicka E.H., The necrotizing vasculitides; Thorax 1987; 42: 913.
3. Alarcon-segovia D., The necrolizing vasculitides; A new pathologenic classification; Clin. North Amer 1977; 61: 241.
4. Dent R.G., *et al.*, Pulmonary hyalinising granuloma in association with reteroperitoneal fibrosis; Thorax 1983: 38: 955.
5. Fanburg B.L., Ed., Lung biology in health and disease; P. Marcel Dekker, N.York; 1983.
6. Epler G.R., *et al.*, BOOP, New Eng. J. Med 1985; 312: 152-58.
7. Sulavik S., The concept of organising pneumonia, Chest 1989; 96: 967-69.
8. Izumi T., *et al.*, BOOP: Clinical features and differential diagnosis, Chest 1992; 102: 7 15-19.
9. Cordier *J.F. et al.*, Idiopathic bronchiolitis obliterating pneumonia. Definition of characteristic clinical profiles in a series of 16 patients, Chest 1989; 999-1004.
10. Barbara J., *et al.*, Haemoptysis as the presenting symptom in bronchiolitis obliterans; Chest 1997; 111: 1775-78.
11. Epstein D.M., Bennet M.R., BOOP with migratory pulmonary infltrates, AJR 1992; 158: 515-17.

12. Bellomo R.I., *et al.,* Clinical spectrum of COP; Thorax 1991; 46: 554-58.
13. Costabel R., *et al.,* BOOP in Europe, Chest 1992; 102: 145-205.
14. Dina R., Sheppared M.N., The histological diagnosis of clinically documented cases of COP diagnostic features in transbronchial biopsies; Histopathology 1993; 23: 541-45.
15. Cordier J., COP: Clinics in Chest Medicine 1993; 14(4): 677-92.
16. Udwadia Z.F. *et al.,* COP—A rare but reversible cause of acute respiratory failure; JAPI 1995; 43 (a): 638-40.

HONEYCOMB LUNG

Introduction

Honeycomb lung is characterised by the presence of numerous small cysts distributed unevenly throughout both the lungs. Interstitial lung diseases generally end up with honeycomb lung. Common causes are listed in the following table.

Common causes of honeycomb lung

Localized	*Diffuse*
• Systemic sclerosis	• Cryptogenic fibrosing alveolitis
• Sarcoidosis	• Rheumatoid lung
• Tuberculosis	• Langerhen's cell histiocytosis
• Asbestosis	• Tuberous sclerosis
• Berylliosis	• Neurofibromatosis

The clinical presentation may be a part of systemic diseases or may present as an isolated pulmonary disease. It can occur in histiocytosis X, tuberous sclerosis, mesodermal dysplasia, Marfan's syndrome, progressive systemic sclerosis, neurofibromatosis and biliary cirrhosis. It is a late event in fibrosing alveolitis.

The cysts may be of 1 cm in diameter and are thin walled and occupy a wide area in the lung, located in the terminal parts of the bronchial tree. The cysts are separated by fibrous septa and they do not take part in the exchange of gases. Though some may have a developmental origin, majority appear to be the result of an acquired inflammatory condition. The peripheral parts of the bronchial tree are affected by granulomatous tissue, inflammatory cell infiltration, hyperplasia of smooth muscle or fibrosis. The alveolar walls are thickened. The surrounding bronchioles show dilatation resulting in cysts, which increase in size due to check-valve obstruction.[1]

Clinical Presentation

It is more common in males, presenting with progressively increasing dyspnoea. Often there is fever, cough and sputum in children. Diagnosis is made because of recurrent pneumothorax and it may even be bilateral. The cysts in contact with pleura are likely to rupture, especially among the younger age group. In adults gradually it leads to right heart failure.[1]

Investigations[1]

X-ray chest shows presence of numerous cysts distributed bilaterally and are associated with reticular shadows throughout the lung. The cysts are seen easily in a partially collapsed lung following pneumothorax. The bronchogram is normal and the radio-opaque material does not get into the cysts even after coughing.

Outcome

The course of the disease is slow and is influenced by the complications as well as the course of the associated systemic diseases.[1] Initially, there may not be any clinical features, even though radiological findings are present.

Marfan's syndrome is a rare but well defined hereditary disorder of connective tissue. It consists of a triad of musculoskeletal, ocular and cardiac abnormalities. However, pulmonary, abnormalities have also been reported.[2,3] The occurrence of spontaneous pneumothorax and other pulmonary changes like interstitial alveolar wall fragmentation with honeycombing, diffuse bullous emphysema, congenital malformation of bronchi, bronchiectasis, pneumothorax are seen in this syndrome.[2-7] Moderate degree of restrictive and obstructive defect is quite commonly seen in most of the cases.[8,9]

The basic defect in the collagen fibres is the presence of fewer side to side linkages, resulting in increased tissue friability.[10,11] Changes in pulmonary elastic tissue in the lungs are seen as patchy abnormal alveolar elastica, scattered all over but more pronounced over emphysematous areas.[12] Elastic fibres are irregular, thickened and fragmented.[6,10]

Pulmonary changes are generally overshadowed by the pronounced changes in the eye, heart and great vessels. At the same time, few recognized features, especially the changes in the bone are accepted as important features of this disorder.[4]

Treatment

No specific treatment is available. Symptomatic treatment is required for the infections, pneumothorax and heart failure. Management of pneumothorax may require intercostal intubation. To prevent recurrent episodes of pneumothorax, pleurodesis or pleurectomy has to be done. Radiotherapy is dangerous as it induces fibrosis.[1]

REFERENCES

1. Shankar P.S., Chest Medicine; Oxford and IBH Publ. Co (P) Ltd., New Delhi; 1994; 4th ed.

2. Bolarde R.P. and Tucker A.S., Pulmonary emphysema and other cardiorespiratory lesions as part of the Marfan's abiotrophy, Pediatrics 1964; 33: 356-66.
3. Dwyer E.J. Jr. and Troncale F., Spontaneous pneumothorax and pulmonary disease in Marfan's Syndrome, Ann Inten Med 1965; 62: 1285-92.
4. Tiwari S.G., Jayaswal R., Jettey R.K. and Rao P.B., Pulmonary bullous disease in Marfan's Syndrome, J. Assn. Phys. India 1990; 38: 587-89.
5. Ahuja R.K., Parkash S.K., Singh. N.P., *et al.,* Multiple aneurysms in Marfan's Syndrome, J. Assn. Phys. India 1989; 37: 414-15.
6. Lipton R.A., Greenwald R.A. and Seriff N.S., Pneumothorax and bilateral honeycomb lung in Marfan's Syndrome, Report of a case and review of pulmonary abnormalities in this disorder, Am. Rev. Respir. Dis 1971; 104: 924-26.
7. Turner J. A McM. and Stanley N.N., Fragile lung in Marfan's syndrome, Thorax 1976; 31: 771-74.
8. Chishold J.C., Chemiack N.S. and Carton R.W., Results of pulmonary function testing in 5 persons with the Marfan's Syndrome, J. Lab. Clin. Med 1968; 71:25-26.
9. Streeten E. A., *et al.,* Pulmonary functions in Marfan's Syndrome; Chest 1987; 91: 408.
10. Reye R.D.K. and Bale P.M., Elastic tissue in pulmonary emphysema in Marfan's Syndrome, Arch Pathol 1973; 96: 427-30.
11. Goodman R.M., Wooley C.F., Frazier R.L. and Covault L., Ehler-Danlos syndrome, N.Engl. J. Med 1965; 273: 514-16.
12. Wood J.R., *et al.,* Pulmonary disease in Marfan's Syndrome; Thorax 1994; 39: 780.

HISTIOCYTOSIS X (LANGERHANS CELL GRANULOMATOSIS)

An uncommon condition involving fat, bones and soft tissues such as lungs, skin, neurohypophysis, liver and spleen, is characterised by granuloma formation with infiltration and proliferation of histiocytes. It includes fulminant Latterer-Siwe disease of infancy, Hand-Schuller-Christian disease of childhood and eosinophilic granuloma seen in adults.[1] It accounts for 1-5% of interstitial lung diseases of unknown aetiology.[2]

Pathology

The lung may be involved frequently in eosinophilic granuloma. There is fibrotic destructive lesion. There is histiocytic, and eosinophilic infiltration of alveolar septa and bronchial walls, granuloma formation and honeycombing. The condition is seen in adult males of 20 to 40 years, especially in those who use tobacco heavily. It can only be differentiated from other interstitial lung diseases when the bony lesions co-exist.[3] Previously proliferation of macrophages (histiocytes) was thought to be the characteristic of this disease but now, the precursor cells—dendritic cells present in the alveolar septa and interstitium are recognized, which are different from tissue macrophages and can evolve into Langerhans cells which have a specific CDI surface antigens that react with monoclonal antibodies called T_6 and by intracytoplasmic organelles called X-bodies or Birbeck granules, as seen under electron microscope.[2] Langerhans cells are normally present in the skin and lungs and these get stimulated by smoking. These cells are not pathognomonic for this disease and can be seen in BAL fluid even in smokers, bronchoalveolar carcinoma and idiopathic pulmonary fibrosis. The term eosinophilic granuloma is a misnomer; because in advanced disease, there is neither typical granuloma as seen in sarcoidosis and hypersensitive pneumonitis, nor any increase in eosinophils.[2]

Clinical Features

The patients present with cough, exertional dyspnoea, fatigue and weight loss. There can be polyuria and polydipsia.[1] Occasionally there may be clubbing and crepitations may be heard. Recurrent pneumothorax may be presenting feature in about 10 per cent of patients. Chest X-ray shows diffuse mottling, reticulonodular or honeycomb shadows predominantly in the upper and mid-zones bilaterally. Hilar adenopathy is uncommon.[4] In advanced cases, chest X-ray may resemble that of chronic obstructive lung disease. Punched out bony defects may be visible in ribs and scapulae. CT shows cysts with intervening normal parenchyma of lung.[5] Associated disorders with histiocytosis X are listed in Table 10.10.

Table 10.10: Histiocytosis X: Associated disorders
Iatrogenic (Lung biopsy, aspiration cannula, external cardiac massage)
Oesophageal rupture
Positive pressure assisted ventilation
Pleural malignancy
Subphrenic abscess, sarcoidosis
Tuberculosis, tuberous sclerosis

There is progressive loss of lung function with a mixed restrictive and obstructive pattern, and decrease in diffusing capacity.[6] Mononuclear phagocytic cells (histiocytes) are demonstrable in BAL and open lung biopsy specimens.[1]

Treatment

Extending fibrocystic lesions cause gradual loss of lung functions. Spontaneous remission and non-progression of disease are frequent. Steroids have shown little benefit in those with significant symptoms and progressive disease.[1] Penicillamine has been tried. Bronchodilators may help in advanced cases with symptoms of airways obstruction.[2]

REFERENCES

1. Shankar P.S., Chest Medicine; Oxford and IBH Co., N. Delhi; 4th ed; 1994.
2. *Harrison's principles of internal medicine:* Wilson J.D., Braunwald E., Isselbacher K.J., *et al.*, (ed), 2nd Vol. 12th ed; McGraw Hill, N.York, 1991.
3. Hance A.J., *et al.*, Pulmonary and extrapulmonary manifestations of Langerhans cell granulomatosis; Seminar Resp. Med 1988; 9: 349.
4. Lacronique J., Roth C. and Battesti J.P., Thorax 1982, 37: 104.
5. Muller N.L., Miller R.R.; Amer Rev Resp Dis 1990; 142: 1440-49.
6. Friedman P.J., Liebow A.A. and Isokoloff J., Medicine, Baltimore 1981; 60:385.

PULMONARY TUBEROUS SCLEROSIS

Development of an abnormal mesodermal tissue that can occur as a genetic defect involving skin and the nervous system is called Bourneville's disease,[1] and manifests features of epilepsy, mental retardation and adenoma sebaceum at an early age which is a hallmark of this disorder and is an angiofibroma, distributed over the cheeks, chin and forehead in a butterfly pattern. The condition is frequently associated with intracranial calcification, tumours of optic disc, retina or kidney and sclerotic bone changes. Very rarely there can be pulmonary involvement.[2] The disorder is an autosomal dominant trait. The mutant gene is located on the chromosome.[3] A Carney's triad of pulmonary hamartomas, gastric leiomyosarcoma, and paraganglionoma has been described.[4]

The lung manifestations are frequent in adult women. These can occur in those with milder defects and normal intelligence. Dyspnoea on exertion may be presenting symptom. Recurrent pneumothorax is frequent.[5]

Pathologically, alveoli and bronchioles are destroyed to form small cavities. There are multiple nodular hamartomas and patchy fibrosis. The radiological abnormalities vary from fine reticular shadows to a honeycomb appearance of the lungs. The pulmonary lesions progress slowly to result in respiratory insufficiency.[2] Death is usually due to non-pulmonary causes like seizures and intercurrent diseases of associated tumors.[6]

REFERENCES

1. Adams R.D., Neurocutaneous diseases; In; Dermatology in general medicine; 3rd ed; Fitzpatrick T.B., *et al.*, (ed), McGraw Hill, New York, 1986.
2. Shankar P.S., Chest Medicine; Oxford and IBH Publ. Co; N. Delhi; 4th ed; 1994.
3. Adams R.D. and Lyon G., *Neurology of hereditary metabolic diseases of children,* McGraw Hill, New York, 1982.
4. Liberman B.A. *et al.*, Tuberous sclerosis with pulmonary involvement; J Cando. Med. Assn 1984; 130:287.
5. Dwyer J.M., Hickie J.B., Carvin J. and Camat J., Med 1971; 40: 115.
6. Harrison's principles of internal medicine, Wilson J.D., Braunwald E., Isselbacher K.J., *et al.*, (ed) 12th ed.Vo1.2; McGraw Hill, N. York 1991.

PULMONARY AMYLOIDOSIS

Amyloid means *starch-like* and the term was originally coined in 1854. Amyloidosis is a rare disorder featuring extracellular deposition of fibrils derived from the light chain of a monoclonal immunoglobulin (AL). The deposits of fibrous amyloid protein occurs at one or more sites of the body.[1] Macrophages play an important role either by converting immunoglobulins into amyloid or by secreting mediators which induce amyloid production.

Lower respiratory tract may have localised involvement or it can be a part of systemic primary amyloidosis. Rarely the respiratory tract is involved in secondary amyloidosis (amyloid A, AA). Pulmonary amyloidosis is noted in elderly males.[2]

Pulmonary tuberculosis or chronic lung abscess can be predisposing aetiological diseases.[3] Amyloid has a variable origin. The AL-type is derived from light chains of immunoglobulin, as described earlier, and AA is derived from a larger precursor protein SAA which is an acute phase reactant, resembling the C-reactive protein. The AL type is derived from a pre-albumin precursor in serum.[3]

AL and AA types can be differentiated histopathologically. AA type amyloid fibrils lose the capacity to stain with congo red following incubation with potassium permanganate while AL-type fibrils retain their capacity. Immuno histochemical techniques and elaborate amino acid sequence studies can also help differentiate the two.[1]

Clinically, the condition may be tracheobronchial or parenchymal. It may be incidentally recognised at bronchoscopy as a pseudotumour in tracheobronchial tree. Multifocal submucosal plaques may cause diffuse narrowing of the tracheobronchial tree resulting in bronchial obstruction and manifest cough and dyspnoea. Lung lesions such as parenchymal nodule that may pose difficulty to distinguish from malignancy or granulomatous conditions and manifest cough and haemoptysis. Diffuse form with multiple localised deposits of amyloid in the vessel wall and alveolar septa may present with dyspnoea. Generally features of congestive heart failure, in which pulmonary manifestations are an incidental finding, may be present.[2]

Atelectasis or linear interstitial shadows can be seen on chest X-ray. There can be associated lung abscesses or thickened pleura in addition to well defined nodules and punctate calcified foci can be demonstrated on CT.[5] Transbronchial biopsy or transcutaneous fine needle aspiration helps in the diagnosis, but appears to be insufficient for specific histological diagnosis.[5] Chances of amyloid diagnosis from tissue diagnosis in terms of percentage positivity includes skin biopsy (50%), gingival biopsy (75%), rectal biopsy (75-85%), abdomial fat tissue aspiration (88%), liver biopsy (90%) and kidneys biopsy (95%).[6,7] Amyloid deposits appear as amorphous, eosinophilic material and exhibit a green birefringence under a polarised light after staining with congo red.

Definite diagnostic criteria for pathological diagnosis of amyloidosis include the following:[3]

1. As described earlier, unique green birefringence when congo red stained sections are seen under polarised microscope.
2. Fine non branching rigid fibrils measuring 100A° in diameter with individual fibril of 70A° in diameter, tending to aggregate laterally are seen by electron microscope.
3. Cross beta pattern is seen in tissues examined with X-ray diffraction technique.

Routine investigations are not contributory, except ESR which is moderately raised. Liver function tests may be altered, as liver is involved in 56-70% cases, but amyloid hepatomegaly is not synonymous with hepatic amyloidosis. At the same time, liver biopsy is relatively contraindicated in cases with massive hepatic amyloid infiltration.[1,8] Monoclonal protein specific IgG can be demonstrated by protein electrophoresis. A restrictive lung disease pattern is observed by lung function tests.

The prognosis is good in a localised form of pulmonary amyloidosis and it is generally unfavourable in systemic form. Endoscopic laser resection is useful when there is diffuse tracheobronchial involvement. Nodular forms do not require treatment as they remain fairly stable or show slow progression for years. Death may come from respiratory failure in cases of diffuse amyloidosis.[2]

Progress of secondary amyloidosis (AA) may be arrested and occasionally reversed by treating the primary disease. In primary (AL) forms, treatment with colchicine and dimethyl sulphoxide has been tried with little benefit. Colchicine helps in slowing the development of amyloidosis in familial mediterranean fever.[3]

Amyloidosis continues to occur in India. Whereas primary forms are becoming more frequent in western countries, secondary forms due to suppurative lung diseases and pulmonary tuberculosis are still the most common forms prevalent in India.[9]

REFERENCES

1. Cohen A.S. and Skinner M., *Amyloidosis of the liver,* In: Schiff E.R., Eds. Diseases of the Liver. Philadelphia, JB Lippincott 1987; 1093-108.
2. Shankar P.S., *Pulmonary amyloidosis,* in Chest Medicine, Oxford and IBH Publ. Co., N. Delhi, 1994, 4th edn.
3. Mohandar K.M., Swaroop U.S. and Advani S.H., A case of massive hepatomegaly due to amyloidosis, J. Assn. Phys. India 1991; 39:711-13.
4. Graham C.M., *et al.,* Amer. J, Radiol 1992; 158:255-57.
5. Charboneau J.W., Reading C.C. and Welch T.J., CT and sonographic guided needle biopsy: Current techniques and innovations, AJR 1990; 154: 1-10.
6. Libby C.A., Skinner M. and Cohen A.S., Use of abdominal fat tissue aspiration in the diagnosis of systemic amyloidosis, Arch Interm Med 1983; 143: 1549-52.
7. Gertz M.A. and Kyle R.A., Hepatic amyloidosis primary (AL), Immunoglobulin light chain fraction. The natural history in 80 patients, Am. J. Med 1988; 85:73-80.
8. Hoffman M.S., Stein B.E., Davidian M.M. and Rosenthal W.S., Hepatic amyloidosis presenting as severe intrahepatic cholestasis: A case report and review of literature, Am, J. Gastroenterol 1988; 83:783-85.
9. Chug K.S., Singhal P.C., Sakhuja V., Datta B.N., Jain S.K. and Dash S.C., Pattern of renal amyloidosis in India, Postgrad Med J 1981; 57:31-35.

IDIOPATHIC PULMONARY HEMOSIDEROSIS

Idiopathic pulmonary hemosiderosis (IPH) is a rare condition characterised by recurrent haemoptysis, fleeting pulmonary infiltrates and iron deficiency due to intrapulmonary haemorrhage.[1]

The condition is noted in childhood and young adults. Though it is more common in male adults, the sex ratio is reversed in childhood. Aetiology of IPH remains disputed even to date. Theories implicating viral infections, cold agglutinins, direct toxins or allergens or exposure to hydrocarbons from fuel and other combustion products have been put forth. However, the intermittent course, lymphoid hyperplasia, observed eosinophilia, an association with celiac sprue and remissions with steroids and immunosuppressants favours an auto immune basis of the disease.[2]

Pathology

It is associated with intra-alveolar and intrabronchial haemorrhage of undetermined aetiology from the pulmonary capillaries. Initially there is hyperplasia and degeneration of the alveolar epithelial cells. The capillaries are damaged leading to haemorrhage. Later there is fibrosis of alveolar walls. The alveoli are filled with haemosiderin-laden macrophages and red blood cells during exacerbation.[3] The ultrastructural criteria include a normal basement membrane and capillary endothelium without IgM, B1c, Clq, and fibrinogen.[4] There is a need to exclude histologies such as vasculitis, capillary proliferation, inflammation, necrosis, thrombosis or embolism in all the cases.[1] There is a need for making definitive diagnosis of IPH as a case of micropolyarteritis presenting as pulmonary haemorrhage as has been detected only by the anti-neutrophil cytoplasmic antibodies (ANCA).[5]

Clinically there is dry cough initially followed by appearance of blood tinged sputum. The bleeding may be periodic or persistent and its amount varies from small to massive quantity. Other clinical features are progressively increasing breathlessness, fatigue, palor, weakness and loss of weight. Pyrexia is noted frequently. Some cases show lymphadenopathy, hepatosplenomegaly and clubbing. Chest examination reveals an impaired percussion note and fine crepitations over bases.[3] Differential diagnosis include bronchiectasis, tuberculosis and schistosomiasis.

Chest X-ray reveals transient shadows after haemorrhagic episodes. Later miliary shadows are noted due to accumulation of blood pigment in the mid and lower zones which may coalesce into patchy shadows. The shadows may simulate those of pulmonary haemosiderosis secondary to chronic congestion of mitral stenosis but do not exhibit septal lines or calcification or alteration in the configuration of cardia. Fine linear shadows appear with the onset of fibrosis. Bleeding into the alveoli following chest trauma, administration of anticoagulants, inhalation of resins containing trimellitic anhydride, bleeding diathesis, pulmonary infarction and haemorrhagic pneumonia may produce patchy radiological shadows.[3] Recurrent haemoptysis may occur due to blood dyscrasias, bronchial adenoma, recurrent pulmonary emboli, arteriovenous malformations and mitral stenosis.[2] The sputum and gastric washings show haemosiderin-laden macrophages. Such a finding is not diagnostic since it may occur in other conditions causing pulmonary haemorrhage. Iron deficiency anaemia is noted with low serum levels of iron. Defective gas transfer leads to reduction in arterial oxygen tension. There are no circulating immune complexes or antibasement membrane antibodies[6] unlike Goodpastuer's syndrome.

Prognosis

The disease has a variable course. The episodes of haemorrhage are interrupted by period of remission. It may slowly progress to chronic cor pulmonale or may terminate with massive fulminant bleeding. It may be self limiting in some adults.[3,7]

Treatment

Splenectomy was the first modality tried but discarded.[1] The treatment is directed towards correction of anaemia by iron therapy. A short course of glucocorticoids in high doses during acute episodes may be beneficial but not a long term remedy for keeping the disease suppressed and preventing its recurrence.

The efficacy of plasmapheresis, azathioprine and chloroquine have been reported[8-10] but lot of difficulties exist in evaluating any form of treatment, as the disease has a tendency for spontaneous remissions and exacerbations.[2]

REFERENCES

1. Soergel K.H. and Sommers S.C., IPH and related syndromes. Amer J Med 1962; 32:499-511.
2. Nair N. and Jindal S.K., IPH: An unusual cause of recurrent haemoptysis; Ind J Chest Dis All Sci 1993; 35:35-39.
3. Shankar P.S., Idiopathic pulmonary haemosiderosis, In; Chest Medicine, Oxford and IBH Pub. Co. (P) Ltd., New Delhi, 1994; 4th ed.
4. Irwin R.S., *et al.,* IPH: An electron microscopic immuno-fluorescent study, Chest 1974; 65: 41-45.
5. Leaker B. *et al.,* IPH: A form of microscopic polyarteritis; Thorax 1992; 47: 988-90.
6. Brambilla C.G., *et al.,* IPH, Chest 1982; 81: 120-23.
7. Wilson J.D., *et al.,* ed., Harrison's principles of Internal medicine; l2th ed; 2nd vol, McGraw Hill, New York, 1991.
8. Pozo-Rodriquez F., *et al.,* IPH treated by plasmapheresis; Thorax 1980; 35: 399.
9. Byrd R.B. and Gracey D.R., Immunosuppressive treatment of IPH; JAMA 1973; 226: 458.
10. Bush A., *et al.,* Chloroquine in IPH, Arch Dis Child 1992; 67: 625-27.

PULMONARY ALVEOLAR PROTEINOSIS (PAP)

Pulmonary alveolar proteinosis is an uncommon condition of uncertain aetiology, characterised by accumulation of periodic acid schiff (PAS) positive lipid rich proteinaceous material in the distal air spaces of the lungs.[1] Because of recent reports of therapeutic efficacy of selective bronchoalveolar lavage and trypsin aerosol treatment, an early diagnosis of this rare disease is important.[2,3]

Pulmonary alveolar proteinosis as a distinct entity was first described by Rosen, *et al.,* in 1958. This disorder is known for its rarity and the largest review of 139 cases by Davidson, *et al.,* recorded a male preponderance (M:F =3: 1) with age ranging from eight months old baby to 75 years old male.[4]

Aetiology and Pathology

Aetiology is undetermined. However various atmospheric pollutants like silica, wood dust, noxious fumes and vapours have been incriminated. There are no distinct haematological abnormalities associated with pulmonary alveolar proteinosis. Hyperlipidaemia, hyperglobulinaemia and elevated LDH levels occur in some patients.[4-7] The alveoli contain periodic-acid-schiff attaining acidophilic material. It is rich in lipoprotein especially palmitoyl lecithin similar to that of surfactant. The material appears to be due to delayed degradation of alveolar lipids, bound to denatured protein. Though there is alveolar hyperplasia, there is no evidence of inflammation and fibrous thickening of the interalveolar septa, but lung alveoli filled with eosinophilic granular material is seen. In between the septal wax and eosinophilic maternal, defected septal cells containing light coloured cytoplasm can be seen, which are strongly PAS positive.

Clinical Features

It is commonly seen in young and middle-aged individuals, affecting males more often than females. It involves the lungs alone with a variable clinical pattern. It may remain asymptomatic or show progressive pulmonary insufficiency. Progressive, exertional dyspnoea is a prominent symptom. It may be preceded by fever. Cough with gelatinous expectoration, chest tightness, weight loss, fatigue and cyanosis appear with the progress of the disease. Clubbing may be present. The physical signs are minimal and fine crepitations are heard.[8] There may be prolonged pyrexia of one and half years duration.[5] Chest pain and haemoptysis are unusual.[6]

Investigations

The radiological picture simulates that of pulmonary oedema. There are symmetrical, diffuse, patchy, bilateral, alveolar and interstitial infiltrates. Unlike pulmonary oedema, the cardia and pulmonary vessels are of normal size. There is no evidence of hilar adenopathy or pleural effusion.[8] CT scan shows a coarse reticular pattern of 2-3 cm diameter. Reticulonodular opacities extending from both hila towards periphery, which are denser than the bases are seen. The surrounding interstitial tissue is thickened as compared to the rest of alveolar tissue and is a diagnostic feature. Initially the diagnosis of alveolar proteinosis was only possible with lung biopsy but now lung lavage findings along with CT scan has made it possible without that.

BAL fluid is rich with phospholipid and glycoprotein.[9] Alveolar washing may show alveolar macrophages filled with PAS attaining material. Electron microscopy of sputum or lung washing reveals granular material and lamellar bodies. Findings on light microscopy and clinical presentation may be confused with these of pneumocystic carinii infection. A bethenamine silver stain excludes this possibility. Lung biopsy gives confirmatory evidence. If lung biopsy is contraindicated, monoclonal antibodies to surfactant apoprotein-A (Sp-A) can be assayed as concentration of more than 400 times higher has been demonstrated and is diagnostic for PAP.[10] Serum lactic acid dehydrogenase may be elevated. Pulmonary function tests reveal restrictive defect with severe hypoxaemia. Often these patients succumb to pulmonary infection due to a poor pulmonary defence mechanism from alveolar macrophages exhibiting decreased phagocytic activity.[8,9]

Treatment

Mucolytic or proteolytic aerosols in gradually increasing doses are used to make the sputum thin. If there is hypoxaemia or secondary infection from less common pulmonary pathogens such as nocardia, bronchopulmonary lavage has to be promptly undertaken with an irrigating solution containing buffered normal saline, heparin (5 units/ml) and 1 per cent acetyl cysteine. The volume of the solution varies from 10 to 20 litres. The primary effect of lavage appears to be mechanical and a large quantity of phospholipid and protein can be removed.[8] It gives a quick improvement in clinical and radiologic picture. Whole lung lavages are quite relieving in cases of dyspnoea and progressive deterioration of arterial oxygenation and gives a long-term relief.[11] The procedure may be repeated. Heparin activates lipoprotein lipase. S/o injection of granulocyte macrophage colony stimulating factor (GM-CSF) therapy is a promising alternative to those requiring repeated whole lung lavage.[12] The outcome of the disease is variable. 25% of patients improve spontaneous, while in 20% of cases the disease runs a fulminant course ending in respiratory failure. It may progress over years, ultimately developing interstitial fibrosis.

REFERENCES

1. Rosen S.H., Castleman B. and Liebow A.A., Pulmonary alveolar proteinosis, N. Engl. J. Med 1958; 258:1123-32.
2. Ramirez R., Alveolar proteinosis, Importance of pulmonary lavage, Am. Rev. Resp. Dis 1971; 103:666-78.
3. Ricker J.B. and Welinsky H., Trypsin aersol treatment of pulmonary alveolar proteinosis, Am. Rev. Resp. Dis 1973; 108: 108-13.
4. Davidson J.M. and Macleod W.M., Pulmonary alveolar proteinosis Br. J. Dis. Chest 1969; 63:13-25.
5. Ramirez R.J., Walenty N. and Mclangheins J., Pulmonary alveolar proteinosis diagnostic technics and observations, N. Eng. J. Med 1963; 268: 165-71.
6. Altose M.D., *Pulmonary alveolar proteinosis in pulmonary diseases and disorders.* Ed. Fishman A.P. McGraw Hill, NewYork 1980; 1341-46.
7. Chauhan M.S., Jayaswal R., Rajan R.S., *et al.,* Pulmonary alveolar proteinosis, J. Assn. Phys. India 1988; 36:445-46.
8. Shankar P.S., Chest Medicine; Oxford and IBH Publ. Co. (P) Ltd., N. Delhi; 4th ed; 1994.
9. Gonzalez-Rothi R.J. and Harris J.O., Chest 1986; 90: 856-64.
10. Masuda T., *et al.,* Lancet 1991; 337: 580-82.
11. Kariman K., *et al.,* Pulmonary alveolar proteinosis, Clinical experience in 23 patients over 15 years, Lung 1984; 162: 223.
12. Shende RP; *et al.,* GM CSF therapy for pulmonary alveolar proteinosis; JAPI 2013; 61: 209-11.

PULMONARY ALVEOLAR MICROLITHIASIS

It is a rare condition of obscure aetiology, often familial, featuring diffuse intra-alveolar deposition of a large number of minute calcific concretions uniformly throughout both the lungs. The condition may be recognised on routine chest X-ray in a child, before the symptoms appear. Pulmonary alveolar microlithiasis was described for the first time in 1918 by Harbitz[1] but the term was coined by Puhr in 1933.[2] Definite description of the disease was published by Sosman, *et al.* in 1957.[3] Recent reports show that it is more common in Turkish population.[4] Almost 300 cases have been documented in world literature.[5]

It is a rare idiopathic disorder.[6] The aetiology is unknown. A local alteration in the cells of alveolar septa appears to predispose to occurrence of calcification. It is postulated that it occurs due to an inborn error of metabolism at the alveolar interface, possibly an enzymatic defect resulting in precipitation of calcium in the presence of undue alkalinity[3,4] Also it is suggested that microlithiasis is a peculiar exudative response to a variety of insults in the form of pneumonia and rheumatic fever.[5] There is no metabolic abnormality, including that of calcium and Vitamin D metabolism nor any calcium deposits elsewhere in the body. Cases have been seen in the age group from 30 to 50 years. There is no sex predilection. Familial occurrence is a notable feature[3] and there is a tendency to appear in the siblings.

The lungs appear like sacks of sand containing innumerable homogeneous intra-alveolar calcific bodies. Microliths range from 0.01 to 2.8 mm in diameter. Energy dispersive X-ray microanalysis reveals presence of calcium and phosphorus in 2:1 ratio, consistent with a $CaPO_3$ composition.[6] Smaller amounts of calcium carbonate and traces of silica, magnesium and iron have also been seen. The calcified shadows may be so profuse as to make the lungs diffusely white, obscuring the cardiac borders.[7-9] The radiological features are chracteristic and diagnosis can solely be based on chest X-ray abnormality. The sand like diffuse micronodulation invovling both the lungs is often described as a *sandstorm appearance.* CT reveals inferior and posterior predominance of deposits.[10] The *Black pleura* sign is quite clearly seen in the CT scan.[11] Sputum specimen may reveal microliths. Microscopic examination of bronchoalveolar lavage fluid also reveals microliths,[12] which may have *onion skin* appearance. Transbronchial lung biopsy has been safe procedure for histopathology.[13,14] Investigations like percutaneous or open lung biopsy are seldom warranted.[9]

X-ray findings of stannosis and calcified miliary histoplasmosis may simulate microlithiasis but these lesions are larger and have different distribution. Pulmonary calcification has also been documented in chronic dialysis patients.[15] Lung biopsy reveals alveolar spaces containing laminated calcific microliths with fibrosis and thickening of the alveolar walls.[9]

Symptoms and signs are sparse with occasional complaint of cough and later on dyspnoea. Most of the patients are asymptomatic initially.[9] There is an increased susceptibility to chest infections. No specific signs are seen. Pulmonary functions studies are normal in early stages but in late stages may show restrictive defect with impaired diffusion. Even obstructive abnormality has been described in some cases.[3,11] Clubbing and cyanosis may occur. The intraalveolar disease in earlier stages develops interstitial fibrosis as it advances.[16] The disease may slowly progress to fibrosis leading to cardiopulmonary failure. There is no known specific treatment. Corticosteroids and chelating agents fail to influence the course of the disease.[17] Therapeutic BAL had been effective in giving relief of dyspnoea.[18] Recently bilateral sequential lung transplantation has been attempted.[19] There is mention of pulmonary alveolar microlithiasis from Indian subcontinent, especially after 1980.[11,20,21] Benign nature of the disease is overemphasised. Physician feels quite helpless in treating such conditions especially in a family setting.[22]

REFERENCES

1. Harbitz F., Extensive calcification of the lungs as a distinct disease, Arch Intern Med 1918; 21:139-46.
2. Puhr L., Mikrolithiasis alveolaris pulmonum, Virchows Arch (Pathol Anat) 1933; 290: 156-60.
3. Sosman M.C., *et al.,* The familial occurrence of pulmonary alveolar microlithiasis, Am. J. Roentgenol 1957; 77: 947-1012.
4. Ulan E.S. *et al.,* Pulmonary alveolar microlithiasis; Review of Turkish reports; Thorax 1993; 48: 171-73.
5. Mariotla S., *et al.,* PAM: Review of Italian reports; Eurp. J. Epidem 1999; 13:587.
6. Kashyap S., *et al.,* Pulmonary alveolar microlithiasis in athimachali women; JAPI 1996; 44(1):56-57.
7. Gayathri Devi HJ; *et al.,* PAM; Lung India 2011; 28: 139-41.
8. Kent G., *et al.,* Pulmonary microlithiasis: Microlithiasis alveolaris pulmonum Arch Pathol 1955,60:556-62.
9. Prakash V.B.S., *et al.,* Pulmonary alveolar microlithiasis: A review including ultrastructural and pulmonary function studies, Mayo Clin. Proceed 1983,58:290-300.
10. Shas MS; *et al.,* Pulmonary alveolar microlithiasis; Ind J Radiol Imaging 2003; 13: 277-79.
11. Boghani A., *et al.,* Pulmonary alveolar microlithiasis revisited with CT scan, bone scan and bronchalveolar lavage; Lung India 1993; 11: 37-39.
12. Palmobini B.C., *et al.,* BAL in alveolar microlithiasis;Chest 1981; 80:242-43.
13. Wallis C., *et al.,* Pulmonary alveolar microlithiasis: Diagnosis by transbronchial biopsy; Paed. Pulmonol 1996; 21:62-64.
14. Hira H.S., *et al.,* Pulmonary alveolar microlithiasis; Role of trans bronchial lung biopsy; JAPI 2000;48:832-33.
15. Shankar P.S., ed. *Chest medicine,* Oxford and IBH Publ Co.(P) Ltd. New Delhi, 4th ed,1994.
16. Barnard N.J., *et al.,* PAM:A new analytical approach; Histopathology 1987;11:639.
17. Tachibane T; *et al.,* Pulmonary alveolar microlithiasis; Review and management; Curr Opin Pulm Med 2009; 15: 486-90.
18. Pracyk J.B., *et al.,* Composition of lung lavage in pulmonary alveolar microlithiasis; Respiration 1996; 63:254-60.
19. Edelman J.D., *et al.,* Bilateral sequential lung transplantation for pulmonary alveolar microlithiasis; Chest 197;112: 1140-44.
20. Gupta S.K., *et al.,* Pulmonary alveolar microlithiasis; Ind J Chest Dis and All Sci 1982; 24: 29-32.
21. Sandhyamani S., *et al.,* Pulmonary alveolar microlithiasis; Ind J Chest Dis. and All Sci 1982; 24: 333-35.
22. Mitra S., Ghosal A.G., A family of PAM; Lung India 2000; 18: 97-99.

BRONCHOLITHIASIS

A calcified fragment of tissue which is loose within the lumen of bronchus is called broncholithiasis. The calcification of lung tissue has lymph node which erodes into the bronchial lumen. Generally calcification follows some infection which leads to granulomatous response as in tuberculosis, coccidioidomycosis, histoplasmosis, etc. This may occur in bronchiectatic necrosis and calcification of bronchial cartilage that protrudes into the lumen[1,2] which gets fragmentated into small pieces called broncholiths. Rarely, calcification of aspirated food may also form a broncholith. With these moving broncholiths in the bronchial lumen, broncholithiasis presents as proxsysmal cough, obstruction, infection and haemoptysis.

The calcareous material may be coughed up (Lithoptysis) as broncholith.[3] Rarely erosion into the oesophagus may occur.

It is commonly noted in 5th to 6th decades, among both sexes. Sputum may show calcified particles. Radiologically it presents as hilar or mediastinal calcification. Calcified deposits may be evident in airways on tomography. The bronchoscopy confirms the presence of broncholith and is useful in its removal. Forceful manipulation may result in fistula formation or massive haemorrhage.[4] Surgical management may be necessary in massive haemoptysis or persistent obstruction.[5] Antibiotics are required for controlling infection.

REFERENCES

1. Galdermans D.J., *et al.*, Resp. Med 1990; 84:155-56.
2. Shankar P.S., Chest Medicine; Oxford and IBH Pub. Co. Pvt. (L); N. Delhi; 1994; 4th ed.
3. Haines J.D., Coughing up a stone, What to do about broncholithiasis? Post Grad, Med 1988; 83:83.
4. Igo D., *et al.*, Resp. Med 1990; 84: 163-65.
5. Cole P.H., *et al.*, Management of broncholithiasis, Is thoracotomy necessary? Ann Thor Surg 1986; 42:255.

PULMONARY INVOLVEMENT IN CONNECTIVE TISSUE DISORDERS

These disorders are characterized histologically by inflammation and necrosis of collagen and blood vessels and clinically by manifestations affecting different systems like skin, joints, vessels and viscera. Lungs get commonly involved in connective tissue disorders and respond to injury by a variety of pathologic changes. It is worth noting that the same clinical syndromes may be associated with different pathologies and several different clinical syndromes may lead to the same pathology in the lung. Key markers in multiple connective tissue disorder syndromes such as SLC, PSS, RA, etc. are essentially immunological. There is a presence of non-organ specific antibodies, immune complexes and markedly raised E.S.R., which help in the diagnosis of the diseases.[1] Routine tests, PFTS, chest X-ray, CT findings help in diagnosing quite a good number of cases; even then diagnostic dilemma persists. That is why holistic approach is considered to be useful in diagnosing pulmonary involvement in connective tissue disorders. The aetiology of these conditions, however, remain undermined.

Rheumatoid Lung[1]

The pulmonary changes in rheumatoid arthritis present mainly as three basic clinical forms, i.e., pleurisy with or without effusion, necrobiotic pulmonary nodules and fibrosing alveolitis, and rarely as bronchiolitis obliterans and rheumatoid laryngitis. Pleuropulmonary manifestations are more simple, and include pleural disease, interstitial fibrosis, pleuropulmonary nodules, pneumonitis and arteritis.[2] Rheumatoid arthritis increases with age and female excessive involvement is observed. Onset may be slow, but stiffness is often decapacitating. Rheumatoid nodules are more common in males, occurring in long standing cases, more so in skin and subcutaneous tissue, also appearing in lung, upper airways and heart.[2]

Revealed in 2% of cases a chest X-ray, and 22% on CT chest. May complicate as empyema, pneumothorax, pleural effusion or bronchopleural fistula.[3] These may occur along with other lesions of rheumatoid arthritis, before or after the appearance of arthritic manifestations. Correlation between the severity of arthritis and lung disease cannot be made. The presence of circulating rheumatoid factor is of diagnostic help.

In rheumatoid lung, pleuropulmonary involvements are common; but pulmonary vasculature is rarely involved.[4,5] Various presentations, clinical manifestations, investigations, pathological features and differential diagnoses are listed in the following Tables I-VI.

Table I: RA related pleuropulmonary involvement

- Involves pleura or diffuse interstitial fibrosis.
- Involves small airways.
- Pulmonary vasculature involvement is extremely rare.
- Pulmonary manifestations in RA are common in 6-10%, having worst outcome due to functional impairment and mortality.
- Rheumatoid arthritis induced ILD is observed in 5-40%, however, clinical ILD observed in 5-10% of RA.
- Usual interstitial pneumonia (UIP) and some (NSIP) forms are seen.
- Cor pulmonale occurs because of hypoxia induced pulmonary vasoconstriction.
- Pulmonary fibrosis and pleural effusion are most common presentations. Others are listed in the table.

Table II: Respiratory manifestations of RA
Pleural effusion/fibrosis
Bronchopleural fistula
Pulmonary nodules and diffuse fibrosis
Caplan's syndrome
Recurrent infections
Bronchiolitis obliterans
Eosinophilic pneumonia
Pulmonary hypertension
Shrinking lung
Bronchocentric granuloma
Bronchiectasis
Cricoarytenoid obstruction

Table III: Pathology in rheumatoid lung

- 5 different groups have been identified
- Rheumatoid pulmonary nodules
- UIP
- NSIP
- BOOP
- Lymphoid hyperplasia and cellular interstitial infiltrates.

Table IV: Clinical presentation

- Cough, wheeze
- Exertional dyspnoea
- Hemoptysis

Table V: Investigations in rheumatoid lung

- **RA factor** +ve in 2/3rd of cases
- **PFTS**- Airways obstruction ↓FEV_1/VC
  or Severe restriction ↓FVC or small airway disease (↓FEF 15-75)
- **Chest X-ray:** Pleural effusion or thickening
  or and/- Necrobiotic nodules
  or and/- Diffuse interstitial fibrosis
  or and/- Caplan's syndrome
  or and/- Pulmonary hypertension
- **DLCO** indicates progress of disease
- **CT :** May show:
  - Reticulations
  - Ground glass opacity
  - Honeycombing
  - Lung nodules
  - Consolidation
  - Bronchiectasis
  - Air trapping
  - Pleural effusion/thickening
  - Lymphadenopathy
  - Pulmonary artery enlargement

Contd

Contd

Categorizing the findings into major CT pattern of:
- Usual interstitial pneumonia (IPF/CFA)
- NSIP
- Bronchiolitis
- Organizing pneumonia (COP)

Table VI: Differential diagnosis

- Mycobacterial infection
- Non mycobacterial infection
  - Nocardia
  - Cryptococcus
  - Histoplasma
  - Aspergillus
- Neoplasms
  - Bronchoalveolar carcinoma
  - Multiple myeloma
- Lymphoma
- Other Conn Tissue disorders
  - SLE
  - SS
  - MCTD
  - PAD
  - DM/Polymyositis

\+ Diagnostic dilemma persists.
++ Holistic approach is helpful in diagnosing pulmonary manifestation.

Pleurisy

Pleurisy is the most common variety of pulmonary involvement in rheumatoid arthritis that is seen in 50% of cases. It presents generally without any underlying lung involvement. Usually it appears after several years of arthritis and mostly in middle aged males. Effusion may be small or large, unilateral or bilateral. It may remain asymptomatic. There may be chest pain or dyspnoea but fever is infrequent.

There is an exudative pleural effusion. It is turbid and yellow in colour with lymphocytes as predominant cells. There may be large, elongated multinuclear giant cell (ragocytes) with cytoplasmic inclusions. Glucose content is extremely low (less than 25 mg/dl). Oral or intravenous glucose administration fails to increase glucose content in the pleural fluid.[3] A selective block for glucose transport into the pleural space probably exists due to inhibition by mediators released from the inflammed pleura.[4] The pleural fluid pH is less than 7.2. The complement levels tend to be low compared with the serum level. Immune complexes and rheumatoid factor are detected in pleural fluid and these may be greater than those present in the serum of the same patient.[5] The level of proteins and lactic dehydrogenase is high (more than 700 IU/l). Often, biospy is non-informative as the rheumatoid nodules are on the visceral surface. The effusion resolves over several months or may persist for years. It may lead to pleural thickening and adhesions. Repeated paracentesis helps in clearing the effusion and if recurs, corticosteroids or pleurodesis may be requried. Chronic effusion appears chyliform due to presence of increased amount of cholesterol. Presence of dyspnoea from thickened pleura may require decortication.

Necrobiotic Granuloma

Necrobiotic granuloma, which is histologically similar to cutaneous rheumatoid nodules, form the least common pulmonary manifestations of rheumatoid arthritis.[6] The condition may exist without any symptoms or may present with cough and haemoptysis, when the nodule undergoes liquefaction and forms a cavity. It may produce pneumothorax and broncho-pleural fistula.[2]

The nodules may be single or multiple and are seen most frequently in the upper zones of the lung. They are generally associated with long-standing rheumatoid arthritis. The nodules may persist or undergo spontaneous resolution. They have to be distinguished from malignancy or infection. The nodules do not require any treatment unless there is infection or bronchopleural fistula. The nodules are often associated with bronchogenic carcinoma.[1]

A variant of rheumatoid nodules may coexist with certain pneumoconiosis such as Caplan's syndrome. Its formation is stimulated by the presence of silica or silicates found in coal or in other organic dusts. Multiple, clearly defined, round opacities develop rapidly in both lungs especially at their peripheries under the background of simple pneumoconiosis. They cause minimal disability. Another differential diagnosis is progressive massive fibrosis which develops slowly with an irregular outline.

Fibrosing Alveolitis

A mural type of fibrosing alveolitis may develop and present with dyspnoea and non-productive cough. Immune complexes have been implicated in its pathogenesis.[7] On chest auscultation, crackles are audible in the basal regions of the lung. Clubbing is less common compared to that seen in *lone* cryptogenic fibrosing alveolitis.[8] Reticular shadows are seen on chest X-ray, which may progress to honeycombing. PFTs show decreased lung volumes, restrictive ventilatory defect and impaired diffusing capacity. Progression of the disease is much slower and the course is more benign than that of idiopathic pulmonary fibrosis.[7]

Interstitial pulmonary fibrosis may occur in rheumatoid arthritis as a complication to gold therapy, requiring discontinuation of gold therapy and in some, giving a short course of corticosteroids.[1] Early intervention is essentially important before extensive fibrotic changes occur.

Rheumatoid Laryngitis

Rheumatoid affection of the cricoarytenoid joints may cause hoarseness and stridor. Cricoarytenoid arthritis or laryngeal nodules may produce upper airway obstruction.[9,10]

Bronchiolitis Obliterans

Due to penicillamine therapy, rapidly progressive bronchiolitis obliterans may develop rarely in patients with rheumatoid arthritis. Bronchioles and small bronchi are obliterated by submucosal inflammation and fibrosis. Clinically it presents with progressively increasing dyspnoea. Chest examination reveals coarse early inspiratory crackles. It is not associated with any radiologic abnormality. Pulmonary function studies show air-trapping and a reduction of flow rates. Steroids do not have much effect.

Pulmonary hypertension due to interstitial fibroris in rheumatoid arthritis and in some cases due to pulmonary arteritis may develop. No therapy is of any value in the natural course of the disease. Upper lobe fibrobullous disease resembling radiologically to ankylosing spondylitis is being recognized in rheumatoid arthritis.

Rheumatoid arthritis is being recognised as an independent risk factor in bronchogenic carcinoma, possibly because of its increased incidence secondary to epithelial metaplasia and hyperplasia in the diffuse fibrotic lungs.[11,12]

Ankylosing Spondylitis

Lungs are affected late in the course of ankylosing spondylitis.[1,13] Pulmonary lesions include chronic fibrotic changes in the upper lobe of the lung with apical pleural thickening. This occurs in 1% of cases. The condition may progress to bronchiectasis or cavitation. Often there are preceding attacks of pneumonia. The condition presents with dry cough, purulent expectoration and recurrent episodes of haemoptysis. Though there is decrease in the vital capacity and maxium voluntary ventilation, the total lung capacity remains normal, unlike other restrictive lung diseases, as the chest is held in an expanded state. The majority of the patients do not demonstrate rheumatoid factor in the serum. There is a high association with HLA-B 27.

Systemic Lupus Erythematosus (SLE)

In 45-64 years of age female incidence and prevalence is in 9:1 ratio : : Female : Male. SLE is a chronic, systemic autoimmune disorder, pulmonary complications include pleurisy, pleural effusion, pneumonitis, pulmonary hypertension, alveolar haemorrhage and interstitial lung disease. Pleuritis with or without pleural effusion, acute non-eosinophilic infiltrates and rarely pulmonary haemorrhage. Progression of disease often ends up in shrinking lung syndrome.[14]

Belimumab is the first biological agent approved for the treatment of SLE; which will be useful for refractory cases, having property of suppressing auto immunity.[15]

Systemic Sclerosis[16,17]

The condition is seen in 3rd to 5th decades, more commonly in females. Pulmonary involvement is more common in patients with systemic sclerosis than in other collagen vascular diseases. The primary complications may be either interstitial or vascular disease. Secondary complications are aspiration pneumonia and lung cancer. Lung cancer and PSS association is well recognized; bronchoalveolar carcinoma, followed by squamous cell carcinoma, oat cell carcinoma and anaplastic carcinoma of lung are in the order of frequency of occurrence. This has been discussed earlier (PSS).

Polymyositis/Dermatomyositis[1]

5 to 10 per cent of patients with polymyositis/dermatomyositis may show radiologic evidence of interstitial lung disease.[18] This was first described by Mills and Mathews in 1956.[19] Clinically there can be an acute onset of fever, dyspnoea and a non-productive cough or with insidious onset of dyspnoea and cough. There is a subacute diffuse interstitial fibrosis, with a component of active inflammation. There is no relation between the severity of interstitial fibrosis and the muscle disease. However, the fibrosis is frequently associated with joint manifestations and Jo-1 antibody.[7,20] Rarely pulmonary manifestations include isolated pulmonary artery hypertension and further pulmonary disorders secondary to muscle dysfunction such as respiratory failure, aspiration pneumonia, atelectasis and cardiac failure, may also manifest. Corticosteroids exhibit a favourable response in pneumonitis. Aspiration pneumonia and respiratory insufficiency are more frequent in severe cases of myopathy.[1]

ILD adversely affects prognosis with 40% mortality in 31-32 months follow-up.

Sjögren's Syndrome

Sjögren's syndrome predominantly affects middle aged women in a 9:1 : Female : Male ratio.[21] This is chronic inflammatory disorder characterised by lymphocytic infiltration of lacrimal and salivary glands, resulting in dryness of eyes and mouth. Those patients develop lymphoproliferative syndrome in the form of lymphadenopathy and increased risk of lymphoma.

Interstitial lung disease resembling idiopathic pulmonary fibrosis may rarely develop in Sjörgen's syndrome. Pulmonary involvement is seen in 9-75% of patients. Usually lung involvement is seen in the form of chronic bronchitis, lymphocytic interstitial pneumonitis and pleural effusion. There is airways' narrowing. Pulmonary function tests show a restrictive pattern with a decreased diffusing capacity.

Interstitial pneumonitis caused by an infiltration of mononuclear cells or a discrete nodular lesion called pseudolymphoma. The former is of little significance and the latter may get infective, inflammatory or neoplastic changes in it (malignant lymphoma).[22] Immune complex vasculitis, and thromboangiitis obliterans in patients with pre existing Raynaud's phenomenon may also occur.[23-25]

Clinically upper mucosal dryness extending upto upper airways may induce dry cough (xerotrachea) or hoarseness, which increases in cold weather.

ESR may be raised, Wimary PA is increased and leucopenic thrombocytosis may be present. None of the features are diagnostic. However, Schirmer's test indicating ocular dryness is a pointer towards Sjögren's syndrome.[26]

No specific treatment is available, steroids may be of help. Immunosuppressive drugs are not required for whole life. Pseudolymphoma should be treated with caution as cytotoxic therapy may convert it into true lymphoma.[2]

Temporal Arteritis

Rarely lungs may be affected due to a primary pulmonary vasculitis. Multiple nodular lesions or diffuse interstitial lung disease,[27] may be the feature. Restrictive ventilatory defect is present. Steroids are useful.

Polyarteritis Nodosa

A multisystem disorder featuring necrosis, inflammation and thrombosis in small and medium sized arteries of various organs. Pulmonary involvement is very rare.[9] The lesions are perivascular and granuloma is not formed. There is a fibrinoid necrosis. Initial inflammatory polymorphic infiltrate is later raplaced by lymphocytes and plasma cells. Thrombosis leads to obliteration of vascular lumen, resulting in aneurysms, ischemia and infarction. Patient may present with wheezing. Peripheral eosinophilia is present. Clinical features of involvement of heart, kidney, skin and nervous system are also present. Steroids and cyclophosphamide induce remissions.[27]

Rheumatic Pneumonia

Pneumonia may develop during acute rheumatic fever, characterised by fibrinoid necrosis of alveolar walls and infilteration by mononuclear cells of the interstitium. Focal pulmonary odema and hyaline membrane formation occurs as a result of increased capillary permeability.[27] Steroids are useful as the condition responds to.

Mixed Connective Tissue Disease (MCD)

It is seen in about 25% of cases where cumulated respiratory clinical features of rheumatoid arthritis, SLE, systemic sclerosis and polymyositis are present. Pleurisy with or without effusion and pulmonary fibrosis are seen.[26] There is reduced co-transfer factor in 75% of cases, pleurisy in 25-30% of cases and pulmonary hypertension in 30% of cases. Diagnostic criteria include co-diffusing capacity less than 70% normal, pulmonary hypertension and proliferative vascular lesions on lung biopsy.[17]

Pulmonary Involvement with Undifferentiated Connective Tissue Disease (UCTD)

Mixed connective tissue disease is multisystem affection, where lung is commonly involved, ranging from consolidation, interstitial pneumonitis, pleural effusion and rarely bronchiolitis obliterans and pneumothorax.[27-29] Other pleuropulmonary problems are shown in the following table.

Pleuro-pulmonary problems in mixed connective tissue disorders (MCTD)
• Pleuritic pain and pleural effusion
• ***Pulmonary HT**
• ILD
• Thromboembolic disease
• Alveolar hemorrhage
• Diaphragmatic dysfunction
• Aspiration pneumonia
• Obstructive airways disease
• Pulmonary vasculitis
• Pulmonary infections
* Main cause of death among patients with MCTD. Some promise by calcium channel blockers, ACE inhibitors, steroids and other immuno suppressive drugs.

Undifferentiated connective tissue disease is seen in young patients having pyrexia, myalgia. Chest pain and having non-specific interstitial pneumonitis (ILD). Termed coined by Le Roy, *et al.* in 1980, criteria of UCTD include:

a. Systemic inflammation.
b. Absence of clinical infection.
c. Absence of criteria for other connective tissue disorder.

Non-pulmonary affections include:

- Arthralgia.
- Raynaud's phenomenon.
- Leukopenia.
- Neuro/Renal involvement is absent.
- Cutaneous affection includes patichiae, risk, calcinosis, aeroscleroderma, purpura, erythema nodosum, telangiectasia.

Pulmonary manifestations[30,31] include:

- Dyspnea.
- Cough/wheeze.
- Pleuritic chest pain.
- Pleural effusion.
- Non-specific interstitial pneumonitis (NSIP) on histopathology.

NSIP can also occur with:

- Scleroderma.
- Polymyositis/dermatomysitis.
- Sjögren's syndrome.

HRCT of NSIP shows:

- 100% ground glass appearance.
- Less than 50% irregular linear opacity.
- More than one third traction bronchiectasis.
- Less than 1/6th consolidation.
- More than 1/7th nodular opacity.
- More than 1/8th emphysema.

Response to oral corticoids and low dose of methotrexate is very good. Patient has to continue low dose corticosteroids.

REFERENCES

1. Shankar P.S., Pulmonary manifestations of connective tissue diseases, In; Dalal P.M., ed: Medicine Update API Bombay 1991;1:137-41.
2. Chitnis N., *et al.,* Case of pulmonary rheumatoid nodules in rheumatoid arthritis; JAPI 2012; 60:46.
3. Tanoue T., Pulmonary manifestations of rheumatoid; Clin Chest Med 1998; 19:667-85.
4. Tanaka N; *et al.,* RA related lung disease: CT findings; Radiology 2004; 232: 81-91.
5. Acharya S; *et al.,* Rheumatoid interstitial lung disease presenting as cor pulmonale; Lung India 2010; 27: 256-59.
6. Payne CR., Pulmonary manifestations of rheumatoid arthritis, Br. J. Hosp. Med 1984; 32: 192-97.
7. Hochberg M.C., Feldman D. and Stevens M.B., Adult onset polymyositis/dermatomyositis. An analysis of clinical and laboratory features and survival in76 patients with are view of the literature. Sem. Arthritis Rheum 1986; 15: 168-78.
8. Turner-Warwick M., Interstitial pulmonary fibrosis with or without associated collagen vascular disease, Amer. Rev. Respir. Dis 1981; 123: 73.
9. Pathan M.I., *et al.,* Upper airway obstruction due to cricoarytenoid arthritis in a case of systemic onset juvenile rheumatoid arthritis; JAPI 2001; 49: 566-67.
10. Langford C.A., Van Waes C., Upper airway obstruction in rheumatic diseases; IN, Life threatening complication of autoimmune disease; Rheum. Clin. North Amer 1999; 23: 345-63.
11. Brannan M.H., *et al.,* Pulmonary disease associated with rheumatoid arthritis; JAMA 1984; 189:914.
12. Helmers R., *et al.,* Pulmonary manifestations associated with rheumatoid arthritis; Chest 1991; 100:235.

13. Shankar P.S., Scott J.A. and Anderson C.L., Pulmonary disease in ankylosing spondylitis positive for rheumatoid factor and HLA-27, Ind. J. Chest. Dis 1977; 19: 27-31.
14. Harpreet Singh; *et al.,* SLE; IN; SR Joshi; ed; Med Update API 2014; 24: 409-17.
15. Rajadhyaksha AG; *et al.,* Biologics in SLE–the current status; JAPI 2013; 61: 262-67.
16. Wooten, Marc M.D., Lung Cancer in PSS; Southern Medical Journal 2008;101:59-62.
17. Kundu S., *et al.,* Squamous cell carcinoma lung with PSS; JAPI 2012:60:52-54.
18. Dickey B.F. and Meyers A.B., Pulmonary disease in Polymyositis and dermatomyositis, Sem Arthritis Rheum 1984; 14: 60-76.
19. Sareen D., Paljor P., Idiopathic polymyositis presenting as interstitial lung disease; JAPI 2000; 48: 654-55.
20. Lakhanpal S., Lie J.T., Conn D.L., *et al.,* Pulmonary diseases in polymyositis/dermatomyositis: A clinicopathological analysis of 65 autospy cases, Ann. Rheum. Dis 1987; 46: 23-29.
21. Mahajan A; *et al.,* Rheumatological manifestations in 40+ women: IN : SR Joshi; ed; Med Update, API 2014; 24: 383-87.
22. Kambolz S., Sher A., Barland P., *et al.,* Sjögren's syndrome in severe upper airways obstruction due to primary malignant tracheal lymphoma developing during successful treatment of lymphocytic interstitial pneumonitis, J. Rheumatol 1987; 14: 588-94.
23. Fox R.I., *et al.,* Primary Sjögren's syndrome, Clinical and immunopathologic features, Semin Arth. Rheum 1984; 14: 77.
24. Talal N., *et al.,* (ed): Sjögren's syndrome, *Clinical and Immunological aspects;* N. York, Springer-Verlag 1987; 299.
25. Tsokos M., *et al.,* Vasculitis in primary Sjögren's syndrome, Histologic classification and clinical presentation, Amer. Clin. Pathol 1987; 88: 26.
26. Bhadoria D.P., *et al.,* Sjörgren's syndrome in north Indian patients of rheumatoid arthritis, JAPI 1988; 38: 650-52.
27. Shankar P.S., Chest Medicine, Oxford IBH Publ Co (P) Ltd. N. Delhi 1994; 4th ed.
28. Mukherjee S., Kar S., MCTD; In: Y.P. Munjal, ed., PG Med. API 1999; 13: 477-86.
29. Jais X; *et al.,* Immunosuppressive therapy in lupus and mixed connective tissue disease associated pulmonary arterial hypertension–A retrospective analysis of 23 cases; Arth Rheum 2008; 58(2): 521-31.
30. Bodolay E; *el al.,* Evaluation of ILD in MCTD; Rheumatol 2005; 44 (5): 656-61.
31. Narsimulu G, Prasad V; MCTDs; IN; MS Rao; ed; Med Update, API 2010; 20: 841-45.
32. Kinder BW; *et al.,* Idiopathic NSIP: Lung manifestations of undifferentiated connective tissue disease (UCTD)? Amer J Resp Crit Care Med 2007; 176: 691-97.
33. Arjun P., *et al.,* UCTD with pulmonary involvement; JAPI 2011; 59: 175-78.

Miscellaneous Lung Disorders and Diseases

11

DRUG-INDUCED PULMONARY DISEASES

INTRODUCTION

Pulmonology has established itself as a subspeciality of medicine, though a little late, in developing countries. Drug-induced respiratory diseases (shown in Table 11.1) are becoming quite increasingly apparent[1] as more than 40 commonly used drugs are reported to cause pulmonary parenchymal tissue injury.[2,3] Drug-induced interstitial lung diseases can be acute or chronic. Due to irreversible damage that may result from drugs, treatment for lethal diseases have to be withdrawn prematurely. It is difficult to estimate the true incidence of drug-induced pulmonary disease because of the lack of specific markers, histologic findings or diagnostic clinical features and also because of sporadic nature of many of these reactions. Pharmacologic agents that may cause pulmonary parenchymal injury can be classified into 2 groups (Table 11.2), cytotoxic drugs and the non-cytotoxic drugs.

Mechanism of Action

The lungs are the only human organs that are exposed to both internal and external insults of various types. There are number of homeostatic mechanisms for maintaining a balance between damaging inflammatory reaction and protective detoxification pathways. Drugs can affect any of these systems resulting in pulmonary injury. Four types of mechanisms have been suggested.

Table 11.1: Drug-induced disorders of respiratory system

Disorders	*Possible drugs*
1. Asthma	Penicillin, Aspirin, Griseofulvin, Tetracycline, Streptomycin, Organic iodides, Iron, Dextran, Vaccines, Antisera, NSAIDs, ACE inhibitors
2. Pulmonary eosinophilia	PAS, Penicillin, Nitrofurantoin, Aspirin, Sulphonamides, Pituitary sniff
3. Lipoid pneumonia	Cod liver oil, Liquid paraffin, Ephedrine nasal drops
4. Alveolar oedema	Long term use of high concentration of oxygen
5. Intra alveolar oedema and fibrosis	Busulphan, Bleomycin, Gold Salts, Methysergide, Nitrofurantoin, Practolol
6. Interstitial alveolitis	Lignocaine
7. Pulmonary oedema	Overdose of salicylates, Amitriptyline and IV fluids, Adrenaline, Phenylbutazone, Beta blockers, Hydro chlorthiazides, Methadone, IV heroin, Angiography dye
8. Goodpasture's syndrome	Penicillamine
9. Pulmonary hypertension	Aminorex fumarate
10. Pulmonary thromboembolism	Amphetamine, Oral contraceptive
11. Mediastinal lymphadenopathy	PAS, Phenytoin, Phenylbutazone, Potassium iodide
12. Pleural effusion and fibrosis	Nitrofurantoin, Methysergide
13. Hydrothorax	Gonadotropins, Practolol
14. Haemothorax	Anticoagulants
15. Pneumothorax	Corticosteroids (in tuberculosis), Adriamycin
16. Lipomatosis	Corticosteroids
17. Respiratory depression	Overdose of sedative
18. Hyperventilation	Overdose of salicylates

Table 11.2: Drugs causing pulmonary parenchymal injury

Cytotoxic drugs	*Non-cytotoxic drugs*
Antibiotics	Antimicrobial agents
Bleomycin	Nitrofurantoin
Mitomycin	Amphotericin
Neocarzinostatin	Sulfasalazine
Alkylating Agents	Analgesics
Busulfan	Aspirin, NSAIDs
Cyclophosphamide	Anticonvulsants
Chlorambucil	Diphenylhydantoin
Melphalan	Carbamazepine
Antimetabolites	Antiarrhythmics
Methotrexate	Amiodarone
Azathioprine	Lidocaine
Mercaptopurine	Tocainide
Cytosine arabinoside	Procainamide
	Disopyramide
Nitrosoureas	Beta adrenergic blockers
Carmustine (BCNU)	Practolol
Semustine (Methyl CCNU)	Propranolol
Lomystine (CCNU)	Pindolol
Chlorozotocin	Diuretics
	Hydrochlorothiazide
	ACE inhibitors
Miscellaneous	Opiates
Procarbazine	Heroin
VM-26	Propoxyphene
Vinblastine	Methadone
Vindesine	Sedatives
	Ethchlorvynol
	Chlordiazepoxide
	Tranquillizers
	Haloperidol
	Fluphenazine
	Miscellaneous
	Gold salts
	Penicillamine
	Isoniazid
	Colchicine

Oxidant-Antioxidant System[2]

Drugs such as bleomycin, cyclophosphamide and amiodarone are capable of producing reactive oxygen species (Oxidants) including the superoxide anion (O_2), hydrogen peroxide (H_2O_2), the hydroxyl radical (OH), singlet oxygen ($1O_2$) and hypochlorous acid (HOCl). These oxidants can cause autologous cytotoxicity, unless they are neutralized by antioxidants such as superoxide dismutase (SOD), catalase, glutathione peroxidase, ceruloplasmin and Vitamin E. These antioxidant systems are present in virtually every cell in the body. Over production of oxidants by the drugs, thus results in an alteration of normal balance between oxidants and antioxidants, resulting in pulmonary toxicity. Oxidant damage can stimulate the immune system and attract neutrophils with protease activity.

Immunologic System[2,4-6]

Normal resident pulmonary cells are alveolar macrophages and lymphocytes. Drugs can activate resident pulmonary cells, resulting in attracting and activating peripheral inflammatory cells such as polymorphonuclear neutrophils (PMN), eosinophils and monocytes. These activated cells liberate cytotoxic mediators. Experimental pulmonary fibrosis induced by agents such as bleomycin, paraquat, N-nitroso-N methylurethane, etc. had shown that fibrosis of the alveolar wall first requires *injury* to the alveolar wall, that is, damage to the existing cells and matrix comprising the lung parenchyma. Most of the injury results from the effector processes of these cell types comprising alveolitis. Bronchoalveolar lavage (BAL) studies[7-9] have demonstrated increased numbers of polymorphonuclear neutrophils in patients with bleomycin, methotrexate, gold salts, amiodarone and nitrofurantoin. Lung eosinophilia have been reported in lung diseases due to bleomycin, procarbazine, nitrofurantoin, gold, etc. The relative potency of the effector cells in regard to their ability to injure the alveolar wall is probably, in descending order, neutrophils, alveolar macrophages, eosinophils and lymphocytes. If the damage is sufficient such that normal alveolar architecture cannot be re-established, a secondary form of *repair,* i.e., replacement of normal parenchyma by fibroblasts and their products, takes over. Activated alveolar macrophages release chemoattractants for neutrophils, leukotriene B4, interleukin 1, possibly interleukin 8, oxidants and a variety of growth signals for mesenchymal cells inclding platelet-derived growth factor (PDGF-B) fibronectin (FN) insulin like growth factor 1 (IGF-1), transforming growth factor—beta (TGF-B), and Tumour Necrosis Factor (TNF). Macrophage derived growth factors are shown in Table 11.3. Neutrophils release oxidants and potent proteinases such as collagens and neutrophil elastase. Eosinophils liberate oxidants, collagese and a variety of other agents such as major basic protein. Lymphocytes release interleukin-2, migration inhibition factor, monocyte chemotactic factor and oxidants.

Fibronectin and alveolar macrophage derived growth factors (AMDGF), and the mediators released by alveolar macrophages play an important role in fibrosis. Fibronectin (FN) recruits fibroblasts to the area of injury. Fibroblast numbers expand as a result of mediators released by macrophages. FN attaches fibroblasts to matrix which is made up of type I and type III collagen. FN also acts as a *competence factor* to move fibroblasts through the early phases of the G_1, portion of the cell cycle (G_1 is the earliest phase of the cell proliferation cycle and precedes DNA synthesis). AMDGF acts as a growth factor and in the presence of the *competence factor* (FN) induces fibroblasts to move, through the late stages of G_1 and proliferate. This ultimately leads to fibrosis by replacement of normal

Table 11.3: Macrophage derived growth factors

Platelet derived growth factor (PDGE)	Insulin-like growth factor (IGF)	Transforming growth factor- Beta (TGF-B)	Inhibitors of proliferation
Competence	Progression G_1	Collagen and matrix production	IL_1 + TNF PGE_2
Resting	GO_2 Gell cycle S M G_2 Mitosis Pre-mitosis	DNA synthesis	

parenchymal cells and matrix by fibroblasts and fibroblast products. However, macrophages are also capable of arresting fibrotic response by releasing two cytokines, TFN-a and IL 1.[9] They interact synergistically to augment production of prostaglandins (PGE 2). PGE 2 is a powerful second messenger that inhibits fibroblast proliferation. Pathogenesis of the fibrotic response is given in Table 11.4.[10,11]

Proteolytic System[6]

Proteolytic enzymes, particularly elastase, are produced by polymorphonuclear leukocytes and alveolar macrophages. There are a number of antiprotease systems in the lower respiratory tract, the most important being the alpha-1-protease inhibitor. Reactive oxygen radicals released by drugs such as bleomycin and cyclophosphamide can inactivate alpha-1-protease inhibitor resulting in enhanced activity of proteolytic enzymes.

Central Nervous System (CNS)[1,6]

A variety of CNS insults can cause neurogenic pulmonary oedema in which there will be an increased capillary protein leak. This may suggest that pulmonary capillary permeability may be, in part, controlled by the central nervous system. Several drugs such as opiates, major tranquilizers, salicylates and methotrexate may cause pulmonary oedema through their effects on CNS. Presence of plentiful opiate receptors near the medullary respiratory centre may support for neural influences in the development of pulmonary oedema.

Risk Factors[6]

Risk factors predisposing to development of drug-induced pulmonary disease are given in Table 11.5. Pulmonary involvement under the effect of drug therapy depends on certain risk factors, which possibly predispose or precipitate. These include the drug dosage which may affect the lungs due to cumulative effect, e.g., bleomycin, amiodarone, etc. or the unit dose may cause the pulmonary disease as seen with many drugs like amiodarone, chlordiazepoxide, colchicine, ethchlorvynol, haloperidol, imipramine etc. Apart from drug dosage, the frequency of drug administration as with bleomycin, also forms important risk factor in developing drug induced pulmonary disease.

Associated radiotherapy with bleomycin, mitomycin and busulfan and oxygen therapy along with bleomycin, cyclophosphamide, nitrofurantoin and mitomycin predispose to pulmonary involvement.

Associated other drug therapy like bleomycin, BCNU, Vinca alkaloids, cyclophosphamide etc., other pre-existing pulmonary disease with BCNU, amiodarone, other systemic illness like renal failure with bleomycin, blood transfusions with amphotericin and mitomycin, pulmonary angiography with amiodarone, steroid therapy with methotrexate may predispose to drug induced pulmonary involvement.

Clinical Manifestations

Six distinct syndromes have been described clinically.

Pneumonitis/Fibrosis[2,6]

Drugs causing pneumonitis/fibrosis are shown in Table 11.6. Symptoms begin insidiously, progressive over several weeks to months, in the form of non-productive cough, dyspnoea on exertion, fatigue and malaise. Significant weight loss can also occur. Clubbing may be present. Bi-basilar end-expiratory crackles can be heard on auscultation. The chest radiograph

Table 11.4: Pathogenesis of the fibrotic response

Neutrophils		Macrophages	Lymphocytes	Eosinophils
PDG F(B) TG_2F-B	+ ve		-ve IL_1 IFN	TNF
			Fibroblast	
Chemotaxis	Proliferation		Collagen and matrix	Wound contraction

Table 11.5: Possible predisposing risk factors for pulmonary toxicity

Risk factors	*Drug(s) implicated*
1. *Dose*	
a. Cumulative dose	Bleomycin carmistine (BCNU), Amiodarone
b. Unit dose	Amiodarone, Heroin, Proproxyphene methadone, Ethchlorvynol, Chlordiazepoxide, Haloperidol, Colchicine, Imipramine
2. *Dispensing*	
a. Route of administration	Bleomycin
b. Frequency of administration	Methotrexate
3. *Other Modes*	
a. Oxygen therapy	Bleomycin, Mitomycin, Cyclophosphamide, Nitrofurantoin
b. Radiotherapy	Bleomycin, Busulfan, Mitomycin
4. *Anti Cancer Drugs*	Bleomycin, BCNU Cyclophosphamide, Mitomycin, Methotreaxate, Vinca alkaloids
5. *Other Factors*	
a. Age	Bleomycin
b. Previous pulmonary diseases	BCNU, Amiodarone
c. Blood component transfusions	Mitomycin, Amphotericin
d. Renal failure	Bleomycin
e. Steroid tapering or adrenalectomy	Methotrexate
f. Pulmonary angiography	Amiodarone

Table 11.6: Drugs causing pneumonitis/fibrositis

Chemotherapeutic agents for cancer	*Other drugs*
Bleomycin	Amiodarone
Busulfan	Gold salts
Cyclophosphamide	Nitrofurantoin
Chlorambucil	Penicillamine
Carmustine (BCNU)	Sulfasalazine
Chlorozotocin	Tocainide
Lomustine (CCNU)	
Mitomycin	
Melphalan	
Methotrexate	
Neocarzinostatin	
Semustine (Methyl CCNU)	

show bilateral reticular infiltrates. Occasionally chest radiograph is normal, even in the presence of pulmonary symptoms and physiologic abnormalities. Pulmonary function may show a restrictive ventilatory defect with a reduced diffusing capacity. Some residual pulmonary impairment is left despite appropriate treatment which includes discontinuation of the offending drug and institution of corticosteroids.

Hypersensitivity Pneumonitis[2,6,12] (Eosinophillic Pulmonary Infiltration)

Drugs that cause hypersensitivity pneumonitis (HP) are shown in Table 11.7. HP is characterised by a subacute onset (within hours to days) of dyspnoea, non-productive cough, chills, myalgia, fever and headache. Skin rash may be present in 50% of patients. Auscultation may reveal crackles. 40% of patients will have peripheral eosinophilia. There may be signs of hepatitis in a few cases. The chest radiograph shows diffuse acinar infiltrates, pleural effusions are more common than those of pneumonitis. Pulmonary function shows restriction with mildly reduced diffusing capacity. Lung biopsy may show interstitial and airway eosinophilia with a paucity of fibrosis. Virtually all patients, except those due to methotrexate, recover with few residual pulmonary dysfunction. Treatment includes withdrawal of the offending drug and institution of corticosteroids.

Table 11.7: Drugs causing hypersensitivity pneumonitis

Azathioprine	Mercaptopurine
Ampicillin	Mephenesin carbamate
Bleomycin	Methylphenidate
Carbamazepine	Mecamylamine
Chlorpropamide	Nitrofurantoin
Cromolyn	Naproxen
Diphenylhydantoin	Procarbazine
Dantrolene	Paraaminosalicyclic acid
Febarmate	Penicillin
Hydralazine	Pyrimethamine
Imipramine	Sulfasalazine
Isoniazid	Sulfadimethoxine
Methotrexate	Salazopyrin

Non-cardiogenic Pulmonary Oedema[1,5]

Symptoms occur acutely (over minutes to hours) and usually are associated with overdose of the offending agents. Drugs that cause non-cardiogenic pulmonary oedema are given in Table 11.8. Prognosis is variable and generally better than other causes of non-cardiogenic pulmonary oedema on removal of the offending agents.

Table 11.8: Drugs causing non-cardiogenic pulmonary oedema

Chemotherapeutic drugs for cancer	*Other drugs*
Cyclophosphamide	Amphatericin
Cytosine arabinoside	Chlordiazepoxide
Mitomycin	Colchicine
Methotrexate	Ethchlorvynol
VM-26	Heroin
	Haloperidol
	Isoxsuprine
	Imipramine
	Lidocaine
	Methadone
	Propoxyphene
	Ritodrine
	Terbutaline

Bronchiolitis Obliterans[13]

This rare complication has been described with drugs like cephalosporin, amiodarone, acetabutol, sulindac and phenytoin and more oftenly with gold salts, sulfasalazine and penicillamine. The underlying disease, particularly rheumatoid arthritis, can cause similar pulmonary pathology in the absence of drugs. Clinical symptoms include insidious onset of cough, dyspnoea and weight loss. Chest radiographs may be normal or show localised infiltrate. Pulmonary function shows an obstructive ventilatory defect. Histology shows areas of inflammation surrounding bronchioles resulting in their obliteration. In a proportion of patients especially due to sulfasalazine and penicillamine, a significant alveolitis is present. Prognosis of this condition is poor. Despite corticosteroid treatment and discontinuation of drugs, residual pulmonary abnormalities remain persisting.

Pulmonary Renal Syndrome[6]

This is a rare complication of penicillamine treatment. Clinical presentation includes hemoptysis, dyspnoea, pleuritic chest pain and uremia. Chest radiographic abnormalities include diffuse acinar, reticular or confluent large round densities. Lung histology shows pulmonary haemorrhage and haemosiderin-laden macrophages. Although similar to Goodpasture's syndrome, there are no typical linear pattern of basement membrane immunoglobulin deposition. Treatment includes immunosuppression and plasmapheresis.

Airways Obstruction

Airways obstruction presenting as cough, chest heaviness and asthma with drugs like beta blockers, NSAIDs,[14,15] Prostaglandin F_2 alpha and ACE inhibitors. This may happen with laxatives and anti-depressants. Even selective beta blockers should be used with caution in asthma patients. Enalapril precipitating bronchial asthma has been documented.[16]

Screening Tests[2,6]

Diffusing Capacity for Carbon Monoxide (TLCO)

TLCO appears to be sensitive, but relatively non-specific tests as a predictor of drug-induced pneumonitis especially in bleomycin or amiodarone-induced pneumonitis. Patients who never develop clinical disease have also shown a reduced TLCO. Baseline readings are always helpful.

Lung Volumes

A reduction in lung volumes as a restrictive ventilatory defect, appears to be a specific test, but is not very sensitive. Patients with lung disease have rarely shown normal lung volumes. Specificity decreases since many lung diseases have reduction in lung volumes.

Computed Tomographic (CT) Scanning

The detection of fibrosis by CT scanning has been correlated with lung volume measurements. CT abnormalities are detected in patients with normal chest radiographs. However, CT may not differentiate reversible pneumonitis from irreversible fibrosis. CT may prove to be sensitive and specific test in predicting development of drug-induced lung disease, slightly more sensitive than chest radiography but is rarely indicated.

Chest Radiographs

Chest radiographs are both non-specific and insensitive in detecting pulmonary disease. However, an abnormal chest radiograph is a late manifestation of drug-induced lung disease.

Gallium Scanning

It is non-specific. However, positive gallium scans, i.e., uptake of gallium-67 in area of acute inflammation, in the absence of abnormal chest radiographs have been reported in drug-induced lung diseases. However, there are no proper studies to evaluate gallium scanning in drug-induced lung disease.

Soluble Mediators

Soluble mediators such as serum angiotensin converting enzyme have been described in all patients receiving bleomycin, but most of them do not develop pulmonary fibrosis. This is a fertile field for future research in drug-induced lung disease. No organ system in the body functions in an isolation and lungs are no exception to this rule. Rather it is interdependent, especially with the heart, e. g., Daunorubicin, cyclophosphamide, radiation therapy or aerosol therapy can cause cardiac failure, myocardial fibrosis, left ventricular dysfunction or pericarditis and propranolol, amiodarone, thiazides, practolol, hydralazine, aspirin etc. can cause bronchospasm, alveolitis, pulmonary oedema, pleural fibrosis, lupus syndrome and bronchial asthma respectively. Even acetaminophen can precipitate allergy, rhino conjunctivitis and asthma.[17] So, it is always wise to use the minimum and most appropriate drugs and keep in mind the interface and the possible drug reactions in the lungs so to act urgently to remove the offending agents and institute the therapy.

Pathology of drug-induced disorders is pretty diverse still. BAL will be unnecessary if there is blood eosinophilia. Nevertheless, it will be contributory if there is lung eosinophilia in the absence of systemic eosinophilia.[18,19]

Recently development of electromechanical dissociation and acute pulmonary oedema has been reported with anti-arrhythmic agent disopyramide.[20]

REFERENCES

1. Vijayan V.K., *Drug-induced respiratory diseases,* In: Chandrasekharan S. (ed); Medicine Update, Assn. Phys. India, Bombay 1993; 3: 177-86.
2. Dinesh Badyal and RS Bhatia; ADRs: Peepee Publ: N Delhi 2006; 103-14.
3. Rosenow E.C., The spectrum of drug-induced pulmonary disease, Ann, Intern Med 1972; 77: 977-91.
4. Bedrossiane C.W.M., Pathology of drug-induced lung diseases, Semin Respir Med 1982; 4: 98-l05.
5. Ginsberg S.J. and Comis R.L., The pulmonary toxicity of antineoplastic agents, Semin Oncol 1982; 9: 34-51.
6. Cooper JAD. Jr. and Mathay R.G. Drug-induced pulmonary disease, DM 1987; 33: 66-120.
7. Davis W.B., Cristal R.G., *Chronic interstitial lung disease,* In: Daniel H. Simons (Ed); Current pulmonology V5. John Wiley and Sons, Inc 1984; 247-473.
8. Sibilee Y. and Reynolds H.Y., Macrophages and polymorphonuclear neutrophils in lung defence and injury, Am. Rev. Respir. Dis 1990; 141: 471-501.
9. Kelley J., Cytokines of the lung, Am. Rev. Respir. Dis 1990; 141: 765-88.
10. Cherniack R.M., Crystal R.G. and Kalica A.R., NHLBL Workshop summary, Current concepts in idiopathic pulmonary fibrosis, A road map for the future, Am. Rev. Respir. Dis 1991; 143: 680-83.
11. Shaw R.J., The role of lung macrophages at the interface between chronic inflammation and fibrosis, Resp. Med 1891; 85: 267-73.
12. Davidson AC., Bateman C, Shovlin C., *et al.,* Pulmonary toxicity of malaria prophylaxis, BMJ 1988; 297: 1240-41.
13. Daga M.K., Arora N.; Bronchiolitis obliterans—An overview; In; M.M. Singh, ed., Med. Update, API 1999; 9:369-76.
14. Mangalvedhekar S.S. *et al.*, Adverse drug reactions postal survey—Bronchial asthma and angioedema with nimesulide, JAPI 2000; 48:548.
15. Gupta D; *et al.*, Near fatal asthma following ingestion of diclofenac sodium tablet; JAPI 2000; 48: 258-59.
16. Bhatia R.S., Enalapril precipitating an attack of asthmaticus bronchitis; JAPI 42: 506.
17. Beasley RW; *et al.,* Amer J Resp Crit Care Med 2011; 183: 171-78.
18. Tattersfield A.E., Personal communication, 1994.
19. Bhatia R.S. and Sibia S.S., BAL: Indications and present status; Lung India 1994; 12:27-29.
20. Sethi K.K., Mohan J.E., Singhal A. and Gupta M.P., Electromechanical dissociation induced by intravenous disopyramide, JAPI 1987; 35:605-07.

RESPIRATORY FAILURE[1-5]

It is defined on the basis of arterial blood gas criteria as a partial pressure of arterial oxygen (PaO_2) of less than 60 mm Hg with or without partial pressure of arterial carbon dioxide ($PaCO_2$) more than 49 mm Hg, at rest and at sea level. It is classified as acute or chronic on the basis of duration of abnormal gas exchange.

Pathophysiology of mechanism includes hypoventilation, mismatching of ventilation-perfusion, shunt and diffusion defect (which is seen only in extensive damage of parenchyma and capillaries).

Hypoventilation in alveoli results in hypercapnia with respiratory acidosis and hypoxemia, due to decreased quantity of inspired oxygen in the alveoli.

Poorly ventilated alveoli due to parenchymal damage have a low *V/Q* ratio, which results in hypoxemia. Areas with high *V/Q* ratio are adequately ventilated but poorly perfused, resulting in wasted ventilation, i. e., increased dead space. However, they release CO_2, preventing the rise in $PaCO_2$. But $PaCO_2$ will rise where there is concomitant depressed respiration preventing rise in minute ventilation.

Intrapulmonary shunt results from ventilation-perfusion mismatch where ventilation is absent but blood flow continues. It differs from VQ mismatch since unventilated alveoli have the same PO_2 as of mixed venous blood irrespective of concentration of oxygen being inspired.

In type I respiratory failure, there is low PaO_2 and low or normal $PaCO_2$; with an increased alveolar-arterial gradient ($PA\text{-}aO_2$). In type II, there is decreased PaO_2 and increased $PaCO_2$ as a result of alveolar hypoventilation. Associated fall in minute volume causes a rise in $PaCO_2$ and fall in PaO_2, but $PA\text{-}aO_2$ remains normal. A combined respiratory failure results in low PaO_2 and high $PaCO_2$, with normal PaO_2.

Parenchymal diseases and diseases affecting airway or lung vasculature result in type I or hypoxemic respiratory failure. Conditions decreasing central respiratory drive can cause hypercapnic respiratory failure (type II), as listed in Table 11.9.

Table 11.9: Causes of respiratory failure

Type I	*Type II*
Pneumonia	*Pulmonary*–COPD
Asthma	*CNS disorder* – Brain injury/CVA, meningitis, encephalitis, diabetic coma
ARDS	*Peripheral nervous system disorder* – Myasthenia gravis, Myopathies, Guillain-Barré Syndrome
COPD	*Muscle disorder* – Polymyositis
Diffuse interstitial lung disease	– Muscle relaxant drugs
LVF	*Rib cage*
Pneumothorax	– Flail chest
Pulmonary embolism	– Kyphoscoliosis

Diagnosis

History of parenchymal damage in the form of fever, cough and dyspnea (in chronic cases) or history of trauma, toxic inhalation to CNS are pointer to diagnosis.

On examination, patient feels exhausted, semiconscious, with facial signs of using accessory respiratory muscles. Central cyanosis of lips and tongue indicates hypoxemia. Muscle twisting may be present. Raised intracranial pressure may cause papilloedema.

Investigations

Plain chest X-ray reveals pneumonic consolidation or fluffy shadows suggestive of ARDS may point towards cause of respiratory failure. Also, COPD, bronchiectatic cystic basal changes, pneumothorax, pleural effusion or cage deformity can also be detected by chest X-ray.

ABG analysis may reveal P_aO_2 less than 60 mm Hg and $PaCO_2$ more than 49 mm Hg. PA-aO_2 is increased indicating ventilation perfusion mismatch, or normal gradient may be indicating ventilation failure.

Treatment

Supplemental oxygen is essential. In case of airway block, decision for endotracheal intubation, tracheostomy or mechanical ventilation may be taken. Intermitted positive pressure ventilation or non-invasive continuous positive pressure have been successfully tried. In COPD cases, long-term oxygen therapy has to be considered. Specific therapy depends on the underlying process that precipitated ARF, general supportive measures are to be applied in most of the situations in ARF. And in case, no apparent aetiology could be identified, it is mainly the supportive treatment than the curative which is carried out. Reversing the primary process, if identifiable, is always rewarding in the management of ARF, e.g., opiate over dose, pneumococcal pneumonia, pulmonary oedema, asthma exacerbation where antidote for overdose drug, antibiotic for infection, diuretic for pulmonary oedema and steroids for asthma can potentially reverse the primary process that has caused ARF. Recognizing acute respiratory failure as a first manifestation of underlying neurological cause such as syringomyelia is a rare observation.[6]

Non-invasive continuous positive pressure ventilation (NIPPU) has become the choice made of non-invasive ventilation (NIV) in outpatient and hospital settings, effectively treating hypercapnic respiratory failure, cardiogenic pulmonary edema and respiratory failure secondary to neuromuscular diseases. Indications and contraindications are given below:

Non-invasive Ventilation (NIV): Indications[7-9]

A. Acute Respiratory Failure

a. *Obstructive airway disease*
- COPD (Acute exacerbation)
- Asthma
- Cystic fibrosis

b. *Hypoxemic respiratory failure*
- Cardiogenic pulmonary oedema.
- Pneumonia.
- ARDS/ALI.
- Chest trauma.
- Post operative respiratory failure.
- Respiratory failure in immunocompromised patient.

B. Chronic Respiratory Failure
- OSA
- Neuromuscular disease
- Kyphoscoliosis

Non-invasive Ventilation (NIV) : Contraindications

- Cardiorespiratory arrest.
- Arrhythmias.
- Upper gastrointestinal bleeding.
- Excessive secretions.
- Facial surgery/trauma.
- Agitated patient.
- Multiorgan system failure.

REFERENCES

1. Rogers R.M., Kriet J. W., Approach to a patient with ARF; In; Atress. S. H. *et al.*, ed., Textbook of Ciritical Care, USA; W. B. Saunders 1994; 680-84.
2. Mahashur A.A., Respiratory failure; In; G. S. Sainani, *et al.*, (ed); API Textbook of Med 1999; 12th ed.; 277-79.
3. Antonelli M., *et al.*, A comparison of NIPPU and conventional mechanical ventilation in patients with ARF; New Eng. J. Med 1998; 339:429.
4. Das P. R., Das., ARF: State of art management; In; Thakur B. B. (ed.); PG Med API 2002; 16: 105-12.

5. Bhatia R.S., Complications of ARF: IN; Mumbai Y.P. (ed) Med Update: API 1997; 7: 783-86.
6. Bashapsha AA, *et al.*, ARF as a first manifestation of syringomyelia; Lung India 2010; 27:93-95.
7. Chawla R; *et al.*, Guidelines for NIV in acute respiratory failure; Ind J Crit Care Med 2013; 17: 42-70.
8. Boldrini R; *et al.*, Non-invasive mechanical ventilation; Curr Opin Crit Care 2012; 18: 48-53.
9. Gupta S; *et al.*, Critical illness in neuromuscular disorders in medical ICU; IN; SR Joshi; ed; Med Update; API 2014; 24: 621-26.

ADULT RESPIRATORY DISTRESS SYNDROME (ARDS)[1]

ARDS is an acute condition with clinical hallmarks as hypoxia and bilateral pulmonary infiltrate due to diffuse inflammatory lung injury which leads to increased pulmonary vascular permeability along with loss of normal lung parenchyma.

ARDS is an acute lung injury (ALI) due to a large number of unrelated massive infarcts. The adult respiratory distress syndrome (ARDS) is a clinical entity of diverse aetiology often complicating trauma or other major medical illnesses. Cardiogenic pulmonary edema can be differentiated from ARDS, clinically, radiologically, by echocardiography using biomarkers (BNP below 100 Pg/ml favours ARDS), right heart catheterization, and rarely by a cautious response to diuretics (ARDS patients relatively hypovolemic).

- ARDS may mimic the following:
  - ILD.
  - Diffuse alveolar hemorrhage.
  - Cryptogenic organizing pneumonia.
  - Idiopathic acute eosinophilic pneumonia.
  - Acute interstitial pneumonia or Hamman Rich syndrome.
  - Leukemia, lymphoma etc.

A partial listing of potential aetiologies and mechanisms of lung injury in ARDS is given in Tables 11.10 to 11.12. Transfusion related acute lung injury is a rare but senous complication of blood transfusion. Diagnosis is made by exclusion. Discontinuation of transfusion and giving respiratory and cardiovascular support may help the patient to recover.[2] ARDS may occur as a pulmonary complication of solid organ and hematopoietic stem cell transplantation.[3] The inciting cause, i.e., ALI of ARDS is often complicated by factors such as superimposed infection, aspiration, overhydration and barotrauma.

Table 11.10

Revised definition of ARDS (2012) include:

1. **Timing:** Acute timeframe specified.
2. **Risk factor:** Identified i.e. ruling out hydrostatic edema due to left atrial HT or fluid overload.
3. **ALI category:** Removed.
4. **Oxygenation:** Minimum PEEP level was added.
5. **Left atrial HT:** PAWP requirement removed.
6. **Chest radiography:** Example chest radiograph set of ARDS is created.

Table 11.11: ARDS: Aetiology

1. Shock: Anaphylaxis, sepsis, haemorrhage, cardiogenic, hemodynamic-hypovolaemic
2. Trauma: Direct pulmonary contusion, fat embolism and non-pulmonary causes like surgery, gun shot wounds, multiorgan blast injury
3. Infections:
   A. Aspiration pneumonia
   B. Bacterial staphylococcal, gram negative septicemia and miliary TB
   C. Viral pneumonia
   D. Fungal
   E. Parasitic
4. Inhaling agents: Chlorine, ozone, SO_2. MIC, phosgene, oxides of nitrogen
5. Drugs and toxins: Barbiturates, methadone, heroin
6. Metabolic: Uraemia, pancreatitis
7. Embolism: Fat, toxic and amniotic fluid emboli
8. Multiple blood transfusion and disseminated intravascular coagulation syndromes
9. Radiation pneumonitis
10. Cardiopulmonary byepass
11. CNS disease

Clinical Tetrad

ARDS was first described by Ashbaugh *et al.* in 1967 but the name ARDS was coined and reported in 1971.[4,5] Following an acute pulmonary illness or injury, a tetrad of clinical features that characterizes ARDS includes progressive respiratory distress; decreased lung compliance and increased work of breathing; acute hypoxaemia not relieved by oxygen breathing; and diffuse radiographic opacification of the lungs. Acute respiratory failure manifests with features of hypercapnoea and hypoxaemia. Clinically hypoxia presents with tachypnoea, dyspnoea, palor and cyanosis in a patient who is restless, disoriented and confused, complaining of headache, lassitude, blurred vision, somnolence, impaired judgement, slow-reaction time and may have manic depressive psychosis and coma.

Hypercapnoea is associated with tachycardia tachypnoea, vasodilation, hypertension, headache, hallucinations, drowsiness, sweating and convulsions. Functional disturbance accompanying ARDS also includes a decrease in functional residual capacity and increase in the ratio of dead-space ventilation to tidal volume and an increase in pulmonary artery pressure and pulmonary vascular resistance (normally <1.0 mmHg/min per liter). In severe ARDS these functional disturbances usually manifest themselves within hours and are present even when cardiac output is normal and hypoxaemia has been corrected. The increase in pulmonary vascular resistance indicates a marked reduction in effective pulmonary

Table 11.12: Potential aetiologies and mechanisms of lung injury in ARDS

Mode	*Examples*	*Potential mechanisms of injury*
Infection (of lungs and other organs)	Bacteria Viruses Mycoplasma Legionnaires' Miliary tuberculosis Endotoxemia	Endothelial injury Microvascular, fluid leakage Disseminated intravascular coagulation
Thromboembolism (Macrothromboembolism and microthromboembolism)	Peripheral venous thrombi Fat/tissue debris Platelets/leukocytes Tumour Amniotic fluid	Endothelial injury Vasoactive substances and/or cytotoxins Lung ischaemia
Trauma (thoracic and extrathoracic)	Pulmonary contusion Multiple long bone fracture	Pulmonary haemorrhage Mechanical cell injury Decreased surfactant Macroemboli/microemboli Overhydration
Aspiration inhalation	Near drawing Gastrointestinal contents Toxic gases such as O_2, phosgene and smoke Heavy metals	Alveolar flooding Hyperosmolarity Cellular necrosis Decreased surfactant Alveolar macrophage activation
Circulating toxins	Heroin Paraquat	Vasculitis Particulate vascular emboli Free-radicals (OH, O_2, H_2O_2 and HOCl) Endothelial injury Vasoactive substances
Immune disorders	Goodpasture's disease Acute vasculitis Opportunistic infection	Basement membrane necrosis Destructive immune complexes Chemical mediators Superimposed infection
Shock	Anaphylaxis Cardiogenic	Hypersensitivity reactions Humoral activation Leukocyte and platelet aggregates Pulmonary venous hypertension
Miscellaneous	Lung radiation Pancreatitis Uraemia High altitude hypoxia Neurogenic oedema	Free radicals Lipases and proteases Cell necrosis Circulating endotoxins Pulmonary vasoconstriction Biventricular failure

vascular cross-section. Mechanism of injury includes infection (endotoxins), inflammation and direct toxicity (independent of inflammation) to lung.[6] Following primary lung injury due to aspiration or inhalation of toxic fumes or secondary pulmonary involvement due to non-pulmonary conditions such as bleeding, shock or septicemia, respiratory dysfunctions set in within 48 hours, with PaO_2/F_1O_2 ratio going down to 200, reduction in lung compliance and appearance of radiological interstitial infiltrations. ARDS is a multi-organ failure disorder, therefore derangements of many other systems will be evident. Aggressive therapeutic interventions prevent ARDS as well as multi-organ system failure.[5]

Salient Features of Acute Lung Injury
(Med Update, API 2010; 20: 777-83)

- ALI is an inflammatory damaging process to alveolar-capillary membrane.
- ARDS describes severe end of ALI.
- Sepsis, pneumonia, aspirations are more risk factors for ARDS.
- Mechanical ventilation is the mainstay of therapy.
- No successful pharmacological intervention available.
- Mortality remains as high as 30%.
- Sequelae include dyspnoea, psycho stress and neuromuscular weakness.

Pulmonary Artery Thrombosis[8]

Angiographic examination of the pulmonary vasculature during the course of ARDS has demonstrated arterial occlusive disease in almost one half of the patients, with an increased pulmonary vascular resistance and disseminated intravascular coagulation. Postmortem studies frequently show evidence of widespread macroscopic and microscopic pulmonary artery thrombosis in patients in whom angiographic pulmonary artery filling defects were found in life. These abnormalities tend to be more frequent in patients with ARDS secondary to pneumonia and trauma and less frequent in patients with ARDS resulting from sepsis. Evidence of pulmonary vascular fibrin thrombi at postmortem following severe extrapulmonary trauma and burns has been seen. The pathogenesis of widespread pulmonary artery thrombosis in ARDS is not yet known.

Coagulopathy[8]

Patients with ARDS frequently have thrombocytopenia and coagulopathy in more than half of the patients. Two thirds of patients with ARDS have evidence of thrombocytopenia (<100000 platelets/mm^3), and doubled platelet turnover rates. Factor VIII antigen levels (a participating molecule in platelet adherence to vessel walls) are also elevated in the serum of patients with ARDS. Factor VIII abnormalities may contribute to some of the bleeding and clotting disturbances that are frequently found. Since factor VIII is synthesized by vascular endothelium, elevation of some of its components may be a signal of endothelial injury. Marked increases in plasma fibrin-(ogen) degradation products, particularly the D-antigen and soluble fibrin complexes (substrata for fibrin formation) are further evidence of coagulopathy in ARDS.

Pathophysiology[8]

The primary pathophysiological abnormality of ARDS is a diffuse alveolar damage (DAD) to alveolar capillary membrane that leads to leakage of proteinaceous and haemorrhagic oedema fluid across the alveolar-capillary membrane. Pathophysiology can be divided into three phases namely exudative, proliferative and fibrotic, without any sharp demarcation. The oedema fluid leaks into the interstitium, and air spaces of the lungs. When plasma freely enters the interstitium there is a loss of transvascular wall colloid osmotic pressure differences which further diminishes the lung's ability to maintain an appropriate transcapillary fluid balance. Fluid flooding of the alveoli and small airways reduces ventilation and increased intrapulmonary venous admixture. Direct intravascular injury leads to endothelial cell swelling and necrosis as well as denudation of the basement membrane. The endothelial injury itself promotes fluid leakage. As ARDS progresses, the microvasculature appears to undergo compression, obstruction and architectural alteration and in the late stages, there is often widespread obliteration of the micro-vasculature. ARDS is an inflammatory disorder with BAL studies confirming the presence of increased acute inflammatory cells (neutrophils and macrophages) and pro-inflammatory cytokines. Direct degeneration of the alveolar lining cells (type I pneumocytes) occurs in lung injuries of diverse aetiologies, including aspiration of gastrointestinal contents and inhalation of toxic gases (for example, phosgene, oxygen, smoke and heavy metals). Such bronchogenic pathway injury directly alters membrane permeability by damaging the normally tight type I pneumocyte intercellular junctions. Elevation of the pulmonary microvascular pressure aggravates the resulting extravascular fluid leakage.

Within hours of acute lung injury, there is intra-alveolar protein coagulation and necrosis of type I pneumocytes. The cellular/protein debris contributes to the formation of hyaline membranes. This is followed by hyperplasia of the surfactant-producing cells (type 2 pneumocytes)[9] which tend to bridge the denuded alveolar surface. Progression of ARDS is marked by fibroblast and other cell activation and proliferation in the oedematous injured interstitial matrix. Abnormally high levels of collagen have been found in patients surviving ARDS for long period. The fibrosis, which begins to develop within a week of the onset of ARDS, tends to centre on alveolar ducts. Interstitial fibrosis encroaching on uninjured or potentially recoverable alveoli may prevent their participation in normal gas exchange. Conversely, fibrosis of non-perfused alveoli may reduce dead-space ventilation. Some fibrosis appear to be reversible since occasional survivors of ARDS show minimal evidence of radiographic abnormalities or restrictive lung disease.

In addition to thrombotic occlusion of the pulmonary vasculature, vasoconstriction may contribute to the decreased effective pulmonary vascular cross-section noted in ARDS. Local lung and circulating vasoactive mediators, such as thromboxane A_2, PGF_2 and the leukotrienes LTC_4 [10] and LTD_4, histamine and serotonin, promote regional vasoconstriction and thereby may contribute to hypoxaemia and acidosis. The rise in interstitial pressure due to microvascular fluid leakage and vasoconstriction contributes to both locally increased pulmonary vascular resistance and reduced blood flow. This resultant vascular stasis may promote the formation of in-situ thrombosis. Once formed, thrombosis may produce further tissue injury through ischaemia and proximal propagation.

Experimental evidence suggests that human polymorphonuclear leucocyte granules, which have a tissue-thromboplastin-like activity, also promote mictothrombosis. Pathogenesis and stages of ARDS are listed in Tables 11.13 and 11.14 respectively.

Table 11.13: ARDS: Pathogenesis

a. Massive complement activation
b. Activation of coagulation system, leading to platelet-fibrin microemboli
c. Fibrinolysis
d. Alveolar and interstitial oedema, due to injury caused to pulmonary capillary endothelium, by free O_2 radicals and inflammatory mediators protease, produced by neutrophils
e. Further damage caused by vasoactive substances like histamine and arachidonic acid
f. Still further damage is done to alveolar membrane by prostaglandins and leukotrienes.

Table 11.14: Stages of ARDS

1. Initial stage of insult to the lung is by marked alkalosis
2. Silent stage, with stable circulation, low PaO_2, low pulmonary compliance and low alveolar-arterial oxygen pressure gradient
3. Pulmonary functions: Progressive deterioration
4. Final stage of ventilatory failure, hypoxia, hypercapnia and death may occur due to cardiac arrest.

There is gross oedema of the lung, septa are thickened, type I pneumocytes are replaced by type II pneumocytes, and hyaline membrane is visible, lining alveolar ducts and membrane. This is responsible for impaired transport of oxygen across the alveolar capillary membrane, increased intra pulmonary shunting and decreased pulmonary compliance.

The lung microvasculature may trap microemboli such as platelet and leukocyte aggregates, other denatured proteins cellular stroma, amniotic fluid, and fat and air emboli. These microemboli further promote pulmonary artery thrombosis and aggravate lung injury directly or through local mediators. Platelets are known to sequester in the lungs during ARDS. Activated platelets release such substances as adenine nucleotides and thromboxane A_2 which cause vasoconstriction and platelet aggregation. This may promote further local accretion of platelets in the microvasculature, exacerbating an initial occlusion.

Cardiopulmonary bypass and haemodialysis can activate plasma complement (C5a) thus causing aggregation of leukocytes which can embolize to the pulmonary microvasculature. However, significant derangements of pulmonary function do not usually occur. Intrabronchial instillation of activated components of the complements system (C3a and C5a) is quickly followed by acute pulmonary injury, leukocyte and platelet aggregates in the pulmonary microvasculature, and invasion of the alveoli by neutrophils. Local chemical mediators implicated in the evolution of increased microvascular leakage include serotonin, histamine, PGF_2, thromboxane A_2, plasma-derived or phagocyte-derived proteases and specific peptides from fibrin (ogen) degradation products. Proper interpretation of PFT is always rewarding.[11]

Lung injury is associated with and aggravated by the liberation of proteases and other toxic products from activated phagocytes. Activated polymorphonuclear leukocytes liberate neutral and acid proteases which can activate the Hageman factor, complement and other plasma proteins, ultimately causing destruction of the structural proteins of the lung, that is collagen and elastin. Vascular basement membrane once denuded of endothelium is vulnerable to injury since it is also a substrate for neutral proteases liberated by these activated polymorphonuclear leukocytes.

Activated interstitial cells may gain access to the alveolar space through holes in the basement membrane made by these proteases and thus initiate intra-alveolar fibrosis. Bronchoalveolar lavage studies have demonstrated that more than two thirds of patients with ARDS have increased neutrophil elastase concentrations. There is evidence for increased proteolytic activity in ARDS and is important in the presence of alpha$_1$ antiprotease inactivation by oxidation and complexing.

The role of oxygen and oxygen radicals in the process of lung cell injury in ARDS has yet to be determined. Rat models of oxygen toxicity with prolonged hyperoxia (PaO_2 of 87 per cent) demonstrate progressive muscularization of precapillary arteries associated with pulmonary artery hypertension. In the presence of hyperoxia certain drugs, such as nitrofurantoin, paraquat and bleomycin, can greatly aggravate an initial hyperoxic injury. Oxygen breathing in rats activates the alveolar macrophage to release chemotactic factors for polymorphonuclear leukocytes. Once activated the leukocytes can release oxygen radicals (OH, O_2, H_2O_2) which further contribute to lung cell injury by oxidation of lipoproteins in cell membranes.[12]

Signs of respiratory distress appear in 1-3 hrs (or hours) or 1-3 days. Patient may not complain of shortness of breath but actually there is a tachypnoea, and tachycardia followed by dyspnoea. Accessory muscles of respiration come in action with increased respiratory effort. Cyanosis appears late. Chest auscultation may not be contributory. Few crepitations may be heard. In ARDS, rise in PCO_2 is accepted till PH falls below 7.2; the strategy called permissive hypercapnoea. Lower tidal volume of 6-8 ml/kg of ideal body weight is considered standard supportive treatment in patients with acute lung injury/ARDS. Refractory hypoxia may be corrected using high FiO_2, high PEEP and inverse I:E ratio. Oxygen toxicity is more prominent in these cases. Prone positioning improves oxygenation in 60-70% of patients through improved ventilation-perfusion matching, changes in lung mass and shape and alteration in compliance of chest wall. Chest X-ray, as described earlier, may show diffuse, rapidly progressive pulmonary infiltrates. The infiltrates are peripheral. BAL fluid may show marked increase in the number of PMN. Specimen for microbiological diagnosis is also obtained. Also, BAL fluid contains potentially toxic mediators of injury such as myeloperoxidases and neutrophil elastase—an enzyme concerned with abnormalities in gas transport.[13] ABG analysis shows rise in $PaCO_2$ as hypoxemia is the hallmark of ARDS.

There can be septicemia, thrombocytopenia, haemorrhagic manifestations like DIC (diffuse intravascular coagulation) due to transient fall in platelets and fibrinogen. Clinical features of ARDS have been listed in Table 11.15.

Table 11.15: Clinical features: ARDS

1. Dyspnoea
2. Cyanosis
3. Hypoxia: PaO_2 below 50 mm, that does not improve despite inhalation of 100% oxygen
4. Chest radiograph: Diffuse pulmonary infiltrate, early interstitial and later alveolar oedema
5. Series of changes like low PaO_2, less than 50 mm, abnormal blood gases, Hypercapnia and reduced pulmonary compliance, intrapulmonary shunting and wide alveolar-arterial pressure gradient.

European American Consensus Committee on ARDS has defined Acute Lung Injury (ALI) as a distinct entity, different from ARDS.[14] The difference rests only in oxygenation. It is difficult to differentiate both the conditions clinically. Further, ARDS is a clinical syndrome and ALI is a pathological entity, in the same spectrum of disease. The Berlin definition has revised the ARDS entity.[15]

Criteria	ALI	ARDS
Timing	Acute onset	Except
Oxygenation	$PaO_2/F_1O_2 < 300$ muntly (regardless of PEEP)	$PaO_2/F_1O_2 < 200$ muntly (regardless of PEEP)
Chest X-ray	Bilateral infiltrates in frontal film	Level

Management[8]

Management includes protective ventilatory strategy with low tidal volume ventilation; treatment targets supportive therapy along with identifying and managing pulmonary and extra-pulmonary organ dysfunction.[16] The aim of supportive management is to maintain airway patency, to provide an acceptable level of arterial oxygenation (PaO_2 of 60-70 mm Hg) at the lowest possible level of administered oxygen concentration (F_1O_2) and to optimize pulmonary and systemic blood flow, i. e., maintaining adequate gas exchange, without compromising haemodynamic stability. The effectiveness of therapy depends on the aetiology and severity of the lung injury. It is of prognostic and therapeutic value to grade the severity of the lung injury. Patients with severe ARDS, who have a mortality rate of 90 per cent, have extensive radiographic lung consolidation, an increased pulmonary venous admixture (>30 per cent) and require mechanical ventilation with positive end-expiratory pressure (PEEP) and high levels of F_1O_2 (that is 0.5-1). Patient with moderate ARDS, having widespread consolidations on chest X-ray, who have a mortality rate of 50 per cent, usually require intubation and mechanical ventilation for more than 24 hours (without PEEP) with an $F_1O_2>0.5$. Patients with mild ARDS, the majority of whom survive, have gas exchange abnormalities and require supplementary oxygen but may or may not need medical ventilation. Important features of management of ARDS are shown in Table 11.16

Table 11.16: ARDS: Management

1. Maintain airway and proper oxygen tension (PaO_2)
2. Shock and hypotension should be corrected
3. Maintaining airway patency, using parenteral bronchodilators
4. Correction of acid-base balance
5. Use of antibiotics; in proper dosage and for proper period
6. Supplementation with metronidazole in case of anaerobic infection
7. Diuretics in case of fluid overload
8. Treatment of complications like gastric haemorrhage and using H_2 receptor antagonists
9. Treating the specific causative factor like antidote in cyanide poisoning

Haemodynamics

Patients with ARDS require intensive monitoring of respiratory and haemodynamic function to assess response to treatment. A thermodilution pulmonary artery catheter is essential for the monitoring of pulmonary haemodynamic function in severe cases of ARDS. This type of catheter can provide measurements of pulmonary artery pressure, pulmonary capillary wedge pressure and cardiac output and be used to obtain mixed venous blood-gas tensions and in the calculation of intrapulmonary venous admixture. The catheter can also be used for local angiography of the pulmonary vasculature. Balloon occlusion pulmonary angiography through thermodilution pulmonary artery catheters can be performed at the bedside with conventional portable radiographic equipment to obtain high definition vascular studies. The presence of pulmonary filling defects can thus be determined.

Mechanical Ventilation[17] and PEEP

In ARDS mechanical ventilation is administered with an approximate tidal volume of 10-15 ml/kg at a respiratory rate necessary to maintain the $PaCO_2$ at 35-40 mmHg. PEEP titrated upto 20 cm H_2O is used as required to maintain oxygenation. One action of PEEP is to restore the functional residual capacity towards normal by inflation of flooded and collapsed air spaces. Parallel increase in PaO_2 has been demonstrated in ARDS with increasing levels of PEEP. It has also been shown that PEEP decreases the percentage of the cardiac output perfusing unventilated alveoli thus decreasing the intrapulmonary venous admixture. However, increasing airway pressure can overdistend peripheral alveoli so promoting the development of subpleural cystic spaces that may lead to pneumothorax and/or pneumoperitoneum. The haemodynamic effects of PEEP include increased pulmonary vascular resistance and decreased cardiac output probably due to direct compression of the heart and the diminished venous return. Transfusion of fluid or administration of inotropic agents may be necessary to continue therapy with PEEP if cardiac output decreases. The ability of modest levels of PEEP to improve oxygenation usually outweigh its adverse effects.

The appearance of chest radiographic lung consolidation apparently improves with administration of PEEP. This radiographic improvement may or may not be accompanied by a physiological improvement in gas exchange. The immediate radiographic improvement in PEEP is due to an increase in the ratio of the gas/solid content of the lungs rather than to any alteration in the quantity of lung water. Non invasive ventilation can be useful in ARDS/ALI when there is hypoxemic respiratory failure.[18]

Extracorporeal Membrane Oxygenation

Partial bypass with extracorporeal membrane oxygenators can aid in carbon dioxide removal and supplement oxygenation. However, the results of a prospective randomized study of extracorporeal membrane oxygenation indicated that the mortality rate from severe ARDS caused by infectious pneumonias was not reduced by this technique.[1] Partial bypass with extracorporeal membrane oxygenators is presently used only by a limited number of skilled teams, primarily in the treatment of carefully selected patients with post-traumatic ARDS.

High Frequency Ventilation

High frequency ventilation (that is frequencies of > 3 Hz) is at present not used in ARDS when increased lung volumes and PEEP are also required. It is most useful in infants with respiratory distress requiring low tidal volumes or in adults with bronchopleural fistulas and good lung compliance.

Cardiac Function

Cardiac dysfunction often accompanies ARDS and is usually manifested by an elevation in pulmonary capillary wedge pressure or central venous pressure or by a fall in cardiac index. ARDS patients can develop acute right ventricular failure due to the increased pulmonary vascular resistance of severely damaged lungs. Inotropic agents such as dopamine, isoprenaline or dobutamine are used to maintain cardiac output. Ventilatory therapy with PEEP may have major effects on both right and left ventricular function. Using right ventricular first-pass nuclear angiography, it has been shown that an increase in PEEP from 5 to 10 cm H_2O can diminish stroke volume and right ventricular end-diastolic volume in patients with ARDS. However, PEEP also tends to increase the right ventricular ejection fraction.

Fluid Therapy

Fluid therapy in ARDS attempts to balance lung capillary leakage and adequate pulmonary and systemic blood flow. There is no clinical method to precisely measuring lung water content in severe ARDS. The numerous techniques thus far employed have proved to be unsatisfactory because they depend on the patiency of vasculature which is frequently deranged in ARDS. In mild ARDS or congestive heart failure the double-indicator technique may be useful because vascular occlusive disease is less frequent. Mechanically ventilated patients tend to have a positive water balance which can be reversed with cautious administration of diuretics and fluid restriction. There is controversy as to whether colloid or crystalloid intravenous fluid administration is more appropriate in ARDS. To enable normal or minimally injured lung units to resorb interstitial fluid, plasma or colloid is often used to augment blood volume.

Antibiotics

Primary pulmonary infection may be associated with ARDS in one third of patients. The risk of secondary infection depends on the length of hospital stay, the underlying aetiology of ARDS and the presence of immunocompromise. Infection can be detected early only if body secretions are regularly cultured. Blood cultures should be obtained persistently in the presence of continuous fever or high leukocyte counts. Prompt treatment with appropriate antibiotics is needed if there is to be a successful outcome. Distal respiratory tract infection or colonization, without proximal contamination, can be diagnosed with insulated bronchial brush catheters inserted via fiberoptic bronchoscopes. In special circumstances open lung biopsy may be required to identify infectious or non-infectious lung conditions.

Platelet Transfusion, Heparin and Fibrinolytic Therapy

Fibrinolysis and disseminated coagulopathy is a common occurrence in ARDS (affecting 60 per cent of patients).

Appropriate therapy for coagulopathy depends on its early detection. Platelet transfusions may be needed when the platelet count falls below 20,000/mm^3. An increased tendency to coagulate should be pre-empted with low dose intravenous heparin (600-1000 u/h) while maintaining the activated clotting time at approximately 100 seconds. Definitive pulmonary thromboembolism, that is pulmonary artery filling defects demonstrated by angiography, may be treated with infusion of fibrinolytic agents (streptokinase or urokinase) into the pulmonary vasculature. It has been demonstrated that patients with uncomplicated pulmonary emboli treated with fibrinolytic agents show improved carbon dioxide diffusion capacity and capillary blood volume 2 weeks and one year after treatment. This suggests that fibrinolytic therapy promotes clearing of microvascular thrombi and may help to increase the gas-exchanging vascular surface area of survivors.

Steroids

Steroid therapy is controversial even when treating the inflammatory reactions caused by gastric acid aspiration and the effects of fat embolism to the lungs. Decreased albumin concentrations have been reported in the bronchoalveolar lavage fluid of patients with ARDS due to sepsis after steroid administration. This finding suggests that steroids may induce a decrease in fluid leakage in ARDS. However, routine treatment of all forms of ARDS with steroids must await further evaluation.

Nutrition

Malnutrition tends to increase susceptibility to infection and decrease lung elasticity, surface forces and lung protein synthesis. Patients with severe ARDS may require parenteral feeding. However, high carbohydrate intake increases carbon dioxide production and necessitates increased ventilation to eliminate carbon dioxide. Fever and other hyperdynamic states also increase the metabolic rate and oxygen consumption, thus altering the response to glucose infusion by failing to suppress fat oxidation. Fat emulsions can be used to supply 50 per cent of calorific intake so decreasing carbon dioxide production. However, fat emulsions may also impair pulmonary diffusing capacity and therefore should not be used routinely in ARDS.

Hypothermia

To decrease the large intrapulmonary venous admixture of preterminal ARDS, it may be necessary to reduce cardiac output, oxygen consumption and carbon dioxide production. Hypothermia produces vasoconstriction and decreases venous return and oxygen consumption. Therefore, external cooling to core temperature of 32-35°C is often employed with deep sedation in patients with severe ARDS. Paralysis is used to avoid the excessive shivering associated with hypothermia treatment.

Investigative Drugs

The proline analogue L_{34}-dehydroproline has been used in clinical trials for upto 3 weeks in an attempt to decrease the extent of acute pulmonary fibrosis. Free radical scavengers, for example superoxide dismutase and catalase, are also being studied in animal models of ARDS in an attempt to find an agent to decrease injury from oxygen therapy by scavenging oxygen radicals released by activated phagocytes. Pulmonary artery hypertension is being addressed with short-term infusions of vasodilators such as nitroprusside and long-term treatment is with cyclo-oxygenase inhibitors (ibuprofen) and selective thromboxane synthetase antagonists. Newer modalities being explored are use of PGI_2 and E_1, beta agonists and fibrinonectin. Aerosolised surfactant to improve lung compliance and oxygenation has been tried; despite heavy cost survival benefits are not established.

Outcome

Severe ARDS can produce a pathological picture of relentless progression of disease with lung remodelling by fibrosis, alveolar consolidation and vascular thromboembolism. Mechanical ventilation with high F_1O_2 prevents death from hypoxaemia. Whether the rate of mortality is significantly cut down by newer modes of ventilation, is yet to be seen in future. Death is frequently due to renal or hepatic failure, systemic sepsis, intractable biventricular failure or severe coagulopathy and haemorrhage.[19] Recovery from ARDS primarily depends on the patient's age, the mechanisms and severity of lung injury and the absence of other organ complications. Common risk factors as listed in Table 11.17 do influence the outcome in ARDS.[20,21] Those who survive first few days, may take 4-6 weeks to recover with full lung repair, these patients are very difficult to manage and require a state of cut in pulmonology. Five points Bruce-Jenner-protocol, of step-up gradual exercise, nutrition, fluid management, proper sleep and emotional support has been suggested for these patients.[13] Abnormal pulmonary function is found in about 40 cent of survivors 6 months after recovery from ARDS. The $PaO_2$with exercise, lung volumes and carbon dioxide diffusing capacity are reduced in survivors but improvement in pulmonary function tends to continue during the first year following ARDS.

Table 11.17: Common risk factors in ARDS

- Sepsis.
- Sepsis with a chronic alcohol abuse.
- Aspiration of gastric contents.
- Community acquired pneumonia.
- Nosocomial pneumonia.
- Severe trauma.
- Massive transfusion.
- Transfusion related acute lung injury.
- Lung and hematopoietic stem cell transplantation.
- Radiologic contrast media in susceptible individuals.

A landmark study showed light tidal volume ventilation not only increased alveolar inflammation but also disseminated inflammatory cytokines. Raised revels of procollagen III peptide in early BAL samples and persisting BAL neutrophilia predicts a prolonged clinical course with progression to pulmonary fibrosis in patients with ARDS. Plasma levels of von Willebrand factor antigen in ARDS patients independently predicts mortality in the clinical course.[22] Geno type for ACE determines development of ARDS and also adversely affects survival.[23] Intensive insulin therapy confecing a distinct survival benefit to critically ill patients is another landmark study.[24] Pro-inflammatory mechanical ventilation when replaced by, unconventional ventilation support (high frequency jet ventilation and oscillatory ventilation liquid ventilation using perfluorocarbons, ECMO etc). devices, may improve survival in ARDS patients. It is hoped that mortality in ARDS may be correctly predicted and survival eventully improved in the near future.[25,26]

CPR (Cardiopulmonary Resuscitation)

CPR—cardiopulmonary resuscitation is a simple life saving procedure. Surprisingly, this essential essentiality does not form a part of the curriculum in all Indian medical schools. But scientifically this is taught in American medical schools.[18] Surprisingly, one of the leading killers of modern days is coronary artery disease also called ischaemic heart disease. In USA every year 1,00,000 people die due to accidents, but deaths due to heart disease amount to 6,00,000. Out of each 100 people dying of heart disease, more than 50 die due to heart attacks. About 2/3rd of the deaths due to heart attacks occur before the victim could not reach the hospital. In USA it was estimated that out of 4.8 lakh persons dying of heart attack per year, around 3.2 lakh would die even before reaching the hospital. In India the death figures due to heart attack are even greater and it is estimated that out of 24 lakh people dying of heart attacks every year, 18 lakh die before reaching the hospital.

With recent advance in hospital management and installation of advanced sophisticated gadgetry in our coronary care units we have been able to save and rehabilitate only those patients who could reach the hospital alive in time. Majority of deaths which occur before reaching the hospital, are unnatural sudden and preventable. The astonishing fact is that majority of these deaths are preventable and a substantial number of them reversible during the first five minutes.

The concept of CPR, i.e., Cardiopulmonary resuscitation which is concerned with the ABCs of basic life support, i.e., keeping a person alive who is the victim of a life threatening problem till medical help is reached or victim is transferred to hospital, has revolutionized the whole scenario. In USA, programmes aimed at training the public in the prehospital emergency care and educating them in basic life support including CPR, has drastically brought down the number of pre-hospital deaths due to heart attack. It is estimated that out of 3. 2 lakh sudden deaths due to heart attack every year, about 2 lakh are revived and saved by CPR alone. Similarly, in India if through a mass CPR training programme we educate our people, bring awareness about the heart disease, impart CPR technique training, we may be able to save about 13.5 lakh people every year from dying unnatural sudden deaths due to heart attacks.

Apart from the heart attack, there are lots of other situations like drowning, electrocution, choking or accident, cause a healthy heart and lungs to stop all of a sudden and if heart and lungs are not put back to action by the rescuer within 4-6 minutes of stoppage of heart, the brain cell damage starts and by 10 minutes of stoppage of heart, the brain death ensues, from which the victim cannot be revived.

In these situations, availability of a doctor or a medical professional trained in CPR technique cannot be ensured within 4 minutes. Further, in Indian set up, whenever such a situation arises, the usual response of the attendants is confusion or emotional breakdown. Our communication system is such that in emergency it usually breaks down. Looking at the transport system and the condition of the roads in our country it is next to impossible to reach the victim within 4-6 minutes. Hence the need is to know and learn yourself the simple techniques of CPR and teach it to others. It requires no equipment or stethoscope, no drugs but the availability of two hands, your mouth and lungs and presence of mind. In fact, to learn CPR you have to relearn your ABC where A stands for Airway and not for apple, B stands for Breathing not for bat and C stands for Circulation and not for cat.

If you only know the proper CPR technique you could probably save the victim and then train your subordinates or your friends who are always with you, you may probably be saved by any one of them if such an unwarranted occasion arises. If each doctor learns it correctly and trains 10 of his friends/relations/patients in this technique and asks each of them to train 10 more the whole population of India at risk can be covered when the need for CPR arises. For example, in the city of Delhi if 80,000 persons are trained in CPR and if each of them trains another 10 persons then 8 lakh population thus trained can cover for 80 lakh population of Delhi assuming that 10 persons are usually gathered in emergency situations. Times to rise to the occasion and initiate a series of *Self Education* followed by Public Education programmes for *CPR.* Who knows tomorrow the *life saved is your own.* In view of all this, the following text has been devoted to. Need for CPR and its management assessment are listed in Tables 11.18 and 11.19.

Table 11.18: Need for cardiopulmonary resuscit ation

1. Loss of consciousness
2. Loss of carotid and femoral pulses
3. Loss of heart sounds
4. Loss of blood pressure
5. Loss of respiration

Table 11.19: Management assessment

1. Vital capacity 30-45 ml/kg: Requires simple chest physiotherapy.
2. Vital capacity 20 ml/kg: Requires deep breathing to counter hypoxia and atelectasis that is starting in the dependent portions of the lungs.
3. Vital capacity 15 ml/kg: Needs elective ventilation and positive ventilation as at this stage atelectasis is prominent and arteriovenous shunting starts.
4. Vital capacity 10 ml/kg: Requires full ventilatory assistance as this is a hypoventilation stage.

Health care providers are required to be skilled enough in practices and procedures of basic life support and advanced cardiac life support, with an aim to restore and maintain cerebral perfusion untill restoration of cardiopulmonary functions as well as neurological functions. Early defibrillation is critical as most of adult cardiac arrests are secondary to ventricular arrhythmias.

So, encountering an unconscious patient, basic life support is properly implemented and defibrillation is done when indicated under the guidance of leader of the attending medical team. Following this: proper endotracheal intubation, and ventilation, intravenous catheter, administration of cardiovascular medicines and diagnosis and treatment of cause of the arrest should be correctly performed. Patient's pulse and heart rhythm should be assessed after every intervention. Temination of resuscitative efforts has to be decided by the team leader.

Basic life support has (A) airway, (B) breathing, and (C) circulation care as its essentials. Encountering an unconscious patient, following should be done:

1. Gently shake the patient.
2. Position the patient on a firm, flat surface.
3. Open the airway by opening patient's mouth and removing dentures (if any). In case of neck injury, take care of avoiding spinal cord injury.
4. Give two breath blows 1-2 seconds/breath, repeat twice, if spontaneous respiration is not present.
5. Assess patient's carotid artery and if pulse is present, continue rescue breathing and if absent, compression of chest 80-100 times per minute.
6. Stop basic life support for 5 seconds, every 1-2 minutes. If pulse returns, check blood pressure and continue ventilation. If patient cannot be ventilated after two attempts, intubate. Active compression and decompression and interposed abdominal compression are experimental techniques that hold promise for increasing cerebral and cardiac blood flow.

Guidelines for Cardiopulmonary Resuscitation

Advanced Life Support[27]

The first guidelines for advanced life support promoted by the Resuscitation Council of the United Kingdom were published in 1994 as consensus from a larger group of European countries.[14]

The use of the precordial thump has been reintroduced but only for witnessed or monitored arrests, in line with published evidence of its efficacy for pulseless ventricular tachycardia or ventricular fibrillation of very recent onset. The risk of exacerbating a ventricular arrhythmia is recognised, but the likelihood of harm is small when the arrest has been witnessed. Before discussing defibrillation, practical tips are given in Table 11.20.

Table 11.20: Practical points

- Advanced cardiac life support consists of basic life support plus the use of special equipment and techniques (e.g., ECG monitoring and the correction of arrhythmias by defibrillation and using drugs).
- Ventricular fibrillation is the most common cause of cardiac arrest outside hospital. A defibrillator should be used as soon as it is available.

Extension of basic life support under guidance of medical team is the advanced cardiac life support.[28]

1. Patient's rhythm and pulse should be assessed and pulse ventricular tachycardia or ventricular fibrillation should immediately be defibrillated.
2. Right paddle in upper right sternal border below clavicle and left paddle on the left mid axillary line alongside left nipple should be placed, after proper application of gelly. No one should touch the patient or the bed and the defibrillation should be executed with firm pressure on the paddles.
3. Ventilation and airways management requiring endotracheal intubation (tube not going into oesophagus—as checked by stethoscope on epigastrium) followed by 100% oxygen is essential. Transtracheal catheterisation may rarely be required in case of obstruction.
4. Proper intravenous line connection is made.
5. Even endotracheal atropine, lidocaine and epinephrine may be given if there is delay in IV connection.
6. Intracardiac injections are not recommended.
7. IV normal saline is given in case of blood loss, hypovolemia or hypotension.
8. Team leader should try to find the cause of cardiac arrest and relevant investigations such as electrolytes, haematocrit, ABG, ECG, and radiographs are ordered.
9. Internal cardiac compression due to penetrating chest trauma, severe hypothermia, ruptured aortic aneurysm, and following thoracotomy should also be considered.
10. Initiation and discontinuation of advanced cardiac life support is the decision of team leader, and may take 15 minutes duration following which asystole or an agonale rhythm persists despite continued resuscitative efforts, end point for resuscitation is reached.

Defibrillation

No modifications have been made to the recommendations for defibrillation. Same equipment still in use will be calibrated in terms of stored energy that correspond only roughly to the figures that are now appropriate. Causes, mechanisms of cardiac arrest, followed by their management are shown in Tables 11.21 to 11.25.

Table 11.21: Cardiac arrest: Aetiology

1. Cardiac: Coronary artery disease, heart failure, Stoke Adams syndrome
2. Pulmonary: Pulmonary embolism, respiratory failure
3. Neurological
4. Systemic: Uremia
5. Allergic: Anaphylaxis

Table 11.22: Cardiac arrest: Mechanism

1. Electromechanical dissociation
2. Ventricular asystole
3. Ventricular fibrillation

Table 11.23: Ventricular fibrillation: Management

VENTRICULAR FIBRILLATION PULSELESS VENTRICULAR TACHYCARDIA
↓
Precordial thump
↓
Direct current shock 200 J (1)
↓
Direct current shock 200 J (2)
↓
Direct current shock 360 J (3)
↓
If not already:
- Intubate
- Intravenous access

→ (loop start)
Adrenaline I mg intravenously
↓
Ten cardiopulmonary resuscitation sequences in a ratio of 5:1 of compression to ventilation
↓
Direct current shock 360 J (4)
↓
Direct current shock 360 J (5)
↓
Direct current shock 360 J (6)
(loop back)

Notes:
- The interval between shocks 3 and 4 should be no longer than 2 min.
- Adrenaline given during loop approx every 2-3 min.
- Continue loops for as long as defibrillation is indicated.
- After three loops consider:
  – An alkalizing agent
  – An antiarrhythmic agent

Algorithm for ventricular fibrillation: Check monitor shows ventricular fibrillation and for absent pulse before each shock.

Table 11.24: Cause of electromechanical dissociation

ELECTROMECHANICAL DISSOCIATION

Investigate for:
Hypovolaemia
Tension pneumothorax
Cardiac tamponade
Pulmonary embolism
Drug overdose/intoxication
Hyphothermia
Electrolyte imbalance

(If present give specific treatment)

→ (loop start)
If not already:
- Intubate
- (Intravenous access)

↓
Adrenaline 1 mg intravenously
↓
Ten cardiopulmonary resuscitation sequences in a ratio of 5: 1 compression to ventilation
(loop back)

Consider:
- Pressor agents
- Calcium
- Alkalizing agents
- Adrenaline 5 mg
- Intravenously

Algorithm for electromechanical dissociation: Think of underlying causes and transfer to hospital without delay.

Order of Drugs

An important change has been made in the order of the drugs that should be given if ventricular fibrillation fails to respond to the first three shocks. Adrenaline has replaced lignocaine as the first pharmacological agent. Lignocaine is of proved efficacy in treating ventricular tachycardia and in the prophylaxis of ventricular fibrillation, and by extrapolation many believe that the drug must be of value as an adjunct to defibrillation. Thus the fourth shock in a series may well defibrillate when others have failed quite irrespective of drug treatment.

While the evidence to command adrenaline as an adjunct to defibrillation is no better than that for lignocaine, it does have one other attribute that led to include it earlier in the algorithm. Animal experiments offer convincing evidence that adrenaline increases the cerebral circulation during basic life support. The main purpose of adrenaline at this point therefore is to maintain cerebral perfusion during a prolonged resuscitation attempt. It

Table 11.25: Asystole: Management

ASYSTOLE
↓
Precordial thump
↓
Ventricular fibrillation exclude
↓ (no)
Direct current shock 200 J
↓
Direct current shock 200 J
↓
Direct current shock 360 J
(yes)
↓
If not already:
- Intubate
- Intravenous access

↓
Adrenaline 1 mg intravenously
↓
Ten cardiopulmonary resuscitation sequences in ratio of 5:1 of compression to ventilation
↓
(Atropine 3 mg intravenously once only)
↓
Electrical activity evident?
(no)
↓ (yes)
Pace

Algorithm for asystole: Remember to check for lead disconnection and turn up the gain to maximum.

enhances the efficacy of a direct current shock is doubtful though many believe that this can occur in some circumstances. Amiodarone 150 mg IV over 10 minutes can be given for recurrent or refractory ventricular fibrillation or ventricular tachycardia (pulseless) and is as effective as bretylium.

The use of sodium bicarbonate is no longer encouraged except in prolonged resuscitation. The carbon dioxide formed by the breakdown of bicarbonate readily crosses cell membranes unless it is removed by respiration. The alkaline moiety, on the other hand, remains predominantly extracellular. Repeated shocks at maximum energy levels are advised if fibrillation is refractory after the initial three shocks and the two drugs (plus the fourth shock) have been administered.

Asystole

An important change has been introduced in the advice offered for victims of apparent asystole. This electrical disorder has grave prognostic implications and treatment is generally disappointing, especially in ischaemic heart disease. Routine defibrillation asystole is detrimental and is not recommended. Errors have occurred owing to the incorrect diagnosis of asystole in victims who are in ventricular fibrillation. This may occur if equipment is faulty, if the gain control of the electrocardiograph has been turned down, if ventricular fibrillation is very fine or, rarely, if the dominant vector of the waveform is at right angles to the bipolar diagnostic lead. Other causes of asystole should also be looked for and treated such as hypoxia, hyperkalemia, hypokalemia, pre existing acidosis, drug-overdose, hypothermia.

The algorithm itself has also been modified, with adrenaline now having precedence over atropine. Isoprenaline is no longer recommended and the possibility of using the intracardiac route for adrenaline has been deleted. Other causes of electromechanical dissociation—special circumstances in which calcium chloride has undoubted value—have now been listed.

Bradycardias—These are treated according to patient's haemodynamic stability and mechanism of bradycardia. For sinus bradycardia, junctional rhythm and type I second degree block, patient is only observed if asymptomatic. Atropine and a pacemaker should be considered for type II second degree and complete AV bock even if patient is asymptomatic. Atropine need be used with caution in treating bradycardia associated with myocardial infarction as it may exacerbate ischemia or induce ventricular tachycardia or fibrillation.

Transcutaneous or transvenous pacing can be considered.

Use of lidocaine may be lethal in case of bradycardia being ventricular escape rhythm. Pulseless Electrical Activity (PEA) requires special attention as it has poor outcome.

Doppler ultrasound reveals blood flow which is not detected by arterial palpation, need aggressive management for severe hypotension. Tachycardias require specific management but immediate cardioversion may not be required for sinus tachycardia of 150 beats per minute.

Haemodynamically stable ventricular tachycardia is treated with lidocaine and if fails, procainamide followed by bretylium may be used. Refractory cases may require synchronised cardioversion.

Stable wide complex tachycardia may require procainamide. Verapamil is not used as it may worsen (WPW syndrome) and if it is supraventricular tachycardia with normal blood pressure, verapamil can be used in the absence of an accessory pathway.

Paroxysmal SVTs may be treated with vagal stimulation, diltiazem or verapamil.

Maintaining Resuscitation

The importance of maintaining cardiopulmonary resuscitation emphasises: no more than 10 seconds should be permitted for any manoeuvre that demands temporary cessation of chest compression. The endotracheal route is now recognised as being an unreliable route for drug administration and should be used only when an intravenous line cannot be established. Repeated doses of adrenaline and sodium bicarbonate are recommended for prolonged resuscitation.

The 1989 recommendations represent the permanent truth, but they can all be justified by reasonable evidence[27] as per 1994 revised consensus.

Basic Life Support[29]

Basic life support refers to maintaining an airway and supporting breathing and circulation without any equipment. Basic life support skills should be learnt by everyone, including school children. The techniques of basic life support are no different when practised by health care professionals, but they should also be expected to practise more complex skills, including the use of airway and ventilatory adjuncts and two rescuer cardiopulmonary resuscitation. Basics, importance of team work and initial measures in CPR are listed in Tables 11.26 to 11.28.

Table 11.26: Basics of therapy in CPR

1. **Basic cardiac life support:** To maintain adequate cerebral oxygen by artificial measures in a patient with cardiopulmonary arrest.
2. **Advanced cardiac life support:** Providing basic life support with artificial ventilation, intravenous canulation, correction of cardiac arrhythmias and practically using resuscitation drugs.

Table 11.27: Team work in CPR

1. Senior physician as a leader.
2. Experienced nurse or junior doctor to perform closed chest cardiac massage and artificial ventilation.
3. Junior physician or a trained nurse each for ready monitors, intra-venous line, drug delivery.
4. Lab assistant to assess blood biochemistry.

Table 11.28: Basic cardiac life support: Initial measures

O*Thump version
A*Airway-clearing
B*Breathing-institution through ventilation
C*Circulation-restoration including cardiac massage

Most cardiac arrests in the community are the result of ischaemic heart disease. Forty per cent of sudden deaths from ischaemic heart disease occur within one hour after the onset of symptoms and the proportion is higher—around 60% — among middle aged and younger men. Over 90% of the deaths which occur outside hospital are due to ventricular fibrillation, a potentially reversible condition.[23]

Survival from cardiac arrest is optimal when:

- The event is witnessed.
- A bystander starts resuscitation.
- The rhythm is ventricular fibrillation.
- Defibrillation is carried out at an early stage.[30]

The emphasis should be on early defibrillation and, irrepsective of other considerations, defibrillators should be made available more widely for the use of suitably trained staff.

Cardiac arrests, particularly in younger people, may be due to causes other than ischaemic heart disease—for example, acute asthma, drug overdose, electrocution, immersion, hypothermia, etc. In some circumstances properly performed cardiopulmonary resuscitation can sustain life for up to an hour while treatment for the underlying condition is being provided. Prolonged resuscitation attempts should be made in cases of drowning, of exposure with hypothermia and in patients who have taken an overdose of hypnotic, narcotic or sedative drugs.

Resuscitation should be started in all patients with sudden loss of consciousness and absent breathing and pulses. It is inappropriate, however, to attempt to resuscitate those patients whose lives are drawing naturally to close because of irreversible disease. Tables 11.29 to 11.31 a show advanced CPR and drugs used in advanced cardiac life support.

Alphabets of CPR are listed in Table 11.32.

Table 11.29: Advanced cardiac life support (Advanced CPR)

1. Basic cardiac life support
2. Endotracheal intubation
3. Cardiac monitoring especially for detecting arrhythmias
4. Defibrillation
5. Intravenous therapy using drugs to prevent or terminate arrhythmias, supporting circulation and correcting acidosis
6. Stabilisation of patient's condition
7. This can, of course, be performed in intensive care units or an equipped hospital van.

Table 11.30: Drugs used in advanced cardiac life support

1. Essential drugs:		Oxygen Epinephrine Morphine Lidocaine Atropine
2. Useful drugs:	Corticosteroids	
	Vasoactives:	Levarterenol Metaraminol
	Isoproterenol Propranolol	
3. Additional methods and drugs:		Cardiac pacing Dopamine Diuretics Brethylium Procainamide
2 Miscellaneous:		Calcium chloride especially for severe hypocalcemia, toxicity of calcium channel blockers and severe hyperkalemia.

Table 11.31: Advanced cardiac life support: Drugs and their dosage

1. Epinephrine—1 mg, to be repeated every 3-4 minutes.
2. Atropine—0.5-1 mg IV, repeated every 3-4 minutes for bradycardia and asystole.
3. Lidocaine—1-1.5 mg/kg—maintenance infusion 2-4 mg/minutes for ventricular tachycardia and ventricular fibrillation.
4. Procainamide—20-40 mg/minute infusion for recurrent ventricular tachycardia.
5. Bretylium tosylate—5 mg/kg bolus for refractory ventricular tachycardia or ventricular fibrillation.
6. Magnesium sulfate—1-2 gm IV in 1-2 minutes for Torsade de pointes.
7. Adenosine—5-6 mg over 2-3 seconds bolus for supraventricular tachycardia.
8. Diltiazem or verapamil in 0.25 mg/kg and 2.5-5 mg as dose for atrial fibrillation and flutter.
9. Sodium bicarbonate—1 meq/kg initial dose for hyperkalemia and acidosis.
10. Calcium—10% IV bolus 5-10 ml (500-1000 mg) for hypocalcemia, hyperkalemia, calcium channel antagonist toxicity.

Table 11.32: Alphabets of CPR

A. Airway
B. Breathing
C. Circulation
D. Drugs
E. ECG
F. (De) Fibrillation

Assessment and Airway Control[31]

Members of the public should be aware of the importance of calling an ambulance immediately in case of sudden collapse. They should be encouraged to summon professional help. The rescuer should demonstrate unresponsiveness by shaking the causalty carefully and asking, *What's happening?* or *Are you all right?* If the patient is unresponsive the rescuer should call for help. The ABC (Airway, Breathing, Circulation) order of assessment and resuscitation is recommended for the lay rescuer. Occasionally a single rescuer's initial attempts may be rewarded by the return of respiration or a spontaneous heartbeat.

The rescuer should *open the airway* by the combined manoeuvre of head tilt and chin lift. In most cases this alone will lift the tongue from the back of the throat.[25] Any obvious obstruction should be removed from the mouth. This includes broken or displaced dentures.

Breathing (Ventilation)

Once the airways has been opened the rescuer should check for breathing by looking for chest movements, listening for breath sounds and feeling for the exhaled air on the back of the hand.

There is now evidence that giving breaths rapidly in expired air respiration causes air to enter the stomach. This increases the likelihood of regurgitation and aspiration of stomach contents.[32] The recommendations of the American Heart Association are that at the beginning of resuscitation of the apnoeic patient there should be two, slow expired breaths of air, each sufficient to cause the chest to rise,[33] rather than the four rapid breaths previously recommended. The chest should be seen to fall between ventilations. Each of the initial breaths should last from one to one and a half seconds. Succeeding ventilations should, likewise, last long enough to allow the chest to rise.

Mouth to mouth respiration is usually preferred, but for resuscitation in water the mouth to nose method may be more practicable. Exhalation with the mouth to nose method should, however, be through the mouth as the nasal tissues often obstruct passive exhalation. There should be no fear that HIV shall be transmitted by saliva. It is important to remember that upto 70% of cardiac arrests occur in the home and involve people who will be known to the rescuer and who might be family members.[29] So, there should not be hesitation in saving a patient by mouth to mouth respiration.

Circulation

Basic life support training materials should emphasise the importance of checking the pulse properly. The carotid pulse should be palpated for at least five seconds. For chest compressions to be effective and delivered without undue fatigue, a rate of 60-80 per minute is recommended.

Recovery Position

The patient whose airways is clear, who is breathing spontaneously, should be turned into the recovery position. This prevents the tongue falling back and reduces the risk of inhalation of gastric contents. There is no universally standard recovery position. The casualty's head, neck and trunk should be kept in a straight line. The position should be suitable for a casualty being carried on a stretcher.[34]

Choking

The management of choking is surrounded by controversy.[35] In the absence of scientific evidence to the contrary, the recommendations of the Resuscitation Council, based on the philosophy of keeping things safe and simple, are as follows. A conscious, choking victim should be encouraged to cough. The victim should be bent forward, for example over a chair to enlist the aid of gravity. If coughing fails to dislodge the obstruction, she or he should lean forward and blows should then be delivered to the middle of the upper back. The trained first aider should also administer a series of abdominal thrusts (Heimlich manoeuvre). Alternating a series of back blows with a series of abdominal thrusts seems to be the most effective procedure. An unconscious victim should be given abdominal or chest thrusts by direct compression. Tables 11.33 and 11.34 show check lists of effective and ineffective CPR.

Table 11.33: Effective CPR: Checklist

1. Feeling of pulse in femoral and carotids
2. Recordable blood pressure and hearable heart sounds
3. Spontaneous return of respiration
4. Constriction of pupils
5. Returning of consciousness
6. Patient feels improvement with returning of peripheral movements

Table 11.34: Ineffective CPR: Checklist

Considering some kind of problem at the following levels:

1. Patient's neck position
2. Evaluate the seal made with patient's mouth or nose
3. Ineffective chest compression: Because of lack of hard surface on which the patient was lying or the rate of cardiac compression may be slow
4. Degree of chest compression may be less than 5 cms
5. Compression may not have been smooth and periodical regularity of 50% compression with 50% release may not have altered.

Resuscitation by Health Care Professionals

In witnessed collapse—for example in hospital—when a primary cardiac arrest can be presumed, professionals might wish to combine the initial assessment of airway, respirations and pulse.

There is evidence that ventricular fibrillation can be successfully terminated by a chest thump,[36] but in a large study of out-of-hospital resuscitation attempts, an appreciable proportion of patients were thumped to an untreatable rhythm.[35] The chest thump seems to have a role in witnessed arrests, perhaps when a defibrillator is not immediately to hand.

Ventilation airways should meet the following requirements:

- They should have a minimum lumen diameter of 5 mm.
- They should incorporate a one way valve to minimise cross contamination.
- They should permit an adequate seal at the casualty's mouth.

Mouth to mask ventilation using a portable facemask (with supplemental oxygen insufflation), together with the use of an oropharyngeal airway, is strongly recommended for the professional rescuer.

Bag valve mask units are incapable of delivering high concentration of oxygen without the addition of an attached oxygen reservoir. This is particularly important for resuscitation in children. When oxygen powered ventilators are used with a facemask, the potential for gastric distension is high; preferably they should be used only in conjunction with a cuffed endotracheal tube.

Training and Retention of Skills

Basic life support is essentially a practical skill and students require practical training for at least two hours devoted mainly to making practice with one instructor to no more than six pupils is required to teach basic life support. Retention of skills is also poor unless regular retraining is carried out.[38,39] The Resuscitation Council strongly endorses the recommendations of the 1987 report of the Royal College of Physicians on the training and organization required to provide effective resuscitation.[40]

Resuscitating Resuscitation

Sudden death is always disturbing, especially when it occurs in the young. Even more distressing is when the death could have been avoided. In hospitals such skills are taken for granted, but they are not always available.[41] Junior hospital doctors and nurses in many hospitals are not much familiar with basic life support techniques. Even hospital should have an on-call resuscitation team skilled in all the disciplines of advanced life support; this team will have to integrate with those on site who start first aid. The resuscitation team must have a designated leader to take complete responsibility to avoid confusion. The team must include a senior physician and an anesthetist and trained ambulance men. An ambulance makes an ideal resuscitation vehicle and it should be equipped with *intelligent* defibrillators.[42]

The old concepts that external compression promotes cardiac output through massage of the heart is no longer accepted. The technique currently advised, therefore, comprises compression-pause-release.

Coughing has been observed to help restore pulse and blood pressure in patients of hypotension resulting from bradycardia or asystole during injection of contrast media. Independent observations support the value of coughing in case of ventricular fibrillation also.

In respect of defibrillation, the ideal strength of the external shock has been widely studied and debated. The consensus favours an initial trail with a shock if 200-300 Watt seconds. A second shock of higher strength can be appointed if required.

Resuscitation in Hospital[43]

In hospital it is important to consider the areas where resuscitation may be required because the logistics of delivery are very different.

Intensive Care Areas

In the intensive care unit, accident and emergency department, coronary care unit, anaesthetic rooms and operating theatres and special care baby units, skilled personnel with appropriate equipment should be readily available to start advanced life support immediately. Most patients will be monitored and many will have established intravenous lines.

General Wards

The emphasis has to be on immediate basic life support, usually by nursing staff, with the cardiac arrest team being summoned to provide advanced life support. Basic life support should be taught to all ward staff, they should appreciate that effective basic life support procedures are essential until the cardiac arrest team arrives and that the survival of patients is greatly affected by the speed at which basic support is started and the adequacy with which it is maintained.

Non-ward Areas

In X-ray, radiotherapy, physiotherapy, nuclear medicine departments, etc., the emphasis is again on basic life support until the cardiac arrest team arrives. In the past very little effort has been made to train paramedical staff, such as physiotherapists, radiographers, medical physicists, in basic life support or even to explain to them how the cardiac arrest call system works.

Other Areas

Other areas where the patient may attend adjacent to the hospital include psychiatric day hospitals and facilities for the physically or mentally handicapped. Again all attending staff should be taught basic life support.

General Thoroughfares of the Hospital

Basic life support should be provided by any staff available. Ideally any person working in a hospital should be able to provide basic life support, so training should ultimately be extended to all grades and categories, to include such groups as clerical, administrative and portering staff. Obviously they must know how to alert the hospital cardiac arrest team, and the patient will then usually be removed to the nearest clinical area for treatment unless the necessary equipment can be brought to the patient.

In a well-run intensive care or coronary care unit it is reasonable to expect the nursing staff to have resuscitated many of the patients, especially those in ventricular fibrillation, well before the doctors arrive.

In all other areas the staff on the spot must immediately initiate adequate basic life support and maintain it until the cardiac arrest team arrives. They will have to dial an emergency telephone number, which should be marked on every telephone and be taught to give a clear message stating the exact location of the cardiac or respiratory arrest.

In many hospitals the cardiac arrest team consists of the duty medical and anaesthetic registrars, a more junior doctor, one or two senior nurses and a porter who will bring the emergency trolley. In multistorey hospitals special emergency keys to the lifts should be provided for the two senior doctors and the porter with the emergency trolley to enable them to commandeer the nearest lift and reach the patient as soon as possible. If patients are known to be suffering from contagious disease on airways or face mask with a non-returnable valve must be used.

Each hospital should have a subcommittee or panel, meeting at least quarterly to discuss problems and general policies. It should report directly to the hospital medical executive committee. Any patient of any age or suffering from any disease will rightly be subjected to an attempt at resuscitation unless a contrary instruction has been left by the medical staff and entered into the medical and nursing records.

The resuscitation training officer will organize and document training courses, take care of training equipment and audit cardiac arrest calls. A suitable person would have had extensive experience in resuscitation either as a sister or charge nurse or as a paramedic in the ambulance service.

Included in the training programme are all junior medical staff, all medical students, all trained nurses, paramedical staff such as physiotherapists, ancillary staff and probably in future, ambulance crews and even the lay public.

Retention of resuscitation skill is known to be poor. It is important that the hospital should be a designated room for resuscitation training. Hospitals should provide regular revision courses.

Post-Resuscitation Care[44]

The restoration of electrocardiographic complexes marks the start and not the end of a successful resuscitation. The true end point is a fully conscious, neurologically intact patient with a spontaneous stable cardiac rhythm and an adequate urine output.

The chances of achieving this are greatly enhanced if the conditions in the Table 11.35 are met.

Table 11.35: Successful resuscitation
1. Arrest was witnessed
2. Underlying arrhythmia was ventricular fibrillation
3. Successful cardioversion achieved in 2-3 minutes and not longer than 8 minutes
4. When defibrillation was delayed for longer than 2-3 minutes, cardiopulmonary resuscitation was started and maintained.

A senior doctor takes a decision about transferring the patient to an intensive care area. Elective ventilation is often necessary. Clearly if the time from the onset of cardiac arrest to return to full consciousness is about two to three minutes elective ventilation may prove unnecessary. Unfortunately this is rare and is likely to occur only when the patient is already under intensive care. On a hospital ward, although the arrest is often witnessed, it may be many minutes before definitive treatment can be started. These patients will invariably need transfer to an intensive care unit for further assessment monitoring and treatment.

Trauma and emergency departments receive patients who have had unwitnessed arrests. In these patients special attention must be given to cerebral resuscitation. All doctors who resuscitate patients must be aware of the consequences when resuscitation is incomplete and brain damage occurs. Nevertheless, more brains are damaged by inadequate than by inappropriate resuscitation. That is why experienced senior doctors must be involved as a leader early in the management of cardiac arrest, ideally from the start though it does not happen. Checklist of post CPR care is given in Tables 11.36.

Table 11.36: Post CPR care: Checklist
1. Look for precipitating factor: Myocardial infarction, rhythm disorder or pulmonary embolism.
2. Assessment of neurological features especially oedema.
3. Assessment of circulatory status and vital organ perfusion.
4. Cardiac monitoring: As another cardiac arrest is likely to occur in post CPR period.

When the heart stops, the brain may be damaged both by the initial ischaemia and by failure of adequate reperfusion. The latter is ultimately the most damaging. The brain may survive a period of hypoxia if cerebral flow is maintained. When cerebral blood flow ceases, the electroencephalogram is flat within 10 seconds and cerebral glucose used up within one minute. Neuronal activity may, however, continue for upto an hour. Unfortunately progressive deterioration of the brain cannot be reversed or halted after about three minutes. A carotid pulse may be restored but the myriad of tiny cerebral vessels cannot be reperfused. Factors implicated are as following:

Vasospasm

Movement of calcium ions is implicated in vasospasm and calcium antagonists have improved cerebral survival in animals. The administration of calcium during cardiac arrest must therefore be questioned and can be endorsed only for electromechanical dissociation.

Cerebral Oedema

Hypoxia leads to cerebral oedema and this is augmented by the high blood levels of carbon dioxide associated with apnoea. Administration of sodium bicarbonate may release yet more carbon dioxide and compound the problem. Hyperventilation and elective lowering of the PCO_2 may reduce cerebral oedema and obviate the need for bicarbonate.

Microthrombus Formation and Sludging

When cerebral flow ceases, the smaller vessels silt up. Once formed, these blockages cannot be removed. Cerebral damage after cardiac arrest can be minimised by the following manoeuvres:

Immediately after restoration of cardiac rhythm, other measures include:

1. With a laryngoscope ensure that the endotracheal tube is correctly placed in the trachea and not in the oesophagus.
2. Ensure that the patient is being adequately ventilated with 100% oxygen. Listen with a stethoscope and confirm adequate and equal air entry. If you suspect pneumothorax insert a chest drain.
3. Estimate arterial pH and gases, preferably from an arterial sample, but use a central venous sample if necessary.
4. Estimate serum potassium.
5. Obtain a chest radiograph. An anteroposterior supine view is adequate.
6. Obtain a 12 lead electrocardiograph.
7. Measure the arterial blood pressure.
8. Measure the central venous pressure.
9. Insert a urinary catheter (under asepsis) and measure the urinary output.
10. Insert a nasogastric tube delicately and aspirate the contents of the stomach.

Rapid Return of Spontaneous Cardiac Output

Cardiopulmonary resuscitation sometimes achieves no more than 5% of normal cerebral flow and minimal cerebral oxygenation. It does, however, prevent total cessation of cerebral blood flow.

Meticulous Control

The pH, blood gases and electrolytes in the period immediately after the arrest, need meticulous control. In most cases this can be achieved only by elective ventilation of a sedated paralysed patient in an intensive care unit. It is also worth considering barbiturate coma, hypothermia, steroid treatment and intracranial pressure monitoring.

Barbiturate Coma

This may prevent the damaging effect of epileptic fits and protects against incomplete ischaemia, possibly by reducing cerebral activity. Barbiturates are mild calcium channel blockers and some are free radical scavengers. However, their effectiveness is not proved or widely accepted.

Hypothermia

This reduces the activity of the brain but may itself induce cardiac arrest. It is technically difficult to achieve and is usually used when the patient is already hypothermic, for example, after near-drowning.

Steroids

There is some evidence that steroids may modify the action of free radicals and so protect an ischaemic brain. They are valuable in controlling cerebral oedema associated with slow growing tumours but may also have a place after an arrest.

Intracranial Pressure

Monitoring may detect changes in intracranial pressure and help evaluate the efficacy of treatment.

Although spontaneous respiratory effort may return quite soon after a heart beat, it is rarely adequate and the gag reflex is usually impaired. A cuffed endotracheal tube will protect the airway and facilitate positive pressure ventilation. 100% oxygen should be used in the early stages to ensure adequate oxygenation of poorly perfused areas. If the patient resists the endotracheal tube, an immediate decision must be made about elective ventilation. This will allow hyperventilation to be used. A reduction of the PCO_2 to about 4kPa (30 mm Hg) will reduce cerebral oedema and control of ventilation will allow some correction of blood gas abnormalities and scrupulous maintenance of the PO_2.

A self expanding bag and valve are inadequate for more than a few minutes of resuscitation. They will allow carbon dioxide to build up, which can lead only to an increase in intracranial pressure and a deterioration in the acid base status. A mechanical ventilator must be used.

External chest compression may create a flail segment. This may be the result of rib fracture, or more commonly, of costochondral or sternal dislocation. Elective ventilation is mandatory for this condition. Do not wean a patient off a ventilator unless you know the rib cage is intact.

Acid Base Balance

When an arrest is witnessed, there is no need to administer sodium bicarbonate immediately. It need be given only when other methods have failed to reverse the acidosis. Even when the arrest is unwitnessed it is wise to administer bicarbonate only when there is a measured acidosis. External chest compression produces poor cerebral blood flow but even less peripheral circulation. There is little effective venous return, so lactic acid builds up but is not returned to the circulation until the heart is restarted. It is in the phase immediately after the arrest that serious acid base problems may occur and continuous monitoring of the blood gases every 15 minutes, possibly for several hours, is essential. Sodium bicarbonate provides a large hyperosmolar sodium load to an extremely compromised circulation. It can produce a precipitous fall in the serum potassium concentration. It neutralises acid by the release of carbon dioxide and a rise in the PCO_2 will lead to increased cerebral oedema. Carbon dioxide will move into the cerebrospinal fluid, making central monitoring of the pH by the brain extremely precarious once cardiac output has been restored. Blood gas and acid base abnormalities should initially be controlled by ventilation and the restoration of renal function. If these prove inadequate then small doses of bicarbonate can be given if blood gases are constantly monitored.

Hypokalaemia may precipitate cardiac arrest, particularly in elderly patients taking digoxin and diuretics. Bicarbonate administration may further lower the serum potasssium value. If the serum potassium concentration is very high, usually as the result of renal failure, then it can be lowered with glucose and insulin.

Each resuscitation attempt must be accompanied by a chest radiograph. Check the position of the central venous line and ensure that the endotracheal tube is not down in a main bronchus. Pneumothorax often occurs and is an important reversible cause of electromechanical dissociation. When electrical activity is recorded by the electrocardiogram but there is no cardiac output it is important to eliminate any other easily reversible condition. Cardiac tamponade may be diagnosed by an enlarged cardiac shadow and a raised central venous pressure. If in doubt obtain an echocardiogram.

Once a rhythm has been restored, it is only of value if it produces an output. If you cannot feel a pulse, continue external chest compression and treat the patient for electromechanical dissociation. If the patient is hypotensive, a dopamine infusion may be required.

If a short period of hypertension ensues, this is not harmful and may even be beneficial to the brain. Consider a lignocaine infusion after ventricular fibrillation. An adequate blood pressure will produce 40-50 ml of urine every hour (i.e., nearly 1 ml/mt). A urinary catheter may be necessary to monitor urine output.

Early attempt at mouth to mouth and bag and mask ventilation will have introduced air into the stomach. An initially misplaced endotracheal tube will also do the same. Gastric distention provokes vomiting and is uncomfortable. It is usually necessary to insert a nasogastric tube. The cause of the arrest and its effects on the heart may be shown by a 12 lead electrocardiogram. Any subsequent changes can be related to this early reading.

If patients are to be protected from the dangers inherent in our decision to resuscitate them, we must accept that a commitment to treating cardiac arrest is a commitment to intensive post resuscitation care. The patient can be managed only in an intensive care unit and will need at least a short period of elective ventilation.

Caution

The pupillary response is of little value immediately after an arrest. Pupils dilate during cardiac arrest for several reasons. Concentrations of circulating endogenous catecholamines are very high immediately before and during an arrest and exogenous catecholamines are likely to have been given. Atropine may also have been administered. Ischaemia to the anterior chamber can dilate the pupils. Only when hypoxia has been corrected and the effect of drugs allowed to wear off, can the tests of brainstem function be employed. This may take several hours.

When feeling for carotid pulses, inserting a nasogastric tube or replacing an endotracheal tube, always watch the electrocardiographic monitor.

Hypoxia augments vagally mediated reflexes and stimulation of the carotid sinus or oropharynx under these circumstances may lead to marked reflex bradycardia and asystole. Table 11.37 features time to terminate CPR.

Table 11.37: Time to terminate CPR

1. Failure to restore cardiac rhythm and adequate pump performance.
2. Evidence of irreversible and severe cerebral damage: Clinical assessment or EEG wise getting flat graph—an evidence of brain death.

Training Manikins[45]

Training cardiopulmonary resuscitation embodies theoretical and practical skills.

Citizen cardiopulmonary resuscitation programmes have quite different requirements from those for professional hospital staff.[46] A guide to skill expectation is given in the Table 11.38, although the division between basic and advanced cardiopulmonary resuscitation is not absolute.

New practices in cardiopulmonary resuscitation may not be demonstrable on manikins designed several years ago—for example, treatment of choking by abdominal thrust, use of the recovery position, management of trauma and haemorrhage, abdominal counterpulsation and application of medical anti-shock trousers. More importantly, recent concern about cross infection poses problems about decontamination of manikins during training,[47] and the current public demand for the use of protective resuscitation airways could not have been anticipated.

Choice of Manikins

In global market, a variety of models of manikins are available. Although not as realistic, torso models are more portable than full size manikins. Ambu's features look rather robotic but are quite functional and easily cleaned. Laerdal manikins have realistic eyes, hair and skin.

Anatomic-Anne is particularly useful for demonstrating anatomical and physiological principles. Although it lacks indicators yet it is an adequate teaching aid.

Resusci-Anne and Baby manikins have lights to indicate adequate ventilation, adequate compression and wrong hand position. Recording Resusci-Anne also has a metronome and a battery operated, pressure sensitive paper strip writer which can provide a permanent record.

Ambu-S can display ventilation and circulation on two pneumatic meters (29×28 cm) and a 230 V AV paperstrip recorder is an optional (extra). Resusci Junior simulates a 5-year-old child capable of resuscitation and suitable for land or water rescue (floating or submerged). Understandably, it lacks electrical indicators. It is particularly suitable for teaching lifesavers, playschool nurses and children. A deep water version of Ambu' ABC torso is also available.

Table 11.38

Skill expectation	Advanced cardiac life support
Basic life support	Resuscitation airways
Airway control (± simple airways)	Suction equipment
Mouth clearance, management of choking	Manual resuscitators (± mechanical devices)
Expired air resuscitation (± adjuncts)	Endotracheal intubation
Pulse detection	ECG diagnosis
External cardiac compression	Defibrillation and cardioversion
Posture including recovery position	Intravenous access and drug therapy
Control of haemorrhage and fractures	Neonatal resuscitation
Paediatric resuscitation	Circulation support (MAST garments, etc.)

For teaching infant resuscitation Laerdal's Resusci Baby is particularly realistic. Other manufacturers also provide baby manikins ranging from the premature baby to infant models (Simulaids).

Some models can also be used for teaching other skills, for example, basic nursing care (Adam Rouilly, CLA, Gaumard) and first aid management of haemorrhage and fractures (Alderson, San Arena). Many of these manikins may be used to test rescue and transportation skills under a wide range of conditions.

Airway Control, Management of Choking and Recovery Position

In all manikins, the neck can be tilted. Laerdal's adult models require excessive neck extension to achieve a patent airway, which might be hazardous in real casualties with associated neck injuries. Resusci Junior requires only a moderate head tilt if jaw thrust is performed simultaneously. Ambu manikins do not allow rotation of the neck (a disadvantage when practising mouth clearance) but do allow for the combination of neck lift and jaw thrust. In both Ambu-S and Resusci Junior, stomach inflation will occur if expired air resuscitation is attempted while the airway is obstructed.

Manikins for basic life support generally have small mouths with rudimentary oral cavities and tongues, which make the practice of mouth sweep and in insertion of resuscitation airways virtually impossible.

The effect of back blows and abdominal thrusts can be shown only in models with the appropriate anatomy (Simulaids). Adoption of the recovery position is impracticable for manikins lacking jointed body and limbs, though the posture can be shown on volunteers. Resusci Junior is notably lifelike in this respect.

Rescue Breathing

For expired air resuscitation considerations include realistic compliance and resistance, suitable display of ventilatory performance and an effective means of avoiding cross infection. Ambu rely on a clean mouthpiece and a disposable bag insert within the head for each rescuer (though lay people may need reminding that a plastic bag is not pushed into the mouth during real cardiopulmonary resuscitation). Laerdal offer disposable face moulds for each rescuer and replaceable lung bags. Both manufacturers incorporate one way valves and recommend a schedule of chemical disinfection.[47]

Mouth to nose ventilation is difficult to perform on these manikins because they have small noses, which are too soft, lack septa and have inadequate nostrils. The noses are designed simply to be pinched closed during resuscitation and access for nasal airways and catheters is impossible. Expired air resuscitation by facemask depends on the quality of seal between mask and face and is best performed using a mask with an inflatable cuff. This is easier to achieve on the smoother faced Laerdal models. Bag and mask ventilation requires a very firm one-handed grip and gas leaks readily occur.

Cardiac Compression

Essential requirements for cardiac compression include appropriate chest wall compliance and recoil and a suitable display of circulatory performance. Ambu-S, with circulation meter or recorder, displays an integrated effect during cardiac compression, simulating a *blood pressure* waveform which decays when compression is interrupted. This has some teaching advantage over Laerdal's recording system, which represents a beat to beat "stroke volume" waveform. However, the latter is more useful for assessing depth and rate of compression. Ambu-S has a valve system and clicking xiphoid plate for detecting incorrect hand placement, while Laerdal's Resusci models have a lighted *wrong hand position,* which can be irritating sensitive.

Carotid pulses can be palpated on several manikins. These are not activated by rescuer compression but require the supervisor to operate a squeeze bulb to simulate the pulse. Ambu offer an optional hand with radial pulse, but current teaching discourages reliance on peripheral pulses.

No single manikin presently tests all the skills required for an interactive or team approach. Kaye has used elements of several models to construct a manikin for teaching his Megacode scheme.[48]

Tracheal Intubation

Tracheal intubation requires an extended head, a large open mouth and accurate pharyngolaryngeal anatomy. Various features offered on the UK models include: posturable head and neck; use of resuscitation airways; the ability to practise oropharyngeal suction and oral and nasal intubation; and audible alarm for excessive jaw force, variable laryngeal position and dental configurations. There is also an infant version.

Ambu's model has a cut away section of the left face and neck to improve visualisation of technique, while Vitalograph provides a second laryngeal assembly alongside the head for a traumatic practice before intubating the manikin. Additional features such as the oesophageal obdurators and bronchoscopy are offered by CLA.

Careful choice of a robust trainer is recommended and lubricant spray should always be used. Damage to mouth, tongue and larynx is common.

Cardiac Rhythm and Defibrillation

Real time electrocardiographic changes on an oscilloscope are more realistic than leisurely inspection of static rhythm strips.

Simulators have been available for years using magnetic tape cartridges, cassettes or solid state filter networks, but micropressor technology offers improved capabilities. Laerdal's new arrhythmia Anne IV comprises a rhythm simulator that uses 15 basic electrocardiograph patterns to provide more than 60 rhythm disturbances. When this is linked to a Recording Resusci-Anne with a special torso skin incorporating paddle electrodes and discharge box training in defibrillation can be practised. Correct technique results in rhythm changes pre-selected by the supervisor. The simulator is designed for use with real defibrillators at 50 J but can withstand repeated discharges of 400 J. It should be remembered that energies of 50-400 J are associated with potentially lethal voltages of 2.5-7 kV.

Intravenous Access

Laerdal's infusion arm allows percutaneous venepuncture to be practised although the simulation of tactile sense and elasticity is disappointing. Several other manufacturers produce similar models and a torso manikin for central nevous cannulation of internal jugular and subclavian veins is also available (Nasco).

Display of Performance

During cardiopulmonary resuscitation the trainee, supervisor and audience need clear, concise and objective indications of performance. It is important to identify inadequate, correct or excessive force. Lights or buzzers can provide only a *yes/no* indication, whereas analogue meters display a quantitative value. The ability to make a permanent record is particularly useful for group teaching, retrospective, analysis and examination.

Evaluation of Process in Resuscitation

None of the UK manikins is capable of *spontaneous* response, although some feature a carotid pulse that can be controlled by the supervisor. Recording Resusci-Anne has a squeeze bulb to change pupil size, but apart from this no model can indicate to the rescuer its *cerebral status.*

There is a need for automated respiratory and circulatory activity and for clinical indicators such as *blood oxygenation, cerebral responsiveness* and *pupil response,* which would enable the trainee to assess progress in resuscitation.

Concurrent Task Performance/Team Interaction

Successful resuscitation requires the integration of multiple tasks, whether performed by a sole rescuer or by a team. Testing of team skills is limited only by the ingenuity of the instructor or physical limitation such as power supply.

Recommendations

Hospitals must be responsible for maintaining resuscitation standards among medical, nursing and auxiliary staff. A 400-600 bedded district general hospital needs one or two full body manikins, such as Ambu-S or Anatomic-Anne. For paediatric training a baby or child manikin or both, should be provided.

For advanced cardiopulmonary resuscitation doctors and nurses in specialised units require access to adult and neonatal intubation trainers and an arrhythmia generator (with or without torso capability).

The burden of teaching has traditionally fallen on anaesthetists, cardiologists and trauma and emergency specialists. The trend to train pulmonologist in the management of criticlly ill patients has increased rapidly in the recent years. The tasks of organisation, training, cleaning and maintenance of equipment are time consuming if performed properly and merit the appointment of a designated resuscitation training officer, probably with a nursing or paramedical background. Such a person will unify and improve the quality of training and should be affordable within a health district's budget.

Future Developments

The use of a microcomputer and video screen to measure performance and display results graphically is already feasible. There is increasing development of sophisticated simulators using computer technology (San Areana, Koken Resim) but these are too costly for most basic cardiopulmonary resuscitation schemes. An ingenious computer operated trainer/tester linked to a video disc is a potential example of a computerised manikin.

Resuscitation at Birth[49]

The priority of all those responsible for the care of babies at birth must be to ensure that adequate resuscitation facilities are available. Unfortunately some babies may have irreversible brain damage by the time of delivery, but it is unacceptable that any damage should occur after delivery because of inadequate equipment or insufficiently trained staff.

Respiratory distress syndrome (RDS) in neonates occur because of lack of surfactant formation in premature lungs. The surfactant contains four proteins, out of which B and C proteins are important as being responsible for structural organization and functional durability of surfactant by rapid dispersion of phospholipids at the air liquid interface which brings about reduction in surface tension that prevents small alveoli from collapsing. Exogenous synthetic surfactant therapy is useful in RDS in neonates; where nebulization is being tried over endotracheal tube delivery for better results.

All babies at increased risk should be delivered in a unit with full respiratory support facilities. These deliveries must always be attended by a doctor who is soley responsible for the care of the baby and skilled in resuscitation. There should also be a trained assistant. The babies at increased risk (as shown in Table 11.39) are about 25% of all deliveries, and will include about two thirds of those requiring resuscitation. The remaining one third of resuscitations occur in babies born after a normal uneventful labour who have no apparent risk factors. Therefore labour ward staff must be trained for an adequate resuscitation until further help can be obtained.

The padded platform on which the baby is nursed can be either flat or have a head down tilt. It is essential to have an overhead heater. Facilities must be available for manual face mask resuscitation, endotracheal tube resuscitation and umbilical vein catheterisation. Additional equipment includes an overhead light, a clock with a second hand, suction equipment, a stethoscope and preferably an electrocardiographic monitor, as shown in Table 11.40.

The standard policy to suck out the pharynx as soon as the face appears, using either a mucous extractor or a suction catheter, is almost always unnecessary, unless the amniotic fluid is meconium or blood stained. Aggressive pharyngeal suction can also delay the onset of spontaneous respiration for a considerable time. As soon as the baby is delivered wipe any excess fluid off the baby, using warm towel to reduce evaporative heat loss along with examining the child for major external congenital abnormalities, such as spina bifida and severe microcephaly. Most babies will start breathing during this period, as the median time for the onset of spontaneous respiration is only 10 seconds. They can then be handed to their parents. If necessary the baby can be encouraged to breathe by skin stimulation—for example, flicking the baby's feet. Those not responding must be transferred immediately to the Resuscitaire.

Table 11.39: High risk deliveries

Delivery	*Fetal*
Fetal distress	Multiple pregnancy
Abnormal presentation	Preterm
	Small for dates
Prolapsed cordi	Rhesus
Antepartum haemorrhage	Isoimmunisation
	Abnormal baby
Meconium staining	
High forceps	
Maternal	
Heavy sedation	
Drug addiction	
Diabetes	
Chronic illness	

Check first for respiratory efforts. If these are present and perhaps vigorous but producing no tidal exchange the airway is obstructed. This can often be overcome by extending the baby's neck. If the baby has choanal atresia or Pierre Robin Syndrome (cleft palate and micrognathia) obstruction will continue until an airway is inserted.

If respiratory efforts are feeble or totally absent, count the heart rate over 10-15 seconds using the stethoscope. When the heart rate is over 80 beats/min it is sufficient to repeat skin stimulation and if this fails, proceed to face mask resuscitation.

Face Mask Resuscitation

Only face masks consisting of a soft continuous ring provide an adequate seal. Most standard neonatal manual resuscitation devices fail to produce adequate tidal exchange when the pressure limiting device is unimpeded. Thus, a satisfactory outcome almost always depends on the inflation pressure stimulating the baby to make inspiratory efforts (Head's paradoxical reflex). This poor performance is related to the short inspiratory time (one third to half a second) provided by the devices. Tidal exchange can be increased by using a 500 ml rather than a standard 250 ml reservoir, which allows inflation pressure to be maintained for one second.

More satisfactory tidal exchange can be achieved by blowing oxygen directly into the face mask at 4-6 l/min and occluding the outlet from the face mask as if it were an endotracheal T piece. Obviously it is essential to incorporate a pressure valve into the inspiratory lines so that the pressures cannot exceed 30 cm. H_2O_2. The baby's lungs can then be inflated at a rate of about 30 per minute, allowing 1 second for each part of the cycle. Listen to the baby's chest within 5-10 inflations to check that there is bilateral air entry and that the heart rate is satisfactory. If the heart rate falls below 80 beats/min, proceed immediately to endotracheal intubation.

Endotracheal Intubation

Most non-anaesthetists find a straight bladed laryngoscope preferably for performing intubation. This must be held in the left hand and the baby's neck gently extended, if necessary, by the assistant. Pass the laryngoscope down, making sure that it

Table 11.40: Equipment for resuscitation

Padded shelf	Clock	Face mask system
Overhead heater	Stethoscope	Endotracheal tube
Overhead light	Electrocardiographic monitor	system (2.0-3.5 mm)
Oxygen cylinder (± wall supply)	Laryngoscope	Umbilical vein catheter set
Suctions (50-100 cm H_2O_2)		Syringes -1, 10, 20 ml

is in the mid line, until the epiglottis come into view. The tip of the blade can then be positioned either proximal to or immediately over the epiglottis so that the cords are brought into view. Gentle backward pressure may need to be applied over the larynx at this stage. As the airway tends to be fluid filled the upper airway may have to be cleared with the suction catheter held in the right hand.

Once the cords are visible, pass the endotracheal tube, using the right hand and remove the laryngoscope blade, taking care that this does not displace the tube out of the larynx. Then attach the endotrachal tube either to a T piece system, incorporating a 30-40 cm H_2O_2 blow off valve in the inspiratory line or to a neonatal manual resuscitation device. If a T piece is used, maintain the initial inflation pressure for two to three seconds, which will help lung expansion. The baby can subsequently be ventilated at a rate of 30 per munute, allowing about 1 second for each inflation.

Inspect the chest during the first few inflations, looking for evidence of chest wall movement and confirm by auscultation that oxygen is entering both lungs. If there is no air entry, the most likely cause is that the endotracheal tube is lying in the oesophagus. If this is suspected, remove the endotracheal tube immediately and reintubate. If auscultation reveals that oxygen is entering only in one lung, usually the right, try withdrawing the endotracheal tube by 1 cm while listening over the left lung. If this leads to dramatic improvement, the tip of the endotracheal tube was lying in the right main bronchus. If there is no improvement the possible causes include pneumothorax, diaphragmatic hernia or pleural effusion.

Severe Bradycardia

If the heart rate falls below 30 beats/min, external cardiac massage must be started by compression over the junction of the lower and middle third of the sternum, using the tips of two fingers or by placing and hand round the chest and compressing it between the thumb and fingers at a rate of 100-120 compressions per minute. This will achieve about compressions for every ventilation. If there is no dramatic improvement within 10-15 seconds the umbilical vein should be catheterised using a 5 French gauge catheter. This is best achieved by transecting the cord 2-3 cm away from the abdominal skin and inserting a catheter until there is a free flow of blood up the catheter. The baby should then be given 3 ml of sodium bicarbonate per kg body weight over two to three minutes. This is best provided by mixing 8.4% solution mixed with an equal volume of 10% dextrose, injecting a total of 20 ml to a term baby and 10 ml to a small baby, while continuing external cardiac massage and intermittent positive pressure ventilation. Those who fail to respond or who are in asystole, require 1 ml of 1 in 10000 adrenaline. This can be given either intravenously or injected directly down the endotracheal tube.

It is reasonable to continue with this regimen for 20 minutes, even in those who are born in apparent asystole, provided a fetal heart beat was noted within 15 minutes of delivery. Resuscitation efforts should not be continued beyond half an hour unless the baby is making at least intermittent respiratory efforts.

Intravenous Naloxone

Intravenous naloxone (40 ug should be given to all babies who become pink and have an obviously satisfactory circulation on resuscitation but fail to start adequate respiratory efforts. There is often a history of recent maternal opiate sedation. Some authorities recommend that an additional 200 ug should be given intramuscularly to prevent relapse.

Meconium Aspiration

Direct laryngoscopy should be carried out immediately after birth whenever there is meconium staining. If this shows meconium in the pharynx and trachea, intubate the child immediately and place a piece of gauze over the open end of the endotracheal tube. Then suck up the free fluid while removing the endotracheal tube and then reintubate. Provided the baby's heart rate remains about 60 beats/min this procedure can be repeated until meconium is no longer recovered.

Babies with a gestation of greater than 32 weeks do not differ from full term babies in their requirement for resuscitation. Under this gestation they may have a lower morbidity and mortality if a more active intervention policy is adopted. There is, however, no evidence that a rigid policy whereby all babies with a gestation of less than 28 or 30 weeks are routinely intubated leads to improved outcome. Indeed, unless the operator is extremely skilful, intervention may produce severe hypoxia in a previously lively pink baby and produce conditions which may well predispose to intraventricular haemorrhage. A reasonable compromise would therefore seem to be to start face mask resuscitation at 15-30 seconds unless the baby has not achieved satisfactory respiratory efforts by 30-60 seconds.

Resuscitation of Infants and Children[50]

In 1984 in England and Wales there were 6037 infant deaths (9.5 per 1000 live births); 281 occurred in the first week of life and 3544 in the first month. At the same time accidents were the second most common cause of death in children aged 14 (92 per million population) and the most common cause of death in children aged 5-14 (86 per million population). If most of these children are considered to be fit and healthy before their accidents it is surprising that paediatric resuscitation does not play a more prominent part in both community and hospital resuscitation programmes.

Hypoxia is the most common cause of cardiac arrest in infants and children. Sudden infant death syndrome, the loss of blood of body fluids, as in gastroenteritis and resulting in circulatory hypovolaemia, congenital heart disease and septicemia are also notable causes. Treatment must be immediate to be effective; delays in recognising or treating a cardiac arrest or therapeutic mistakes may seriously affect the outcome.

Resuscitation must begin immediately and should not await the arrival of equipment. This is essential in infants and children as just the simple manoeuvre of opening the airway may be all that is needed and may certainly prevent any further progress of the event.

As in any resuscitation, the airway, breathing, circulation sequence is most appropriae. Table 11.41 shows features of management in Infantile Respiratory Distress Syndrome.

Airway

Opening the airway is achieved by tilting the head and supporting the lower jaw.

Precaution suggested include (a) not to overextend the neck as this may cause the soft trachea to kink and obstruct and (b) not to press on the soft tissues in the floor of the mouth, as this will force the tongue into the airway and cause obstruction.

The small infant has an obligatory nose breather, so the patency of the nasal passages must be checked and maintained.

Maintaining the paediatric airway is a matter of trying various positions until the most satisfactory one is found. The rescuer must be flexible and willing to adapt his technique. The obstructed airway in infants and children is one example of a cause of collapse which is often immediately treatable. Obstruction may be caused by a foreign body (food or a toy) or by vomit. Careful removal of a foreign body is essential so as not to make the situation worse. An indifferent technique, such as blind probing or finger sweeps, may result in trauma, haemorrhage and oedema of the upper airway or further impaction of the foreign body. Inverting the child and applying back blows is an effective way of clearing an obstruction. The abdominal thrust procedure (Heimlich manoeuvre) should be applied only to older children.

Infectious diseases of the upper airway may cause serious and even fatal obstruction if not dealt with properly. The term croup is used to describe such disease and simply diagnosed as an inspiratory stridor.

The child may prefer to sit up and lean forward. Breathing a humidified atmosphere may also help, but further active interference may lead to a rapid worsening of the condition. These children must be moved, with care and supervision, into hospital to be dealt with by an expert team with the proper equipment.

Breathing

The patency of the airway is checked by listening and feeling for breaths over the nose and mouth of the child. The rescuer must look to see if the child has normal chest movement or if there is intercostal recession or a see saw movement of the chest or abdomen, indicating residual airway obstruction. Small children may also show flaring of the nares.

Expired air resuscitation must be started immediately if the child is not breathing. With the airway held open, the rescuer should cover the child's mouth (or mouth and nose) with his mouth and breath gently into the child until the chest rises. The correct volume can be simply judged by watching the chest movement. Ventilation may be increased by raising the rate of breathing and not by increasing the tidal volume.

Four individual breaths should be given initially. If the child requires only ventilation then breathing is continued at a rate of 15 to 30 breaths a minute according to the size of the child.

Circulation

The circulation is best assessed by palpating the brachial pulse. The femoral or carotid pulses may also be used depending on the experience of the rescuer. The pulse should be assessed not only for adequacy of volume but also for heart rate. Bradycardias occasionally accompany hypoxia and they are best treated by establishing adequate ventilation. Knowledge of the relevant pulse rates of infants and children is essential to make this diagnosis.

Table 11.41: Infantile respiratory distress syndrome: Management

a. Oxygen to give arterial PO_2 of 50-90 mm Hg (6.7-12 k Pa) b. If acidotic, give mechanical ventilation c. Maintain calorie and fluid intake d. Prevention of sepsis e. Check coagulopathies and anaemia f. Prevent hypothermia	
	1. Can be prevented by antenatal corticosteroids to mother. 2. Recovery or death: Within three days. 3. Prolonged high pressure arterial PO_2 may cause reterolental fibroplasia.

If an adequate pulse is not found, external chest compressions must be started. The heart lies under the lower part of the sternum in children and thus chest compressions should be applied to the junction of the lower and middle third of the sternum. The optimal position is found by measuring either two fingers breadth below the internipple line or the same distance above the xiphisternum.

The small baby is best served by encircling the baby's chest with both hands; the sternum is compressed by the thumbs and additional support provided by the interlaced fingers behind the infant's back. In toddlers and small children compressions can be applied by the tips of two fingers, while the larger child may require compressions applied by the heel of one hand.

The rate and depth of compressions also depend on the child's size. Compressions should be smooth and the compression phase last at least half the cycle. The accuracy of the rate and depth of compression is not vitally important; again the rescuer should be flexible and able to adapt his technique to achieve the best result. The rate of compressions should be fast enough to provide a circulation, the depth of compression deep enough to feel a pulse on palpation. Although the ideal is to match the normal physiological rates, a compression rate of at least 100 per minute is recommended.

A ratio of five compressions to one ventilation is recommended for infants and children. It is essential that adequate ventilation be achieved and a pause in the chest compressions may be required to ensure this. The adult ratio of two ventilations to 15 compressions should be used in older children.

Advanced Life Support

Table 11.42 shows sizes of endotracheal tubes and bag volumes in relation to different paediatric age groups.

The use of equipment in paediatric resuscitation is fraught with difficulties. Not only must a wide range of equipment be available to correspond with the variety of sizes of child but also the rescuer must be skilled enough to be able to choose and use the equipment efficiently.

Airway

The simplest airway adjunct is the Guedel oropharyngeal airway, but even here there is a choice of sizes from 000 to 4. Too small an airway will not overcome the obstruction of the tongue and may force it to the back of the pharynx. Too large an airway may injure the posterior pharyngeal wall. Nasopharyngeal airways are often a simple solution in children—for example, an endotracheal tube of suitable nasal diameter cut to a short length.

If the paediatric airways is to be guaranteed, the child must be intubated. Intubation requires skill acquired only through training and practice. A complete range of sizes of endotracheal tubes must be available and the choice is made by using either a table or a simple formula. The endotracheal tube must be cut to an appropriate length and after intubation the position of the tip of the tube should be checked by auscultation to ensure that the left or right main bronchi have not been inadvertently entered, resulting in the ventilation of one lung only.

Once the tube is correctly positioned it should be firmly secured to prevent accidental movement or inadvertent extubation.

Table 11.42

Age	*Endotracheal tube internal diameter (mm)*	*Length (cm)*		*Suction catheter (F)*
		Oral	*Nasal*	
Premature	2.5-3.0	11	13.5	6
Newborn	3.5	12	14	8
1 Year	4.0	13	15	8
2 Years	4.5	14	16	8
4 Years	5.0	15	17	10
6 Years	5.5	17	19	10
8 Years	6.0	19	21	10
10 Years	6.5	20	22	10
12 Years	7.0	21	22	10
14 Years	7.5	21	23	10
16 Years	8.0	23	24	12

Age and weight	*Bag volume (ml)*	*Tidal volume (ml)*
< 2 Years (< 7 kg)	240	205
2-10 Years (7-30 kg)	500	350
>10 Years (> 30 kg)	1600	1000

There is a wide variety of ancillary intubation equipment. The straight blade laryngoscope is usually recommended for infants and children but in emergencies an adult curved blade can be used with extreme care.

There is also a choice of endotracheal tube connections. The simplest answer is to pick the system which fits most of the ventilation equipment available. A range of sizes of suction catheters must also be available to keep the airway clear.

Breathing

Supplemental oxygen by facemask, head box, nasal cannulae or an oxygen tent is a simple and useful initial solution. If the child is not breathing then ventilation can be achieved with a resuscitation bag attached to a mask or an endotracheal tube.

The resuscitation bags usually used are self inflating and made in three sizes. The two smaller bags have a pressure limiting device preset to 45 cm H_2O_2 to prevent overpressurisation of the child's lungs. This can be overridden where the lungs have become non-compliant. Spontaneous respiration is possible through such bags. It is always worth adding supplemental oxygen to a resuscitation bag.

There are a variety of designs and sizes of masks to be used in association with a resuscitation bag. The design is often favoured for its shape that minimises apparatus dead space. Recently circular masks, made of soft plastic, have been found to be successful, especially by inexperienced users. A snug fit is essential when selecting the size of mask. Clear plastic masks are recommended so that the child's colour can be observed without having to remove the mask during resuscitation.

Automatic resuscitators are, at present, not recommended for use with children. Paediatric ventilation requires repeated re-evaluation and adaptation of techniques and a false sense of security may be developed which can result in inadequate or excessive ventilation.

Circulation

The administration of fluids and drugs to support the circulation usually requires intravenous access. Fluids can be administered via the interosseous route and some drugs can be given down the endotracheal tube for absorption in the lungs. If the latter route is used a short period of hyperventilation is required to aid distribution absorption of the drug by the pulmonary vascular bed.

One of the major problems in paediatric resuscitation is establishing intravenous access. The choice of which cannula to use and what route to select is a matter of personal preference and experience. Central venous access is better than peripheral access because of the poor peripheral blood flow during resuscitation. Central venous access may be gained via the femoral, subclavian, or internal or external jugular veins. Whichever route is chosen, central or peripheral, it must be remembered that it is the venous access which is important and not the size of the cannula. Most resuscitations can be carried out by drug administration through a 20 or 22 SWG cannula.

Fluids should be administered sparingly as fluid overload can be a problem in resuscitation attempts. Peripheral venous administration often necessitates the flushing of drugs centrally. Repeated administration via this route can easily result in fluid overload. A record of all fluids given either as drugs or as fluid loading should be maintained. In hypovolaemic conditions, such as trauma or gastroenteritis, it may be necessary to give blood, plasma or a plasma substitute in appropriate volumes. Children do not tolerate hypovolaemia and the rescuer must bear in mind their normal circulating blood volume.

Heart rate and cardiac rhythm are best assessed by attaching the child to an electrocardiographic monitor. A stethoscope allows auscultation of the heart and breath sounds. Blood pressure measurements depend on using the right size of paediatric blood pressure cuff together with a machine capable of measuring young children's relatively low but normal blood pressures. The width of the cuff should be two thirds of the length of the child's upper arm.

Ventricular fibrillation and ventricular trachycardia are not often a problem in paediatric resuscitation. Should they occur, defibrillation is the treatment of choice. Two joules/kg is the recommended energy level. Some defibrillators can be charged only to preset levels (20, 50, 100, 200 or 400) whereas others have a maximum output of 100 J when the paediatric paddles have been connected. The paddle size and position are chosen as being those which provide the best contact with the child's chest wall. Paddles are available in two sizes, 4.5 or 8 cm in diameter.

Drugs

Drugs may be given intravenously or via the endotracheal tube. The correct dose requires knowledge of the recommended dose in mg/kg (surface areas are inappropriate in resuscitation). Thus the rescuer must know the body weight of the child as shown in Table11.43. Most children who have been admitted to hospital before the resuscitation attempt have usually been weighed. If the child is particularly ill and likely to need cardiopulmonary resuscitation, the drug doses should be precalculated both in mg of drug required and in ml of drug solution to be administered.

Table 11.43: Body weight in childhood: Expected value
Infants double their birthweight in 5-6 months
Infants treble their birthweight in 1 year
Between 1 and 7 years weight (kg) = (age+4) × 2
Between 7 and 12 years weight (kg) =age × 3

In an emergency the child may not present with a known accurate body weight. It is usually easier to obtain or estimate the child's age and the weight can then be estimated by using a paediatric nomogram. An alternative is to use the accompanying approximate rules of thumb.

The simplest solution is to use a table which relates age, weight and drug dosage.

Temperature

It is vitally important to maintain or restore the child's body temperature during resuscitation. Hypothermia causes additional strain on the cardiovascular system. Warm blankets, infra red heaters and incubators should all be available as part of the paediatric resuscitation equipment.

Care After Resuscitation

Like adults, children require intensive post resuscitation care. Ventilation may be needed and monitoring of the arterial and central venous pressures may require invasive techniques. Investigations should include a chest radiograph and measurement of plasma electrolyte and blood sugar concentrations. Arterial pH and blood gases may indicate a cause of the collapse and require further correction to prevent a recurrence.

The Airway at Risk[51]

Failure to maintain a patient airway is a common cause of avoidable death in unconscious patients. The principles of airway management after cardiac arrest are the same as those used during anaesthesia or resuscitation after major trauma. Patency of the airway may be impaired by loss of normal muscle tone or by obstruction, including contamination by foreign material from the mouth, nasopharynx, oesophagus or stomach.

Airway Clearance

Opening the Airway

In the unconscious patient relaxation of the tongue, neck and pharyngeal muscles causes soft tissue obstruction of the supraglottic airway. Correction using long established manoeuvres includes head tilt and jaw lift or jaw thrust. The use of neck lift to produce head tilt is widely recommended in first aid manuals, but it leaves one hand committed behind the neck and it may be dangerous in the presence of an unstable injury of the cervical spine. Head tilt will relieve obstruction in 80% of patients and jaw lift or jaw thrust will further improve overall patency but tends to oppose the lips. In some of these patients airway obstruction may persist, particularly during expiration, probably because of nasal airway obstruction caused by a *flapvalve* effect of soft palate and nasopharyngeal tissues, as in the snoring subject.

Recovery Posture

Patients with adequate spontaneous ventilation and circulation but who cannot safeguard their own airway will be at risk in the supine position. Turning the patient laterally into the *coma or recovery* position allows the tongue to fall forward, with less risk of pharyngeal obstruction and fluid in the mouth can drain out instead of soiling the trachea and lungs.

Recovery positions range from a true lateral posture (with either upper or lower leg flexed) to the semiprone, depending on the relative tilt of the pelvis and shoulders and the attitude of the arms. Several authorities favour the lower arm extended behind the back to prevent reverse roll. The semiprone posture has been preferred as producing better airway patency and drainage and greater stability during transport. However, it is more difficult to observe the casualty's face, colour and chest movement in this position and ventilation may be impaired. Moreover, the patient is inconveniently positioned if he has to be turned supine again for further resuscitation.

The subject may lie on either side. Some argue that emergency tracheal intubation may be performed more easily with the patient lying on his left rather than right side, but a full stomach is more liable to compression and regurgitation in this position. First aid texts recommend that unconscious patients with associated chest injuries are best positioned with the uninjured lung uppermost. The complex pathophysiology of thoracic injury suggests that there may be some circumstances in which this may not be appropriate.

Casualties with spinal injuries need careful handling and should be managed in the supine aligned position with constant attention to the airway. If the recovery posture has to be adopted, the patient should be turned into a true lateral position by several rescuers in unison to avoid spinal rotation. The semiprone position is not suitable in these circumstances because considerable rotation of the neck is required to prevent the subject lying on his face.

Vomiting and Regurgitation

Rescuers should always be aware of the hazard of contamination of the unprotected airway by fluid or solid debris and attempt to forestall it. Vomiting and regurgitation are subtly different.

Vomiting happens more commonly during light levels of unconsciousness and may occur as the level of consciousness improves during successful resuscitation. It is an active process of stomach contraction and retrograde propulsion up the oesophagus. Prodromal stretching may allow time to put the patient in the lateral recovery position or head down

(Trendelenburg) tilt and prepare for suction or manual removal of debris from the mouth and the pharynx.

Regurgitation is a passive and often silent flow of stomach contents (typically fluid) up the oesophagus, with the risk of unprotected inhalation and soiling of the lungs. Acidic gastric fluid may cause a severe chemical pneumonitis. Failure to maintain a clear airway during spontaneous respiration may also encourage regurgitation because the excessive negative intrathoracic pressure developed during obstructed inspiration may aspirate gastric contents across a weak mucosal flap valve from the stomach to oesophagus. Recent food or fluid ingestion, obesity, hiatus hernia, intestinal obstruction and late pregnancy all make regurgitation more likely to occur during resuscitation. Cardiac compression and the use of abdominal binders or counterpulsation also add to the hazard of regurgitation.

Gaseous distension of the stomach increases the likelihood of regurgitation and restricts lung expansion. Inadvertent gastric inflation may arise during artificial respiration when rapid lung ventilation with large tidal volume and high inflation pressures are used. This is particularly likely when gas powered resuscitations are used with a facemask. The current emphasis on rapid incremental breaths and synchronous combined ventilation-compression can also produce high inspiratory pressures.

The cricoid pressure manoeuvre, recommended by Sellick in 1961, is well known. Compressing the oesophagus between the cricoid ring and the sixth cervical vertebra prevents passive regurgitation, but it should not be applied during active vomiting. It also serves a useful purpose during resuscitation in preventing undesired gastric inflation but will require the help of another rescuer.

Choking

Asphyxia due to impaction of food or a foreign body in the upper airway is a dramatic and frightening event and may closely resemble a heart attack. It requires urgent action to avert a catastrophe. In the conscious patient back blows and Heimlich abdominal thrusts have been widely recommended. Attempts may be made to provoke coughing or vomiting. If these are not successful the patient will become unconscious and collapse. The supine casualty may be given further abdominal thrusts and manual attempts at pharyngeal disimpaction should be undertaken. Visual inspection of the throat with a laryngoscope and the use of Magill forceps or suction is desirable, but such equipment is seldom available at the time of need.

If resuscitation so far has been unsuccessful, the ultimate hypoxic arrest may be indistinguishable from other causes of cardiac arrest and treatment should be along standard lines, although ventilation may be difficult or impossible to perform. On the other hand, the act of forceful chest compression may clear the offending object from the laryngopharynx.

The desperate and heroic manoeuvre of cricothyrotomy (laryngotomy) may be lifesaving and should not be unduly delayed. Any strong sharp knife, scissor point, large bore cannula or similar instrument can be used to create an opening through the cricothyroid membrane, although purpose designed cricothyrotomy devices are best if available. Once created, the opening needs to be maintained by some means. Artificial ventilation may be applied directly to this orifice.

The formal procedure of tracheostomy is technically difficult and should not be undertaken under adverse conditions.

Suction

Equipment for suction clearance of the oropharynx and airways is essential for comprehensive life support. When reviewing the many devices available, consideration of cost, portability and power supply are paramount. Devices powered by electricity or compressed gas are susceptible to exhaustion of the power supply at a critical time and battery-operated devices need regular recharging or battery replacement. Hand or foot operated pumps are particularly suitable for field use and for the occasional user. Ease of cleaning and simple reassembly are important factors. The use of rigid, wide bore plastic or metal suction cannulae can be supplemented by soft plastic suction catheters when necessary. A *suction booster,* which traps fluid debris in a reservoir close to the patient, may improve suction capability.

The Airway During Artificial Ventilation

If, despite adequate clearance of the patient's airway, spontaneous respiration is absent, artificial ventilation must be started. Earlier manual methods have been uninversally superseded by intermittent positive pressure techniques which produce better ventilation.

Expired Air Ventilation

Expired air ventilation exploits the rescuer's expired air to achieve good lung expansion and although less rich in oxygen than ambient air (16% v 21%), the resulting oxygenation is adequate.

The mouth to mouth technique is widely acclaimed and can be successfully applied by relatively unskilled rescuers. Nevertheless, during its performance it is difficult for the rescuer concurrently to maintain airway patency, but the rescuer can effect an airtight seal with his lips, pinch the nose and also deliver an adequate ventilatory volume.

An alternative route is mouth to nose ventilation which until recently has been popular only with water life-savers. This method permits maximum head extension and jaw thrust while usefully effecting lip closure. It may be the only option for small mouthed rescuers. Contact with vomit, saliva, etc., is reduced, which may take mouth to nose ventilation more acceptable and lessen the risk of infection. Natural nasal resistance limits high inspiratory flow, which might otherwise lead to gastric inflation. If nasopharyngeal obstruction is noted during expiration the rescuer may need to open the casualty's mouth to allow exhalation.

Ventilation Masks

Ventilation masks offer some protection to the rescuer. The rescuer blows through a mask firmly applied to the casualty's face. An example is the transparent Laerdal pocket masks, which has a rescuer mouthpiece and a pneumatic cuff. During expired air resuscitation the rescuer uses two hands to maintain airtight seal with the mask on the face while also lifting the jaw.

Air flow generally occurs through the nose. Unless oral or nasal airway support devices are used, obstructed expiration may go unrecognised in some subjects.

A self refilling bag can be attached to the mask to deliver ambient air and this can be enriched with oxygen if a source of compressed oxygen is available. The technique requires additional training because it is difficult to apply the mask and lift the jaw with one hand while squeezing the bag with the other.

Airway Support and Ventilation Devices

Artificial airways can be used to maintain patency and improve spontaneous breathing and may also provide a mouthpiece for artificial ventilation if required. Some afford protection to the rescuer against infection and some isolate the airway against pulmonary soiling from gastric aspiration.

The classic Guedel airway used in anaesthesia improves patency but often requires supplementary jaw support. In slightly comatose patients it may cause oropharyngeal stimulation and vomiting. Soft nasopharyngeal tubes are less stimulating but may cause nasopharyngeal bleeding and they need some skill in insertion. These simple airways are also suitable for use with mask ventilation.

Rescuer Protection

There is concern about the risk of infection associated with mouth to mouth ventilation and an increasing public demand for small and inexpensive airway adjuncts which will protect against communicable disease. A simple expedient is to blow through a handkerchief moulded over the patient's face. A plastic sheet incorporating a central bite block with a one way patient valve can also be used.

The Safar S shaped reversible double airway consists of a medium and a large Guedel airway placed back to back. The uninserted airway provides a port for expired air ventilation if required and provides some protection for the rescuer.

To provide rescuer protection, an airway using a non-return valve has been brought out. An ingenious Dual-Aid airway capable of airway support and ventilation has the advantage of optional use through the nose or mouth.

Airway Isolation

The ultimate in airway management in deeply unconscious patients is tracheal intubation, which requires experience and specific equipment. Traditionally the forte of anaesthetists, this skill has been learnt by emergency medical staff, specialists nurses and skilled paramedics such as ambulance crews. The technique essentially involves flexing the subject's neck, extending his head, exposing the epiglottis with a laryngoscope, forward elevation of the jaw and base of tongue to expose the larynx and inserting a curved tube into the trachea. Inflation of the tracheal cuff isolates the airway and enables safe ventilation to be performed. The risks are those of stimulating vomiting in the semi-conscious patient, trauma to mouth and larynx, unilateral bronchial intubation and unrecognised intubation of the oesophagus.

If attempts at tracheal intubation are unsuccessful, they must be abandoned without delay and alternative methods of airway control chosen. Techniques for tracheal intubation have been advocated which avoid formal laryngoscopy but these have limited success even in experienced hands. They include blind nasal intubation, digital manipulation of the tube in the laryngopharynx or trans-illumination using lighted tube stylets.

Oesophageal Obdurators

Oesophageal obdurators are popular in the USA. The obdurator is a long cuffed tube attached to a facemask. The tube is passed blindly into the oesophagus and the cuff is then inflated to isolate the oesophagus and stomach from the airway. In the original version the oesophageal obdurator tube is blocked distally and a series of holes at laryngeal level permit air blown down the tube to pass from the tube into the larynx. In a later version the oesophageal tube is not terminally sealed and this allows for aspiration or pressure relief of gastric contents. A second orifice in the mask is used for ventilation. Hazards in the use of these tubes include trauma to the oesophagus and stomach, the risk of inducing vomiting and gastric rupture, and paradoxically, the rare occurrence of unrecognised tracheal intubation.

Training and Retention of Skills[52]

Resuscitation training is essentially a practical skill and student need practical training to acquire it. This has been made possible since 1960 by the development of various manikins and training aids. However in most hospitals teaching of resuscitation is haphazard and medical and nursing students are perhaps taught only once during their courses.

Better Teaching of Skills

A recognised national training programme for basic or advanced life support in medical and nursing schools, should be included as per issued guidelines on basic and advanced life support.

Retaining Skills

This is true even six weeks after training and severe loss of skills occurs after about 12 months, when hardly 20% or fewer trainees can perform basic life support proficiently. Reason is simple that skills that are not regularly practised are not retained. Attaining and retaining cardiopulmonary resuscitation skills may also depend on course content and time devoted to manikin practice.

It is estimated that only12% of those trained are capable of carrying out effective cardiopulmonary resuscitation. There is a rapid and linear decay in resuscitation skills over time, with fewer than 20% of the subjects achieving a score of 75% on performance only six months after training. A regular update and recurrent practice under the supervision of guide or trainer may improve retension of skills in resuscitation.

Advanced Life Support

Teaching methods which can be used for basic life support and advanced cardiac life support training are the following.

Verbal Instruction

Clarity, accuracy and repetition are necessary.

Visualisation

Techniques and procedure can be visualized in the form of demonstrations, blackboard pictures, charts, projected slides, films and videos.

Practice

It is the most important aspect of cardiopulmonary resuscitation training. Training manikins must be used for practising lung ventilations and chest compressions. These should be as realistic as possible, to enhance motivation and physiologically correct learning. Each student should have enough time for manikin practice to reach perfection in performance.

Self-Training System

This has many advantages over traditional lectures and manikin practice supervised by an instructor. People learn at different rates, so training programmes should allow for individualised learning.

Recommendations for Improving the Quality of Cardiopulmonary Resuscitation Training

1. Practical training on a manikin is better.
2. Feedback is essential, especially via a recording monitoring manikin.
3. Practice after initial training.
4. Refresher training.
5. Periodic refresher training within a year of training.
6. Guidelines for training should be as uniform throughout the world.
7. Schools should play a great part in disseminating knowledge about first aid and cardiopulmonary resuscitation and in teaching proficiency to the public at large.
8. Ideally every hospital should have a resuscitation training room equipped with all the appropriate training aids for basic and advanced life support. Trainees should be encouraged to visit the room in small groups to use the equipment at their own pace and under the direction and supervision of a resuscitation training officer.
9. A designated resuscitation training officer is vital if standards of skills are to be maintained.

Drowning and Near Drowning[53]

Near drowning poses several problems in resuscitation which are not commonly encountered in hospital practice and which, if not handled correctly, may reduce the chances of survival without brain damage. In hospital patient monitoring is relatively simple. Whether or not the breathing can be established with ease and an electrocardiogram provides instant evidence of cardiac activity. In contrast, making a firm diagnosis of cardiac arrest or even respiratory arrest at the scene of a drowning/ accident can be very difficult. This, coupled with the knowledge of miraculous survival after prolonged periods of submersion in water, makes the decision when to abandon attempts at resuscitation formidably difficult.

Survival After Prolonged Submersion

In hospital, circulatory arrest usually occurs as a result of ventricular fibrillation and breathing stops soon afterwards. During drowning this sequence of events is reversed. Breathing stops as soon as the head becomes immersed but the heart continues to beat for some time. Just how long blood circulation continues is unknown but clearly this is a crucial factor in determining how much damage is done to the brain. Human beings have been recovered from the water apparently dead but been revived without evidence of brain damage after as long as 40 minutes' total submersion. Since no victim of cardiac arrest in hospital could possibly have survived that length of time without intervention, important protective mechanisms must be at work beneath the water.

The Diving Reflex

Survival after prolonged submersion has been attributed to a diving reflex. Aquatic mammals can hold their breath beneath the water for as much as 10 times longer than man. They do this by shunting blood from tissues that can metabolise anaerobically and redistributing it to the brain and heart, which have little or no anaerobic reserve. Slowing in the heart rate and vasoconstriction of vessels in skeletal muscle occurs as a reflex via sensory afferents from the trigeminal nerve stimulated in turn by face immersion. This reflex is reinforced by increasing hypoxia via afferents from the carotid body chemoreceptors.

An additional advantage, unique to some diving mammals and unrelated to the diving reflex, is a large store of myoglobin, which provides a sizeable reserve of oxygen. Although a diving response is demonstrable in many non-diving mammals, it has yet to be shown in man that the diving reflex is anything but vestigial.

Protective Effect of Hypothermia

For at least 40 years it has been known that in an individual made sufficiently cool circulation can be stopped for around 30 minutes and then restarted without any apparent damage to the brain. The cooler the body, the longer the safe period for which circulation can be stopped, the only limiting factor being the development of ventricular fibrillation (which is very difficult to terminate in deep hypothermia). Circulatory arrest resulting from ventricular fibrillation occurs in children at a lower cardiac temperature than in adults, thus permitting more profound cerebral cooling. This might perhaps explain why so many miraculous recoveries from near drowning have been reported in children or infants.

Practical Problems with Resuscitation

Whatever the mechanisms influencing survival, rescuers have been trained to assume that every patient is potentially recoverable, however gloomy things may at first appear. They are trained to continue resuscitation for at least an hour before giving up.

Water poured into fresh cadavers can be retrieved from the stomach by inverting the corpse, but not from the lungs. Most rescue services have therefore abandoned drainage procedures. Notwithstanding this, data collected from actual resuscitation attempts indicate that in around two thirds of them, rescuers experience difficulty in clearing the upper respiratory tract of water. An abdominal thrust, which decants some water from the patient's mouth and promptly clears the obstruction. Despite this, the practical value of abdominal thrusts or back blows remains to be proved.

Because of the difficulties encountered in finding the pulse, rescuers are recommended to palpate the carotid artery for at least 10 seconds, having first successfully inflated the chest. If no pulse is felt then combined heart-lung resuscitation proceeds along standard lines for at least one hour without interruption.

The problem of exhaustion can be eased by using two rescuers, one performing mouth to mouth resuscitation and one performing chest compression, changing roles from time to time. Considerable practice is required to perfect this technique and the importance of training cannot be overstated. It is almost impossible to continue chest compression while transporting the patient over even short distances, so it is now routine to try to re-establish pulse at the accident site before moving the patient.

Fresh and Salt Water and Serum Electrolytes

Clinically important changes in serum electrolyte concerntrations, do not occur, after either fresh or salt water immersion. Hypokalaemia is seen after both salt and fresh water aspiration and hypernatraemia is a constant feature of salt water immersion, perhaps due to ingestion from the stomach. Marked hyponatraemia is seen in infants who suffer near drowning in fresh water.

Secondary Drowning, Dry Drowning and Pulmonary and Cerebral Oedema

The teaching of cardiopulmonary resuscitation to medical trainees has been inadequate in the past and inability of junior doctors to carry out effective basic life support had been prevalent. All medical students need to be training in accordance with the guidelines set down by the Resuscitation Council of the United Kingdom.[54] Resuscitation skills erode with time and may return to pertaining standards on repeat testing after 12 months.

Active Compression-Decompression[55]

Despite the nearly universal application of standard cardiopulmonary resuscitation (CPR), most out-of-hospital cardiac arrest patients do not survive.[56] In an effort to improve the chances of survival, a number of techniques have been investigated. The standard method of manual CPR, first described by Kouwenhoven, *et al.*[57] more than four decades ago, relies on the active compression and passive decompression of the chest wall. The importance of an active decompression phase of CPR has been recently suggested by an anecdotal report of successful cardiac resuscitation using a *plumber's helper* (household drain plunger) applied to the anterior chest wall.[58] To test the hypothesis that a simple suction device could assist chest wall expansion and improve the hemodynamics during CPR, active compression-decompression (ACD) resuscitation was compared with standard CPR in a canine model of cardiac arrest.[59] In eight dogs, cardiac output, systolic aortic pressure, coronary artery perfusion pressure and minute ventilation were significantly augmented with ACD resuscitation compared with standard CPR. (ACD) CPR has been used as a simple manual technique in 10 patients during cardiac arrest. Although (ACD) CPR may have produced a return of spontaneous circulation in three patients refractory to standard measures, its impact on survival when used early in cardiac arrest remains to be deterrnined.[55] Where rational team work, in a resuscitation team for each hospital has been stressed, the guidelines for CPR training have also been laid down,[31] stressing the need to standardize the reporting and correlation of the details of resuscitation attempts.

REFERENCES

1. Todi SK; Current classification and early diagnosis of ARDS; IN M. Panja; ED; Pa Med, API 2013; 27: 226-31.
2. Sherif L., *et al.*, A suspected case of transfusion-related acute lung injury; Lung India 2011; 28:216-18.
3. Kotloft RM; *et al.,* Pulmonary complications of solid organ and hematopoietic stem cell transplantation; Amer J Respir Crit Care Med 2004; 170: 22.
4. Ashbaugh D.G., *et al.,* Acute respiratory distress in adults; Lancet 1967; ii: 319.
5. Petly T.L., Ashbaugh D.G., ARDS: Clinical features, factors influencing prognosis and principles of management; Chest 1971;70: 233.
6. Khilnani O.C., ARDS; In., M.M. Singh; ed; Med. Update; API 1999; 9: 255-63.
7. Rama Rao D., MOSF; In; Y. P. Munjal; ed.; PG Med.; API 1999; 13: 148-54.
8. Boggis C.R.M. and Greene R., Adult respiratory distress syndrome, J. Appl. Medicine 1983; 9: 749-57.
9. Morton N.S., Exogenous surfactant treatment for ARDS? A historical perspective, Thorax 1990; 45: 825.
10. Bernard G.R., *et al.,* Persistent generation of peptide leukotrienes in patients with ARDS; Amer. Rev. Resp. Dis 1991; 144: 263.
11. Iyer V; PFT interpretation: Clinical pearls using a case based approach; IN; SR Joshi; ed; Med Update; API 2014; 24: 565-72.
12. Varani *et al.,* Pulmonary endothelial cell killing by human neutrophils; possible involvement of hydroxyl radical; Lab Invest 1985; 53: 665.
13. Hyers T.M., *et al.,* Tumor necrosis factor levels in serum and BAL fluid of patients with ARDS; Amer. Rev. Resp. Dis 1991; 144: 268.
14. Bernard G.R., *et al.,* Report of American-European Consensus Conference on ARDS: Definitions, mechanisms, relavant outcome and clinical trial coordination; Interns Care Med 1994; 20: 225-32.
15. ARDS Definition Task Force; Ranieri VM; *et al.;* ARDS : The Berlin Definition; JAMA 2012; 307: 2526-33.
16. Jain NP; *et al.,* ARDS; IN; SR Joshi; ed; Med Update; API 2014; 24: 602-05.
17. Barthwal MS; ARDS; IN; MS Rao; ed; Med Update 2010; 20: 777-83.
18. Choudhary D, Roshan R; Non-invasive ventilation; IN; SR Joshi; ed; Med Update, API 2014; 24: 588-94.
19. Stapleton RD; *et al.,* Causes and timing of death in patients with ARDS; Chest 2005; 128: 525.
20. Soni NK, Ohri K; Nosocomial infections in ICU; IN; SR Joshi; ed; Med Update, API 2014; 24:627-43.
21. Jani CK; Ventilator associated pneumonia; IN; SR Joshi; ed; Med Update; API 2014; 24: 606-13.
22. Ware L.B., *et al.* von Willebrand factor antigen is an independent marker of poor outcome in patients with acute lung injury; Crit Care Med 2001; 29:2325-31.
23. Marshall R.P., *et al.* ACE insertion/deletion polymorphism is associated with susceptibility and outcome in ARDS; Amer J Resp Crit Care Med 2002; 166: 646-50.
24. Van den Berghe G. *et al.* Intensive insulin therapy in critically ill patients; New Eng J Med 2001; 345: 1359-67.
25. Udwadia Z.F., ARDS; predicting mortality and improving survival; JAPI 2003; 51: 849-50.
26. Ware LB, Matthay MA; Clinical practice–Acute pulmonary odema; N Eng J Med 2005; 353: 2788.
27. Chamberlain D.A., Advanced life support, Brit, Med. Jour 1989; 299: 446-48.
28. Ian Kendall, *et al.,* Advanced cardiac life support; Medicine Update 1993; 1(7): 553-59.
29. Marsden A.K., Basic life support BMJ 1989; 299: 442-45.
30. Weaver W.D., Cobb L. A., Hallstrom A. P., *et al.,* Factors influencing survival after out-of-hospital cardiac arrest, J. Am. Col. Cardiol 1986; 7; 752-57.
31. Gupta S.B., Bhattacharya A.K., Cardiopulmonary resuscitation—Newer insights; In; Thakur B. B. ed; PG Med; API 2002; 16: 65-76.
32. Wenzel Y., *et al.,* Effects of smaller tidal volumes during basic life support ventilation in patients with respiratory arrest; Good ventilation, less risk? Resuscitation 1999; 43: 25.
33. Guidelines 2000 for Cardiopulmonary Resuscitation and Emergency Cardiovascular Care; Part 3; Adult Basic Life Support; The American Heart Assn. in collaboration with the International Liaison Committee on Resuscitation; Circulation 2000; 102: 122.
34. Chandra N.C., *et al.,* Instructor's Manual for Basic Life Support; American Heart Assn., Dallas, 1997.
35. Montoya D., Management of the choking victim. Can. Med. Assoc. J. 1986; 135: 305-10.
36. Caldwell G., Millar G., Quinn E., *et al.,* Simple mechanical methods for cardioversion, defence of the precordial thump and cough version. Br. Med 1. 1985; 291: 627-30.
37. Miller J.M., Tresch D., Horowitz L., *et al.,* The precordial thump, Ann. Emerg Med 1984, 13: 791-94.

38. Wynne., Training and retention of skills. In: Evans TR, ed. ABC of Resuscitation, London, British Medical Journal 1986; 32-35.
39. McKenna S.P. and Glendon A. I., Occupational first aid training; Decay of CPR skills, Journal of Occupational Psychology 1985; 58:109-17.
40. Royal College of Physicians, Resuscitation from cardiopulmonary arrest. Training and organisation. J. R. Coil, Physicians Lond 1987; 21: 1-8.
41. Royal College of Physicians, *Resuscitation from cardiopulmonary arrest. Training and organisation,* London, RCP, 1987.
42. Johnson R.W.G., Resuscitating resuscitation, BMJ 1987; 295: 71.
43. Evans T.R., Resuscitation in hospital, BMJ 1986; 292: 1377-79.
44. Redmond A.D., Post resuscitation care, BMJ 1986; 292: 1444-46.
45. Simmons R.S., Training manikins, BMJ 1986; 292:1509-13.
46. Safar P., Stavanger 1981; 183-203. (Distribution by W B Saunders and available from Laerdal).
47. Committee for evaluation of sanitary practices in CPR training recommendations for decontaminating manikins used in cardiopulmonary resuscitation training. Resp. Care 1984; 29:1250-52.
48. Kaye W., Linhares K.C., Breault R.V., Norris P.A., Stamoulis C.C. and Khan A. H., The Mega-Code for training the advanced cardiac life support team. Heart Lung 1981; 10: 860-65.
49. Milner A.D., Resuscitation at birth, BMJ 1986; 292: 1657-59.
50. Zideman D., Resuscitation of infants and children, BMJ 1986; 292:1584-88.
51. Simons R.S. and Howells H., The airway at risk, BMJ 1986; 292: 1722-26.
52. Wynne G., Training and retention of skills, BMJ 1986; 293: 30-32.
53. Harries M., Drowning and near drowning, BMJ 1986; 293: 122-24.
54. Morris F., Tardoff S.G., Wallis D. and Skinner D. V., Cardiopulmonary resuscitation skills of pre registration house officers. Five Years on, BMJ 1991; 302: 626-27.
55. Cohen T.J., Tucker K.J., Lurie K.G., *et al.,* Active compression-decompression, JAMA 1994; 267: 2916-23.
56. Curry L. and Gass D., Effects of training in cardiopulmonary resuscitation on competence and patient outcome. Can. Med. Assoc. J 1987; 137: 49 1-96.
57. Kouwenhoven W.B., Jude J.R. and Knickerbocker G.G., Closed chest cardiac massage, JAMA 1960; 173: 1064-67.
58. Lurie K.G., Lindo C. and Chin J., C.P.R., The P stands for plumber's helper. JAMA 1990; 264: 1661.
59. Cohen T.J., Tucker K.J., Redberg R.F., *et al.,* Active compression-decompression resuscitation, Circulation 1991; 84:11-19.

MECHANICAL VENTILATION[1-10]

Introduction

Apart from intensive pulmonary care units, in modern intensive care management of critical problems, most of the patients need artificial respiration during some stage of their illness. With the availability of variety of ventilators and increasing medical expertise, mechanical ventilation has become easier today. Any patient who is in respiratory failure (i.e.) his arterial PO_2 is less than 60 mm of Hg, PCO_2 more than 50 mm Hg, needs ventilatory support.

The first recorded account of resuscitation by artificial respiration is by the Prophet Elisha in the old Testament. During the great epidemic of Poliomyelitis in Copenhagen in 1952 artificial respiration was used using Water's Canister and reservoir bag which was manually compressed by relays of medical students even upto three months. This method of *bag ventilation* has been extensively developed and replaced by mechanical ventilators. Artificial ventilation by intermittent positive pressure applied mechanically via a tracheostomy tube or endotracheal tube is a standard method of treatment today for respiratory failure from various causes.[1,2]

Causes of Respiratory Failure

Muscular

Tetanus.
Myasthenia.

Lungs

COPD, ARDS, Asthma, Post Operative, Drowning.

CNS

Drugs, Poisoning, Head Injuries, Infection, CVA, Status Epilepticus, Polio, Polyneuritis.

Bony Structures

Crush Injury, Thoracoplasty, Severe Scoliosis.

Guidelines to Ventilatory Support (Tables 11.44 and 11.45)

Vital capacity – < 10 ml/kg of ideal body weight.
PaO_2 – < 60 mm Hg.
Respiration rate – > 35/minute.
Inspiration force – < -25 cm H_2O_2.

The above are the criteria based on which mostly ventilatory support is initiated. But in centres, where facilities for estimating arterial blood gas or lung function are not available the following criteria are used:

a. Inability to count upto 10 in a single breath.
b. Weak cough.
c. Chest expansion less than 1 cm.
d. Tachycardia.
e. Sweating and restlessness.
f. Accessory muscles working.
g. Cyanosis and convulsions are late signs.

Table 11.44 shows different criteria for institution of mechanical ventilation.

Table 11.44: Criteria for institution of mechanical ventilation

1. Decreasing levels of consciousness
2. Vital capacity less than 15 ml/kg
3. PaO_2 less than 70 torr with fraction of inspired concentration of oxygen (FIO_2) of 0.4
4. Alveolar to arterial diffusion of oxygen (A-aDO) greater than 400 torr with FIO^2 of 1.0
5. $PaCO_2$ greater than 50 torr (in a previously homocapnic patient)
6. Dead space/Tidal volume ratio (Vd/Vt) greater than 0.6
7. Inspiratory force less than 25 cm H_2O.

Table 11.45: Guidelines indicating the use of respirator

1. Respiratory rate: More than 35/minute
2. Vital capacity: Less than 15 ml/kg body weight
3. Inspiratory force: Less than 25 cm of water
4. PaO_2: Less than 50 mm
5. pH: More than 7.25
6. Compliance: Less than 10 ml/cm of water

Ventilators are specially designed pumps to support ventilatory functions of respiratory system through oxygen provision. They offer physiologic support to stabilize patients with respiratory failure for the time they are being treated. However, in addition to lungs, mechanical ventilation also affects cardiovascular, gastrointestinal, and renal systems, other complications include decubitus ulcers, muscle deconditioning, malnutrition, venous thrombosis, depression, etc., when used for prolonged periods.[3]

Ventilatory Methods

Mouth to Mouth Breathing

Most satisfactory method available for emergency use. Being taught to medical men and public, to be exercised in time of need usually outside the hospital.

Brook Airway

An improved and pleasant way of performing mouth to mouth breathing.

Ambu Resuscitator

One of the efficient ways of initiating ventilatory support in the hospital set up and in the mobile intensive care. Performed till the patient is properly connected to the ventilator. Needs adequate training for the persons to use the Ambu's bag ventilation effectively.

Mechanical Devices

In the recent years a number of mechanical devices have been developed to maintain artificial ventilation.

Negative Pressure Ventilation

Until the mid 1950s mechanical ventilation was of the negative pressure variety—*Iron lung* or tank ventilators. Variants of tank ventilators are still employed today especially in paediatrics and rarely in adults with COPD. Iron lung ventilator encases all the patient's body except the head and negative external pressure is applied to the thoracic cage to induce inspiratory flow. Though this method obviates the need to intubate and routine nursing care, and secretions are main problems.

Positive Pressure Ventilation

In today's acute care positive pressure ventilators are preferred. These ventilators create a super atmospheric pressure in the upper airway create a pressure gradient between upper airway and lungs so that air pushes through the airways. In modern positive pressure ventilators, respiratory rates up to 60/mt is possible and when we administrate air of higher frequency rates, it is called as *Higher Frequency Positive Pressure Ventilation (HFPPV).*

High Frequency Jet Ventilation (HFJV)

Gases are delivered into the trachea by means of a narrow cannula at rates between 100 to 350 breaths per minute.

High Frequency Oscillation (HFO)

Here ventilation is done at much higher frequencies in the order of 1200 breaths per minute.

The advantages of HFPPV is that adequate gas exchange can be maintained with lower mean airway pressure. This lower airway pressure interferes less with cardiac output, reduces the risk of barotrauma and reduces leakage of air through bronchopleural fistulas. HFPPV is used in the following indications today:

i. In patients with bronchopleural fistula.
ii. During airway endoscopic procedures.
iii. In ventilator dependent patients undergoing surgeries.

Type of Ventilators[4]

Generally two types of positive preserve ventilators are available —Pressure preset and volume preset ventilators.

Volume Pressure Ventilation

These machines deliver a pre-fixed volume with each breath regardless of the pressure generated. A reduction in lung compliance or an increase in airway resistance will result in increase in pressure. These are the commonly preferred ventilators.

E.g., Bennett, Bear, Emerson, Servo Ventilators.

Pressure Preset Ventilator

With these machines, the inspiratory air pressure is preset and volume delivery depends upon the airway resistance and lung compliance. They are not preferred for continuous ventilation of patients. When used, must be carefully monitored for inadvertent hypoventilation. Chosen in certain case of COPD.

How to Connect the Patient to the Ventilators[4,5]

Steps to begin ventilatory support and patient's evaluation during mechanical ventilation are listed below in Tables 11.46 and 11.47.

Table 11.46: Steps in beginning ventilatory support
1. Patient preparation.
2. An airway establishment.
3. Manual ventilation by ambu bag to monitor patient's own breathing efforts.
4. Cardiovascular stabilization: Cardic dysarrhythmias due to hypoxia and myocardial ischaemia; hypotention due to sedatives, narcotics, muscle paralysing agents.
5. Checking the ventilatory needs.
6. Treating the cause of respiratory failure. If mechanical ventilation is used in treating respiratory failure, hypoxemia has to be corrected and alveolar ventilation must be maintained.

Table 11.47: Patient evaluation during mechanical ventilation: Check list
1. Heart rate and systemic blood pressure.
2. Temperature.
3. Venous pressure and pulmonary artery pressure.
4. Airway care: Sputum and airway infection check.
5. Physical examination of chest.
6. Fluid balance and aerosolized medication.
7. Measuring lung function tests like vital capacity and maximum inspiratory pressure.
8. Assessment of psychologic and neurological status.
9. Bladder care, patient comfort, safety and general nursing.

Having chosen the patient and types of ventilator, the physician must connect the patient to the ventilator. Though this job is done in many intensive care units by anaesthesia colleagues, internist must know to intubate himself and connect the patient to ventilator in emergencies. Patient can be connected to ventilator by the following methods:

Face Mask

Here ventilation is not efficient. Secretions clearing and abdominal distension are problems, cannot be maintained for long time.

Endotracheal Tube

The method of choice today is to initiate ventilatory support. Correctly fitting rubber or PVC tubes are introduced into trachea using a laryngoscope and connected to the ventilators. Can be maintained for 7-10 days.

Tracheostomy Tube

Rarely done these days as the first procedure except in severe neck injuries. Usually needed in prolonged ventilation where endotraecheal tubes are not advisable as, they can cause damage to oral mucosa, laryngeal and tracheal damage and difficulties in feeding. A tracheostomy tube of appropriate size is introduced through the tracheostomy and connected to the ventilator. This is a safe and convenient method. Patient can be made to sit up and take solid food. Wearing is also easier with tracheostomy than with endotracheal tube. Ventilator can be maintained for any length of time with tracheostomy.

Through the Cricothyroid Membrane

In case of emergency or failed intubation, needle or catheter can be passed through cricothyroid membrane and ventilation initiated efficiently till alternate methods are done.

Observing a Patient on Mechanical Ventilation

a. Adequacy of oxygenation checked continuously by oximetry or arterial blood gas analysis.
b. Patency of endotracheal tube (ET), Blocks in ET tube are usually reflected by a rise in inspiratory pressure. Prompt and periodic attention to secretions will maintain the patency.
c. Warning signs and trigger in the machine.
d. Air entry in the bases to be observed.
e. Blood pressure and heart rate.
f. Alertness of the patient.

Mechanical Ventilatory Modes[2,6]

Conventional Positive Pressure Ventilatory Modes

a. Control mode.
b. Assist-control mode.
c. Intermittent mandatory ventilation (IMV).
d. Synchronized IMV (SIMV).

Currently Used Modes

a. Pressure support.
b. Continuous flow apneic.
c. Airway pressure release.
d. Inverse ratio.
e. Mandatory minute.
f. Negative pleural pressure.
g. Extracorporeal CO_2 removal.

Merits of a few modes of ventilation are considered here. In modern ventilators many modes of ventilation are combined.

Controlled Ventilation

Routine mode of ventilation. The ventilator delivers breaths at intervals set on the machine. Both tidal volume and respiratory rate are programmed on the respirator. Prolonged use of this mode will lead to disuse atrophy of respiratory muscles.

Assisted Ventilation

Tidal volume is preset and respiratory frequency is determined by the patient who triggers the machine by making an inspiratory effort and the ventilator gives a positive pressure breaths. Useful to prevent respiratory muscle atrophy.

Assist Control Ventilation

Though the volume and rate are preset the machine is sensitised to respond to the patient's inspiratory effort. Accordingly the timer is automatically reset.

Intermittent Mandatory Ventilation (IMV)

IMV combines spontaneous and controlled ventilation. Between the mechanical controlled breaths, the patient can breath spontaneously. Respiratory-alkalosis is less and useful for weaning the patients.

Synchronised IMV (SIMV)

SIMV is a combination of spontaneous and assist controlled ventilation. It is assured to be more comfortable to the patient.

Pressure Support Ventilation

This is a form of pressure preset ventilation. IPP breathing is delivered at the time the patient makes an inspiration effort. A present fixed amount of pressure is applied throughout inspiration. This may not be adequate for unstable ill patient, though it may be useful for weaning.

Inverse Ratio Ventilation (IRV)

Inspiratory time is prolonged. IE Ratio is raised upto 4:1. This leads to improved oxygenation in selected case of ARDS. Very much uncomfortable for the patient and hence needs sedation.

Independent Lung Ventilation

Each lung is ventilated separately according to its requirements for ideal volume PEEP etc. A bifid endotracheal tube is connected by a single ventilator with two circuits or two ventilators.

Choice of Mode of Ventilation[6,7]

Commonly employed type is controlled mode of ventilation. Assist control and IMV are the best available, as they cause least respiratory muscle atrophy.

Ventilator Settings

Tidal Volume and Inspiration Rate

Usually tidal volume is set at a rate of 10 ml/kg of body weight. Respiratory frequency is selected to coincide with the patients normal respiratory rate. For infants it is set around 30 breaths/mt and 15 breaths/mt for adults.

Inspiratory/Expiratory Ratio

Set at a ratio of 1:1.5 or 1:2. After making the initial settings arterial blood gas estimation is done and based upon pH and PCO_2 further adjustments made.

Fraction of Inspired Oxygen (FiO_2)

All patients started on mechanical ventilation should receive initially 100% oxygen and later adjusted as per ABG results. Indiscriminate use of oxygen will lead to lung toxicity.

Sighing

Periodic hyperinflation is a reflex, normally done to prevent atelectasis. Many ventilators incorporate a *sigh mode.* In the absence, periodic Ambu ventilation will help the manoeuvre.

Inspiratory Flow Rate

Depending upon the clinical indication, the inspiratory flow rate is adjusted by trial and error and clinical assessment of the individual patient. Low flow rate may prolong inspiration, thereby decreasing cardiac output. High flow rate may improve gas exchange in COPD patient but may be uncomfortable for the patient.

Positive End Expiratory Pressure (PEEP)[8]

PEEP is the artificial maintenance of positive pressure after passive exhalation is complete.

This technique will increase end expiratory lung volume or functional residual capacity, thereby leading to opening of airways and recruitment of alveoli. Indicated in severe refractory hypoxemia, defined as PaO_2 below 50 cms Hg with the patient breathing greater than 60% oxygen for atleast 30 minutes. Advantages and disadvantages of PEEP are shown in Table 11.48.

Table 11.48: Advantages and disadvantages of PEEP

Advantages
1. It improves lung compliance.
2. Stabilizes fluid filled and atelectic alveoli.
3. Thereby prevents collapse during expiratory cycle and hence improves oxygenation.

Disadvantages
It may reduce cardiac output with hypotension, that can be countered by intravenous fluid administration.

Indications[9]

Useful in patient with ARDS and cardiogenic pulmonary oedema, improving the matching of ventilation and perfusion. Used in post surgical cases to prevent post operative atelectasis.

Application of PEEP

The approximate pressure needed has to be carefully evolved by the bed side by estimating the lung compliance, cardiac output, blood pressure and arterial blood gases. Started with 3-5 cms of water and may be increased upto 30-40 cm of water. While reducing PEEP, the procedure has to be gradually done, assessing the PaO_2.

Complications of PEEP[10-15]

Cardiovascular: PEEP may reduce cardiac output by decreasing venous return. In many cases, this reduction of cardiac output with hypotension can be managed with volume replacement and pressor drugs and may need rarely discontinuation of PEEP. Other complications include water retention in the lungs, jaundice due to portal congestion and ischaemic bowel due to reduction in splanchnic circulation.

Pulmonary: Pulmonary complications are a sequelae to barotrauma leading to pneumomediastinum, pneumothorax, subcutaneous emphysema, pneumoretroperitoneum and pneumoperitoneum. The frequency of pneumothorax may be as high as 23%. PEEP also increases the work of breathing in patients and may hinder with weaning.

Renal: Renal effects appears to be multifactorial, through direct effect on decreased cardiac output, redistribultion of renal blood flow and altered venous pressure and indirectly by sympathetic stimulation and hormonal changes in the form of increased antidiuretic hormone, altered renin-angiotension-aldosterone and decline in atrial natriuretic factor.

Gastrointestinal: Gastrointestinal complications include gastrointestinal haemorrhage, stress-related mucosal damage and oesophagitis. Other complications are given in Table 11.49.

Table 11.49: Gastrointestinal complications

Organ	*Complications*
a. Oesophagus and stomach	Oesophagitis (erosive) GER Stress ulcer Impaired gastric emptying
b. Small intestine and colon	Ileus Stress ulcer Diarrhoea Pseudo colonic obstruction Altered microflora Luminal toxins
c. Gallbladder	Atonic gallbladder Acalculous cholecystitis
d. Liver	Increased bilirubin or transaminase levels Impaired drug metabolism
e. Pancrease	Acute pancreatitis

Weaning From the Ventilator

Having connected the patient to the ventilator physician must know when to detach the patient from it and how. Most of the patients on short term ventilation are easy to wean and the problem is with long term ventilated patients for more than a month. Premature attempts of weaning will make subsequent attempts more difficult. Weaning will be considered when the patient is able to trigger the ventilator by dropping the intratracheal pressure. Guidelines for weaning and its assessment are shown in Tables 11.50 and 11.51 respectively.

Table 11.50: Guidelines for weaning

1. Verbal explanation to the patient, especially regarding reconnection to the ventilator if necessary.
2. Baseline measurement of (Airways) of respiratory rate, BP, pulse and arterial blood gases.
3. Deflation of tracheal cuff, ET tube or tracheostomy tube. Supplemental oxygen with humidified air is given through T tube adaptor, keeping FiO_2 10 mm Hg higher than when the patient was on ventilator.
4. Look for vital signs for half an hour, perform arterial blood gases analysis and if patient can tolerate an hour spontaneous breathing.

Table 11.51: To assess weaning of ventilated patient

1. *Clinical factors:* a. Electrolytes, blood sugar, fluid balance and acid base balance b. Body temperature, anemia, malnutrition, pain, renal functions, psychological condition and state of consciousness c. Cardiac output, cardiac arrhythmias, blood pressure, exercise tolerance and infection.
2. *Respiratory evaluation:* Respiratory rate less than 25 per minute Tidal volume more than 3-5 ml/lb of body weight Minute volume less than 10 l/minute Vital capacity more than 15-20 ml/kg Oxygen status, dynamic compliance more than 25 m/cm of H_2O_2 MVV should be atleast 2X minute volume Ventilatory pattern synchronous and stable.
3. *Signs measuring increase workload of breathing:* Using accessory muscles, asynchronous breathing, disphoresis, tachypnoea, substernal or intercostal retraction, 1.8 kg/minute (measured work of breathing) or 15% of total VO_2.

Indications

When the following criteria are fulfilled, successful weaning will usually be possible. For weaning, the patient must be conscious, well oriented and cooperative.

Inspiratory Force: The patient should be able to generate a negative pressure of greater than 20 cm of H_2O_2.

Vital Capacity: Vital capacity must be equal to or exceeding 10 ml/kg.

Minute Ventilation: Resting minute ventilation must be 10 litre per minute and should be able to double it with a maximum ventilatory effort.

Respiratory Muscles During Spontaneous Breathing: Diaphragm, chest muscles and abdominal muscles must be watched for their rate, depth and pattern of movement. Any fatigue or paradoxical abdominal movement indicate unsuccessful weaning.

Methods

Tube or Trial and Error Method—Conventional Method

T-tube is connected to endotracheal or tracheostomy tube through which O_2 is administered and patient is closely watched.

IMV Technique

The technique allows the patient to assume respiratory work gradually. Ventilatory breaths are regularly interspersed between patient's spontaneous breathing. This is advantageous over conventional weaning.

Other Weaning Techniques

1. Pressure support ventilation.
2. Continuous positive airway pressure (CPAP) breathing.

When to Stop Weaning Attempt

1. PAO_2 falls below 55 mm Hg.
2. Acute hypercapnia.
3. Clinical deterioration —Muscle failure, change in vital sign, etc.
4. Patient requests for ventilator.

Failure to Wean (Table 11.52)

Table 11.52: Causes of weaning failure

1. Premature attempts
2. Defective acid base balance
3. Disturbed ventilatory control
4. Muscular dysfunction

I. Attempts to increase respiratory muscle strength
   a. Reverse malnutrition.
   b. Reverse metabolic deficiencies—Calcium, magnesium, potassium etc.
   c. Discontinue all sedation.
   d. Use theophylline as direct respiratory centre and diaphragmatic stimulator.
   e. Use sitting posture —Diaphragm may function better.
   f. Consider use of progesterone as a respiratory centre stimulant.
   g. Evaluate for the presence of organic neuromuscular disease.
   h. Consider drug induced neuromuscular dysfunction. E.g. Aminoglycosides.

II. Attempts to decrease respiratory muscle demand
   a. Treat infection adequately and decrease metabolic requirements.
   b. Keep the lung dry and less stiff.
   c. Decrease airway resistance by use of theophylline and beta agonists.
   d. Try with large size endotracheal tube.
   e. Try a course of steroids in COPD.
   f. Calorie intake must be met more by fats and not by carbohydrates.
   g. Underlying cardiac disorder is looked for and corrected.

h. IMV may be discontinued and conventional method tried.

Weaning from Intra Tracheal Intubation

After weaning the patient from the mechanical ventilator, either endotracheal tube or tracheostomy tube must be extubated. Before removing either tube, keep another endotracheal tube ready so that reintubation can be immediately done in case of emergency.

Before removing the tracheostomy tube, assess whether he can breath without, it by plugging it. Before doing it check whether it is a fenestrated tube and fenestrations are patent.

Complications of Mechanical Ventilation

Complication of Intubation and Extubation

Injury to cervical spine, cornea, nasal and oral mucosa. Damage to teeth, pharynx, larynx and oesophagus. Dislocation of arytenoids and aspiration.

Stimulation of nerves of pharynx, larynx and trachea may cause laryngeal spasm, bronchospasm, cardiac arrhythmias or hypotension.

Extubation may cause trauma to glottis and airway obstruction from oedema.

Complication of Endotracheal and Tracheostomy Tubes

Early: Ventilatory obstruction, aspiration, bleeding, pneumothorax and rarely rupture of trachea.

Late: Sore throat, dysphagia, vocal cord paralysis, laryngitis, sinusitis, pneumonia, tracheal stenosis.

Though all these complications are theoretically possible, careful attention to selection of size and material of the tube, cuff inflation pressure and keeping the ventilation parameters to minimum, will result in safe intubation, ventilation and extubation.

Complications Due to Ventilator

Machine failure, alarm failure, inadequate humidification, overheating of inspired air and bacterial contamination. All these complications can be prevented or minimised by efficient care.

Medical Complications During Assisted Ventilation

Pulmonary: Alveolar hypoventilation and hyper ventilation can occur. Barotrauma causing pneumomediastinum and pneumothorax, and atelectasis and pneumonia can occur.

Cardiac: Hypotension due to reduction in cardiac output and decrease in venous return. Water retention due to increased circulating ADH and various arrhythmias can occur.

Gastric: Gastric dilatation, ulcerations and bleeding can occur. Sucralfate is very much effective in preventing stress ulcer and can cause lesser incidence of pneumonia. Causes of sudden respiratory distress during mechanical ventilation are shown in Table 11.53.

Table 11.53: Causes of sudden respirato ry distress during mechanical ventilation
1. *Airway problems:* Bronchospasm, pulmonary oedema, pneumothorax, hyperinflation, abnormal respiratory drive.
2. *Ventilator related causes*: Circuit malfunction, inadequate FiO_2, inadequate ventilatory support, patient ventilator asynchrony.
3. *Miscellaneous:* Abdominal distension, anxiety, drug induced problems.

Mechanical ventilation is a life-saving procedure.[10] This procedure needs a team work by intensive care physician, anaesthetists, internists, nursing staff and physiotherapist and also involves lot of equipments like ventilators, ABG analyser etc. In places where adequate facilities do not exist, the physician incharge must be able to intubate and connect the patient to a volume preset ventilator. Care in selecting the patient, endotracheal tube or tracheostomy tube, type of ventilator, time of weaning and aseptic nursing with watchful expectancy for ventilator complication are the sheet anchors of favourable outcome. With these cautions the mortality has been reduced in modern Intensive Respiratory Care units from 30-40% to 10-20%.

REFERENCES

1. James M. Rippe., *Mechanical Ventilation*, Manual of Intensive Medical Care 1989; 160-180.
2. Arulraj S., *Mechanical ventilation* In, Chandrasekharan S., ED, Medicine Update API; Bombay 1993; 3: 129-39.
3. Daga M. K., Tiwari N., Non-pulmonary complications of mech. ventilation; In; Gupta S.B.; ed.; Med Update 2002; 12: 697-703.
4. Stock M.C., Mechanical Ventilation, Old Vs New, Critical Care Medicine 1987; 15:462.
5. Stone P. A., *et al.*, How to perform tracheal intubation, Journal of Applied Medicine 1991; 17:6 373.
6. Kulpati D. D. S., Newer modes of ventilation in critical cases; In; Y. P. Munjal (Ed.); PG Med., API 1999; 13:130-41.
7. Bhagwati A. M., PEEP and its complications; In; Gupta S. B. ed., Med. Update API 2002; 12: 693-96.
8. Bhagwati A. M., Oxygen therapy; In; Gupta S. B. ed., Med. Update; API 2002; 12: 686-92.
9. Marini J. J. Evolving concepts in ventilatory management of ARDS; In; Recent advances in mechanical ventilation; Clinics in Chest Med. 1996; 17: 555-76.
10. Welsh D. A. *et al.*, Haemodynamic consequences of mech ventilation; Clin. Pulm. Med 1999; 6:52-65.

11. Liolios A., *et al.*, GI complications in ICUS; Chest Med 1999; 20: 329-45.
12. Wilmer A., *et al.*, Duodenogastro-esophageal reflux and oesophageal mucosal injury in mechanically ventilated patients; Gastroenterology 1999; 116: 1293-99.
13. Melin M. M., *et al.*, Percutaneous cholecystostomy—A valuable technique in high risk patients with presumed acute cholecystitis; Br. J. Surg 1995; 82: 1274-77.
14. Gommonpila 5., *et al.*, Effect of positive and negative expiratory pressure on renal function; B. J. Anasth 1997; 49: 199-205.
15. Guidelines 2000 for Cardiopulmonary Resuscitation and Emergency Cardiovascular Care; Part 3; Adult Basic Life Support; The Amer. Heart Assn. in collaboration with the International Liaison Committee on Resuscitation; Circulation 2000; 102:122.

RESPIRATORY PROBLEMS IN NEUROMUSCULAR DISORDERS

Respiratory muscles may be involved in the disease of the peripheral nerves, neuromuscular junction and muscles.[1] The involvement is generally symmetrical. The diaphragm, intercostal muscles or abdominal muscles may be affected to a variable extent.[2] There can be kyphoscoliosis due to involvement of axial muscles. The respiratory centre may also be damaged in poliomyelitis. All these affect pulmonary functions.

Neuromuscular disorders affecting the respiratory muscles are as follows:

Neural:	Poliomyelitis; Infective polyneuritis; Acute intermittent porphyria; and Motor neurone disease.
Neuromuscular junction:	Myasthenia gravis; Tetanus; Botulism; Organophosphorous insecticides; and curare like drugs.
Muscle:	Muscular dystrophy; Myotonias; and Polymyositis.

There may be sufficient ventilatory dysfunction to cause dyspnoea. Severe disorders result in respiratory failure, hypoventilation, hypoxaemia and hypercapnia. The volume capacity and capability during both inspiration and expiration is decreased. There is decrease in vital capacity, voluntary ventilation and total lung capacity (TLC) although there is no obstruction to the expiratory flow. This all occurs due to weakness of respiratory muscles. RV may be slightly increased due to increased pressure. Despite reduction in vital capacity, distribution of inspired gas in the lung remains normal. The diffusion capacity is not affected. The arterial blood gases are maintained within normal limits, except in severe cases. The sedatives, narcotics and muscle relaxants are better avoided in these patients. Administer aminoglycoside antibiotics, polymyxin, quinidine and propranolol with caution.[1]

Hypoventilation with increasing hypercapnia may occur with acute neuromuscular weakness. The respiratory failure may develop rapidly in some acute neuromuscular disorders and it is self-limited. The respiratory muscle weakness can be monitored by repeated measurement of the vital capacity or inspiratory force. If the patient is unable to count upto 20 without catching his breath, it implies imminent respiratory failure.[2] Frank hypercapnia may require to ventilatory assistance; relieve dyspnoea, to give rest to the respiratory muscles and to allow sleep.

In acute conditions such as myasthenia gravis, infective polyneuritis or poliomyelitis where ventilatory abnormalities are potentially reversible, it is advisable to offer ventilatory assistance as soon as the progressive fall in respiratory muscle function is noticed. There is progressive diminution in muscle force. It can be determined by inspiratory force (MIF) and by vital capacity. The patient is also not able to generate sufficient force for an effective cough. The secretions get accumulated in the airways and result in areas of atelectasis.[1]

In patients with chronic neuromuscular diseases (motor neurone disease, muscular dystrophy and poliomyelitis), respiratory failure may be precipitated by pulmonary infection and abdominal operation. There is decrease in TLC and pulmonary compliance. These patients use much of the reserve capacity and are compensated without being aware of chronic hypoventilation and hypoxaemia. Ultimately it leads to pulmonary hypertension and cor pulmonale.[1]

Pulmonary Involvement in Poliomyelitis[3,4]

It is an acute infectious disease caused by enterovirus and has global prevalence. Clinically the illness may be varying from a mild attack to extensive paralytic attack involving any group of muscles, respiratory failure and may prove fatal. Varieties type (1) being quite common and type (3) being least common cause of paralytic poliomyelitis. Orofaecal route is the most common mode of infection and patient passes poliovirus into the faeces 6-8 weeks after the onset of illness.

The virus multiplies in the intestine and travels to the regional lymph nodes, with a transitory viremia. As a result, antibodies are produced which counteraffect the illness, neutralise the virus and hence the illness is aborted. In the absence of host defence, steroid therapy, other illnesses etc. the virus involves the nervous system either via neural pathway or through haematogenous route.

Pathology includes the nervous system involvement depending upon the area involved by neural injury, perivascular infiltration and nuclear changes in the cells. Upto this stage the process is reversible and later on perivascular cuffing occurs. The symptoms depend on the areas affected in the nervous system.

Clinical features occur after 1-2 weeks of incubation period. Minor illness may go away by itself with non-specific symptoms, sore throat, bodyachc, abdominal and generalised pains, headache, vomiting etc. And there is no neurological involvement. Major illness includes: (1) Aseptic meningitis, (2) Paralytic poliomyelits, (3) Respiratory symptom involvement.

In paralytic poliomyelitis, tremors and weakness of tendon reflexes occurs before the muscle paralysis in spinal form. Respiratory difficulty occurs in involvement of diaphragm and intercostal muscles. In bulbar or bulbospinal form, which is generally life threatening illness, weakness of soft palate, pharynx and vocal cords occurs following paralysis of vagus nerve. Voice becomes hoarse, acquiring nasal tone, secretions get pooled in the pharynx and aspiration of secretions causing aspiration pneumonia and atelectasis.

Respiration becomes shallow and irregular following involvement of respiratory center. Respiratory involvement occurs because of paralysis of intercostal muscles, bulbar paralysis and aspiration of secretion into the lungs. These complications are seen in 5 to 10% of cases. Table 11.54 shows respiratory care suggested in inflammatory neuropathies.

Prevention

Prevention lies in proper vaccination under natural immunization programme and improving sanitary conditions. Infectious diseases including poliomyelitis pose bigger threat than AIDS in the developing countries even today.[5] National programme to give polio vaccine 2 booster doses orally, irrespective of immunization status, is a good step for healthier India. Recent 2011 reports show the greatest effort by India in getting the nation polio free.

Treatment

Complete rest, care of the paralysed limb, good nursing, nutrition care and physiotherapy are important measures of general management of the disease; respiratory failure is managed by mechanical ventilators through assisted respiration. Prevention of aspiration and intensive care by a team of pulmonologist, anaesthetist and general physician generally benefits.

REFERENCES

1. Shankar P.S., *Chest Medicine,* 4th Ed. Oxford and IBH Publi. Co. N. Delhi, 1994.
2. Wartery R. V., Assessment of respirtatory failure in poliomyelitis BMJ 1959; 2: 82.
3. Hill R., *et al.,* Sleep apnoea syndrome after poliomyelitis: Amer Rev Resp Dis 1983; 127: 129.
4. Ghai O.P., *Essential paediatrics,* 2nd ed, Interprint, N. Delhi, 1990.
5. Bhatia R.S., Typhoid-changing trends in presentation and treatment; Curr, Med. Pract 1992; 36:109.

RESPIRATORY DISORDERS RELATED TO SLEEP

Sleep is a non-homogeneous phenomenon having two distinct forms called rapid-eye movement (REM) and non-rapid-eye movement (NREM) sleep. REM sleep shows bursts of rapid eye movements and the skeletal muscle tones is decreased. NREM sleep exhibits four stages demonstrating a progression into deeper stages of sleep. REM and NREM sleeps alternate in a cyclic fashion throughout the night in a normal adult and are governed by the 100 minute ultradian rhythm.[1] Various stages are listed in Table 11.55.

Table 11.55: Classification of sleep stages by Rechtschaffen and Kales

1. 1st stage: NREM (Non-rapid eye movement) sleep
2. 2nd stage: NREM sleep
3. 3rd stage: NREM sleep
4. 4th stage: NREM sleep and REM sleep

Table 11.54: Respiratory care in inflammatory neuropathies

1. 10-20% of patients develop respiratory insufficiency, requiring assisted ventilation.			
2. Bed side assessment of adequacy of respiratory capacity can be made by respiratory rate, single breath count, breathholding time, chest expansion and blood pressure recording.			
3. Assessment of vital capacity is superior to arterial blood gas analysis: Vital normal capacity in males, females and children respectively.	25 ml × height in cm	20 ml × height in cm	200 × age in years

Breathing and Sleep[2,3]

The two forms of sleep affect the breathing patterns by influencing the respiratory stability and its drive. During REM sleep, the breathing is irregular with short periods of central apnoea of 10 to 20 seconds duration, due to phasic automatic and neuromuscular discharges. The central nervous system exhibits fluctuation between a stage of wakefulness and sleep during light stages (stages 1 to 2) of NREM sleep. It is due to variation in neural stimuli to the medullary respiratory neurones. The neural stimuli and the chemical respiratory stimuli interact to bring about an instability in the respiratory drive, manifested with waxing and waning of ventilation (periodic breathing). The periodic breathing is absent during deeper stages of sleep (stages 3 and 4), as there is a significant fall in the neural inputs. During those stages, breathing is regulated by the metabolic control system in the brainstem and respiration is regular.

The respiratory drive is weak during sleep than during wakefulness. The reduction in the skeletal muscle tone seen in REM sleep is associated with a decrease in intercostal and accessory muscle activity and partial collapse of the rib cage without affecting the diaphragm. During NREM sleep there is a decrease in the diaphragmatic drive and it is associated with a small reduction in ventilation and a decrease in PaO_2 of 5 to 10 mm Hg.

Sleep also has an effect on the upper respiratory passages. The upper airway resistance is significantly increased during NREM sleep compared with the wakeful state. The muscle tone and the phasic respiratory discharges of the upper airway dilator muscles are lost during REM sleep thereby further increasing in the upper airway resistance.[3]

The influence of sleep on breathing is not of much consequence in health, its effect on individuals with chronic obstructive pulmonary diseases, primary alveolar hypoventilation syndrome and diaphragmatic paralysis has significant clinical consequences.[2]

Sleep Apnoea

Normal individuals exhibit one or two apnoeic episodes at the onset of sleep or during periods of REM sleep. Apnoea is of brief duration and is not repetitive.

Sleep Apnoea Syndrome

Sleep apnoea syndrome is said to affect 1% of population, refers to disturbed sleep and respiration. It may be potentially life-threatening.[4] The nocturnal events produce features, both during sleep and during daytime. It is characterised by intermittent absence of airflow at the nose and mouth for more than 15 seconds during sleep.[5] The apnoeic episodes are repetitive and result in sleep arousal. They occur at a rate greater than 20 per hour of sleep and are associated with marked fall in arterial oxygen saturation (SaO_2). Sleep fragmentation and hypoxia are responsible for the clinical abnormalities.[2]

Types of Sleep Apnoeas

Sleep apnoea syndrome is more common in adult males especially the idiopathic variety. Three types of apnoeas have been described: central, obstructive and mixed depending on the existence of respiratory effects.[1] Often the apnoeic episodes are mixed. Different types are listed in Table 11.56.

Table 11.56: Types of sleep apnoea

1. Obstructive apnoea in which oronasal airflow is blocked and diaphragmatic efforts continue.
2. Central apnoea in which diaphragmatic and intercostal efforts cease.
3. Mixed apnoea in which periods of obstructive apnoea follow periods of central apnoea.
4. Sleep related changes in patients with chronic obstructive airflow obstruction and asthma are increasingly being recognised.

Respiratory efforts of the chest in central apnoea are stopped. Drive to the diaphragm and the intercostal muscles is absent and they do not contract during the period of apnoea and there are intermittent respiratory arrests. Obstructive sleep apnoea is most common.

In obstructive sleep apnoea, extrathoracic upper airway is obstructed at the level of oropharynx. The cyclical respiratory efforts of the diaphragm and chest wall muscles are present throughout the episodes of apnoea. But they are ineffective and do not result in airflow. There is paradoxical collapse of the chest during respiratory attempts.[2]

Mixed apnoeas begin as central events and are followed by obstructive patterns of apnoea in the same individuals,[6] as a variant of obstructive apnoea.

Central Apnoea

Central apnoea is encountered in drowsy patients who are going to sleep or during REM sleep in persons over the age of 50 years.

Periodic alteration in respiration with apnoea appears to be due to an instability in the automatic control of respiration (periodic or Cheyne-Stokes respiration) in an otherwise intact respiratory control system. There is periodic fluctuation in muscle one and power in REM sleep due to transient abolition of central drive to the ventilatory muscles. The sequence of events are similar to those occurring in obstructive apnoea.[7] Decreased muscle tones during bursts of rapid eye movement are associated with apnoea. In high altitude, hyperventilation alkalaemia results in an imbalance of respiratory control between central and peripheral chemoreceptors. Such an imbalance is also seen in congestive heart failure. Brainstem disorders body affect respiratory control. The automatic control of breathing can be severely affected in supratentorial mass lesion and in Ondine's curse. The later condition exhibits failure of automatic ventilation with intact voluntary control. It results following bilateral cervical cordotomies.[2]

The patients may be asymptomatic. Sleep is fragmented or deprived when the apnoeic episodes are frequent or long. The patient will wake up frequently. There is insomnia that affects patient's activities during the day time and make him lethargic. The most frequent instability is transient fall in PCO_2 levels below the critical PCO_2 value required for systromic respiration.[8] Hence, an apnoea develops.[5]

There may be features of myxoedema, congestive heart failure or brainstem disease. Clinical examination may be non-contributory.

Obstructive Apnoea

This is generally due to occlusion of nasopharynx and oropharynx and is commonly seen in male patients after 30-60 years presenting with history of snoring.[5] Recumbency increases airways resistance. The posterior displacement of the tongue and soft palate bring about their apposition with the posterior pharyngeal wall.[9] The air flow stops at the mouth and nose for periods of 10 seconds or more (apnoea), accompanied by continuing repiratory movements is called obstructive apnoea. And occurrence of more than 5 apnoeas per hour or more than 35 per night, during sleep, with frequent arousals, unrestful sleep, followed by daytime hypersomnolence constitutes obstructive sleep apnoea syndrome (OSAS).[10-12] It results in obstruction to airflow, decreased alveolar ventilation and progressive asphyxia. Then apnoea is terminated by a brief arousal from sleep. Wakefulness is associated with activation of upper airways muscles, restoration of patency of the upper airway and resumption of airflow. The decreased pharyngeal muscular tone due to effect of sleeping predisposes to an inspiratory collapse of the upper airways.[13] Obesity, thick neck and small pharynx with or without tonsils and adenoids are other predisposing factors. Again the patient goes back to sleep and there is repetition of sequence of events often 400 to 500 times per night.[3] OSA and systemic disorders are shown in Tables I to VII.

Table I
OSA and Hypertension

OSA
- One of the important causes of reversible hypertension.
- 25% of hypertensives have obstructive sleep apnea.
- Long term use of CPAP results reduction of HT both in awake and during sleep. Even cardiovascular events get substantial reduction.

Table II
Sleep Apnea and Coronary Artery Disease

- Greater risk of CAD in sleep related disorders.
- 20 fold risk of developing MI in untreated OSA.
- Almost one third of CAD patients have sleep related disorder.
- Concomitant CAD and sleep apnea patients experience myocardial ischemia atleast in 30% of patients.

Table III
OSA and Diabetes

- OSA and insulin resistance are closely associated.
- CPAP treated OSA in diabetic patients results in favourable control of hyperglycemia.

Table IV
OSA and Stroke

- 50% reduction in central blood flow during apneic and hypoapneic events.
- Factors pointing stroke in OSA are nocturnal desaturations, autonomic instability and increased intracranial pressure which reduce cerebral perfusion pressure.
- Elevated catecholamines in OSA also promote thrombosis.
- Higher prevalence of OSA in acute stroke has also been observed.
- Morning headache in OSA patients occurs as a consequence of cyclic hypoxemia.
- Treatment of OSA collects basic defect i.e. cyclic hypoxia and accompanying cardiovascular and metabolic consequences.

Table V
OSA and Mood

- OSA and depression are closely associated.
- Depression promotes daytime sleepiness.

Table VI
OSA and Fatty Liver

- Obesity and insulin resistance are in the centre stage but factors for progression and transformation are still eluding.
- Cyclic hypoxemia and sympathetic stimulation in OSA cause liver injury.
- Recurrence in liver insult possibly transform hepatic steatosis to hepatic inflammation and subsequently cirrhosis.

Table VII
OSA and Pregnancy

- Sleep disordered breathing in pregnancy adversely affects both mother and foetus.
- Low birth weight babies constitute almost one fourth in India and is associated with elevated glucocorticoid levels in later life.

A majority of obstructive apnoeic episodes are encountered in patients where already some degree of upper airways obstruction is existing. There may be some structural defect causing airways size reduction creating *pharyngeal crowding* or high upstream airways resistance causing *upper airways* collapse.[14] The obstruction may be in the nose (deviated nasal septum, blocked nose, rhinitis, nasopharyngeal stenosis), pharynx (macroglossia, micrognathia, hypognathia, large uvula, vertical mucosal folding of pharyngeal mucosa, enlarged tonsils and adenoids, lingual and pharyngeal cysts, retropharyngeal masses, swelling of epiglottis, infiltration of the soft tissues with fat as in obesity or myxomatous tissue as in myxoedema or acromegaly, mucopolysacchariodoses and myotonic dystrophy) or larynx (Shy-Dragger syndrome associated with decreased abduction of the vocal cords due to brainstem damage).[12] Alcohol is often a co-factor. Apnoea is associated with oxygen desaturation and a marked fall in tissue oxygen concentration during sleep. Recently an increased risk of OSA among COPD/Bronchial asthma has been suggested.[15] A link between obstructive sleep apnoea and insulin resistance, independent of obesity, has also been documented.[16,17] The clinical features noted during night time are severe snoring, excessive motor activity in the form of flailing of the limbs and thrashing about in bed, recurrent awakenings and insomnia. The intermittent snoring and frequent arousals occur due to a combination of hypoxia and hypercapnia. There can be impotency. There are day time manifestations in the form of awakening unrefreshed in the morning, day-time hypersomnolence, intellectual deterioration in the form of personality disturbance, memory loss and poor judgement.[1] Weight reduction is not helpful in all adult snorers.[18]

Progressive asphyxia is associated with acute pulmonary vasoconstriction and pulmonary hypertension. Though pulmonary artery pressure returns to normal level during wakefulness in a majority of the patients, the nocturnal event may be accentuated in patients with obstructive airways diseases associated with sustained day time hypoxaemia, hypercapnia and polycythemia in 10-15% of patients.[5] Such an event leads to the right heart failure. All such patients are obese and may well fit into pickwickian syndrome.[5] Cardiac arrhythmias (ventricular premature beats and ventricular tachycardia) may be noted, which may cause death during sleep[12] but further corroborative data is lacking.[3] Following Tables show OSA and its untoward effects.

Obstructive Sleep Apnoea (OSA)

i. OSA is a condition of cessation of airflow in air tube during sleep, because of collapse of airway walls, leading to obstruction.
ii. 5% of adult population suffers from the condition.
iii. Higher risk in snorers.

Untoward Effects of OSA

1. Lethargy and daytime drowsiness.
2. Higher risk of road traffic and industrial accidents.
3. Reduced concentration, memory and judgement.
4. Excess of carbondioxide in circulation and retension of the same lead to morning headache.
5. OSA is associated with refractory hypertension, ischemic heart disease, arrhythmia, heart failure and even higher risk of occlusive stroke from hypercoagulable state.
6. Obesity, insulin resistance, lysine resistance and higher serum levels of homocysteine are associated with OSA.
7. Polysomnography is gold standard for diagnosis of OSA.
8. Nasal CPAP is widely used effective therapy. Surgery and placement of intraoral devices have limited role.

Investigation

To look for the site of obstruction, local examination of the nose and pharynx by indirect is useful.[1] The lateral radiogram and CT scanning of the nasopharyngeal region may reveal the presence of small oropharyngeal lumen.[9] The existence of the upper airways obstruction is confirmed by pulmonary function tests and the patients with obstructive apnoea demonstrate a characteristic saw tooth appearance of the flow volume loop.[12] Table 11.57 gives the parameters used for determining the sleep stages.

Table 11.57: The parameters used for determination of sleep stages[19]

1. Electroencephalogram (EEG)
2. Electro-Oculogram (EOG)
3. Electro-Myogram (EMG)

The diagnostic findings in obstructive apnoea are episodes of cessation of airflow at nose and mouth despite evidence of continuing respiratory efforts, and can be investigated definitely by gold standard investigation polysomnography, which includes (a) detailed recording of ECG variables during sleep and its various stages; (b) ventilatory variables identifying both obstructive and central apnoeas; and (c) heart rate. Monitoring of movements of rib cage and abdomen is done with impedence plethysmography. The negative pressure applied at the nose to cause obstruction of the upper airway may be -3 cm H_2O_2 in cases of obstructive sleep apnoea (normal -15 cm H_2O). Monitoring of oxygen saturation with an ear lobe oximeter or in-dwelling arterial line, demonstrates presence of recurrent episodes of arterial oxygen desaturation (fall in SaO_2 of 4 per cent or more from the preceding stable SaO_2 when asleep). Overnight Holter cardiac monitoring is helpful to demonstrate cyclical fluctuations of the heart rate.[12] Berlin questionnaire is found to be a better screening tool than Epworth sleepiness scale for Indian patients with sensitivity of 92% and 68% respectively in screening OSA.

Treatment

Respiratory depressants, hypnotics and anti-histaminics should be stopped. The intake of alcoholic beverages must be stopped.[20] It is necessary to treat congestive heart failure and the hypothyroid state. Replacement therapy with thyroxin may lead to a reduction of pharyngeal myxoid tissue. Weight reduction is essential for obese patients. Great care has to be taken while administering general anaesthetics to the patients with sleep apnoea.[21]

The symptoms may be relieved in specific cases by removal of nasal polyp, correction of deviated nasal septum, lengthening of a short mandible and removal of tonsils and adenoids.[2]

Nasal sprays of nasal decongestants can be used in acute and chronic rhinitis. Drugs with respiratory stimulating action (acetazolamide, progesterone) or general neuroactive effects (tricyclic antidepressants) may be useful. Acetazolamide in a dose of 125 to 250 mg at bed time increases breathing by producing metabolic acidosis.[22] It relieves apnoeic episodes especially in central apnoea. Breathing can be improved by drugs which produce carotid body stimulation such as intravenous prochlorperazine (a dopamine blocking agent) or oral almitrine in a dose of 200 mg daily.[23] Medroxyprogesterone acetate (60 to 120 mg a day) acts a respiratory stimulant in patients with central apnoea. It reduces duration of apnoea and day time sleepiness. Strychnine may help to increase the muscle tone in a small number of patients. Tricyclic antidepressant such as protriptyline, is useful in obstructive sleep apnoea.[24] It acts by increasing the tone of the upper airway muscles. It reduces the amount of REM sleep and the time during which obstruction may occur.

Inconsistent results have been obtained with nocturnal oxygen therapy in sleep apnoea syndrome as it helps to reduce the total duration of apnoea and the number of cardiac arrhythmias. Use of nasopharyngeal airways has been tried as a simple, inexpensive and yet an effective mode of therapy.[12,25]

A continuous positive airways pressure with a mask in the from of nasal CPAP to the nose helps in prevention of airway collapse in nearly 80% cases.[5] It has shown to be beneficial in the treatment of central and obstructive sleep apnoea and in prevention of snoring.[26] The precise mechanism by which CPAP provides relief in central apnoea is not clear.[5] A lower pressure of 3 to 6 cm H_2O applied to upper airway may help in relieving apnoea in all stages of sleep and daytime somnolence and it is possible to eliminate snoring by a higher pressure of 5 to 13 cm H_2O. The treatment may not be necessary every night. Nasal CPAP has made tracheostomy virtually obsolete. CPAP is useful to add life to life in OSA patients. Additionally it reduces blood pressure, improves cardiovascular functioning, reverse metabolic syndrome, reduce albuminuria and reduce day time sleepiness.[27] Although tracheostomy has shown to be useful in the treatment of individuals in whom nasal CPAP cannot be used or has been found not to be effective providing immediate relief. It helps in bypassing the obstruction during sleep.[2] It interferes with speech and patient suffers from chronic cough.[28]

Extensive surgical resection of soft tissue in the oropharynx in the form of uvulopalatopharyngoplasty may help in eliminating the obstruction[29] in more than 50% of cases. The procedure consists of submucosal resection of redundant tissue from the tonsillar pillars to aryepiglottic folds. Other surgical procedures include expansion hyoidplasty to increase the size of the hypopharynx. The unacceptable method—tracheostomy and the unpredictable method-uvulo-palato-pharyngoplasty, are still prevalent as attractive modes of treatment in this part of tropic.[2] Those who do not get benefit from operation, are unlikely to derive benefit from the CPAP as CPAP fails to open the closed upper airways.[30] Sleep clinics help early diognosis and after effective management to lead a better social life. Various modes of management are shown in the following table.

Management of OSA[31,32]

1. **General measure**
   1. Sleep on one side
   2. Reduce obesity
2. **CPAP–Choice treatment**
   - Safe, effective
   - Acceptable
   - Portable
   - Immediately relieving
3. **Non-CPAP management**
   a. Surgery–Uvulopalatopharyngoplasty (UPPP)
   b. Oral appliances
   c. Tracheostomy

REFERENCES

1. Shankar P. S., Sleep apnoea/hypoapnoea syndrome, Ind J Clin Pract 1993; 4: 34-36.
2. Shankar P. S., Chest Medicine; Oxford and IBH Publ. Co.; N. Delhi 1994; 4th ed.
3. Mathew C. P. and Remmers J. E., Respiratory function of upper airway. In: N. A. Saunders and C. E. Sullivans (eds), Sleep and Breathing. Lung Biology in health and disease. New York, Marcel Dekker, XX 1984; 21: 163-200.
4. Nasser S., Rees P.J. Sleep apnoea; Causes, consequences and treatment; Brit J. Chin. Pract 1992;46(1):39-43.
5. Wilson J. D., *et al.*, (ed), Harrison's Principles of internal medicine, 12th ed, Vol. 2, McGraw Hill, New York, 1991.
6. Cherniack N. S., Sleep apnoea and its causes, J Clin Invest 1984; 73: 1501-06.
7. Plum F. Leigh R.J., Abnormalities of central mechanisms, In: Regulation of Respiration, Hornbein T.F. (ed): Lung Biology

in Health and Disease, Vol (17), Marcel Deckker, N. York, 1981.
8. Cherniack N. S., Longobardo G. S., Abnormalities in respiratory rhythm, In: Hand Book of Physiology, The Resp. System, Vol. 2. Control of breathing, Cherniack N. S., Widdecombe J. G., (ed), Bethesda M. D., Amer. Phys. Soc., 1986.
9. Suratt P. M., Dee P., Atkinson R. L., *et al.*, Fluorscopic and CT features of the pharyngeal airway in obstructive apnoea, Amer Rev Resp Dis 1983; 127: 487-92.
10. NHLB Workshop summary, Respiratory disorders of sleep, Amer Rev Res Dis 1987; 136: 755-61.
11. Lavie P., Incidence of sleep apnoea in a presumably healthy working population; Sleep 1983; 136: 312-18.
12. Kalra S., *et al.*, Obstructive sleep apnoea syndrome, Ind J Chest Dis and All Sci 1990; 32: 189-92.
13. Lopes J. M., *et al.*, Total airways resistance and repiratory muscle activity during sleep, J Appl Physiol 1983; 54: 773-77.
14. Thawley S. E., Ed, Sleep apnoea disorders, Med Clin N, Amer 1985; 169: 6.
15. Kumar R; *et al.*, OSA and atopy among middle aged COPD and bronchial asthma patients; JAPI 2013; 61: 615-18.
16. Punjabi N.M. *et al.*, Sleep disordered breathing and insulin resistance in middle aged and overweight men; Amer J Resp Crit Care Med 2002; 165: 677-82.
17. IP S.M. *et al.*, OSA is independently associated with insulin resistance; Amer J Resp Crit Care Med 2002; 165: 670-76.
18. Shukla AD; *et al.*, Does weight reduction help all adult snorers? Lung India 2013; 30: 16-19.
19. Shneerson J., Modern management of excessive sleepiness; Med Update 1999; 7: 905-09.
20. Taasan V. C., Block J. A., Boyson P. G., *et al.*, Alcohol increases sleep apnoea and oxygen desaturation in asymptomatic men, Amer J Med 1981; 71: 240-45.
21. Strohl K. P., Bedline S., Nasal CPAP therapy, Upper airway muscle activation and obstructive sleep apnoea, Amer Rev Resp Dis 1986; 134: 555-58.
22. Debacker W.A., *et al.*, Central apnoea index decreases after prolonged treatment with acetazolamide; Amer J Resp Crit Care Med 1995; 151: 87-91.
23. Krieger J., Mangin P., Kuntz D., Effects of almitrine in the treatment of sleep apnoea syndrome, Bull Europ Physiopathy Resp 1983; 19: 631.
24. Brownwell I.G., West P., Sweatman P., *et al.*, Protripathyline in obstructive sleep apnoea, N Engl J Med 1982; 307: 1037-42.
25. Nahmias J. S., Karetzky M.S., Treatment of OSAS using a nasopharyngeal tube; Chest 1988; 94: 1142-47.
26. Bhatia RS; Sleep Apnoea syndrome: Pathophysiology and management; Curr Med Trends 2005; 9: 1769-74.
27. Sharma SK; *et al.*, Sleep disordered breathing disorders; IN; A Muruganathan; ED; Med. Update, API 2013; 23: 473-78.
28. Chhajed PN; *et al.*, OSA: Therapies other than CPAP; JAPI 2004; 52: 143-51.
29. Fujita S., Conway W., Zorcock F., *et al.*, Surgical correction of anatomical abnormalities in obstructive sleep apnoea syndrome uvulopalatopharyngoplasty, Otolaryng Head Neck Surg 1981; 89: 923-34.
30. Douglas N. J., Systematic review of efficacy of nasal CPAP; Thorax 1998; 53: 414-15.
31. Iyer SR; Iyer RR; OSA–Clinical Spectrum and management; IN; MS Rao; ed; Med Update 2010; 20: 802-05.
32. Iyer SR, Iyer RR; Sleep, Ageing and stroke–Newer directions in management of stroke; JAPI 2010; 58: 442-46.

PICKWICKIAN SYNDROME

This obesity-hypoventilation syndrome was noted by Wadd in 1810 in the form of relationship between massive obesity, periodic breathing and daytime somnolence and the term Pickwickian syndrome was coined by Osler in 1918. Originally, it was described by Burwell in 1956. In obese persons, an increased work of breathing associated with alveolar hypoventilation, cyanosis, hypoxaemia, hypercapnia and policy- thaemia may be noted.[1] Pulmonary hypertension and right sided heart failure may occur. Often they have day time somnolence; and somnolent, resembling the fat boy of pickwick papers, hence referred to as pickwickian syndrome. Obstructive sleep apnoea is a prominent feature and even in those without sleep apnoea, sleep-induced hypoventilation is another important element of the disorder.[2,3]

Pathophysiology

Obesity adds mechanical load on the rib cage and abdomen has to serve to reduce chest compliance. Thus breathing occurs at low lung volumes, basal lung airways remain closed, thus resulting in underventilation. So, there is a shallow breathing and small lung volumes. Obesity restricts chest expansion. However, in majority of patients, the respiratory centre exhibits an insensitivity to inhaled CO_2 and there is often a decrease in central respiratory drive[1,4] which may be inherent or acquired. In small number of patients, chronic hypercapnia, hypoxemia and eventually polycythemia, pulmonary hypertension and right sided heart failure develops. Often there is airflow obstruction possibly related to associated smoking.

Clinical Presentation

Both the sexes are equally affected, often in their middle age. There is marked obesity, somnolence, periodic respiration, twitching, cyanosis, secondary polycythemia and right sided heart failure.

Chest X-ray reveals cardiomegaly and ECG shows evidence of right ventricular hypertrophy.

Weight reduction is very important part of treatment. Cessation of smoking and elimination of obstructive sleep apnoea also helps. Treatment with progesterone 100 mg I. M. daily[5] or medroxy progesterone acetate 20 mg sublingually[1] every eight hours have been shown to enhance the respiratory drive.[6] Frequent episodes of obstructive sleep apnoea may require mechanical device to maintain ventilation.[7]

REFERENCES

1. Shankar P. S., Chest Medicine; Oxford and IBH Publ Co (P) Ltd. N. Delhi, 4th ed, 1994.
2. Wilson J. D., *et al.,* (ed), Harrison's Principles of Internal Medicine, 12th ed. Vol. 2; McGraw Hill New York.
3. Phillipson E. A., Hypoventilation syndromes, In; Textbook of Respiratory Medicine, Murrey J. F., Nadel J. A., (ed), Saunders Philadelphia, 1988.
4. Gastant H., Tassinari C. A., Duron B., Polygraphic study of diurnal and nocturnal manifestations of Pickwickian syndrome; Brain Res 1966; 1: 167.
5. Crofton and Douglas, Resp. Diseases; Seaton A., Seaton D. and Gardon Leitch A., ed, 4th ed, 1989, Oxford University Press, Delhi.
6. Mathew O. P. and Remmers J. E., Respiratory function of upper airway. In: N. A. Saunders and C. E. Sullivan (eds). Sleep and Breathing. Lung Biology in Health and Disease, New York, Marcel Dekker 1984; 21: 163-200.
7. Mahashur A. A., Disorders of ventilation; In; Sainani G. S., *et al.*, API; Textbook of Med 1999; 6th ed.; 275-77.

LUNG TRANSPLANTATION

Introduction

From 1963 through 1974, at least 36 lung transplants were performed in medical centers throughout the world[1,2] following the first human lung transplantation by James Hardy in 1963 for carcinoma of the lung. Because of poor survival and deaths due to respiratory failure, multiorgan failure, pneumonia, rejection and dehiscence of the airway anastomosis, for the next 10 years only a few attempts at human lung transplantation were made. However, the development of the bronchial omentopexy technique to restore circulation to the donor bronchus,[3,4] a better understanding of the potential adverse effect of corticosteroid therapy on the healing of the bronchial anastomosis,[5] and the introduction of cyclosporine set the stage for successful lung transplantation in the 1980s.

Since the first successful single-lung transplant was reported in patients with pulmonary fibrosis,[6] the indications for lung transplantation has subsequently been extended to patients with chronic obstructive pulmonary disease (COPD)[7] primary pulmonary hypertension,[8] and coupled with concomitant repair of the cardiac defect, some forms of Eisenmenger's syndrome. Double-lung transplantation, originally described in relatively young patients with severe obstructive lung disease,[9] has been offered to patients with cystic fibrosis and other types of bronchiectasis.[10] Thus lung transplantation is a successful therapeutic intervention to selected patients with end stage pulmonary parenchymal and vascular diseases without other significant illnesses and unresponsive to other forms of management.

Despite the transplantation of human organ act passed in Indian Parliament in 1994, only few transplantations are being undertaken since it is the option of organ donation of brain-dead heart-beating patient's attending family members. Higher rate of cadaver organ donation can be achieved in India[11] and enhanced by encouraging families to not to go waste the invaluable opportunity to register victory after death.[12]

Indications

The indications for lung transplantation are: irreversible, progressively disabling, end-stage pulmonary disease exhibiting respiratory failure, unresponsive to conventional medical treatment and a poor quality of life. Most of the patients require oxygen 24 hours a day. There should be evidence of disease progression with a life expectancy of 12 to 18 months or less without transplant intervention.[13] The conditions may be restrictive (idiopathic pulmonary fibrosis), obstructive (end stage emphysema especially alpha-1 antitrypsin deficiency), infection (cystic fibrosis) or those associated with high pulmonary vascular resistance caused by primary pulmonary hypertension or Eisenmenger syndrome.[14] Transplantation is advocated for individuals exhibiting mixed venous oxygen saturation of pulmonary arterial blood less than 63%, cardiac index of less than 1.5 l/min/m^2 in primary pulmonary hypertension[15] or right ventricular failure refractory to diuretic therapy and arterial oxygen desaturation on exercise.[16]

Heart lung transplantation (HLT) advocated as a treatment of pulmonary vascular disease offers better tracheal anastomotic healing as the mediastinal collateral blood supply is preserved. Double lung transplantation (LT) is advised in patients aged less than 50 years, with end stage emphysema or cystic fibrosis, provided they have no previous surgery or pleurodesis or pleurectomy, because these may increase technical difficulties and operative risk of lung transplantation.

Cardiothoracic

The lung is a delicate organ with intimate approximation of its peripheral gas exchanging areas and capillaries, whose integrity has to be preserved while undertaking its transplantation.[13]

The transplant lung must start functioning immediately. The success of a lung transplant depends on the healing of the sutured airway without stricture formation. The occurrence of dehiscence of bronchial anastomosis proves fatal. The bronchial circulation must be anastomosed properly to provide systemic blood supply to the donor bronchus, otherwise it will cause ischaemia of the airway. Bronchial omentopexy (wrapping bronchial anastomosis with a pedicle of greater omentum at the time of reimplantation) restores arterial circulation to the bronchus by collateral vessels from the omentum and protects against dehiscence.[17] It has reduced the chances of bronchial necrosis, infection and fistula formation.[13] Airborne contamination makes the lung more susceptible to infections.

Meticulous suture technique has to be adopted to avoid narrowing of the pulmonary arteries and venous connections. It helps in maintenance of normal pulmonary vascular resistance in the reimplanted lung. Post-operative immunosuppression with cyclosporin-A, facilitates normal collagen organization and bronchial wound healing. Cyclosporin acts by blocking the production of interleukin-2 and inhibiting the function of the T-helper lymphocytes.[18]

Donor Selection

There is scarcity of suitable lungs for implantation. Unilateral lung transplantation makes economic use of donor organs as both donor lungs can be used for separate recipients and the heart for a cardiac transplant. Bronchiolitis obliterans is less common in isolated lung transplantation. The donor lung must have no radiologic abnormality and the age must be less than 55 years. Arterial oxygen tension must be 300 mm Hg on 100% oxygen and PEEP of 5 cm H_2O_2. There should not be any significant thoracic trauma. They should not have had any surgery on the side of harvest. There should not be any pulmonary of systemic infections and the chest radiograph must be normal. Bronchoscopy should not demonstrate any purulent secretions or aspiration. The size of the donor lung must match properly with the recipient's chest and there should be ABO compatibility.[13]

While harvesting the donor lung, cardiectomy is done before removal of the lung en bloc. The left atrial incision be done in such a way that it leaves an adequate cuff on both the heart and lung bloc. A transverse incision of the pulmonary artery has to be made half way between the pulmonary valve and bifurcation of the pulmonary artery. The lungs are to be flushed with colloid based cold preservative solution via pulmonary artery. It should be preceded by injection of prostacycline (PGI^2) in a dose of 500 micrograms into the pulmonary artery. It helps in dilatation of the donor's pulmonary vascular bed.[19] The lungs are to be ventilated during the pulmonary artery flush. The trachea must be divided as far proximal to the carina as possible. The lungs removed from the donor can be preserved for four to six hours.

Recipient

The recipients should not have other systemic diseases or coronary artery disease or evidence of contraindications for immunosuppression. They must be psychologically stable and must be ambulatory and must not be on steroids. They must be able to carry on with the post-operative medication regimen. They should not be steroid dependent because steroids therapy has an adverse effect on healing and strength of bronchial anastomosis.

Though transplantation can be performed on either side with equal success, the left side is often preferred as it is easier to achieve adequate recipient left atrial cuff. The recipient pulmonary artery branches are larger and easier to prepare. An oversized lung may be more easily accommodated in the left chest because of mediastinal shift and easier descent of the left hemidiaphragm. The gastrocolic omentum should be mobilized from the transverse colon. The arterial anastomosis is done first and the bronchial anastomosis is performed later. Double lung transplantation requires total cardiopulmonary bypass. Fluid overload should be avoided in the transplant lung as there is total disruption of pulmonary lymphatics.[13]

The lung implanted is larger than the native lung in pulmonary fibrosis and in COPD the implanted lung is smaller. A larger lung causes mediastinal shift, descent of diaphragm and expansion of thorax to accommodate the donor lung. Following transplantation, in COPD, the over-inflated chest cavity decreases in size as air trapping no longer exists.

Immunosuppression which is described in details in the following text, is done with cyclosporine 4 mg/hr, azathioprine 2 mg/kg/day and anti-lymphocytic globulin 15 mg/kg/day intravenously. Later, cyclosporin is administered orally on starting of functioning of the gastrointestinal tract. Steroids are to be used only after first three weeks, so that their deleterious effect on bronchial wound healing is avoided. Steroids are to be given when immunologic rejection is suspected.[13]

Procedures

The single-lung transplant operation has not changed significantly since its first description,[20] but the indications have expanded substantially. Pulmonary fibrosis, the original indication, was ideally suited to single-lung transplantation because of the low lung compliance and high vascular resistance in the remaining native lung, which preferentially directed ventilation and perfusion to the allograft. Excellent results have been reported from the Toronto series.[21]

The early attempts at single-lung transplantation for obstructive lung disease were plagued by problems of over-inflation of the compliant native lung, compression of the allograft and ventilation-perfusion imbalance between the two lungs. In the last 2 years, the results of single-lung transplantation for patients with COPD have been reassessed and the outcome measures are favourable.[7,8]

The latest advancement has been single-lung transplantation for primary pulmonary hypertension and certain forms of Eisenmenger's syndrome, principally atrial or ventricular septal defects that can be repaired simultaneously with transplantation.[9,10] Traditionally, these pulmonary vascular diseases have been treated by heart-lung transplantation. However, single-lung transplantation can normalize pulmonary arterial pressure and relieve the afterload on the right ventricle.

The operative procedure for double-lung replacement has been revised significantly since its introduction in 1986. In the present technique, bilateral sequential lung transplants are performed through a transverse thoracosternotomy. Exposure of the pleural spaces is improved and cardiopulmonary bypass can be avoided in the majority of cases. Perioperative morbidity and mortality have been substantially reduced.[12]

Bilateral, rather than single, lung transplantation is mandatory in patients with generalized bronchiectasis, including cystic fibrosis and for any other disease characterized or complicated by chronic infection of both lungs. Both bilateral and single-lung transplantation currently are being performed on patients with COPD. The choice of procedure has been dictated by individual circumstances and by donor organ availability. International guidelines have been laid down for patient selection have been listed indications and contra- indications in Tables 11.58 to 11.61.[22,23]

Table 11.58: Potential recipient's selection
Severe obstructive or restrictive lung disease or severe pulmonary hypertension.
Medical therapy ineffective or unavailable.
Substantial limitation in activities of daily living.
Limited life expectancy.
Ambulatory with rehabilitation potential.
Adequate cardiac function without significant coronary artery disease.
Acceptable nutritional status.
Satisfactory psychosocial profile and emotional support system.

Table 11.60: Lung transplant recipients
Common Diagnosis
Chronic obstructive pulmonary disease
Alpha-l antitrypsin deficiency emphysema
Cystic fibrosis
Primary pulmonary hypertension
Pulmonary fibrosis
Bronchiectasis
Sarcoidosis
Eosinophilic granuloma
Eisenmenger's syndrome
Lymphangiomyomatosis

Table 11.61: Heart and lung transplant r ecipients
Common Diagnosis
Cryptogenic fibrosing alveolitis
Cystic fibrosis
Emphysema
Sarcoidosis
Histiocytosis X
Bronchiectasis

Only recently pulmonary transplant with a bi-pulmonary partition has been successfully performed where one lung of the donor was surgically separated and implanted as two small lung grafts in the thoracic cavity of the recipient, recreating arteries, veins and bronchi in certain portion of the lung. Lung grafting is particularly useful in children ailing from cystic fibrosis. But patient has to remain on immunosuppressive drugs throughtout the life. Bipulmonary partition increases the availability of transplants as well as may be of help in serving patients suffering from pulmonary hypertension, pulmonary fibrosis, chronic bronchitis and emphysema.

The cause of death could be progression of their underlying disease. Important complication could be respiratory failure. The most common diagnoses among recipients include COPD and alpha antitrypsin deficiency and emphysema with severe obstructive lung disease.

Table 11.59: Contraindications to lung transplant ation

Absolute	*Relative*
Acute illness or unstable clinical status	— Symptomatic osteoporosis
Active pulmonary or extrapulmonary infection	— Poor nutritional status
Active malignancy in the past 2 years	— Kyphoscoliosis
Systemic disease with non-pulmonary end-organ involvement	— High dose steroids therapy
Significant coronary artery disease or left ventricular dysfunction	— Ventilator dependence
Significant liver or kidney disease of any cause	— Prior cardiothoracic surgery
Current systemic steroid therapy	— Pleurodesis or pleurectomy
Progressive neuromuscular disease	— Active collagen vascular disease
Current cigarette smoking	
HIV infection	
Significant psychosocial problems, drug or alcohol abuse, or history of medical non-compliance.	

Lung functions are markedly improved after both single-lung and bilateral lung transplantation. A mild-to-moderate obstructive pattern may persist after single-lung transplantation. During the last decade, lung transplantation has come of age.[24] While many problems remain to be solved, lung transplantation is now a viable option for appropriately selected patients with end-stage lung disease as it provides 1 year actuarial survival in 80% approx.

Heart and Lung Transplantation

Human heart and lung transplantation was first reported in 1982.[25] The patients had severe pulmonary vascular disease, either primary or secondary to cardiac disease.[26,27] Despite the long term problems in diagnosing rejection or infection in the transplanted lung,[26-28] this treatment may be beneficial for patients with other lung diseases.

Combined heart and lung transplantation was initially used to treat pulmonary vascular disease. Current review places lung transplantation for lung disease in perspective.[29] Success, however, has lagged behind that with other organs for various reasons.

Major clinical problems have been cytomegalovirus infection and rejection. The cytomegalovirus infections were primary, occurring shortly after the operation and are assumed to have been acquired by previously seronegative recipients from the donor.[30] This has led to a change in practice. Donors are now serotyped for cytomegalovirus and the recipient is matched. In future it may be possible to vaccinate the seronegative recipients for cytomegalovirus to extend the potential range of donors.

Serious rejection episode may follow with conventional antibiotics as antibiotics are known to reduce the efficacy of cyclosporin.[31] A full response to increased immunosuppression, including relief of symptoms, the disappearance of abnormal physical signs and an increase in pulmonary function, may be good sign of transplantation.

Bacterial bronchitis may be potentially dangerous. Three factors may have contributed to these infections: a reduction in the efficacy of the cough reflex, impaired mucociliary clearance and interruption of the mucociliary *escalator* at the tracheal anastomosis. These patients can cough because the larynx and trachea are innervated.[32] The airways below the anastomosis, however, are denervated, preventing the initiation of the cough reflex from the bronchial tree. Mucociliary clearance may also be impaired in these regions as a result of denervation,[33,34] although this has not yet been studied. The interruption of the mucociliary escalator at the tracheal anastomosis may also be important.

The size of the donor lungs and the recipient's thoracic cavity must be matched. If the donor lungs are too large, atelectasis and right to left shunt may occur.[28] Thoracic vertebral height and width of the rib cage in the chest radiograph has been suggested to be measured. All patients should have a normal total lung capacity after operation.

Patients with pulmonary vascular disease who undergo heart and lung transplantation have a restrictive ventilatory defect.[35] This probably reflects changes in the mobility of the chest wall after median sternotomy,[36] which is also seen in patients after coronary artery bypass grafting and which resolves with time.[37]

Combined heart and lung transplantation for lung disease may not be superior to transplantation of both lungs or of a single lung.[38] It is easier to transplant the heart and lungs together.[28] But it is no longer thought that the transplanted heart offers a means of diagnosing rejection through an endomyocardial biopsy.[39] The transplanted heart and lungs reject independently of one another.[40]

Single lung transplantation is valuable for fibrotic lung disease,[41] but earlier experience with a wide range of lung disease was disappointing.[42] This reflects the poorer healing of a bronchial anastomosis compared with a tracheal anastomosis, which has a better collateral blood supply.[43] Patients who have suppurative lung disease, will infect the transplanted single lung and ventilation and perfusion mismatch may occur in emphysema.[44] Combined heart and lung transplantation should therefore be offered to these patients.

Theoretically, alpha-1 antitrypsin deficient recipients may be prone to develop emphysema in the transplanted lungs during periods of pulmonary inflammation,[45] this might occur with episodes of infection or rejection.

More patients with cystic fibrosis than with other diseases are likely to benefit from combined heart and lung transplantation, particularly as most now survive until adult life.[46] Selection is important, relative contraindications would be extrapulmonary disease—for example, insulin dependent diabetes mellitus and liver disease with portal hypertension. It is now possible, however, to combine transplantation of the liver with transplantation of heart and lungs. Extensive pleural fibrosis from surgical treatment of recurrent pneumothorax may be an important contraindication. Recurrent pneumothorax is common in the older patients with cystic fibrosis.[47] Pulmonary infection in cystic fibrosis is not a problem since it is usually confined to the lungs. Pleural and systemic infections are rare.[48] Transplantation offers the removal of the main source of sepsis. The presence of aspergillus fumigatus is of concern as a possible opportunistic infection after transplantation.[49]

There is still the problem of diagnosis and treatment of rejection.[27] Transbronchial lung biopsies may help to solve this. In addition, there remain difficulties in using cyclosporin, particularly in determining adequate treatment for the patient and avoiding nephrotoxicity.[50]

Complications

These can occur in early or late period following transplantation due to ischaemia, infection and rejection.

Primary graft failure occurs in 15% of cases of freshly transplanted allograft due to ischaemia-reperfusion injury within 72 hours of operation, resulting in severe hypoxemia and appearance of widespread infiltrates on chest X-ray film. Treatment is supportive with mechanical ventilation.

Anastomotic stenosis develops after several weeks of transplantation, as a result of stricture, granulation tissue or bronchomalacia and is recognized by presence of focal wheezing and recurrent lower respiratory tract infections. Bronchoscopic stent replacement is the treatment.[50]

Exposure of allograft to external environments enhances the rate of infection among the recipients, in the form of sinusitis and even pneumonia, both in early as well as late period following transplantation. Most common organism is P. aeruginosa, requiring prompt treatment. Immunosuppression, poor lymphatic drainage, depressed cough reflex, impaired mucociliary clearance, narrowing of bronchial anastomosis and even passive transfer of microorganisms along with the donor's lung are the predisposing factors for infection.

Single episode of acute rejection is seen in most of the patients, incidence being higher in first three months of transplantation. The condition manifests by low-grade fever, malaise, cough and dyspnoea and often accompanied with leucocytosis and hypoxemia. Chest X-ray reveals alveolar, nodular or interstitial opacities, with or without pleural effusions. Vital capacity and $FEVI_1$ falls. Often it becomes difficult to distinguish acute rejection from that of an infection as these abnormalities are seen in infection also.

Bronchoscopic transbronchial biopsy helps in recognising acute rejection, which is manifested by a perivascular and subendothelial lymphocytic infiltration accompanied by varying degree of alveolar spaces being flooded with air causing loss of aeration.[51] Repeated transbronchial biopsy through the fiberoptic bronchoscope helps in its recognition.[52] Bronchoalveolar lavage reveals an increase in absolute number of lymphocytes[53] and the cell mediated lymphocytic activity is increased during rejection.[54] There is an increase in soluble interleukin-2 receptor.[55] Radionucleotide perfusion scan shows reduced perfusion to the transplant lung due to increased vascular resistance accompanying rejection.[56] Acute rejection and infection are associated with a significant fall in vital capacity and in forced expiratory volume in one second.[57]

Rejection is characterised by fever, hypoxaemia, decreased exercise tolerance and presence of fluffy hilar infiltrates radiologically. Often, it is difficult to distinguish it from infection. There will be resolution of infiltrates on administration of 500 mg methyl prednisolone sodium succinate. Pulse therapy with 250 to 500 mg methyl prednisolone sodium succinate is given on succeeding two days.[13] However, 1/3rd of cases may continue to exhibit permanent rejection.

Opportunistic lung infections from viruses (cytomegalovirus, herpes simplex virus), protozoa (pneumocystis carinii) and fungus (invasive aspergillosis) occur frequently in the first few months after lung transplantation.[15] Cytomegalovirus infection in the transplant lung is avoided by use of prophylactic cytomegalovirus hyperimmune globulin (100 mg/kg/week) or by administering Gancyclovir 5 mg/kg twice a day if infection has occurred. Herpes simplex virus (HSV) infection is treated with intravenous acyclovir 5 mg/kg thrice a day. Prophylactic oral acyclovir 200-400 mg thrice a day may prevent HSV infection. Pneumocystis carinii pneumonia needs treatment with intravenous sulphadimidine 1 g 6 hourly and trimethoprim 4-6 mg per kg per day in divided doses. Intravenous amphotericin B is useful in controlling invasive aspergillosis. It is given intravenously in a dose of 0.25 mg/kg and it is increased to 1 mg/kg daily if tolerated. The total dose given is 1.2 to 1.5 g over 2 to 3 months. Chronic rejection is a constant problem manifesting as bronchiolitis obliterans histologically.

Small airways are the seat of fibro proliferative process. There is dense submucosal scarring that completely obstruct the lumen of bronchioles. Transbronchial biopsy cannot establish the diagnosis unlike acute rejection. PFTS, however, establish the evidence of airflow limitation. Chronic rejection is noted after 6 months after transplantation in 69:70% of survivors (for five years). It is immunologically mediated,[58] insidiously developing into bronchiolitis obliterans syndrome, that presents with cough, dyspnoea and purulent expectoration. This progressive condition has airflow obstruction. Chest X-ray is mormal. PFT shows fall in mid-expiratory flow rates in early phase, later on followed by fall in FEV_1 and in the ratio of FEV_1 to forced vital capacity (FVC). HRCT of lungs reveals decreased peripheral vascular markings, peripheral bronchiectasis and evidence of air trapping on expiratory images. The late morbidity and mortality is due to progressive airway obstruction with a histologic picture of bronchiolitis obliterans. It appears to be a manifestation of chronic rejection and is noted in those who have repeated early rejection episodes. Treatment lies in augmentation of immunosuppressive therapy. And in case failure occurs, reimplantation of the lung can be considered in selected patients. Through lung transplantation is advocated as a successful therapeutic intervention for selected group of patients, chronic rejection is still a major hurdle for long-term patient survival. Therefore, it has to be utilised only when other options are exhausted or an improved life is expected following transplantation of lung.

Cyclosporine

Organ transplants brought in an era of a new form of surgery. However, rejection of the graft by the body's immune mechanism brought this type of surgery to a standstill. This system of defence had to be overcome for a successful transplant operation.

Cyclosporine was discovered in 1969 by a naturalist researcher. Lately a mutant species of tolypocladium inflatum that is, tolypocladium terricola has been discovered. It is reported to have a higher bioavailability and retains an increased therapeutic blood level even after 24 hours. The future potential of this immunosuppressant is enormous and will continue to have an impact in clinical medicine.

Mechanism of Action

Cyclosporine inhibits T lymphocyte activation and proliferation but is not cytotoxic. Unlike corticosteroids, azathioprine and other cytotoxic drugs, it inhibits selectively both antigen induced activation of $CD4^{+}$ (T helper) lymphocytes and the production by these cells of interleukin[2] and other cytokines,[59,60] cyclosporine can also interrupt active immune responses, as shown by its efficacy in treating autoimmune diseases—presumably by blocking the secretion of cytokines by lymphocytes. The drug inhibits the in vivo transcription of genes encoding interleukin 2 and interferon[61] and blocks the expression of interleukin 2 receptors, whose induction is essential to T cell proliferation.

It is now clear that cyclosporine reversibly inhibits early, calcium dependent events in T lymphocyte activation and that there are probably several molecular targets within the cell membrane, cytosol and nucleus.[59] The most exciting new developments concern the uptake and concentration of cyclosporine in cystolic and nuclear target sites mediated by cyclophilin, a recently discovered enyzyme (peptidylprolyl isomerase). The relation between T cell activation and the function of this enzyme is unknown, but, by interfering with cyclophilin's role in the folding of regulatory peptides, the drug may prevent the formation or function of nuclear factors that regulate the expression of cytokine genes.[62] Recent evidence suggests that cyclosporine blocks the function of a gene termed NF-AT (nuclear factor of activated T cells), which may be the immediate or early regulator of T cell activation.[63] These properties of cyclosporine are shared by the novel anti-T cell agent FK-506, which may also have important clinical potentia l.[64,65]

Among the guidelines for its safe use are an initial dosage of no more than 5 mg/kg day, unless a rapid effect is critical and the maintenance of through blood concentrations of cyclosporine at 200 mg/ml or less (as measured by radio-immunoassay). If serum creatinine concentrations rise more than 30% above baseline, the dose should be reduced.

Cyclosporine was first used for bone marrow transplantation in the late 1970's. Graft versus Host disease (GVHD), an autoimmune like disorder developing 3 to 15 months after marrow transplantation is a major clinical complication of allogenic bone marrow transplanation. Cyclosporine used alone or with other immunosuppressive agents was found to be of benefit in the prevention and treatment of acute GVHD. Cyclosporine is now established as the principal immuno-suppressant in renal transplantation, with a graft survival of 85 per cent to 95 per cent following cadaveric or living donor transplantation, with a subsequent failure rate of two to three per cent per year. A similar evolution has occurred in the cardiopulmonary transplantation with a patient survival rate exceeding 75 per cent at five years. Though liver transplantation involves various surgical and pharmacological complexities, patient survial is around 60 per cent by five years.

Immunosuppressive therapy when compared with a combination of azathioprine and corticosteroids showed that the graft survival rates are higher in patients receiving cyclosporine with or without corticosteroids.

Therapeutic Monitoring

If cyclosporine is administered in doses below the recommended dose, it causes insufficient immunosuppression resulting in allograft rejection. High doses can cause toxicity to the patient due to erratic absorption of the drug. These include undesired events such as hepatotoxicity, renal toxicity, hypertension and neuro toxicity. Hence to ensure that the concentration of cyclosporine remains within the therapeutic window, close monitoring of blood levels of the drug is mandatory.

Several analytical methodologies have emerged for the monitoring cyclosporine A. These include:

1. High pressure liquid chromatography (HPLC).
2. Selective radioimmunoassay (RIA).
3. Selective fluorescence polarization immunoassay (FPIA).

HPLC, though is a very sensitive and specific assay, requires expensive instrumentation, trained personnel and is time consuming. Hence, it has been replaced by selective RIA and FPIA.

Adverse Effects

It produces reversible nephrotoxic effects which are generally dose dependent. Hypertension occurs frequently in renal and cardiac transplant patients. Seizures may occur. Adverse dermatologic, hematologic and neurologic effects have also been reported. However most of the side effects are reversible on discontinuance of the drug.

Current research is on presently in Snider's Laboratory to develop a totally implantable membrane lung, while at the same time solving problems associated with these current devices like blood clotting and infections. Presently the research is pointed towards a device which is to be inserted percutaneously into the favoral artery and to go up the vena cava through right ventricle and into the pulmonary artery to achieve the gas exchange. The device is positioned near the heart to enable it to receive nearly all the heart's oxygen-depleted blood supply. This century, advanced lung replacement technology would be available.[66]

Cancer After Transplantation

Skin cancer and lymphomas are the cancers most commonly described in patients who received transplanted organs.[67-73] Evidence for a significant increase in cancer of other organs is, however, conflicting and depends on data from few patients.[70,71,74] Whether there is an increase in overall tumour incidence is also not clear.[75,76]

The importance of viral infections as a risk factor for cancer in transplant recipients is not clear. Squamous cell carcinoma of the skin, which is believed to be caused by a virus, occurs more often than basal cell carcinoma in transplant recipients,[68,70] whereas the opposite is true in the normal population. Moreover, the genome of human papillomavirus has been detected in one third of squamous carcinomas from transplant recipients.[70] Skin warts, which are common in transplant recipients, are not, however, observed to become malignant and the incidence of specific infections with herpes virus or human papillomavirus is similar in transplant recipients whether or not they develop skin cancer.[77]

Immunosuppressive treatment may be a further risk factor. Patients who had heart transplants and are given high doses of immunosuppressive drugs are more likely to develop malignancies, particularly lymphoma than patients given lower doses.[72,73]

Because transplantation is a new procedure, the problem of malignancy may largely lie ahead. Cancer occurs more often in older patients and in those with long surviving grafts.[67,68,70]

Controlled multicentre studies are necessary to determine if tumours other than skin tumours occur more often in transplant recipients, followed for at least five years. In short term, the risks seem small and do not detract from the benefits of successful transplantation, even in the elderly.[78]

Stem cell research as regenerative medicine has emerged; advisory issued regarding good lab practice, good tissue practice, good manufacturing and good clinical practices along with standard operative procedure. We strongly need a good regulatory mechanism to ensure compliance by investigators.[79]

REFERENCES

1. Wildevuur C. R. H. and Benfield J. R., A review of 23 human lung transplantations by 20 surgeons, Ann Thorac. Surg 1970; 9: 489-515.
2. Veith F. and Koerner S. K., Problems in the management of human lung transplant patients, Vasc Surg 1974; 8:273-82.
3. Trulock E. P., Lung transplantation: State of the art; Amer. J. Resp. Crit. Care Med 1997; 155: 789-818.
4. Morgan E., Lima O., Goldberg M., Ferdman A., Luk S. K. and Cooper J. D., Successful revascularization of totally ischemic bronchial autografts with omental pedicle flaps in dogs. J. Thorac Cardiovasc Surg 1982; 84:204-10.
5. Lima O., Cooper J. D., Peters W.J., *et al.*, Effects of methylprednisolone and azathioprine on bronchial healing following lung autotransplantation, J. Thorac Cardiovasc Surg 1981; 82: 211-15.
6. The Toronto Lung Transplant Group. Unilateral lung transplantation for pulmonary fibrosis, N Engl J Med 1986; 314: 1140-45.
7. Trulock E. P., Egan T. M., Kouchoukos N., *et al.,* Single lung transplantation for severe chronic obstructive pulmonary disease, Chest 1989; 96: 738-42.
8. Trulock E. P., Cooper J. D., Kaiser L. R., Pasque M. K. and Ettinger N. A., Washington University Lung Transplantation Group. Unilateral lung transplantation for pulmonary hypertension, Am Rev. Respir, Dis 1991; 143: A467.
9. Cooper J. D., Patterson G. A., Grossman R. and Maurer J., Toronto Lung Transplant Group, Double-lung transplant for advanced chronic obstructive lung disease, Am. Rev. Respir Dis 1989; 139: 303-07.
10. Pasque M. K., Cooper J. D., Kaiser L. R., Haydock D. A., Triantafillou A. and Trulock E. P., Improved technique for bilateral lung transplantation, Ann Thorac Surg 1990; 49: 785-91.
11. Raut I; Organ donation for transplantation: Hurdles imposed by thoughtless officials: Natl Med J India 2010; 23: 186-87.
12. Desai HG; Organ donation: Victory after death; JAPI 2011; 59: 509-10.
13. Shankar P. S., Chest medicine; Oxford and IBH Publ. Co. (P) Ltd., N. Delhi; 1994; 4th ed.
14. Barr M. L., *et al.*, Recipient and donor outcomes in living related and unrelated lobar transplantation; Transplant Proc 1998; 30: 2261-63.
15. Fuster V., Steele P. M., Edwards W. D., Gersh B.J., McGoon M.D. and Frye R. L., Primary pulmonary hypertension, a natural history and the importance of thrombosis, Circulation 1984; 70: 580-87.

16. Smyth R. L., Higenbottam T., Scott J. P. and Wallwork J., Transplantation of the lungs, Resp Medicine 1989; 459-66.
17. Dubois P., Cheiniere L. and Cooper J. D., Bronchial Omentopexy in canine lung allotransplantation, Ann Thorac Surg 1984; 38: 211.
18. Van Buren C. T., Cyclosporin progress, problems and perspectives, Surg. Clin North Am 1986; 66: 435-39.
19. Hakin M., Higenbottam T., Bethune D., *et al.,* Selection and procurement of combined heart and lung grafts for transplantation, J. Thorac Cardiovasc Surg 1988; 66: 435-39.
20. Cooper J. D., Pearson F. G., Patterson G. A., *et al.,* Technique of successful lung transplantation in humans. J. Thorac Cardiovasc Surg 1987; 93: 173-81.
21. The Toronto Lung Transplant Group, Experience with single-lung transplantation for pulmonary fibrosis, JAMA 1988; 259: 2258-62.
22. American Thoracic Society; International Guidelines for the selection of lung transplant candidates; Amer. J. Resp. Crit. Care Med 1998; 158: 335-39.
23. Maurer J. R. *et al.*, International Guidelines for the selection of lung transplant candidates; J. Heart Lung Transplant 1998; 17: 703-09.
24. Theodore J. and Jewiston N., Lung transplantation comes of age, N. Eng 1. J. Med 1990; 322: 772-74.
25. Reitz B. A., Wallwork J., Hunt S. A., *et al.*, Heart-lung transplantation, a successful therapy for patients with pulmonary vascular disease, N. Engl. J. Med 1982; 306: 557-63.
26. Jamieson S. W., Baldwin J. Reitz B. A., *et al.*, Combined heart and lung transplantation, Lancet 1983; i: 1130-32.
27. Burkee C.M., Theodore J., Baldwin J. C., *et al.,* Twenty-eight cases of human heart-lung transplantation, Lancet 1986; i: 517-19.
28. Reitz B. A., Heart-lung transplantation, a review, Heart Transplantation 1982; 1: 291-97.
29. Veith F. J., Lung transplantation in perspective, N. Engl. J. Med 1986; 314: 1186-87.
30. Hakim M., Wreghitt T. G., English T. A. H., Stovin P. G. I., Cory-Pearce R. and Wallwork J., Significance of donor transmitted disease in cardiac transplantation, Heart Transplantation 1985; 4: 302-06.
31. Jones D. K, Hakim M., Wallwork J. and Higenbottam T. W., A serious interaction between cyclosporine A and sulphadimidine, Br Med J 1986; 292: 728-29.
32. Jamieson S. W., Stinson E. B., Oger P. E., Baldwin J. C., Shumway N. E., Operative techniques for heart lung transplantation, J. Thorac Cardiovasc Surg 1984; 87:930-35.
33. Camner P., Strandberg K. and Philipson K, Increased mucociliary transport by adrenergic stimulation, Arch Environ Health 1976; 31:79-82.
34. Camner P., Strandberg K and Philipson K., Increased transport by cholinergic stimulation, Arch Environ Health 1974; 29: 220-24.
35. Theodore J., Jamieson S. W., Burke C.M., *et al.*, Physiologic aspects of human heart-lung transplantation, pulmonary function status of the post-transplanted lung, Chest 1984; 86: 349-57.
36. Locke T. J., Griffiths T. L., Sutton A. and Gibson G. J., Rib cage expansion after median sternotomy, Thorax 1987; 42: 227-28.
37. Braun S. R., Birnbuam M. L. and Chopra P. S., Pre- and post-operative pulmonary function abnormalities in coronary artery revascularization surgery, Chest 1978; 73: 316-20.
38. Dark J. H., Patterson F A., Al-Jalahauri A.N., Hsu H., Egon T. and Cooper J. D., Experimental en-bloc double-lung transplantation, Ann Thorac Surg 1986; 42: 394-98.
39. Caves P. K., Stinson E. B., Billingham M., Rider A. K. and Shumway N. E., Diagnosis of human cardiac allograft rejection by serial cardiac biopsy, J Thorac Cardiovasc Surg 1973; 66: 461-64.
40. McGregore C. G. A., Baldwin J. C., Jamieson S. W., Bullingham M. E. and Yousen S. A, Isolated pulmonary rejection after combined heart and lung transplantation, J. Thorac. Cardiovasc Surg 1985; 99: 623-26.
41. Toronto Lung Transplant Group, Unilateral lung transplantation for pulmonary fibrosis. N. Engl. J. Med 1986, 314: 1140-45.
42. Veith F. J., Montefusco C., Kanholz S. L. and Millenkopf F. P., Lung-transplantation, Heart Transplantatioñ 1983; 2: 155-64.
43. Nelens J. M. B., Rebuck AS., Cooper J. D., Goldberg M., Halloran P. F and Vellend H., Human lung tranplantation, Chest 1980; 78: 569-73.
44. Stevens P. M., Johnson P. C., Bell R. L., Beal A. C. and Jenkins D. E., Regional ventilation and perfusion after lung transplantation in patients with emphysema, N. Engl. J. Med 1970; 282: 245-49.
45. George P. M., Vissers M. C. M., Travis J., Winterbourn C. C. and Carrell R. W., A genetically engineered mutant of alpha-1 antitrypsin protects connective tissue from neutrophil damage and may be useful in lung disease, Lancet 1984; ii: 1426-28.
46. Wood R. E., Boat T. T. and Doershuk C.F., State of the art, cystic fibrosis, Am Rev. Respir. Dis 1976; 113: 833-78.
47. Penketh A. R. L., Knight R. K, Hodson M. E. and Batten J. C., Management of penumothorax in adults with cysticfibrosis, Thorax 1982; 37: 850-53.
48. McCarthy M., Rourk M. H. and Spock A., Bacteraemia in patients with cystic fibrosis, Clin Paediatr 1980; 19: 746-48.
49. Nelson C. A, Caccerame M. L. and Shwartz R. A., Aspergillus and atopy in cystic fibrosis, Am. Rev. Respir. Dis 1979; 120: 863-65.
50. Susanto I., *et al.*, Use of balloon-expandable metallic stents in the management of bronchial stenosis and bronchomalacia after lung transplantation; Chest 1998; 114: 1330-35.
51. Christie J. D., *et al.*, Primary graft failure following lung transplantation; Chest 1998; 114:51-60.
52. Higenbottam T., Stewart S. and Wallwork J., Transbronchial lung biopsy to diagnose lung rejection and infection of heart-lung transplants, Transplant Proc. 1988; 20 (Suppl 1): 767-69.
53. Herlan D., Kormos R., Zeevi A., *et al.*, Dynamics of bronchoalveolar lavage in the canine lung transplant, Transplant Proc 1988; 20 (Suppl 1): 832-35.
54. Griffith B. P., Detection of rejection in the tramplanted lungs and immunology. In: Wallwork J (ed), Heart and Heart-Lung Transplantation, Philadelphia, WB Saunders Co 1989; 507-521.

55. Lawrence E. C., Brousseau K. P., Kurman C. C., *et al.*, Soluble interleukin-2 receptor levels in serum as a marker of rejection in heart-lung transplantation, Chest 1986; 89: 5526.
56. Pio Roda C. L., Strandberg J. D., Baker J. W., *et al.*, Serial changes in pulmonary blood flow occurring during acute rejection of the lung allograft. J. Thorac Cardiovasc Surg 1973; 65: 88-93.
57. Ofulans B. A., Higenbottam T. W., Scott J. P., Clelland C. Hutter J. A. and Wallwork J., Pulmonary function monitoring allows diagnosis of rejection in heart lung transplant recipients, Transplant Proc 1989; 21: 2583-84.
58. Heng D., *et al.*, Bronchiolitis obliterans syndrome: Incidence, natural history, prognosis and risk factors; J. Heart Lung Transplant 1998; 17: 1255-63.
59. Ryffel B., Pharmacology of cyclosporine, 6 Cellular activation, regulation of intracellular events by cyclosporine, Pharmacol Rev 1989; 41: 407-22.
60. Borel J. F., Pharmocology of cyclosporine (Sandimmune), 4. Pharmacological properties in vivo. Pharmacol Rev 1989; 41: 259-371.
61. Granelli-Piperno A. Lymphokine gene expression in vivo is inhibited by cyclosporine A.J., Exp. Med 1990; 171: 533-44.
62. Crabtree G. R., Contingent genetic regulatory events in T lymphocyte activation, Science 1989; 243: 355-60.
63. Gallagher R. B. and Ambier J. C., Signal transmission pathways and lymphocyte function, Immunology Today 1990; 11:. 187-89.
64. Thomson A. W., FK-506. Profile of an important new immuno-suppressant, Transplantation Reverses 1990; 4: 1-13.
65. Starzl T. E., Todo S., Fung J., Demetris A.J., Venkataraman R. and Jain A., FK-506 for liver, kidney and pancreas tansplantation, Lancet 1989; ii: 1000.
66. Goldsmith M. F., After two decades Pan State Researchers may be near performing replacement of hearts and lungs, JAMA, India 1993; 13: 25-32.
67. Sheil A. G. R., Cancer in renal allograft recipients in Australia and New Zealand, Transplant Proc 1977; 9: 1133-36.
68. Hardie I. R., Strong R. W., Hartley L. C. J., Woodruff P. W. H. and Clunie G. J. A., Skin Cancer in Caucasian renal allograft recipients living in as ubtropical climate, Surgery 1980; 87: 177-83.
69. Sheil A. G. R., Mahony J. F., Horvath J. S., *et al.*, Cancer following successful cadaveric donor renal transplantation, Transplant Prog 1981; 13: 733-35.
70. Sheil A. G. R., Cancer after transplantation, World J. Surg. 1986; 10: 389-96.
71. Hoover R. and Fraumeni J. F., Risk of cancer in renal transplant recipients, Lancet 1973; ii: 55-57.
72. Bieber C. P., Hunt S. A., Schwinn D. A., *et al.*, Complications in long-term survivors of cardiac transplantation, Transplant Proc 1981; 13: 207-11.
73. Kinlen L., Doll R. and Peto J., The incidence of tumours in human transplant recipients, Transplant Proc 1983; 15: 1039-42.
74. Kinlen LJ., Sheil A. G. R., Peto J. and Doll R., Collaborative United Kingdom. Australasian study of cancer in patients treated with immunosuppressive drugs, Br. Med. J 1979; ii: 1461-66.
75. Wing A. J., Broyer M., Brunner F. P., *et al.*, Combined report on regular dialysis and transplantation in Europe, XII, 1982. In: Davison A. M., ed. Proceeding of the European Dialysis and Transplant Association-European Renal Association. Vol. 20 London, Pitman 1983;5-75.
76. Birkeland S. A., Malignant tumours in renal transplant patients, Cancer 1983; 51: 1571-75.
77. Kelly G. E., Mahoney J. F., Sheil A. G. R., Meikle W. D., Tiller D. S. and Horvath J., Risk factors for skin carcinogenesis in immunosuppressed kidney transplant recipients, Clinical Transplantation 1987; 1: 271-77.
78. Macleod A. M. and Catto G. R. D., Cancer after transplant, BMJ 1988; 297: 4-5.
79. Bajaj JS; Regenerative Medicine; in Gupta SB; ed; PG Med; API 2004; 28: 3-13.

EOSINOPHIL-RELATED PULMONARY DISORDERS

Recently synonymity in pulmonary eosinophilia and eosinophilic pneumonia has been purposed[1] signifying that these terms provide a pathological diagnosis of eosinophilic infiltration of the lung (with or without radiological shadows, with or without peripheral blood eosinophilia). Its subgroup clinical entity is pulmonary infiltration with eosinophils syndrome (PIE) in which radiological lung shadows are accompanied with peripheral blood eosinophilia. This will exclude conditions with peripheral eosinophilias with radiological lung shadows that are not due to eosinophilic pulmonary infiltration such as TB, carcinoma lung, Hodgkin's disease, histoplasmosis, brucellosis, sarcoidosis and rheumatoid arthritis and are grouped as extrinsic pulmonary eosinophilias.

The various eosinophil-related pulmonary disorders may be discussed on the basis of blood eosinophilia under the following heads: [1,2]

I. Low eosinophilia
   - Bronchial asthma
   - Hypersensitivity vasculitis
   - Acute eosinophilic pneumonia.

II. Moderate eosinophilia
   - Loffler's syndrome
   - Prolonged pulmonary eosinophilia syndrome
   - Chronic eosinophilic pneumonia
   - Bronchocentric granulomatosis.

III. High eosinophilia
   - Bronchopulmonary aspergillosis (Sometimes may not have high eosinophilia)
   - Tropical eosinophilia
   - Pulmonary vasculitis
   - Hypereosinophilic syndrome.

Eosinophilic pneumonias can also be grouped as shown in Table 11.62.

Table 11.62: The eosinophilic pneumonias

Known cause	*Idiopathic*
Allergic bronchi pulmonary aspergillosis	Loeffler's syndrome
Chronic eosinophilic pneumonia	
Parasitic infestations	Churg and Strauss
Drug reactions	hypereosinophilia syndrome

Low Eosinophilia

Bronchial Asthma

Bronchial asthma can indeed be regarded as eosinophilic bronchitis. There is a close relationship between eosinophil count in bronchoalveolar lavage fluid (BALF) and airway hyper-responsiveness.[3,4] Eosinophils release a variety of mediators, including leukotrienex C_4, PAF, oxygen radicals and also basic proteins, such as major basic protein which are toxic to airway epithelium. The mediators are responsible for airway hyper-responsiveness are in Chapter 7.

Hypersensitivity Vasculitis

Hypersensitivity vasculitis is characterised by fibrinoid necrosis and cellular inflammation of small branches of arteries, veins and capillaries which may involve the whole vessel wall. Organs other than lungs may be involved, e. g., skin, heart, spleen, joints, kidney, liver, etc. Asthma and pulmonary symptoms are only infrequently present. Chest radiograph may show migratory infiltrates, cavitating nodules and pleural effusion. There is low to moderate increase in serum IgE levels.

Acute hypersensitivity lung diseases secondary to drugs are described earlier. Acute eosinophilic pneumonia needs a mention here. The condition appears to be due to acute hypersensitivity phenomenon, although peripheral eosinophilic count is not that high.[5]

Moderate Eosinophilia

Loeffler's syndrome is defined as an asymptomatic or minimally symptomatic self limiting condition with peripheral blood eosinophilia and transient migratory infiltrates in the chest radiograph. This is believed to be the manifestation of allergic reaction generally to a drug or a helminth. The condition revolves itself in 3-4 weeks. Pathologically there is infiltration of alveolar septa and spaces with eosinophil cells and histiocytes. There is a moderate increase in the serum IgE level.

Prolonged Pulmonary Eosinophilia Syndrome[2]

In prolonged pulmonary eosinophilia syndrome, the pulmonary infiltrates persist longer than 3-4 weeks and are accompanied by moderate symptoms; these are the distinguishing features from Loeffler's syndrome. The various aetiologic factors associated with this condition—characterised by allergic reaction—are parasitic, fungal or bacterial infections or drug reactions. Pathologically there is cellular infiltration of alveolar walls and interstitial tissue. There is moderate increase in serum IgE levels.

Chronic Eosinophilic Pneumonia

Described with ILDS.

Bronchocentric Granulomatosis

Described with ILDS.

High Eosinophilia

Bronchopulmonary Aspergillosis[2]

Bronchopulmonary aspergillosis is clinically characterised by chronic asthma, fever, expectoration of mucoid plugs containing eosinophil cells and fungal hyphae, demonstrable hyper-sensitivity to aspergillus. Bronchi are dilated and filled with inspissated mucus and exudate containing hyphae. There is infiltration of bronchial wall with eosinophils, lymphocytes and plasma cells along with eosinophilic pneumonia of surrounding pulmonary parenchyma. Serial chest radiographs show recurrent changing shadows usually bilateral and in upper zones, homogeneous but may by mottled, nodular, ring or unusually shaped, proximal segmental bronchiectasis and lobar skinkage. Serum IgE levels are very high.[6]

Infestations with helminths (cestodes, nematodes and trematodes) are the most common causes of pulmonary eosinophilia in tropical countries.[7-9] Other causes of pulmonary eosinophilia include Allergic Broncho-Pulmonary Aspergillosis (ABPA),[10] chronic eosinophilic pneumonia,[11] cryptogenic pulmonary fibrosis[12] Wegener's granulomatosis,[13] lympho-matoid granulomatosis,[14] eosinophilic granuloma of lung,[15] Churg-Strauss syndrome,[16] drug hypersensitivity reactions[17] and infections such as brucellosis,[18] coccidioidomycosis.[19] corynebacterium pseudotuberculosis[20] and tuberculosis.[21]

Pulmonary Eosinophilia due to Helminths

One of the most common forms of pulmonary eosinophilia in tropical countries is due to hypersensitivity reaction to an occult form of filariasis termed as tropical (filaria) eosinophilia[22] or Tropical Eosinophilia (TE).[23-26] TE presents with symptoms suggestive of bronchial asthma such as cough, dyspnoea, nocturnal wheezing and chest discomfort, occasionally associated with such constitutional symptoms as weight loss, anorexia and fever.[23,27] Physical examination reveals rhonchi and rales.[27] Chest radiographs show a variety of abnormalities, including diffuse miliary mottling, pleural effusions and uncommonly cavitation and large areas of consolidation.[28] High levels of blood and lung eosinophils with elevated serum and lavage fluid levels of IgE and filaria-specific IgE and IgG antibodies[23,29,30] have also been demonstrated. Pulmonary function studies have shown airway obstruction in addition to reduced lung volumes and reduced diffusing capacity.[27,31-33] Following a three-week course of diethylcarbamazine (DEC), there is incomplete reversal of clinical, haematological, radiological and physiological changes one month after starting treatment.[31] In conformity with these findings, a chronic respiratory tract inflammation as evidenced by a persistent eosinophilic alveolitis with lower respiratory tract inflammatory cells spontaneously releasing exaggerated amounts of O_2 and H_2O_2 has also been demonstrated.[34] It has also been shown that, at one year, patients with eosinophilic alveolitis had a significantly reduced diffusing capacity despite three weeks treatment with DEC.[27] It has also been reported that bronchiectasis can occur during and persists after clinical attacks of TE.[35] Therefore, there is an urgent need to undertake controlled clinical trials in TE to assess the role of corticosteroids in preventing the occurrence of irreversible radiological and lung function changes.

A similar syndrome of pulmonary eosinophilia with respiratory symptoms can result from infestations with other helminths such as Ascaris,[36] Ancylostoma species,[37] Strongy loides stercoralis[38] and Toxocara species.[39,40] Currently available immunological investigations of antibody assays[40] may not differentiate the eosinophilic syndromes due to various helminthic infections because of antigenic similarities. Allergy may or may not be in the background of all these cases. And eosinophilia may be noted in many cases of helminthic infestation during their "circulatory tour".[5] Because of the probable broad-spectrum anti-helminthic action of DEC, patients with pulmonary eosinophilia due to various helminthic infections, respond to treatment with DEC. Thus it appears that the syndrome of tropical eosinophilia is an end result of common pathogenesis resulting from infestations helminths. Though the syndrome of tropical eosinophilia is common in tropical and sub-tropical countries, it has also been described in subjects from temperate countries on exposure to appropriate infections in endemic areas.[42] Therefore, it will be ideal to have a better name for this syndrome based on aetiology and research should be directed to identify tests that may differentiate various types of pulmonary eosinophilia.

Allergic Broncho-Pulmonary Mycosis

A similar disease resulting from a hypersensitivity reaction to fungal antigens (Aspergillus species) has been termed Allergic Broncho-Pulmonary Aspergillosis (ABPA).[10] ABPA also manifests as asthma with elevated serum levels of total IgE and specific antibodies to aspergillus antigens.[43] Pulmonary function tests have revealed both obstructive and restrictive ventilatory defects.[44] Irreversible lung changes including proximal bronchiectasis can occur if ABPA is left untreated,[45] since other fungi such as Candida.[46,47] Helminthosporium,[48] Stemphylium[49] and curvularia[50] can cause a similar syndrome, it is suggested that the term *Allergic Broncho-Pulmonary Fungal diseases* can be a better name for the disease.[51]

Allergic Broncho-Pulmonary Mycosis

Allergic Broncho-Pulmonary Aspergillosis
Allergic Broncho-Pulmonary Candidiasis
Allergic Broncho-Pulmonary Helminthosporiasis
Allergic Broncho-Pulmonary Stemphyliosis
Allergic Broncho-Pulmonary Curvulariasis

Comparison of ABPA and TE (Tropical Eosinophilia)

Thus, there appears to be a similarity in pathogenesis of pulmonary eosinophilia resulting from hypersensitivity reactions to fungi and helminthis. A comparison of two diseases viz. ABPA and TE which are prototypes of pulmonary eosinophilia due to fungi and helminths is given in Table 11.63.

Table 11.63

	ABPA	*TE*
1. Features of asthma	+	+
2. Blood and sputum eosinophilia	+	+
3. Lung eosinophilia	+	+
4. Chest radiographic infiltrations	+	+
5. Total IgE	++	++
6. Specific IgG and IgE	++	++
7. Pulmonary function	Obstruction + Restriction	Obstruction + Restriction
8. Irreversible lung damage including bronchiectasis	Can occur	Can occur
9. Antigens	Fungus	Helminths
10. Treatment	Corticosteroids	DEC Corticosteroids

Both result from exaggerated immune responses to respective antigens as evidenced by elevated levels of total IgE and specific antibodies.[23,41,43] Both have bronchial and lung parenchymal abnormalities as revealed by similar pulmonary function abnormalities.[31,44] These may be due to type I and type III hypersensitivity reactions. Lung eosinophils in both diseases can cause irreversible lung changes if left untreated.[23,35,45] Therefore, it is suggested that the term *Allergic Broncho-Pulmonary Helminthiasis* is a better term for pulmonary eosinophilia due to helminthic infections. Terminologies that are appropriate for pulmonary eosinophilia resulting from various helminthic infections, are given.

Allergic Broncho-Pulmonary Helminthiasis

Suggested list of infestations:
1. Allergic Broncho-Pulmonary Filariasis.
2. Allergic Broncho-Pulmonary Ascariasis.
3. Allergic Broncho-Pulmonary Ancylostomiasis.
4. Allergic Broncho-Pulmonary Strongyloidiasis.
5. Allergic Broncho-Pulmonary Toxocariasis.

Tropical eosinophilia can then be termed as *Allergic Broncho-Pulmonary Filariasis.*

In case of an incorrect diagnosis in a patient with pulmonary eosinophilia due to strongyloidiasis and if this patient is treated with steroids, the parasite may become disseminated.[52] This emphasises the need for an aetiologic diagnosis in patients with pulmonary eosinophilia,[53] a suggested hypothesis.

Tropical Eosinophilia

Tropical pulmonary eosinophilia (TPE), a filarial disorder found throughout the tropical world but especially in the Indian subcontinent results from an exaggerated immune response to human filarial parasites, Wuchereria bancrofti and Brugia malayi[22,54,55] and is characterized by paroxysmal nocturnal cough, dyspnoea and wheezing, diffuse reticulonodular shadows in chest skiagram with marked peripheral blood eosinophilia.[23] Apart from TPE the other most commonly encountered pulmonary eosinophilia (PE) in this part of the country is one associated with worm infestations in the gut. Elevated serum levels of IgE along with levels of blood eosinophils have been reported in both tropical and worm infestation pulmonary eosinophilia.[56] Chest X-ray may be normal in 25% of cases. There is no correlation between radiologic changes, severity of the disease and eosinophilic count.[57]

High serum levels of IgE in normal Indians than in North Americans have been observed.[34] Extreme elevation of serum IgE levels in patients with TPE as well as in patients with worm infestation PE are observed.[58] Total blood eosinophil count of patients with TPE is higher than those with worm infestation PE. However, there was no significant correlation between the degree of blood eosinophilia and the levels of the serum IgE,[56,59] both in TPE and TE with worm infestaion.[58]

Lung diseases are often induced by a variety of circulating helminths and elevation of serum IgE is maximum when parenchymal tissues are involved.[60] Distinction between the two categories of PE to be made. Determination of filaria specific IgE in TPE and helminth specific IgE in cases with worm infested PE would be essential.[58] Besides quantitation, qualitative characterisation[61] of specific IgE may also become necessary. Response to DEC is very well-known. Nevertheless, refractory cases have also been documented. Relapses are to be treated with DEC and steroids may be beneficial in preventing interstitial fibrosis.

Pulmonary Vasculitis[2]

Allergic granulomatosis with anigiitis (Churg-Strauss syndrome) is a rare condition characterised by necrosis, fibrinoid deposition and leukocyte infiltration of small and medium sized arteries with extravascular granulomatus nodules. While pulmonary involvements are consistent, heart, skin and central nervous system may also be involved. Pulmonary symptoms are those of asthma, bronchitis and pneumonia and often precede systemic dissemination of vasculitis. Chest radiograph may be normal or shows usually diffuse but sometimes focal infiltrates, multiple areas of consolidation with occasional cavitation, changing pattern with resolution of same lesions and involvement of new areas, and is described with diseases of unknown aetiology.

Polyarteritis nodosa and Wegener's granulomatosis are other eosinophilic lung diseases associated with connective tissue disease and vasculitis. These are described under (diseases of unknown aetiology).

Hypereosinophilic Syndrome[62]

It is characterised by a multisystem organ dysfunction[63] with evidence of eosinophils, more than 1500/microlitre and without evidence of any parasitic, allergic or other known cause of eosinophilia. Bone marrow has rich infiltration with mature eosinophils. Heart, lung, speen, liver, nervous system and skin are affected. These varieties include predominant pulmonary, predominant cardiac or CNS involvement and eosinophilic leukaemia. Steroids with or without hydroxyurea or interferon are useful. Treatment of cardiac dysfunction is essential otherwise, it may add to agony of morbidity and may be responsible for mortality.

Significant respiratory impairment is seen in 5% cases. Dyspnoea may be due to pneumonitis, pulmonary odema or pulmonary fibrosis. Low grade fever, Raynaud's phenomenon and arthralgia may also be present. Chest X-ray shows minimal transient pulmonary infiltrates but progression to interstitial fibrosis occurs in later stages.[64]

Any case with eosinophil-related pulmonary involvement must be investigated.[2] Some of these cases will definitely require tissue biopsy before treatment. Common causes are given in Table 11.64.

Table 11.64: Common causes of eosinophilia: To revise

1. Allergic: Asthma hypersensitivity, drugs, angio oedema
2. Drugs: Penicillin, streptomycin
3. Infection: Scarlet fever, a post infection convalescence
4. Leukaemia: Chronic myeloid leukaemia, eosinophilic leukaemia, myeloproliferative syndrome
5. Malignancy: Hodgkin's disease, carcinoma
6. Pulmonary : Ascaris, toxocara, aspergillus involvement of the lung
   : Tropical eosinophilia
   : Polyarteritis nodosa, Rheumatid arthritis, SLE, Churg-Strauss syndrome
7. Parasitic infestation: Hookworm, tapeworm, ascaris, hydatid cyst, bilharzia, strongyloides, filaria, trichinia, toxocara, larva migraneing (visceral)
8. Skin diseases: Pemphigus, eczema, exfoliative dermatitis, psoriasis, dermatitis herpetiformis
9. Miscellaneous: Post splenectomy, idiopathic neutropenia, familial neutropenia

REFERENCES

1. Mirchandani L.V., Joshi J.M., Pulmonary eosinophilia; JAPI 1997; 45: 292-301.
2. Jain S. K., Eosinophil-related pulmonary disorders; Ind. J. Clin Pract 1993; 3: 13-14.
3. De Monchy J. G. R., Kufman H. F., Venge P., *et al.*, Bronchoalveolar eosinophils during allergen-induced late asth matic reactions, Am. Rev. Respir. Dis 1985; 131: 373.
4. Shankar P. S., Personal Communication, 1995.
5. Greenberger P. A., Allergic bronchopulmonary aspergillosis. J. Allergy Clin. Immun 1984; 74: 645.
6. Singh N, Singh V; Clinical presentation and investigations in asthma; JAPI (S) 2014; 62: 7-11.
7. Crofton J. W., Livingstone J. L., Oswald N. C. and Roberts A. T. M. Pulmonary eosinophilia, Thorax 1952; 7: 1-35.
8. Spry C. J. F., Lung Disease associated with eosinophils, In: Current perspectives in Allergy, Edinbugh. Churchill Livingston 1982; 67-77.
9. Sharma O.P., Pulmonary eosinophilia, Lung India 1988; 6: 39-47.
10. Hinson K.F.W. Moon A. J. and Plummer N. S., Bronchopulmonary aspergillosis, a review and a report of eight new cases, Thorax 1952; 7: 317-33.
11. Carrington C., Addington W., Goff A, Madoff L., Marks A., Schwaber J. and Gaensler E., Chronic eosinophilic pneumonia, New Engl, J. Med 1969; 280:787-98.
12. Tumer-Warwick M. and Haslam P. L., The value of serial bronchoalveolar lavages in assessing the clinical progress of patients with cryptogenic fibrosing alveolitis, Am. Rev. Respir. Dis 1987; 135:26-34.
13. Hunninghake G. W and Fauci A. S., State of the art, Pulmonary involvement in the collagen vascular diseases. Am. Rev. Respir. Dis 1979; 119: 471-503.
14. Leibow A. A., Carrington C.R., B., and Friedman P. J., Lymphomatoid granulomatosis, Hum. Pathol 1972; 3:457-558.
15. Case Records of the Massachusettes General Hospital Weekly Clinico-Pathological exercises, Case 8-1986. A 39-year-old woman with bilateral pulmonary infiltrates, New Engl. J.M. ed 1986; 314:564-74.
16. Churg J. and Strauss L., Allergic granulomatosis allergic angiitis and polyarteritis nodosa, Am J. Pathol 1951; 27: 277-301.
17. Rosenow E., C., III, The spectrum of drug-induced pulmonary disease, Ann. Intern. Med 1972; 77: 977-91.
18. Elsom K. A. and Ingelfinger F.J., Eosinophilia and pneumonitis in chronic brucellosis, A report of two cases, Ann Intern. Med 1942; 16: 995-1002.
19. Lombard C. M., Tazelaar H. D. and Krasne D. L., Pulmonary eosinophilia in coccidioidal infections, Chest 1987; 91: 734-36.
20. Keslin M. H., McCoy E. L., McCusker J. J. and Lutch J. S., Corynebacterium pseudotuberculosis. A new cause of infectious and eosinophilic pneumonia, Am J. Med 1979; 67: 228-302.
21. Bhatia R.S., Update management of tuberculosis; The Ind. Pract 1991; 44:527-32.
22. Neva F.A. and Ottesan E. A., Tropical (filarial) eosinophilia, New Engl. J. Med 1978; 298: 1129-31.
23. Udwadia F.E., Tropical Eosinophilia, In: Pulmonary eosinophilia, Progress in Respiration Research, Vol. 7, Basal, Karger 1975; 35-155.
24. Viswanathan R., Pulmonary eosinophiliosis, Natural history, aetiology and pathogenesis, Ind. J. Chest. Dis 1963; 5: 213-30.
25. Kamat S. R., Warrier N. V. U. Store S. D., Kavandikar E. D. and Hoskote V. R., Clinical studies in pulmonary eosinophilia, Comparative study of response to diethylcarbamazine and corticosteroid drugs, Ind. J. Chest. Dis 1976; 18: 221-32.
26. Ray D., Relapsing tropical eosinophilia, Ind. J. Chest Dis 1977; 19: 65-71.
27. Bhatia R. S., Tropical eosinophilia—atypical presentation; Curr. Med. Pract 1990; 34: 321-24.
28. Jain V. K. and Beniwal O. P., Unusual presentation of tropical pulmonary eosinophilia, Thorax 1984; 39: 634-35.
29. Pinkston P., Vijayan V. K., Nutman T. B., Rom W. N., O'Donnell K. M., Cornelius M.J., Kumaraswamy V., Ferrans V. J., Yenokida G., Thiruvengadam K. V., Tripathy S. P. Ottesen E. A. and Crystal. R, G., Iropical eosinophilia, characterisation of the lower respiratory tract inflammation and its response to therapy, J. Clin. Invest 1987; 80:216-25.
30. Nutman T. B., Vijayan V. K., Pinkston P., Kumaraswamy V., Steel C., Crystal R. B. and Ottesen E. A., Tropical Pulmonary eosinophilia, analysis of antifilarial antibody localized to the lung, J. Infect. Dis 1989; 160: 1042-50.
31. Vijayan V. K., Kuppurao K. C., Sankaran K., Venkatesan P. and Prabhakar R., Tropical eosinophilia, Clinical and physiological response to diethylcarbamazine, Respiratory Medicine 1991; 85: 17-20.

32. Poh S.C., The course of lung function in treated tropical eosinophilia, Thorax 1974; 29: 710-12.
33. Mann J. M. and Heurich A.E., Response of diffusion capacity in the treatment of tropical eosinophilia, Chest 1991; 99: 776-77.
34. Rom W. N., Vijayan V. K., Cornelius M. J., Kumaraswamy V. Prabhakar R., Ottesen E. A. and Crystal R.G., Persistent lower respiratory tract inflammation associated with interstitial lung disease in patients with tropical pulmonary eosinophilia following conventional treatment with diethylcarbamazine, Am. Rev. Respir. Dis 1990; 142: 1088-92.
35. Rab S. M., Nurul Haq A. Q. M. and Chaudhary G. M., Tropical eosinophilia and bronchiectasis, Brit J. Dis. Chest 1963; 57: 103-106.
36. Loffler W., Zur Differential-Diagnose der Lungeninfiltrierugen I. Fruhinfiltrate unter besonderer Beruchsichtigung der Ruckbildungzeten. II Uber fluschitage succedan infiltrate (mit eosinophilie). Beitrage zur klinik der Tuberkulose and Spezifischen Tuberkulose Forschung 1932; 79: 338-82.
37. Butland R. J. and Coulson I. H., Pulmonary eosinophilia associated with cutaneous larva migrans, Thorax 1985; 40: 76-77.
38. deMessias I.T., Telles F. Q., Boaretti A. C., Silva S., Guimarres L. M. and Genta R. M., Clinical immunological and epidemiological aspects of strongyloidiosis in an endemic area of Brazil. Allergol. Immunopathol. (Madr) 1987; 15: 37-41.
39. Chaudhari R. N. and Saha T. K., Tropical eosinophilia, Experiments with toxicara canis, Lancet 1959; 2: 493-94.
40. Beaver P. C., Toxocariasis (Visceral larva migrans) in relation to tropical eosinophilia, Bull Soc. Patho. Extol 1963; 55: 555-76.
41. Saha K., Sarkar N., Paul D. N. and Ray D., Serum immunoglobulins and complement profile in parasitic diseases, Ind. J. Med. Res 1979; 70: 22-32.
42. Hodes P. J. and Wood. R. D., Eosinophilic Lung (Tropical eosinophilia); Am J. Med. Sci 1945; 210: 288-95.
43. Rosenberg M., Patterson R., Mintzer R., Cooper B. J., Roberts M. and Harris K. E., Clinical and immunologic criteria for the diagnosis of allergic bronchopulmonary aspergillosis, Ann. Intern. Med 1977; 86: 405-14.
44. Malo J. L., Hawkins R. and Pepys J., Studies in chronic Allergic bronchopulmonary aspergillosis, Clinical and physiological findings, Thorax 1977; 32: 254-61.
45. Chapman B., Capewell S., Gibson R., Greining A. P. and Crompton G. K., Pulmonary eosinophilia with and without allergic bronchopulmonary aspergillosis, Thorax 1989; 44: 919-24.
46. Pepys J., Hypersensitivity disease of the lungs due to fungi and organic dusts, Monogr. Allergy 1969; 4: 63-68.
47. Slavin K.G., Stanczyk D. J., Lonigro A. J. and Broun G. O., Allergic bronchopulmonary aspergillosins—A North American rarity, Clinical and immunologic characteristics, Am J. Med 1969; 47: 306-13.
48. Dolan C. T., Weed L. A. and Dines D. E., Bronchopulmonary helminthosporiosis, Am. J. Clin Path 1970; 53: 235-42.
49. Benatar S. R., Allar B., Hewitson R. P. and Don P. A., Allergic bronchopulmonary stemphyliosis, Thorax 1980; 35: 515-18.
50. Mcheer R., Kroenert D. B., Elder J. L. and Fondist J. H., Allergic bronchopulmonary disease caused by Curvularia lunata and Drechslera hawailensis, Thorax 1981; 36: 338-44.
51. Glancy J. J., Elder J. L. and McAleer R., Allergic bronchopulmonary fungal disease without clinical asthma. Thorax 1981; 36: 345-49.
52. Case records of Massachusetts General Hospital. Weekly Clinico-Pathological exercise. Case 47-1987. A 79-year-old Cuban native with asthma, weight loss, vomiting, eosinophilia and post meningitis, New Engl. J. Med 1987; 317: 1332-42.
53. Vijayan V. K., ABPH, Lung India 1991; 9: 145-148.
54. Ottesen E. A., Filariasis and tropical eosinophilia, In: Warren K. S., Mahmond A. R., eds, Tropical Geographical Medicine, New York, McGraw-Hill 1984; 390-412.
55. Spry C. J. F. and Kumaraswami V., Tropical eosinophilia, Semin Hematol 1982; 19: 101-15.
56. Saha K., Sarkar N., Paul D. N. and Ray D., Serum Immunoglobulin and complement profile in parasitic diseases, Indian J. Med. Res 1979; 70: 22-32.
57. Vijayan V.K., Changes in respiratory functions and lung inflammation in patients with tropical eosinophilia one year treatment with DEC; IJCP and T 1997; 18: 24-28.
58. Debidas Ray and Sri Krishna K., Serum immunoglobulin E levels in tropical and worm infestation pulmonary eosinophilia, Lung India 1992; 10: 7-9.
59. Takenaka T., Okuda M., Kubo K. and Uda H., Studies on interrelation between eosinophilia, serum IgE and tissue mast cells, Clin. Allergy 1975; 5: 175-80.
60. Warwick M. T., Immunology of the respiratory tract, In: Recent Advances in Medicine, 16th edition, London, Churchill, Linvingstone 1973; 143-47.
61. Hussain R. and Ottesen E. A., IgE response in human filariasis II. Qualitative characterization of filaria-specific IgE, J. Immunol 1983; 131: 1516-21.
62. Weller P.F., Bubley G. J., The idiopathic hypereosinophilic syndrome; Blood 1994; 83: 2759.
63. Rohtagi A., Singh N. P., The idiopathic hypereosinophilic syndrome; JAPI 1995; 43(3): 207-10.
64. Londhey V.A., *et al.*, Idiopathic hypereosinophilic syndrome manifesting as pulmonary oedema; JAPI 2003; 51: 414-15.

ATELECTASIS (LUNG COLLAPSE)

Introduction

Lung collapse can be associated with a variety of conditions like infection, effusion, trauma, malignancy, pneumothorax, etc. Patchy atelectasis may be seen in smokers. Rounded atelectasis may be associated with pleural effusion. The term, pulmonary atelectasis, as it is, is controversial. Etymologically, the word is from Greek language, which means Ateles-incomplete and ektasis=extension.[1] It is applied to denote diminished air within the lung, associated with reduced lung volume. Various causes have been listed in Table 11.65. Resorption atelectasis is seen in bronchial obstruction mostly, but can occur without obstruction as in bronchiectasis. Compression type is seen with pleural effusion or pneumothorax.

Table 11.65: Causes of pulmonary collap se (Atelectasis)

1. Bronchial obstruction
2. Pneumothorax or pleural effusion
3. Fibrosis of a lobe, usually following tuberculosis
4. Bronchiectasis
5. Pulmonary embolus.

Lung collapse[2] is imperfect expansion of lung, confined to segment, lobe or whole lung. It can be due to congenital causes—neonatal collapse—which may be due to non-aeration of lungs at birth or under development of lungs in low birth babies. It can also be due to neonatal hyaline membrane disease. Acquired causes include compression collapse during thoracoplasty or due to diseases such as pleural effusion, pneumo/haemothorax or absorption collapse due to bronchial obstruction, as a result of intraluminal causes such as tumour, mucus, foreign body or external pressure by lymphadenopathy, aortic aneurysm or enlarged left atrium.

Pathogenesis

In pressure collapse, the bronchopulmonary are not obstructed. Therefore complications due to infections are quite delayed. Collapsed alveolar walls develop excess of reticulum and later on collagen fibres.

In absorption collapse, bronchial obstruction results in atelectasis, distal to obstruction. Hence site and degree of obstruction and extent of collateral ventilation will determine the ultimate outcome. Secondary infections may lead to progressive destruction of bronchial walls and bronchiectasis may result.

Clinically

Breathlessness and cough are present in lobe atelectasis and tachycardia, restlessness, cyanosis and even circulatory collapse occurs in massive atelectasis. Fever may be present even without infection.

Shift of trachea and heart towards affected side, with an impaired percussion note and diminished bronchial sounds are pointer towards lung collapse. Whispering pectoriloquy may be heard. Acute respiratory failure may result in massive atelectasis.

Investigations

X-ray chest usually confirms the diagnosis of shrunken lung lobe or segment.

Bronchoscopy is mandatory in all obstructive collapse. Aspirates of bronchoscope should be sent for cytology and micro-organisms including AFB. PFT shows restrictive defect. CT scan helps to locate a mass or lymph node.

Treatment

Specific treatment depends upon the cause and nature of collapse. Bronchoscopic removal of foreign body and mucus plug and often vigorous efforts at cough, deep breathing, steam inhalation and percussion may facilitate expansion. Surgical intervention may be required to treat lung abscess, bronchiectasis and recurrent chest infections.

Pulmonary Rounded Atelectasis

Rounded atelectasis is an unusual, localised form of lung collapse, associated with pleural effusion, described for the first time by Loeschke in 1928. The lower edge of the lung is seen folded on itself due to pressure exerted by the pleural fluid.[3] It was 1966 when Blesovsky described it under the heading *Folded lung.*[4] These lesions are generally coiled ones which are seldom round, hence the term *helical atelectasis* is suggested which is more descriptive and informative regarding pathogenesis as well.[2] It generally occurs following pleural effusion but may follow complicated pneumothoraces.[3]

Pathogenesis

It is thought to be secondary to pleural effusion. Hypothesis regarding its formation is as follows:

a. The two pleural surfaces are separated by pleural effusion causing an area of atelectasis within the compressed lung lobe. A cleft is created between the atelectatic and aerated parts of the lung lobe. This occurs mostly at the lung base because of more pressure (positive) at the base of the pleural space, relative to the apex as well as effect of the gravity.
b. The atelectatic part of lung lobe, as it floats over the effusion, tilts at the cleft and the enfolding process begins in one direction. This then gets fixed in the same position by the progressive fibrinous deposition, over the surface of the lobe, especially at the cleft.
c. The normal lung tissue expands, following resorption of effusion but the tilted portion remains atelectatic and gets further engulfed within the pleural viscera of the re-expanding lobe. This is further exaggerated by retraction of subpleural fibrotic lung tissue. Further gentle enfolding occurs due to normal respiration, giving it an oval, spherical or angular shape.

Absence of free fluid or presence of very small amount of pleural fluid[5,6] before atelectasis develops and pleural involvement in the form of irregular thickening, has brought forward another hypothesis regarding the formation of rounded ateletasis, which is as under:

a. The lesion begins as a local process in the visceral pleura (possibly due to irritant effect of asbestos, lime, silica or smoking), in the form of local reaction, which leads to formation of thick fibrotic coating, over a specified area of the lung.

b. The fibrotic coating consequently shrinks, causing folding of lung surface. Formation of the new fibrotic coating and shrinkage of old plaque occur simultaneously.

c. This pleural shrinkage leads to development of atelectasis of the underlying lung parenchyma. The shrinkage of perpendicular septa along with, gives the collapsed area a round form and is sometimes termed as shrinking pleuritis with atelectasis.[6]

Pathology

Central area contains lung parenchyma and visceral pleura is dipped into the lung, much twisted into a curl. The bronchi as well as blood vessels supplying the collapse area are retracted towards the lesion and pulled close together.[7] Visceral pleura shows fibrous thickening. The folded pleura has blood vessels, elastic fibres and moderate infiltration of inflammatory cells but mesothelial cells are absent.[5] Lung parenchyma underneath the thickened pleura is atelectatic with minimal interstitial fibrosis and scattered infiltration of lymphocytes and plasma cells. Pulmonary vessels may be sclerotic. Asbestos bodies may be present.

Investigations

Chest X-ray reveals a rounded, oval, angular or comma shaped density, generally seen at the lungs bases posteriorly, although it has been described in other parts of the chest also.[8,9] Alelectasis occurring due to bronchial obstruction, the causes of which are listed in Table 11.66.

Table 11.66: Causes of bronchial obstruction

1. Bronchial wall lesions
   a. Usually primary carcinoma
   b. Rarely endobronchial tuberculosis
   c. Rarely bronchial adenoma
2. Intraluminal occlusion
   a. Mucus plugging, particularly in post operative pneumonia or asthmatic patients
   b. Foreign body
3. Invasion or compression by an adjacent mass
   a. Malignant tumour
   b. Enlargement of lymph nodes.

CT findings of rounded atelectasis include seven major signs:[10]

1. A rounded mass lying at the lung periphery, measuring 4-7 cms in diameters.
2. Mass is most dense at the periphery since it is the area of most atelectasis.
3. Mass forms an acute angle with the pleura.
4. Presence of pleural scarring, thickest adjacent to the mass.
5. Presence of at least 2 sharp margins caused by the curving lung structures.
6. *Comet tail* appearance of entering vessels.
7. Presence of air bronchogram, usually in the central part of the mass.

Five minor signs include:[10]

1. Hyperinflation of lung adjacent to the mass.
2. Posterior displacement of right main bronchus (in right-sided lesions.
3. Thickening and displacement of interlobar fissure.
4. Bilateral lesions may be present.
5. Unchanged appearance over a period of one year.

Differential Diagnosis

Differential diagnoses include loculated empyema, haematoma, mesothelioma, carcinoma lung, metastasis, fibrin ball, mineral oil granuloma and conglomerate shadow of pneumoconiosis.

Management

There are no uniform management criteria laid down for rounded atelectasis. Regression of pleural thickening, spontaneous atelectatic reduction and even disappearance of mass in[6] 'toto' may occur over a period of one year. Such patients may remain symptom-free,[11] but should be followed up regularly as not much is known about the natural history of the condition.[6] Surgical management includes decortication and is indicated (a) when diagnosis of atelectasis is in doubt, (b) in advanced cases where restoration of atelectatic part cannot be done, requiring limited resection. Thoracotomy reveals lung which is not adhered to chest wall, plaques are seen on the parietal pleura, close to the lung lesion, that consists of subpleural palpable mass, covered with localised greyish white coating. The coating is made up of many layers of fibrous tissue, responsible for folding and ultimate atelectasis of the lung tissues. After removing these coating layers, the atelectatic part of the lung is allowed to expand to restore normal appearance. The surrounding lung tissue is generally emphysematous. However, recurrence of the mass may occur after thoracotomy.[6]

REFERENCES

1. Fraser R. G., *et al., Diagnosis of the diseases of the chest,* 3rd ed, 2nd Vol, WB Saunders Co. 1988; 487-90.
2. Guleria J. S., Atelectasis and pulmonary fibrosis; In; Sainani G. S., *et al.,* ed., API Textbook of Medicines 1999; 6th ed.; 295-98.
3. Cho S. R., *et al.,* Round (helical) atelectasis, Brit J Rad 1981; 54: 643-50.
4. Blesovsky A., The folded lung, Brit J Dis Chest 1966; 60: 19-22.

5. Mintzer R. A., Cugel G. W., The association of asbestos, induced pleural disease and rounded atelectasis, Chest 1982; 81: 457-60.
6. Derneik L., *et al.*, Shrinking pleuritis with atelectasis, Thorax 1982; 37: 252-58.
7. Hilgenberg A. D., Mark E.J., A 61years old man with a peripheral lung mass, N Engl J Med 1983; 308: 1466-72.
8. Schneider A.J., *et al.*, Rounded atelectasis, Amer J Rad 1980; 134: 225-37.
9. Fadhli H., Derrick J.R., Twisted lingula—a case of solitary pulmonary nodule, Ann Thoracic Surg 1965; 6: 753-54.
10. Doyle T.E., Lawler G. A., CT features of rounded atelectasis of the lung; Amer J Radiol 1984; 143: 225-28.
11. Gaude Gajanan S., Pinto Maria J. W., Rounded atelectasis, Lung India 1993; 11: 56-59.

PULMONARY FIBROSIS[1]

Pulmonary fibrosis is a pathological than clinical entity, as a sequele of a number of pulmonary disorders.

Aetiology

Localised or widespread causes of pulmonary fibrosis are listed below:
1. Infections: Pulmonary tuberculosis, bronchopulmonary suppurations, fungal and parasitic diseases.
2. Allergic (chronic): Extrinsic allergic alveolitis.
3. Chronic venous congestion from long standing left ventricular failure.
4. Following radiation therapy, to lung, breast, oesophagus and mediastinum malignant tumours.
5. Occupational diseases: Asbestosis, silicosis, anthracosis, siderosis, berylium pneumonitis, bauxite and graphite fibrosis.
6. Collagen diseases: Systemic sclerosis, polyarteritis nodosa, dermatomyositosis and rheumatoid disease.
7. Drug induced: Methotrexate, bleomycin, busulphan, nitrofurantoin, hydralazine, haemothorium.
8. Granulomas like sarcoidosis, eosinophilic granuloma.
9. Idiopathic: Acute diffuse interstitial fibrosis or the Hamman-Rich Syndrome and chronic diffuse interstitial fibrosis.

Pathology

Affected portion of the lung appears shrunken, airless and firm to feel. It gives a dark mottled tissue after cut section, with an evidence of original or causative disease. Pleural adhesions may be seen. Unaffected pulmonary areas may show compensatory emphysema.

Clinical Presentation

It is always variable with cough and expectoration usually present. Dyspnoea of varying degree is present depending upon degree of pulmonary parenchyma involvement. Cyanosis and right heart failure may be seen in few. Chest is retracted on the affected side, with trachea and heart also being pulled due to fibrotic changes. Vocal fremitus may be present. Percussion note may be hyper resonant in the areas of compensatory emphysema. Breath sounds are diminished; moist rales and rhonchi are present. Thorax on the affected side is small with loss of volume and tracheal and mediastinal shift is seen towards the affected side on plain X-ray chest. PFTs show restrictive defect. CT scan and bronchoscopic studies help in establishing the diagnosis.

Diagnosis

Diagnosis is easy. But it is important to assess the extent of fibrosis and the primary cause.

Treatment

Symptomatic management and treatment of original disease form the mainstay. Surgery can be contemplated if the disease is localized. Steroids, azathiaprine or cyclosporine has been used with varying results. Deriphylline and non-invasive intermittent oxygen therapy at home may offer some help.

Prognosis

Limited fibrosis can be compatible with routine activities of life. Complications such as emphysema, lung abscess, bronchiectasis and right heart failure, when present, or extensive pulmonary disease often shorten life span.

REFERENCE

1. Guleria J. S., Pulmonary fibrosis; In; Sainani G. S., *et al.*, (ed.); API Textbook of Med 1999; 6th. ed; 295-98.

ENDOCRINES AND RESPIRATORY SYSTEM[1]

Pulmonary physiology is significantly influenced by various endocrinopathies as discussed below:

A. Lungs in Diabetes Mellitus

- Both ventillatory mechanism and gas diffusion are altered.
- Chest infections are increased in case of uncontrolled diabetes due to vasculopathy, reduced tissue perfusion, reduced tissue healing, impaired cell mediated immunity and reduced IL_1 and IL_2 production. Patients become 3-4 times more susceptible to tuberculous infection, because of vascular insufficiency, malnutrition, dehydration, hormonal factors and impaired phagocytosis.
- Respiratory epithelium is more prone to infection because of lowered resistance due to factors like hypovitaminosis,

tissue hyperglycemia, enhanced growth of bacteria reduced immunity and defective in vitro lymphocyte transformation.

- Treatment in diabetics should be done only with switching over to insulin.
- Life threatening bacterial and fungal infections are common in uncontrolled diabetics.
- Type 2 diabetes mellitus, obesity and obstructive sleep apnoea is quite common; autonomic neuropathy adds more problem; vagal pathways when involve may increase risk of cardiorespiratory arrest.
- Pleural effusion pneumothorax, aspiration pneumonia, respiratoy failure, ARDS in diabetic beta acidosis, pulmonary odema and plugging of airways with mucous are more common in diabetics.
- Risk of neonatal respiratory distress syndrome is more in newborn basis of diabetic mothers.

B. Thyroid and Lungs

I. Hyperthyroidism

- Respiratory muscle strength and vital capacity are reduced.
- Cardiopathy and CCF may occur.

II. Hypothyroidism

- Exertional dyspnoea, alveolar hypoventilation, respiratory failure, pleural effusion and central/ obstructive sleep apnoea may occur.

C. Parathyroid Disease and Lungs

- In secondary hyperparathyroidism with end stage renal disease, diffuse metastatic calcification of lungs is observed.
- PFTs show ventilatory restriction with hypoxemia and low diffusion of carbon monoxide.
- Rarely it can occur in primary hyperparathyroidism.

D. Adrenals and Lungs

- Hypercortisolism from endogenous Cushing's syndrome offers risk for fungal and other opportunistic infections.
- Adrenal insufficiency makes low birth weight babies more susceptible to bronchopulmonary dysplasia.

E. Pituitary Adenoma

May cause acromegaly due to increased growth hormone secretions. These patients have oropharyngeal narrowing, increased total and vital lung capacity, sleep apnoea syndrome and vocal cord dysfunction.

F. Female Endocrines and Lungs

Cyclic decrease precipitate premenstrual asthma. Fibroma ovary may produce ascitis and pleural effusion called Meig's syndrome. Restrictive pulmonary defects are seen in Klinefelter syndrome. In male endocrinopathies, cystic lung disease may be associated with Marfan's syndrome.

REFERENCE

1. Bhatia R.S., Respiratory consequences of metabolic disorders; Lung India 2000;18 : 81-83.

BRONCHIAL COLLATERAL CIRCULATION: PHYSIOLOGICAL AND CLINICAL IMPORTANCE[1]

Introduction

Two different circulations supply blood to a normal lung, namely (a) pulmonary, bringing the deoxygenated blood from the right heart and (b) systemic, bringing the oxygenated blood from the left heart through the bronchial arteries. In contrast to pulmonary circulation, the bronchial circulation is a high pressure, high resistance circulation and is also known as *pulmonary collateral circulation.* Besides bronchial arteries there are other smaller systemic arteries supplying the lungs, e.g., intercostals.[1] Galen observed systemic blood supply to lungs as early as 2nd century AD,[2] but it was only in 1808, when their functional importance as nutrient arteries of the lungs was realised.[3] Philosophically, these vessels could be considered as the coronaries of the lungs. Bronchial circulation though diminutive in health, is significant in disease. That is why it continues to interest both physiologists as well as clinicians especially in conditions with diminished or absent pulmonary circulation.[1]

Functional Anatomy

Bronchial arteries are usually multiple, having variable origin and course in human beings. They arise from the intercostal branches or directly from the aorta. As they enter the hilum of the lung, they form a communicating arc around the main bronchi, from which main arterial divisions are formed, which go along the bronchial tree, adhering closely to their walls. Usually there are two divisions along the bronchus intercommunicating with each other. Smaller twigs penetrate the bronchial walls and form a similar submucosal network for the respiratory bronchioles. The bronchial arteries supply blood to the bronchial tree, pulmonary lymph nodes, pulmonary vessels, the vagi and the supporting tissue of the alveolar septa and the pleura. Routes of the bronchial venous blood for its drainage include:

a. Venous blood from the proximal bronchial tree drains through the bronchial veins into the vena azygos which terminates in the superior vena cava—the *true* venous drainage since it goes to the right heart.
b. Venous blood from the distal bronchial tree and lung

parenchyma enters the pulmonary circulation through bronchopulmonary vascular anastomoses. Those anastomoses which exist at the post capillary level of pulmonary microcirculation, add deoxygenated venous blood to the pulmonary veins. The mixing results in a minor *physiological shunt* which normally exists-the non-gas-exchanging portion of the circulation. Blood which enters the pulmonary circulation at capillary and precapillary levels gets oxygenated since it takes part in *gas exchange* at the alveolar capillary membrane—the effective portion of bronchial blood flow.[1] There is much interspecies variation in the bronchopulmonary anastomoses. They are present in man and horse.[4] Physiological studies in dog demonstraes anastomoses on both sides of the alveolus.[5] About one third of bronchial blood now (QBr) drains into the vena azygos and two thirds into the pulmonary circulation.[6]

Bronchial Blood Flow

Physiological measurements of bronchial blood now (QBr) are difficult and in most instances, extensive surgery is required.[1] Dog has been the most studied animal for QBr using a variety of techniques. After ligation of the pulmonary artery and vein of a lobe, the retrograde flow of blood from that lobe is measured through an outflow canula placed proximal to the venous legation. This now represents QBr since no pulmonary flow exists to the lobe.[6,7]

Role in Health and Disease

Nutrient Function

The bronchial circulation serves the nutritive functions for the tracheobronchial tree and the supporting framework of the lungs in a healthy person. That is why the bronchial vessels are called *vasa privata* in contrast to *vasa publica*—the pulmonary vessels.[8]

Pulmonary artery occlusion (PAO): Occlusion of a pulmonary artery by ligations or by embolus is not usually followed by pulmonary infarction.[9] Clinically infarction occurs in less than 10% of pulmonary embolism cases.[10] The continued supply of oxygen and substrate for the viability of the tissues is maintained through bronchopulmonary anastomoses.[11] Increased dilation and proliferation of bronchial circulation and increase in QBr after PAO[11-15] which starts within minutes of PAO.[16] However, the mechanisms of this increase have long been debated. A fall in the microvascular pressure distal to the PAO would open up the anastomotic vessels.[17] Hypocapnia, resulting from a disease in alveolar PCO_2 that occurs in the pulmonary embolism area may also dilate bronchial vessels.[7] Alterations in CO_2 on the occuluded side initiate a vagally mediated reflex.[18] In dogs there are nerve fibres and terminal autonomic axons close to the bronchial venules influencing the diametres of these vessels directly by neurogenic stimuli. Bilateral cervical vagotomy attenuated the acute increase in QBr which occurs after PAO.[19] This increase was blocked completely by arachydonic acid inhibitors like indomethacin and sodium salicyclate. There is a rise in both thromboxane—a vasoconstrictor—and prostacycline—a vasodilator—after PAO, which is also inhibited by indomethacin. The increased level of arachidonic acid metabolites may play an important role in mediating the increase in QBr. The prolonged compensatory bronchial vessel's enlargement keeps the areas viable and does not allow infarct to occur.[11,13,14,17,20] However, necrosis and infarction after PAO do occur when the QBr is not allowed to increase due to lowering of systemic arterial pressure chronically.[20] Long-term expansion occurs due to vascular proliferation and neovascularization by angiogenetic factors.[14]

Congenital abnormality of pulmonary artery: Pulmonary artery abnormality (congenital) like pulmonary artery atresia[21] and pulmonay stenosis in Fallot's tetralogy.[21,22] Where there is diminished pulmonary blood flow, bronchial circulation gets markedly expanded.

Ischemic pulmonary disease: It is hypothesized that compromising the nutrient functions of bronchial vessels results in emphysema, but whether this is the cause or a consequence is difficult to decide.[23] Moreover, bronchial circulation has been reported to rather increase in certain cases of COPD and emphysema.[24]

Primary bronchogenic carcinoma: Primary lung cancer is generally deprived of blood supply from pulmonary artery. In that case, the adjacent bronchial arteries get enlarged, supplying oxygenated blood, which not only influence the growth pattern of the tumour but also may become source of brisk haemoptysis in these cases.[1,25]

Lung transplantation: Bronchial complications following lung allotransplantation include necrosis and bleeding at the site of bronchial anastomosis, aspiration pneumonia, focal stricture and transient narrowing of the airways, possibly because of interruption of bronchial vascular supply. Complications reduce on reconstitution of bronchial artery.[26]

Haemodynamic Effects

The communications between low pressure pulmonary and high pressure systemic circulations—the bronchopulmonary anastomosis, serve as low resistance conduits, delivering arterial blood into the pulmonary circulation in chronic destroyed lungs by chronic suppurative lung disease, with sufficient force to divert mixed venous blood away from the anastomotic sites.[27] These are suggested to be sphincteric vessels under control of systemic vasomotor nervous system.[28] The haemodynamic effect can be seen in right-sided heart failure. With enhanced right atrial pressure and insufficient bronchial venous valves, the proximal bronchial venous drainage which normally occurs to right atrium through vena azygose is rerouted to the left atrium through these anastomoses. Thus haemodynamic burden on left heart is increased when the collateral circulation is expanded in diseases like chronic cor pulmonale.[1]

Role in Gas Exchange

The expanded collateral circulation following PAO_2 does participate in alveolar-capillary gas exchange in part.[29] The lung with ligated pulmonary artery barel contributes to oxygen uptake under ordinary conditions of ambient air breathing. The component of *QBr* which reaches the alveolar capillary surface of the lung to participate in gas exchange is the *effective QBr,* which may be quite large in patients with diminished or absent pulmonary circulation. *Non-effective QBr* is measured, otherwise in the normal human lung.[21] The gas exchange pathways, in which QBr participates, may have a significant tissue diffusion limitation, as has been studied in dog using trace quantities of six inert gases.[30]

Pathogenesis of Haemoptysis

The expanded bronchial vessles in patients with tuberculosis,[31] bronchiectasis,[32] lung abscess,[33] bronchogenic carcinoma[34] and mitral stenosis[35] may be responsible for massive haemoptysis. The expanded circulation may be involved in the resolution and repair during infection.[33] Bronchial artery embolization by transcatheter technique is well accepted now-a-days to stop and prevent haemoptysis.[36]

Lung Oedema

Transudate fluid in pulmonary oedema is chiefly from pulmonary circulation; but bronchial circulation may play an important role in chemically induced oedema as has been demonstrated in dogs and rats.[19] Histamine and bradykinin administration by different routes produces peribronchial interstitial oedema. Bronchial venules of both submucosa and peribronchial plexus also become permeable. In hydrostatic oedema the role of bronchial circulation is not that clear. However, dense bronchial microvascular plexus in the peribronchial spaces has been observed where early oedema occurs. Because this plexus drains into the capillary network, pressure in the pulmonary micro-vasculature is likely to be carried forward to the bronchial vessels, which may leak into the pulmonary veins due to increased hydrostatic pressure, thereby contributing partly to the interstitial lung oedema.[37] Similarly enhanced right atrial pressure may cause leakage from the bronchial veins draining into right atrium through vena azygos.[1] In non-cardiac lung oedema in adult respiratory distress syndrome (ARDS) QBr may increase to serve the role of inflammation and repair,[38] since pulmonary vessels in ARDS are constricted, occluded or destroyed. This increase in QBr in ARDS simulating lung injury in dogs has been demonstrated.[38] This increase is perhaps mediated at least in part by cycloxygenase products of arachidonic acid, since the increase was blocked by indomethacin.[39] However, it is difficult to evaluate clinical importance of QBr in ARDS.[1] It is suggested to sustain QBr by maintaining systemic arterial pressure and since positive end exp. pressure assisted ventilation has markedly reduced QBr,[5] to limit PEEP strictly to that level that is necessary to improve oxygenation. The healing in ARDS is usually dramatic possibly due to maintenance of an adequate QBr.[1]

Bronchoconstriction

The subserosal and submucosal bronchial vascular plexus communicate with intercommunicating branches through gaps in the cartilages and muscle fibre bundles of the airway wall. QBr is affected with any alterations in bronchomotor tone, bronchoconstriction increasing QBr directly or due to accompanying hypocapnia.[7] Similarly, vagal stimulation acetylcholine and histamine increase QBr and epinephrine and sympathetic stimulation decrease QBr and all these effects are blocked by appropriate antagonists.[40] QBr has been demonstrated to increase following methacholine aerosol inhalation,[41] which was partly reversed by atropine and prostaglandin F2 alpha in a study on ioslated *in situ* LLL in open chested dog.[42] In both situations, indomethacin was found to block the increase.[41,42] The increase in QBr in bronchoconstriction is possibly mediated by the releases of arachidonic acid metabolites and serves the actively contracting airway muscle.[1] Bronchial circulation remains less known, yet equally important collateral circulation.[43]

REFERENCES

1. Jindal S. K., Functional and clinical significance of the collateral circulation, Ind J Chest Dis & All Sci 1985; 27: 236-46.
2. Miller W. S. The Lung; Ed 2 Charles C Thomas Publ. Springfield III, 1947.
3. Von Sommering S. T. Resseissen F. D., Ueber den Bau der Lungen Voss, Berlin, 1808.
4. Mclaughilin R. F. Jr. Bronchial artery distribution in various mammals and in humans, Amer, Rev Resp Dis 1983; 128: 557-58.
5. Modell H. I., *et al.,* Functional aspects of canine bronchial pulmonary vascular communications, J App. Physiol Resp Environ Exer Physiol 1981; 50: 1045-51.

6. Aramendia P., *et al.,* Response of the bronchial veins in a heart lung bronchial preparation, Circ Res 1962; 10: 3-10.
7. Aviado D. M., The lung circulation; In: Physiol. and Pharm, New York, Pergamon, vol I, 1965.
8. Von Luschka H.D., *Die anatomie des Menschen* L, Pt 2; In: Rucksicht auf die Bedurtnisse der Prakhchen Heilkunde. Tubingen, West Germany: Laupp, 1963.
9. Virchow R.L., Gasamelte Werke; In: Abhand lungen zur wissensch laftlichen Medizin. Frankfurt: Mcdingr 1856; 285-96.
10. Moser K. M., Pulmonary embolism; Amer Rev Resp Dis 1977; 115: 829-52.
11. Huber G. H., Edmunds L.J., Pulmonary artery occlusion II Morphological studies; J App Physiol 1967; 22:1002-11.
12. Schalepfer K., Ligation of the pulmonary artery of one lung with and without resection of phrenic nerve; AMA Arch Surg 1924; 9: 25-94.
13. Ellis F. H. Jr., *et al.,* The bronchial arteries III, Structural changes after division of the rat's left pulmonary artery; Amer J Path 1952; 28: 89-103.
14. Weibel E. R., Early stages in the development of the collateral circulation to the lung in rat, Cir Res 1960; 8: 353-76.
15. Malik A. B., Tracy S. E., Bronchovascular adjustments after pulmonary embolism, J App Physiol Resp, Environ Exer Physiol 1980; 49: 476-81.
16. Jindal S. K., *et al.,* Acute increase in anastomotic bronchial blood flow after pulmonary arterial obstruction, J App Physio, Resp Environ Exer Physiol 1984; 57: 424-28.
17. Leibow A. A., *et al.,* The genesis and functional implications of collateral circulation of the lung; Yale J Biol Med 1950; 22: 637-50.
18. Hertz C., *et al.,* Reflektorisce beeinflussing der atmung durch Anderung der CO_2, Konzentration in den lungen allveoloii bzw. Lungencapillaren: Ein bispher unbeckannter Atemrefle; Klin Wschr 1961; 39:650-51.
19. Jindal S. K., *et al.,* Effect of cervical vagotomy on anastomotic bronchial blood flow after pulmonary artery obstruction in dogs, Ind J Med Res 1985; 81: 83-85.
20. Haworth S. G., *et al.,* How the left lung is perfused after ligating the left pulmonary artery in the pig at birth, Clinical implications for the hypoperfused lung, Cardiovasc Res 1981; 15: 214-26.
21. Fishman A. P., *et al.,* The effective pulmonary collateral blood flow in man, J Clin Invest 1958; 37: 1071-86.
22. Nakamura T., Bronchopulmonary circulation, its systemic and functional implications, The Jap Circ 1958; 22: 427.
23. Strawbridge H. T. G. Chronic pulmonary emphysema, An experimental study, Amer J Path 1960; 37: 161-74.
24. Boushy S. F., *et al.,* The bronchial arteries in COPD, Amer J Med 1969; 46: 506-15.
25. Cudkowicz L., Armstrong J. B., The blood supply of malignant pulmonary neoplasms, Thorax 1953; 8:152.
26. Mills N. L., *et al.,* The significance of bronchial circulation in lung transplantation, J., Thoracic Cardiovas Surg 1970; 60: 866-74.
27. Alley R. D., *et al.,* Demonstration of bronchial pulmonary artery reverse flow in suppurative pulmonary disease, Clin Res 1958; 6: 41.
28. State D., *et al.,* Physiologic and pharmacologic studies of collateral pulmonary flow, J Thoracic Surg 1957; 34:599-60.
29. Bloomer W. E. H., *et al.,* Respiratory function and blood flowing the bronchial artery after ligation of the pulmonary artery, Amer J Physiol 1949; 157: 317-28.
30. Robertson H. T., *et al.,* Gas exchange properties of the bronchial circulation in a dog lobe maintained in zone I condition, Amer Rev Res Dis 1984; 129: A229.
31. Katori R., *et al.,* Bronchial blood flow in pulmonary tuberculosis, Tohuko J. Exp. Med 1970; 100: 135-42.
32. Cocketa F. B., Vtss C.C.N., A comparison of role of the bronchial arteries in bronchiectasis and in experimental ligation of the pulmonary artery, Thorax 1951; 6: 268.
33. Charan N. B., *et al.,* The role of bronchial circulation in lung abscess, Amer Rev Res Dis 1985; 131: 121-24.
34. Wright R. D., The blood supply of abnormal tissues in the lungs, J Path 1938; 47: 489-99.
35. Shedd D. P., *et al.,* Observations of the haemodynamics of bronchial pulmonary vascular communications; J Thoracic Surg 1951; 22: 537-48.
36. Uflacker R., *et al.,* Management of massive haemoptysis by bronchial artery embolization, Radiol 1983; 146: 623-34.
37. Charan N. B., *et al.,* Gross and subgross anatomy of bronchial circulation in sheep, J App Physiol Resp Environ Exercise Physiol 1984; 57: 658-64.
38. Lakshmi S., *et al.,* Bronchial blood flow increases in inflammatory lung oedema (Abstr), Physiolo 1983;, 26: A56.
39. Deffebach M., *et al.,* Arachidonic acid metabolites and anastomotic bronchial blood flow in generalised lung injury, Clin Res 1985; 33: 76A.
40. Baile E. M., *et al.,* Effect of PEEP on bronchial blood flow and bronchial vascular resistance in dogs, Physiolo 1982; 25: 203.
41. Jindal S. K., *et al.,* Methacholine increases anastomotic bronchial blood flow in dogs, Physiolo 1983; 26: A56.
42. Jindal S. K., *et al.,* Prostaglandin F2 alpha increases bronchial blood flow in dogs, Clin Res 1984; 32: 63A.
43. Bhatia R. S., Bronchial circulation, clinical review, Lung India 1995; 13(i): 29-31.

PLEUROPULMONARY DENGUE HAEMORRHAGE SYNDROME

Introduction

Dengue fever is a public health problem. Dengue haemorrhagic fever is a serious manifestation, occurring in a person, previously infected with dengue on reinfection with different subtypes. Four subtypes have been recognized, infection with a subtype is followed by immunity to that subtype for rest of the life. However, reinfection with other subtype is dangerous with pleuropulmonary affection with haemorrhages and manifests with haemoptysis, pulmonary haemorrhages, pneumonitis and pleural effusion.

Clinically, patients present with history of fever of 4-7 days, with non productive cough, skin rash and with or without haemoptysis. Cutaneous petechial haemorrhages, purpuric lesions and even ecchymosis may be seen. Chest examination may reveal bilateral few inspiratory crepitations. Routine investigations reveal lower platelet count, $\pm$ 40,000/mm^3.Chest X-ray may show bilateral fluffy shadows. HRCT chest show bilateral patchy ground glass opacities in central and basal lung fields, consistent with pulmonary haemorrhage. Large consolidation and pleural effusion may also be detected. Therapeutic bronchoscopy if applied, should never be extended to attempt diagnostic biopsy because of haemorrhagic manifestations.[1] Dengue serology for IgM and IgG is positive.

Pathogenesis of bleeding in dengue haemorrhagic fever which is reported in 1.4% of dengue infection, is not clearly understood. Perhaps many factors such as abnormalities in coagulation cascade, platelet dysfunction, thrombocytopenia, disseminated intravascular coagulation, vascular defects and increased vascular permeability possibly histamine mediated are responsible.[3] Unnecesary, irrational drugs such as antibiotics, NSAIDS, and antimalarials to combat fever may precipitate haemorrhage.[4]

Conservative Line of Management

With cautious intravenous fluids and platelets transfusion should be choice treatment. HRCT thorax follow up can be used for evaluation and recovery.

Cutaneous petechiae or ecchymosis are sufficient to alert the physician for aggressive management. Epistaxis, bleeding gums, haematuria, gastrointestinal and even intracranial haemorrhage may be less frequently encountered in dengue fever. Pulmonary haemorrhage, haemoptysis, pneumonitis and pleural effusion are rare manifestations of dengue haemorrhagic fever.[2]

REFERENCES

1. Sharma SK; *et al.,* Pulmonary haemorrhage syndrome associated with dengue haemorrhagic fever; JAPI 2007; 55: 729-30.
2. Liam CK; *et al.,* Dengue fever complicated by pulmonary haemorrhage manifesting as haemoptysis; J Trop Med Hygiene 1993; 96: 197-200.
3. Setlik, Robart F; Pulmonary haemorrhage syndrome associated with an autochthonous case of dengue haemorrhagic fever; Southern Med Journal 2004; 97: 688-91.
4. Badyal Dinesh, Bhatia RS; Adverse drug reactions; Peepee Publ, 2006.

ROLE OF VITAMIN D IN CHEST DISORDERS

Since decades, role of vitamin D has been appreciated in prevention of rickets and osteomalacia. Also, its role is very much time tested in calcium and skeletal homeostasis.[1] One nutrient–one disorder has been aside, searching the role of vitamin in various respiratory disorders.[2]

Therapeutic use of vitamin D rich cod liver oil was popularly prescribed in fifties before the advent of streptomycin. However vitamin D toxicity hampered the use and research in the areas of non-skeletal indications of vitamin D.

Again, the interests and utilizations of vitamin D has surfaced with promise being observed in these newer concepts. Nevertheless, the utilisation has to be taken with critical appraisal with a constant watch, patiently observing these newer existing areas of research to advent newer horizon of vitamin D effects.[3] But the enthusiasm must have judicious caution, learning a prudent lesson from our past follies.

Areas of possible indication/utilization/research of vitamin D in various chest diseases/disorders[4] being currently applied are shown in Table 11.67.

Table 11.67: Potential role of vitamin D or its metabolites in chest disorders

	Disorder	*Evidence based*	*Possible role*
1.	Tuberculosis	Moderate/Direct	Promising/ Cautious
2.	URIs	Moderate/Indirect	"
3.	Viral respiratory infections	Moderate/Indirect	"
4.	HIV-Lung disease	Moderate/Indirect	"
5.	Asthma	High/Indirect	"
6.	Respiratory diseases and diabetes	High/Direct and indirect	Convincing/ Cautious
7.	Lung cancer	High/Direct and indirect	"

Modified from Ref.[2]

REFERENCES

1. Heaney RP; Vitamin D–How much do we need and how much is too much? Osteoporosis Intern 2000; 11: 553-55.
2. Rao DS; Vitamin D–It's not just for bones any more; Med Update; Rao MS; (ed) 2010; 20: 446-48.
3. Holick MF; Vitamin D deficiency; NEJM 2007; 357: 266-81.
4. De Luca HF, Cantorna MT; Vitamin D–Its role and uses in immunology; FASEB Journ 2001; 15: 2579-85.

PULMONARY DISORDERS CAUSING SYNDROME OF INAPPROPRIATE SECRETION OF ANTIDIURETIC HORMONE (SIADH)[1,2]

Apart from underlying etiology of CNS disorders, drugs. AIDS/ HIV disease and metabolic disorders, pulmonary diseases such as pneumonia cavitary aspergillosis, tuberculosis, lung abscess and carcinoma can lead to electrolyte abnormality, causing symptomatic or asymptomatic hyponatremia. Pulmonary and other causes of SIADH are listed in Table 11.68. Generalized tonic clonic seizures may pointer towards underlying neurologic disorder, but in lieu of normal MRI brain, other causes of seizures were looked for. Chest X-ray may be normal and chest CECT may give clue of presence of consolidation, accompanied with hyponatremia, suspecting SIADH of pulmonary origin. Treatment of pneumonitis with broad spectrum antimicrobial along with hypertonic saline infusion at the rate of 1 meq/L/hour to avoid precipitation of osmotic demyelination syndrome due to rapid correction of hyponatremia.

Table 11.68: Pulmonary and other disorders causing SIADH

Pulmonary disorders	: Tuberculosis
	Pneumonia
	Lung abscess
	Cavitary aspergillosis
	Carcinoma.
CNS disorders	: Head trauma
	Enciphalitis, meningitis
	CV ovulation
	CV haemorrhage
	Cavernous sinus thrombosis
	Guillain-Barre syndrome
	Hydrocephalus
	Multiple sclerosis
	Psychosis
	Peripheral neuropathy
	Congenital malformations such as cleft lip/palate
Malignant disorders	: Ca lung
	GI neoplasms
	Ovarian carcinoma
	Thymoma
Drugs	: Vasopressin
	Vincristin
	Cyclophosphamide
	Carbamazepine
	Chlorpropamide
	Nicotine
	MAO inhibitors
	Tricyclic antidepressants
	Phenothiazines
Miscellaneous	: Legionella infection
	HIV infection
	Acute intermittent porphyria

Acute severe hyponatremia urgently require saline infusion; while chronic SIADH require, if not severe, only fluid restriction and loop diuretics; and if severe, demechocycline or fludrocortisone. Vasopressin antagonists such as tolvaptan, lixivaptan, conivaptan help free water excretion without altering excretion of sodium and potassium.

REFERENCES

1. Siragy HM; Hyponatrenia, fluid-electrolyte disorders and SIADH secretion: Diagnosis and treatment options; Endocr Pract 2006; 12 : 446-57.
2. Aggarwal A; *et al.*, Causes of seizures: Lungs, not the brain; Lung India 2011; 28: 65-66.

SUMMARY

Utility of stem cells in lung diseases has seen tremendous forward leap in the last decade. Potential use of embryonic, endogenous and adult stem cells is being studied for different lung disorders such as emphysema, cystic fibrosis, lung cancer, ARDS, pulmonary artery hypertension etc. Various biomaterials and biomimetic microsystems are being developed to be utilized in experimental labs in place of animal models for studying drugs and their toxic effects. Nevertheless potential role of stem cells in lung disorders is still in its infancy and may become reality in the near future.

Stem Cell Therapy in Pulmonary Disorders

Stem cells are defined as the cells of clonogenic and renewing capabilities and that can differentiate into linages of multiple cells. Before the stem cell therapy becomes a reality, few points which deserve consideration are: (a) the diverse pathology of lung diseases to be targeted; (b) need to consider boosting endogenous regenerative mechanisms in comparison with exogenous stem cell transplantation; and (c) importance and value of selecting the stem cells, particularly their source and potential to differentiate.

These can be intrinsic or extrinsic[1] as shown in Table 11.69.

Features of Stem Cells include:

- Undifferentiated cells.
- Ability for unlimited self-renewal.
- Infrequent proliferation.
- Replenish progenitor cells.

Table 11.69: Stem cells

Intrinsic	*Extrinsic*
• Basal epithelial cells in trachea/ larger airways	• Adult stem cells
• Clara cells in smaller airways	• Embryonic sterna cells.
• Type II pneumocytes in parenchyma of lung	

Capability of proliferation must be accompanied with at least one of the progeny retaining the stem cell parent character, helps for long term maintenance of stem cells and also through this capability, these can play an important role in reparative and regenerative process in the lungs.[2]

Potency of Stem Cells

It can be termed as unipotent i.e. cells can produce one cell type e.g. spermatogonial stem cells can form sperms only; multipotent i.e. adult stem cells having ability to produce multiple cell types of one lineage e.g. Hematopoietic stem cells; pluripotent stem cells are capable of producing all lineages of body, e.g., embryonic stem cells; and totipotent stem cells having ability to (re)generate an organism in total, e.g., zygote and first cleavage blastomeses in mammals are totipotent.[3] Ideal stem cells for transplantation would be the one generated from renewable source which can be differentiated along a specific lineage/function and are immunocompatible, survive and integrate after engraftment and function till the recipient survives.

Use of pluripotent human embryonic stem cells have ethical issues and also requires recipient's immunosuppression. Induced pluripotent stem cells form a viable alternative which are engineered by expressing a stereotypic selection of genes in somatic cells derived from the patient. Although, these are histocompatible but have their limitation in case of genetic disorders as normal cells are likely to carry the same genetic defect.

Umbilical cord blood, adult hematopoietic and mesenchymal stem cells are being extensively researched.

Lung specific cell phenotypes from embryonic stem cells can be derived using small airways growth medium. However, embryonic cells, apart from capability of proliferation and replication, that can form tissues during embryonic development are different from adult cells that are capable of repair and maintenance after birth.[4] At the same time, majority of genes expressed in multipotent embryonic progenitors are not expressed in endogenous lung stem cells or in adult lung. Eventual organ formation results from rapid proliferation of embryonic cells and undergoing shape-changes that mediate branching morphogenesis and patterning in terms of tissue development.[5] Nevertheless, consistent differentiation directed proficiently towards a single cell lineage is lacking. Other ethico-moral objections regarding potential malignant transformations and immune rejection in host are also raised.

Phenotypic characterization of *adult stem cells* into lung epithelial stem cells can be obtained from patients' own cells in culture and then reintroduced into the patient. Autologus cells help avoid immunologic rejection. Adult stem cells of mesenchymal, hematopaietic, neural, hepatic, cutaneous, pancreatic and skeletal muscle can also be characterized.

After a number of studies favouring and against the engraftment of bone marrow derived stem cells as airway and alveolar epithelium,[6] the controversy focuses on the actual degree of chimerism or engraftment of adult marrow derived cells.[7,8] Accumulating evidence confirms that bone marrow derived stem cells contribute to fibroblasts/myofibroblasts in the lungs via circulating fibrocyte cells, which express the HSC marker CD 34 and collagen. In a bleomycin induced lung fibrosis in a mouse, 80% of type 1 collagen-expressing firbroblasts were observed to be of marrow (donor) origin.[9] Other marrow progenitors such as endothelial progenitor cells have been found in engraftment of pulmonary vasculature.

Endogenous stem cells are responsible for tissue maintenance and repair in all the tissues. These cells can produce unspecific as well as daughter cells called progenitor cells which are transit amplifying cells. These are currently being used for targeting with gene transfer vectors to obtain sustained expression. Three distinct regions[10] that support lung tissue stem cells are (a) Intercartelaginous regions of tracheobronchial airways (b) neuroepithelial bodies in bronchioles; and (c) bronchoalveolar duct junction.

These progenitor cells have finite life span with more robust proliferative potential, e.g.; a toxin-resistant cells, clara cells, basal cells etc.

Therapeutic potential that can be utilized is shown in Table 11.70.

Table 11.70: Therapeutic capabilities of stem cells in lung disorders[2]

1. Regenerating extracellular matrix	• Emphysema • ARDS • Lung fibrosis
2. Regeneration of alveoli	• Emphysema
3. Stem cell acting as genetic vectors	• Cystic fibrosis
4. Endogenous progenitor cells transducted with nitric oxide synthetase	• Pulmonary artery hypertension
5. Targeting endogenous stem cells with potential for malignant transformation by identifying with specific surface marker	• Lung cancer

Lung is a complex tissue with specifically aligned airspace and vasculature for exchange of gases where extracellular matrix plays a major role in this structural organization. Lung tissue elasticity and elastic recoil seriously affect the mechanical propers if injured/diseased; such as restrictive conditions following tissue scar, sarcoidosis or IPF.

Role of biomaterials in providing structural frame (Scaffold) for grafted stem cells to orderly integrate and provide functional connections is also being currently investigated. Both natural and synthetic biomaterials are being used to create tissue engineered lung, though, development of lung tissue using these materials has not been substantial.[11] For implantation of a relatively unvascularized engineered tissue lungs form the best site where oxygen enriched pleural cavity environment offers direct diffusion of O_2 or other gases even without the support of blood flow. Thus decellularized lung itself offers the best possible matrix to support engineering of lung tissue. Studies are being conducted using cells stripped off the cells that possibly cause organ rejection, followed by infusion of this extracellular matrix with lung specific stem cells to culture for eight days. Results have shown that the natural extra cellular matrix could direct the cells to their correct locations, essentially training them for appropriate functioning. This tissue on replantation in rats has functioned for two hours, fulfilling the basic criterion of key lung function of gas exchange, i.e., O_2 for CO_2.[12] Others have also utilized the same approach using embryonic-like stem cells called induced pleuripotent stem cells which could differentiate into key type of lung cells when grown on decellularized matrices.[13,14] However, the matrix structurally gets weakened/degraded during decellularization itself.

Biomimetic microsystem is also in the offing that reconstitutes the functional alveolar-capillary interface of human lung and responds to bacteria as well as inflammatory cytokines when introduced into alveolar spaces. This offers a low cost lab model, alternative to animal model, for conducting clinical research regarding drug use, drug screening and toxicological behaviour.[15] This great achievement may become reality in near future; stem cell therapy remains still in its infancy as regards lung disease in man. That stem cell based protocols would achieve the goal in the coming years, is the optimism that is growing in scientific circles and is sending exciting message to general population. It is important that an effective critique of what is not biologically sound and not evidence based is absolutely essential and an absolute sure stress test must be undertaken before releasing the clear-cut benefit of the scientific research in stem cell therapy to avoid unfounded higher expectations as well as disappointments. Continuous efforts in stem cell research along with alternative newer pathways and better optional modalities should be made keeping in mind the transparency in effects and adverse effects of stem cell therapy with regards to cultural/religious as well as scientific/ethical aspects/implications.

Public and profession must be continuously informed through internet and medical journals so that scientists have wide variety of selecting right source of stem cells for the appropriate pathology, utilizing biomedical engineering, all time real addressal of ethical issues as far as utilization of certain varieties of stem cells and legislative safeguard regarding in cell experimental and commercial exploitation in diverse pathological situations.

REFERENCES

1. Stripp BR, Shapiro SD; Stem Cells in Lung disease: Repair and the potential for therapeutic interventions; Amer J Resp Cell Mol Biol 2006; 34: 517-22.
2. Singhal S; *et al.*, Stem cells and lung diseases; JAPI 2011; 59: 433-36.
3. Weiss DJ; *et al.*, Stem cells and cell therapies in lung biology and lung disease; NHLB1/Cystic fibrosis foundation workshop; Proc Am Thorac Soc 2008; 5:637-67.
4. Varanou A; *et al.*, Human embryonic stem cells and lung regeneration; Brit J Pharm 2008; 155: 316-25.
5. Lu P; Werb Z; Patterning mechanisms of branched organs; Science 2008; 322; 1506-09.
6. Krause DS; Engraftment of bone marrow-derived epithelial cells; Anu NY Acad Sci 2005; 1044: 117-24.
7. Zander DS; *et al.*, Bone marrow-derived stem cell repopulation contributes minimally to the type II pneumocyte pool in transplanted human lungs; Transplantation 2005; 80: 206-12.
8. Kotton DN; *et al.*, Failure of bone marrow to reconstitute lung epithelium; Amer J Resp Cell Mol Biol 2005; 33: 328-34.
9. Hashimoto N; *et al.*, Bone marrow-derived progenitor cells in pulmonary fibrosis; J Clin Invest 2004; 113: 243-52.
10. Giangreco A; *et al.*, Terminal bronchioles harbor a unique airway stem cell population that localizes to the bronchoalveolar duct junction; Amer J Pathol 2002; 161:173-82.
11. Andrade CF; *et al.*, Cell-based tissue engineering for lung regeneration: Amer J Physiol Lung Cell Mol Physiol 2007; 292: 510-18.
12. Paterson TH; *et al.*, Tissue-engineered lungs for in vivo implantation; Science advance online publication Doi: 10.1126/ Science 118 9 345 (2010).
13. Price AP; *et al.*, Development of a decellularized lung bioreactor system for bioengineering the lung: The matrix reloaded. Tissue engineering–Part A advance online publication: Doi: 10.1089/ ten. tea 2009; 0 659 (2010).
14. Cortiella J; *et al.*, Influence of acellular natural lung matrix on murine embryonic stem cell differentiation and tissue formation: Tissue engineering: Part A advance online publication Doi; 10. 1089/ten. tea 2009; 0730 (2010).
15. Hug D; *et al.*, Reconstituting Organ-level lung functions on a chip; Science 2010; 328: 662-68.

IMPORTANT SYNDROMES, CLINICAL FEATURES, INVESTIGATIONS AND TREATMENT

Table 11.71: Pulmonary manifestation of certain diseases

Disease	*Lung involvement*
Syphilis	Diffuse consolidation
	Gummata in airways or lungs
	Cavitation, diffuse pulmonary fibrosis
Acute pancreatitis	Pleural effusion, atelectasis, ARDS
Neurofibromatosis	Chest wall neurofibroma
	Bullous emphysema
	Pneumothorax
	Diffuse interstitial fibrosis
Tuberous sclerosis	Multiple hamartomas
	Carney's triad of pulmonary harmartoma, gastric leiomyosarcoma and paraganglio-noma
Marfan's syndrome	Mild scoliosis, pneumothorax, upper lobe bullae and fibrosis
Ehlers-Danlos syndrome	Recurrent sinusitis
	Haemoptysis
	Pneumonitis
	Pneumothorax
	Tracheomegaly and pectus excavatum
Hermansky-Pudlak syndrome	Interstitial lung fibrosis
	– Albinism
	– Platelet aggregation defect
	– Chromolipids in macrophages

Table 11.72: Kartagener's syndrome

Presentation:	Dextrocardia, sinusitis, bronchiectasis, with or without transposition of viscera.
Investigation:	Chest X-ray and barium meal are helpful.
Aetiology:	Hereditary.
Treatment:	Surgical correction of defects; antibiotics and symptomatic management of pulmonary and sinus problems.

Table 11.73: Irukandji syndrome

Cause:	Jelly fish sting.
Clinical presentation:	Severe pain, shaking, profuse sweating, tachycardia, systemic hypertension, acute respiratory failure, acute pulmonary oedema.
Pathogenesis:	Massive release of catecholamines.
Treatment:	Intravenous marcotics in high doses, phenotolamine, diuretics, nitrates, endotracheal intubation and intermittent positive pressure ventilation.

Table 11.74: Hamman-Rich syndrome

Presentation:	Diffuse progressive interstitial lung fibrosis.
Investigation:	Chest X-ray: Diffuse reticulation.
Management:	Not effective.
Prognosis:	Usually fatal.

Table 11.75: Hand-Schuller-Christian syndrome

Synonymus:	Histiocytosis X.
Presentation:	Diabetes insipidus, exophthalamos, otitis externa, skull bone absorption, with or without gingivitis and skin rash.
Investigations:	Skin biopsy and bone marrow (Foam cells).
	Skull X-ray (Map like areas of decreased density).
	Chest film (Mottled or honeycomb appearance).
Treatment:	Chemotherapy and radiotherapy
	It is usually seen in children and is a non-familial syndrome.

Table 11.76: France's triad

1. Asthma
2. Aspirin sensitivity
3. Allergic rhinitis

Table 11.77: Cervical rib syndrome

Synonymus:	Naffzigar's syndrome: Thoracic outlet syndrome.
Features:	Pain and parasthesias in arm and hand along the ulnar nerve distribution, reduced pulsations of radial and ulnar arteries, Horner's syndrome.
Investigations:	Addison' s test +ve.
Chest X-ray:	Cervical rib present.
Management:	Problem is slowly progressive, follows an intermittent course; rest, traction and surgical excision of rib are helpful.

Table 11.78: Important points: Management of sleep apnoea

1. Rule out myxoedema and other pathology.
2. In obese patients, weight reduction is advised.

Table 11.79: Tietze's syndrome

Synonymus:	Anterior chest wall syndrome, costochondral syndrome.
Presentation:	Pain and tenderness of costochondral junctions. Commonly seen in 30-50 years age group. Self limiting; may need analgesics.

Table 11.80: Pancoast's syndrome

Features:	Shoulder and chest pain, ipsilateral Horner's syndrome.
Investigation:	Chest X-ray, lung biopsy and sputum cytology helpful.
Treatment:	Surgery, radiotherapy and chemotherapy.
Prognosis:	Survival rate is poor.

Table 11.81: Meig's syndrome

Synonymus:	Demons-Meig's syndrome.
Features:	Ascitis, hydrothorax, ovarian fibroma.
Investigations:	Sex hormone levels helpful.
Treatment:	Surgical removal of ovarian fibroma.

Table 11.82: Mendelson's syndrome

Features:	Bronchospasm and chemical pneumonitis associated with coma or general anaesthesia.
Management:	Intubation and oxygen.
	Hydrocortisone, bronchodilators and antibiotics.
	Artificial ventilation.
	Acid-base balance maintenance.

Table 11.83: Loeffler's syndrome

Synonymus:	Pie syndrome.
Features:	Wheeze, cough, fever, pulmonary infiltrates with eosinophilia.
Investigation:	Lung biopsy is diagnostic.
Management:	Need to treat underlying cause (drugs, allergens, microfilaria) (PIE).
	Prone to syndrome are asthmatics.

COMMON RESPIRATORY PROBLEMS

Signs and Symptoms (Important Features)

Table 11.84: Pleural friction rub

On auscultation:	A grating sound with each breath.
Positive in:	Pleurisy, Pulmonary thrombosis, Lung carcinoma, Empyema.

Table 11.85: Features of ventilation

Hyperventilation
Cause: Due to low pO_2, high pCO_2or direct cerebral action.
Respiratory rate: Rapid more than 35/min.
Seen: In conditions like anxiety, pain, fever, hysteria, metabolic acidosis, sepsis, anoxia, cerebral haemorrhage, pneumothorax, drugs (adrenaline).
Hypoventilation
Due to direct action on respiratory centre or physical limitation of lung expansion.
Low, less than 10 breaths/min.
Seen: In conditions with raised intracranial pressure (tumour, abscess, haemorrhage), drugs like sedatives, asthma, lung collapse, pleural effusion, pneumonia, pneumothorax, neuromuscular disorder, bronchiectasis.

Table 11.86: Scarlet fever (Streptococcal throat)

Features: Circumoral pallor, strawberry tongue, tachycardia
Investigations: Throat swab +ve
ASO: Raised titre
Total leucocyte count: High
ESR: High
Differential diagnoses:
Viral URI
Vincent's angina
Infectious mononucleosis
Diphtheria
Rubella
Measles
Drug rash, agranulocytosis, SJS, Roseola infantum

Table 11.87: Causes of wheeze (Syndromewise)

1. Carcinoid syndrome (flushing, diarrhoea, abdominal cramps)
2. France's triad (aspirin sensitivity, asthma, allergic rhinitis)
3. Loeffler's syndrome (cough, fever, pulmonary eosinophilia)
4. Mendelson's syndrome (pneumonitis, bronchospasm)

Table 11.88: Causes of cough (Syndromewise)

1. *Goodpasture's syndrome:* Haemoptysis, dyspnoea, anaemia
2. *Kartagener's syndrome:* Dextrocardia, sinusitis
3. *Loeffler's syndrome:* Wheeze, fever, pulmonary eosinophilia
4. *Louis-Bar syndrome:* Telangiectasia of face and flexures

Table 11.89: Common causes of wheeze

Asthma, anaphylaxis, acute left ventricular failure, Alpha-1-antitrypsin deficiency (in children), aspergillosis
Bronchitis, bronchiolitis, bronchiectasis, bronchial carcinoma
Cystic fibrosis
Emphysema, echinococcosis
Gastroesophageal reflex
Hypoparathyroidism
Pneumonitis

Table 11.90: Pulmonary causes of syncope

Pulmonary embolism (Cough, shock, chest pain)
Anoxia from any cause (Cyanosis, bradycardia)
Hypoventilation due to tetany or fright
Drugs like narcotics and hypnotics

Table 11.91: Causes of stridor (Harsh whistling with inspiration)

Croup, congenital cysts, tumours and membranes
Diphtheria
Epiglottitis
Foreign body in larynx or trachea
Infectious mononucleosis
Laryngo-tracheitis-bronchitis (in children), laryngitis, laryngeal papillomata
Laryngomalacia (congenital)
Retropharyngeal abscess (rare)
Subglottic haemangioma

Table 11.92: Differential diagnosis of stridor wheezing

	Sudden	Inspiratory	Foreign body in the larynx
	Paroxysmal	Expiratory (Mixed)	Bronchial asthma Cardiac asthma
	Acute	Inspiratory	Acute inflammation of the larynx (acute laryngitis, diphtheria, false croup) Oedema of the larynx (laryngospasm, laryngeal oedema) Acute inflammation of the pharynx (retropharyngeal abscess, peritonsillar abscess)
		Mixed	Acute bronchiolitis
Stridor/ wheezing		Inspiratory	Nasal disease, palatine tonsil hypertrophy, adenoids (nasal stridor/wheezing, pharyngeal stridor/wheezing) Benign or malignant tumor of the pharynx or larynx, cicatricial stenosis, tuberclulosis, syphilis, bilateral paralysis posticus Congenital laryngeal stridor (soft epiglottis, epiglottic abnormally, congenital vocal cord paralysis, glottic or subglottic membrane)
	Chronic	Mixed	Benign or malignant tumor of the trachea or bronchi, cicatricial stenosis, external pressure (goiter, vascular abnormality, thymic hyperplasia, lymph adenoma, tumour of the mediastinum, oesophageal carcinoma) Foreign body in the bronchi Tuberculosis of the trachea or bronchi, syphilis Diffuse bronchiolitis Hyperventilation syndrome
		Expiratory	Chronic bronchitis, pulmonary emphysema with asthma Tracheobronchomalacia

Table 11.93: DPLD (History-wise)

Episodic Eosinophilic pneumonia Vasculitides/pulmonary haemorrhage Churg-Strauss syndrome Extrinsic allergic alveolitis Cryptogenic organizing pneumonia *Acute, episodic or chronic* Eosinophilic pneumonia Cryptogenic organizing pneumonia Wegener's granulomatosis BOOP	*Acute or chronic* Drug induced pulmonary injury *Acute history with fever* Hypersensitivity pneumonia *Acute* and *typical history* Cryptogenic fibrosing alveolitis DPLD and connective tissue disorder

Table 11.94: Six main groups of DPLD

1. Collagen vascular/connective tissue diseases and pulmonary renal syndrome
2. Idiopathic pulmonary fibrosis
3. Granulomatous disease
   a. Unknown aetiology
      - Sarcoidosis
      - Histiocytosis
   b. Known aetiology
      - Hypersensitivity pneumonitis
      - Drug induced
4. Inhalation
   - Occupational dusts: Organic
     Inorganic
   - Environmental pollutions: Indoor
     Outdoor
   - Gases, fumes, aerosols: Pet animals, birds
5. Inherited causes: Familial –IPF
   - Sarcoid
   - Tuberous sclerosis
   - Hermansky-Pudlak syndrome
   - Neurofibromatosis
   - Hypocalciuric hypercalcemia
   - Metabolic storage disorders
6. Miscellaneous
   - Bronchiolitis obliterans with or without organizing pneumonia
   - Eosinophilic pneumonia
   - Iatrogenic (drug, irradiation)
   - Lymphangioleiomyomatosis
   - Alveolar proteinosis
   - Veno-occlusive disease
   - Lymphangitic carcinomatosis
   - Idiopathic pulmonary hemosiderosis

Raghu G., Interstitial lung disease —A diagnostic approach; Amer. J. Crit. Care Med 1995; 151: 909-14.

Table 11.95: Diffuse parenchymal lung disease (Indian dat a)

1. Cryptogenic fibrosing alveolitis
2. Collagen vascular disease
   - PSS
   - Overlap syndrome
   - RA
   - SLE
   - Sica syndrome
3. Sarcoidosis
4. Others
   - Pulmonary eosinophilia
   - Extrinsic allergic alveolitis
   - Wegener's granulomatosis
   - Drug induced interstitial pulmonary fibrosis

Mahajan R., *et al.*, DPLD: An approach to diagnosis; JAPI 2002; 50: 1285-94.

Table 11.96: Pulmonary oedema

Left ventricular failure, atrial fibrillation, hypertensive heart disease.
Severe asthma, diffuse pulmonary infections, aspiration, ARDS, high altitude.
Shock, neurogenic causes, heroin toxicity.

Table 11.97: Hyperbaric oxygen therapy

(A) Beneficial effects	*(B) Complications*	*(C) Toxic effects on respiratory system*
1. Correction of hypoxia	1. Pain in ears	1. Irritating cough
2. Inhibition of bacterial growth by affecting their metabolism	2. Rupture of tympanic membrane	2. Dyspnoea
	3. Haemorrhage in the ear	3. Substernal pain
3. Enhancing fibroblastic activity	4. Surgical emphysema of mediastinum	4. Breathing discomfort
4. Promoting gas exchange in the appropriate direction	5. Pneumothorax	5. Broncho pneumonia (Prolonged exposure)
	6. Rupture of pulmonary cavities	
	7. Arterial air embolism	

Table 11.98: Classification of hypoxia

1. *Arterial hypoxemia*: Hypoventilation and ventilation perfusion imbalance, high altitude, diffusion defect, right to left shunt as in congenital heart disease and increased physiological shunt in lungs.
2. *Circulatory:* Cardiac failure, arrhythmias, myocardial infarction, shock.
3. *Cellular:* Cyanide poisoning.
4. *Abnormal blood oxygen transport*: Carboxyhaemoglobinemia, abnormal Hb.
5. *Increased demand, as in hypermetabolic states*: Thyrotoxicosis, hyperpyrexia, exercise.

Table 11.99: Risk factors for acute lung injury

A. Direct/Pulmonary Injury
1. Infectious/Pneumonia/Aspiration gastric sac
2. Pulmonary contusion
3. Inhalational injury
4. Fat emboli
5. Near-drowning

B. Indirect/Extrapulmonary Injury
1. Sepsis
2. Shock
3. Severe trauma
4. Haemoproduct hyperperfusion
5. DIC
6. Drug overdose
7. Acute pancreatitis
8. Anti-phospholipid syndrome

Table 11.100: Acquired bronchoesophageal fistula (ABEF)

I. Characteristic Features
- a. Bouts of cough while eating/drinking (Ohno's sign)
- b. Recurrent pulmonary infections

II. Complications
- a. Pneumonia
- b. Life threatening hemoptysis
- c. Respiratory failure

III. Gold Standard Test
- a. Conventional barium oesophagography (fistulography) Diagnostic sensitivity is 78% (Gasography CT)
- b. Bronchoscopy, esophagoscopy
- c. CT and MRI non-invasive tests

IV. Varieties

a. Congenital	- Diagnosed in neonatal period - May remain silent till adulthood
b. Acquired	- Mostly in adults

V. Causes

1. Malignancy of esophagus or adjacent structures	
2. Infections	- TB, syphilis, histoplasmosis, actinomycosis, candidiasis
In AIDS	- Candidiasis and TB
3. Traumatic	- Blunt chest injury - Prolonged endotracheal intubation - During endoscopic intervention for denture/foreign body
4. Autoimmune disorders	- Crohn's disease - Behcet's disease
5. Corrosive ingestion	
6. Broncholithiasis	

VI. Management
- a. Surgical repair in acquired non-malignant cases
- b. Bypass or stenting is best option in malignant fistula

Table 11.101: Thoracic manifestations of multiple myeloma

1. Boney involvement of thoracic cage
2. Pneumonia
3. Intraparenchymal mass lesions
4. Mediastinal lymphadenopathy
5. • Reticulonodular shadows
   • Intrapulmonary calcification
   • Interstitial pattern
6. Incurable, despite high dose chemotherapy with
   - Vincristine
   - Melphalan
   - Cyclophosphamide
   - Prednisone
7. Recently thalidomide, lenalidomide and bortezomib have been used.

Differential Diagnoses*
- Metastatic carcinoma
- Lymphoma
- Bone neoplasm
- Chronic lymphocytic leukemia.
- Prognosis is poor
- Associated occurrence with primary pulmonary plasmacytomas of lung with multiple myeloma has been reported; former has long survival rate, latter having poor prognosis.

* Prasad R; *et al.* Multiple myeloma with lung plasmacytoma; Lung India 2011; 28: 136-38.

Table 11.102: Complications of bronchoscopy

a. Complications Due to Anaesthesia
1. Hypoxemia
2. Hypoventilation
3. Hypotension/Hypertension
4. Tachycardia
5. Arrhythmias
6. Bronchospasm
7. Laryngospasm
8. Laryngeal edema

b. Complications Associated with Procedure
1. Dislodgement of tooth
2. Gum trauma/Trauma of lips, pharynx, oral cavity, glottis
3. Luxation/laceration of vocal cords and arytenoids
4. Airway wall/oesophageal perforation
5. Spinal cord injuries in patients with cervical spine disease/ severe osteoporosis
6. Severe haemorrhage following biopsy, pneumothorax etc.

Table 11.103: Diagnosis of hepatopulmonary syndrome

- a. Normal chest X-ray
- b. Chronic liver disease present
- c. Gas exchange abnormality present
- d. Positive contrast enhanced echocardiogram or abnormal intravenous radiolabelled perfusion lung scan or both.

Table 11.104: Common findings of chest diseases on plain chest X-ray

A. *Chronic bronchitis*
- Prominent linear shadows
- Ill-defined opacities
- Altered lung markings
- Emphysematous changes

B. *Bronchiectasis*
- Bilateral basal involvement
- Dilated bronchi may be visualised
- Cystic or honeycomb appearance
- Secondary infection (pneumonitis) may be coexisting

C. *Pulmonary tuberculosis*
- Discrete mottled shadows
- Mediastinal glandular enlargement absent
- Occasionally consolidation present
- Lung destruction and fibrosis present
- Cavity lesion (in acute phase)
- Irregular cluster of calcified foci (caseation and calcification)

D. *Primary childhood type of tuberculosis*
- Hilar nodes enlarged
- Ghon's focus–a simple pneumonic consolidation, undergoes fibrosis and may calcify
- Cavitation rare/pleural effusion may be small

E. *Miliary TB*
- 1-2 mm dots and opacities in the lung fields, may coalesce to form a patchy density
- Mediastinal glands enlargement–absent
- Emphysema or fibrosis–absent

F. *Emphysema*
- Horizontal ribs with widened intercostal spaces and depressed diaphragm
- Narrow heart shadow
- Hilar shadows—prominent

G. *Pneumonia*
- Lung volume unaffected
- Hazy and indistinct shadow of consolidation
- Hilar glands not affected
- Pleural effusion may be present

H. *Lung abscess*
- Fluid level in consolidation
- Defined cavity with 2-3 mm wall of the cavity
- Lung marking increased
- Hilar glands not enlarged

I. *Pulmonary oedema*
- Fluffy cotton wool opacities within lungs-diurnal variations
- Air bronchogram present

J. *Pneumothorax*
- Radiolucent pleural cavity devoid of lung markings
- Lungs are separated by white line of visceral pleura
- Mediastinal shift (larger pneumothorax)

K. *Pleural effusion*
- Homogenous opacity in pleural cavity
- Lungs retracted towards hilum
- Costophrenic angle-obscured

L. *Hodgkin's disease*
- Paratracheal glands are affected rather than hilar
- Pulmonary appearances are pleomorphic
- Coarse line variety of pulmonary fibrosis

Contd.

Contd.

M. *Lung metastasis*
- Pleural effusion common (pleural nodular metasis—infrequent)
- Erosion or pathological fracture of ribs
- Mediastinal glands enlarged
- Cannon ball pulmonary metastasis

N. *Hilar enlargement*

Unilateral	*Bilateral*
Bronchogenic carcinoma	Sarcoidosis
Lymphoma	Silicosis
Primary TB	Histoplasmosis
Histoplasmosis	Pulmonary
Perihilar pneumonia	Arterial hypertensoion

O. *Shifting of mediastinum*

Same side	*Opposite side*
Scar formation	Massive pulmonary tumour
Massive atelectasis	Massive pleural effusion
Pulmonary emphysema	Tension pneumothorax
Bilateral pneumothorax	Obstructive emphysema
Thoracoplasty	Mediastinal tumour

P. *Honeycomb appearance*
- Cystic bronchiectasis
- Cystic fibrosis
- Rheumatoid lung
- Idiopathic interstitial fibrosis

Q. *Bilateral pulmonary odema*
- Cardiac failure
- Head injury/raised intracranial pressure
- Fluid overload
- Transfusion reaction
- Overdose of morphine

R. *Raised diaphragm*
- Decrease in size of hemithorax
- Abdominal mass
- Colonic distension
- Hepatomegaly
- Abscess

S. *Multiple mottling* (Bilateal)
- MiliaryTB
- Coal miner's pneumoconiosis
- Fungal infection
- Sarcoidosis
- Silicosis
- Haemosiderosis

T. *Increased insterstitial lung markings*
- Sarcoidosis
- Histiocytosis
- Pneumoconiosis
- Haemosiderosis
- Interstitial fibrosis
- Lymphangitis carcinomatosis

Differential Diagnosis in Bilateral Dense Peripheral Opacities on Chest X-ray

- Chronic/eosinophillic pneumonia.
- Bronchiolitis obliterans organizing pneumonia.
- Radiation lung injury.
- Sarcoidosis.

Table 11.105: Chest X-ray in trauma to the chest

1. RIB FRACTURE can be diagnosed by noting a break or step in the cortex of a rib. Extrapleural soft tissue swelling due to bruising or crack haematoma may be visible. Rib fractures are frequently multiple and may result in a flail segment (Easily diagnosed on oblique view).
2. PLEURAL EFFUSION often accompanies rib fractures, the fluid frequently being blood.
3. PNEUMOTHORAX occur if the lung is punctured by the direct injury or by sharp edge of a rib fracture. And a fluid level in the pleural cavity is common in such situations.
4. SURGICAL EMPHYSEMA of the chest wall may indicate the escape of air from the lungs. The presence of mediastinal emphysema may indicate the unusual phenomena of rupture of a bronchus.
5. PULMONARY CONTUSION: Localised traumatic alveolar haemorrhage and oedema may be seen, whether or not a rib fracture can be identified.
6. ADULT RESPIRATORY DISTRESS SYNDROME (ARDS) may follow severe trauma to any part of the body. There is diffuse widespread airspace filling often closely resembling pulmonary oedema. Radiological abnormality may only develop some 12-24 hours after the onset of tachypnoea, dyspnoea and hypoxaemia.
7. RUPTURE OF THE DIAPHRAGM due to penetrating injury or compression of the abdomen may permit herniation of the stomach or intestine into the chest. Such herniation is much commoner on the left than the right. Gas shadows of the stomach or intestines are seen above the presumed position of the diaphragm. Barium meal and follow through may be indicated to establish the diagnosis.
8. RUPTURE OF AORTA: The injury to the aorta is usually at the level of the ligamentum arteriosum. Bleeding may occur into the pleural cavity and mediastinal bleeding may be evident by mediastinal widening. Aortography may be useful. Even CT scanning may be required as widening of the mediastinum can be a very difficult sign to assess. It may be noted that mild trauma may cause aortic rupture and fractures of ribs or sternum but there can be aortic rupture without any damage to the thoracic cage.
9. RUTURE OF THE TRACHEO BRONCHIAL TREE: Occurs with major chest injury. Pneumomediastinum or pneumothorax, that is not responding to chest tube suction, are the important features. Subsequent complication includes bronchostenosis.

Thoracic Ultrasound Guided Interventions[1]

Advances in medical imaging indicate that a new age of imaging in biomedicine is on its way. The advent of new technologies especially the non-invasive techniques are quite promising but the risk associated with their use, restricts their use and recommendation for routine clinical use. However, image guided procedures have become primary tools in the diagnosis and management of various thoracic lesions. Sonographic guided modality is the choice as it is relatively safe, inexpensive and accurate. CT guidance is required in very small or deep seated lesions. Also it cannot be realtime especially in percutaneous procedures where needle tip has to be checked after each advance. Other disadvantages of CT guidance are listed in the Table 11.106.

Table 11.106: CT guidance: Disadvantages

1. May require several needle punctures, before needle can be placed in the region of interest.
2. As needle stays there during respiratory excursions, may cause more trauma to the tissues.
3. Radiation exposure to the patient and the operator cannot be ruled out.

Sonographic studies of chest and its uses are given in Tables 11.107 to 11.110.

Table 11.107: Image guidance: Preferred mode

a. Sonographic modality is the preferred mode.
b. CT guidance is reserved for those lesions which are not visible on sonography.
c. Fluoroscopy may be of use in checking position and manipulating indwelling catheter or for performing contrast studies.

Table 11.108: Preparation of patient

1. Chest radiograph.
2. Ultrasound study to localize and characterise the lesion.
3. Haemogram and coagulation profile.
4. Decision about the patient's position during the procedure.
5. Availability of local anaesthesia, pentazocine and diazepam for uncooperative patients.

Table 11.109: Techniques commonly followed

1. Biopsy a. Fine needle aspiration (FNAC)—2G needle. b. Core biospy—18G meningeal cutting needle.
2. Needle aspiration of fluid collection—18/20G long needle with stilette.
3. Catheter drainage: 8F pigtail angiographic catheters are used, with insertion by single step catheter—over needle or seldinger technique.

Table 11.110: Sister Mary Joseph's Nodule (Umbilical and metastasis)

That occurs in primary tumour of
- Gastrointestinal tract 65%
- Urinary
- Respiratory

} System malignancipes 25-30%

Table 11.111: Radiological differential diagnoses of lung consolidation include

Pneumonia
Infarction
Alveolar haemorrhage
Bronchoalveolar carcinoma

Table 11.112: Differential diagnoses on chest X-ray of lung collapse include

Pleural effusion
Pleural thickening
Consolidation
Mass lesion

Table 11.113: Direct signs of collap se

Displaced septa
Loss of aeration
Bronchovascular crowding

Table 11.114: X-ray-chest suggestive of large pleural effusion without mediastinal shift

- Fixed mediastinum by malignant lymph nodes
- Malignant mesothelioma
- Extensive tumour infiltration of ipsilateral lung
- Carcinoma bronchus causing collapse

Table 11.115: Chest X-ray showing p arapneumonic effusion

A pleural effusion associated with:
- Bacterial pneumonia
- Lung abscess
- Bronchiectasis

Table 11.116: Causes of disseminated miliary nodes on plain chest X-ray include

TB
Fungal disease
Malignant tumour
Tropical pulmonary eosinophilia
Sarcoidosis
Pneumoconiosis
Interstitial fibrosis
Rheumatoid arthritis

Table 11.117: Unilateral hyperlucency on plain chest X-ray seen in

- Large bulla
- Pneumothorax
- Unilateral mastectomy
- Pulmonary arterial embolism
- Hypoplastic pulmonary artery
- Ball-valve obstruction in main bronchus
- Swyer-James syndrome

Table 11.118: Chest X-ray without pulmonary oedema seen in

Focal radiation insult
Sarcoidosis
Boop

Table 11.119: Opacities in radiographic zones preferable dif ferential diagnoses

Upper zone	*Mid zone*	*Lower zone*	*Generalized*
- TB - Subacute silicosis - Chronic sarcoidosis - Progressive massive fibrosis - Extrinsic allergic alveolitis - Langerhan's cell histiocytosis	- Pulmonary oedema - Pneumocystis - Carinii pneumonia - Alveolar proteinosis	- Asbestosis - Bronchopneumonia - Cryptogenic fibrosing alveolitis - Tropical eosinophilia - Collagen lung disease HIV - Microlithiasis - Haemosiderosis	- Miliary TB - Pneumoconiosis - Sarcoidosis - Metasis - Cystic fibrosis - Opportunistic lung infection - ADRs - Drug reaction - Lymphangitis carcinomatosis

REFERENCE

1. Sawney S; Ultrasound guided interventions in the chest. In: Manoria P.C., ed: Sonography Updates; Ind Fed of US and Med Bio 1993; 2: 46-49.

Table 11.120: Migratory pulmonary infiltrates seen on plain chest X-ray in

Chronic eosinophilic pneumonias
ABPA
Loeffler's syndrome
Churg-Strauss syndrome

Table 11.121: Overpenetrated films of chest X-ray are useful in

- Calcified lesions
- Bone lesions
- Lesion hidden below
  - Clavicle
  - Mediastinum
  - Diaphragm

Table 11.122: Use of ultrasonography in chest disease

- Pleural space examination
- Pleural effusions: Diagnosis
- Pneumothorax
- Diagnostic thoracocentesis
- Lung parenchyma evaluation
  a. Consolidation
  b. Abscess
  c. Lung tumor
- Lung biopsy: Percutaneous transthoracic (under fluoroscopic guidance)

Table 11.123: CT scan thorax: Indications

a. Mediastinal mass
b. Staging of Ca lung
c. Chest wall/pleural abnormality
d. ILDs
e. Pulmonary metastases
f. Planning of radiation therapy
g. CT guided transthoracic biopsy

Table 11.124: CT scan patterns of lungs

- Honeycomb
- Interlobular septal thickening
- Cystic
- Tree-in-Bud
- Nodular
- Ground glass
- Mosaic lung attenuation

Table 11.125: CT signs of lung disease

Diagnosis
Bronchoalveolar Ca
Lymphoma: Air bronchogram
Intra cavity mass mycetoma: Air crescent sign
ABPA : Finger in glove sign
Bronchoalveolar Ca:
Lymphoma:
Infections (Pneumonia): CT angiogram sign
Ca lung: Golden S sign
Invasive pulmonary aspergillosis: Halo sign
Pulmonary infarction: Hampton thump sign
Resolving pulmonary infarct: Melting ice cube sign
Pneumo-mediastinum: Ring around the artery sign
Empyema: Split pleura sign
Pulmonary embolism: Westermark sign (Focal oliguria in sight lung)
Thrombus in the main and right pulmonary arteries

Table 11.126: Indications of bronchoscopy

1. Pulmonary infections in immunocompromised host.
2. Pulmonary TB.
3. Fungal infection.
4. Viral infection.
5. Pneumocystis carinii infection.
6. Bacterial pneumonia.
7. Bronchiectasis and lung abscess.
8. For removing impacted/viscious secretions.

Therapeutic Uses

1. Brush biopsy/Protected specimen brushing.
2. Bronchial washing.
3. Bronchoalveolar lavage.
4. Protected BAL.
5. Endobronchial biopsy.
6. Transbronchial lung biopsy.
7. Transbronchial needle aspiration of mediastinal lymph nodes.

Table 11.127: Indications of thoracoscopy

a. **Diagnostic**
   - An unexplained exudative effusion
   - Staging of lung cancer
   - Assessing/staging of pneumothorax
   - Chest wall lesions
   - Local/diffuse lung disease
b. **Therapeutic**
   - Pleurodesis
   - Intrapleural therapy
   - Removing foreign body

Table 11.128: Uses of echocardiography in pulmonary disorders

1. Parenchymal lung disease e.g. COPD
2. ILDs
3. Pulmonary vascular disease
4. Primary pulmonary hypertension
5. Pulmonary thromboembolic disease
6. Acute respiratory distress syndrome

INDEX